Textbook of Melanoma

Textbook of Melanoma

Edited by

John F Thompson MD FRACS FACS
Professor of Melanoma and Surgical Oncology,
The University of Sydney, NSW Australia

Donald L Morton MD FACS
Medical Director and Surgeon-in-Chief, John Wayne Cancer
Institute at Saint John's Health Center
Santa Monica, CA, USA

Bin BR Kroon MD PhD FRCS
Professor of Surgery, Department of Surgery,
The Netherlands Cancer Institute,
Antoni van Leeuwenhoek Hospital, Amsterdam, The Netherlands

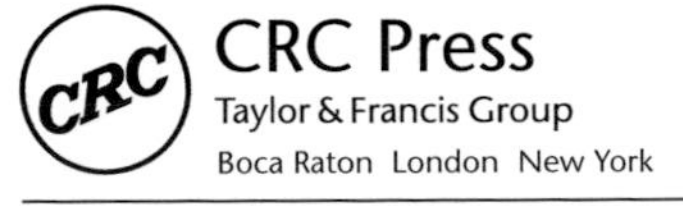

CRC Press is an imprint of the
Taylor & Francis Group, an **informa** business

CRC Press
Taylor & Francis Group
6000 Broken Sound Parkway NW, Suite 300
Boca Raton, FL 33487-2742

First issued in paperback 2019

ISBN-13: 978-1-901865-65-3 (hbk)
ISBN-13: 978-0-367-39497-4 (pbk)

Visit the Taylor & Francis Web site at
http://www.taylorandfrancis.com

and the CRC Press Web site at
http://www.crcpress.com

Contents

Contributors

Joanne Aitken SM PhD
Director, Epidemiology Unit, Queensland Cancer Fund, Queensland Australia

Bruce Armstrong AM FAA
Head, School of Population Health and Health, Services Research, The University of Sydney, NSW, Australia

Philippe Autier MD MPH
Head, Centre for Research in Epidemiology and Health Information Systems; Luxembourg Health Institute, Luxembourg

Charles M Balch MD, FACS
Professor of Surgery and Oncology, John Hopkins Medical Institutions, Baltimore, Maryland; Excecutive Vice-President and Chief Executive Officer, American Society of Clinical Oncology, Alexandria VA, USA

Alfonsus JM Balm MD PhD FRCS FACS
Otorhinolaryngologist and Head and Neck Surgeon, The Netherlands Cancer Institute, Amsterdam, The Netherlands

Therese M Becker BSc PhD
Research Officer, Westmead Institute for Cancer Research, Sydney University, Westmead Hospital, Westmead NSW 2145, Australia

Filiberto Belli MD
Department of Surgery, National Cancer Institute, Milan, Italy

Anton J Bilchik MD PhD FACS
Assistant Director of Surgical Oncology, and Director of Gastrointestinal Research, John Wayne Cancer Institute, Santa Monica CA, USA

Michael Binder MD
Dermatologist, Department of Dermatology and Decisions System Group, Harvard Medical School; Associate Professor, University of Vienna Medical School, New General Hospital (AKH), Vienna, Austria

Mathieu Boniol MS
Centre Leon Berard, Lyon, France

Robert C Burton MD PhD BS BA BMedSci FRACP FRACS FAFPHM
Director, Anti-Cancer Council of Victoria, Carlton, Victoria, Australia

Antonio C Buzaid MD
Executive Director, Oncology Centre, Hospital Sirio-Lebanes, Sao Paulo, Brazil

Dominique S Byrne MB ChB MPhil FRCS
Consultant Surgeon, Department of General and Vascular Surgery, Gartnavel General Hospital, Glasgow, UK

Natale Cascinelli MD
Department of Surgery, National Cancer Institute, Milan, Italy

Alistair J Cochran MD
Professor of Pathology and Director of Surgical Pathology, Department of Pathology and Laboratory Medicine, UCLA Medical Center, Center for the Health Sciences, Los Angeles CA, USA

Daniel G Coit MD FACS
Attending Surgeon and Chief, Gastric and Mixed Tumour Service, Memorial Sloan-Kettering Cancer Center, New York NY, USA

Kerry Crotty MBBS
Department of Anatomical Pathology, Royal Prince Alfred Hosptial, Camperdown NSW, Australia

Piero Dalerba MD
Research Fellow, Unit of Immunotherapy of Human Cancer, Department of Experimental Oncology, Istituto Nazionale Tumori, Milan, Italy

Neville C Davis AO MD DS(Hon) FRACS FACS FRCS Hon(Eng) Hon FRCS (Edin)
Foundation Coordinator, Queensland Melanoma Project, Honorary Consultant Surgeon, Princess Alexandra Hospital, Brisbane, Queensland, Australia

Jakob DH de Vries MSc
Department of Surgery, The Netherlands Cancer Institute, Antoni van Leeuwenhoek Hospital, Amsterdam, The Netherlands

Johannes HW de Wilt MD PhD
Surgeon, Erasmus Medical Center Rotterdam, Daniel den Hoed Cancer Center, Department of Surgical Oncology, Erasmus MC, Rotterdam, The Netherlands

Jean-François Doré PhD
INSERM Research Director, Centre Leon Berard, Lyon, France

Alexander MM Eggermont MD PhD
Surgical Oncologist, University of Rotterdam, Department of Surgical Oncology, Rotterdam Hospital, Den Hoed Cancer Center Rotterdam, The Netherlands

Mark Elwood MD DSc MBA FRCPC FAFPHM
Director, National Cancer Control Initiative, Melbourne, Carlton VIC, Australia

Richard Essner MD
Assistant Director Surgical Oncology, John Wayne Cancer Institute, Santa Monica CA, USA

Erin A Felger MD
Department of Anatomical Pathology, Royal Prince Alfred Hospital, Camperdown NSW, Australia

Kate Fife MD MRCP FRCR FRANZCR
Consultant Clinical Oncologist, Addenbrooke's NHS Trust, Cambridge, UK

Jeffrey E Gershenwald MD
Associate Professor of Surgery and Cancer Biology, Department of Surgical Oncology and Cancer Biology, The University of Texas, MD Anderson Cancer Center, Houston TX, USA

Michael E Giblin MB BS FRANZCO
Ophthalmic Surgeon, VMO Sydney Eye Hospital, Lindfield NSW, Australia

Gary M Halliday BSc PhD DSc
Associate Professor, Melanoma and Skin Cancer Institute, University of Sydney Melanoma Unit, Department of Medicine (Dermatology), Sydney NSW, Australia

Michael Henderson MB BS BMed Sci FRACS
Associate Professor of Surgery, University of Melbourne, Department of Surgery, St Vincents Hospital, Fitzroy; Head, Peter MacCallum Cancer Institute, Victoria, Australia

Peter Hersey MBBS FRACP DPhil
Conjoint Professor, Immunology and Oncology, Newcastle Melanoma Unit; Senior Staff Specialist, Newcastle Mater Hospital; Consultant Immunologist, Sydney Melanoma Unit, NSW, Australia

Cornelis A Hoefnagel MD PhD
Head of Department of Nuclear Medicine, The Netherlands Cancer Institute, CX Amsterdam, The Netherlands

Harald J Hoekstra MD PhD
Associate Professor of Surgical Oncology, Groningen University, Groningen, The Netherlands

Elizabeth A Holland BSc
Senior Research Officer, Westmead Institute for Cancer Research, Sydney University, Westmead NSW, Australia

Dave SB Hoon MSc PhD
Director, Department of Molecular Oncology, John Wayne Cancer Institute, Santa Monica CA, USA

Eddy C Hsueh MD
Assistant Director of Surgical Oncology, John Wayne Cancer Institute, Santa Monica CA, USA

T Michael D Hughes MBBS(Hons) FRACS
Surgical Oncologist, Head of Melanoma and Sarcoma Service, Westmead Hospital, Sydney NSW, Australia

Peter C A Kam FANZCA FRCA FCARCSI FHKCA (Hon)
Professor of Anaesthetics, University of NSW, St George Clinical School, St George Hospital, Kogarah NSW, Australia

Constantine P Karakousis MD PhD
Professor of Surgery, Chief of Surgical Oncology,, State University of New York at Buffalo and Kaleida Health, Kaleida Health, Millard Fillmore Hospital, Buffalo NY, USA

Richard F Kefford PhD MBBS FRACP
Consultant Medical Oncologist, Sydney Melanoma Unit, and Professor and Head, Department of Medicine, Westmead Hospital, Westmead NSW, Australia

David Khayat PhD
Professor, Medical Oncology, Pitié-Salpêtrière Hospital, Paris, France

Joost M Klaase MD PhD
Academic Medical Center, Department of Surgery, Amsterdam, The Netherlands

David N Krag MD
University of Vermont School of Medicine, Burlington Vermont, USA

Bin BR Kroon MD PhD FRCS
Professor of Surgery, Department of Surgery, The Netherlands Cancer Institute, Antoni van Leeuwenhoek Hospital, Amsterdam, The Netherlands

Richard GB Langley MD FRCPC
Director of Research, Divison of Dermatology, Department of Medicine, Dalhousie University, Halifax, Nova Scotia, Canada

Ferdy J Lejeune MD PhD
Professor and Director Multidisciplinary Oncology Centre, Centre Hospitalier Universitaire Vaudios (CHUV), Lausanne, Switzerland

Leonardo Lenisa MD
Dept of Surgery, Casa di Cura San Pio, Milan, Italy

Per Lindnér MD PhD
Associate Professor, Consultant in Surgery, Sahlgrenska University Hospital, Grotegorg, Sweden

Graham J Mann MBBS PhD
Department of Medicine, Westmead Hospital, Westmead NSW, Australia

William H McCarthy MBBS
Sydney Melanoma Unit, Royal Prince Alfred Hospital, Camperdown NSW, Australia

Stanley McCarthy AO MBBS DCP(Syd) FRACP FFOP FRCPA
Senior Staff Specialist, Department of Anatomical Pathology, Royal Prince Alfred Hospital, Camperdown NSW, Australia

Brian C McCaughan MBBS (Hons) FRACS
Clinical Associate Professor, Department of Cardiothoracic Surgery, Royal Prince Alfred Hospital, Camperdown, NSW, Australia

Alan J McKay MBChB MPhil FRCS Glas FRCSEd
Consultant General and Vascular Surgeon, Department of General and Vascular Surgery Gartnavel General Hospital, Glasgow, UK

Scott Menzies MBBS PhD
Senior Lecturer, Department of Surgery, University of Sydney, Sydney Melanoma Unit, Royal Prince Alfred Hospital, Camperdown NSW, Australia

Jean-Baptiste Meric MD
Medical Oncology, Pitié-Salpêtrière Hospital, Paris, France

Martin C Mihm Jr MD
Department of Dermatopathology, Massachussetts General Hospital, Boston MA, USA

Michael J Millward MBBS MA FRACP
Head of Clinical Research, Sydney Cancer Centre, Royal Prince Alfred Hospital, Camperdown NSW, Australia

Gerald W Milton MBBS FRCS FRACS MD (Hons) MS
Emeritus Professor, Skin and Cancer Foundation, Darlinghurst NSW, Australia

Wolter J Mooi MD
Professor of Pathology and Consultant Pathologist, Department of Pathology, The Netherlands Cancer Institute, Amsterdam, The Netherlands

Donald L Morton MD FACS
Medical Director and Surgeon-in-Chief, John Wayne Cancer Institute at Saint John's Health Center, Santa Monica CA, USA

Julia Newton Bishop MBChB
Department of Medicine, Marsden Hospital, Westmead NSW, Australia

Omgo E Nieweg PhD MD
Surgeon, Department of Surgery, The Netherlands Cancer Institute, Antoni van Leeuwenhoek Hospital, Amsterdam, The Netherlands

Christopher J O'Brien MS
Royal Prince Alfred Hospital, Medical Centre, Newtown, NSW, Australia

David W Ollila MD
Assistant Professor of Surgery; Director, Sentinel Lymph Node Program, The University of North Carolina, Department of Surgery, Division of Surgical and Endocrine Surgery, Chapel Hill NC, USA

John A Olson Jr MD PhD
Memorial Sloan-Kettering Cancer Center, New York NY, USA

Ian N Olver MD BS PhD FRACP RACMA FAChPM
Clinical Director, Royal Adelaide Hospital, Director of Medical Oncology, Clinical Professor University of Adelaide, Medical Oncology, Adelaide SA, Australia

Giorgio Parmiani MD
Deputy Scientific Director, Head, Unit of Immunotherapy of Human Cancer, Department of Experimental Oncology, Istituto Nazionale Tumori, Milano, Italy

Richard Perry MB BS FRANZCR
Consultant Radiologist, Hornsby Ku-ring-gai Hospital, Hornsby NSW, Australia

Michael Quinn MBBS(Hons) FRACS (Plast and Reconstr)
Associate Surgeon Sydney Melanoma Unit, Royal Prince Alfred Hospital, Newtown NSW, Australia

Douglas Reintgen MD
Program Leader Moffitt Cancer Center, Tampa FL, USA

Jason K Rivers BSc MD FRCPC
Professor, Department of Medicine, Division of Dermatology, University of British Columbia; British Columbia Cancer Agency, Vancouver BC, Canada

Olivier Rixe MD
Medical Oncology, Pitié-Salpêtrière Hospital, Paris, France

Helen Rizos BSc (Hon) PhD
Senior Research Officer, Westmead Institute for Cancer Research, Sydney University, Westmead Hosiptal, Westmead NSW, Australia

Merrick I Ross MD
Professor of Surgery, Chief, Section of Melanoma/Sarcoma Surgery, Department of Surgical Oncology, The University of Texas, MD Anderson Cancer Center, Houston TX, USA

Dirk J Ruiter MD PhD
Professor and Clinical Chairman of Pathology, Department of Pathology, University Medical Center St. Radboud, Nijmegen, The Netherlands

John D Sadoff MD
Attending, Williamsport Hospital, Williamsport PA, USA

Mario Santinami MD
Director Melanoma and Sarcoma Unit,, Istituto Nazionale Tumori, Milano, Italy

Heimen Schraffordt Koops MD PhD
Associate Professor of Surgical Oncology, Groningen University, Groningen, The Netherlands

Jatin P Shah MD
Memorial Sloan-Kettering Cancer Center, New York NY, USA

Helen M Shaw PhD
Senior Research Fellow, Department of Surgery, University of Sydney, Sydney Melanoma Unit, Royal Prince Alfred Hospital, Camperdown, NSW Australia

Carol L Shields MD
Ocular Oncology Service, Wills Eye Hospital, Associate Professor of Ophthalmology, Thomas Jefferson University, Philadelphia, USA

Jerry A Shields MD
Director, Ocular Oncology Service, Wills Eye Hospital, Professor of Ophthalmology, Thomas Jefferson University, Philadelphia, USA

B Mark Smithers MBBS FRCS(Eng) FRACS
Associate Professor, Department of Surgery, University of Queensland, Princess Alexandra Hospital, Brisbane, QLD, Australia

Seaver L Soon MD
Research Fellow, Clinical Pharmacology Unit, Department of Dermatology, Emory University, Atlanta, GA USA

Seng-jaw Soong PhD
Professor of Biostatistics and Biomathematics, University of Alabama School of Medicine, Birmingham, AL, USA

Graham Stevens BSc MD FRANZCR
Clinical Leader Oncology Unit, Dunedin Hospital and Clinical Associate, Professor University of Otago, Dunedin, New Zealand

Wilhelm Stolz MD
Department of Dermatology, University of Regensburg, Regensburg, Germany

Bret Taback MD
Department of Surgical Oncology, Molecular Oncology, John Wayne Cancer Institute, Santa Monica CA, USA

John F Thompson MD FRACS FACS
Professor of Melanoma and Surgical Oncology, The University of Sydney; Royal Prince Alfred Hospital, Camperdown NSW, Australia

Roger F Uren MD FRACP DDU
Clinical Associate Professor, Department of Medicine, University of Sydney; Nuclear Medicine and Diagnostic Ultrasound, RPAH Medical Centre, Newtown NSW, Australia

Goos NP van Muijen PhD
Associate Professor of Pathology, Department of Pathology, University Medical Center, St. Radboud, Nijmegen, The Netherlands

Bart C Vrouenraets MD PhD
Surgical Registrar, Department of Surgery, The Netherlands Cancer Institute, Antoni van Leeuwenhoek Ziekenhuis, Amsterdam, The Netherlands

Foreword

Over the past decade, major progress has been made in achieving a better understanding of the development and progression of melanoma. As molecular biology comes of age, we stand poised on the threshold of even more important advances in knowledge and may soon be in the position to solve some of the many remaining mysteries that are associated with this tumour. An added sense of urgency has been injected by the recognition that there is a worldwide epidemic of melanoma, with inexorably rising incidence rates in most countries populated by fair-skinned people. In countries such as Australia, the disease has already become a major public health problem, and a similar situation is emerging in Europe, North America, and South America.

The melanoma problem is being tackled on many fronts, and this is reflected by the wide range of international authors, all experts in their respective fields, who have contributed chapters to this book. The result is a comprehensive review of current knowledge, a guide to what is currently regarded as best clinical practice, and a pointer to likely future developments. We hope that the book will serve not only as a useful reference work for all those who have an interest in melanoma, but that it will also assist in promoting the highest possible standards of multidisciplinary clinical care for melanoma patients worldwide.

John F Thompson, Donald L Morton, Bin BR Kroon

1

Melanoma: an historical perspective

Neville C Davis, Helen M Shaw, William H McCarthy

ANTIQUITY

By dating with radiocarbon 14, the antiquity of melanoma has been estimated to be at least 2400 years.[1] This information was obtained from nine pre-Colombian Inca mummies of Peru, seven from Chancay and two from Chongo in the Ica region of the Andean foothills. Diffuse metastases to bones, particularly the skull and extremities, were present. In the mummies' skin there were hair follicles and rounded melanotic masses, which seemed to be melanoma satellites. The deposits in the skull were distributed mostly throughout the subperiosteal layer. The number of Inca mummies with skeletal melanotic involvement is paradoxical in view of the low incidence of melanoma in darker-skinned individuals today.

Urteaga and Pack suggest that the first accredited mention of 'melanoma' was probably by Hippocrates in the 5th century BC.[1] It was not until the 1st century AD that the next annotation by the Greek physician Rufus of Ephesus could be found by these authors.

CHANGING PERCEPTIONS OF SUNLIGHT

Sun worshippers have always been in existence. Sun gods were considered the source of all goodness and life in some ancient cultures. Solar mythology placed the sun at the centre of religion and myth. Sunday was set aside as the day to worship the sun. The Greeks further established the link between the sun and health with Apollo, god of the sun, and his son Aesculapius, god of medicine. Sunbathing was used extensively in the Aesculapian health clinics 2000 years ago as a method of restoring good health.

In 17th and 18th century Europe and the New World, there was a bizarre fascination with pigmented lesions, which had magical and religious connotations.[2,3] At the time porcelain paleness was the epitome of stylishness, and pale skin helped distinguish rich social classes from common, outdoor manual labourers. By the 20th century, the stereotype associated with skin colour began to shift. A dark tan became a sign of distinction associated with sufficient wealth to enjoy leisure pursuits in warm and sunny climates.

The first recorded warnings of the potentially harmful effects of sunlight were given in 1894 by Unna.[4] He described degenerative skin changes in sailors ('seamen's skin') and attributed them to the sun. In 1906 Cleland first commented on how common skin cancer was in Australia.[5] In 1907, Dubreuilh observed that grape pickers in Bordeaux had many skin cancers, predominantly on areas exposed to sunlight.[6] He showed there was a strong association between squamous cell carcinoma and solar keratoses and working outdoors. Lancaster and Nelson noted in 1957 that persons most commonly affected by melanoma in Australia were those with fair skins, who did not tan on exposure to the sun but who burned and freckled.[7] They made the first attempts to delineate the role of sunlight in the causation of melanoma.

FIRST REPORT OF A MELANOMA

The first published account of a patient with melanoma (a secondary deposit) was by John Hunter in 1787, although Hunter never described the disease as such (Figure 1.1). Hunter's original specimen, No. 219, preserved in the Hunterian Museum of the Royal College of Surgeons of England, was from a 35-year-old man with a recurrent mass behind the angle of the lower jaw. The lump was excised, only to recur locally 3 years later. The metastasis enlarged slowly until it was struck with a stick during a drunken brawl, after which it doubled in size over the next few weeks. After removing the lump, John Hunter described that 'part of it was white and part spongy, soft and black'; he labelled it as a 'cancerous fungous excrescence'. In 1968, Bodenham reported that microscopic examination of the specimen confirmed that it was a melanoma – presumably a secondary deposit from an unknown primary tumour (Figure 1.2).[8]

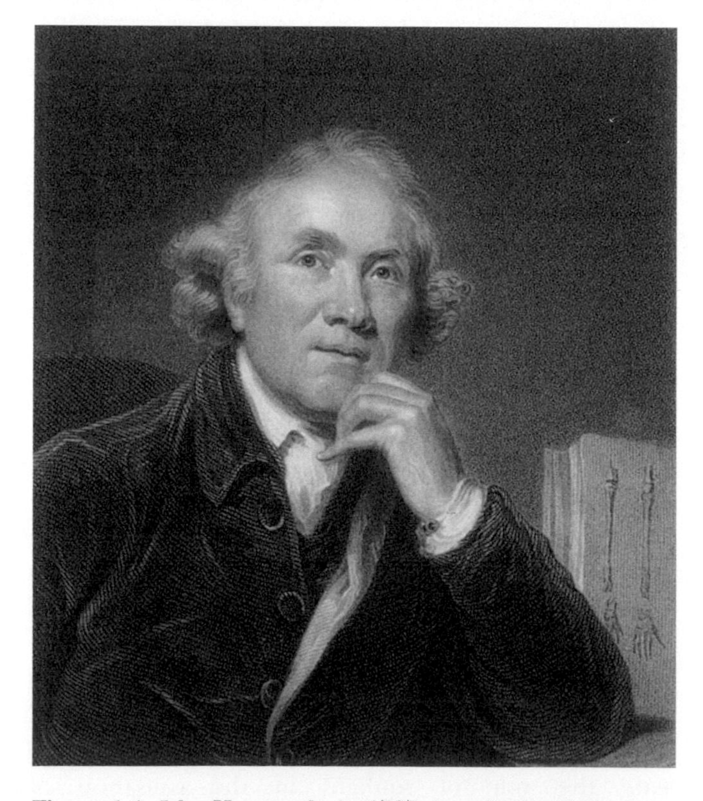

Figure 1.1 *John Hunter who in 1787, is credited with the first published account of a melanoma (a secondary deposit).*

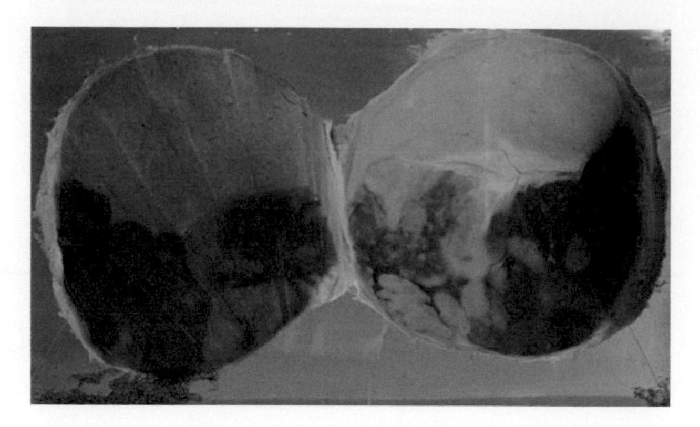

Figure 1.2 *A recurrent mass from the angle of the lower jaw in a man aged 35 years. This is John Hunter's original specimen of 1787, preserved in the Hunterian Museum of the Royal College of Surgeons of England.*

PROGRESS IN THE 19TH CENTURY

First description of a melanoma

There is some argument about who was the first person to describe melanoma. Breschet and Pemberton gave credit to Dupuytren, and he certainly claimed it.[9–11] Dupuytren was an exacting and innovative surgeon but was said to be cold, hard and contemptuous of his colleagues. Percy, a lifelong friend of the French surgeon Larrey, described Dupuytren as the first of surgeons and the last of men. He is said to have believed that operations should not be performed on melanoma patients as the condition was hopeless.

Most authorities, however, credit Rene Laennec with being the first to describe melanoma as a disease entity (Figure 1.3). His description was first presented as a lecture to the Faculté de Médecine de Paris in 1804, and was subsequently published in 1806 in that faculty's bulletin, although he did not use the word 'melanosis' (from the Greek word meaning 'black') until 1812.[12] Laennec stated that the condition had apparently escaped the notice up to then 'of anatomists and of doctors who ordinarily do post mortems'. He noted that melanoma metastases in the mediastinal and hilar lymph nodes were different from the more common black bronchial glands, the colour of which he recognized resulted from a large quantity of carbon. He also described melanomas involving the liver, lungs, eye, pituitary gland, stomach wall, and surface of the peritoneum and noted that melanotic deposits in the lungs did not cause the

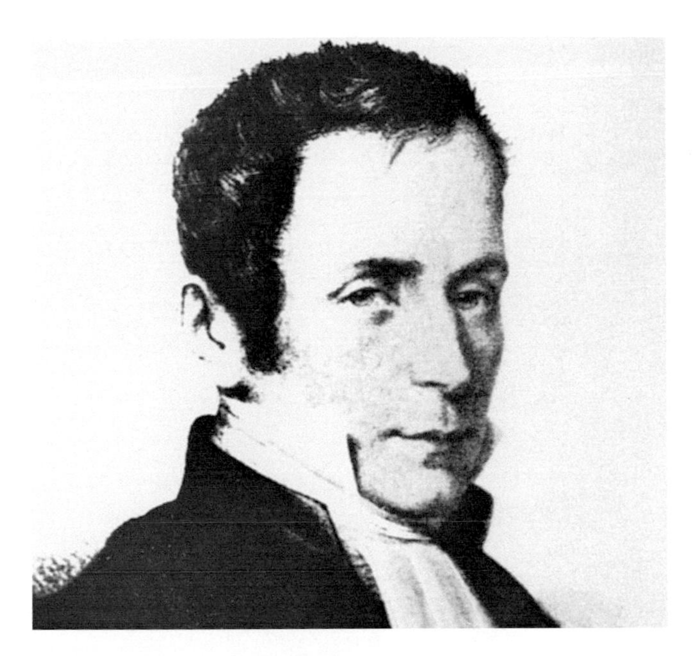

Figure 1.3 *Rene Laennec, who in 1806 was the first to describe melanoma as a disease entity and in 1812, to use the term 'melanosis'.*

same hectic fever as tuberculosis, a common cause of death at the time.

William Norris – the first case in England

In 1820, William Norris reported the first case of melanoma recorded in the English literature.[13] He referred to it as a case of fungoid disease, but he actually described a patient who died from disseminated melanoma. Subsequently, he declared that this patient was 'the first genuine good case of melanoma', as the following description indicates (Figure 1.4).

> 'Mr D., aged 59 years, of light hair and fair complexion, presented to Dr Norris on February 6, 1817 with a tumour of his abdominal wall midway between umbilicus and pubis. There had always been a mole on this position, but nine months previously, it began to grow and tumour developed. It was half the size of a hen's egg, of a deep brown colour, of a firm and fleshy feel, ulcerated, and discharging a highly foetid ichthorous fluid. The apex of the tumour was broader than its base. Some months after the tumour appeared, several distinct brown nodules sprang up around it (satellites).
>
> The primary tumour was removed by the knife but then recurred in the scar in less than six weeks. The glands of the groin were swollen and slightly tender to the touch. In spite of the disseminated nature of the tumour the general health of the patient was not so much impaired as to interfere with his exercise or business. Multiple subcutaneous deposits developed with a distressing cough and dyspnoea before he died.'

Norris performed the autopsy himself and found the residual primary tumour to be 'dark brown and reddish, not unlike the internal portions of a nutmeg'. A thick, black fluid discharged from the subcutaneous deposits after they were punctured. Metastases were found in the sternum and throughout the abdomen, which contained a quart of ascitic fluid. The 'lumbar glands' were 'in a shockingly morbid condition'; the liver was enlarged and 'studded with large oval masses of disease'. The spleen and bladder were the only abdominal organs free of disease. The lungs were grossly involved, and the heart was literally encrusted with numerous specks varying in size from a pin's head to that of a pea. The dura mater was studded with metastases, but the brain itself was apparently uninvolved.

Mr Causer, a surgeon in the town and a previous house surgeon of John Hunter, was told by Dr Norris that this patient's father had also died of melanoma. He remarked that he was not acquainted with any case affording so strong a probability of the hereditary nature of the disease.

Norris subsequently reported in 1857 eight cases of melanosis with pathological and therapeutical remarks on that disease, and this included a report on the first patient previously seen in 1820.[14] In this paper, Norris referred to the condition as 'melanosis', a term still used in the literature, although Robert Carswell had earlier coined the term 'melanoma' in 1838.[15]

In his article in 1857 Norris stated that melanoma often occurred in those persons who have moles on various parts of the body.[14] He noted that most of his cases occurred in patients residing in very smoky iron and coal districts ... in men, who have smoked immoderately. He referred to a case he reported in former years, where melanosis affected almost every organ, the first tumour was not black – it was more of a scirrhous character. A second tumour sprang from the cicatrix, and, during life put on a similar appearance to the first, yet after death, it looked perfectly black. The patient's daughter had a cancer of the breast and his son a cancer of the lip and mouth. He claimed that there was a strong tendency to hereditary predisposition, and that melanosis was a disease allied to cancer.

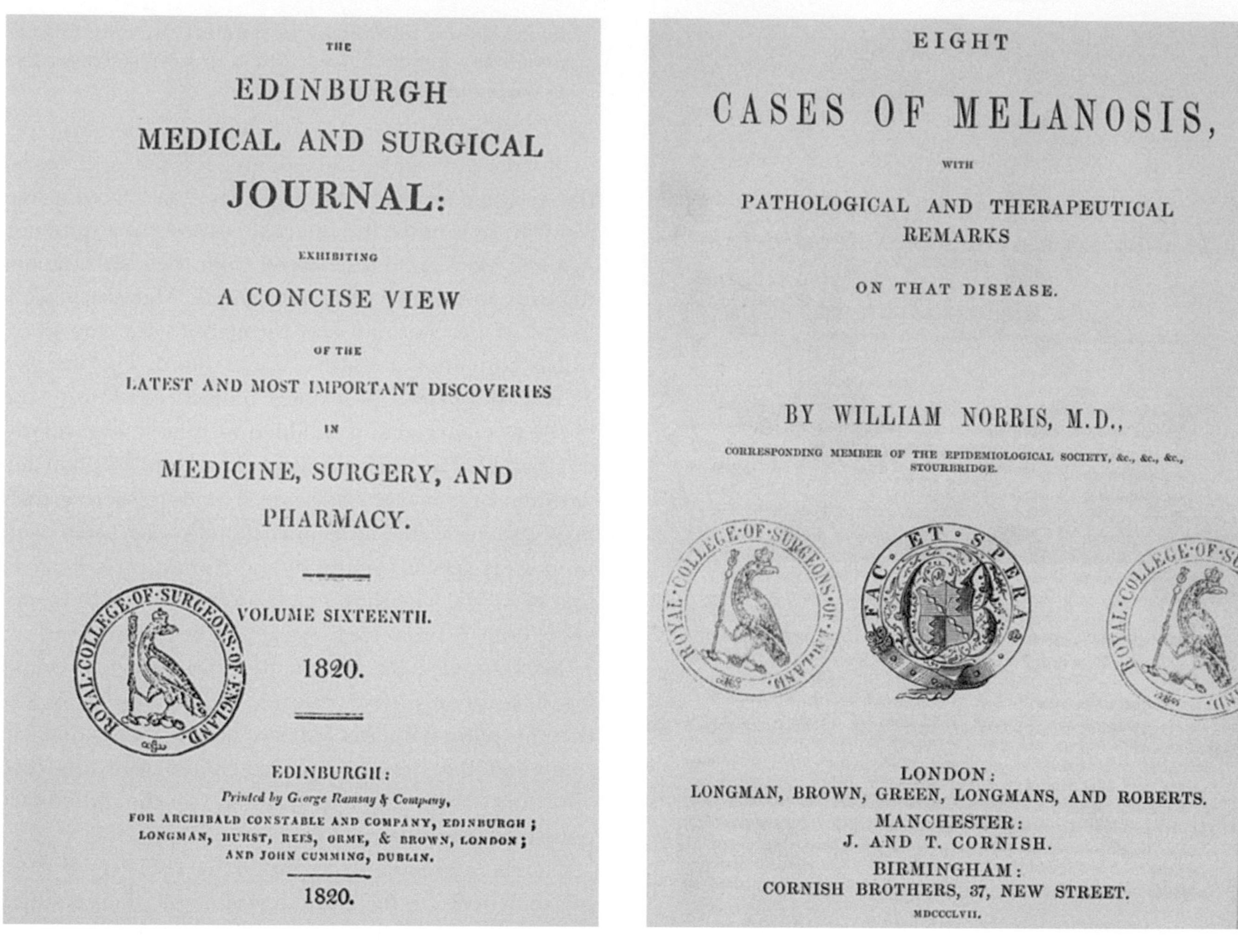

THE

EDINBURGH
MEDICAL AND SURGICAL
JOURNAL:

EXHIBITING

A CONCISE VIEW

OF THE

LATEST AND MOST IMPORTANT DISCOVERIES

IN

MEDICINE, SURGERY, AND
PHARMACY.

VOLUME SIXTEENTH.

1820.

EDINBURGH:
Printed by George Ramsay & Company,
FOR ARCHIBALD CONSTABLE AND COMPANY, EDINBURGH;
LONGMAN, HURST, REES, ORME, & BROWN, LONDON;
AND JOHN CUMMING, DUBLIN.

1820.

EIGHT

CASES OF MELANOSIS,

WITH

PATHOLOGICAL AND THERAPEUTICAL
REMARKS

ON THAT DISEASE.

BY WILLIAM NORRIS, M.D.,

CORRESPONDING MEMBER OF THE EPIDEMIOLOGICAL SOCIETY, &c., &c., &c.,
STOURBRIDGE.

LONDON:
LONGMAN, BROWN, GREEN, LONGMANS, AND ROBERTS.
MANCHESTER:
J. AND T. CORNISH.
BIRMINGHAM:
CORNISH BROTHERS, 37, NEW STREET.
MDCCCLVII.

Figure 1.4 *William Norris' description in 1820 of the first case of melanoma recorded in the English literature contained in the first comprehensive study of a series of melanoma patients.*

One of his patients, a 26-year-old woman of fair and freckled appearance, provided him with 'the most perfect specimen of melanotic tumour I had ever seen, which originated in a mole.' Three years before, her brother, who was much annoyed at the mole's unsightly appearance, 'ran a pair of scissors through it with the hope of removing it'. Three months later the mole began to grow and was 'oval, flat, black and soft, situated between the shoulders. There was also a small tumour, the size and colour of a black grape near its upper surface.' Norris removed 'all the disease with abundance of the surrounding substance.' The wound healed satisfactorily, and there was no return of the disease within 8 years.

If Norris suspected a malignant change in a mole, he recommended that the physician or surgeon 'should immediately not only remove the disease, but cut away some of the healthy parts. I would, after excising the part, touch the wound with caustic so as not to leave an atom of the disease, if possible, and occasionally apply the same remedy to the skin in the vicinity.' He used arsenic in this third case of melanosis, and the disease had not returned for 8 years. 'In the present state of our knowledge, when the disease appears in several parts of the body, physic will, I fear, uniformly fail and surgery will be foiled.'

Norris was jealous of his priority in describing the first case of melanoma, and he complained about subsequent authors not alluding to his case. 'It is singular that Cullen, Carswell and Fawdington should have written on the disease some years after I first published and never alluded to my case.' He claimed that he had seen more cases of melanosis than most provincial medical men and thought it was probably 'owing to my residing near the great coal and iron districts in England, where persons are frequently breathing air clouded with black smoke'.

Several principles involving the clinical management and the epidemiology of melanoma were pointed out by Norris 150 years ago. Some of these tenets are as follows.

First, the epidemiological features included: (1) that there was a relation between moles and melanomas, (2) that most patients had light-coloured hair and a fair complexion (3), that there was a family history in some cases and probably a hereditary disposition to the disease, and (4) that trauma may accelerate growth of the tumour.

Second, some pathological features included: (1) while melanoma was often black in colour, the degree of pigmentation varied, and it could be amelanotic, (2) it was often nodular or pedunculated, (3) satellite tumours might develop around the primary growth, (4) subcutaneous deposits might develop elsewhere, and (5) widespread dissemination could involve the lungs, liver, bone, heart, and dura mater.

Third, clinical features of the patients included: (1) they were more often men and heavy smokers, (2) they usually remained in good health until a very late stage of the disease, and (3) fever was not a feature, in contrast to tuberculosis.

Finally, regarding treatment, Norris (1) reported that local recurrence occurred after minimal excision, (2) was the first to advocate wide excision of the tumour and surrounding tissues, and (3) noted that neither medical nor surgical treatment was effective when the disease was widely disseminated.

Jean Cruveilier

Cruveilier is credited by Denkler and Johnson with having made original descriptions of primary melanomas of the hand, foot, and vulva and metastatic melanoma of the breast and bowel in his Anatomie Pathologique du Corps Human between 1829 and 1842.[16]

First description of a superficial spreading melanoma

In 1834, David Williams described a primary tumour in the following manner.[17] On his right shoulder he had a purple or dark brown stain like connate (i.e. congenital) spot or spilus (i.e. mole) about the size of a section of a pea; his wife noticed this mark was increasing in size.

The spilus continued to spread gradually, and after it had attained the circumference of a shilling, an excrescence, similar in colour to itself, began to rise in its centre. Williams's observation may be the first description of what we now refer to as horizontal and vertical growth phases of a superficial spreading melanoma.

First case in the United States of America

In 1837, Isaiah Parrish formally reported the first case of melanoma in America.[18] It concerned a 43-year-old woman with a 'fungous tumour on the ball of the great toe ... about half the size of a pigeon's egg. It had a red ... smooth ulcerated surface. On the upper surface of the toe, about half an inch from the nail, there was a black tubercule, slightly elevated above the skin and about the size of a shilling. The lymphatic glands [were] tender and inflamed. At autopsy, melanose bodies [were] scattered over the surface of the peritoneum.'

In 1838 Robert Carswell described melanoma in his *Illustrations of the Elementary Forms of Disease.*[15] He illustrated melanotic tumours in the liver, brain, small intestine, and omentum.

No known remedy

In 1840, Samuel Cooper gave a good description of the 'black cancer'.[19] Cooper remarked that 'no remedy is known for melanosis. The only chance for benefit depends upon the early removal of the disease by operation, when the situation of the part affected will admit of it.' It is interesting that this observation remains pertinent to present day treatment strategy, some 160 years later. Cooper continues that 'an eye affected by melanosis has been extirpated without any relapse having followed the operation at the end of two or three years; so have melanotic tumours of the skin and cellular tissue.'

First excision of metastases in lymph nodes

A case report published in 1851 in the *Lancet* describes secondary melanoma in the groin of a 45-year-old woman, occurring 2 years after excision of a dark tumour on the mons veneris.[20] Mr Fergusson removed the secondary deposit, 'the patient having been rendered insensible by chloroform. The tumour was about the size of an orange and when cut into presented all the characters of melanosis. The patient progressed favourably and was discharged well about six weeks after the operation.' This is apparently the first recorded case involving surgical excision of metastatic melanoma.

Sir James Paget – amelanotic melanoma

In 1853, Sir James Paget wrote in one of his best works, *Lectures on Surgical Pathology*, that 'spurious melanosis' described by previous authors were 'blackenings of various structures whose only common character is that they are not tumours'.[21] He emphasized that 'melanotic cancers [were] ... medullary cancers modified by the formation of black pigment in their elemental structures.' He referred to amelanotic tumours: 'Even in cancers that look colourless to the naked eye, I have found, with the microscope, single cells or nuclei having the true melanotic characters.' Paget was the first to report a comparatively large series of patients (25) with 'melanoid cancer'. Paget described what we now call superficial spreading melanoma in the following words. 'The patient is usually aware of a time at which a mole, observed as an unchanging mark from birth or infancy, began to grow. In some instances the growth is superficial, and the dark spot acquires a larger area and appears slightly raised by some growth beneath it: in other cases, the mole rises and becomes very prominent or nearly pendulous.'

Oliver Pemberton – variation in colour and first description in a black person

In 1858, Pemberton referred to melanosis in his *Observations on the History, Pathology and Treatment of Cancerous Diseases.*[10] He noted that melanotic cancer is very frequently 'located near a congenital mole or wart, or the congenital marks themselves undergo melanic degeneration'. He was the first to note the variation in colour within a melanoma. He remarked that 'in colour, melanosis has many shades. In its primary form in the skin it is almost always brownish. Later the brown shade assumes every intensity of black. Sometimes, especially in the alteration of warts, the first change is of a slate colour.' He noted that 'it is a disease of adult, middle-aged and even advanced life, rather than of childhood.' Pemberton also reported the first case of melanoma in a black man, a 29-year-old native of Madagascar. It is not surprising to learn that the lesion was located on the foot, a common site in dark-skinned melanoma patients. The patient died of disseminated disease, despite amputation below the knee.

Sir Jonathan Hutchinson – subungual melanoma and Hutchinson's melanotic freckle

Sir Jonathan Hutchinson is given credit for the first description of subungual melanoma.[22] Hutchinson referred to this entity of melanotic 'whitlow' again in 1886, stating that 'early amputation is demanded'.[23]

In 1892 and 1894, Hutchinson described and illustrated a series of cases, from which the name Hutchinson's melanotic freckle has been applied.[24,25] He described 'Sir A.D... (aged 56 years) with a large black stain on his left cheek, present for many years but increasing in size of late.' It was not one continuous patch but a 'number of separate spots, many of them confluent. An ugly nonpigmented ulcer developed above the black patch, close to the edge of the eyelid. This ulcer was epitheliomatous in some cases, and sarcomatous in others.' The pathological diagnosis was made by his son.

Cahn wrote some notes on Hutchinson.[26] He said that Osler described Hutchinson as the greatest generalized specialist of his generation, the last of the polymaths, (i.e. one varied and diversely learned, according to *Webster's New International Dictionary*). He became known as a syphilogist, a dermatologist, an ophthalmologist, a neurologist, and a surgeon. He probably recorded more clinical observations than anyone in the history of medicine. It is of interest, for example, that he was the first to describe a kerato-acanthoma. Most amazing of all, however, are his *Archives of Surgery*, which appeared as quarterly journals and were published over a period of 11 years. *He wrote every word of them.* McGovern believed that he was the first to recognise that melanomas could arise in lesions acquired in adult life.[27] His surgical ability culminated in his election as president of the Royal College of Surgeons of England.

Black urine

In 1885, Tennent reported that 'the urine has presented a somewhat peculiar colour, a greenish black tint' in a patient with advanced melanoma.[28] He believed that the peculiar colour of the urine was probably caused by the absorption of melanin. He also noted that the colour of multiple secondary tumours varied considerably in degree. He mentioned that a few of the tumours had no appearance of colour or pigmentation of any kind. Tennent noted that 'meddlesome interference with a mole has been spoken of as highly dangerous.'

First melanoma recorded in an American black man

In 1899 Gilchrist reported the first case of a microscopically confirmed melanoma in an American black man.[29] It commenced on the sole of the foot and disseminated widely.

First guidelines for surgical treatment

In 1885, Joseph Coats advocated extensive excision of primary melanomas.[30] Subsequently, in 1892, Herbert Snow recommended in addition to wide excision, a radical regional lymph node dissection.[31] This will be further discussed later in this chapter.

EARLY 20TH CENTURY REPORTS

Frederick Eve

In 1903, Frederic Eve delivered a lecture, in which he reported details of 45 melanoma patients treated at the London Hospital over the previous 20 years.[32] Eve described a melanoma on the sole of the foot and illustrated one on the palm of the hand. He remarked that 'it is generally stated that the melanomata are the most malignant of tumours' but referred to 'certain remarkable exceptions', including one patient who survived 20 years. The clinical management at that time also addressed surgery of the primary melanoma with elective removal of the regional lymph nodes. In his words: 'The treatment of melanoma of the skin can be given in a few words (i.e. free excision or amputation), in accordance with the position and extent of the disease. The removal of the nearest chain of lymphatic glands, whether palpably enlarged or not, should never be omitted; for it may be taken as a matter of certainty that in the great majority of cases they are infected.'

Melanoma arising in blemish free skin

In 1906, Fox noted that melanoma could arise on blemish free skin, 'although moles are by far the commonest situations from which melanotic growths arise, yet they can originate in a skin entirely devoid of naevus tissue'.[33]

Radical surgery – William Sampson Handley

In 1907, William Sampson Handley gave two Hunterian lectures on 'the pathology of melanotic growths in relation to their operative treatment'.[34] He showed both the anatomical pathways involving the spread of melanoma and centrifugal lymphatic permeation. He based his study on a single autopsy examination of a patient with a very advanced melanoma. On the basis of this slender database, he advocated wide local excision of the primary lesion, regional lymph node dissection, and amputation in selected cases. This is an important historical document, for Handley's recommendations formed the basis of melanoma treatment for the ensuing 60 years or more, until extensive resections of the primary melanoma and the effectiveness of elective regional lymphadenectomy began to be questioned (Figure 1.5).

Handley recommended and illustrated operations for 'melanotic sarcoma of the skin'. He stated 'When malignant melanoma arises in the digits, amputation should be performed at once. The flaps should never be cut so as to include any skin within, at least, one inch of the tumour.' For tumours elsewhere Handley recommended that 'a circular incision should be made through the skin around the tumour at what is judged by present standards to be a safe and practicable distance. The incision, situated as a rule about an inch from the tumour, should be just deep enough to expose the subcutaneous fat. The skin with a thin attached layer of subcutaneous fat is now separated from the deeper structures for about two inches in all directions around the skin incision. At the extreme base of the elevated skin flaps, a ring incision down to

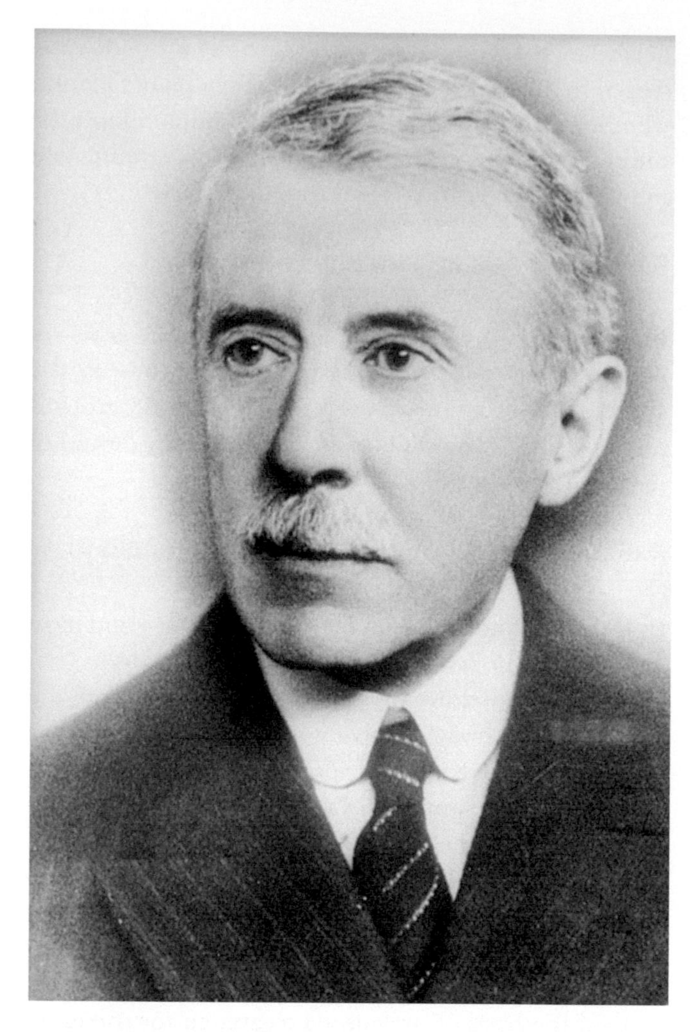

Figure 1.5 *William Sampson Handley, whose 1907 recommendations formed the basis for the treatment of melanoma for the following 60 years.*

the muscles surrounds and isolates the area of deep fascia and overlying deeper subcutaneous fat to be removed. This fascial area is next to be dissected up centripetally from the muscles beneath up to a line which corresponds with that of the circular skin incision. Finally, the whole mass with the growth at its centre is removed by scooping out with a knife a circular area of the muscle immediately subjacent to the growth. The excision of the (lymphatic) gland must ... be carried out on exactly the same principles as the excision of the primary tumour. In late cases it may even be right to remove an area of skin over the infected glands.'

It is of interest that, by 1935, Sampson Handley had treated 'only eight or ten cases in all, apart from hopelessly inoperable ones'. Three of these had long term survival.[35]

Hogarth Pringle

In 1908 Hogarth Pringle from Glasgow advised, in addition, the excision of a broad strip of subcutaneous tissue and deep fascia up to and including the nearest anatomical group of lymph nodes.[36] 'All that is removed should be in one continuous strip as far as possible.'

He based his advice on only three cases, but provided a follow up article in the *Lancet* in 1937.[37] Two of the three patients were alive 30 and 38 years after operation. The other patient developed widespread metastases. What he was trying to do was to avoid in-transit metastases, examples of which he had seen clinically.

William Dubreuilh

In 1912, Dubreuilh referred to pigmented lesions appearing in the skin during adult life.[38] McGovern later separated these into two distinct entities:[27]

1. The spreading macular pigmented lesions of the cheek and temple of elderly persons. In about 1800, Goya painted Carlos IV's family, a member of which had this type of lesion on her right temple. Hutchinson later descibed these as senile freckles and lentigo melanoses, subsequently known as Hutchinson's melanotic freckles (lentigo maligna) (Figure 1.6).
2. All other spreading macular pigmented lesions of the skin and mucosae. McGovern called these premalignant melanosis, now referred to as superficial spreading melanomas.

It is important to distinguish between these two groups, as the first rarely give rise to metastases whereas invasive nodules of malignant melanoma appearing in premalignant melanosis often lead to widespread metastases.

Advanced nature of melanoma

It must be remembered that melanoma was usually very advanced when diagnosed in the early 20th century and the prognosis was therefore poor. Crude 5-year survival rates are shown in Table 1.1, but comparison is not really valid since it is difficult to ascertain just what

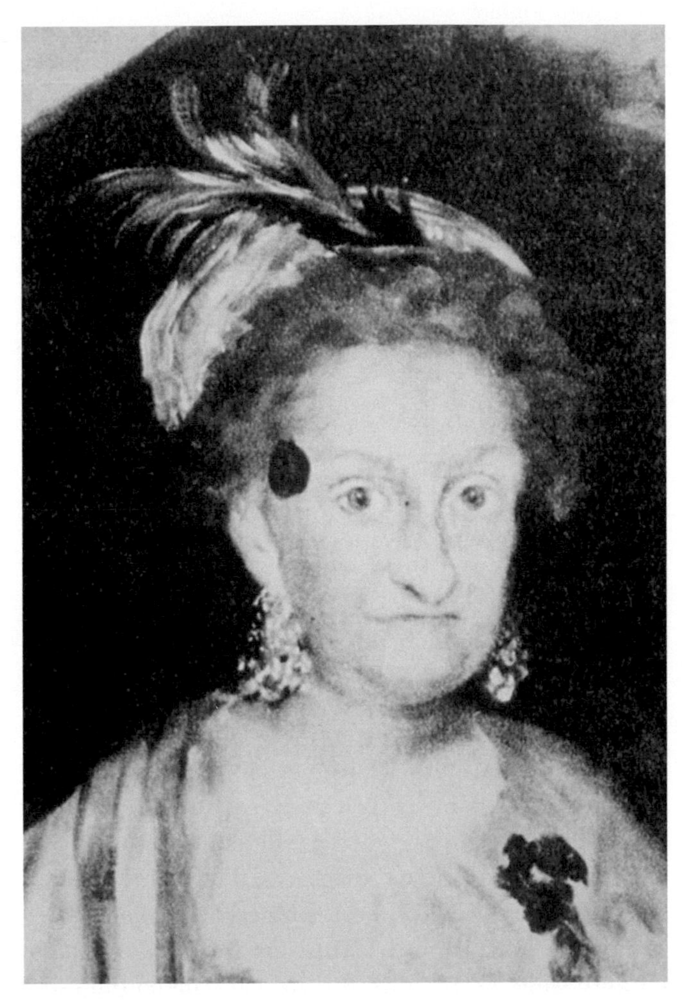

Figure 1.6 *Goya's painting of the Infanta Dona Maria Josefa, on the right temple of whom is a lesion that is almost certainly what we now call a Hutchinson's melanotic freckle or lentigo maligna.*

proportion of patients who first presented for treatment already had metastatic melanoma.

In 1916, Broders and MacCarty reported that 'the prognosis of melanotic tumours has been regarded as hopeless'.[39] Again in 1916, Coley and Hoguet stated that 'the prognosis of melanotic tumours has been regarded as hopeless. Unfortunately, the surgeon rarely sees a primary melanoma when surgery might offer some hope of permanent cure. The family physician fails to appreciate the gravity and either ties off the mole with a silk ligature or applies some caustic-like nitrate of silver or liquid air which not only increases the irritation but hastens its transformation into a highly malignant tumor.'[49] They used Coley's toxins but reported no case of permanent cure. However, they stated that there had been a marked retardation in a number of cases where toxins had been used.

Table 1.1 *Crude 5-year survival rates*

Source	No. of cases	Survival (%)
Broders and MacCarty (1916)[39]	70	13
Bloodgood (1922)[40]	200	<1
Gleave (1929)[41]	22	10
Scharnagel (1933)[42]	70	28
Adair (1936)[43]	105	33
Affleck (1936)[44]	170	10
Daland and Holmes (1939)[45]	61	21
Cholnoky (1941)[46]	75	42
Sylven (1947)[47]	151	48
Pack, Scharnagel and Morfit (1952)[48]	575	21

As late as 1932 Farrell from the Mayo Clinic stated that 'The prognosis in cases of melanoma is more unfavorable than that of any other type of neoplasm. Many investigators have maintained that treatment of any kind is of little value and believe that the lesions are better left entirely alone.'[50] He reviewed 265 cases and found that, in 30% of cases, there was a recurrence at the site of primary lesion excision. Only 26 patients presented at the Mayo Clinic without previous treatment and without metastases. Only 11 of these 26 survived 5 years, or, in other words, there was a 58% mortality. He believed deep x ray treatment was indicated rather than excision when the regional nodes were extensively involved. Of those treated in this manner, 95% were dead at 5 years.

In 1933, Amadon reported a series of 27 cases treated by electrocautery with 100% recurrence at the site of the primary, and early regional and distant metastases in most cases.[51]

ANATOMICAL SITE OF PRIMARY MELANOMAS

In the 19th and early 20th century there was a relatively low incidence of cutaneous melanoma compared with ocular melanoma (Table 1.2). The presumption is that ultraviolet radiation in those years was not a major factor in the aetiology of cutaneous melanoma. This left an apparently high proportion of non-cutaneous

Table 1.2 *Anatomical site of primary melanomas*

Source	No. of cases	Cutaneous (%)	Ocular (%)
Paget (1853)[21]	52	65	35
Pemberton (1858)[10]	23	61	39
Coley and Hoguet (1916)[49]	79	86	14
Broders and MacCarty (1916)[39]	70	94	6
Cooke (1928)[53]	43	77	23
Gleave (1929)[41]	40	55	45
Howes and Birnkrant (1943)[54]	26	77	23
US National Cancer Data Base (1985–94)[55]	77,370	94	6

melanomas such as ocular melanomas, the aetiology of which is not influenced by ultraviolet radiation.[52]

ANATOMICAL SITE OF CUTANEOUS MELANOMAS

It is interesting to note that the anatomical location of primary cutaneous melanomas in the early 20th century was considerably different from the present day. Then there was a high percentage on the feet, especially the toe (Table 1.3).

Table 1.3 *Anatomical site of cutaneous primary melanomas*

Source	No. of cases	Foot (%)	Other (%)
Coley and Hoguet (1916)[49]	68	13	87
Broders and MacCarty (1916)[39]	56	25	75
Cooke (1928)[53]	22	32	68
Horwitz (1928)[56]	45	38	62
Gleave (1929)[41]	13	23	77
Driver and McVicar (1943)[57]	60	23	77
Sydney Melanoma Unit (1999)	765	2	98

EVOLUTION OF SURGERY FOR MELANOMA

General considerations

Epidemiological studies have questioned the biological significance of many early lesions, suggesting that what was regarded as a melanoma epidemic was really an epidemic of 'melanoma' diagnosis, that included many lesions which would never progress or metastasize, regardless of treatment.[58] Thus the previous treatment of very wide excision of the primary melanoma and elective lymph node dissection has given way to a more precise, evidence supported policy of more limited local treatment, based on specific clinical and histological parameters, supported by careful investigation and precise definition of each patient's specific situation.

From 1970 to the present day the management of melanomas has undergone a series of important changes. Many of these changes have resulted from a changing pattern of disease presentation. In most countries nowadays, most patients with melanomas now presenting for treatment have early lesions with a tumour thickness <1 mm, thus rendering largely irrelevant the historical approaches developed for locally advanced melanomas.

TREATMENT OF THE PRIMARY LESION

The radical surgical management of primary melanoma developed initially in response to the almost universal presentation of locally advanced primary lesions. Coats in 1885 recommended that 'the operation should be so executed as to remove the tissue for some distance outside the apparent limits of the growth'.[30] In 1892 Snow recommended, in addition to wide excision, radical regional node dissection.[31] In 1907 Handley strongly urged the need for very wide excision of the tumour, guidelines which were adhered to for over 60 years.[34] A subsequent report by Olsen of 'atypical melanocytes found within 5 cm of the primary' advanced the wide excision approach.[59] Both these papers, and the other supporting documentation, suggested that not only was it likely there would be free melanoma cells in the vicinity of a primary melanoma, but also that activated melanocytes were present well clear of the primary lesion. Unless all these atypical melanocytes were removed, local recurrence was deemed to be very likely. Thus excisions of 10 cm in diameter ('dinner plate' excisions), with large skin grafts, were regularly performed for melanomas in many parts of the world. However, over the next 20 years, it became clear that these deforming operations did not substantially influence survival. In recent years, controlled clinical studies have confirmed that margins >2 cm are unnecessary and that for early lesions, a 1 cm clearance is adequate.[60,61] Thus a generally accepted policy, based on tumour thickness, has been developed and is standard practice in most countries of the world. A margin of 5 mm for in situ lesions, 1 cm for all T1 tumours <1 mm thick, and 2 cm for all other melanomas is now generally accepted as appropriate. Although there is as yet no evidence that margins >1 cm have any influence on survival, they do appear to influence the rates of local recurrence.

It has been shown that desmoplastic melanomas, particularly if neurotropism exists, have a substantially increased rate of local recurrence, so a 3 cm margin is advocated for these lesions.[62]

Treatment of regional lymph nodes

The controversy regarding the surgical management of regional lymph nodes began over 100 years ago. In 1892 Herbert Snow in his lecture on melanotic cancerous disease advocated wide excision of the primary lesion and elective lymph node dissection to control lymphatic permeation of metastases.[31] He writes about 'the utter futility of operative measures which are addressed to the primary lesions only. We further see the paramount importance of securing, whenever possible, the perfect eradication of those lymph glands which will necessarily be first infected before enlargement takes place, radical removal ... is a safe and easier measure.' This was based on the premise that metastatic melanoma progresses sequentially from primary site to regional lymph nodes. In his Hunterian lectures in 1907, Sampson Handley also advocated wide excision of the primary melanoma together with a regional lymphadenectomy.[35] One year after Handley's paper, Hogarth Pringle emphasized that wide excisions should be performed in continuity with regional lymph nodes.[36] These principles established the basis of melanoma treatment for more than 60 years. In the last 20 years, a number of major studies have questioned the value of elective lymph node dissection while the technique of selective lymphadenectomy (sentinel node biopsy) has provided a credible alternative to the procedure.[63–66] These matters are discussed in detail in other chapters of this book

EARLY PUBLIC AND PROFESSIONAL EDUCATION ABOUT MELANOMA

It has been known for several decades that Australia, and particularly its northern state, Queensland, has the highest incidence of skin cancer in the world. The Queensland Health Department was producing literature in the early 1960s describing the early signs of skin cancer and warning the public against excessive sun exposure.

An important part of the Queensland melanoma project, which started in 1963, has been its public and professional education campaign.[67] The educational programme has comprised lectures on melanoma, newspaper articles, discussions on radio and television, movie films, pamphlets, and posters. The 'slip, slap, slop' campaign proved to be a great success, with school aged children and adults being urged to slip on a shirt, slap on a hat, and slop on some sunscreen. Perhaps the most effective public educational activity in Australia was a nationally televised programme devised by the Sydney Melanoma Unit, portraying a young man's death from melanoma. Without doubt, this, and the efforts of the New South Wales State Cancer Council, have led to an increased diagnosis of melanoma at an early biological stage in Australia. In other parts of the world, public and professional education programmes are still generally less well developed, but the need for them is gradually becoming apparent.

REFERENCES

1. Urteaga OB, Pack GT, On the antiquity of melanoma. *Cancer* 1966; 19: 607–10.
2. Ariel MM, Is the beauty mark a mark of beauty or a potentially dangerous cancer? In: *Malignant melanoma*, (Ariel, M, ed.) New York: Appleton-Century-Crofts, 1981: 3–8.
3. Cameron JRJ, Melanoma of skin. *J R Coll Surg Edinb* 1968; 13: 233–54.
4. Unna PG 1894, quoted by Randle HW, Suntanning: differences in perceptions throughout history. *Mayo Clin Proc* 1997; 72: 461–6.
5. Cleland JB, Some remarks on the causes of cancer. *Australas Med Gazette* 1906; 25: 279–83.
6. Dubreuilh W, Epitheliomatose d'origine solaire. *Ann Dermatol Syphiligr (Paris)* 1907; 8: 387–91.
7. Lancaster HO, Nelson J, Sunlight as a cause of melanoma: a clinical survey. *Med J Aust* 1957; 1: 452–6.
8. Bodenham DC, A study of 650 observed malignant melanomas in the South West Region. *Ann R Coll Surg Engl* 1968; 43: 218–39.
9. Breschet G, *Considérations sur une altération organique appelee dégénérescence noire melanose, cancer melane, etc.* Paris: Bechet, 1821.
10. Pemberton O, *Observations on the history, pathology and treatment of cancerous diseases.* London: Churchill, 1858.
11. Dupuytren G, Anatomie pathologique. *Bulletin de la Faculté de Médecine de Paris, 1806.* Premier serie 1804–1808 (Tome Premier): 2–22.
12. Laennec RTH, Sur les melanoses. *Bulletin de la Faculte de Médecine de Paris, 1806.* Premier serie 1804–1808 (Tome Premier): 24–6.
13. Norris W. Case of fungoid disease, *Edinb Med Surg J* 1820; 16: 562–5.
14. Norris W, *Eight cases of melanosis with pathological and therapeutical remarks on that disease.* London: Longman, Brown, Green, Longman and Roberts, 1857.
15. Carswell R, *Illustrations of the Elementary Forms of Disease.* London: Longman, Orme, Brown, Green and Longman, 1838.
16. Denkler K, Johnson J, A lost piece of melanoma history. *Plast Reconstr Surg* 1999; 104: 2149–53.
17. Williams D, quoted in Silvers DN, On the subject of primary cutaneous melanoma: an historical perspective. In: *Progress in surgical pathology.* (eds Fenoglio CM and Wolff M). Vol.6. New York: Masson, 1982; 277–91.
18. Parrish I, Case of melanosis. *Am J Med Sci* 1837; 20: 266–8.
19. Cooper S, *First lines of theory and practice of surgery.* London: Longman, Orme, Brown, Green and Longman, 1840.
20. Mr Fergusson, Recurrence of melanotic tumour. *Lancet* 1851; 1: 622–3.
21. Paget J, *Lectures on surgical pathology.* Vol.2. London: Longman, Green, Longman, Roberts and Green, 1853.
22. Hutchinson J, Melanotic disease of the great toe, following a whitlow of the nail. *Trans Pathol Soc London* 1857; 8: 404.
23. Hutchinson J, Melanosis often not black: melanotic whitlow. *Br Med J* 1886; 1: 491.
24. Hutchinson J, One tissue dotage. *Arch Surg* 1892; 3: 315–22.
25. Hutchinson J, Lentigo melanosis. *Arch Surg* 1894; 5: 253–6.
26. Cahn LR, Some notes on Sir Jonathan Hutchinson (1828–1913). *Am J Surg Pathol* 1979; 3: 563–6.
27. McGovern VJ, Melanoma. In: *Malignant melanoma: clinical and histological diagnosis.* New York: John Wiley & Sons, 1976: 55–84.
28. Tennent GP, On a case of multiple melanotic sarcoma. *Glasg Med J* 1885; 24: 81–91.
29. Gilchrist TC, Are malignant growths arising from pigmented moles of a carcinomatous or sarcomatous nature? *J Cutan Dis* 1899; 17: 117–31.
30. Coats J, On a case of multiple melanotic sarcoma with remarks on the mode of growth and extension of such tumours. *Glasg Med J* 1885; 24: 92–7.
31. Snow H, Melanotic cancerous disease. *Lancet* 1892; 2: 872–4.
32. Eve F, A lecture on melanoma. *Practitioner* 1903; 70: 165–74.
33. Fox W, Research into the origin and structure of moles and their relation to malignancy. *Br J Dermatol* 1906; 18: 83–103.
34. Handley WS, The pathology of melanotic growths in relation to their operative treatment. *Lancet* 1907; 1: 927–33, 996–1003.
35. Handley WS, Prognosis of simple moles and melanotic sarcoma. *Lancet* 1935; 1: 1401–2.
36. Pringle JH, A method of operation in melanotic tumours of the skin. *Edinb Med J* 1908; 23: 496–9.
37. Pringle JH, Cutaneous melanoma: two cases alive 30 and 38 years after operation. *Lancet* 1937; 1: 508–9.
38. Dubreuilh W, De la melanose circonscrite précancereuse. *Ann Dermatol Syphiligr (Paris)* 1912; 3: 129–51.
39. Broders AC, MacCarty WC, Melano-epithelioma. *Surg Gynecol Obstet* 1916; 23: 28–32.
40. Bloodgood JC, Excision of benign pigmented moles. *JAMA* 1922; 79: 576.
41. Gleave HH, Prognosis in malignant melanoma. *Lancet* 1929; 2: 658–9.
42. Scharnagel T, Treatment of malignant melanomas of the skin and vulva at the Radiumhemmet, Stockholm. *Acta Radiol* 1933; 14: 473–90.
43. Adair F, Treatment of melanoma. *Surg Gynecol Obstet* 1936; 62: 406–9.
44. Affleck DE, Melanomas. *Am J Cancer* 1936; 27: 120–38.
45. Daland EM, Holmes JA. Malignant melanomas: clinical study, *N Engl J Med* 1939; 220: 651–60.
46. Cholnoky T, Malignant melanoma: clinical study of 117 cases. *Ann Surg* 1941; 113: 392–410.
47. Slyven B, Malignant melanoma of the skin. *Acta Radiol* 1947; 32: 33–59.
48. Pack GT, Scharnagel I, Morfit M, The principle of excision and dissection in continuity for primary and metastatic melanoma. *Surgery* 1945; 17: 849–61.
49. Coley WB, Hoguet JP, Melanotic cancer. *Ann Surg* 1916; 64: 206–41.
50. Farrell HJ, Cutaneous melanomas with special reference to prognosis. *Arch Dermatol Syph* 1932; 26: 110–24.
51. Amadon PD, Electrocoagulation of melanoma and its dangers. *Surg Gynecol Obstet* 1933; 56: 943–6.
52. Woll E, Bedikian A, Legha SS, Uveal melanoma: natural history and treatment options for metastatic disease. *Melanoma Res* 1999; 9: 575–81.
53. Cooke HH, Location of primary lesion in 53 cases of malignant melanomata. *Southern Med J* 1928; 21: 117–21.
54. Howes WE, Birnkrant M, Melanoma. *Am J Surg* 1943; 60: 182–9.
55. Chang AE, Karnell LH, Menck HR, The national cancer data base report on cutaneous melanoma. *Cancer* 1998; 83: 1664–78.
56. Howitz A, Melanotic tumors. *Ann Surg* 1928; 87: 917–32.
57. Driver JR, McVicar DN, Cutaneous melanomas. *JAMA* 1943; 121: 413–20.
58. Burton RC, Armstrong BK, Non-metastasizing melanoma? *J Surg Oncol* 1998; 67: 73–6.
59. Olsen, G, The malignant melanoma of the skin. New theories based on a study of 500 cases. *Acta Chir Scand Suppl* 1966; 365: 1–222.
60. Bono A, Bartoli C, Clemente C, et al, Ambulatory narrow excision for thin melanoma (<2mm): results of a prospective study. *Eur J Cancer* 1997; 33: 1330–2.
61. Ringborg U, Andersson R, Eldh J, et al, Resection margins 2 versus 5 cm for cutaneous malignant melanoma with a tumor thickness of 0.8 to 2.0 mm. *Cancer* 1996; 77: 1809–14.
62. Quinn MJ, Crotty KA, Thompson JF, et al, Desmoplastic and desmoplastic neurotropic melanoma: experience with 280 patients. *Cancer* 1998; 83: 1128–36.
63. Reintgen D, The role of elective lymph node dissection: who should undergo this nodal staging procedure. *J Am Coll Surg* 1999; 189: 224–32.
64. Cascinelli N, Moribito A, Santinami M, et al, Immediate or delayed dissection of regional nodes in patients with melanoma of the trunk: a randomized trial. *Lancet* 1998; 351: 793–6.
65. Morton DL, Wen DR, Wong JH, et al, Technical details of intraoperative lymphatic mapping for early stage melanoma. *Arch Surg* 1992; 127: 392–9.
66. Morton DL, Thompson JF, Essner R et al, Validation of the accuracy of intraoperative lymphatic mapping and sentinel lymphadenectomy for early-stage melanoma. *Ann Surg* 1999; 220: 453–65.
67. Davis NC, Herron JJ, Queensland melanoma project: organisation and a plea for comparable surveys. *Med J Aust* 1966; 1: 643–4.

2

Cell cycle regulation in the melanocyte

Helen Rizos, Therese M Becker, Elizabeth A Holland

INTRODUCTION

The principal function of epidermal melanocytes is the production of photoprotective melanin pigments. This activity does not require high cell turnover, and melanocytes in adult skin are only intermittently mitotic. In certain situations, however, such as wound healing or after exposure to ultraviolet (UV) radiation, there are additional requirements for melanin and the mitotic rate of melanocytes increases several fold. This proliferative response requires a delicate balance between negative and positive cell cycle regulatory signals. Any alteration in these signals can result in unlimited cell division, which is the hallmark of malignancy. Genetic alterations in hundreds of different genes may contribute to tumour formation, but the role of the negative cell cycle regulator $p16^{INK4a}$ in melanoma susceptibility indicates that cell cycle regulatory events are critical in the genesis of this cancer. To identify the precise links between $p16^{INK4a}$ inactivation and melanoma development the specific molecular mechanisms controlling the melanocytic cell cycle need to be defined. The regulation of the cell cycle in the normal melanocyte is the focus of this chapter.

Note: The nomenclature of molecules controlling cell cycle progression is complex, and names are frequently derived from named homologues isolated from earlier studies in yeast cells. The terms and abbreviations are gathered for convenience in the glossary at the end of the chapter.

CELL CYCLE CONTROL IN MAMMALIAN CELLS

A cell cultured in the laboratory requires up to 48 hours to complete one cell division cycle. This cycle is divided into four phases, a DNA synthesis phase (S phase), a mitotic cell division stage (M phase), and two intervening phases called 'Gap 1' (G1) and 'Gap 2' (G2) (Figure 2.1). Progression through these cell cycle phases is associated with the sequential expression and activation of cyclin/cyclin dependent kinase complexes.[1] There are at least 16 different mammalian cyclins (including A, B1, B2, D1, D2, D3, and E) and 12 different cyclin dependent kinase (cdk) molecules (including cdk1, cdk2, cdk4, and cdk6).[2,3] D-type cyclins act as growth factor sensors, and as cells enter the cell cycle from quiescence (G0) they are induced in response to growth factor stimulation. The association of D-type cyclins with their catalytic partners, cdk4 and cdk6, promote transition through the G1 phase and into the S phase of the cell cycle (Figure 2.1).[4] Specific INhibitors of cdK4 and cdk6 – the INK4 proteins – inhibit cyclin D associated kinase activity and induce potent G1 cell cycle arrest. The four INK4 protein members ($p15^{INK4b}$, $p16^{INK4a}$, $p18^{INK4c}$, and $p19^{INK4d}$) bind and inhibit cdk4 and cdk6, but not other cdks (Figure 2.1) (reviewed in[5,6]). The $p16^{INK4a}$ inhibitor can also induce cell cycle arrest in the G2 phase by inhibiting the cyclin D3/cdk4 complex (Figure 2.1).[7,8]

The primary substrates of the cyclin D dependent kinases are the retinoblastoma family of proteins, which include the retinoblastoma protein (pRb), p107, and p130 (reviewed in[9,10]). These functionally and

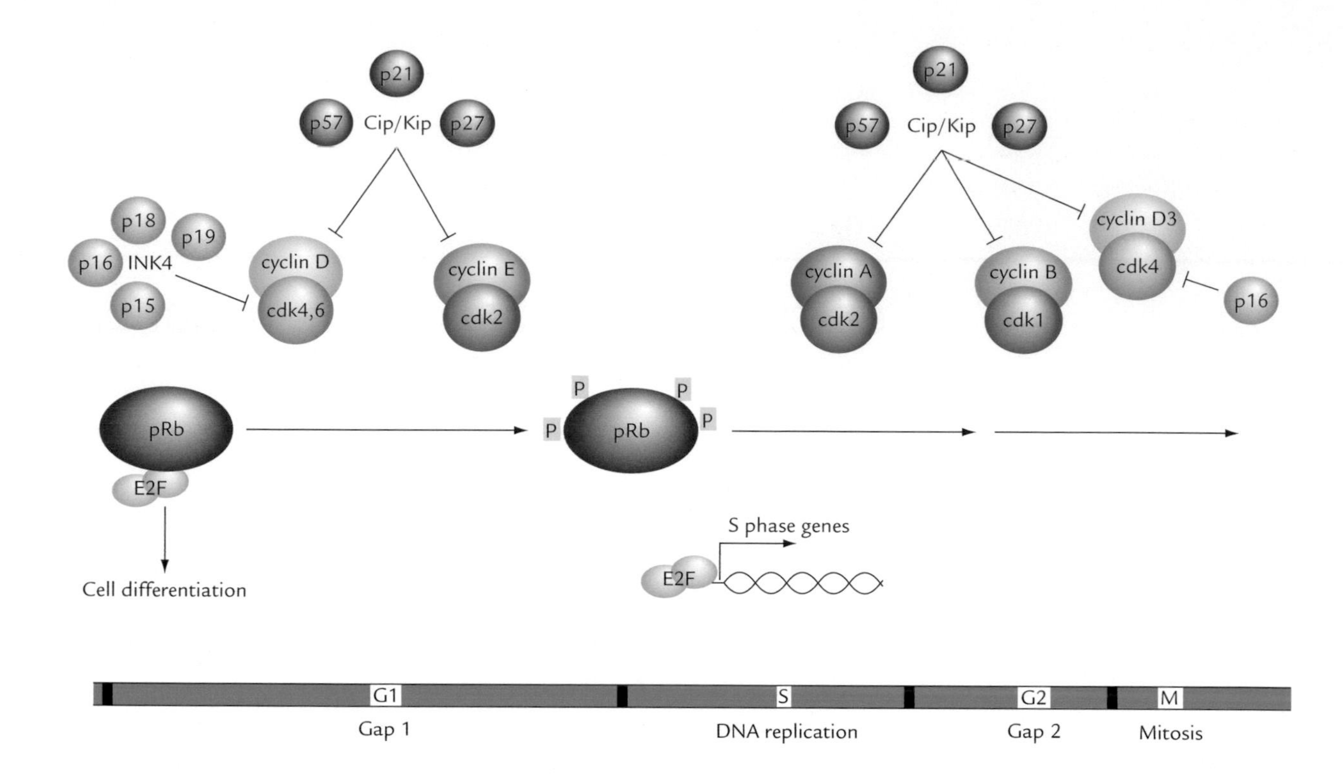

Figure 2.1 *Regulation of the eukaryotic cell cycle. Active, hypophosphorylated pRb binds E2F transcription factors in early G1 and suppresses the expression of specific target genes. In late G1, cyclin D/cdk 4,6 and cyclin E/cdk2 complexes phosphorylate pRb. This leads to the release of E2Fs and the expression of S phase target genes. Cyclin A associated kinase activity is required for entry and completion of DNA synthesis (S phase) and entry into mitosis (M phase) of the cell cycle. Cyclins are inhibited by two classes of cyclin dependent kinase inhibitors, INK4 (p15, p16, p18, p19) and Cip/Kip (p21, p27, p57).*

structurally related pocket proteins bind and regulate a large number of cellular proteins, including members of the E2F family of transcription factors.[11] E2Fs are heterodimers containing a subunit encoded by the E2F gene family (E2F-1 to E2F-6) and a subunit encoded by the DP family of genes (DP-1 and DP-2). E2F factors control the transcription of many genes that encode proteins involved in cell cycle progression (for example, p107, E2F-1, E2F-2, cyclin E, cyclin A), DNA metabolism (dihydrofolate reductase, thymidine kinase, thymidylate synthase, histone H2A), the p53 pathway ($p21^{Cip1}$, p14ARF[12]) and proto-oncogenes (Myc, Myb) (reviewed in[10]). Binding of pocket proteins to the E2Fs inhibits the transactivation activity of E2F factors, and in some instances converts E2Fs from transcriptional activators to transcriptional repressors.[13] The end result of this binding is to restrict the cell in the resting G1 phase of the cell cycle. Clearly, alteration of this biochemical cascade will perturb the regulation of the cell cycle, with a tendency to precipitate cells into unregulated cell division.

Phosphorylation of pRb and the other two family members is initiated by the cyclin D dependent kinases and then accelerated by the cyclin E/cdk2 complex in mid to late G1 (Figure 2.1).[4] pRb hyperphosphorylation results in the release of E2F transcription factors and the expression of the above mentioned E2F regulated genes. Cyclin E is itself E2F responsive and cyclin E/cdk2 acts through positive feedback in progressive rounds of pRb phosphorylation and E2F release.[14] Although all three pocket proteins are likely to be phosphorylated by the cyclin D/cdk complexes, pRb is the critical cell cycle regulator.

DNA replication and transition into the G2 phase of the cell cycle requires cyclin A/cdk2 kinase and the proliferating cell nuclear antigen (PCNA).[15–17] Cyclin A associated kinases maintain pRb in its hyperphosphorylated state and phosphorylate the E2F heterodimerization partner DP1, resulting in inhibition of E2F transactivation capacity (reviewed in[2]). PCNA stimulates the activity of both DNA polymerase δ and ε and is required for DNA replication and for nucleotide excision repair.[18–21] Regulators of the G2/M transition include cyclin B/cdk1 and cyclin D3/cdk4 complexes (Figure 2.1).[8,22] The cyclin B/cdk1 complex phosphorylates cytoskeletal proteins including lamins, and cyclin D3/cdk4 phosphorylates p130.[23,24] Any perturbation of these regulators will arrest the cell cycle at the G2/M checkpoint.

Most cyclin/cdk complexes can be inhibited by the Cip/Kip (Cyclin dependent kinase Interacting Protein-1/Kinase Inhibitory Protein) family of cdk inhibitors, $p21^{Cip1}$, $p27^{Kip1}$ and $p57^{Kip2}$ (Figure 2.1).[22] $p21^{Cip1}$ can also interact with PCNA to inhibit DNA replication, but not the DNA repair function of PCNA (Figure 2.2).[25–27] In normal cells the Cip/Kip inhibitors are gathered into complexes that contain a cyclin and a cdk molecule, and a PCNA molecule in the case of $p21^{Cip1}$. The level of cyclin/cdk inactivation is determined by the fraction of kinase molecules complexed with the cdk inhibitor.[28] The expression of the Cip/Kip proteins can delay the cell cycle at the G1 and G2 phases and permits the repair of damaged DNA before DNA replication (S phase) or before cell division (M phase).

The most important feature of $p21^{Cip1}$, in terms of tumourigenesis, is its inducibility by the p53 tumour suppressor. p53 is rapidly activated in response to cellular stress signals, and it can induce delays in the G1 and

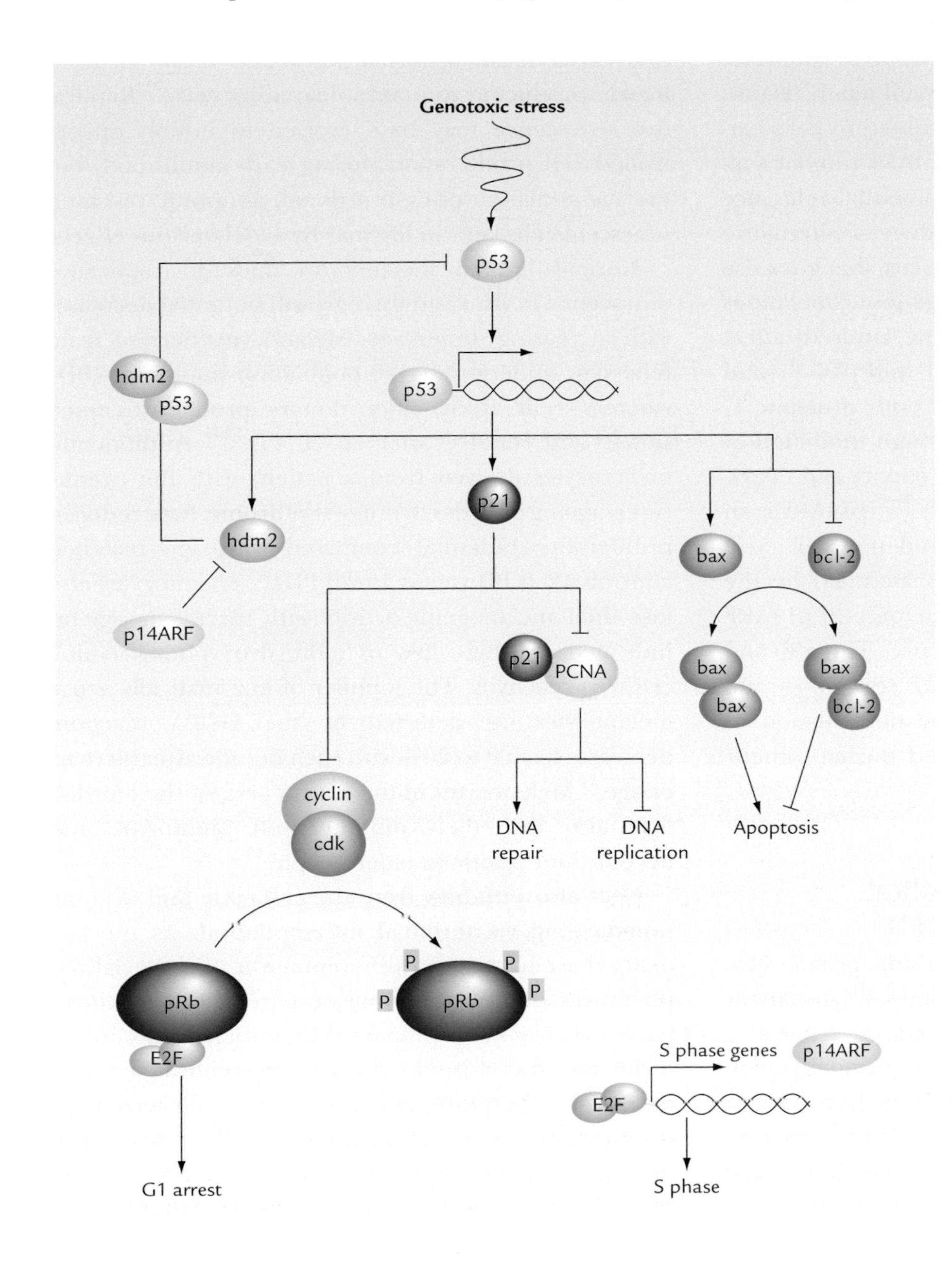

Figure 2.2 *Regulation of growth arrest and apoptosis by p53. Cellular DNA damage induces p53 accumulation by post-translational stabilization. p53 increases the expression of (1) hdm2, which operates in a feedback loop to limit p53 function; (2) $p21^{Cip1}$, which induces growth arrest and repair by inhibiting cyclin/cdk complexes and interacting with the proliferating cell nuclear antigen (PCNA); and (3) bax, an activator of apoptosis. p53 also downregulates the survival gene, bcl-2. Cell cycle arrest in the G1 phase is mediated by the inhibition of cyclin/cdk complexes and the maintenance of pRb in an hypophosphorylated state (Figure 2.1). p53 induced apoptosis involves a shift in the levels of bcl-2 and bax proteins, favouring bax accumulation (adapted from[106]).*

G2 phases of the cell cycle, or apoptotic cell death if cellular damage is irreparable. Induction of G1 arrest by p53 is mediated largely by the transcriptional activation of the $p21^{Cip1}$ cdk inhibitor (Figure 2.2). The p53 regulated G2 arrest also involves p53 regulated genes. Several of these, including $p21^{Cip1}$, Gadd45, and 14-3-3σ, inhibit the activity of cyclin B/cdk1 (reviewed in[29]). Cells exposed to high doses of radiation often undergo rapid apoptotic cell death via p53 dependent and independent pathways. p53-mediated apoptosis does not depend on $p21^{Cip1}$, and p53 directly induces apoptosis promoting genes, such as bax and downregulates survival genes, such as bcl-2.[30–32] The relative level of bcl-2 and bax in a stressed cell determines its fate; accumulation of bax/bcl-2 heterodimers will suppress apoptosis, while bax homodimers will promote cell death (Figure 2.2). The p53 checkpoint is also activated in cells harbouring active oncogenes, via the p14ARF tumour suppressor.[33,34] p14ARF has particular potential relevance to melanoma because it is the product of alternative splicing from the CDKN2A genetic locus, that gives rise to $p16^{INK4a}$ (see Chapter 5). Certain genomic mutations in this locus in hereditary melanoma kindreds affect the amino structure of both p14ARF and $p16^{INK4a}$ and alter the subcellular localization of both proteins.[35,36] p14ARF causes p53 stabilization through inhibition of hdm2, which promotes the nuclear export and degradation of the p53 protein (Figure 2.2).[37–44] p14ARF is an important link between the pRb and p53 cell cycle pathways. Expression of p14ARF is activated by the pRb-regulated E2F-1 transcription factor, and p14ARF enhances the stability and activity of p53. The pRb and p53 pathways are closely linked in regulating and maintaining the cell cycle, and the deregulation of both pathways is commonly observed during tumour evolution.

AGEING OF MELANOCYTES: TERMINAL DIFFERENTIATION AND SENESCENCE

Most normal diploid cells have a finite proliferative capacity and will eventually enter a state of permanent growth arrest, referred to as cellular or replicative senescence. Senescent cells remain viable and metabolically active in culture but are completely refractory to physiological mitogenic stimuli (reviewed in[45,46]). Expression of senescence associated pH 6.0 β-galactosidase activity in human skin cells has provided evidence that cells also undergo replicative senescence in vivo.[47] The physiological significance of this terminal non-dividing state remains controversial. It is thought to be an important, albeit flawed, tumour suppressive mechanism; tumours often contain immortal cells or cells with an extended replicative lifespan.[48] Senescence may also contribute to ageing of the organism. Skin biopsies from older individuals have a greater proportion of senescent cells in situ and a lesser proliferative capacity in culture.[49] Senescent cells can become resistant to apoptotic cell death, by overexpressing bcl-2 (see Figure 2.2 and Cell cycle control in mammalian cells above for more detail), and display changes in differentiated functions.[50] So for example, the onset of senescence induces normal fibroblasts to switch from matrix producing to matrix degrading cells.[51] Replicative senescence may have evolved to inhibit uncontrolled cell proliferation during early adulthood, but the accumulation of dysfunctional, apoptotic resistant, senescent cells later in life may have deleterious effects.

Normal human melanocytes undergo replicative senescence in vitro and their growth potential decreases with increasing donor age. Melanocytes derived from fetal skin undergo 90–120 population doublings (PD) whereas cells from older donors proliferate much slower and senesce after 20–30 PD.[52,53] Additionally, melanocytes derived from a patient with the prematurely ageing disorder, Werner's syndrome, have reduced proliferative potential compared with age matched controls (2–3 PD versus 15–20 PD).[53] Melanocytes also lose their melanogenic activity with increasing age, as indicated by their loss of α-dihydroxyphenylalanine (DOPA) reactivity. The number of enzymatically active melanocytes, as detected by the DOPA reaction, decreases from 8 to 20% with each decade after 30 years of age.[54] Melanocytes in the matrix area of the hair follicle also lose their differentiated phenotype and become amelanotic in older people.[55]

Cells also withdraw from the cell cycle and become non-dividing via terminal differentiation. As the cell nears the end stage of differentiation, the specialized phenotype of the cell becomes apparent, and its mitotic potential ceases.[56] Terminally differentiated cells do not divide and therefore do not undergo replicative senescence.[57] Furthermore, unlike senescent cells terminally differentiated cells accumulate low levels of bcl-2 (Figure 2.2) and are consequently susceptible to apoptosis.[56] Proliferating melanocytes and melanoma cells accumulate high levels of bcl-2 whereas the differentiation of melanocytes in culture is associated with the downregulation of this apoptotic inhibitor.[58–60] Thus, the decrease in melanocyte numbers as humans age may result from the programmed cell death of the accumulating, terminally differentiated melanocytes.

The onset of replicative senescence and terminal differentiation involves the negative cell cycle regulatory genes $p27^{Kip1}$, $p21^{Cip1}$ and $p16^{INK4a}$ (Figure 2.1). The $p21^{Cip1}$ and $p16^{INK4a}$ kinase inhibitors participate in the regulation and/or maintenance of cellular senescence and terminal differentiation of keratinocytes, myocytes, lymphocytes and neuronal cells.[48,61–66] Discovery of inactivating $p16^{INK4a}$ gene mutations in hereditary melanoma kindreds and the differential expression of $p21^{Cip1}$ during the growth of melanoma suggest that these proteins also participate in regulating the senescent or differentiation pathways in normal melanocytes.[67–73]

Melanocytes terminally differentiate when grown in medium supplemented with the cAMP inducer cholera toxin. In this culture system, melanocytes accumulate high concentrations of melanin and prematurely withdraw from the cell cycle. Terminally differentiated and senescent melanocytes are similar in that they maintain pRb in its active, hypophosphorylated state, thus preventing the activation of transcription factors and cell cycle progression (Figure 2.1). The hypophosphorylation of pRb is maintained via the accumulation of various cdk inhibitors and the subsequent inhibition of cdk4 and cdk2. In terminally differentiated melanocytes expression of the cdk inhibitor $p27^{Kip1}$ is dramatically increased, the level of $p21^{Cip1}$ and $p16^{INK4a}$ is only moderately enhanced and the expression of cyclin D1 is reduced (see summary panel).[53,74] In contrast, senescent melanocytes accumulate high levels of $p21^{Cip1}$ and $p16^{INK4a}$, rather than $p27^{Kip1}$.[53] The specific role of $p27^{Kip1}$ in the onset of terminal differentiation is not well understood. It has been suggested that the process of differentiation requires a function of $p27^{Kip1}$ other than the inhibition of cyclin associated activities, and that this requirement may reflect a novel pRb kinase activity present in $p27^{Kip1}$ complexes.[75]

Senescent and terminally differentiated melanocytes also differ from proliferating melanocytes in their mitogen-activated protein kinase (MAPK) and UV response pathways. The MAPK pathway is necessary for melanocyte proliferation and is stimulated by many growth factors. This signal transduction pathway is not active in senescent or terminally differentiated melanocytes, which do not activate the critical MAP kinase, ERK2.[76] The inability to activate ERK2 may maintain high levels of melanin synthesis as ERK2 phosphorylates and thereby activates the degradation of the microphthalmia associated transcription factor

Summary panel *Ageing of melanocytes: terminal differentiation and senescence*

Senescent melanocytes	Terminally differentiated melanocytes
• Non-dividing	• Non-dividing
• Cdk inhibitors inactivate cyclin/cdks	• Cdk inhibitors inactivate cyclin/cdks
High concentrations of $p21^{Cip1}$ and $p16^{INK4a}$	Modest increase in $p21^{Cip1}$ and $p16^{INK4a}$
No increase in $p27^{Kip1}$ levels	High concentrations of $p27^{Kip1}$
	Reduced cyclin D1
• pRb remains hypophosphorylated	• pRb remains hypophosphorylated
• E2F factors remain bound to pRb	• E2F factors remain bound to pRb
• Inactive ERK2	• Inactive ERK2
• Delayed p53 response after UV	• Delayed p53 response after UV
No further increase in $p21^{Cip1}$	No further increase in $p21^{Cip1}$
• Resistant to apoptosis (high bcl-2)	• Susceptible to apoptosis (low bcl-2)

(MITF).[77] This transcriptional regulator stimulates tyrosinase and tyrosinase related protein-1 (TRP-1), which are involved in the enzymatic process that converts tyrosine to melanin pigments.[74] As a result, senescent and terminally differentiated melanocytes, with inactive ERK2, may have constitutive MITF expression, high levels of MITF induced melanogenic enzymes, and increased melanin production. The accumulation of inactive ERK2 in senescent and terminally differentiated melanocytes may also affect p53 stabilization after UV irradiation. MAP kinases have a direct role in the UVB induced phosphorylation of p53 at serine 15.[78] Phosphorylation of this residue stabilizes p53 by reducing its interaction with hdm2 (Figure 2.2). Consequently, whereas UVB irradiation of normal melanocytes induces the expression of the cdk inhibitor, $p21^{Cip1}$, in a p53 dependent manner (discussed in more detail under Modulation of the melanocyte cell cycle by ultraviolet radiation below), senescent and terminally differentiated melanocytes have a delayed induction of p53, after UVB light exposure, and no further increase in $p21^{Cip1}$ levels (see summary panel). In addition, senescent melanocytes express high levels of the apoptotic inhibitor bcl-2 and are more resistant to UVB induced apoptosis than young, proliferating melanocytes.[52] Thus, although senescence prevents melanocytes from dividing indefinitely, exposure to DNA damaging agents, such as UV radiation, may produce a population of viable but genetically damaged melanocytes, keenly predisposed to malignant progression.

MODULATION OF THE MELANOCYTE CELL CYCLE BY ULTRAVIOLET RADIATION

UV irradiation of skin stimulates melanocyte division and promotes the production and release of photoprotective melanin pigments.[79–81] The number of melanocytes and melanin synthesis activity returns to normal after radiation exposure ceases.[82]

The stimulation of melanin synthesis after UV irradiation involves the α-melanocyte stimulating hormone (α-MSH) receptor system and the p53 transcription factor (Figure 2.3). UV radiation enhances the synthesis and release of α-MSH and other paracrine factors, including adrenocorticotropic hormone by the human epidermis.[83,84] These factors act via the melanocortin-1 receptor, on melanocytes, to activate the cAMP pathway (Figure 2.3). Activation of this pathway initiates a series of events that culminate in increased melanin synthesis. The cAMP cascade involves the activation of protein kinase A, which phosphorylates and activates the cellular transcription factor CREB, leading to the transcriptional activation of MITF. Activation of MITF enhances the expression of melanogenic enzymes and thereby increases melanin synthesis (Figure 2.3).[77,85–87] Specific variants in the human melanocortin-1 receptor (Arg151Cys, Arg160Trp and Asp294His) influence the response to UV radiation and are associated with red hair, fair skin, poor tanning, and melanoma.[88–90] UV light is also a potent inducer of p53 expression and, like MITF, p53 directly stimulates tyrosinase and TRP-1.[91]

In addition to melanin accumulation, melanocytes in culture respond to UV radiation with a dose-dependent decrease in cell cycle progression and cell survival. The UV induced apoptosis of melanocytes involves accumulation of p53 and reduction in the levels of the survival promoting bcl-2 (Figures 2.2 and 2.3). The decrease in melanocyte cell cycle progression is due to transient delays in the G1 phase, after one UVB dose, or in the G2 phase, after multiple doses.[92] Melanocytes exposed to a single dose of UVB radiation respond, within 15 hours of irradiation, with an accumulation in G1, which is accompanied by a reduction in the percentage of cells undergoing DNA synthesis.[93] In these cells, p53 rapidly accumulated 4 hours after UVB exposure and remained elevated for at least 48 hours. The accumulation of p53 in UVB irradiated cells correlated with increased expression of the cdk inhibitor $p21^{Cip1}$, which continued to accumulate 48 hours after irradiation. As expected, hyperphosphorylation of pRb was strongly and persistently inhibited in UVB irradiated melanocytes, consistent with the observed UVB induced G1 cell cycle arrest. It is possible that cdk inhibitors, such as $p16^{INK4a}$, initiate the block in pRb phosphorylation, since $p21^{Cip1}$ accumulation was detected 16 hours after pRb phosphorylation was inhibited.[92]

Melanocytes exposed to multiple doses of UV irradiation can arrest in the G2 phase of the cell cycle. This arrest is associated with post replication repair of damaged DNA and, since melanocytes express maximal α-MSH activity in this phase, a delay in G2 may stimulate melanin synthesis in an autocrine fashion.[94–96] The induction of UV induced G2 cell cycle arrest involves the INK4 cdk inhibitor, $p16^{INK4a}$ (Figures 2.1 and 2.3). In response to UV radiation epidermal melanocytes in vivo expressed elevated concentrations of $p16^{INK4a}$ (Figure

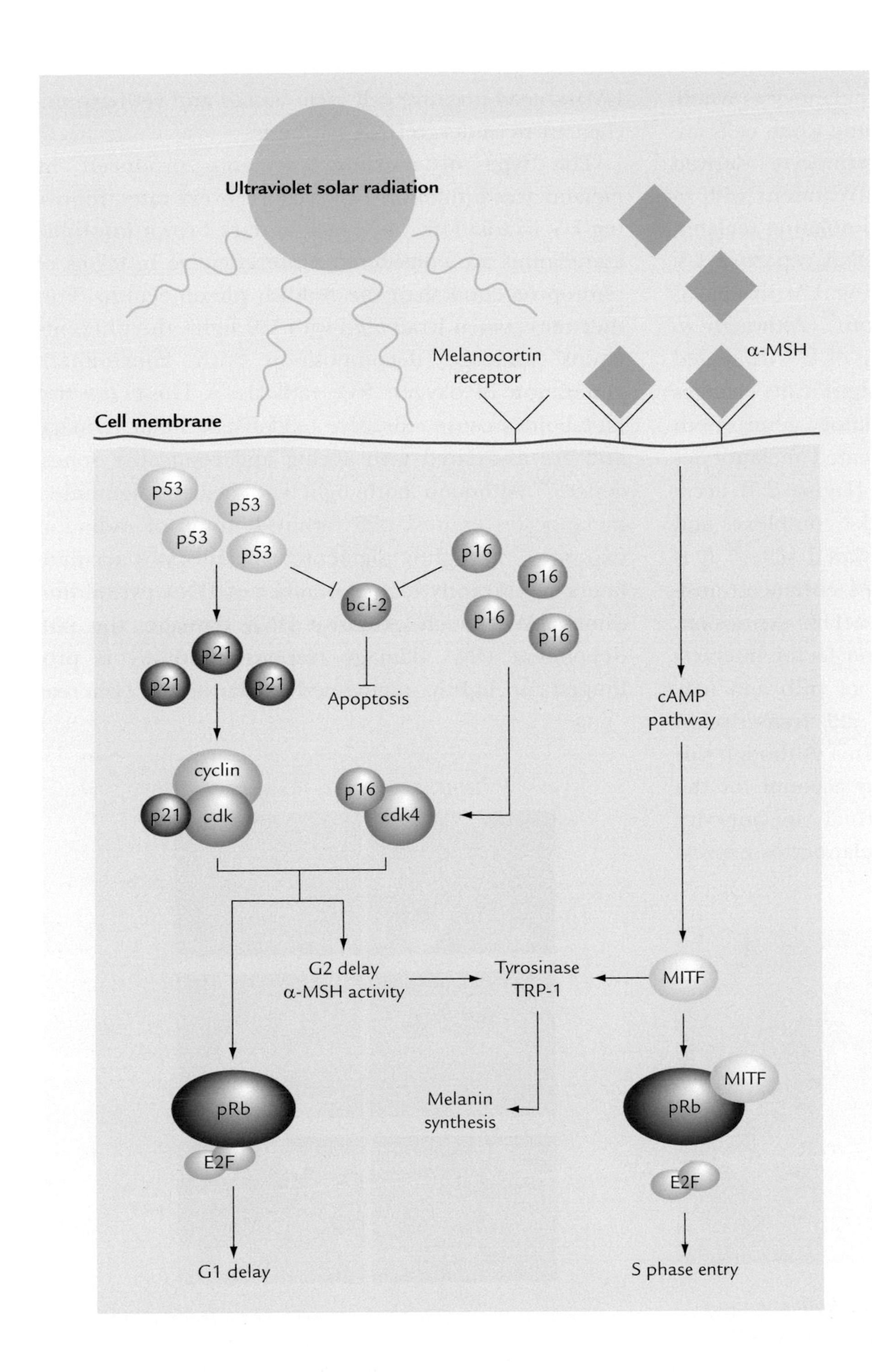

Figure 2.3 *UV response pathways active in epidermal melanocytes. UV irradiation induces the activation of the α-MSH pathway, the accumulation of the cdk inhibitor p16^INK4a^ and the p53 tumour suppressor in melanocytes. These proteins initiate a complex cascade of events that culminates in increased melanin synthesis. The transient cell cycle delays in the G1 and G2 phases, allows DNA repair to occur before DNA synthesis (S phase) or mitosis (M phase) occur (see text for details).*

2.4).[97] The accumulation of p16^{INK4a} in melanocytes was delayed compared with p53, peaking between 24 and 48 hours after irradiation and decreasing by 72 hours.[97] The increase in p16^{INK4a} after irradiation of HeLa cells correlated with S and G2 phase delays.[7] The radiation induced G2 cell cycle delay was absent in HeLa and melanoma cell lines that did not express p16^{INK4a}. The loss of functional p16^{INK4a} also correlated with an increase in DNA damage after radiation exposure.[98] In HeLa cells exposed to UV light, p16^{INK4a} bound and inhibited the cyclin D3/cdk4 (Figures 2.1 and 2.3). This complex is necessary for cell cycle progression through G2 phase into mitosis and its inhibition, by p16^{INK4a}, delays G2 phase progressing after UV exposure.[8] This may provide the mechanistic link between UV exposure, p16^{INK4a} function, and melanoma.

The cell cycle delay observed in melanocytes irradiated with UV light is partially overcome when cells are treated with α-MSH or the keratinocyte derived paracrine factor, endothelin-1.[99,100] Treatment with α-MSH provides photoprotection by stimulating melanin production and may enhance the DNA repair of UV induced photoproducts, thus allowing UV irradiated melanocytes to resume proliferation.[99] Although α-MSH treatment enhances the cycling of UV irradiated melanocytes, it does not cause any significant changes in the expression of cell cycle regulatory genes. Both UVB-minus and UVB-plus α-MSH-treated melanocytes express high levels of p53 and $p21^{Cip1}$ (Figure 2.5), accumulate inactive $p21^{Cip1}$-cyclin D1/cdk4 complexes and maintain pRb in an hypophosphorylated state.[99] It is possible that α-MSH and endothelin-1 enhance transition into S phase by upregulating MITF expression. This melanocyte specific transcription factor interacts with the hypophosphorylated form of pRb and may therefore induce the release of the E2F transcription factors and S phase entry (Figure 2.3).[101] Although this model remains to be proved, it may account for the continued cell cycling of epidermal melanocytes exposed to UV radiation. These melanocytes express UV induced negative cell cycle signals and yet have the capacity to undergo DNA synthesis.

The type of melanin pigments produced by melanocytes influences cell cycle recovery rates, following UV irradiation. The black to dark brown insoluble eumelanins are considered more effective in terms of photoprotection than the reddish pheomelanins. Furthermore, when irradiated with UV light, the pheomelanins undergo decomposition with concomitant generation of oxygen free radicals.[102] These reactive metabolites cause extensive oxidative cellular damage and are associated with ageing and replicative senescence.[103] Although both light and heavily pigmented melanocytes express p53 within 4 hours of radiation exposure, the lightly pigmented melanocytes accumulate a significantly higher number of DNA pyrimidine dimers. With such extensive DNA damage, the p53 dependent DNA damage response pathway is prolonged in lightly pigmented melanocytes, whereas

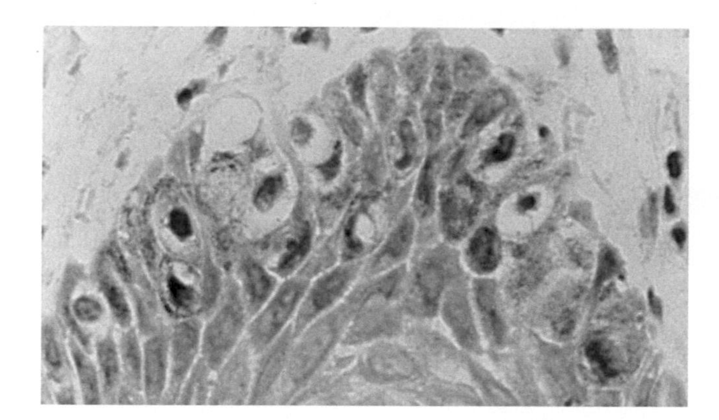

Figure 2.4 *Exposure of human skin to UV radiation induces the accumulation of the cdk inhibitor $p16^{INK4a}$. Organ cultures established from neonatal foreskins were irradiated with 250 J/m^2 UVB (0.3 minimal erythemal dose). Immunostaining was conducted 24 hours after irradiation using a rabbit polyclonal $p16^{INK4a}$ antibody. Sections were lightly counterstained with haematoxylin. Control unirradiated skin samples expressed very low to undetectable concentrations of $p16^{INK4a}$. UV irradiation induced the accumulation of $p16^{INK4a}$ in keratinocytes and melanocytes located in the basal layer of the epidermis. This figure was kindly provided by S Pavey and B Gabrielli, University of Queensland, Australia.*

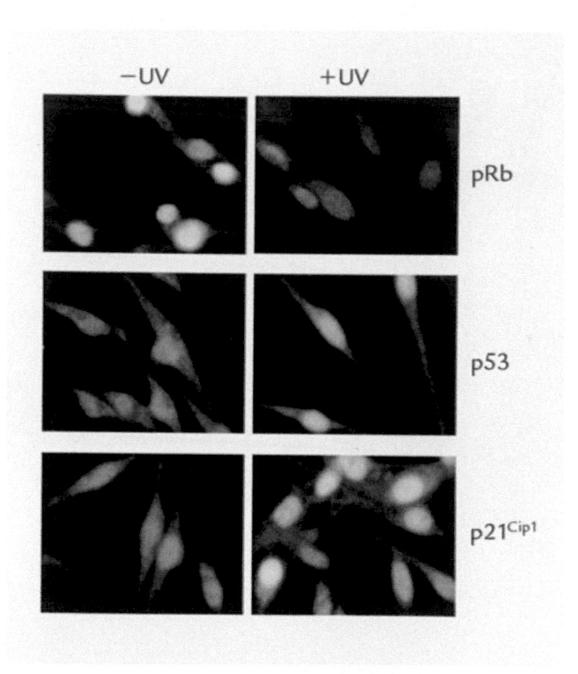

Figure 2.5 *UV induced alterations in cell cycle regulatory genes in normal human epidermal melanocytes. Cultured melanocytes at early passage numbers (9–14) were immunostained for pRb, p53 and the cdk inhibitor $p21^{Cip1}$, before or after pulse UV irradiation (150 J/m^2). Melanocytes in vitro respond to UV exposure by upregulating p53 and $p21^{Cip1}$ and downregulating pRb. The net effect of these changes in gene expression is potent cell cycle arrest. This work was conducted in collaboration with Dieter Kaufmann, University of Ulm, Germany.*

heavily pigmented melanocytes resume proliferation sooner, enabling them to accumulate and release high concentrations of photoprotective melanins (Figure 2.6).[93] This is in accord with the strong genetic and epidemiological evidence indicating that red hair (due to a predominance of pheomelanin) is the strongest risk factor for melanoma development (reviewed in[102]).

The increased number of epidermal melanocytes established under UV irradiation are slowly reduced to normal concentrations, after cessation of irradiation, via apoptotic cell death.[82] This may also involve the UV induced accumulation of p16^{INK4a}. Specifically, p16^{INK4a} mediates apoptosis in non-small cell lung carcinoma cell lines by directly downregulating pRb and indirectly reducing the expression of bcl-2 (Figure 2.3).[104] Both bcl-2 and pRb are downregulated in UV irradiated melanocytes.[92,105] Thus p16^{INK4a} plays a critical part in regulating the proliferation, repair, and death of human melanocytes after exposure to UV radiation (Figure 2.3).

CONCLUSIONS

The regulation of their growth, differentiation and death is fundamental to all eukaryotic cells. Any disruption in these processes compromises the integrity of the cell cycle and can promote cell transformation. Of the many proto-oncogenes and tumour suppressors identified, most impact either directly or indirectly on the machinery controlling passage through the cell cycle. An example is the disruption of cell cycle progression by genetic alterations affecting the negative cell cycle regulator p16^{INK4a}. These alterations are frequent in human cancer and strongly associated with melanoma susceptibility.

Research into the regulation of the cell cycle has clarified the role of p16^{INK4a} in the melanocytic cell cycle and UV response pathways. Following UV irradiation the increase in p16^{INK4a} expression induces potent arrest in the G2 phase of the cell cycle. Melanocytes transiently delayed in G2 undergo rapid DNA repair prior to cell division and are stimulated to produce melanin pigments. These pigments are secreted to neighbouring keratinocytes and protect the skin against UV irradiation. The inactivation of p16^{INK4a} prevents the UV induced G2 arrest and may permit the replication of damaged DNA. Melanocytes regularly traverse the G1-S checkpoint after UV irradiation and thus the G2 cell cycle block is crucial for maintaining DNA integrity. Once breached melanocytes with UV induced DNA damage may undergo cell division.

Defining the intricate pathways and the components involved in regulating cell cycle progression is central to understanding the continuous cycling of tumour cells. With this information, the course of a tumour can be predicted and treatments that target particular components of specific cell cycle pathways can be engineered to induce rapid cell cycle exit.

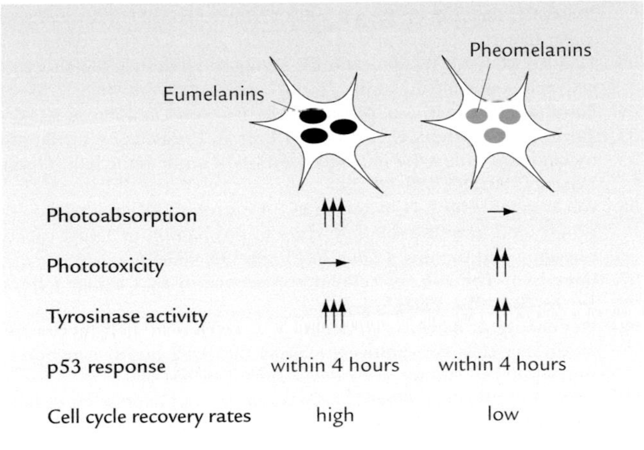

	Eumelanins	Pheomelanins
Photoabsorption	↑↑↑	→
Phototoxicity	→	↑↑
Tyrosinase activity	↑↑↑	↑↑
p53 response	within 4 hours	within 4 hours
Cell cycle recovery rates	high	low

Figure 2.6 *Ultraviolet responses of light and heavily pigmented melanocytes. →, no change in function, ↑↑ significant increase in function, ↑↑↑ very significant increase in function (adapted from[107]).*

ACKNOWLEDGEMENTS

We thank Richard Kefford for critical reading of the manuscript and James Indsto for photography.

REFERENCES

1. Morgan DO, Principles of CDK regulation. *Nature* 1995; 374: 131–4.
2. Johnson DG, Walker CL, Cyclins and cell cycle checkpoint. *Annu Rev Pharmacol Toxicol* 1999; 39: 295–12.
3. van den Heuvel S, Harlow E, Distinct roles for cyclin-dependent kinases in cell cycle control. *Science* 1993; 262: 2050–4.
4. Sherr CJ, G1 phase progression: cycling on cue. *Cell* 1994; 79: 551–5.
5. Sherr CJ, Roberts JM, Inhibitors of mammalian G1 cyclin-dependent kinases. *Genes Dev* 1995; 9: 1149–63.
6. Roussel M, The INK4 family of cell cycle inhibitors in cancer. *Oncogene* 1999; 18: 5311–17.
7. Wang XQ, Gabrielli BG, Milligan A, et al, Accumulation of p16^{CDKN2A} in response to ultraviolet irradiation correlates with late S-G(2)-phase cell cycle delay. *Cancer Res* 1996; 56: 2510–14.

8. Gabrielli BG, Sarcevic B, Sinnamon J, et al, A cyclin D-Cdk4 activity required for G2 phase cell cycle progression is inhibited in ultraviolet radiation-induced G2 phase delay. *J Biol Chem* 1999; 274: 13961–9.
9. Weinberg RA, The retinoblastoma protein and cell cycle control. *Cell* 1995; 81: 323–30.
10. Graña X, Garriga J, Mayol X, Role of the retinoblastoma protein family, pRB, p107 and p130 in the negative control of cell growth. *Oncogene* 1998; 17: 3365–83.
11. Johnson DG, Schneider-Broussard R, Role of E2F in cell cycle control and cancer. *Front Biosci* 1998; 27: d447–8.
12. Bates S, Phillips AC, Clark PA, et al, $p14^{ARF}$ links the tumour suppressors RB and p53. *Nature* 1998; 395: 124–5.
13. Luo RX, Postigo AA, Dean DC, Rb interacts with histone deacetylase to repress transcription. *Cell* 1998; 92: 463–73.
14. Sherr CJ, Cancer cell cycles. *Science* 1996; 274: 1672–7.
15. Walker DH, Maller JL, Role for cyclin A in the dependence of mitosis on completion of DNA replication. *Nature* 1991; 354: 314–17.
16. Girard F, Strausfeld U, Fernandez A, et al, Cyclin A is required for the onset of DNA replication in mammalian fibroblasts. *Cell* 1991; 67: 1169–79.
17. King RW, Jackson PK, Kirschner MW, Mitosis in transition. *Cell* 1994; 79: 563–71.
18. Bravo R, Frank R, Blundell PA, et al, Cyclin/PCNA is the auxiliary protein of DNA polymerase-δ. *Nature* 1987; 326: 515–17.
19. Burgers PMJ, Saccharomyces cerevisiae replication factor C. II. Formation and activity of complexes with proliferating cell nuclear antigen and with DNA polymerases d and e. *J Biol Chem* 1991; 266: 22698–706.
20. Shivji MK, Grey SJ, Strausfeld UP, et al, Cip1 inhibits DNA replication but not PCNA-dependent nucleotide excision-repair. *Curr Biol* 1994; 4: 1062–8.
21. Shivji MK, Podust VN, Hubscher U, et al, Nucleotide excision repair DNA synthesis by DNA polymerase epsilon in the presence of PCNA, RFC, and RPA. *Biochemistry* 1995; 34: 5011–17.
22. Graña X, Reddy EP, Cell cycle control in mammalian cells: role of cyclins, cyclin dependent kinases (CDKs), growth suppressor genes and cyclin-dependent kinase inhibitors (CKIs). *Oncogene* 1995; 11: 211–19.
23. Dessev G, Iovcheva-Dessev C, Bischoff JR, et al, A complex containing p34cdc2 and cyclin B phosphorylates the nuclear lamin and disassembles nuclei of clam oocytes in vitro. *J Cell Biol* 1991; 112: 523–33.
24. Dong F, Cress WD Jr, Agrawal, D et al, The role of cyclin D3–dependent kinase in the phosphorylation of p130 in mouse BALB/c 3T3 fibroblasts. *J Biol Chem* 1998; 273: 6190–5.
25. Li R, Waga S, Hannon GJ, et al, Differential effects by the p21 CDK inhibitor on PCNA-dependent DNA replication and repair. *Nature* 1994; 371: 534–7.
26. Waga S, Hannon GJ, Beach D, et al, The p21 inhibitor of cyclin-dependent kinases controls DNA replication by interaction with PCNA. *Nature* 1994; 369: 574–8.
27. Medema RH, Klompmaker R, Smits VA, et al, $p21^{waf1}$ can block cells at two points in the cell cycle, but does not interfere with processive DNA-replication or stress-activated kinases. *Oncogene* 1998; 16: 431–41.
28. Hengst L, Göpfert U, Lashuel HA, et al, Complete inhibition of cdk/cyclin by one molecule of $p21^{Cip1}$. *Genes Dev* 1998; 12: 3882–8.
29. Amundson SA, Myers TG, Fornace Jr AJ, Roles of p53 in growth arrest and apoptosis: putting on the brakes after genotoxic stress. *Oncogene* 1998; 17: 3287–99.
30. Miyashita T, Reed JC, Tumour suppressor p53 is a direct transcriptional activator of the human bax gene. *Cell* 1995; 80: 293–9.
31. Miyashita T, Krajewski S, Krajewski M, et al, Tumor suppressor p53 is a regulator of bcl-2 and bax gene expression in vitro and in vivo. *Oncogene* 1994; 9: 1799–805.
32. Miyashita T, Harigai M, Hanada M, et al, Identification of a p53–dependent negative response element in the bcl-2 gene. *Cancer Res* 1994; 54: 3131–5.
33. Palmero I, Pantoja C, Serrano M, $p19^{ARF}$ links the tumour suppressor p53 to Ras. *Nature* 1998; 395: 125–6.
34. de Stanchina E, McCurrach ME, Zindy F, et al, E1A signaling to p53 involves the $p19^{ARF}$ tumor suppressor. *Genes Dev* 1998; 12: 2434–42.
35. Darmanian A, Rizos H, Kefford R, et al, A subset of melanoma-associated INK4a/ARF mutations disrupts the localisation of the p14ARF and $p16^{INK4a}$ tumour suppressors. *Third Peter MacCallum Symposium, Melbourne, Australia*, 1999.
36. Rizos H, Darmanian A, Mann G, et al, Two arginine rich domains in the p14ARF tumour suppressor mediate nucleolar localisation. *Oncogene* 2000; 19: 2978–85.
37. Kamijo T, Weber JD, Zambetti G, et al, Functional and physical interactions of the ARF tumor suppressor with p53 and mdm2. *Proc Natl Acad Sci USA* 1998; 95: 8292–7.
38. Pomerantz J, Schreiber-Agus N, Liégeois NJ, et al, The Ink4a tumor suppressor gene product, $p19^{Arf}$, interacts with MDM2 and neutralizes MDM2's inhibition of p53. *Cell* 1998; 92: 713–23.
39. Zhang Y, Xiong Y, Yarbrough WG, ARF promotes MDM2 degradation and stabilizes p53: ARF-INK4a locus deletion impairs both the Rb and p53 tumor suppression pathways. *Cell* 1998; 92: 725–34.
40. Stott FJ, Bates S, James MC, et al, The alternative product from the human CDKN2A locus, p14ARF, participates in a regulatory feedback loop with p53 and MDM2. *EMBO J* 1998; 17: 5001–14.
41. Weber JD, Taylor LJ, Roussel MF, et al, Nucleolar Arf sequesters Mdm2 and activates p53. *Nat Cell Biol* 1999; 1: 20–6.
42. Kubbutat MHG, Jones SN, Vousden KH, Regulation of p53 stability by mdm2. *Nature* 1997; 387: 299–303.
43. Fuchs SY, Adler V, Buschmann T, et al, Mdm2 association with p53 targets its ubiquitination. *Oncogene* 1998; 17: 2543–7.
44. Haupt Y, Maya R, Kaza A, et al, Mdm2 promotes the rapid degradation of p53. *Nature* 1997; 387: 296–9.
45. Campisi J, The biology of replicative senescence. *Eur J Cancer* 1997; 5: 703–9.
46. Stein GH, Dulic V, Molecular mechanism for the senescent cell cycle arrest. *J Invest Dermatol Symp Proc* 1998; 3: 14–18.
47. Dimri GP, Lee X, Basile G, et al, A biomarker that identifies senescent human cells in culture and in aging skin in vivo. *Proc Natl Acad Sci USA* 1995; 92: 9363–7.
48. Huschutscha LI, Reddel RR, $p16^{INK4a}$ and the control of cellular proliferative life span. *Carcinogenesis* 1999; 20: 921–6.
49. Bayreuther K, Francz PI, Gogol J, et al, Terminal differentiation, aging, apoptosis, and spontaneous transformation in fibroblast stem cell systems in vivo and in vitro. *Ann N Y Acad Sci* 1992; 663: 167–79.
50. Campisi J, Replicative senescence: an old lives' tale? *Cell* 1996; 84: 497–500.
51. West MD, Pereira-Smith OM, Smith JR, Replicative senescence of human skin fibroblasts correlates with a loss of regulation and overexpression of collagenase activity. *Exp Cell Res* 1989; 184: 138–47.
52. Medrano EE, Aging, replicative senescence, and the differentiated function of the melanocyte. In: *The pigmentary system.* (Nordlund JJ, Boissy RE, Hearing VJ, King R, eds), Oxford: Oxford University Press, 1999: 151–8.
53. Haddad MM, Xu W, Medrano EE, Aging in epidermal melanocytes: cell cycle genes and melanins. *J Invest Dermatol Symp Proc* 1998; 3: 36–40.
54. Nordlund JJ, The lives of pigment cells. *Dermatol Clin* 1986; 4: 407–18.
55. Takada K, Sugiyuma K, Yamamoto I, et al, Presence of amelanotic melanocytes within the outer root sheath in senile white hair. *J Invest Dermatol* 1992; 99: 629–33.
56. von Wangenheim K-H, Peterson H-P, Control of cell proliferation by progression in differentiation: clues to mechanism of aging, cancer causation and therapy. *J Theor Biol* 1998; 193: 663–78.
57. Campisi J, The role of cellular senescence in skin aging. *J Invest Dermtol Symp Proc* 1998; **3**: 1–5.
58. Plettenberg A, Ballaun C, Pammer J, et al, Human melanocytes and melanoma cells constitutively express the Bcl-2 proto-oncogene in situ and in cell culture. *Am J Pathol* 1995; 146: 651–9.
59. Selzer E, Schlagbauer-Wadl H, Okamoto I, et al, Expression of Bcl-2 family members in human melanocytes, in melanoma metastases and in melanoma cell lines. *Melanoma Res* 1998; 8: 197–203.
60. Sermadiras S, Dumas M, Joly-Berville R, et al, Expression of Bcl-2 and bax in cultured normal human keratinocytes and melanocytes: relationship to differentiation and melanogenesis. *Br J Dermatol* 1997; 137: 883–9.
61. Hara E, Smith R, Parry D, et al, Regulation of $p16^{CDKN2}$ expression and its implications for cell immortalization and senescence. *Mol Cell Biol* 1996; 16: 859–67.

62. Noda A, Ning Y, Venable SF, et al, Cloning of senescent cell-derived inhibitors of DNA synthesis using an expression screen. *Exp Cell Res* 1994; 211: 90–8.
63. Guo K, Wang J, Andrés V, et al, MyoD-induced expression of p21 inhibits cyclin-dependent kinase activity upon myocyte terminal differentiation. *Mol Cell Biol* 1995; 15: 3823–9.
64. Jiang H, Lin J, Su ZZ, et al, Induction of differentiation in human promyelocytic HL-60 leukemia cells activates p21, WAF1/CIP1, expression in the absence of p53. *Oncogene* 1994; 9: 3397–406.
65. Lois AF, Cooper LT, Geng Y, et al, Expression of the p16 and p15 cyclin-dependent kinase inhibitors in lymphocyte activation and neuronal differentiation. *Cancer Res* 1995; 55: 4010–13.
66. Missero C, Di Cunto F, Kiyokawa H, et al, The absence of p21Cip1/WAF1 alters keratinocyte growth and differentiation and promotes ras-tumor progression. *Genes Dev* 1996; 10: 3065–75.
67. Hussussian CJ, Struewing JP, Goldstein AM, et al, Germline p16 mutations in familial melanoma. *Nat Genet* 1994; 8: 15–21.
68. Holland EA, Beaton SC, Becker TM, et al, Analysis of the p16 gene, CDKN2, in 17 Australian melanoma kindreds. *Oncogene* 1995; 11: 2289–94.
69. FitzGerald MG, Harkin DP, Silva-Arrieta S, et al, Prevalence of germline mutations in p16, p19ARF, and CDK4 in familial melanoma: Analysis of a clinic-based population. *Proc Natl Acad Sci USA* 1996; 93: 8541–5.
70. Holland EA, Schmid H, Kefford RF, et al, CDKN2a ($p16^{INK4a}$) and CDK4 mutation analysis in 131 Australian melanoma probands: Effect of family history and multiple primary melanomas. *Genes Chromosom Cancer* 1999; 25: 339–48.
71. Soufir N, Avril M-F, Chompret A, et al, Prevalence of p16 and CDK4 germline mutations in 48 melanoma-prone families in France. *Human Mol Genet* 1998; 7: 209–16.
72. Kamb A, Shattuck-Eidens D, Eeles R, et al, Analysis of the p16 gene (CDKN2) as a candidate for the chromosome 9p melanoma susceptibility locus. *Nat Genet* 1994; 8: 23–6.
73. Jiang HP, Lin J, Su ZZ, et al, The melanoma differentiation-associated gene mda-6, which encodes the cyclin-dependent kinase inhibitor p21, is differentially expressed during growth, differentiation and progression in human melanoma cells. *Oncogene* 1995; 10: 1855–64.
74. Haddad MM, Xu W, Schwahn DJ, et al, Activation of a cAMP pathway and induction of melanogenesis correlate with association of $p16^{INK4}$ and $p27^{KIP1}$ to CDKs, loss of E2F-binding activity, and premature senescence of human melanocytes. *Exp Cell Res* 1999; 253: 561–72.
75. Hauser P, Agrawal D, Flanagan M, et al, The role of p27Kip1 in the in vitro differentiation of murine keratinocytes. *Cell Growth Differ* 1997; 8: 203–11.
76. Medrano EE, Yang F, Boissy R, et al, Terminal differentiation and senescence in the human melanocyte: repression of tyrosine-phosphorylation of the extracellular signal-regulated kinase 2 selectively defines the two phenotypes. *Mol Biol Cell* 1994; 5: 497–509.
77. Busca R, Ballotti R, Cyclin AMP a key messenger in the regulation of skin pigmentation. *Pigment Cell Res* 2000; 13: 60–9.
78. She Q-B, Dong Z, ERKs and p38 kinase phosphorylate p53 protein at serine 15 in response to UV radiation. *J Biol Chem* 2000; 275: 20444–9.
79. Youn J, Lee A, Lee Y, The effect of ultraviolet irradiation on epidermal melanocytes and the influence of sunscreen: A histochemical and ultrastructural study. *Seoul J Med* 1990; 31: 253–62.
80. Nordlund JJ, Collins CE, Rheins LA, Prostaglandin E2 and D2 but not MSH stimulate the proliferation of pigment cells in the pinnal epidermis of the DBA/2 mouse. *J Invest Dermatol* 1986; 86: 433–7.
81. Nakagawa H, Rhodes A, Momtaz T, et al, Morphologic alterations of epidermal melanocytes and melanosomes in PUVA lentigines: A comparative ultrastructural investigation of lentigines induced by PUVA and sunlight. *J Invest Dermatol* 1984; 82: 101–7.
82. Bacharach-Buhles M, Lubowietzki M, Altmeyer P, Dose-dependent shift of apoptotic and unaltered melanocytes into the dermis after irradiation with UVA1. *Dermatology* 1999; 198: 5–10.
83. Imokawa G, Yada Y, Miyagishi M, Endothelins secreted from human keratinocytes are intrinsic mitogens for human melanocytes. *J Biol Chem* 1992; 267: 24675–80.
84. Halaban R, Langdon R, Birchall N, et al, Basic fibroblast growth factor from human keratinocytes is a natural mitogen for melanocytes. *J Cell Biol* 1988; 107: 1611–19.
85. Bertolotto C, Abbe P, Hemesath T, et al, Microphthalmia gene product as a signal transducer in cAMP-induced differentiation of melanocytes. *J Cell Biol* 1998; 142: 827–35.
86. Hunt G, Kyne S, Wakamatsu K, et al, Nle^4DPhe^7–α-MSH increases the eumelanin: pheomelanin ratio in cultured human melanocytes. *J Invest Dermatol* 1995; 104: 83–5.
87. Suzuki I, Cone R, Im S, et al, Binding of melanocortin hormones to the melanocortin receptor MC1R on human melanocytes stimulates proliferation and melanogenesis. *Endocrinology* 1996; 137: 1627–33.
88. Valverde P, Healy E, Jackson I, et al, Variants of the melanocyte-stimulating hormone receptor gene are associated with red hair and fair skin in humans. *Nat Genet* 1995; 11: 328–30.
89. Valverde P, Healy E, Sikkink S, et al, The Asp84Glu variant of the melanocortin 1 receptor (MC1R) is associated with melanoma. *Hum Mol Genet* 1996; 5: 1663–6.
90. Smith R, Healy E, Siddiqui S, et al, Melanocortin 1 receptor variants in an Irish population. *J Invest Dermatol* 1998; 111: 119–22.
91. Nylander K, Bourdon JC, Bray SE, et al, Transcriptional activation of tyrosinase and TRP-1 by p53 links UV irradiation to the protective tanning response. *J Pathol* 2000; 190: 39–46.
92. Medrano EE, Im S, Yang F, et al, Ultraviolet B light induces G1 arrest in human melanocytes by prolonged inhibition of retinoblastoma protein phosphorylation associated with long-term expression of the p21Waf-1/SDI-1/Cip-1 protein. *Cancer Res* 1995; 55: 4047–52.
93. Barker D, Dixon K, Medrano EE, et al, Comparison of the responses of human melanocytes with different melanin contents to ultraviolet B irradiation. *Cancer Res* 1995; 55: 4041–6.
94. Wong G, Pawelek J, Sansone M, et al, Response of mouse melanoma cells to melanocyte stimulating hormone. *Nature* 1974; 248: 351–4.
95. Varga JM, DiPasquale A, Pawelek J, et al, Regulation of melanocyte-stimulating hormone action at the receptor level: discontinuous binding of hormone to synchronized mouse melanoma cells during the cell cycle. *Proc Natl Acad Sci USA* 1974; 71: 1590–3.
96. Bolognia JL, Sodi SA, Chakraborty AK, et al, Effects of ultraviolet irradiation on the cell cycle. *Pigment Cell Res* 1994; 7: 320–5.
97. Pavey S, Conroy S, Russell T, et al, Ultraviolet radiation induces $p16^{CDKN2A}$ expression in human skin. *Cancer Res* 1999; 59: 4185–9.
98. Milligan A, Gabrielli BG, Clark JM, et al, Involvement of $p16^{CDKN2A}$ in cell cycle delays after low dose UV irradiation. *Mutat Res* 1998; 422: 43–53.
99. Im S, Moro O, Peng F, et al, Activation of the cyclic AMP pathway by a-melanotropin mediates the response of human melanocytes to ultraviolet B radiation. *Cancer Res* 1998; 58: 47–54.
100. Tada A, Suzuki I, Im S, et al, Endothelin-1 is a paracrine growth factor that modulates melanogenesis of human melanocytes and participates in their responses to ultraviolet radiation. *Cell Growth Differ* 1998; 9: 575–84.
101. Yavuzer U, Keenan E, Lowings P, et al, The microphthalmia gene product interacts with the retinoblastoma protein in vitro and is a target for deregulation of melanocyte-specific transcription. *Oncogene* 1995; 10: 123–34.
102. Jimbow K, Quevedo Jr WC, Prota G, et al, Biology of melanocytes. In: *Fitzpatrick's dermatology in general medicine.* (eds, Freedberg IM, Eisen AZ, Wolff K, et al,) 5th edn, Vol. 1. New York: McGraw-Hill. 1999; 192–220.
103. Sohal RS, Weindruch R, Oxidative stress, caloric restriction, and aging. *Science* 1996; 273: 59–63.
104. Kataoka M, Wiehle S, Spitz F, et al, Down-regulation of bcl-2 is associated with $p16^{INK4a}$-mediated apoptosis in non-small lung cancer cells. *Oncogene* 2000; 19: 1589–95.
105. Pedley J, Ablett E, Pettit A, et al, Inhibition of retinoblastoma protein translation by UVB in human melanocytic cells and reduced cell cycle arrest following repeated irradiation. *Oncogene* 1996; 13: 1335–42.
106. Hainaut P, The tumor suppressor protein p53: a receptor to genotoxic stress that controls cell growth and survival. *Curr Opinion Oncol* 1995; 7: 76–82.
107. Hearing VJ, Biochemical control of melanogenesis and melanosomal organization. *J Invest Dermatol Symp Proc* 1999; 4: 24–8.

GLOSSARY

CREB cAMP-responsive transcription factor.

14–3–3σ Induced by p53. Induces G2/M cell cycle arrest by preventing the activation of cdk1.

Bax Bax is a p53 induced member of the bcl-2 family of proteins. Bax homodimers promote apoptosis.

Bcl-2 Bax/bcl-2 heterodimers suppress apoptosis. p53 inhibits the expression of bcl-2.

Cdk Cyclin Dependent Kinase. A family of protein kinases that control cell cycle progression.

Cdk4/cdk6 Cyclin D dependent kinases whose primary substrate is the retinoblastoma protein (pRb).

CDKN2A The INK4a/ARF genomic locus which encodes the $p16^{INK4a}$ and p14ARF tumour suppressors.

Cip/Kip Cyclin dependent kinase Interacting Protein-1/Kinase Inhibitory Protein. A family of three cyclin-dependent kinase inhibitors ($p21^{Cip1}$, $p27^{Kip1}$, $p57^{Kip2}$) that inhibit the activity of all cyclin dependent kinases.

Cyclins A family of proteins that interact and activate cyclin dependent kinases.

E2Fs A family of transcription factors consisting of a subunit encoded by the E2F gene family (E2F-1 to E2F-6) and a subunit encoded by the DP family of genes (DP-1 and DP-2). E2F factors interact with hypophosphorylated pRb and when released activate the transcription of many genes.

ERK2 A kinase in the mitogen-activated protein kinase (MAPK) pathway.

Gadd45 Inhibits the activity of cyclinB1/cdk1 and induces G2 cell cycle arrest in a p53 dependent manner.

Hdm2 Binds p53 and promotes p53 nuclear export and degradation.

INK4 INhibitors of cdK4. A family of cyclin-dependent kinase inhibitors ($p15^{INK4b}$, $p16^{INK4a}$, $p18^{INK4c}$, $p19^{INK4d}$), that exclusively bind to and inhibit the D-type cyclin dependent kinases, cdk4 and cdk6.

MAPK Mitogen-Activated Protein Kinases are involved in signal transduction pathways activated by a range of stimuli and mediate a series of physiological changes in cell function.

MITF The MIcrophthalmia-associated Transcription Factor plays a critical role in the differentiation of various cell types, including melanocytes.

p107 Functionally and structurally related to pRb and p130.

p130 Functionally and structurally related to pRb and p107.

p14ARF Interacts with hdm2 to stabilize and enhance the activity of the p53 tumour suppressor.

$p15^{INK4b}$ Member of the INK4 family of cyclin dependent kinase inhibitors.

$p16^{INK4a}$ Member of the INK4 family of cyclin dependent kinase inhibitors.

$p18^{INK4c}$ Member of the INK4 family of cyclin dependent kinase inhibitors.

$p19^{INK4d}$ Member of the INK4 family of cyclin dependent kinase inhibitors.

$p21^{Cip1}$ Member of the Cip/Kip cyclin dependent kinase inhibitors. Also binds to and inhibits the DNA replication function of proliferating cell nuclear antigen (PCNA). Downstream effector of p53.

$p27^{Kip1}$ Member of the Cip/Kip cyclin dependent kinase inhibitors.

p53 Transcriptional regulator that is frequently altered in cancer.

$p57^{Kip2}$ Member of the Cip/Kip cyclin dependent kinase inhibitors.

PCNA Proliferating Cell Nuclear Antigen is required for replication of DNA by the polymerase δ and ε.

pRb Retinoblastoma tumour suppressor, acts as a signal transducer connecting the cell cycle with transcriptional machinery.

TRP-1 Tyrosinase Related Protein-1 is a melanocyte differentiation product involved in the production of melanin pigments.

3

Skin immunity and melanoma development

Gary M Halliday

INTRODUCTION

The skin has a highly evolved and coordinated immune system. There are regional aspects to the immune response of the skin, but lymphoid organs beyond the skin, including the lymph nodes and spleen, are important in the coordinated immunological control of the skin. Skin immunity is regulated at many levels, locally by cytokines and adhesion molecules produced by many different cell types in the skin. This creates the local microenvironment in which the immune response occurs. Regulatory T cells and antibody production at sites other than the skin also determine whether or not an immune response occurs to a particular antigen. Migration of antigen presenting cells (APC) from the skin to lymph nodes, and of T lymphocytes from the lymph nodes to the skin, are also critical events.

Extrinsic environmental influences have a profound effect on immunity in the skin. The most important of these is exposure to ultraviolet (UV) radiation. The skin is particularly vulnerable to the environment because of its location at the interface between internal organs and the outside world. UV radiation and chemical carcinogens are immunosuppressive and alter cytokine production by cells of the skin, therefore disrupting the local homoeostasis.

These factors all influence melanoma development. Modulation of the immune microenvironment influences the development of immunity to melanoma and expression of ongoing immunity. Additionally, these same changes will provide a range of factors such as cytokines, growth factors, and adhesion molecules, which will have an impact on other aspects of melanoma progression such as cell growth and angiogenesis.

THE IMMUNE SYSTEM OF THE SKIN

Langerhans cells (LC) are dendritic cells (DC) found in the epidermal layer of the skin (Figures 3.1 and 3.2). The dermis also contains an array of DC that have been less well characterized than LC. DC are the most potent cells at activating a primary immune response.[1] In the absence of DC it is unlikely that primary immunity

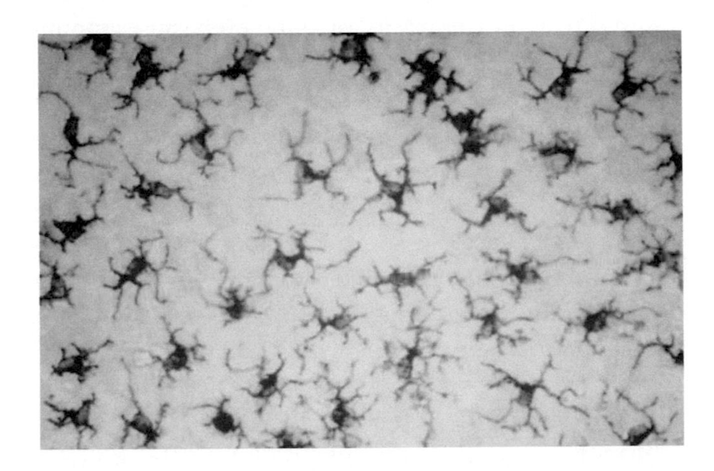

Figure 3.1 *Horizontal view of Langerhans cells in epidermal sheets showing characteristic highly dendritic shape of cells. Cells are evenly distributed throughout the epidermis. Cells stained with anti-MHC class II antibodies.*

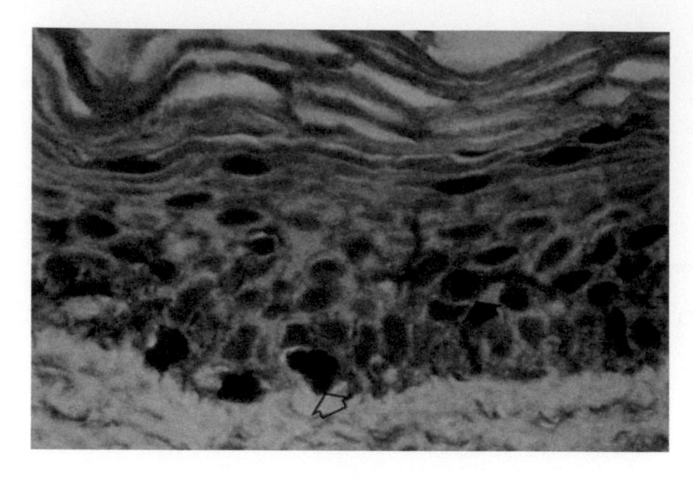

Figure 3.2 *Vertical section of skin showing dendritic Langerhans cells (brown, closed arrow head) in the suprabasal layer of the epidermis, and melanocytes (black, open arrow head) at the basal layer of the epidermis. Langerhans cells stained with anti-S 100 antibodies, and melanocytes with L-DOPA.*

would be induced. Thus these cells play a central part in immunological control of skin immunity. When naive T cells are produced in the thymus with a range of specificities for extrinsic or self antigens, they primarily localize to the secondary lymphoid organs, including the lymph nodes, and traffic between these organs via the circulation. They do not leave this trafficking pattern and enter the skin until they have been activated. T cell activation is stringently regulated to prevent initiation of unrequired immune responses. Such unnecessary immune activation could waste body resources, preventing immunity being directed towards more threatening antigens, or could even cause autoimmunity. It is therefore critical that only naive T cells specific for antigenic epitopes on agents that threaten the body are activated. This seems to be largely the function of DC such as LC (Figure 3.3). Once a naive T cell has been activated and returns to the resting state, its reactivation to generate a secondary immune response is less tightly regulated. It is likely that cells in addition to DC, including macrophages and B cells, can activate a secondary immune response.

Langerhans cells and other dendritic cells of the skin

DC are produced from progenitors in the bone marrow, from where they traffic via the blood to other tissues. It has been recognized for many years that epidermal LC are of bone marrow origin.[2,3] Since procedures were developed for production of DC from mouse bone marrow cultured with granulocyte macrophage colony stimulating factor (GM-CSF),[4] knowledge of DC ontogeny, the factors involved, and the range of pathways by which these cells can develop has increased enormously. It is now recognized that DC can arise from different pathways and that there are different subsets of these cells. CD34+ haemopoietic progenitors give rise to immature non-dividing DC that migrate out into tissues. Some DC progenitors give rise to LC, whereas others form different types of DC.[5] Additionally, monocytes can differentiate into either macrophages or DC depending on the appropriate range of cytokines supplied.[6] Monocytes can differentiate into DC in vivo on migration to lymph nodes or on migration across endothelium.[7,8] Another population of DC has been identified, which expresses high concentrations of interleukin (IL)-3Rα.[9] Distinct from the myeloid related DC this is a further population which arises from a precursor that can also give rise to T lymphocytes. These lymphoid related DC have so far been conclusively identified only in mice, where they express CD8α.[10] It is unclear whether this DC lineage also occurs in humans. The relative roles of these different DC in immunity, and particularly in development of immunity to tumours, is as yet unknown.

Of these DC populations, LC are likely to be important for the progression of primary epidermal melanoma as this is the tissue to which they traffic. However, other types of DC are likely to influence metastasis at sites other than the epidermis. LC seem to differ from other DC subpopulations. During development from CD34+ progenitors, CD1a+ CD14– precursors are thought to give rise to LC, whereas CD1a– CD14+ precursors form other types of DC in the absence of transforming growth factor (TGF) β1, but in its presence form LC.[11] Additionally, the LC precursor expresses the skin homing receptor cutaneous leukocyte antigen (CLA), whereas precursors of other types of DC do not express this molecule.[12] CLA directs cells to migrate into the skin. It therefore seems that during development, DC diverge into cells capable of migrating into the skin (CLA+), which then differentiate into LC, and those that are unable to do this (CLA–), and these later cells differentiate into other types of DC.

The dermis also contains populations of dendritic cells.[13,14] These have a range of phenotypes, and it is not

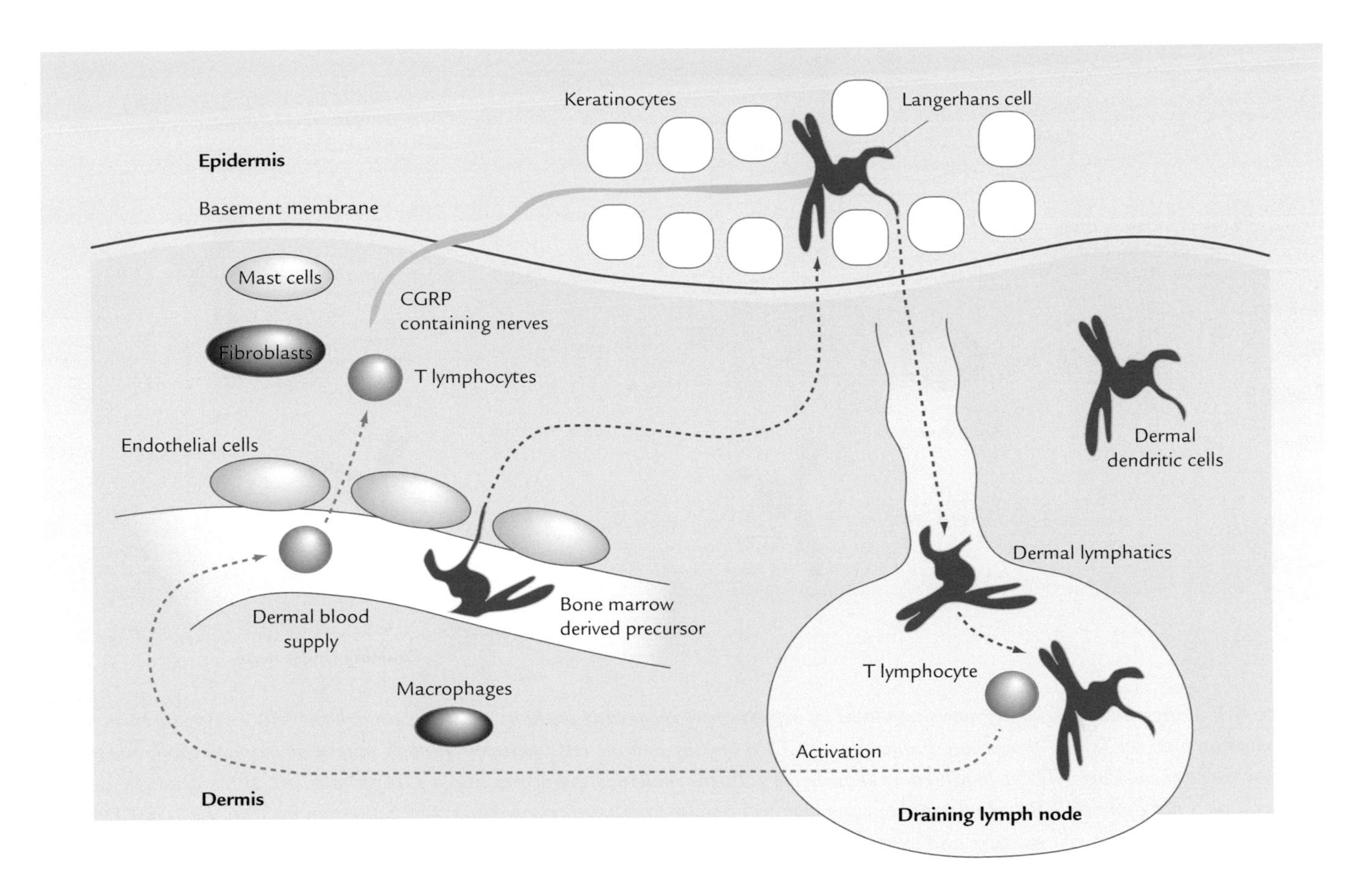

Figure 3.3 *Langerhans cell activation of T lymphocytes. Langerhans cells in the epidermis form tight junctions with keratinocytes and calcitonin gene related peptide (CGRP) containing nerves. In response to cytokines such as TNF and IL-1β they will migrate from the epidermis via dermal lymphatics to draining lymph nodes. During this process they will become activated and express high concentrations of co-stimulatory molecules, which are required to stimulate T cells. In the lymph node they will activate T cells. Because these activated T cells now express the skin homing receptor CLA, they can migrate out of dermal blood vessels into the skin, where they can mediate cellular immunity. Cytokines produced by keratinocytes, mast cells, fibroblasts, and endothelial cells will create a microenvironment that will support or inhibit these processes.*

clear whether there are single or multiple DC subpopulations within the dermis. However, it is likely that they have a similar function to the epidermal DC in the induction of immunity to antigens within the dermis and therefore could be important for development of melanomas that have invaded the dermis.

Migration of DC into tissues and from the tissues to local lymph nodes is regulated by DC expression of chemokine receptors (CCR) (Figure 3.4). Immature DC express a range of CCR, including CCR1 and CCR5, which enables them to respond to chemokines such as monocyte chemotactic protein (MCP)-1, macrophage inflammatory protein (MIP)-1α and regulated upon activation, normal T cell expressed and secreted (RANTES).[15] In contrast to other types of DC, LC precursors also express CCR6, which enables them to be attracted by MIP-3α produced by keratinocytes and therefore migrate into the epidermis.[16] Once a LC precursor has migrated into the epidermis, it matures and forms a network of cells evenly distributed between neighbouring keratinocytes (Figure 3.1) with long dendrites extending between neighbouring cells. In the epidermis they form tight junctions with neighbouring keratinocytes mediated by E-cadherin, and with calcitonin gene related peptide (CGRP) containing nerves.[17,18]

LC do not induce an immune response while located in the epidermis. T cells are in a different location, the secondary lymphoid organs. LC take up antigen and migrate via the dermal lymphatics to draining lymph nodes, where they present the antigen to T cells and provide other signals necessary for their activation (Figure 3.3).[19,20] It has been shown that T cells specific for

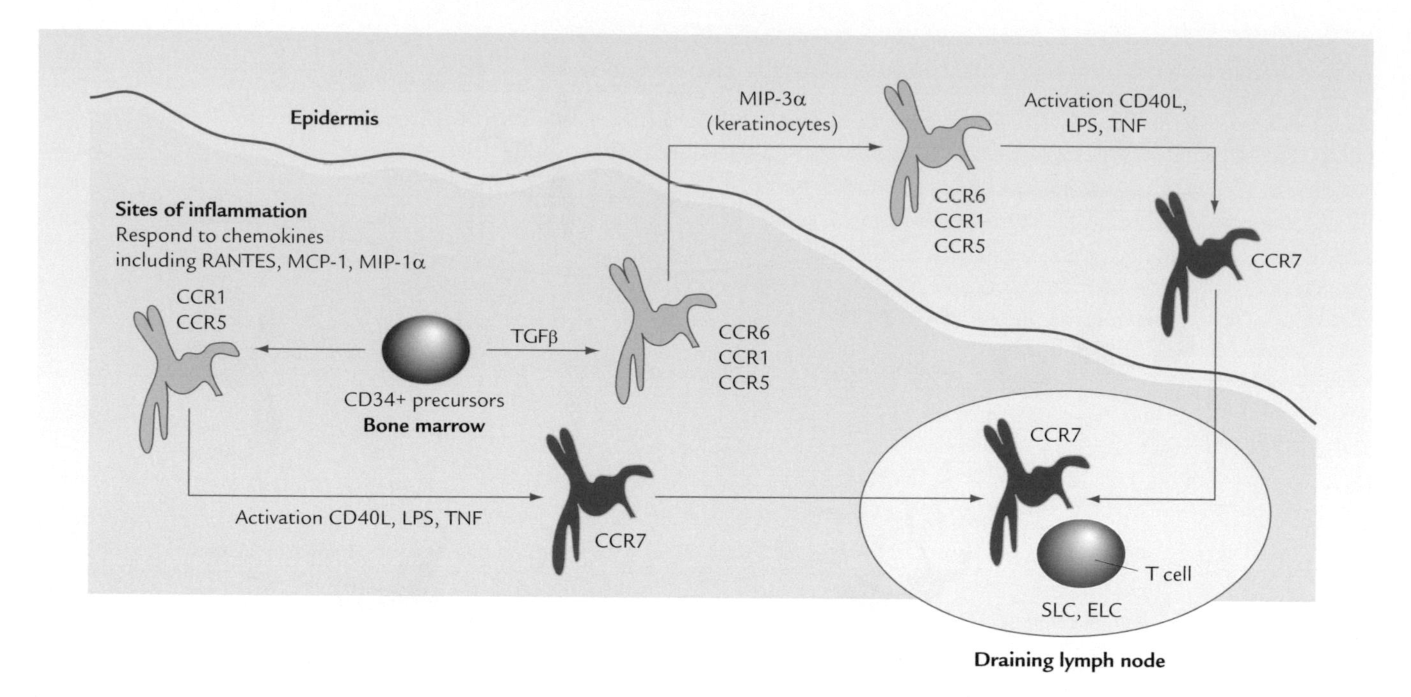

Figure 3.4 *Langerhans cell migration is regulated by expression of chemokine receptors (CCR). Langerhans cells are produced in the bone marrow from a CD34+ progenitor. Expression of CCR6 on Langerhans cell precursors enables migration into the epidermis in response to the chemokine MIP-3a produced by keratinocytes. In the epidermis it matures into a Langerhans cell. If the dendritic cell precursor does not express CCR6, it migrates to other sites in response to different chemokines. On activation by TNF, LPS, or CD40 Ligand, the Langerhans cell matures and expresses CCR7 but loses CCR6. Expression of CCR7 enables the Langerhans cell to migrate to draining lymph nodes in response to the chemokines SLC or ELC. In this way coordinated expression of CCRs and chemokine production controls the induction of cell mediated immunity in the skin.*

tumour antigens are activated in the draining lymph node, thus implying an important role for LC migration to lymph nodes for induction of antitumour immunity.[21] The signals that initiate LC migration from the epidermis to local lymph nodes are not completely understood. Tumour necrosis factor (TNF) and IL-1 are two cytokines that can initiate this trafficking to local lymph nodes.[22–24] Lipopolysaccharide (LPS) can also activate this migratory process in LC.[25] When activated to migrate from the epidermis, LC lose CCR6 surface expression and instead express CCR7, which enables them to respond to secondary lymphoid tissue cytokine (SLC) and EBV-induced molecule 1 ligand chemokine (ELC), which direct them to migrate to the T cell areas of lymph nodes (Figure 3.4).[16,26]

During this development of LC from CD34+ progenitors, migration into the epidermis, and trafficking to local lymph nodes, LC undergo continual maturation. They change their function and phenotype. On migration from the skin to local lymph nodes, LC upregulate major histocompatibility complex (MHC) class I and II, as well as molecules which transduce stimulatory signals to T cells such as CD80 and CD86.[5] Integrins involved in migration of these cells to the lymph node also change.[27,28] Associated with this is a loss of ability to ingest, process, and present antigen.[29] The final result of this maturation is that LC that have matured and migrated to lymph nodes are more proficient activators of T cells.[30]

The maturational state of LC is likely to be important for the induction of immunity to melanomas. It has been shown that immunological tolerance rather than immunity results from antigen exposure to skin during the promoter phase of carcinogenesis.[31] This seems to result from a reduction in the number of epidermal LC so that only those immature LC that remain in the epidermis during tumour promotion present antigen to T cells.[32,33] It has been suggested that mature DC are more efficient at the induction of protective immunity to tumours.[34] DC found infiltrating tumours have been reported to be immature and defective in their ability to mature normally.[35–37]

T lymphocytes

Like most T cells in other tissues, T cells in the skin express the αβ T cell receptor for antigen and either CD4 or CD8 and therefore recognize antigen in an MHC class II or class I restricted manner, respectively.[38] However, unlike most T cells at other sites, T cells in the skin have an activated or memory phenotype and express CLA, the skin homing receptor.[39–41] Thus it seems that naive T cells remain restricted to recirculating through secondary lymphoid organs and the blood. After activation by LC that have migrated to local lymph nodes with antigen, the T cells can leave these sites and enter the skin if they have been induced to express CLA.[41] T cells rapidly migrate through lymph nodes in the body.[42] As there is only a small number of naive T cells with receptors specific for individual antigens, rapid T cell recirculation through the lymph nodes, and delivery of antigen to lymph nodes on an activated dendritic cell ready to stimulate the T cells enables a specific immune response to be initiated with as short a delay as possible after antigen exposure. If the T cells surveyed all tissues of the body and were activated after meeting with antigen in that tissue, immune responses would take much longer to be induced.

Cytokines

Cytokines, growth factors, and chemokines are produced by many cell types, including cells of the immune system as well as keratinocytes, mast cells, fibroblasts, endothelial cells, and others. Melanoma cells can also produce a large array of these factors.[43] These cytokines can modulate the immune system at various levels, by directly affecting the function of immune cells, by altering the expression of adhesion molecules, homing receptors, or other molecules on different cell types. Thus these factors can influence the immune response to melanoma, but they can also have direct effects on melanoma growth and invasion.[44,45] Considering the large number of these factors and the multitude of direct and indirect effects they are capable of exerting, it is difficult to ascertain their individual importance in melanoma development.

Cytokines produced by T lymphocytes have been used to loosely categorize T cells into Th1 cells, which produce interferon (IFN)-γ and are important for cell mediated immunity, and Th2 cells, which produce IL-4 and predominately play a helper part in antibody production by B cells.[46,47] Thus the array of cytokines produced by cells of the immune system, or tissue cells have important effects on the immune system as they regulate it at all levels.

THE IMMUNE SYSTEM CAN INFLUENCE MELANOMA DEVELOPMENT

Observations that (1) melanoma cells express antigens that T cells recognize, (2) T cells can destroy melanoma cells, (3) melanoma spontaneously regresses because of immune destruction, and (4) immunosuppression caused by UV radiation or pharmaceuticals enhances melanoma development all show that the immune response can cause melanoma rejection and thus has an important effect on development of this tumour.

Whether the induction of immunity to melanoma occurs in a similar manner to what has been described for simple chemical antigens or infectious agents is unknown. Our understanding of immunity in the skin is based largely on experiments involving contact sensitizers or other antigens. Skin tumour development probably occurs over many years, hence, as opposed to immunization with other forms of antigen, initially there would be few tumour cells and therefore very little antigen. The tumour then divides and progresses so that there would be a continual increase in antigen concentration over a comparatively long period of time, and the tumour antigens are likely to change during melanoma development. Additionally, melanomas produce their own range of cytokines and adhesion molecules, which will affect the immune response.

Expression of antigens on melanomas that can be recognized by T cells

Many melanoma antigens that can be recognized by T cells have been identified.[48,49] These antigens can be divided into several categories.

(1) Tumour specific shared antigens are specifically expressed on a range of different tumour types, including melanomas from many individuals. These include MAGE, BAGE, and GAGE.

(2) Differentiation antigens whose expression is limited to normally differentiated melanocytes as well as melanoma cells from many individuals. These include tyrosinase, Melan-A/Mart-1, gp100, and gp75.

(3) Antigens specific for individual tumours. These are antigens that are not expressed on a large percentage of a particular type of tumour but arise from individual mutations and therefore occur only in that particular tumour.

The demonstration of targets for T cells on melanoma cells meets an important criterion that the immune system can recognize melanoma cells, and therefore affects its development.

Melanoma reactive T cells

Cytotoxic T cells have been identified and cloned from the blood of patients with melanoma, indicating that melanoma patients have T cells capable of specifically recognizing and destroying melanoma cells.[50] CD4+ cytotoxic T cells that were, unexpectedly, MHC class I restricted, have also been cloned from the blood of a melanoma patient.[51] Most melanoma patients have been found to have antimelanoma cytotoxic T cells in their blood, although a wide range of numbers has been observed.[52]

Spontaneous regression of melanoma

Spontaneous regression occurs when a primary or secondary tumour regresses, or dies, in the absence of treatment capable of causing tumour destruction. Regression can be complete, where the entire lesion disappears, or focal, where the regressive process is incomplete so that only a portion of the tumour disappears. It is difficult to estimate the frequency of complete or partial regression, as complete regression before metastasis could occur without being noticed. In 7–10% of internal cancers, metastasis are found without evidence of the primary lesion, even at autopsy, indicating that at least 10% of primary tumours undergo spontaneous regression.[53,54] It has been reported that 5–8% of patients with melanoma metastasis have no detectable primary lesions suggesting that at least 5–8% of primary melanomas undergo complete regression.[55,56] Primary regressed melanoma has been reported in patients presenting with metastasis.[57] A primary biopsy proven superficial spreading melanoma has been observed to undergo complete regression in a patient who refused treatment.[58]

Partial regression is more common but is usually not reported by the pathologist. We find that about 50% of primary melanomas removed for surgical intervention have focal regions of clinically and histologically identifiable regression, which is consistent with other studies.[59–62] As this represents a single random time point in the development of this tumour, it is likely that most melanomas undergo at least focal regression during their development. Thus melanoma regression seems to be a common occurrence and is likely to shape the development of most melanomas by causing destruction of some clones of melanoma cells while enabling others to progress.

Spontaneous regression of melanoma metastasis has been estimated to occur in 0.25% of melanoma patients and although this seems to be lower than the reported incidence in primary lesions it is likely to be an underestimate.[63] However, it remains likely that metastasis more effectively evade immunological destruction than do primary lesions, and therefore regress spontaneously less frequently.

There is no difference in survival of patients with spontaneous regression compared with those without regression.[62,64] However, regression is usually only identified at the single time point of surgical excision, and it remains likely that all melanomas develop focal regions of regression at some stage during their development. Also, active regression is likely to interfere with histological assessment of Breslow thickness as deeper parts of the tumour may have been destroyed, complicating the prognostic indicators. For regression to have an effect on survival the primary would need to completely regress before metastasis. For these reasons it is difficult to meaningfully assess the lack of prognostic significance of spontaneous regression.

Melanoma regression can be observed clinically as replacement of the pigmented tumour with scar tissue (Figure 3.5). The histological features have been defined as a leukocytic infiltrate spreading into the tumour and dividing the tumour into small clumps.[56] The tumour cells undergo degeneration, probably by apoptosis, with an eosinophilic cytoplasm and a pyknotic nucleus. Later in the process scar tissue is present with proliferation of fibroblasts and new blood vessels.

Spontaneous regression of melanoma appears to be immunologically mediated.[65] In an immunohistological study we found a significant increase in the number of T cells infiltrating regressing melanomas compared with those with no evidence of regression.[59] These T cells infiltrating the tumour were mainly CD4+ and

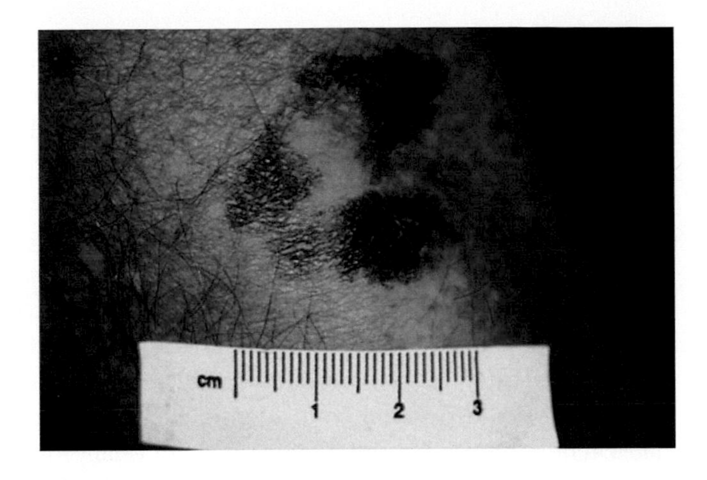

Figure 3.5 *Spontaneously regressing melanoma. A central area of spontaneous regression can be seen as loss of tumour and depigmentation.*

were activated as they expressed the receptor for IL-2. These differences were observed only within the tumour, not at the margins or within surrounding tissues, indicating that the T cells needed to migrate into the melanomas. No differences were observed with eight melanoma associated differentiation antigens, indicating that a different stage of differentiation cannot account for regression of melanoma. CD4+ T cells can mediate melanoma cytotoxicity. MHC class II molecules are mostly expressed only by dendritic cells or other cells of the immune system, where they present antigen to CD4+ T cells. Melanoma cells can also express functional MHC class II, which is capable of presenting antigen to CD4+ T cells and inducing their proliferation.[66] CD4+ T cells activated by MHC class II+ melanoma cells can kill melanoma cells by a mechanism that does not depend upon direct cell contact.[67] Hence once activated by dendritic cells, or MHC class II+ melanoma cells, CD4+ T cells could kill MHC class II− melanoma cells as direct contact between CD4+ T cells and melanoma is not required. This is supported by the observation that murine melanomas transfected with MHC class II molecules can present antigen to CD4+ T cells, augmenting immunity against these tumours.[68] However, MHC class II expressing melanoma cells have also been reported to induce anergy in melanoma reactive CD4 T cells by enabling antigen specific signalling in the absence of co-stimulation.[69]

Quantitation of cytokine message using a non-competitive reverse transcriptase polymerase chain reaction (RT-PCR) showed regressing melanomas to have increased concentrations of the Th1 cytokines lymphotoxin, IL-2, and IFN-γ, without any differences from non-regressing lesions in IL-10, IL-13, IL-1α, IL-1β, IL-6, IL-8, TNF, bFGF, TGF-β, or GM-CSF.[60] Another study found increased concentrations of IL-2, IL-15, and GM-CSF in regressing compared to non-regressing melanoma.[70] Thus these data indicate that Th1 CD4+ T cells are likely to be important for spontaneous regression of melanoma. CD4 Th1 but not Th2 clones isolated from human melanomas have been shown to enhance antimelanoma cytotoxic T cell responses, showing that an increase in CD4 Th1 cells could provide increased help to cytotoxic T cells, and thus be important for tumour regression.[71] The characterization of T cell clones isolated from metastatic lesions as Th2 suggests that conversion from Th1 to Th2 responses may aid progression towards metastasis.[72] In contrast to these studies with regressing primary melanomas, metastatic lesions do not appear to contain mRNA for cytokines which are involved in T cell activation, suggesting that the T cells in metastasis are not actively secreting immunoenhancing cytokines.[73] Hence spontaneous regression of primary melanomas is likely to be mediated by localized cell mediated immunity within the tumour, but metastatic lesions seem to be infiltrated with T cells that are less active or of the Th2 type.

The above studies were all performed on melanomas that were actively regressing at the time of tumour sampling and therefore give information on the process mediating the regression, not the events involved in initiation of regression, which would have occurred at an earlier time point. Similar studies in basal cell carcinoma (BCC) have also implicated local inflammatory CD4+ Th1 secreting cells in regression of this skin tumour indicating that this is likely to be important for other types of skin cancer.[74–76]

Further evidence that melanoma regression is immunologically mediated comes from studies showing that human leukocyte antigen (HLA)-B22 is positively, whereas HLA-B27 and HLA-DR-1 are negatively correlated with regression.[77] This implies immunological control over melanoma regression. Compared with the diverse T cell receptor usage in a non-regressing metastasis, the limited diversity of T cell antigen receptors used by T cells infiltrating regressing melanomas suggests selective clonal expansion of specific T cells and implicates the immune system as being responsible for regression.[78–80] T cells cytotoxic for autologous tumour with restricted T cell receptor usage have also been cloned from regressing melanomas, showing that these cells are capable of melanoma destruction and that protective immunity can naturally develop against melanoma.[80–82] An antibody raised against the specific receptor used by a T cell clone in a regressing melanoma was used to show the presence of these clonal T cells in apposition to the melanoma cells within the lesion.[83]

From these studies it is clear that the immune system can destroy focal regions of melanomas, perhaps removing some clones of cells that have developed. The remaining regions, which escape immune destruction, will then develop further. It is also possible that metastases differ from the primary lesions in either their susceptibility to immune destruction or their ability to evade immune destruction. Nevertheless the immune system is a large factor in melanoma development.

Immunosuppression enhances melanoma development

Extrinsic agents influence the skin immune system. UV radiation suppresses the initiation and elicitation of immunity.[84–86] UV radiation can induce local immunosuppression resulting from contact with antigen at the skin site that received the UV rays, or systemic immunosuppression when antigen contact is on skin distal to the site that was irradiated. The mechanisms by which this occurs are not completely understood, but local immunosuppression at least partly involves depletion of LC from the skin.[87,88] Systemic immunosuppression results from isomerisation of a photoreceptor in the epidermis, *trans*-urocanic acid, or UV-induced genetic damage.[89,90]

UV radiation has been implicated as a causative agent for melanoma.[91] UV immunosuppression contributes to the development of melanoma, at least in a mouse model.[92] UV radiation enhances growth of melanoma lines in immunocompetent but not immunodeficient mice, inhibits the effector phase of the immune response and inhibits melanoma infiltration by T cells, thereby enabling tumour outgrowth.[93,94]

Immunosuppression caused by HIV infection may enhance melanoma development, as there has been some indication that patients with decreased CD4+ T cell counts have increased systemic symptoms and that lower CD4 T cell numbers correlate with tumour stage at presentation. However it is unclear whether melanoma is more frequent in HIV infected individuals.[95–97]

Pharmacological immunosuppression to enhance graft survival has been reported to increase the incidence of new melanomas and recurrence of melanomas which were present before organ transplantation.[98,99] The melanoma incidence in these patients is four times the expected rate.[100] A large number of melanomas have been observed to develop from identifiable dysplastic naevi in immunosuppressed patients, with unusually low concentrations of infiltrating lymphocytes, suggesting that immunosuppression enables precursor lesions to develop into melanomas.[101]

ROLE OF COMPONENTS OF THE IMMUNE SYSTEM IN MELANOMA DEVELOPMENT

As melanomas develop, many clones of cells are destroyed by the immune system; those that are able to survive have a selective advantage and grow. Those that survive immune attack tend to be those that are able to escape immune destruction so that as melanomas progress they become less susceptible to immune destruction. Melanoma cells have evolved many strategies for escaping immune attack. Thus immune control of melanoma results in the selection of melanoma cells that are able to evade immune destruction. This complicates studies into the immune components and their relative roles in melanoma development as it gives the immune system a two-edged sword.

Langerhans cells and other dendritic cells

The successful use of DC for immunotherapy of melanoma indicates that these cells are able to induce protective immunity against melanoma. DC pulsed with tumour antigen were found to activate anti-melanoma immunity and induce tumour regression.[102,103] DC pulsed with melanoma antigens have also been shown to activate cytotoxic T cells in mice.[104] Studies in mice have also indicated that DC can induce protective immunity against skin cancer, including melanoma.[105–107]

DC isolated from melanoma metastasis undergoing regression caused by chemoimmunotherapy were found to be more potent activators of T cell stimulation than DC from progressively growing melanomas, which anergised CD4+ T cells.[37] This suggests that DC within melanomas that are regressing are functionally different from those within lesions that are not regressing.

Compared with normal skin, LC numbers are unchanged above naevi and Clark levels I, II, and III melanomas, but depleted above the more deeply invasive Clark levels IV and V melanomas, suggesting that melanoma progression is associated with a decrease in LC.[108,109] LC have also been reported to be reduced above melanomas in another study.[110] Whereas no differences in LC numbers have been observed between melanomas actively undergoing spontaneous regression and non-regressing tumours the induction of immunity by these cells would probably have occurred before clinical or histological indications of regression.[59] In contrast to these studies, dermal dendritic cells were found to be increased in melanoma compared with compound naevi, with no difference as melanomas progress from the radial to the vertical growth phase.[111]

Human and murine melanomas have been observed to induce apoptosis of DC, indicating that this may be one mechanism by which melanomas inhibit DC.[112] DC treated with IL-10 were found to anergise a CD8 T cell line reactive with the melanoma antigen tyrosinase.[113] Thus IL-10 produced by melanoma cells may inhibit the induction of protective immunity via effects on dendritic cells. Squamous cell carcinomas have also been observed to inhibit LC migration from the tumour to the local lymph node, therefore interfering with the induction of protective immunity, although this has not been investigated for melanoma.[114] It therefore seems that, as melanomas progress, they interfere with dendritic cell function.

LC have been proposed to have an important function in the process of skin carcinogenesis. LC are depleted from skin in response to UV radiation and chemical carcinogens.[115–117] Antigen presentation by LC that have drained from carcinogen treated skin to local lymph nodes activates long lived suppressor lymphocytes.[32,118] This occurs during the promoter but not the initiator stage of carcinogenesis.[31,119] Thus agents that promote the development of melanoma or products of melanomas themselves that have deleterious effects on local dendritic cells are likely to be important for melanoma progression.

T lymphocytes

In a study of 285 primary melanomas in the vertical growth phase, which were divided into groups based on the magnitude of the T cell infiltrate, patients with a brisk infiltrate had a 5-year survival of 77%. This was reduced to 53% for those with a non-brisk infiltrate and to 37% for those in which T cell infiltration was absent. The 10-year survival rates were 55%, 45%, and 27%, respectively, with decreasing concentrations of T cell infiltrate.[120] Multivariate analysis found the presence of tumour infiltrating lymphocytes to be a significant and independent positive prognostic factor, supporting a role for inflammatory T cells in eradication of melanoma. In another study a strong correlation was observed between the degree of lymphocyte infiltration of melanoma and patient survival, but no association was found between non-infiltrating lymphocytes that surrounded the tumour and patient survival.[121] This suggests that inflammatory lymphocytes inhibit the formation of melanoma metastases.

The predominant T cell infiltrating early lesions of superficial spreading melanoma (<0.75 mm) were CD4+, whereas CD8 T cells predominated in more advanced metastatic lesions. Additionally, T cells infiltrating cutaneous melanoma expressed CLA, the skin homing receptor, whereas those in metastasis at non-cutaneous sites did not express this receptor.[122] Therefore there is a change in the T cell populations that infiltrate melanomas as they progress.

CD40 (a member of the TNF receptor family) cross linking by CD40L on T cells provides important co-stimulatory signals for T cell activation. This molecule has been shown to be present on cell lines from metastatic and primary melanoma.[123] Cross linking of CD40 with antibody increased melanoma cell proliferation indicating that, although it may be capable of contributing to T cell activation, it may also enhance melanoma growth by an independent mechanism. Other evidence indicates that CD8 T cell eradication of melanoma is dependent on the CD4+ T cell help which results following CD40/CD40L interactions.[124]

Fas (CD95), a member of the TNF receptor family, transduces a signal leading to apoptosis when it is activated by Fas Ligand. T cells use Fas Ligand to kill Fas expressing target cells. However, tumour cells can also express Fas Ligand and thus kill Fas positive infiltrating lymphocytes. Melanoma cell lines have been found to express both Fas and Fas Ligand, and although Fas Ligand on melanoma cells has been reported to cause apoptosis of T cells, the expressed Fas was found not to be functional.[125] This suggests that some melanomas may escape the immune system by causing Fas Ligand mediated T cell destruction, while developing resistance to the same pathway via a defect in their Fas triggered apoptotic pathway. Fas Ligand is more strongly expressed on metastases than primary melanomas, indicating that Fas Ligand is increased during melanoma development, but not all metastasis were positive for Fas Ligand.[126]

Melanoma cells inhibit the expression of vascular cell adhesion molecule 1 (VCAM-1) by endothelial cells.[127] This adhesion molecule enables T cells to migrate across the endothelial cells into tissues and therefore this may inhibit T cell migration out of the blood into the tumour.

As melanomas progress, some cells cease expressing antigens recognized by cytotoxic T lymphocytes. This antigen loss gives these clones a developmental advantage as they have decreased immunogenicity, enabling them to avoid recognition by T cells. It is likely that selective pressures from the T cells enables antigen loss clones to survive, while those which express the antigens are destroyed by the immune response.[128,129] Downregulation of the peptide-transporter protein TAP-1, which is required for expression of MHC class I associated antigen complexes on the target cell surface, is another mechanism by which melanoma cells evade T cell recognition.[128–130] The selective pressure of cytotoxic lymphocytes has also been shown to result in the growth of melanoma metastasis that fail to express MHC class I molecules.[131] The developing MHC class I deficient metastases then fail to be recognized by class I restricted cytotoxic lymphocytes and therefore evade immunological destruction.[132,133]

Cytokines, growth factors, and chemokines (Table 3.1)

IL-1β injection induced augmented immunity to melanoma in mice, increasing mouse survival, but this cytokine has also been shown to enhance melanoma metastasis possibly via upregulation of adhesion molecules that increase adhesion with endothelial cells.[134–136] Transfection of melanoma cells with IL-1 has confirmed that production of this cytokine by melanoma cells can increase their adhesiveness.[137] IL-1β transduced melanoma cells have also been shown to have reduced growth in vivo but not in vitro, and to be infiltrated with increased numbers of macrophages, CD4+ cells and dendritic cells, suggesting that this cytokine is able to augment immunity to melanoma.[138] Thus melanoma production of IL-1 could increase immune control of the tumour but also metastatic potential.

IL-2 treatment of patients with metastatic melanoma caused complete and partial regression in 7% and 10% of patients, respectively.[139] Immunization of human patients with IL-2 transfected autologous melanoma cells caused delayed type contact sensitivity and some signs of regression in three out of 15 patients.[140] IL-2 transfection of melanoma cells resulted in protective immunity that was due, at least in part, to activation of NK cells.[141] The IL-2 transfected melanoma cells activated protective immunity, which was able to destroy a subsequent challenge with untransfected melanoma cells, indicating that IL-2 can enhance the activation of immunological memory.[142] Thus IL-2 can activate protective antitumour immunity.

IL-6 is a pro-inflammatory cytokine, which has many effects on the immune system and may also directly inhibit melanoma growth. Whereas early radial growth phase melanomas are sensitive to IL-6, cells from advanced metastatic lesions are no longer inhibited by this cytokine.[143] There is also an inverse relationship between IL-6 production and growth of murine melanomas. Overexpression of IL-6 by transfection of murine melanomas reduced their growth rate in syngeneic as well as athymic mice, suggesting that this inhibitory effect of IL-6 was independent of cell mediated immunity.[144] Thus as melanoma cells progress they appear to lose their sensitivity to growth inhibition by IL-6.

IL-8 is a chemokine for neutrophils, T cells, and basophils. It is also chemotactic for keratinocytes and induces these cells to express MHC class II.[145] There is increased expression of IL-8 in thick compared with thin (less than 0.76 mm depth) melanomas, and it correlates with metastatic potential. It is also increased by exposure to UVB radiation.[146,147] Transfection of human melanoma with IL-8 increases metastasis in athymic mice that lack cell mediated immunity and also increases angiogenesis. These studies suggest that

Table 3.1 *Role of cytokines, growth factors, and chemokines in melanoma development*

Factor	Abbreviation	Function in immune systems	Role in melanoma development		
			Immune protective	Immune inhibitory	Other
Interleukin 1β	IL-1β	Pro-inflammatory	X		Increases adhesion and metastasis
Interleukin 2	IL-2	T cell growth and differentiation	X; NK activation		
Interleukin 6	IL-6	Pro-inflammatory			Melanoma cell growth inhibition
Interleukin 8	IL-8	Chemokine			Increases angiogenesis
Interleukin 10	IL-10	Inhibits cell mediated but promotes humoral immunity	X; NK activation	X; Inhibits Th1 responses	Inhibits macrophage production of angiogenic factors. Enhances melanoma cell growth
Interleukin 15	IL-15	T cell growth		X; Inhibits MHC I expression	
Interferon α	IFNα	Pro-inflammatory	X; CD4 and CTL		
Granulocyte-macrophage colony stimulating factor	GM-CSF	Growth and differentation of dendritic cells and macrophages	X; T cell, CTL, DC, Mac		
Tumour necrosis factor	TNF	Pro-inflammatory	X		Cytotoxic for melanoma cells
Regulated upon activation, normal T cell expressed and secreted	RANTES	Chemokine			Enhances melanoma progression

See text for references and details. CTL, cytotoxic T lymphocytes; DC, dendritic cells; Mac, macrophages; NK, natural killer cells

IL-8 affects melanoma development by increasing angiogenesis as opposed to having a role in immune control.[147]

Human metastatic melanoma cells produce the Th2 cytokine IL-10, which suppresses cell mediated immunity, and this cytokine has been found to be produced preferentially by metastatic compared with primary lesions suggesting that it may have a role in melanoma progression.[148,149] Melanoma derived IL-10 has been shown to be immunosuppressive and decrease expression of MHC class I and II on melanoma cells.[150,151] This suggests that production of this cytokine by melanomas may enable the tumour to escape destruction by the immune system and subvert protective Th1 into Th2 responses.

However transfection of human melanoma cells with IL-10 reduced growth and metastasis formation upon inoculation into immunodeficient athymic mice. IL-10 prevented macrophage production of angiogenic factors, thus slowing melanoma growth.[152] Other studies confirmed that melanomas transduced with IL-10 have reduced growth in athymic mice. These mice contain NK cells and therefore are not totally devoid of protective immunity. IL-10 did not inhibit metastasis formation in NK deficient mice, showing that IL-10 activation of NK cells inhibits melanoma metastasis.[153] In another study IL-10 transfection of melanoma induced protective immunity, thus inhibiting melanoma development in syngeneic but not immunodeficient athymic mice.[154] IL-10 also enhances proliferation of melanoma cells in culture.[151] Thus whereas IL-10 production by melanoma does seem to be related to its progression, its mechanism of action remains unclear. IL-10 appears capable of inhibiting cell mediated immunity, but in the process inhibits macrophage production of angiogenic factors. IL-10 can also activate NK cells and melanoma cell growth. Therefore it can both inhibit and enhance melanoma development.

IL-15, which has many similar biological activities to IL-2, has been detected in melanoma cell lines but did not seem to be secreted.[155] Antibody neutralization suggested that IL-15 is not an autocrine growth factor but inhibits MHC class I expression, which could therefore provide a mechanism for escape from CD8 T cell mediated cytotoxicity.

IFN-α treatment improves survival of melanoma patients.[156] A correlation between the extent of IFN-α induced tumour regression and infiltration with CD4+ T lymphocytes has been observed, and IFN-α increases the generation of antimelanoma cytotoxic lymphocytes.[157,158] Thus this cytokine may function, at least in part, by enhancing immune responses against melanoma.

GM-CSF also has an important role in the immune system, being a growth or differentiation factor for macrophages and dendritic cells. GM-CSF is produced by thin melanomas (<0.76 mm depth) but not by deeper tumours, indicating that a loss of GM-CSF could be associated with melanoma progression.[146] GM-CSF transfected murine melanomas have reduced growth than untransfected tumours, induce protective immunity, and are infiltrated with large numbers of lymphocytic, monocytic, and dendritic cells, suggesting that GM-CSF acts via augmenting the immune system.[159,160] Immunization of patients with autologous human melanoma cells transfected with GM-CSF increased infiltration with T cells and dendritic cells, and caused tumour destruction and activation of cytotoxic T cells.[161,162] This indicates that GM-CSF is able to induce an immune response in humans that is able to cause at least focal tumour loss. As discussed earlier, there is a decrease in LC as melanomas progress, and GM-CSF is able to increase the number of LC in skin.[163] Therefore it is possible that reduced production of GM-CSF as melanomas progress leads to a reduction in LC numbers, which in turn causes a reduced immune response to melanoma. Intralesional injection of GM-CSF into melanoma metastasis has been found to increase the number of infiltrating dendritic cells.[164]

TGFβ comprises a family of highly conserved immunosuppressive cytokines. Usually they are produced and secreted in an inactive form so that activation, probably by proteolytic enzymes such as plasmin, is an important regulatory event. Human melanoma cells have been shown to produce both latent and active TGFβ.[45,165] TGFβ expression has been observed to increase during progression of melanoma from thin to thick and to metastatic lesions.[166–168] The growth of melanoma cell lines has been found to be variably affected by TGFβ, but NK activity was suppressed, suggesting that it enables melanoma development by having an immunosuppressive effect.[165] There is a loss of growth inhibition to TGFβ as melanocytes progress to primary tumours and then to metastatic cells.[169] This may enable the developing melanoma to produce this cytokine without suffering from its growth inhibitory properties. TGFβ neutralization with antibodies, in combination with IL-2, inhibits melanoma metastasis in mice, possibly associated with increased leukocyte infiltration of the tumours.[170] We have recently shown that TGFβ inhibits dendritic cell mobilization from tumours, suggesting another immunosuppressive action of this cytokine.[171]

TNF (which used to be called TNFα to differentiate it from TNFβ that is now called lymphotoxin), has a major role in inflammation and activation of the immune system and can induce apoptosis in tumour cells. It can also target tumour vasculature, causing haemorrhagic necrosis of the tumour. It is produced by human melanoma cells and leukocytes infiltrating the tumours.[172,173] Isolated limb perfusion with TNF with melphalan induces 70–80% remission of melanoma.[174,175] The observation that TNF with melphalan does not affect growth of human tumours in immunodeficient nude mice suggests that this effect may be via activation of the immune system.[176] Human melanoma cells express the receptor for TNF showing that they are potentially sensitive to this cytokine.[177] Melanoma cells from a metastasis that subsequently underwent regression were found to express high concentrations of the TNF receptor. TNF was cytotoxic for these cells in vitro and in vivo in athymic mice.[178] Melanoma cells also secrete soluble receptors to bind and inhibit its activity. Patients with melanoma have increased concentrations of serum TNF receptors, which may inhibit immune effector functions, contributing to tumour progression.[179] These studies indicate that TNF produced by melanoma cells or cells of the immune system, and expression of the receptors by melanoma cells are likely to be important for immune responses to melanoma. Additionally, as TNF is an important mediator of LC migration to local lymph nodes, production of this cytokine by melanoma cells could regulate the ability of LC to induce protective immunity to skin tumours.[180]

RANTES is a chemokine for leukocytes that is secreted by melanoma cells and is associated with the ability to form tumours on subcutaneous inoculation into athymic mice.[181] Although RANTES seems to aid melanoma progression, it is unclear whether this involves effects on the immune system.

SUMMARY

The immune response is a potent force in shaping melanoma development. It reduces the incidence of new melanomas, and influences progressing lesions. The observations that melanoma cells express molecules which the immune system can recognize and use as targets for destruction of the tumour and that melanoma patients have tumour reactive lymphocytes infiltrating their tumours meet the basic requirements for melanoma protective immunity. It is also clear that the immune response can cause tumour destruction. Spontaneous regression occurs commonly in melanoma, and there is considerable evidence that this results from immune mediated destruction of tumour foci. Occasionally, this spreads throughout the whole tumour, causing immune destruction of the entire lesion. It is likely that most, if not all, melanomas undergo localized loss of some tumour regions during their development. This is observed clinically and histologically as focal spontaneous regression. Immunosuppression caused by exposure to UV radiation or pharmacological control of graft rejection increases melanoma incidence, showing that the immune system prevents the development of many new melanomas, in addition to exerting control over clinically detectable lesions.

Skin immunity is regulated at many levels, and is dependent on not only cells resident in the skin but also cells that traffic into and out of the skin. Resident skin cells such as keratinocytes and mast cells produce cytokines, chemokines, and growth factors, which influence the ability of the immune system to mount protective immunity, as well as trafficking of inflammatory cells into and from the skin. Furthermore, although Th1-like immunity is likely to protect from melanoma, subversion of immunity into Th2-like responses may not be protective, and locally produced cytokines or other factors seems to be important in determining the qualitative nature of these responses. The induction of immunity is dependent on bone marrow derived dendritic cell precursors migrating into the skin, and receiving the appropriate stimuli to mature and migrate to lymph nodes where they can activate Th1-like or cytotoxic T cells. The T cells then need to express skin homing receptors so that they can migrate to the tumour site, infiltrate the tumour, and maintain an activation state via interactions with local antigen presenting cells, cytokines, and adhesion molecules to effectively destroy the tumour. Melanomas that have metastasized to sites outside the skin are likely to be under quite different immunological control to those that remain within the skin. The dendritic cells that initiate the response seem to be unique to the skin, and the T cells that infiltrate the skin express different homing receptors to those found at other sites.

For melanomas to develop they need to evade immune destruction (Figure 3.6). An indication that the immune system has a major effect on melanoma development is that, as melanomas progress, they activate genes that enable the avoidance of immune detection or destruction. If the immune system did not exert such a strong influence on melanoma development this would not be necessary. It seems likely that during melanoma progression, those clones of tumour cells that are unable to evade immune destruction are killed, while those that express protective measures survive and develop. Thus the immune system puts selective pressure on developing melanomas, with less immunogenic foci of tumour cells developing. There are many regulatory checks on the immune system, any of which can be used by melanomas. Melanomas interfere with dendritic cell activation of T cell mediated immunity by producing cytokines such as IL-10 which inhibit dendritic cell maturation. They also decrease the number of local dendritic cells, possibly because they downregulate production of GM-CSF, a growth and differentiation factor for these cells. Melanomas may also interfere with dendritic cell migration to local lymph nodes. Melanomas also inhibit T cell extravasation and infiltration of the lesion. Melanoma clones that fail to express rejection antigens or do not present them on their surface because of downregulation of MHC class I or TAP will also have a survival advantage and outgrow neighbouring tumour clones. Melanoma cells may also express molecules such as Fas Ligand, that induce apoptosis of inflammatory T cells.

The complex interplay of growth factors, cytokines, chemokines, and adhesion molecules, which regulate the immune process, can also affect melanoma cell

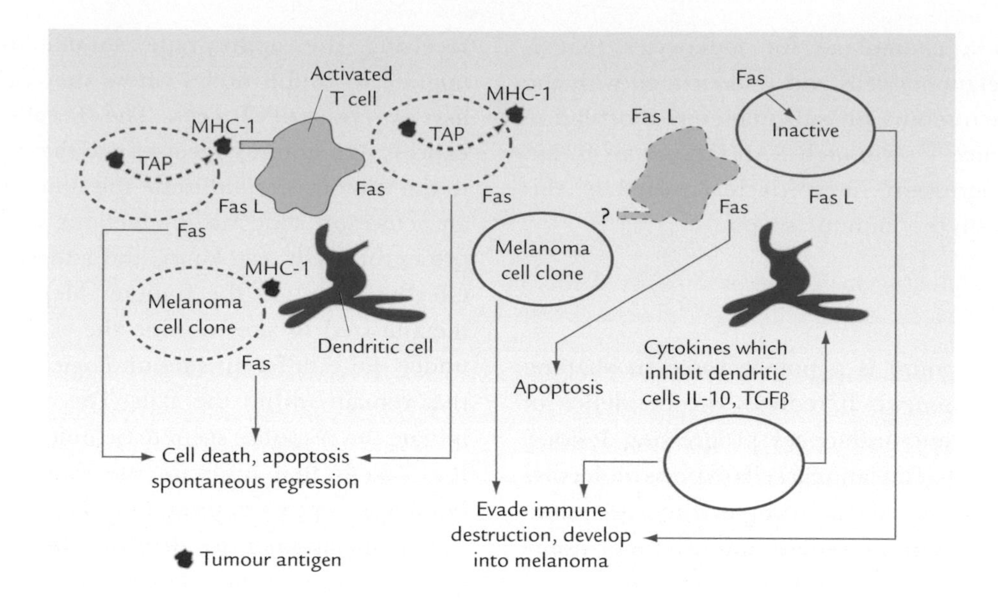

Figure 3.6 *Role of the immune system in melanoma development. During melanoma development the immune system becomes activated and will destroy some lesions before they become clinically apparent. Some clones in the melanomas will avoid immune destruction and therefore develop; clones that do not do this spontaneously regress. Melanomas will produce cytokines that inhibit dendritic cell maturation or migration to lymph nodes, or will induce these cells to undergo apoptosis, preventing activation of T cells. Melanomas will avoid recognition by T cells by loss of antigens, TAP transportation of antigen, or MHC class I expression. Melanomas will avoid T cell destruction by preventing infiltration into the lesion, inducing apoptosis of T cells, or subverting Th1 immunity to a Th2 response. Melanomas will also produce immunosuppressive cytokines while developing resistance to the growth inhibitory effects of these cytokines. As the lesion progresses, the clones that express these protective measures develop.*

growth or production of angiogenic factors, therefore having a secondary effect on melanoma development. It has been suggested that whereas vigorous immune responses destroy tumours, weak responses may enhance their growth.[182] A cell mediated immune response can attract macrophages, which in turn produce angiogenic and other growth factors that the melanoma can use for its advantage. Melanomas may respond to many of the immune cytokines by expressing adhesion molecules or proteolytic enzymes, which aid metastasis. They also increase production of immunosuppressive cytokines such as TGFβ and IL-10, and downregulate their own responsiveness to these cytokines. The requirement of melanoma cells to downregulate or evade the immune response drives selection of melanoma clones with these characteristics, thus effecting melanoma development.

REFERENCES

1. Steinman RM, The dendritic cell system and its role in immunogenicity. *Annu Rev Immunol* 1991; 9: 271–96.
2. Katz SI, Tamaki K, Sachs DH, Epidermal Langerhans cells are derived from cells originating in bone marrow. *Nature* 1979; 282: 324–6.
3. Frelinger JG, Hood L, Hill S, Frelinger JA, Mouse epidermal Ia molecules have a bone marrow origin. *Nature* 1979; 282: 321–3.
4. Inaba K, Inaba M, Romani N, et al, Generation of large numbers of dendritic cells from mouse bone marrow cultures supplemented with granulocyte/macrophage colony-stimulating factor. *J Exp Med* 1992; 176: 1693–702.
5. Banchereau J, Steinman RM, Dendritic cells and the control of immunity. *Nature* 1998; 392: 245–52.
6. Shortman K, Caux C, Dendritic cell development—multiple pathways to natures adjuvants. *Stem Cells* 1997; 15: 409–19.
7. Randolph GJ, Inaba K, Robbiani DF, et al, Differentiation of phagocytic monocytes into lymph node dendritic cells in vivo. *Immunity* 1999; 11: 753–61.
8. Randolph GJ, Beaulieu S, Lebecque S, et al, Differentiation of monocytes into dendritic cells in a model of transendothelial trafficking. *Science* 1998; 282: 480–3.
9. Olweus J, Bitmansour A, Warnke R, et al, Dendritic cell ontogeny – a human dendritic cell lineage of myeloid origin. *Proc Natl Acad Sci USA* 1997; 94: 12551–6.
10. Wu L, Li CL, Shortman K, Thymic dendritic cell precursors – relationship to the T lymphocyte lineage and phenotype of the dendritic cell progeny. *J Exp Med* 1996; 184: 903–11.
11. Jaksits S, Kriehuber E, Charbonnier AS, et al, CD34(+) cell-derived CD14(+) precursor cells develop into Langerhans cells in a TGF-beta 1–dependent manner. *J Immunol* 1999; 163: 4869–77.
12. Strunk D, Egger C, Leitner G, et al, A skin homing molecule defines the Langerhans cell progenitor in human peripheral blood. *J Exp Med* 1997; 185: 1131–6.
13. Meunier L, Immune dendritic cells in human dermis. *Eur J Dermatol* 1996; 6: 327–31.
14. Meunier L, Gonzalez-Ramos A, Cooper KD, Heterogeneous populations of class-II MHC+ cells in human dermal cell suspensions – identification of a small subset responsible for potent dermal

antigen-presenting cell activity with features analogous to Langerhans cells. *J Immunol* 1993; 151: 4067–80.

15. Cyster JG, Chemokines and the homing of dendritic cells to the T cell areas of lymphoid organs. *J Exp Med* 1999b; 189: 447–50.
16. Charbonnier AS, Kohrgruber N, Kriehuber E, et al, Macrophage inflammatory protein 3 alpha is involved in the constitutive trafficking of epidermal Langerhans cells. *J Exp Med* 1999; 190: 1755–67.
17. Tang AM, Amagai M, Granger LG, et al, Adhesion of epidermal Langerhans cells to keratinocytes mediated by E-cadherin. *Nature* 1993; 361: 82–5.
18. Hosoi J, Murphy GF, Egan CL, et al, Regulation of Langerhans cell function by nerves containing calcitonin gene-related peptide. *Nature* 1993; 363: 159–63.
19. Kimber I, Dearman RJ, Cumberbatch M, Huby RJD, Langerhans cells and chemical allergy. *Curr Opin Immunol* 1998; 10: 614–19.
20. Johnston LJ, Halliday GM, King NJC, Langerhans cells migrate to local lymph nodes following cutaneous infection with an arbovirus. *J Invest Dermatol* 2000; 114: 560–8.
21. Marzo AL, Lake RA, Lo D, et al, Tumor antigens are constitutively presented in the draining lymph nodes. *J Immunol* 1999; 162: 5838–45.
22. Cumberbatch M, Kimber I, Dermal tumour necrosis factor-alpha induces dendritic cell migration to draining lymph nodes, and possibly provides one stimulus for Langerhans' cell migration. *Immunology* 1992; 75: 257–63.
23. Cumberbatch M, Dearman RJ, Kimber I, Langerhans cells require signals from both tumour necrosis factor-alpha and interleukin-1–beta for migration. *Immunology* 1997; 92: 388–95.
24. Rambukkana A, Pistoor FHM, Bos JD, et al, Effects of contact allergens on human Langerhans cells in skin organ culture – migration, modulation of cell surface molecules, and early expression of interleukin-1–beta protein. *Lab Invest* 1996; 74: 422–36.
25. Roake JA, Rao AS, Morris PJ, et al, Dendritic cell loss from nonlymphoid tissues after systemic administration of lipopolysaccharide, tumor necrosis factor, and interleukin 1. *J Exp Med* 181: 2237–47.
26. Cyster JG, Chemokines – chemokines and cell migration in secondary lymphoid organs. *Science* 1999a; 286: 2098–102.
27. Aiba S, Nakagawa S, Ozawa H, et al, Up-regulation of alpha4 integrin on activated Langerhans cells – analysis of adhesion molecules on Langerhans cells relating to their migration from skin to draining lymph nodes. *J Invest Dermatol* 1993; 100: 143–7.
28. Ioffreda MD, Whitaker D, Murphy GF, Mast cell degranulation upregulates alpha-6-integrins on epidermal Langerhans cells. *J Invest Dermatol* 1993; 101: 150–4.
29. Dai RP, Grammer SF, Streilein JW, Fresh and cultured Langerhans cells display differential capacities to activate hapten-specific T-cells. *J Immunol* 1993; 150: 59–66.
30. Streilein JW, Grammer SF, Yoshikawa T, et al, Functional dichotomy between Langerhans cells that present antigen to naive and to memory/effector T lymphocytes. *Immunol Rev* 1990; 117: 159–83.
31. Halliday GM, Odling KA, Ruby JC, Muller HK, Suppressor cell activation and enhanced skin allograft survival after tumor promotor but not initiator induced depletion of cutaneous Langerhans cells. *J Invest Dermatol* 1988b; 90: 293–7.
32. Halliday GM, Wood RC, Muller HK, Presentation of antigen to suppressor cells by a dimethylbenz(a)anthracene resistant, Ia-positive, Thy-1-negative, I-J-restricted epidermal cell. *Immunology* 1990; 69: 97–103.
33. Woods GM, Doherty KV, Malley RC, et al, Carcinogen-modified dendritic cells induce immunosuppression by incomplete T-cell activation resulting from impaired antigen uptake and reduce CD86 expression. *Immunology* 2000; 99: 16–22.
34. Labeur MS, Roters B, Pers B, et al, Generation of tumor immunity by bone marrow-derived dendritic cells correlates with dendritic cell maturation stage. *J Immunol* 1999; 162: 168–75.
35. Chaux P, Favre N, Martin M, Martin F, Tumor-infiltrating dendritic cells are defective in their antigen-presenting function and inducible B7 expression in rats. *Int J Cancer* 1997; 72: 619–24.
36. Nestle FO, Burg G, Fah J, et al, Human sunlight-induced basal-cell-carcinoma-associated dendritic cells are deficient in T cell co-stimulatory molecules and are impaired as antigen-presenting cells. *Am J Pathol* 1997; 150: 641–51.
37. Enk AH, Jonuleit H, Saloga J, Knop J, Dendritic cells as mediators of tumor-induced tolerance in metastatic melanoma. *Int J Cancer* 1997; 73: 309–16.
38. Foster CA, Elbe A, In: *Skin immune system (SIS)* (ed. Bos J D), Boca Raton: CRC Press, 1997: 85–108.
39. Picker LJ, Treer JR, Ferguson-Darnell B, et al, Control of lymphocyte recirculation in man. II Differential regulation of the cutaneous lymphocyte-associated antigen, a tissue selective homing receptor for skin-homing T cells. *J Immunol* 1993; 150: 1122–36.
40. Spetz AL, Strominger J, Grohspies V, T cell subsets in normal human epidermis. *Am J Pathol* 1996; 149: 665–74.
41. Picker LJ, Martin RJ, Trumble A, Newman LS, et al, Differential expression of lymphocyte homing receptors by human memory/effector T cells in pulmonary versus cutaneous immune effector sites. *Eur J Immunol* 1994; 24: 1269–77.
42. Sprent J, Circulating T and B lymphocytes of the mouse. I. Migratory properties. *Cell Immunol* 1973; 7: 10–39.
43. Mattei S, Colombo MP, Melani C, et al, Expression of cytokine/growth factors and their receptors in human melanoma and melanocytes. *Int J Cancer* 1994; 56: 853–7.
44. Wang JM, Deng XY, Gong WH, Su SB, Chemokines and their role in tumor growth and metastasis. *J Immunol Methods* 1998; 220: 1–17.
45. Rodeck U, Melber K, Kath R, et al, Constitutive expression of multiple growth factor genes by melanoma cells but not normal melanocytes. *J Invest Dermatol* 1991; 97: 20–6.
46. Mosmann TR, Schumacher JH, Street NF, et al, Diversity of cytokine synthesis and function of mouse CD4+ T cells. *Immunol Rev* 1991; 123: 209–29.
47. Kelso A, Th1 and Th2 subsets: paradigms lost? *Immunol Today* 1995; 16: 374–9.
48. Kawakami Y, Rosenberg SA, Human tumor antigens recognized by T-cells. *Immunol Res* 1997; 16: 313–39.
49. Boon T, Vanderbruggen P, Human tumor antigens recognized by T lymphocytes. *J Exp Med* 1996; 183: 725–9.
50. Pandolfino MC, Viret C, Gervois N, et al, Specificity, T-cell receptor diversity and activation requirements of CD4+ and CD8+ clones derived from human melanoma-infiltrating lymphocytes. *Eur J Immunol* 1992; 22: 1795–802.
51. Darrow TL, Abdelwahab Z, Quinnallen MA, Seigler HF, Recognition and lysis of human melanoma by a CD3(+), CdD4(+), CD8(−) T-cell clone restricted by HLA-A2. *Cell Immunol* 1996; 172: 52–9.
52. Mazzocchi A, Belli F, Mascheroni L, et al, Frequency of cytotoxic T lymphocyte precursors (CTLp) interacting with autologous tumor via the T-cell receptor: Limiting dilution analysis of specific CTLp in peripheral blood and tumor-invaded lymph nodes of melanoma patients. *Int J Cancer* 1994; 58: 330–9.
53. Stewart JF, Tattersall MHN, Woods RL, Fox RM, Unknown primary adenocarcinoma: incidence of overinvestigation and natural history. *BMJ* 1979; 1: 1530–3.
54. Greco FA, Hainsworth JD, Tumors of unknown origin. *CA-A Cancer J Clin* 1992; 42: 96–115.
55. Nathanson L, Spontaneous regression of malignant melanoma: a review of the literature on incidence, clinical features and possible mechanisms. *Natl Cancer Inst Monogr* 1976; 44: 67–76.
56. McGovern VJ, Spontaneous regression of melanoma. *Pathology* 1975; 7: 91–9.
57. Avril MF, Charpentier P, Margulis A, Guillaume JC, Regression of primary melanoma with metastases. *Cancer* 1992; 69: 1377–81.
58. Menzies SW, McCarthy WH, Complete regression of primary cutaneous malignant melanoma. *Arch Surg* 1997; 132: 553–6.
59. Tefany FJ, Barnetson RSC, Halliday GM, et al, Immunocytochemical analysis of the cellular infiltrate in primary regressing and non-regressing malignant melanoma. *J Invest Dermatol* 1991; 97: 197–202.
60. Lowes MA, Bishop GA, Crotty K, et al, T Helper 1 cytokine MRNA is increased in spontaneously regressing primary melanomas. *J Invest Dermatol* 1997; 108: 914–19.
61. Cooper PH, Wanebo HJ, Hagar W, Regression in thin malignant melanoma. Microscopic diagnosis and prognostic importance. *Arch Dermatol* 1985; 121: 1127–31.

62. McGovern VJ, Shaw HM, Milton GW, Prognosis in patients with thin malignant melanoma: influence of regression. *Histopathology* 1983; 7: 673–80.
63. Maurer S, Kolmel KF, Spontaneous regression of advanced malignant melanoma. *Onkologie* 1998; 21: 14–18.
64. Kelly JW, Sagebiel RW, Blois MS, Regression in malignant melanoma. A histologic feature without independent prognostic significance. *Cancer* 1985; 56: 2287–91.
65. Halliday GM, Barnetson RSC, In: *Malignant tumors of the skin* (eds A C Chu, R L Edelson). Arnold, London: 1999: 411–24.
66. Brady MS, Eckels DD, Ree SY, et al, Mhc class II-mediated antigen presentation by melanoma cells. *J Immunother* 1996; 19: 387–97.
67. Brady MS, Lee F, Petrie H, et al, CD4(+) T cells kill HLA-class-II-antigen-positive melanoma cells presenting peptide in vitro. *Cancer Immunol Immunother* 2000; 48: 621–6.
68. Chen PW, Ullrich SE, Ananthaswamy HN, Presentation of endogenous tumor antigens to CD4+ T lymphocytes by murine melanoma cells transfected with major histocompatibility complex class II genes. *J Leukocyte Biol* 1994a; 56: 469–74.
69. Becker JC, Brabletz T, Czerny C, et al, Tumor escape mechanisms from immunosurveillance – induction of unresponsiveness in a specific MHC-restricted CD4+ human T-cell clone by the autologous MHC class-II+ melanoma. *Int Immunol* 1993; 5: 1501–8.
70. Wagner SN, Schultewolter T, Wagner C, et al, Immune response against human primary malignant melanoma – a distinct cytokine MRNA profile associated with spontaneous regression. *Lab Invest* 1998; 78: 541–50.
71. Lee KY, Goedegebuure PS, Linehan DC, Eberlein TJ, Immunoregulatory effects of CD4(+) T helper subsets in human melanoma. *Surgery* 1995; 117: 365–72.
72. Kharkevitch DD, Seito D, Balch GC, et al, Characterization of autologous tumor-specific T-helper 2 cells in tumor-infiltrating lymphocytes from a patient with metastatic melanoma. *Int J Cancer* 1994; 58: 317–23.
73. Luscher U, Filgueira L, Juretic A, et al, The pattern of cytokine gene expression on freshly excised human metastatic melanoma suggest a a state of reversible anergy of tumor-infiltrating lymphocytes. *Int J Cancer* 1994; 57: 612–9.
74. Hunt MJ, Halliday GM, Weedon D, et al, Regression in basal cell carcinoma – an immunohistochemical analysis. *Br J Dermatol* 1994; 130: 1–8.
75. Halliday GM, Patel A, Hunt MJ, et al, Spontaneous regression of human melanoma/non-melanoma skin cancer: Association with infiltrating CD4+ T cells. *World J Surg* 1995; 19: 352–8.
76. Wong DA, Bishop GA, Lowes MA, et al, Cytokine profiles in spontaneously regressing basal cell carcinomas. *Br J Dermatol* 2000; 143: 91–8.
77. Lowes MA, Dunckley H, Watson N, et al, Regression of melanoma, but not keratoacanthoma, is associated with increased HLA-B22 and decreased HLA-B27 and HLA-DR1. *Melanoma Res* 1999; 9: 539–44.
78. Ferradini L, Romanroman S, Azocar J, et al, Analysis of T-cell receptor-alpha/beta variability in lymphocytes infiltrating a melanoma metastasis. *Cancer Res* 1992; 52: 4649–54.
79. Ferradini L, Mackensen A, Genevee C, et al, Analysis of T-cell receptor variability in tumor-infiltrating lymphocytes from a human regressive melanoma – evidence for in situ T-cell clonal expansion. *J Clin Invest* 1993; 91: 1183–90.
80. Zorn E, Hercend T, A MAGE-6–encoded peptide is recognized by expanded lymphocytes infiltrating a spontaneously regressing human primary melanoma lesion. *Eur J Immunol* 1999a; 29: 602–7.
81. Mackensen A, Ferradini L, Carcelain G, et al, Evidence for in situ amplification of cytotoxic T-lymphocytes with antitumor activity in a human regressive melanoma. *Cancer Res* 1993; 53: 3569–73.
82. Zorn E, Hercend T, A natural cytotoxic T cell response in a spontaneously regressing human melanoma targets a neoantigen resulting from a somatic point mutation. *Eur J Immunol* 1999b; 29: 592–601.
83. Mackensen A, Carcelain G, Viel S, et al, Direct evidence to support the immunosurveillance concept in a human regressive melanoma. *J Clin Invest* 1994; 93: 1397–402.
84. Kripke ML, Immunologic unresponsiveness induced by UV radiation. *Immunol Rev* 1984; 80: 87–102.
85. Damian DL, Halliday GM, Barnetson RS, Broad-spectrum sunscreens provide greater protection against ultraviolet-radiation-induced suppression of contact hypersensitivity to a recall antigen in humans. *J Invest Dermatol* 1997; 109: 146–51.
86. Damian DL, Halliday GM, Taylor CA, Barnetson RSC, Ultraviolet radiation induced suppression of Mantoux reactions in humans. *J Invest Dermatol* 1998; 110: 824–7.
87. Bergstresser PR, Toews GB, Streilein JW, Natural and perturbed distributions of Langerhans cells: responses to ultraviolet light, heterotopic skin grafting, and dinitrofluorobenzene sensitization. *J Invest Dermatol* 1980; 75: 73–7.
88. Aberer W, Romani N, Elbe A, Stingl G, Effects of physicochemical agents on murine epidermal Langerhans cells and Thy-1–positive dendritic epidermal cells. *J Immunol* 1986; 136: 1210–16.
89. Noonan FP, De Fabo EC, Immunosuppression by ultraviolet B radiation: initiation by urocanic acid. *Immunol Today* 1992; 13: 250–4.
90. Kripke ML, Cox PA, Alas LG, Yarosh DB, Pyrimidine dimers in DNA initiate systemic immunosuppression in UV-irradiated mice. *Proc Natl Acad Sci USA* 1992; 89: 7516–20.
91. Armstrong BK, Kricker A, How much melanoma is caused by sun exposure? *Melanoma Res* 1993; 3: 395–401.
92. Donawho C, Romerdahl CA, Kripke ML, Effects of UV radiation on immunity to murine melanomas. *Cell Immunity Immunother Cancer* 1990;135: 333–42.
93. Donawho CK, Kripke ML, Evidence that the local effect of ultraviolet radiation on the growth of murine melanomas is immunologically mediated. *Cancer Res* 1991; 51: 4176–81.
94. Donawho CK, Muller HK, Bucana CD, Kripke ML, Enhanced growth of murine melanoma in ultraviolet-irradiated skin is associated with local inhibition of immune effector mechanisms. *J Immunol* 1996; 157: 781–6.
95. Wang CY, Brodland DG, Su W, Skin cancers associated with acquired immunodeficiency syndrome. *Mayo Clin Proc* 1995; 70: 766–72.
96. McGregor JM, Newell M, Ross J, et al, Cutaneous malignant melanoma and human immunodeficiency virus (HIV) infection – a report of three cases. *Br J Dermatol* 1992; 126: 516–9.
97. Aboulafia DM, Malignant melanoma in an HIV-infected man: A case report and literature review. *Cancer Invest* 1998; 16: 217–24.
98. Penn I, Malignant melanoma in organ allograft recipients. *Transplantation* 1996; 61: 274–8.
99. Sheil AG, Cancer after transplantation. *World J Surg* 1986; 10: 389–96.
100. Sheil AG, Flavel S, Disney AP, et al, Cancer incidence in renal transplant patients treated with azathioprine or cyclosporine. *Transplant Proc* 1987; 19: 2214–6.
101. Greene MH, Young TI, Clark WH Jr, Malignant melanoma in renal-transplant recipients. *Lancet* 1981; 1: 1196–9.
102. Nestle FO, Alijagic S, Gilliet M, et al, Vaccination of melanoma patients with peptide- or tumor lysate-pulsed dendritic cells. *Nature Med* 1998; 4: 328–32.
103. Thurner B, Haendle I, Roder C, et al, Vaccination with Mage-3A1 peptide-pulsed mature, monocyte-derived dendritic cells expands specific cytotoxic T cells and induces regression of some metastases in advanced stage IV melanoma. *J Exp Med* 1999; 190: 1669–78.
104. Abdel-Wahab Z, Dematos P, Hester D, et al, Human dendritic cells, pulsed with either melanoma tumor cell lysates or the gp100 peptide((280–288)), induce pairs of T-cell cultures with similar phenotype and lytic activity. *Cell Immunol* 1998; 186: 63–74.
105. Cavanagh LL, Sluyter R, Henderson KG, et al, Epidermal Langerhans cell induction of immunity against an ultraviolet-induced skin tumour. *Immunology* 1996; 87: 475–80.
106. Mayordomo JI, Zorina T, Storkus WJ, et al, Bone marrow-derived dendritic cells serve as potent adjuvants for peptide-based antitumor vaccines. *Stem Cells* 1997; 15: 94–103.
107. Wan YH, Emtage P, Zhu Q, et al, Enhanced immune response to the melanoma antigen gp100 using recombinant adenovirus-transduced dendritic cells. *Cell Immunol* 1999; 198: 131–8.

108. Stene MA, Babajanians M, Bhuta S, Cochran AJ, Quantitative alterations in cutaneous Langerhans cells during the evolution of malignant melanoma of the skin. *J Invest Dermatol* 1988; 91: 125–8.
109. Toriyama K, Wen DR, Paul E, Cochran AJ, Variations in the distribution, frequency, and phenotype of Langerhans cells during the evolution of malignant melanoma of the skin. *J Invest Dermatol* 1993; 100: S269–73.
110. Schreiner TU, Lischka G, Schaumburglever G, Langerhans' cells in skin tumors. *Arch Dermatol* 1995; 131: 187–90.
111. Fullen DR, Headington JT, Factor XIIIa-positive dermal dendritic cells and HLA-DR expression in radial versus vertical growth-phase melanomas. *J Cutan Pathol* 1998; 25: 553–8.
112. Esche C, Lokshin A, Shurin GV, et al, Tumor's other immune targets: dendritic cells. *J Leukocyte Biol* 1999; 66: 336–44.
113. Steinbrink K, Jonuleit H, Muller G, et al, Interleukin-10–treated human dendritic cells induce a melanoma-antigen-specific anergy in CD8(+) T cells resulting in a failure to lyse tumor cells. *Blood* 1999; 93: 1634–42.
114. Lucas AD, Halliday GM, Progressor but not regressor skin tumours inhibit Langerhans' cell migration from epidermis to local lymph nodes. *Immunology* 1999; 97: 130–7.
115. Toews GB, Bergstresser PR, Streilein JW, Epidermal Langerhans cell density determines whether contact hypersensitivity or unresponsiveness follows skin painting with DNFB. *J Immunol* 1980; 124: 445–53.
116. Odling K, Halliday G, Muller H, Effects of low or high doses of short wavelength ultraviolet light (UVB) on Langerhans cells and skin allograft survival. *Immunol Cell Biol* 1987; 65: 337–43.
117. Halliday GM, Muller HK, Sensitization through carcinogen-induced Langerhans cell-deficient skin activates specific long-lived suppressor cells for both cellular and humoral immunity. *Cell Immunol* 1987; 109: 206–21.
118. Halliday GM, Cavanagh LL, Muller HK, Antigen presented in the local lymph node by cells from dimethylbenzanthracene-treated murine epidermis activates suppressor cells. *Cell Immunol* 1988a; 117: 289–302.
119. Halliday GM, Mac Carrick GR, Muller HK, Tumour promotors but not initiators deplete Langerhans cells from murine epidermis. *Br J Cancer* 1987; 56: 328–30.
120. Clemente CG, Mihm MG, Bufalino R, et al, Prognostic value of tumor infiltrating lymphocytes in the vertical growth phase of primary cutaneous melanoma. *Cancer* 1996; 77: 1303–10.
121. Elder DE, Vanbelle P, Elenitsas R, et al, Neoplastic progression and prognosis in melanoma. *Semin Cutan Med Surg* 1996; 15: 336–48.
122. Strohal R, Marberger K, Pehamberger H, Stingl G, Immunohistological analysis of anti-melanoma host responses. *Arch Dermatol Res* 1994; 287: 28–35.
123. Thomas WD, Smith MJ, Si Z, Hersey P, Expression of the co-stimulatory molecule CD40 on melanoma cells. *Int J Cancer* 1996; 68: 795–801.
124. Lode HN, Xiang R, Pertl U, et al, Melanoma immunotherapy by targeted IL-2 depends on CD4(+) T-cell help mediated by CD40/CD40L interaction. *J Clin Invest* 2000; 105: 1623–30.
125. Ferrarini M, Imro MA, Sciorati C, et al, Blockade of the Fas-triggered intracellular signaling pathway in human melanomas is circumvented by cytotoxic lymphocytes. *Int J Cancer* 1999; 81: 573–9.
126. Terheyden P, Siedel C, Merkel A, et al, Predominant expression of Fas (CD95) ligand in metastatic melanoma revealed by longitudinal analysis. *J Invest Dermatol* 1999; 112: 899–902.
127. Piali L, Fichtel A, Terpe HJ, et al, Endothelial vascular cell adhesion molecule 1 expression is suppressed by melanoma and carcinoma. *J Exp Med* 1995; 181: 811–6.
128. Maeurer MJ, Gollin SM, Martin D, et al, Tumor escape from immune recognition–lethal recurrent melanoma in a patient associated with downregulation of the peptide transporter protein tap-1 and loss of expression of the immunodominant mart-1/melan-a antigen. *J Clin Invest* 1996; 98: 1633–41.
129. Jager E, Ringhoffer M, Karbach J, et al, Inverse relationship of melanocyte differentiation antigen expression in melanoma tissues and CD8(+) cytotoxic-T-cell responses: evidence for immunoselection of antigen-loss variants in vivo. *Int J Cancer* 1996; 66: 470–6.
130. Wang Z, Margulies L, Hicklin DJ, Ferrone S, Molecular and functional phenotypes of melanoma cells with abnormalities in HLA class I antigen expression. *Tissue Antigens* 1996; 47: 382–90.
131. Lehmann F, Marchand M, Hainaut P, et al, Differences in the antigens recognized by cytolytic T cells on two successive metastases of a melanoma patient are consistent with immune selection. *Eur J Immunol* 1995; 25: 340–7.
132. Ferrone S, Marincola FM, Loss of HLA Class I antigens by melanoma cells – molecular mechanisms, functional significance and clinical relevance. *Immunol Today* 1995; 16: 487–94.
133. Gervois N, Guilloux Y, Diez E, Jotereau F, Suboptimal activation of melanoma infiltrating lymphocytes (Til) due to low avidity of TCR/MHC-tumor peptide interactions. *J Exp Med* 1996; 183: 2403–7.
134. Neville ME, Pezzella KM, Anti-tumour effects of interleukin 1 beta: In vivo induction of immunity to B16 melanoma, a non-immunogenic tumour. *Cytokine* 1994; 6: 310–7.
135. Garofalo A, Chirivi RGS, Foglieni C, et al, Involvement of the very late antigen 4 integrin on melanoma in interleukin 1-augmented experimental metastases. *Cancer Res* 1995; 55: 414–9.
136. Burrows FJ, Haskard DO, Hart IR, et al, Influence of tumor-derived interleukin-1 on melanoma-endothelial cell interactions in vitro. *Cancer Res* 1991; 51: 4768–75.
137. Chirivi RGS, Chiodoni C, Musiani P, et al, IL-1-alpha gene-transfected human melanoma cells increase tumor-cell adhesion to endothelial cells and their retention in the lung of nude mice. *Int J Cancer* 1996; 67: 856–63.
138. Bjorkdahl O, Wingren AG, Hedlund G, et al, Gene transfer of a hybrid interleukin-1-beta gene to B16 mouse melanoma recruits leucocyte subsets and reduces tumour growth in vivo. *Cancer Immunol Immunother* 1997; 44: 273–81.
139. Rosenberg SA, Yang JC, Topalian SL, et al, Treatment of 283 consecutive patients with metastatic melanoma or renal cell cancer using high-dose bolus interleukin 2. *JAMA* 1994; 271: 907–13.
140. Schreiber S, Kampgen E, Wagner E, et al, Immunotherapy of metastatic malignant melanoma by a vaccine consisting of autologous interleukin 2 transfected cancer cells: Outcome of a phase I study. *Human Gene Ther* 1999; 10: 983–93.
141. Schneeberger A, Koszik F, Schmidt W, et al, The tumorigenicity of IL-2 gene-transfected murine M-3D melanoma cells is determined by the magnitude and quality of the host defense reaction: NK cells play a major role. *J Immunol* 1999; 162: 6650–7.
142. Zatloukal K, Schneeberger A, Berger M, et al, Elicitation of a systemic and protective anti-melanoma immune response by an IL-2-based vaccine–assessment of critical cellular and molecular parameters. *J Immunol* 1995; 154: 3406–19.
143. Rak JW, Hegmann EJ, Lu C, Kerbel RS, Progressive loss of sensitivity to endothelium-derived growth inhibitors expressed by human melanoma cells during disease progression. *J Cell Physiol* 1994; 159: 245–55.
144. Armstrong CA, Murray N, Kennedy M, et al, Melanoma-derived interleukin-6 inhibits in vivo melanoma growth. *J Invest Dermatol* 1994; 102: 278–84.
145. Kemeny L, Ruzicka T, Dobozy A, Michel G, Role of interleukin-8 receptor in skin. *Int Arch Allergy Immunol* 1994; 104: 317–22.
146. Hensley C, Spitzler S, McAlpine BE, et al, In vivo human melanoma cytokine production–inverse correlation of GM-CSF production with tumor depth. *Exp Dermatol* 1998; 7: 335–41.
147. Bar-Eli M, Role of interleukin-8 in tumor growth and metastasis of human melanoma. *Pathobiology* 1999; 67: 12–18.
148. Sato T, McCue P, Masuoka K, et al, Interleukin 10 production by human melanoma. *Clin Cancer Res* 1996; 2: 1383–90.
149. Dummer W, Bastian BC, Ernst N, et al, Interleukin-10 production in malignant melanoma–preferential detection of IL-10-secreting tumor cells in metastatic lesions. *Int J Cancer* 1996; 66: 607–10.
150. Chen QY, Daniel V, Maher DW, Hersey P, Production of IL-10 by melanoma cells–examination of its role in immunosuppression mediated by melanoma. *Int J Cancer* 1994b; 56: 755–60.
151. Yue FY, Dummer R, Geertsen R, et al, Interleukin-10 is a growth factor for human melanoma cells and down-regulates HLA Class-1, HLA Class-II and ICAM-1 molecules. *Int J Cancer* 1997; 71: 630–7.

152. Huang SY, Xie KP, Bucana CD, et al, Interleukin 10 suppresses tumor growth and metastasis of human melanoma cells: potential inhibition of angiogenesis. *Clin Cancer Res* 1996; 2: 1969–79.
153. Zheng LM, Ojcius DM, Garaud F, et al, Interleukin-10 inhibits tumor metastasis through an NK cell-dependent mechanism. *J Exp Med* 1996; 184: 579–84.
154. Gerard CM, Bruyns C, Delvaux A, et al, Loss of tumorigenicity and increased immunogenicity induced by interleukin-10 gene transfer in B16 melanoma cells. *Human Gene Ther* 1996; 7: 23–31.
155. Barzegar C, Meazza R, Pereno R, et al, Il-15 is produced by a subset of human melanomas, and is involved in the regulation of markers of melanoma progression through juxtacrine loops. *Oncogene* 1998; 16: 2503–12.
156. Kirkwood JM, Strawderman MH, Ernstoff MS, et al, Interferon alfa-2b adjuvant therapy of high-risk resected cutaneous melanoma – the eastern cooperative oncology group trial est 1684. *J Clin Oncol* 1996; 14: 7–17.
157. Hakansson A, Gustafsson B, Krysander L, Hakansson L, Tumour-infiltrating lymphocytes in metastatic malignant melanoma and response to interferon alpha treatment. *Br J Cancer* 1996; 74: 670–6.
158. Palmer KJ, Harries M, Gore ME, Collins MKL, Interferon-alpha (IFN-alpha) stimulates anti-melanoma cytotoxic T lymphocyte (CTL) generation in mixed lymphocyte tumour cultures (MLTC). *Clin Exp Immunol* 2000; 119: 412–8.
159. Botella R, Sarradet MD, Potter LE, et al, Inhibition of murine melanoma growth by granulocyte-macrophage colony stimulating factor gene transfection is not haplotype specific. *Melanoma Res* 1998; 8: 245–54.
160. Armstrong CA, Botella R, Galloway TH, et al, Antitumor effects of granulocyte-macrophage colony-stimulating factor production by melanoma cells. *Cancer Res* 1996; 56: 2191–8.
161. Dranoff G, Soiffer R, Lynch T, et al, A phase I study of vaccination with autologous, irradiated melanoma cells engineered to secrete human granulocyte-macrophage colony stimulating factor. *Human Gene Ther* 1997; 8: 111–23.
162. Soiffer R, Lynch T, Mihm M, et al, Vaccination with irradiated autologous melanoma cells engineered to secrete human granulocyte-macrophage colony-stimulating factor generates potent antitumor immunity in patients with metastatic melanoma. *Proc Natl Acad Sci USA* 1998; 95: 13141–6.
163. O'Sullivan GM, Halliday GM, Modulation of MHC class II+ Langerhans cell numbers in corticosteroid treated epidermis by GM-CSF in combination with TNF-alpha. *Exp Dermatol* 1997; 6: 236–42.
164. Nasi ML, Lieberman P, Busam KJ, et al, Intradermal injection of granulocyte-macrophage colony-stimulating factor (GM-CSF) in patients with metastatic melanoma recruits dendritic cells. *Cytokines Cell Mol Ther* 1999; 5: 139–44.
165. Bizik J, Felnerova D, Grofova M, Vaheri A, Active transforming growth factor-beta in human melanoma cell lines – no evidence for plasmin-related activation of latent TGF-beta. *J Cell Biochem* 1996; 62: 113–22.
166. Schmid P, Itin P, Rufli T, In situ analysis of transforming growth factor-beta s (TGF-beta 1, TGF-beta 2, TGF-beta 3), and TGF-beta type II receptor expression in malignant melanoma. *Carcinogenesis* 1995; 16: 1499–503.
167. Moretti S, Pinzi C, Berti E, et al, In situ expression of transforming growth factor beta is associated with melanoma progression and correlates with KI67, HLA-DR and beta-3 integrin expression. *Melanoma Res* 1997; 7: 313–21.
168. Vanbelle P, Rodeck U, Nuamah I, et al, Melanoma-associated expression of transforming growth factor-beta isoforms. *Am J Pathol* 1996; 148: 1887–94.
169. Krasagakis K, Kruger-Krasagakes S, Fimmel S, et al, Desensitization of melanoma cells to autocrine TGF-beta isoforms. *J Cell Physiol* 1999; 178: 179–87.
170. Wojtowicz-Praga S, Verma UM, Wakefield L, et al, Modulation of B16 melanoma growth and metastasis by anti-transforming growth factor beta antibody and interleukin-2. *J Immunother* 1996; 19: 169–75.
171. Halliday GM, Le S, Transforming growth factor-beta produced by progressor tumors inhibits, while IL-10 produced by regressor tumors enhances, Langerhans cell migration from skin. *Int Immunol* 2001; 13: 1147–54.
172. Sander B, Boeryd B, Tumor necrosis factor-alpha expression in human primary malignant melanoma and its relationship to tumor infiltration by CD3(+) cells. *Int J Cancer* 1996; 66: 42–7.
173. Bergenwald C, Westermark G, Sander B, Variable expression of tumor necrosis factor alpha in human malignant melanoma localized by in situ hybridization for mRNA. *Cancer Immunol Immunother* 1997; 44: 335–40.
174. Lejeune FJ, Ruegg C, Lienard D, Clinical applications of TNF-alpha in cancer. *Curr Opin Immunol* 1998; 10: 573–80.
175. Lejeune F, Lienard D, Eggermont A, et al, Efficacy of tumour necrosis factor-alpha (rTNF-alpha) associated to interferon-gamma (IFN-gamma) and to chemotherapy in isolated limb perfusion for inoperable malignant melanoma, soft tissue sarcoma and epidermoid carcinoma: a 4 year experience. *Bull Cancer* 1995; 82: 561–7.
176. Furrer M, Altermatt HJ, Ris HB, et al, Lack of antitumour activity of human recombinant tumour necrosis factor-alpha, alone or in combination with melphalan in a nude mouse human melanoma xenograft system. *Melanoma Res* 1997; 7: S43–9.
177. Carrel S, Hartmann F, Salvi S, et al, Expression of type A and B tumor necrosis factor (TNF) receptors on melanoma cells can be regulated by dbc-AMP and IFN gamma. *Int J Cancer* 1995; 62: 76–83.
178. Gilhar A, Ullmann Y, Kalish RS, et al, Favourable melanoma prognosis associated with the expression of the tumour necrosis factor receptor and the alpha(1)beta(1)integrin – a preliminary report. *Melanoma Res* 1997; 7: 486–95.
179. Viac J, Vincent C, Palacio S, Schmitt D, Claudy A, Tumour necrosis factor (TNF) soluble receptors in malignant melanoma – correlation with soluble ICAM-1 levels. *Eur J Cancer* 1996; 32A: 447–9.
180. Rubel DM, Barnetson RSC, Halliday GM, Bioactive tumor necrosis factor alpha but not granulocyte-macrophage colony-stimulating factor correlates inversely with Langerhans cell numbers in skin tumours. *Int J Cancer* 1998; 75: 210–16.
181. Mrowietz U, Schwenk U, Maune S, et al, The chemokine RANTES is secreted by human melanoma cells and is associated with enhanced tumour formation in nude mice. *Br J Cancer* 1999; 79: 1025–31.
182. Prehn RT, Stimulatory effects of immune reactions upon the growths of untransplanted tumors. *Cancer Res* 1994; 54: 908–14.

4

Environmental influences on cutaneous melanoma

Jean-François Doré, Mathieu Boniol

INTRODUCTION

An individual's risk of melanoma depends on two sets of factors: host related factors such as pigmentation characteristics and skin reaction to sunlight, and environmental factors.[1, 2]

The only well established environmental factor for melanoma development is sun exposure. Studies conducted in the 1980s have established a relation between sun exposure and melanoma, and it is now considered that sun exposure is a major cause of the disease. A monograph published by the International Agency for Research on Cancer exhaustively reviewed available human evidence and concluded that there is sufficient evidence in humans for the carcinogenicity of solar radiation. Solar radiation causes both cutaneous melanoma and non-melanocytic skin cancer.[3]

But the relation between sun exposure and melanoma is not a simple one. It is not only the total accumulated dose of solar radiation that contributes to the induction of melanoma, but the pattern of sun exposure according to age seems to play an important part. Although there is evidence that ultraviolet (UV) radiation contributes to melanoma induction, the wavelengths of solar radiation contributing to the development of melanoma are currently not clearly known. This may hamper any attempt at predicting the possible effects on melanoma incidence of an increase in solar UV radiation reaching the surface of the earth as a consequence of the observed reduction in the stratospheric ozone layer that absorbs the shortest UV wavelengths.

ENVIRONMENTAL INFLUENCES ON MELANOMA INCIDENCE

Sun exposure is a risk factor for melanoma

The factors underlying the rapid increase in incidence of melanoma in recent decades are still far from being completely understood, but it is clear that both the increase in sun exposure of white-skinned populations and altered patterns of exposure are strongly involved. The risk of melanoma is higher in fair-skinned people, especially those with blonde or red hair who sunburn and freckle easily, than in people with darker complexions.[4]

The conclusion that solar radiation causes melanoma is based on the positive association between melanoma incidence and residence at lower latitudes, evidence from migrant studies showing that the risk of melanoma is related to sun exposure at the place of residence in early life, a body site distribution which favours sites regularly or usually exposed to the sun, and evidence from case–control and cohort studies that melanoma is related to residence in sunny climates, is correlated with cutaneous sun damage, and is positively associated with intermittent exposure to the sun including a history of sunburn.[3]

The incidence of melanoma among whites is inversely related to latitude of residence.[2] The incidence is highest in countries such as Australia, a subtropical country with a largely Celtic population,[5] and in hotter regions of the United States. The risk for melanoma is related to latitude of residence in

Australia and in the US; white populations living near the equator are at higher risk than those living near the poles.[6] The situation is less clear in Europe where rates in Scandinavia and Switzerland are higher than those in France or Italy,[7] probably reflecting different skin pigmentation and the importance of intermittent or recreational sun exposure (Table 4.1). Conversely, melanoma is uncommon in darker skinned people; in the US, the incidence among blacks is only 1/10 that among whites.[7] Melanomas in blacks and Asians tend to occur at sites not exposed to sun, such as the nail bed and the sole of the foot.[9] Furthermore, although the incidence of melanoma has increased annually in white people in Europe, the US, Canada, and Australia, there has been very little increase in incidence among pigmented peoples of African and Asian origin.[2]

The risk of melanoma increases for North European migrants to Australia and Israel. In both countries increasing incidence is related to duration of residence, but for superficial spreading melanoma, migration to Australia after the age of 20 is not accompanied by an increased risk, the highest risk being associated with migration before the age of 10.[10,11] The increase of melanoma risk associated with the length of residence in Israel confirms the importance of environmental factors in the aetiology of melanoma, and it has been suggested that, in addition to the possibility of sun exposure, linked to residence in Israel, there may have been an increase in the actual exposure, probably related to an increase in leisure activities.[11]

Several case–control studies have reported that subjects who had a short period of high sun exposure, such as residence or occupation in a tropical or subtropical area, have an increased risk of melanoma (Table 4.2). Interestingly, men who had served in the US forces during the second world war in the Pacific area were found to present a significant excess of melanomas (relative risk 7.7, 95% confidence interval 2.8 to 21.3) compared with those who had served in the US or in Europe. Furthermore, tumours in men who had served in the Pacific were more frequently pathologically associated with pre-existing naevi.[13] More recently, it has been shown in a case–control study in Europe that the risk of melanoma is increased by residence in a sunny area (adjusted odds ratio 2.7, 95% CI 1.4 to 5.2), this risk being further increased if subjects sought a suntan when residing in sunny climates (OR 4.7, 95% CI 1.4 to 13.5), and if subjects arrived before the age of 10 in the sunny area (OR 4.3, 95% CI 1.7 to 11.1).[17]

Numerous case–control studies, conducted in Australia, the US, Canada, and Europe, have assessed the association between the incidence of cutaneous melanoma, intermittent, occupational, and total sun exposure, and history of sunburn at different ages.[1] A full review of these studies has been published by the International Agency for Research on Cancer.[3] Elwood and Jopson have recently conducted a systematic review using results of 29 published case–control studies that have assessed incident melanoma, sun exposure and sunburn (Table 4.3).[18] Overall, there was a significant positive association for recreational intermittent exposure such as sunbathing (OR 1.71), a significantly reduced risk for heavy occupational exposure (OR 0.86) and a small, marginally significant risk for total exposure (OR 1.18). There was a significantly increased risk with sunburn at all ages or in adult life (OR 1.91) and similarly elevated relative risks for sunburn in adolescence (OR 1.73) and in childhood (OR 1.95). These results show the specificity of the positive association between melanoma risk and intermittent sun exposure (reflected by sunburns), in contrast to a reduced risk with high levels of occupational exposure.

It is worthy of note that a history of sunburn indicates unusually intense sun exposure and skin sensitivity. Three large studies from Canada, Australia, and Europe showed that the association was primarily with a tendency to burn rather than with the history of sunburn itself.[19–21]

In addition to patterns of sun exposure, age at exposure is an important risk factor for melanoma. Studies

Table 4.1 *Annual incidence of melanoma in European countries for the period 1983–1987 (rate per 100.000, standardized on the European population). Data from de Vathaire et al., 1996*[8]

Country	Men	Women
France	4.4	5.9
United Kingdom	3.9	6.4
Denmark	10.1	12.5
Switzerland (Geneva)	13.3	12.8
Spain	2.8	3.2
Italy	5.2	5.3

Table 4.2 *Risk of melanoma associated with short periods of high potential sun exposure*

Author/reference	Year	Place	Exposure	Relative risk	95% CI	*P* value
Paffenbarger et al.[12]	1978	USA	Outdoor work recorded at college medical examination (retrospective cohort study)	3.9		0.01
Brown et al.[13]	1984	New York	Service in the US forces in the Pacific versus in US or Europe	7.7	2.8–21.3	0.0002
Elwood et al.[14]	1986	Nottingham, UK	Residence ≥1 year in tropical or subtropical area	1.8	0.6–5.1	
Mackie et al.[15]	1989	Scotland	Residence ≥5 years in tropical or subtropical area	Males 2.6 Females 1.8	1.3–5.4 0.8–4.0	
Beitner et al.[16]	1990	Stockholm	Residence >1 year in Mediterranean, tropical or subtropical area in past 10 years	1.9	1.0–3.6	
Autier et al.[17]	1997	Europe	Residence >1 year in Mediterranean, tropical or subtropical area	2.7 Before age of 10 years: 4.3	1.4–5.2 1.7–11.1	

Table 4.3 *Risk of melanoma and sun exposure. Data from 29 case–control studies (Elwood, Jopson, 1997)[18]*

Sun exposure	Odds ratio
Intermittent	1.71
Professional	0.86
Total sun	1.18
Sunburns (all ages)	1.91
adolescence	1.73
childhood	1.95

These data show the specificity of the positive association with intermittent exposure (reflected by sunburns), and the reduction of risk associated with professional exposure.

in migrants and case–control studies have provided evidence for the role of sun exposure in childhood or adolescence. The analysis of a case–control study in Europe recently showed that the melanoma risk associated with a given level of sun exposure during adulthood increased with higher sun exposure during childhood, but the increase in risk was higher than the simple addition of melanoma risk associated with sun exposure during childhood or adulthood. High sun exposure during adult life constituted a significant risk factor for melanoma only if there had been substantial sun exposure during childhood (Figure 4.1).[22] In addition, consideration of the body site distribution of melanomas in relation to patterns of sun exposure shows that intermittent sun exposure has a greater potential for producing melanoma at ages below 50, whereas at older ages melanoma is more common on areas of continuous sun exposure.[23]

Thus, risk of melanoma is associated with an environmental factor: sun exposure. But while showing a similar geographic and ethnic distribution, melanoma strikingly differs from squamous cell carcinoma in terms of socioeconomic gradient, sex and age distribution, body site distribution, and pattern of sun exposure. These differences gave rise in the early 1980s to the hypothesis of intermittent exposure, as opposed to cumulative sun exposure.[24]

Hence, it is not surprising that there is no clear dose effect relation between sun exposure and melanoma risk. This relation may seem different according to the country where the study has been conducted, such as an area of high solar irradiance or a more temperate climate. Thus, in Queensland, risk increases with increasing total dose, whereas in Western Australia or in Western Canada, risk increases then declines with increasing sun exposure, finally to increase at the highest total exposure levels.[1] The relation between melanoma risk and the dose of sun exposure received is

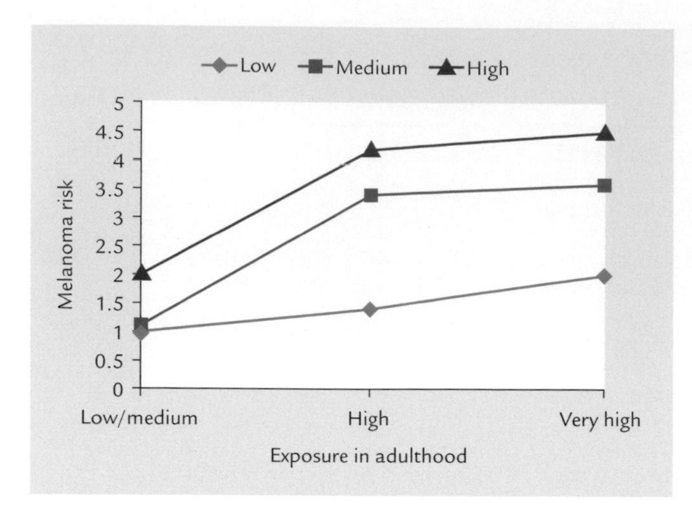

Figure 4.1 *Sun exposure in childhood determines melanoma risk in adulthood (data from[22]).*

complex and seems likely to vary according to the intermittency of the dose, the age at which the dose is received, and the host characteristics. Intermittent and constant exposure may be intrinsically different, with conflicting effects, so that the risk for an individual depends on the relative contribution of accumulated and acute sun exposures.

Exposure to solar ultraviolet radiation is a risk factor for melanoma

The epidemiological evidence implicating sun exposure in the causation of melanoma is supported by biological evidence that damage caused by UV radiation, especially damage to DNA, plays a central part in the pathogenesis of melanoma.

Patients with xeroderma pigmentosum, a rare disease (there are about 800 patients identified and followed worldwide) associated with a grossly deficient repair of DNA photoproducts induced by ultraviolet radiation, suffer from an ultrasensitivity to ultraviolet light and have a greatly increased risk of melanoma and squamous cell and basal cell carcinomas.[25–27] Among these patients, malignant skin neoplasms were present in 70% at a median age of 8 years: 57% had non-melanoma skin cancers and 22% had a malignant melanoma.[27] This median age is 50 years younger than the general population. These findings clearly show the importance of DNA repair mechanisms in the aetiology of melanoma.

It has been shown that the capacity to repair UV induced DNA lesions is reduced in peripheral blood lymphocytes from patients with basal cell carcinomas, a condition that confers a highly elevated risk of melanoma.[28] There is a relation between sensitivity to environmental mutagens or carcinogens and environmental carcinogenesis.[29] Sensitivity to mutagens is related to the capacity for DNA repair and can be measured by means of a genetic instability test based on the induction and repair of chromatid breaks induced in peripheral blood lymphocytes exposed to a mutagen.[30] By using this test, it has recently been shown in a case–control study that patients with melanoma display an increased sensitivity to the induction of chromatid breaks in peripheral blood lymphocytes exposed to 4-nitro-quinoline oxide, an ultraviolet-mimetic mutagen (Table 4.4).[31]

Melanomas can be induced by exposure to UV radiation in animals such as the South American opossum *Monodelphis domestica* and freshwater fishes.[32,33] Moreover, melanomas have recently been induced in human skin grafted on to immunologically tolerant mice by a single exposure to a chemical carcinogen followed by UVB irradiation.[34]

Hence it is believed that the UV component of sunlight is involved in the induction of melanoma.[3] There is a gradient of UV radiation in the sunlight, increasing from the poles towards the equator (Figure 4.2). It should also be noted that the intensity of UV radiation for a given location varies with the elevation of sun above the horizon – the season and the hour – the maximum being observed at the summer solstice, around the middle of the day, when the sun is at its

Table 4.4 *Induction of chromatid breaks in peripheral blood lymphocytes from melanoma patients and controls exposed to 4-nitro-quinoline oxide. Data from Wu et al., 1996[31]*

	Cases (n=71)	Controls (n=137)	Odds ratio
Mean breaks/cell	0.81 ± 0.43	0.48 ± 0.29	
Breaks/cell ≥ 0.62	45	35	5.0
< 0.62	26	102	
Quartiles			
< 0.26	5	36	1.0
0.26–0.39	7	30	1.7
0.26–0.39	7	30	1.7
0.40–0.61	14	36	2.8
≥ 0.62	45	35	9.3

Table 4.5 *Factors affecting terrestrial ultraviolet irradiation (UVR) at a given location*

Factor	Influence	Comments
Latitude	UVR increases from poles to the equator	UVR increases with decreasing sun–earth distance, with increasing zenith angle of sun at noon Variation in UVB greater than variation in UVA
Season	UVR higher in summer than in winter	UVR in summer higher in the southern hemisphere than in the northern hemisphere
Hour	UVR increases with increasing zenith angle	UVR maximum at solar noon 3/4 of daily UVR are delivered between (solar) 10 am and 2 pm
Altitude	UVR increases with increasing altitude	Increase in the proportion of erythemal radiation
Stratospheric ozone layer	Absorption of shorter wavelengths	Solar ultraviolet radiation reaching earth restricted to 290–400 nm. Affects much more UVB than UVA
Reflection/diffraction	Increases ambient UVR	Reflection on water, sand, may significantly contribute to UVR exposure
Clouds	Absorb UVR	UVB penetrate through clouds (sunburn)

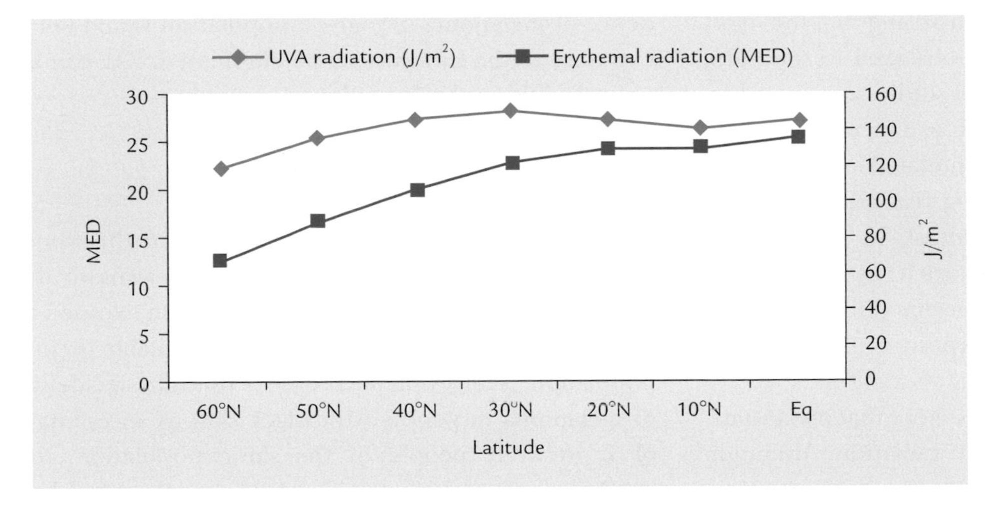

Figure 4.2 *Ambient erythemal and UVA radiation doses (sunrise to 6.30pm) for clear skies during the month of maximum insolation for the northern hemisphere (data from[35]).*

highest elevation (zenith). There is almost a three-fold difference in erythemal intensity (mostly UVB) in the one hour period around solar noon from 60 degrees latitude to the equator, but the daily erythemal dose varies by only a factor two because the length of the day in summertime increases with latitude. For UVA (315–400 nm), there is a smaller variation with latitude, the reason being that the stratospheric ozone layer absorbs part of the ultraviolet radiation and affects erythemal radiation much more than UVA radiation. Actually, the ozone layer absorbs the totality of the UVC radiation (100–280 nm) and part of the UVB radiation (280–315 nm), so that the spectrum of UV radiation reaching the surface of the earth is restricted to 290–400 nm.[35] The intensity of solar UV radiation also increases with the altitude, and because of the shorter distance between sun and earth at high altitude the spectrum of solar UV radiation in mountain regions is shifted towards the shortest wavelengths. In addition, the intensity of solar UV radiation at a given location is influenced by reflection and diffraction (albedo) by snow, water, and sand. Hence, on a sunny summer day on a sandy beach, under a parasol, while being protected from the direct radiation, one can be actually exposed to up to 80% of the incident UV radiation. Furthermore, terrestrial UV radiation is influenced by clouds. Although the influence of clouds on UV radiation is extremely complex, it is possible to express the effect on UV levels using a cloudiness factor 1–0.5 C, where C is the fraction of sky covered by clouds. The size of the liquid droplets (2–60 μm) constituting the clouds is considerably greater than the wavelengths of ultraviolet, and therefore the transmission of ultraviolet radiation through clouds is independent of wavelength and it is possible to catch sunburn when the sun is masked by mist. This may occur, for example, in places such as San Francisco in summer.

Because the distance between sun and earth is shorter during the austral summer than during the summer in the northern hemisphere, and because of variations in ozone thickness, the highest ambient erythemal radiation and UVA radiation are observed at 20–30 degrees latitude south in December or January (Figure 4.2). It is therefore not surprising that the maximum incidence of melanoma is observed in southern latitudes and that epidemiological studies conducted in areas of high UV irradiation such as Queensland tend to indicate an effect of total accumulated sun exposure on melanoma risk, thus reflecting the high UV exposure all the year round. By contrast, in studies conducted in temperate climates, such as Canada or Europe, high UV exposure only occurs during holidays and is reflected by intermittent exposure of sun seeking people.

There is currently little disagreement that melanoma is caused by exposure to solar UV radiation. Although there are complex interactions with the host's susceptibility factors and behaviour (for example intermittent versus continuous exposure), it is likely that melanoma is caused primarily by high intensity UV exposure. Gilchrest et al. have proposed a mechanism to explain the difference in the induction of melanoma and squamous cell carcinoma by ultraviolet radiation.[36] According to their hypothesis, after ultraviolet irradiation, the more damaged keratinocytes trigger apoptosis, while the less damaged repair their DNA almost perfectly. Mutations are 'fixed' in the basal layer of the epidermis and may give rise to clonal expansion. Repeated exposures at low doses cause the accumulation of mutations and give rise to actinic keratoses and cancers. By contrast, in melanocytes, a high initial UV dose causes substantial lesions but no apoptosis, mutated melanocytes survive and divide (ephelids, naevi are clones of mutated melanocytes), and intermittent exposure at high dose gives rise to melanoma.

How much melanoma is caused by sun exposure?

Although melanoma may be caused by other yet poorly characterized causes, it may be important for public health purposes to calculate how much melanoma is caused by sun exposure. Armstrong and Kricker have made estimates of the proportion of cutaneous melanomas caused by sun exposure by comparing the observed incidence of melanoma with estimates of the incidence in the absence of sun exposure.[37]

Determining the proportion of melanoma caused by sun exposure requires estimation of the population attributable fraction (PAF) of melanoma in relation to sun exposure, namely the fraction by which the incidence of melanoma in a given population would fall if exposure to the sun were to be eliminated. PAF can be estimated using the formula:

$$PAF = (I_p - I_u) / I_p$$

where I_p is the incidence of melanoma in the whole population and I_u the incidence of melanoma in the fraction of the population that has not been exposed to sun. Since no accurate measure of I_u is available for any population, Armstrong and Kricker used the incidence of melanoma in people with black skin as an estimate of I_u in white people in the same population, the incidence of melanoma in white people who had migrated in adult life from an area of low to an area of high solar irradiation as an estimate of I_u in the white population born in the area to which they had migrated, and the incidence of melanoma on parts of the body not exposed to the sun (for example, scalp in females and buttocks) as an estimate of I_u in the population from which these site specific data had been derived.

The estimated proportions varied from 0.97 in males and 0.96 in females in Queensland, Australia, when the incidence on the whole body was compared with that on unexposed sites, to 0.68 when incidence in people born in Australia was compared with that in migrants to Australia from areas of lower sun exposures. A comparison of US blacks and whites, in which the melanoma incidence in blacks was taken as an estimate of the incidence in unexposed whites, gave estimates of 0.96 in males and 0.92 in females. It was further estimated that a minimum of 65% of the 91,700 new cases of melanoma that occurred in seven regions of the world in 1985 were caused by exposure to the sun, while 20% of the world's melanomas were estimated to occur in black African and Asian populations and were not considered to be due to sun exposure.[37]

Seasonal variations in melanoma incidence

An intriguing phenomenon is the existence of seasonal variations in melanoma incidence. This was first reported about 20 years ago by Scotto and Nam in a study analyzing the monthly incidence of melanoma in the United States.[38] Using data from the third national cancer survey (1969–1971), seasonal patterns were studied in detail by anatomical site, sex, age, and geographical region in 2490 cases of skin melanoma arising in whites. A strong seasonal pattern with a summertime peak (June, July) was observed for females. This was most pronounced for women younger than 55 years, and for women of all ages with melanomas of the upper and lower extremities. Among men, a seasonal pattern with a summertime peak was observed only for melanomas of the upper extremities. In both women and men of all ages, melanomas of the trunk or of the face and head showed no significant seasonal trends. For the upper and lower female extremities, the seasonal patterns were most striking in the southern states (Georgia, Alabama, Texas), while the mid latitudinal regions (Colorado, San Francisco) showed no significant seasonal trend.

This observation was soon confirmed by Holman and Armstrong, from data derived from a survey of 541 cases of preinvasive and invasive melanomas incident in Western Australia in the 2-year period 1975–1976;[39] the largest numbers of cases were diagnosed in the early summer months, November (females) and December (males).

Seasonal variations in the diagnosis of melanomas, with a summertime incidence peak, were further reported in Hawaii, upstate New York, the Oxford area, the nine population based cancer registries that compose the National Cancer Institute SEER (Surveillance, Epidemiology and End Results) programme and include approximately 10% of the US population, Norway, and Germany, and most recently the Burgundy region in France (Figure 4.3).[40–47]

In most studies, the ratio between melanomas diagnosed in summer and those diagnosed in winter was of the order of 1.6, and the seasonality was more marked for melanomas of the lower limbs in females and of the trunk in males. Interestingly, a seasonal pattern of melanoma diagnosis resembling that of the general population was noticed among members of melanoma prone families.[44] No such seasonal variation was observed for melanomas of the eye and for common cancers such as cancers of the lung, breast, colon, or prostate.[44,48]

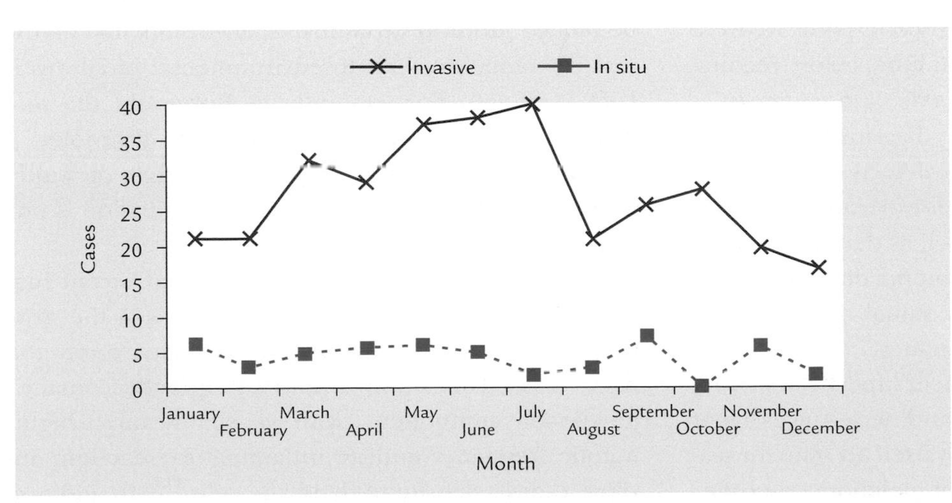

Figure 4.3 *Seasonal variation in melanoma incidence in Burgundy, France (data from[47]).*

The finding of complementary seasonal trends in melanoma diagnosis in the northern and southern hemispheres certainly adds weight to the reality of their existence. The problem of their interpretation is, however, not an easy issue. Scotto and Nam undertook their study bearing in mind that an association between occurrence of melanoma and the degree of solar insolation might provide new insights into the mechanics of the biological action spectrum and the dose response relation suspected in this disease.[38] They speculated that the summertime peaks in the diagnosis of melanoma, most marked in the southern states, were related to the promotion of tumour growth by high intensity UV radiation over short periods of time. But they also noted that, from their data, it was difficult to determine whether the seasonal pattern of melanoma could result from the promoting effects of UVB exposure or from enhanced recognition during the summer months. A commonly advanced hypothesis to explain the existence of seasonal variations in melanoma diagnosis is that the change in clothing habits in summertime enables a better detection of skin lesions.[46] This latter hypothesis was apparently favoured by Holman and Armstrong, who suspected that the phenomenon was due to an increased awareness of the skin in summer.[39] But if this is true, then one would expect lesions diagnosed in summer to be, on average, at an earlier development stage than those diagnosed in winter.

It is unlikely that seasonality of diagnosis of melanoma could simply be an artifact resulting from delay in diagnosis and increased ascertainment during the summer months since a seasonal pattern resembling that of the SEER programme data was noticed among prospectively followed members of melanoma prone families, and since no clear seasonal patterns were observed for cancers of the breast, lung, colon, rectum, stomach, prostate, testis, ovary, cervix, and pancreas.[44]

Is seasonality of melanoma diagnosis occurring because of a greater likelihood of detection during the warm months, when less clothing is worn and more skin is visible? In a tropical climate, such as that of Hawaii, it is unlikely that seasonality of melanoma diagnosis could be entirely due to the type of seasonal differences in attire that occur in temperate climates.[40,44] Presence of seasonal variation in the incidence of superficial spreading melanoma of the head, face, and neck suggests that increased ascertainment cannot by itself account for seasonal variation in the incidence of melanoma on other parts of the body.[43] In Burgundy, during the period 1996–99, there was no difference in the proportions of melanomas diagnosed on the head and neck and on the trunk in winter and summer months: 7 and 22, versus 12 and 34, respectively, $P = 0.92$.[47]

Several lines of evidence would actually indicate the possibility that the seasonality of melanoma diagnosis represents a biological process and accounts for promoting effects of UV exposure, acting on the late stages of malignant transformation of initiated melanocytes. Firstly, the amplitude of the seasonal variation of melanoma incidence is greater in regions of lower latitude than in regions of mid or higher latitude.[38] Second, it is striking to note that no significant seasonal patterns were noticed for preinvasive in situ melanomas in regions of mid or high latitude such as Burgundy and Norway.[46,47] Third, Polednak in 1984 noticed that melanomas diagnosed with a higher frequency in summer on women's legs were not only early tumours but presented with all stages of development.[41] Furthermore, in Burgundy, the analysis of the thickness of invasive melanomas as a function of season of clinical diagnosis showed that melanomas diagnosed in summer were significantly thicker (mean 1.99 mm, SD 2.23, median 1.07) than melanomas diagnosed in winter (mean 1.24 mm, SD 1.79, median 0.7), $P = 0.002$ (Mann-Whitney U test).[47]

The current evidence therefore does not support the hypothesis that melanomas are diagnosed more frequently in summer owing to variation in clothing; on the contrary, it is in line with the hypothesis that seasonal variation in melanoma incidence results at least in part from a biological process such as recent sun exposure. Seasonal variation in melanoma incidence could be related more to variations in environmental erythemal UV radiation than to environmental variations in UVA radiation. For example, in Burgundy, the total daily amount of ambient erythemal ultraviolet in summer is seven times greater than that of winter, whereas the difference in daily UVA irradiation is only three times greater.

There is some biological evidence that recent high UV exposure may result in rapid changes in the structure of melanocytic lesions. It has been shown that naevi excised in summer more frequently contain a junctional component with a significantly higher mitotic frequency and an inflammatory reaction, and show a lower density of dendritic cells.[49,50] In addition, dermatoscopic examination shows that the distribution of pigment in naevi in summer differs from that observed in winter, and that pigmentation characteristics may be modified after intense solar exposure.[51,52] Furthermore, a seasonal variation of DNA damage and repair has been recently shown in non-melanoma skin cancer patients and in normal healthy individuals: in a study conducted in Denmark, it was shown that 'spontaneous' DNA damage (assessed by the comet assay) and DNA repair (assessed by unscheduled DNA synthesis) in peripheral blood lymphocytes were significantly associated with the season in which blood sampling took place, and significantly correlated to the mean daily flux of solar radiation during seven days before blood sampling.[53]

Which wavelength(s) of solar radiation cause melanoma?

Although it has been shown both from experiments in animals and studies in humans that UVB (280–315 nm) is responsible for the induction of squamous cell carcinomas, and that there is a dose effect relation (increasing dose or exposure period results in an increased induction of tumours), there is currently no proof implicating a particular solar radiation wavelength in the induction of melanoma.[3]

There is currently no satisfactory experimental model mimicking the induction of human melanoma by ultraviolet radiation. The induction of melanomas in rodents following ultraviolet irradiation remains exceptional. In these species (guinea pigs and mice), naevi and melanomas are induced by topical application of chemical carcinogens such as dimethylbenz(a)anthracene, a cause not suggested by epidemiological studies in humans, and it has been shown using such an experimental model that UVB irradiation may act as a promoter.[54] Naevi and melanomas have been induced in the South American opossum after repeated UVB irradiations.[32] This model is, however, not representative of the intermittent exposure that is the main risk factor in human populations, but rather represents the induction of melanomas by cumulative exposure, and irradiation with visible light immediately after UVB irradiation reduces the rate of induction of melanoma, a photoreactivation reaction due to the activation of a DNA photolyase, an enzyme that does not operate in humans.

More recently, melanomas have been induced in transgenic mice (see[55] for review), using activated oncogenes under the control of the tyrosinase promoter which ensures the tissue specific expression of the oncogene, or using the cooperation between the tumour suppressing activity of the CDKN2 gene and the melanocyte specific expression of an activated H-ras oncogene.[56,57] In these mouse transgenic models, naevi and melanomas spontaneously develop in the absence of ultraviolet irradiation. But, in these mice with either high or low melanoma susceptibility, melanomas can be induced after UVB irradiation.[57,58] The induction of melanomas in transgenic melanoma prone mice after UVB irradiation offer novel possibilities for the experimental analysis of melanoma-promoting activities of UV radiation.[59]

The publication of an action spectrum for melanoma induction in hybrid *Xiphophorus* fishes initiated a discussion of whether or not UVA radiation is a significant carcinogen for melanoma in humans.[60] A single ultraviolet exposure of *Xiphophorus* fishes aged 7 days induces melanomas that are observable by 4 months. The action spectrum, for exposures at 302, 313, 365, 405, 436, and 547 nm, does not look like the spectrum for light absorption by DNA (mostly in the UVB range), but shows appreciable sensitivities in the UVA and even the visible regions. Under these conditions, it was extrapolated that up to 90% of melanoma induction in humans could arise from UVA and visible exposures, assuming the human spectrum is similar to the fish spectrum. This has important implications, since it can be predicted from this action spectrum that

(1) depletion in stratospheric ozone which mainly absorbs UVB would not affect melanoma incidence,

(2) an increase in sun exposure time as a result of using UVB sunscreens could increase melanoma risk, and

(3) the use of high UVA sun tanning devices could increase melanoma risk.

It has recently been shown that UVA irradiation induces mutations in hamster and human cells in vitro.[61,62] It has been further hypothesized that ultraviolet radiation absorbed by melanins in the melanocytes generates products that may activate carcinogenesis: products formed in the upper layer of the epidermis cannot diffuse down and hence are protective, whereas those formed in the melanocytes may be carcinogenic, thus explaining why well tanning persons may be protected while poor tanning ones may be at risk when exposed to UV radiation.[63] Another argument in favour of a carcinogenic role of UVA is derived from the observation that the relative latitude gradient for UVA is much smaller than that for UVB and that the same apparently holds true for the relative latitude gradients of melanoma and squamous cell carcinoma.[63]

But melanoma incidence in Norway is closely related to local levels of UVB radiation independent of other factors. The analysis of melanoma incidence in the 19 counties of Norway, which has the highest melanoma incidence in Europe, for each 5-year period from 1955 to 1989 showed a highly significant association between melanoma incidence and UVB radiation for each of the time periods studied; foreign holidays showed a significant positive association in the 1980s, but not earlier. Changes in melanoma incidence between 1955–69 and 1985–89 were significantly positively associated with holidays abroad and negatively with income levels.[64]

In addition, it should be noted that if it is true that artificial UVA tanning does increase melanoma risk in fair-skinned persons, most of the ultraviolet tanning devices emit appreciable proportions of UVB. Similarly, it has been suggested that use of sunscreens is associated with an increased risk of melanoma.[65] But, rather than an increased exposure to UVA, this may be related more to a change in behaviour leading to an increase in time of exposure. It has recently been shown in a double blind prospective study using personal dosimeters that volunteers using a high sun protection factor sunscreen tend to prolong the duration of sunbathing activities, especially in the hot hours of the day, and are exposed to higher doses of UVB irradiation.[66]

Attilasoy et al. induced atypical melanocytic lesions and melanoma in human foreskin grafted onto immunodeficient mice and treated either with a single treatment with 7,12-dimethyl(a)benzanthracene (DMBA), with UVB (500 J/m^2, three times weekly), or a combination of DMBA and UVB.[34] Twenty three per cent of normal skin grafts treated with UVB only and 38% of grafts treated with a combination of DMBA and UVB developed solar lentigines within 5–10 months of treatment. Melanocytic hyperplasia was found in 73% of all UVB treated grafts. Lentigo and lentigo maligna were seen in several skin grafts treated with both DMBA and UVB, and in one graft, a human malignant melanoma of the nodular type developed. Thus, chronic UVB irradiation with or without an initiating carcinogen can induce human melanocytic lesions including melanoma.

Therefore, it seems likely that melanoma, like other skin cancers, might be influenced by exposure to UVB radiation. But the possibility that exposure to UVA radiation may carry a significant risk for melanoma cannot be excluded.

Possible effects of stratospheric ozone depletion

As mentioned above, the stratospheric ozone layer absorbs the shortest ultraviolet wavelengths from the solar radiation.

Since the hole in the ozone layer above the Antarctic was recognized and the ozone trend panel claimed a negative trend for the ozone levels of the northern hemisphere in the period 1969–1986, there has been considerable concern and speculation about whether there might be an increase of the influence of ultraviolet radiation from the sun due to ozone depletion and if the increasing trend in incidence rates of skin cancers, both melanoma and non-melanoma, might be related to such an increase.[67–69]

Recent analyses of satellite, ground based, and balloon measurements allow updated estimates of trends in the vertical profile of ozone since 1979.[70] The results show overall consistency among several independent measurement systems, particularly for mid latitudes in the northern hemisphere. Combined trend estimates over these latitudes for the period 1979–96 show significant negative trends at all altitudes between 10 km and 40 km, with two local extremes: $-7.4+/-2.0\%$ per decade at 40 km and $-7.3+/-4.6\%$ per decade at 15 km altitude. There is a strong seasonal variation in trends over northern mid latitudes in the altitude range 10 km to 18 km, with the largest ozone loss during winter and spring.

Although the inverse relation between ozone concentration and UV radiation is well established, the determination of trends in UV radiation due to ozone loss is more problematic, since ground level UV radiation is actually influenced by many factors other than ozone, including solar zenith angle, volcanic impacts, tropospheric aerosols, cloud cover, and albedo. Nevertheless, recent measurements have confirmed an increase in UV radiation, especially in the southern hemisphere, where, for example in the summer 1998–99, in Lauder, New Zealand (45°S), the peak sunburning UV radiation (mostly UVB) was 12% higher than in the first years of the decade. Larger increases were seen for DNA damaging radiation and plant damaging ultraviolet radiation, whereas UVA, which is insensitive to ozone, showed no increase, in agreement with model calculations.[71]

Numerous attempts have been made to estimate the possible effects of an increase in UV radiation due to ozone loss on melanoma incidence, mostly in North America. These calculations are based on the comparison between ground level UV radiation measurements or extrapolations for UVB irradiation derived from differences in latitude and data from local registries of incidence or mortality. Earlier estimates suggested percentage increases in melanoma incidence of 22% and in mortality of 14% for a 10% reduction in ozone.[1]

In Europe, detailed studies have used data from six areas in Norway and from Sweden and Finland. A 10% ozone depletion was found to give rise to a 19% increase in the incidence of melanoma in men and a 32% increase in the incidence rate of melanoma in women.[72] These estimates are higher than other estimates (for Australia an increase in incidence of 11 to 17% was calculated). More recently, in Norway, it has been calculated that melanoma incidence would probably increase by 1.6% if ozone depletion led to 1% enhanced UVB flux.[64]

The calculations made so far show considerable variation, but it seems reasonable to predict that a 1% decrease in ozone will result in a 2% increase in ground UVB level, and it is estimated that a 1% increase in UVB might result in an increase in melanoma incidence of 0.5–2%.

ENVIRONMENTAL INFLUENCES ON MELANOMA PROGRESSION

Exposure to UV radiation could also play a part in melanoma growth and progression. Like other tumours, melanomas progress through a series of sequential steps, from activated melanocyte, to naevus, to in situ melanoma, and to invasive and metastatic melanoma. There is evidence that progression through some of these transformation steps may be driven or enhanced by ultraviolet radiation.

Animal studies indicate that UV radiation stimulates melanocytic proliferation, conversion to an invasive phenotype or a combination of such effects. Notably, ultraviolet radiation promotes the proliferation of melanoma cells after initiation by a chemical carcinogen, and may increase the expression of autocrine growth factors by melanocytes.[54]

Exposure to ultraviolet radiation causes both local and systemic inflammation that could be involved in the growth promotion of melanoma.[73] Experimental work has shown that the local UV irradiation of mice increases the growth of a transplanted melanoma and that this effect can be partially the result of local induction of interleukin-10. Interestingly, several local effects induced by UVB irradiation can be suppressed by a UVB filter, but not the melanoma growth enhancement effect.[74,75] Moreover, it has been shown that UVB irradiation of human melanoma cells increases their tumourigenicity and metastatic ability in nude mice.[76]

A recent International Agency for Research on Cancer/Deutscheskrebsforchung Zentrum workshop has proposed that naevi could be used as exposure and intermediate effect biomarkers in the development of melanomas, and observed that the anatomical distribution of large (>5 mm) naevi in children reflects the anatomical distribution of melanomas in adults younger than 50 years and is likely to be influenced by UVB.[77] A recent case–control study in Europe has shown that melanomas associated with a naevus and melanomas occurring de novo may differ in their risk factors: a history of sunburn was found to be a risk factor only for naevus associated melanomas, suggesting a possible role of high UVB irradiation (sunburn) in the neoplastic transformation of naevi.[78]

CONCLUSIONS

Cutaneous melanoma is essentially a disease of white-skinned people, fair skin being more susceptible to the damaging effects of sunlight. Exposure to sunlight, an environmental carcinogen, is clearly a cause of melanoma. The relation between sun exposure and risk of melanoma is not a direct one, however, and there are interactions with host susceptibility factors and behaviour such as intentional sun exposure.

A minimum of 65% of the melanomas occurring worldwide have been estimated to be caused by sun exposure, but in some estimates, this proportion may be as high as 97%.

The exact wavelengths inducing melanoma in humans are not currently known. It seems likely, however, that UVB and UVA play an important part.

Although melanoma initiation may be most frequent in childhood, the existence of seasonal variation in invasive tumours suggests that sunlight may also act as a short term promoter of early melanomas. In this respect, it would be of great interest to study the influence of ultraviolet exposure on the risk of developing a second primary melanoma.

Adequate protection from ultraviolet radiation may thus prove to be important not only to prevent melanoma initiation in childhood but also to inhibit the progression of small and curable tumours in adults.

The effect of stratospheric ozone depletion on the incidence of melanoma is difficult to estimate. It is, however, generally accepted that ozone depletion will increase melanoma risk: a 1% decrease in ozone will result in a 2% increase in ground UVB level, and it is estimated that a 1% increase in UVB might result in an increase in melanoma incidence ranging from 0.5 to 2%.

REFERENCES

1. Elwood JM, Gallagher RP, Sun exposure and the epidemiology of melanoma. In: *Epidemiological aspects of melanoma.* (eds Gallagher RP, Elwood JM). Norwell, Mass: Kluwer, 1994: 17–66.
2. Boyle P, Maisonneuve P, Doré JF, Epidemiology of malignant melanoma. *Br Med Bull* 1995; 51: 523–47.
3. International Agency for Research on Cancer, IARC monographs on the evaluation of carcinogenic risks to humans, Vol. 55: *Solar and ultraviolet radiation.* Lyon: IARC, 1992.
4. Berwick M, Epidemiology: current trends, risk factors and environmental concerns. In: *Cutaneous melanoma,* 3rd ed. (eds Balch CM, Houghton AN, Sober AJ, Song SJ) St Louis: Quality Medical Publishing, 1998: 551–71.
5. MacLennan R, Green AC, McLeod GRC, Martin NG, Increasing incidence of cutaneous melanoma in Queensland, Australia. *J Natl Cancer Inst* 1992; 84: 1427–32.
6. Jelfs PL, Giles G, Shugg D, et al, Cutaneous malignant melanoma in Australia. *Med J Aust* 1994; 161: 183–9.
7. Parkin M, Muir CS, Whelan SL, et al, eds, *Cancer incidence in five continents.* Vol. 6. 1 vol. Lyon: IARC, 1992.
8. De Vathaire F, Koscielny S, Rezvani A, et al, eds, *Estimation de l'incidence des cancers en France.* Paris: INSERM, 1996
9. Koh HK, Cutaneous melanoma. *NEJM* 1991; 325: 171–82.
10. Holman CDJ, Armstrong BK, Cutaneous malignant melanoma and indicators of total accumulated exposure to the sun: an analysis separating histogenetic types. *J Natl Cancer Inst* 1984; 73: 75–82.
11. Steinitz R, Parkin DM, Young JL, et al, *Cancer incidence in Jewish migrants to Israel.* IARC Scientific Publication n° 98. Lyon: IARC,1989.
12. Paffenbarger RS Jr, Wing AL, Hyde RT, Characteristics in youth predictive of adult-onset malignant lymphomas, melanomas and leukaemias. *J Natl Cancer Inst* 1978; 60: 89–92.
13. Brown J, Kopf AW, Rigel DS, Friedman RJ, Malignant melanoma in World War II veterans. *Int J Dermatol* 1984; 23: 661–3.
14. Elwood JM, Williamson C, Stapleton PJ. Malignant melanoma in relation to moles, pigmentation and exposure to fluorescent and other lighting sources. *Br J Cancer* 1986; 53: 65–74.
15. MacKie RM, Freudenberger T, Aitchison TC, Personal risk-factor chart for cutaneous melanoma. *Lancet* 1989; 2: 487–90.
16. Beitner H, Norell SE, Ringborg U, et al, Malignant melanoma: aetiological importance of individual pigmentation and sun exposure. *Br J Dermatol* 1990; 122: 43–51.
17. Autier P, Doré JF, Gefeller O, et al, EORTC Melanoma Cooperative Group. Melanoma risk and residence in sunny areas. *Br J Cancer* 1997; 76: 1521–4.
18. Elwood JM, Jopson J, Melanoma and sun exposure: an overview of published studies. *Int J Cancer* 1997; 73: 198–203.
19. Elwood JM, Gallagher RP, Davidson J, Hill GB, Sunburn, suntan and the risk of cutaneous malignant melanoma: the Western Canada Melanoma Study. *Br J Cancer* 1985; 51: 543–9.
20. Holman CDJ, Armstrong BK, Heenan PJ, Relationship of cutaneous malignant melanoma to individual sun exposure habits. *J Natl Cancer Inst* 1985; 76: 403–14.
21. Autier P, Doré JF, Lejeune FJ, et al, EORTC Malignant Melanoma Cooperative Group. Recreational exposure to sunlight and lack of information as risk factors for cutaneous malignant melanoma. Results of an EORTC case–control study in Belgium, France and Germany. *Melanoma Res* 1994; 4: 79–85.
22. Autier P, Doré JF, EPIMEL and EORTC Melanoma Cooperative Group, Influences of sun exposures during childhood and during adulthood on melanoma risk. *Int J Cancer* 1998; 77: 533–7.
23. Elwood JM, Gallagher RP. Body site distribution of cutaneous malignant melanoma in relation with patterns of sun exposure. *Int J Cancer* 1998; 78: 276–80.
24. Holman CDJ, Armstrong BK, Heenan PJ, A theory of the etiology and pathogenesis of human cutaneous melanoma. *J Natl Cancer Inst* 1983; 71: 651–6.
25. Setlow RB, Regan JD, German J, Carrier WL. Evidence that xeroderma pigmentosum cells do not perform the first step in the repair of ultraviolet damage to their DNA. *Proc Natl Acad Sci USA* 1969; 64: 1035–41.
26. Kraemer KH, Lee MM, Scotto J, Xeroderma pigmentosum. Cutaneous, ocular, and neurologic abnormalities in 830 published cases. *Arch Dermatol* 1987; 123: 241–50.
27. Kraemer KH, Lee MM, Andrews AD, Lambert WC, The role of sunlight and DNA repair in melanoma and non-melanoma skin cancer – the xeroderma paradigm. *Arch Dermatol* 1994; 130: 1018–21.
28. Wei Q, Matanoski GM, Farmer ER, et al, DNA repair capacity for ultraviolet light-induced damage is reduced in peripheral lymphocytes from patients with basal cell carcinoma. *J Invest Dermatol* 1995; 104: 933–6.
29. Hsu TC, Johnston DA, Cherry LM, et al, Sensitivity to genotoxic effects of bleomycin in humans: possible relationship to environmental carcinogenesis. *Int J Cancer* 1989; 15: 403–9.
30. Wei Q, Spitz MR, Gu J, et al, DAN repair capacity correlates with mutagen sensitivity in lymphoblastoid cell lines. *Cancer Epidemiol Biomarkers Prev* 1996; 5: 199–204.
31. Wu X, Hsu TC, Spitz MR, Mutagen sensitivity exhibits a dose-response relationship in case–control studies. *Cancer Epidemiol Biomarkers Prev* 1996; 5: 577–8.
32. Ley RD, Applegate LA, Padilla RS, Stuart TD, Ultraviolet radiation-induced malignant melanoma in Monodelphis domestica. *Photochem Photobiol* 1989; 50: 1–5.
33. Setlow RB, Woodhead AD, Grist E, Animal model for ultraviolet radiation-induced melanoma: platyfish swordtail hybrid. *Proc Natl Acad Sci* 1989; 86: 8922–6.
34. Attilasoy ES, Seykora JT, Soballe PW, et al, UVB induces atypical melanocytic lesions and melanoma in human skin. *Am J Pathol* 1998; 152: 1179–86.
35. Diffey BL, Elwood JM, Tables of ambient solar ultraviolet radiation for use in epidemiological studies of malignant melanoma and other diseases. In: *Epidemiological aspects of malignant melanoma.* (eds Gallagher RP, Elwood JM) Norwell, Mass: Kluwer, 1994: 61–105.
36. Gilchrest BA, Eller MS, Geller AC, Yaar M, The pathogenesis of melanoma induced by ultraviolet radiation. *NEJM* 1999; 340: 1341–8.

37. Armstrong BK, Kricker A, How much melanoma is caused by sun exposure? *Melanoma Res* 1993; 3: 395–401.
38. Scotto J, Nam JM, Skin melanoma and seasonal patterns. *Am J Epidemiol* 1980; 111: 309–14.
39. Holman D, Armstrong B, Skin melanoma and seasonal patterns. *Am J Epidemiol* 1981; 112: 202.
40. Hinds MW, Lee J, Kolonel LN, Seasonal patterns of skin melanoma incidence in Hawaii. *Am J Public Health* 1981; 71: 496–9.
41. Polednak AP, Seasonal patterns in the diagnosis of malignant melanoma of skin and eye in upstate New York. *Cancer* 1984; 54: 2587–94.
42. Swerdlow AJ, Seasonality of presentation of cutaneous melanoma, squamous cell cancer and basal cell cancer in the Oxford region. *Br J Cancer* 1985; 52: 893–900.
43. Schwartz SM, Armstrong BK, Weiss NS, Seasonal variation in the incidence of cutaneous malignant melanoma: an analysis by body sites and histologic type. *Am J Epidemiol* 1987; 126: 104–11.
44. Braun MM, Tucker MA, Devesa SS, Hoover RN, Seasonal variation in the frequency of diagnosis of cutaneous malignant melanoma. *Melanoma Res* 1994; 4: 235–41.
45. Akslen LA, Seasonal variation in melanoma progress. *J Natl Cancer Inst* 1995; 87: 1025.
46. Blum A, Ellwanger U, Garbe C, Seasonal patterns in the diagnosis of cutaneous melanoma: analysis of the data of the German central malignant melanoma registry. *Br J Dermatol* 1997; 136: 968–9.
47. Sallin J, Boniol M, Chignol MC, Doré JF, Seasonal variation in melanoma incidence in Burgundy.(in press).
48. Schwartz SM, Weiss NS, Absence of seasonal variation in the diagnosis of melanoma of the eye in the United States. *Br J Cancer* 1988; 58: 402–4.
49. Armstrong BK, Heenan PJ, Caruso V, et al, Seasonal variation in the junctional component of pigmented naevi. *Int J Cancer* 1984; 34: 441–2.
50. Azizi E, Schwaaf A, Lazarov A, et al, Decreased density of epidermal dendritic cells in melanocytic naevi: the possible role of in vivo sun exposure. *Melanoma Res* 1999; 9: 521–7.
51. Stanganelli I, Rafanelli S, Bucchi L, Seasonal prevalence of digital epiluminescence microscopy patterns in acquired melanocytic nevi. *J Am Acad Dermatol* 1996; 34: 460–4.
52. Stanganelli I, Bauer P, Bucchi L, et al, Critical effects of intense sun exposure on the expression of epiluminescence microscopy features of acquired melanocytic nevi. *Arch Dermatol* 1997; 133: 979–82.
53. Møller P, Knudsen LE, Frentz G, et al, Seasonal variation of DNA damage and repair in patients with non-melanompa skin cancer and referents with and without psoriasis. *Mutation Res* 1998; 407: 25–34.
54. Berkelhammer J, Oxenhandler RW, Hook RR, Hennessy JM, Development of a new melanoma model in C57Bl/6 mice. *Cancer Res* 1982; 42: 3157–63.
55. Bardeesy N, Wong KK, DePinho RA, Chin L, Animal models of melanoma: recent advances and future prospects. *Adv Cancer Res* 2000; 79: 123–56.
56. Mintz B, Silvers WK, Transgenic mouse model of malignant skin melanoma. *Proc Natl Acad Sci USA* 1993; 90: 8817–21.
57. Chin L, Pomerantz J, Polsky D, et al, Cooperative effects of INK4a and ras in melanoma susceptibility in vivo. *Genes Dev* 1977; 11: 2822–34.
58. Klein-Szanto AJP, Silvers WK, Mintz B, Ultraviolet radiation-induced malignant skin melanoma in melanoma-susceptible transgenic mice. *Cancer Res* 1994; 54: 4569–72.
59. Kelsall SR, Mintz B, Metastatic cutaneous melanomas promoted by ultraviolet radiation in mice with transgene-initiated low melanoma susceptibility. *Cancer Res* 1998; 58: 4061–5.
60. Setlow RB, Grist E, Thomson K, Woodhead AD, Wavelengths effective in induction of malignant melanoma. *Proc Natl Acad Sci USA* 1993; 90: 666–70.
61. Drobetsky EA, Turcotte J, Chateauneuf A, A role for ultraviolet A in solar mutagenesis. *Proc Natl Acad Sci USA* 1995; 92: 2350–4.
62. Robert C, Muel B, Benoit A, et al, Cell survival and shuttle vector mutagenesis induced by UVA and UVB radiation in a human cell line. *J Invest Dermatol* 1996; 106: 721–8.
63. Moan J, Dahlback A, Setlow RB, Epidemiological support for an hypothesis for melanoma induction indicating a role for UVA radiation. *Photochem Photobiol* 1999; 70: 243–7.
64. Bentham G, Aase A. Incidence in malignant melanoma of the skin in Norway, 1955–1989: association with solar ultraviolet radiation, income and holidays abroad. *Int J Epidemiol* 1006; 25: 1132–8.
65. International Agency for Research on Cancer, *Sunscreens.* IARC Handbooks of cancer chemoprevention. Vol. 5. Lyon: IARC 2001.
66. Autier P, Doré JF, Reis AC, et al, Sunscreen use and intentional exposure to ultraviolet A and B radiation: a double blind randomized trial using personal dosimeters. *Br J Cancer* 2000; 89: 1243–8.
67. Farman JC, Gardiner H, Shanklin JD, Large losses of total ozone in Antarctica reveal seasonal reveal seasonal ClOx/Nox interaction. *Nature* 1985; 315: 207–10.
68. Stolarski RS, The antarctic ozone hole. *Sci Am* 1988; 258: 20–6.
69. Lindley D, CFCs cause part of global ozone decline. *Nature* 1988; 323: 293.
70. Randel WJ, Stolarski RS, Cunnold DM, et al, Trends in the vertical distribution of ozone. *Science* 1999; 285: 1689–92.
71. McKenzie R, Connor B, Bodeker G, Increase summertime UV radiation in New Zealand in response to ozone loss. *Science* 1999; 285: 170–1.
72. Moan J, Dahlback A, The relationship between skin cancers, solar radiation and ozone depletion. *Br J Cancer* 1992; 65: 916–21.
73. Kripke ML, Ultraviolet radiation and immunology: something new under the sun. *Cancer Res* 1994; 54: 6102–5.
74. Donawho CK, Wolf P, Kripke ML, Enhanced development of murine melanoma in UV-irradiated skin: UV dose response, waveband dependence, and relation to inflammation. *Melanoma Res* 1994; 4: 93–100.
75. Wolf P, Donawho C, Kripke ML, Effect of sunscreens on UV radiation-induced enhancement of melanoma growth in mice. *J Natl Cancer Inst* 1994; 86: 99–105.
76. Singh RK, Gutman M, Reich R, Bar-Eli M, Ultraviolet B irradiation promotes tumourigenic and metastatic properties in primary cuta neous melanoma via induction of interleukin-8. *Cancer Res* 1995; 55: 3369–74.
77. International Agency for Research on Cancer, *Biomarkers in cancer chemoprevention.* IARC Scientific Publication. Lyon: IARC, 2001.
78. Carli P, Massi D, Santucci M, et al, Cutaneous melanoma histologically associated with a nevus and melanoma de novo have different profile of risk: Results from a case–control study. *J Am Acad Dermatol* 1999; 40: 549–57.

5

Genetic predisposition to melanoma

Richard F Kefford, Graham J Mann, Julia Newton Bishop

INTRODUCTION

The observation that there are families with a higher than expected incidence of melanoma has been made repeatedly for nearly 200 years.[1] In the past two decades this observation has been refined by the application of modern population and molecular genetics, culminating in the identification of specific genes, which, when inherited in altered form, confer on an individual a high risk of developing cutaneous melanoma.

However, in a manner parallel to that seen in other hereditary human cancers, these so called highly penetrant genes are responsible for only a small proportion of the hereditary component in melanoma predisposition. They have come to light first because of the dramatic effect they have in selected multiple case families. Possibly of even greater significance are those genes of much lower penetrance, but higher prevalence in the population, which, themselves, may confer only slight elevations in relative melanoma risk, but which may interact with ultraviolet radiation in causing a high population incidence for certain racial and geographic groups. The identification and analysis of these genes remain the subject of intense research. These genes may include those that, for example, may determine gradations in skin pigmentation and other racial characteristics.

There are two reasons for the current high level of interest in further research into the genetic basis of a melanoma. Firstly, the mapping and identification of melanoma susceptibility genes have pinpointed specific biochemical pathways that are aberrant in melanoma cells, opening new directions for specifically targeted reagents in diagnosis, staging, prognosis, and treatment. Secondly, the refining of our understanding of the genetic and racial risk factors for melanoma will be of major assistance in the identification of specific populations at high risk. In turn, this will permit the design of effective programmes of targeted prevention, screening, and surveillance.

PHENOTYPIC CORRELATES OF MELANOMA RISK

Phenotypic features

Phenotypes associated with melanoma risk include fair skin that fails to tan, red hair, blue eyes, and freckling.[2,3] This constellation of features is characteristic of people of Celtic origin. In converse, factors associated with a very low risk of melanoma include dark skin that tans readily, black hair, and dark brown eyes. These features are characteristic of native Africans and aboriginal Australians. When melanoma does occur in native Africans or aboriginal Australians it is mostly in non-pigmented skin, such as the plantar surface.[4]

The presence of atypical or dysplastic melanocytic naevi* are major markers for melanoma risk across all

* Atypical naevi may be distinguished by their Asymmetry, Border (indistinct irregular margins), Colour (presence of unevenness of pigmentation, red-brown colour), and Diameter ≥5 mm ('ABCD' rules). Multiple naevi of atypical appearance are called dysplastic naevi (DN), the atypical mole syndrome (AMS) or familial atypical multiple mole melanoma (FAMMM) syndrome.

continents, both in high risk families and in the general population.[5–7] The atypical mole syndrome (AMS)/dysplastic naevus syndrome (DNS) phenotype confers potent risk, carrying in the United Kingdom, for example, a relative risk of around 10 for melanoma in the general population.[8,9]

The presence of multiple (non-dysplastic) moles is also an independent risk factor for melanoma.[10]

The inheritance of moles and atypical naevi

There is some evidence for clustering of the AMS/DNS phenotype in relatives of melanoma cases, and this suggests genetic control of the naevus phenotype.[11] That the same phenotype seems to characterize certain, but not all, melanoma families provides further evidence for genetic control of the naevus phenotype.[1,8,12–14]

In certain families with a large number of cases of melanoma, there are also large number of individuals with the so called DNS.[12,13] In these families, the presence of large numbers of dysplastic naevi carries a very high risk for the development of melanoma.[13] In some of these families, the presence of melanoma correlates with the presence of mutations in the CDKN2A gene (discussed below). Even in those families carrying such a mutation, however, the presence of dysplastic naevi correlates poorly with the presence of mutations.[15] This suggests that the specific genetic basis for melanoma is separate from that for the DNS, and that the presence of these naevi is an independent risk factor for melanoma.[16] It is possible, however, that there are complex interrelations between these genetic abnormalities, and that certain modifier genes may influence the expression of both the melanoma and the dysplastic naevus phenotype.

Around the world probably fewer than one third of all families with multiple melanoma affected members have the DNS. The relation between this syndrome, melanoma, and the CDKN2A gene is shown diagrammatically in Figure 5.1.

One of the most elegant and powerful demonstrations of the strength of genetic determination of mole number was the study of monozygotic (genetically identical) and dizygotic (non-identical) sets of twins in Queensland.[17] In contrast to the strong correlation in mole number found between the members of sets of monozygotic twins, sets of dizygotic twins showed no such correlation, despite, presumably, very similar sun exposure histories. This shows that in individuals with presumably comparatively identical sun exposure, genetic constitution is the major determinant of one of the principal phenotypic correlates of melanoma risk, cutaneous naevi.

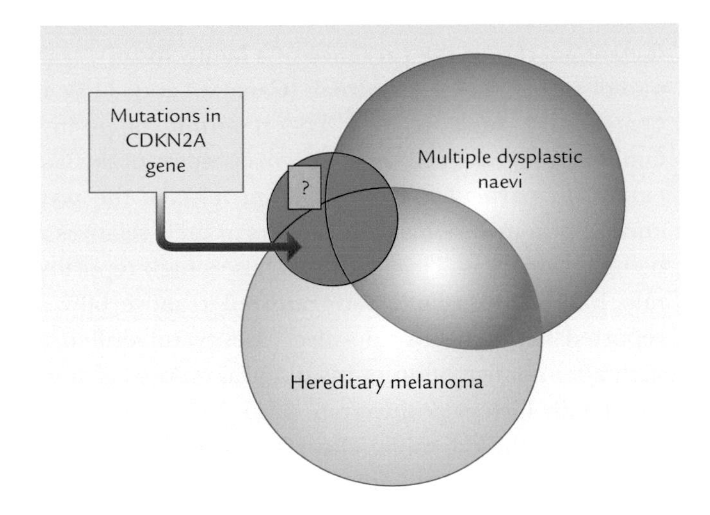

Figure 5.1 *The relation between hereditary melanoma, 'dysplastic naevus syndrome', and the presence of mutations in the melanoma susceptibility gene, CDKN2A.*

Environmental determination of moles and atypical naevi

There is also evidence for a strong environmental influence on the development of moles. Epidemiological studies in Australia, Canada, and the United States show that the development of moles may be induced by exposure to excessive sunlight, and that mole number correlates with sun exposure in childhood.[18–20] Even in those families that display a strong inheritance of dysplastic naevi and melanoma, there is clear evidence for a strong influence of sun exposure on naevus count and melanoma incidence.[21]

These phenotypic data are consistent with the hypothesis that genetic predisposition to melanoma is in part expressed as a UV vulnerable skin type and/or abnormal naevi or 'moliness', but that this predisposition also interacts strongly with sun exposure.

MELANOMA AND FAMILY HISTORY

The degree of familial clustering of melanoma varies roughly in parallel with local geographical incidence rates. For example, in the UK 5.2% of people with melanoma report the presence of a family history, compared with 7% in Montreal, Canada, and 11% in Queensland, Australia.[8,22,23] The reporting of positive family history by melanoma patients is notoriously inaccurate. In particular, patients often mistake the presence of non-melanoma skin cancers in their relatives as being melanomas. This leads to a falsely high reporting rate. In the Queensland study referred to above, 60% of reported family history positive cases were verified as such after confirmation of histological reports, giving a true family history positive rate of 11%.[23]

Some of these familial clusters will be due solely to chance, but heterogeneity analyses have shown that at least one in five familial cases, and at least 2% of all melanoma cases, are caused by inheritance of a high penetrance mutation in a major melanoma susceptibility gene(s), at least in populations experiencing intense UV exposure such as in Queensland, Australia.[24] It is not yet clear what proportion of the remaining familial clusters, or of 'sporadic' (family history negative) cases, results from inherited germline mutations in such genes, the inheritance of more prevalent melanoma susceptibility gene mutations that have a weaker effect, or of non-genetic familial factors. The data from the large Queensland population based study are consistent with genetic heterogeneity in melanoma inheritance, suggesting that other familial factors, such as pigmentation, skin type, and sun exposure habits, play an important part in the familial clustering of melanoma, at least at low latitudes.[24]

MELANOMA SUSCEPTIBILITY GENES

The proportion of all cutaneous melanoma that is attributable to inherited mutations in melanoma susceptibility genes is unknown, but is estimated by the Melanoma Genetics Consortium to be less than 1–2%.[25] Families in which these genes are inherited have members who may be distinguished by the presence of some, but not necessarily all of the features shown in Box 5.1. Of particular interest is that in certain, but not all, of these families there seems to be an association with the presence of multiple unusual or atypical moles. Although certain kindreds have ocular and/or cutaneous melanoma in particular members, none of the families with members affected by ocular melanoma show linkage to the 9p chromosome. A study of seven patients with ocular melanoma and a positive family history of melanoma patients revealed none with constitutional mutations in the CDKN2A or CDK4 genes.[26]

Box 5.1 ***Features associated with genetic susceptibility to melanoma***

Multiple cases of cutaneous melanoma on the same side of the family
Multiple primary cutaneous melanomas in the same individual(s)
Earlier age of onset of cutaneous melanoma
Multiple naevi
Other cancers, particularly pancreatic cancer

Inherited genetic mutations are referred to as 'constitutional' or 'germline', to distinguish them from the very commonly found 'somatic' mutations found in tumour cells themselves. Somatic mutations are found in most melanomas but are not passed on from generation to generation. So far, constitutional mutations have been found in two genes that confer a high risk for the development of melanoma. These are the genes CDKN2A, and CDK4. Both genes play a critical part in the regulation of the cell cycle (see also Chapter 2).

The CDKN2A ('p16') gene and its function

The CDKN2A gene is located on the short 'p' arm of chromosome 9. The gene was mapped and identified by analyzing the inheritance of known, mapped, polymorphic, genetic markers in families with multiple members affected by melanoma. CDKN2A is an unusual gene in that it codes for two separate proteins. One of these proteins, p16INK4A, (colloquially known as 'p16'), is of known relevance to melanoma susceptibility, and the other, p14ARF, remains under investigation.

p16 is one of a family of molecules known as cyclin dependent kinase (CDK) inhibitors. The CDKs and their inhibitors act to regulate many steps in the sequence of biochemical reactions regulating passage of cells through the cell cycle. p16 binds to CDK4, inhibiting the ability of that protein to phosphorylate the retinoblastoma (Rb) protein.[27] The consequence of this is restriction of the cell cycle at the G1–S interface. Mutations in the CDKN2A gene prevent p16 from binding to CDK4. The consequence is phosphorylation of the retinoblastoma protein, release of the E2F transcriptional regulator, and unrestricted passage of cells through the G1–S restriction point. This is discussed in greater detail in Chapter 2.

A second transcript derived from an alternative first exon of the CDKN2A gene encodes the protein p14ARF, which stabilizes p53 levels through interaction with HDM2 (Figure 5.2) (see Chapter 2).[28,29] There is now evidence for the involvement of p14ARF in the genesis of melanoma. Certain hereditary melanoma families with a normal p16 gene structure nevertheless display aberrations in the relative expression of the two gene products.[30] Although mutations which uniquely alter the structure of p14ARF have not yet been described in families, many mutations alter both the amino acid sequence of p16 *and* p14ARF, since both proteins contain segments encoded genetically by a common second exon. These mutations have been shown to alter the subcellular localization of the p14ARF protein,[31] with potential functional significance.

CDKN2A MUTATIONS IN HEREDITARY MELANOMA

Approximately one third of hereditary melanoma families containing three or more affected first degree relatives show inheritance of mutations in the CDKN2A gene.[32] Mutations in the CDKN2A gene occur throughout the first two of the three exons, and a mutation in the 5′-untranslated region has also been described.[33,34] Because current information on each mutation is limited and confined to data from large families, specifically ascertained for the presence of multiple affected members, the confidence limits on current estimates of the penetrance of mutations in the CDKN2A gene are extremely wide. This penetrance appears to be strongly influenced by levels of sun exposure, birth cohort (possibly a proxy for sun exposure), and possibly by modifier genes, which, in certain families, may also be responsible for the presence of multiple moles.[16,21,35]

There are few data on the prevalence of CDKN2A mutations in the population. In a large population based study in Queensland, the prevalence of CDKN2A mutations was 9/87 (10.3%) in the subgroup of kindreds exhibiting the strongest familial clustering, and the overall prevalence in the population was estimated to be 0.2%.[36]

Highly penetrant genes other than CDKN2A

Two families in the United States and one in France have been shown to have mutations in the CDK4 gene on chromosome 12q. This is a biologically fascinating rare mutation whose effects in terms of melanoma carcinogenesis are mediated by the same CDKN2A pathway, as the mutations in CDK4 are located at the p16 protein binding site.[37,38]

The majority of kindreds with multiple affected members that are negative for CDKN2A mutations have been tested by the Melanoma Genetics Consortium for these specific CDK4 mutations and have proved

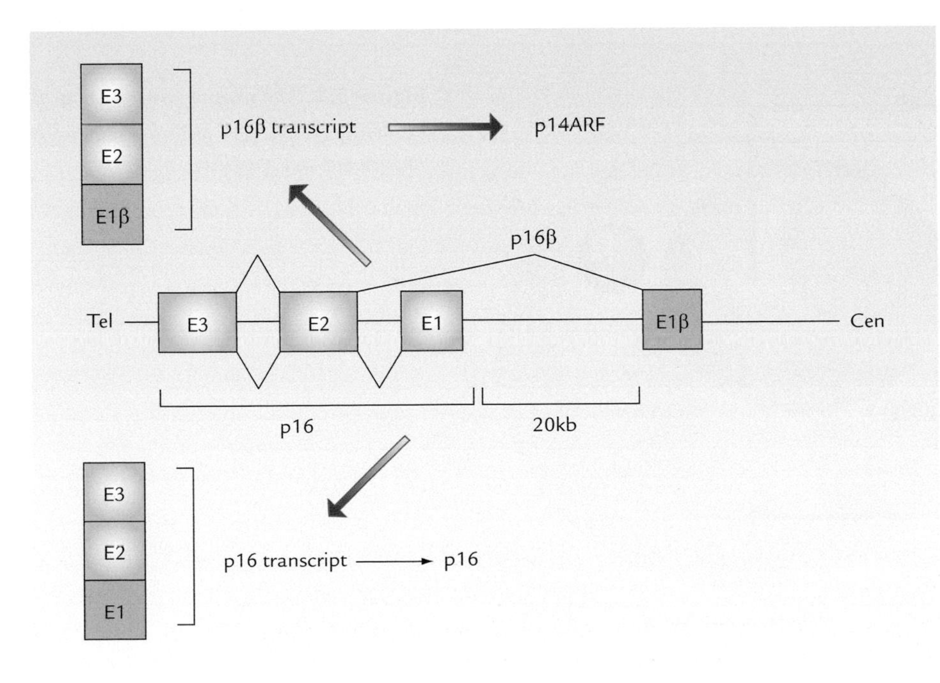

Figure 5.2 *Diagrammatic representation of the INK4A/ARF locus on chromosome 9p. Alternate splicing using one of two alternate first exons, gives rise to two different transcripts, p16, and p14ARF. In the case of p14ARF the genetic code of exon 2 is read differently to that for p16, that is, it is read in* ***A****lternate* ***R****eading* ***F****rame (ARF)*

negative. Inherited mutations in CDK4 therefore seem to be a very rare, although biologically fascinating, cause of melanoma susceptibility.

The genetic basis for the remaining 60–80% of families, in which highly penetrant genes may be operating is the subject of intense research by the International Melanoma Genetics Consortium (Figure 5.3) which is always pleased to be notified of new families.[25]

Low penetrance melanoma susceptibility genes, and 'modifier' genes

Alleles of CDKN2A

Mutations in CDKN2A that alter the function of p16^{INK4A} protein or p14ARF are extremely rare in the population. Certain sequence alterations in the region of the gene that do not alter protein structure are referred to as polymorphisms. A Queensland twin study has demonstrated that polymorphic variation at the CDKN2A locus might explain about 25% of the total variance in naevus count.[17] This might be due to subtle interindividual differences in the regulation of expression of the gene. Alternatively, these allelic variations on chromosome 9p might be indicative of the presence of another neighbouring locus that also determines aspects of melanocyte proliferation and differentiation.

Melanocortin receptor (MC1R)

Variation in human pigmentation is at least in part due to differences in the relative proportions of brown-black eumelanins and reddish pheomelanins produced. This is partly determined by variations in the structure of the receptor for melanocortin (alpha-melanocyte stimulating hormone, MSH). This receptor is located on the surface of melanocytes and is termed the melanocortin type-I receptor (MC1R). MC1R gene variants have been shown to be more frequent in skin types characterized by reddish or fair colour, poor tanning, and tendency to sunburn.[39] One specific variant (asp84glu) has been claimed to confer a relative risk for melanoma of 3.9 in a small case–control study in Britain.[40] In a large Queensland study, among pale-skinned individuals alone, an association between melanoma risk and MC1R variants was absent, but it persisted among those reporting a medium or olive/dark complexion.[41] This suggests that the effect that MC1R variant alleles have on melanoma susceptibility is partly mediated via determination of pigmentation phenotype, but that inheritance of certain MC1R variants may negate the protection normally afforded by darker skin colouring in some members of a predominantly white population. Preliminary data from carriers of a specific CDKN2A mutation commonly found in the south west Netherlands indicate that

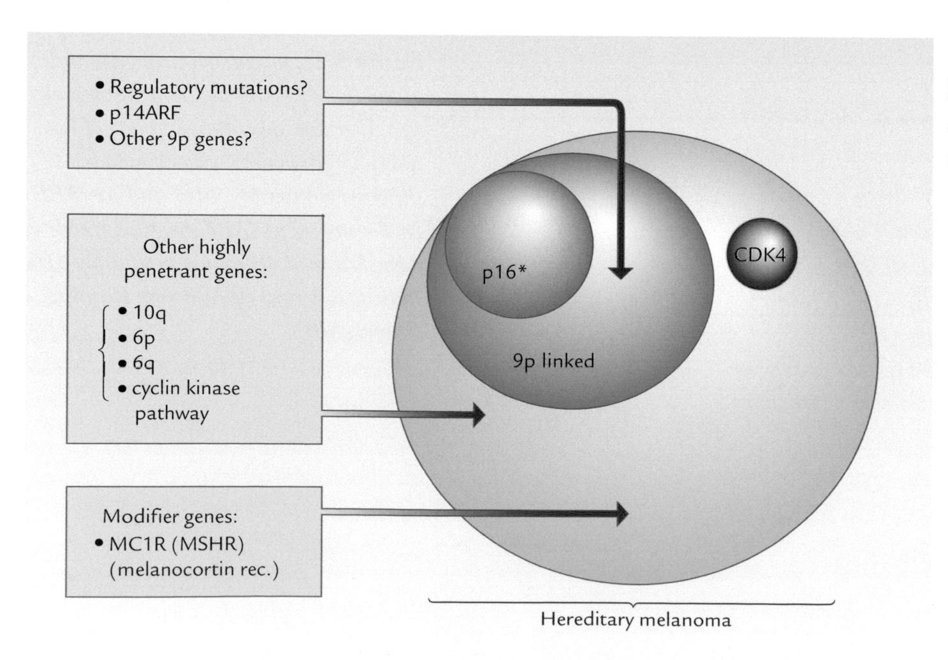

Figure 5.3 *The relative contribution of known, possible, and postulated genes in melanoma susceptibility.*

MC1R variants may modify the risk of melanoma conferred by inheriting a mutant CDKN2A.[42]

INTERACTION BETWEEN GENES AND ENVIRONMENT IN MELANOMA CAUSATION

Evidence for an effect of sun exposure on the penetrance of melanoma susceptibility genes

There is now evidence that the penetrance of mutations in the CDKN2A gene is strongly influenced by sun exposure. This relation between genetic predisposition and environmental sun was investigated in 124 chromosome 9p linked putative mutation carriers in three multiple case melanoma families in Utah.[21] Melanoma affected presumptive mutation carriers were found to have had more sun exposure within each skin type than mutation carriers without melanoma. Presumptive mutation carriers were also found to have higher naevus counts and naevus densities (partial surrogates for sun exposure) than non-carriers.

Additional indirect evidence that sunlight exposure enhances the penetrance of CDKN2A mutations is gained from analyses of the age incidence in melanoma kindreds through periods of changing population habits in recreational sun exposure. In a study of the age at onset of melanoma among different birth cohorts in 18 melanoma kindreds linked to chromosome 9p, the cumulative incidence of melanoma was 21-fold higher (95% confidence interval 5.2 to 84.6) among subjects born after 1959 than in those born before 1900.[35] This supports the notion that penetrance of the CDKN2A gene is increasing, presumably as a result of effect of sunlight exposure on mutation carriers at this locus. There is also some evidence that the predominant mutations found in CDKN2A in melanoma tumour samples from individuals without a family history carry the hallmark of UV induction.[43] Taken together, these data strongly support potent interactions between the effects of sunlight and genes in the determination of melanoma risk. This is now the subject of systematic evaluation in populations with differential exposure to sunlight.

Biological basis for gene–UV interactions in melanoma causation

There are biological explanations for the interaction of the cell cycle control genes, CDKN2A and CDK4, with ultraviolet light and with the genesis of naevi (reviewed in detail in Chapter 2). UV exposure stimulates melanocytes, certainly to melanogenesis, and possibly to proliferation. CDKN2A defective melanocytes in the laboratory proliferate for very much longer than do normal melanocytes, and seem to fail to senesce normally. This seems to mirror the phenotypic changes seen in many patients carrying germline mutations in the gene, having the AMS phenotype, in that their melanocyte population seems dramatically expanded, and they develop naevi in much greater numbers and in more unusual sites than do non-carriers. However, the relation between the AMS and CDKN2A mutations is unclear. Detailed phenotype/genotype studies in UK families have provided strong evidence that the CDKN2A gene is naevogenic, but the correlation between mutation carrier status and the AMS was incomplete.[44,45] Other groups have shown a similar lack of correlation.[46] The likelihood is that there are environmental determinants (for example, mutation carriers with early sun exposure may be more likely to exhibit the AMS) or that there may be variants of modifier genes co-segregating in the families. These would be putative low penetrance melanoma susceptibility genes.

ADVICE TO PATIENTS CONCERNING GENETIC TESTING

It is possible to identify certain pointers to the presence of constitutional mutations in melanoma susceptibility genes in an individual. The best predictor at present is the presence in a melanoma affected person of a strong family history of melanoma.[32] Other pointers include a history of multiple primary melanomas, and an early age of onset of first melanoma.[47–49]

Despite these known correlations with genetic susceptibility, at present, predictive genetic testing for melanoma susceptibility in unaffected individuals should only be performed very rarely outside of a research setting.[25] The reasons for this are as follows:

- Only approximately one third of multiple affected member melanoma kindreds are accounted for by currently known melanoma susceptibility genes.[16,25] While the hunt for other genes continues, DNA testing in most of such families will be uninformative.
- Even where a defined mutation in a known melanoma susceptibility gene has been identified in

one affected family member, this information is often of little value to other family members because of current lack of knowledge about the penetrance of such mutations. In the case of the CDKN2A gene, penetrance seems to be partly influenced by exposure to sunlight. It is therefore not possible to offer even near accurate estimates of the lifetime risk of melanoma in individuals carrying a constitutional mutation in a melanoma susceptibility gene such as CDKN2A. In certain cases, for example, gene carriers have survived to advanced years without developing melanoma.[50] Such lack of precision confounds attempts at accurate predictive DNA testing even within the context of such comparatively rare multiple case families.

- While certain CDKN2A mutations have a clear and demonstrable functional effect on the $p16^{INK4A}$ protein, others do not and may represent population polymorphisms of no predictive value with respect to melanoma occurrence.[51]
- It is not uncommon to find atypical naevi and even melanoma in non-mutation carriers in high risk melanoma kindreds.[15,16,44] This may be due to common environmental exposure by family members, or to the common inheritance of less highly penetrant melanoma susceptibility genes, or modifier genes. Whatever the reason, the practical clinical result is that all members of such families should be subjected to the same protocol of prevention and surveillance.
- There are currently only limited data on the efficacy of prevention and surveillance strategies for melanoma.[6]

Given current gaps in knowledge about the expression of melanoma susceptibility genes in the population, DNA testing cannot be used as a guide to clinical practice of prevention and surveillance. All individuals deemed to be at high risk of melanoma should be managed with the same attention to the following measures.[52] In the absence of randomized controlled clinical trial based data, the evidence for each of these measures is Level IV.*

- Education of all family members about the need for sun protection is essential. Parents in particular should be educated about sun protective measures during infancy and childhood.[54–56] This should include advice on the use of sun protective clothing, hats and sunglasses, broad spectrum UVA and UVB protective sunscreens.[57,58] Avoidance of peak ultraviolet conditions, and absolute avoidance of sunburns are other imperatives.
- From the age of 10 years, family members should have a baseline skin, scalp, iris, and genital examination with characterization of moles. Overview photographs of the entire skin surface and close up photographs of atypical naevi are useful.
- Individuals should be taught about routine self examination in the hope that this will prompt earlier diagnosis and removal of melanomas. Patients may be given their own copy of photographs and shown how to use these in self examination. The significance of change in size or shape of pigmented lesions should be understood and the ABCD rules are often helpful in this regard. In particular, patients should be aware of the importance of new pigmented lesions as one third of melanomas in those with multiple atypical naevi may arise de novo, rather than from existing naevi.[59] Colour photographs of early melanomas and atypical moles may be given to the patient as an aid.
- Self examination should be supplemented where possible with examination by a similarly trained parent, partner, or family member.
- A dermatologist should carry out 6-monthly skin examinations until the naevi are stable and the patient is judged competent in self surveillance. Subsequently the individual should be seen annually or have prompt access to that dermatologist as necessary. During puberty or pregnancy, when the naevi may be unstable, more frequent dermatological examinations may be indicated. Examination should include adequate examination of the scalp and genitalia. Skin surface microscopy (epiluminescence microscopy) may be helpful in a surveillance programme.[60,61]
- The indication for surgical removal of a pigmented lesion is the same as in the general population, namely suspicion of malignant change. There is no justification for prophylactic excision of moles since the probability of a single naevus becoming

* Level IV: Evidence obtained from case series, either post-test or pretest and post-test.[53]

melanoma is low and, with time, most naevi will mature and disappear. Furthermore melanomas may occur on previously entirely normal skin so that 'prophylactic' excision of all moles would not change guidelines on surveillance by the patient or the healthcare provider.[59]

- Screening and surveillance guidelines for other cancers should be carried out as in the general population. Rarely, melanoma occurs in the context of the Li-Fraumeni syndrome. The hallmark for this syndrome is the presence of sarcomas and other early onset cancers, particularly breast cancer, in the pedigree. Screening should be conducted in accordance with guidelines for this condition. Certain hereditary melanoma families carrying CDKN2A mutations have an increased incidence of pancreatic adenocarcinoma.[62,63] At present there is no reliable screening method for early operable pancreatic carcinoma, and survival is poor even with optimal treatment of early disease.[64]
- Where cases of ocular melanoma have occurred in the family, annual fundoscopy is recommended, although it is of unproved efficacy in screening or early detection. The risk in any individual of developing this tumour is likely to be low.

REFERENCES

1. Norris W, A case of fungoid disease. *Edinburgh Med Surg J* 1820; 16: 562.
2. Osterlind A, Tucker MA, Hou-Jensen K, et al, The Danish case–control study of cutaneous malignant melanoma. I. Importance of host factors. *Int J Cancer* 1988; 42(2): 200–6.
3. Bliss JM, Ford D, Swerdlow AJ, et al, Risk of cutaneous melanoma associated with pigmentation characteristics and freckling: systematic overview of 10 case–control studies. The International Melanoma Analysis Group (IMAGE). *Int J Cancer* 1995; 62(4): 367–76.
4. Rippey JJ, Rippey E, Epidemiology of malignant melanoma of the skin in South Africa. *S Afr Med J* 1984; **65**(15): 595–8.
5. Tucker MA, Halpern A, Holly EA, et al, Clinically recognized dysplastic naevi. A central risk factor for cutaneous melanoma (see comments). *JAMA* 1997; 277(18): 1439–44.
6. Tucker MA, Fraser MC, Goldstein AM, et al, The risk of melanoma and other cancers in melanoma-prone families. *J Invest Dermatol* 1993; 100: 350S-5S.
7. Berwick M, Halpern A, Melanoma epidemiology. *Curr Opin Oncol* 1997; 9(2): 178–82.
8. Newton JA, Bataille V, Griffiths K, et al, How common is the atypical mole syndrome phenotype in apparently sporadic melanoma? *J Am Acad Dermatol* 1993; 29(6): 989–96.
9. Bataille V, Bishop JA, Sasieni P, et al, Risk of cutaneous melanoma in relation to the numbers, types and sites of naevi: a case–control study. *Br J Cancer* 1996; 73(12): 1605–11.
10. Grulich AE, Bataille V, Swerdlow AJ, et al, Naevi and pigmentary characteristics as risk factors for melanoma in a high-risk population: a case-control study in New South Wales, Australia. *Int J Cancer* 1996; 67(4): 485–91.
11. Newton Bishop JA, Bataille V, Pinney E, Bishop DT, Family studies in melanoma: identification of the atypical mole syndrome (AMS) phenotype. *Melanoma Res* 1994; 4(4): 199–206.
12. Bergman W, Palan A, Went LN, Clinical and genetic studies in six Dutch kindreds with the dysplastic naevus syndrome. *Ann Hum Genet* 1986; 50(Pt 3): 249–58.
13. Greene MH, Tucker MA, Clark WH, et al, Hereditary melanoma and the dysplastic naevus syndrome: the risk of cancers other than melanoma. *J Am Acad Dermatol* 1987; 16(4): 792–7.
14. Carey WP Jr, Thompson CJ, Synnestvedt M, et al, Dysplastic naevi as a melanoma risk factor in patients with familial melanoma. *Cancer* 1994; 74(12): 3118–25.
15. Gruis NA, Sandkuijl LA, van der Velden PA, et al, CDKN2 explains part of the clinical phenotype in Dutch familial atypical multiple-mole melanoma (FAMMM) syndrome families. *Melanoma Res* 1995; 5(3): 169–77.
16. Goldstein AM, Falk RT, Fraser MC, et al, Sun-related risk factors in melanoma-prone families with CDKN2A mutations. *J Natl Cancer Inst* 1998; 90(9): 709–11.
17. Zhu G, Duffy DL, Eldridge A, et al, A major quantitative-trait locus for mole density is linked to the familial melanoma gene CDKN2A: a maximum-likelihood combined linkage and association analysis in twins and their sibs. *Am J Hum Genet* 1999; 65(2): 483–92.
18. Harrison SL, MacLennan R, Speare R, Wronski I, Sun exposure and melanocytic naevi in young Australian children. *Lancet* 1994; 344(8936): 1529–32.
19. Green A, Siskind V, Green L, The incidence of melanocytic naevi in adolescent children in Queensland, Australia. *Melanoma Res* 1995; 5(3): 155–60.
20. Dennis LK, White E, Lee JA, et al, Constitutional factors and sun exposure in relation to naevi: a population-based cross-sectional study. *Am J Epidemiol* 1996; 143(3): 248–56.
21. Cannon-Albright LA, Meyer LJ, Goldgar DE, et al, Penetrance and expressivity of the chromosome 9p melanoma susceptibility locus (MLM). *Cancer Res* 1994; 54(23): 6041–4.
22. Cutler C, Foulkes WD, Brunet JS, et al, Cutaneous malignant melanoma in women is uncommonly associated with a family history of melanoma in first-degree relatives: a case–control study. *Melanoma Res* 1996; 6(6): 435–40.
23. Aitken JF, Youl P, Green A, et al, Accuracy of case-reported family history of melanoma in Queensland, Australia. *Melanoma Res* 1996; 6(4): 313–7.
24. Aitken JF, Duffy DL, Green A, et al, Heterogeneity of melanoma risk in families of melanoma patients. *Am J Epidemiol* 1994; 140(11): 961–73.
25. Kefford RF, Newton Bishop JA, Bergman W, Tucker MA, Counseling and DNA testing for individuals perceived to be genetically predisposed to melanoma: a consensus statement of the Melanoma Genetics Consortium. *J Clin Oncol* 1999; 17(10): 3245–51.
26. Soufir N, Bressac-de Paillerets B, Desjardins L, et al, Individuals with presumably hereditary uveal melanoma do not harbour germline mutations in the coding regions of either the P16INK4A, P14ARF or cdk4 genes. *Br J Cancer* 2000; 82(4): 818–22.
27. Serrano M, Lee H, Chin L, et al, Role of the INK4a locus in tumor suppression and cell mortality. *Cell* 1996; 85(1): 27–37.
28. Zhang Y, Xiong Y, Yarbrough WG, ARF promotes MDM2 degradation and stabilizes p53: ARF-INK4a locus deletion impairs both the Rb and p53 tumor suppression pathways. *Cell* 1998; 92(6): 725–34.
29. Pomerantz J, Schreiber-Agus N, Liegeois NJ, et al, The Ink4a tumor suppressor gene product, p19Arf, interacts with MDM2 and neutralizes MDM2's inhibition of p53. *Cell* 1998; 92(6): 713–23.
30. Rizos H, Becker TM, Holland EA, et al, Differential expression of p16INK4a and p16beta transcripts in B-lymphoblastoid cells from members of hereditary melanoma families without CDKN2A exon mutations. *Oncogene* 1997; 15(5): 515–23.
31. Rizos H, Darmanian AP, Holland EA, et al, Mutations in the INK4a/ARF melanoma susceptibility locus functionally impair p14ARF. *J Biol Chem* 2001;276:41424–34.
32. Goldstein AM, Tucker MA, Screening for CDKN2A mutations in hereditary melanoma (editorial; comment). *J Natl Cancer Inst* 1997; 89(10): 676–8.

33. Hayward NK, The current situation with regard to human melanoma and genetic inferences. Curr Opin Oncol 1996; 8(2): 136–42.
34. Liu L, Dilworth D, Gao L, et al, Mutation of the CDKN2A 5′ UTR creates an aberrant initiation codon and predisposes to melanoma. *Nat Genet* 1999; 21(1): 128–32.
35. Battistutta D, Palmer J, Walters M, et al, Incidence of familial melanoma and MLM2 gene. *Lancet* 1994; 344(8937): 1607–8.
36. Aitken J, Welch J, Duffy D, et al, CDKN2A variants in a population-based sample of Queensland families with melanoma. *J Natl Cancer Inst* 1999; 91: 446–52.
37. Zuo L, Weger J, Yang Q., et al, Germline mutations in the p16INK4a binding domain of CDK4 in familial melanoma. *Nat Genet* 1996; 12(1): 97–9.
38. Soufir N, Avril MF, Chompret A, et al. Prevalence of p16 and CDK4 germline mutations in 48 melanoma-prone families in France. *Hum Mol Genet* 1998; 7(2): 209–16.
39. Valverde P, Healy E, Jackson I, et al, Variants of the melanocyte-stimulating hormone receptor gene are associated with red hair and fair skin in humans (see comments) Val92Met variant of the melanocyte stimulating hormone receptor gene (letter). *Nat Genet* 1995; 11(3): 328–30.
40. Valverde P, Healy E, Sikkink S, et al, The Asp84Glu variant of the melanocortin 1 receptor (MC1R) is associated with melanoma. *Hum Mol Genet* 1996; 5(10): 1663–6.
41. Palmer JS, Duffy DL, Box NF, et al, Melanocortin-1 receptor polymorphisms and risk of melanoma: is the association explained solely by pigmentation phenotype? *Am J Hum Genet* 2000; 66(1): 176–86.
42. van der Velden PA, SandKuijl LA, Bergman W, et al, Melanocortin-1 receptor variant R151C modifies melanoma risk in Dutch families with melanoma. *Am J Hum Genet* 2001; 69: 774–9.
43. Pollock PM, Pearson JV, Hayward NK, Compilation of somatic mutations of the CDKN2 gene in human cancers: non-random distribution of base substitutions. *Genes Chromosomes Cancer* 1996; 15(2): 77–88.
44. Wachsmuth RC, Harland M, Bishop JA, The atypical-mole syndrome and predisposition to melanoma (letter). *NEJM* 1998; 339(5): 348–9.
45. Bishop JA, Wachsmuth RC, Harland M, et al, Genotype/phenotype and penetrance studies in melanoma families with germline CDKN2A mutations. *J Invest Dermatol* 2000; 114(1): 28–33.
46. Bergman W, Gruis NA, Frants RR, The Dutch FAMMM family material: clinical and genetic data. *Cytogenet Cell Genet* 1992; 59(2–3): 161–4.
47. Monzon J, Liu L, Brill H, et al. CDKN2A Mutations in Multiple Primary Melanomas. *NEJM* 1998; 338(13): 879–87.
48. Burden AD, Newell J, Andrew N, et al, Genetic and environmental influences in the development of multiple primary melanoma (see comments). *Arch Dermatol* 1999; 135(3): 261–5.
49. Goldstein AM, Fraser MC, Clark WH Jr, Tucker MA, Age at diagnosis and transmission of invasive melanoma in 23 families with cutaneous malignant melanoma/dysplastic naevi. *J Natl Cancer Inst* 1994; 86(18): 1385–90.
50. Holland EA, Beaton SC, Becker TM, et al. Analysis of the p16 gene, CDKN2, in 17 Australian melanoma kindreds. *Oncogene* 1995; 11(11): 2289–94.
51. Ranade K, Hussussian CJ, Sirkosi RS, et al, Mutations associated with familial melanoma impair p16INK4 function. *Nat Genet* 1995; 10: 114–6.
52. Kefford RF, Guidelines for the management of those at high risk for developing cutaneous melanoma. In: *Melanoma: critical debates.* (eds Newton Bishop J, Gore M), London: Blackwell 2002: 70–7.
53. Guide to clinical preventive services: an assessment of the effectiveness of 169 interventions. In: *US Preventive Services Task Force.* (ed Fisher M.) Baltimore: Williams and Williams; 1989: Appendix A. p388.
54. National Institutes of Health Consensus Development Conference Statement on Diagnosis and Treatment of Early Melanoma, January 27–29, 1992. *Am J Dermatopathol* 1993; 15(1): 34–43; discussion 46–51.
55. Ferrini RL, Perlman M, Hill L, American College of Preventive Medicine practice policy statement: skin protection from ultraviolet light exposure. The American College of Preventive Medicine. *Am J Prev Med* 1998; 14(1): 83–6.
56. Gasparro FP, Mitchnick M, Nash JF, A review of sunscreen safety and efficacy. *Photochem Photobiol* 1998; 68(3): 243–56.
57. Setlow RB, Grist E, Thompson K, Woodhead AD, Wavelengths effective in induction of malignant melanoma. *Proc Natl Acad Sci USA* 1993; 90(14): 6666–70.
58. Krien PM, Moyal D, Sunscreens with broad-spectrum absorption decrease the trans to cis photoisomerization of urocanic acid in the human stratum corneum after multiple UV light exposures. *Photochem Photobiol* 1994; 60(3): 280–7.
59. Kelly JW, Yeatman JM, Regalia C, et al, A high incidence of melanoma found in patients with multiple dysplastic naevi by photographic surveillance. *Med J Aust* 1997; 167(4): 191–4.
60. Kenet RO, Kang S, Kenet BJ, et al, Clinical diagnosis of pigmented lesions using digital epiluminescence microscopy. Grading protocol and atlas. *Arch Dermatol* 1993; 129(2): 157–74.
61. Menzies SW, Ingvar C, McCarthy WH, A sensitivity and specificity analysis of the surface microscopy features of invasive melanoma. *Melanoma Res* 1996; 6(1): 55–62.
62. Goldstein AM, Fraser MC, Struewing JP, et al, Increased risk of pancreatic cancer in melanoma-prone kindreds with p16INK4 mutationssee comments. *NEJM* 1995; 333(15): 970–4.
63. Hille ET, van Duijn E, Gruis NA, et al, Excess cancer mortality in six Dutch pedigrees with the familial atypical multiple mole-melanoma syndrome from 1830 to 1994. *J Invest Dermatol* 1998; 110(5): 788–92.
64. Nitecki SS, Sarr MG, Colby TV, van Heerden JA, Long-term survival after resection for ductal adenocarcinoma of the pancreas. Is it really improving? *Ann Surg* 1995; 221(1): 59–66.

6

Epidemiology of cutaneous melanoma and current trends

Bruce Armstrong

INTRODUCTION

Cutaneous melanoma (referred to hereafter as melanoma) is comparatively uncommon worldwide. The facts, however, that its incidence is steadily increasing in many populations of European origin, that cure is probable if it is diagnosed early, and that the bulk of it is probably attributable to a single, modifiable risk factor (sun exposure) mark melanoma as an important global public health issue.

Summary Box ***Melanoma as a public health issue – key facts***

- An estimated 105,500 new cases of and 32,800 deaths from melanoma occurred worldwide in 1990. These were estimated to be 1.3% of cancers (except non-melanocytic skin cancers) diagnosed and 0.63% of deaths from cancer in that year.[1,2]
- Between the mid 1960s and the mid 1980s, the incidence of melanoma rose between 3% and 8% a year in most populations of European origin for which data were available.[3]
- There is little if any loss of life expectancy if melanoma is diagnosed at 0.75 mm thickness or less. Recent Australian figures show that just under a half of newly diagnosed melanomas are this thick and that overall 5-year survival from melanoma is 92.8%.[4,5]
- Sun exposure is estimated to cause 65% of melanomas worldwide and 95% in populations of European origin with high sun exposure.[6]

In reviewing the epidemiology of and current trends in melanoma, this chapter will cover the following topics.

- Worldwide incidence patterns.
- Relation of population characteristics (age, sex, ethnic origin, socioeconomic status, etc.) to incidence.
- Relation of constitutional characteristics (body site, pigmentary characteristics, number of cutaneous naevi, freckling, etc.) to individual risk.
- Relation of environmental exposures to individual risk.
- Current trends in incidence, mortality, and survival.

WORLDWIDE INCIDENCE PATTERNS

At the global level, melanoma is largely a disease of people living in developed countries; an estimated 77% of newly diagnosed cases and 66% of deaths occur in these populations. The estimated incidence, standardized to the age distribution of the 'world' population, averages seven per 100,000 person years in the more developed regions and 0.6/100,000 in the less developed regions.

When estimated incidences are distributed by region, the highest rates are seen in Australia and New Zealand, with an estimated average rate in males and females in 1990 of 26.5/100,000 person years. The next highest rates were in North America (9.3/100,000), Northern and Western Europe (7.0 and 6.3), Southern Africa (4.5), Southern Europe (4.3), Polynesia, Melanesia and Micronesia (about 3.5), South America and

Eastern Europe (3.1) (Figure 6.1). These are all areas populated by a substantial minority or more of people of European origin, and they include the most affluent peoples of the world.

These patterns probably reflect the far greater susceptibility to melanoma of people of European origin with light skin than people of dark skin and people of Asian origin. This issue will be addressed in more detail below.

Focusing on individual countries, the highest incidences of melanoma are found in Australia. The highest rates for 1988–92 reported in *Cancer Incidence in Five Continents Volume VII* were in the Australian state of New South Wales (33.1/100,000 in males and 25.7 in females) and the non-Maori population of New Zealand (25.0 in males and 29.8 in females).[7] The most recently reported incidences for the whole of Australia[8] were 36.1/100,000 in males and 28.0/100,000 in females. The lowest incidence rates are generally found in Asian countries, both northern and southern, with rates near or below 0.5/100,000.

When we focus on European populations, a complex pattern appears when incidence rates are plotted against latitude.[9] In Europe, rates are highest in populations at high latitudes (for example, Norway), fall to a minimum at about 52° north, and rise at lower latitudes. If the lower latitude North American populations and those of Australia and New Zealand are added, rates rise further with progressively falling latitude.

These anomalies may be due, at least in part, to lack of a perfect correlation between latitude and exposure of human skin to ultraviolet (UV)B. Other factors may include the tendency for racial skin colour to increase in darkness with increasing proximity to the equator and a highly intermittent pattern of sun exposure from, for example, summer vacations in southern Europe in populations resident in northern Europe.[9]

RELATION OF POPULATION CHARACTERISTICS TO INCIDENCE

Age

In comparison with other cancers in adults, melanoma is more frequent in the young and middle aged. Incidence rates generally rise steeply until about 50 years of age. The pattern thereafter depends on the population under observation and the sex of the subjects (Figure 6.2).

These gross patterns of incidence mask two different age patterns depending on body site. Melanomas occurring on the head and neck show a near exponential increase in incidence with increasing age.[10,11]

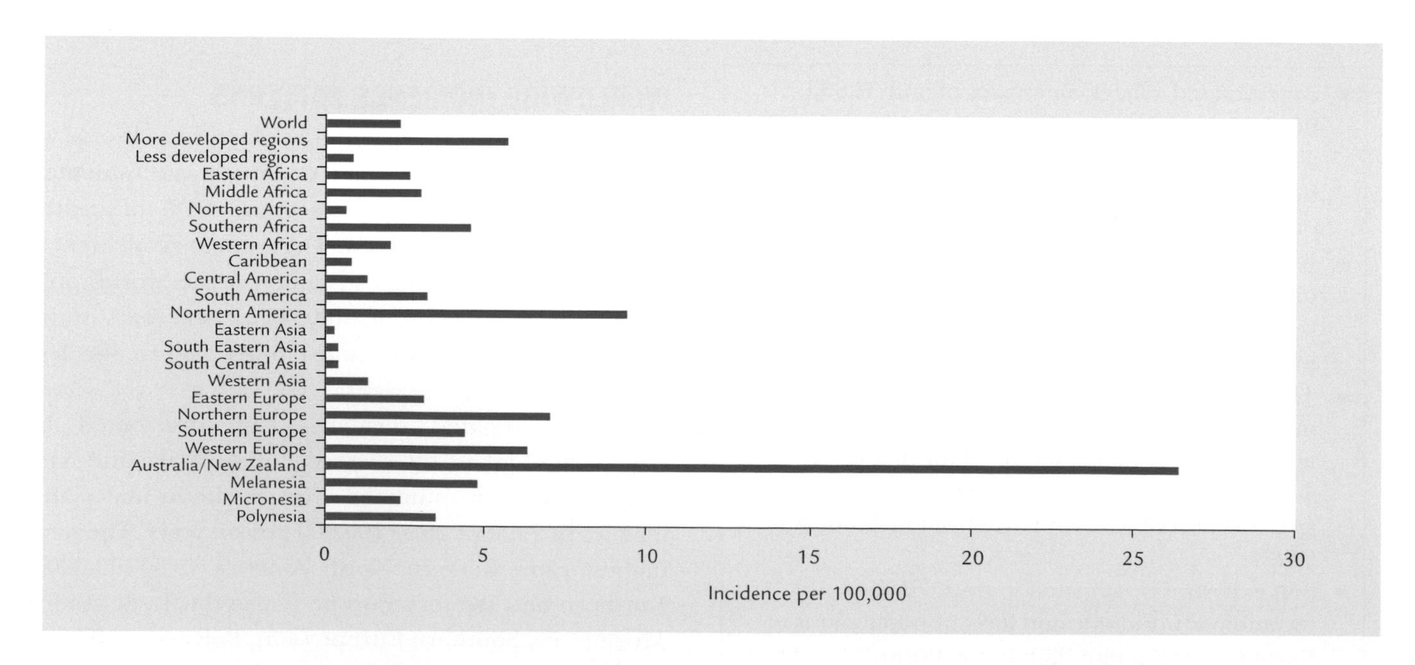

Figure 6.1 *Estimated age standardized incidence rates of melanoma in the major regions of the world in 1990.*[1]

On other body sites, the incidence is highest among the middle to older middle aged and is comparatively stable or falls thereafter, depending on site and sex.

Sex

Age standardized incidences of melanoma in European populations are, on average, about 1.0/100,000 person years higher in women than men.[12] There are though, quite different patterns of increase in incidence with age in the sexes depending on the population. In European populations per se (as exemplified in Figure 6.2 by the South Thames cancer registry population in England) rates in women exceed those in men at most ages. In North America and Australia, however, (as exemplified by the Staging, Epidemiology, and End Results (SEER) cancer registries in the United States and the New South Wales (NSW) cancer registry in Australia – Figure 6.2) rates in men exceed those in women from about 50 years of age. In both these populations, the male to female ratio increases to just over two in the oldest age groups. Interestingly, the populations in Europe with higher incidence rates (for example, Norway and Zurich, the two European cancer registry populations with the highest rates) also show this increasing sex ratio after 50 years of age.[7]

Socioeconomic status

Melanoma incidence rates are generally higher among people of higher socioeconomic status as assessed from occupation, education, income, or characteristics of residential areas.[10,13]

This pattern, however, is not totally consistent. For example, outside Sydney, the capital of the Australian state of New South Wales, risk of melanoma falls with increasing socioeconomic status, as assessed by characteristics of residential areas; the opposite applies in Sydney.[4] In a similar analysis of census tracts in western Washington State, United States, melanoma incidence increased with increasing socioeconomic status overall, but the opposite was true in men older than 70 years.[14] The latter effect was largely confined to melanomas occurring at sun exposed sites. It may be that the positive gradient with socioeconomic status is seen where recreational sun exposure is dominant and the opposite is seen where occupational sun exposure is dominant.

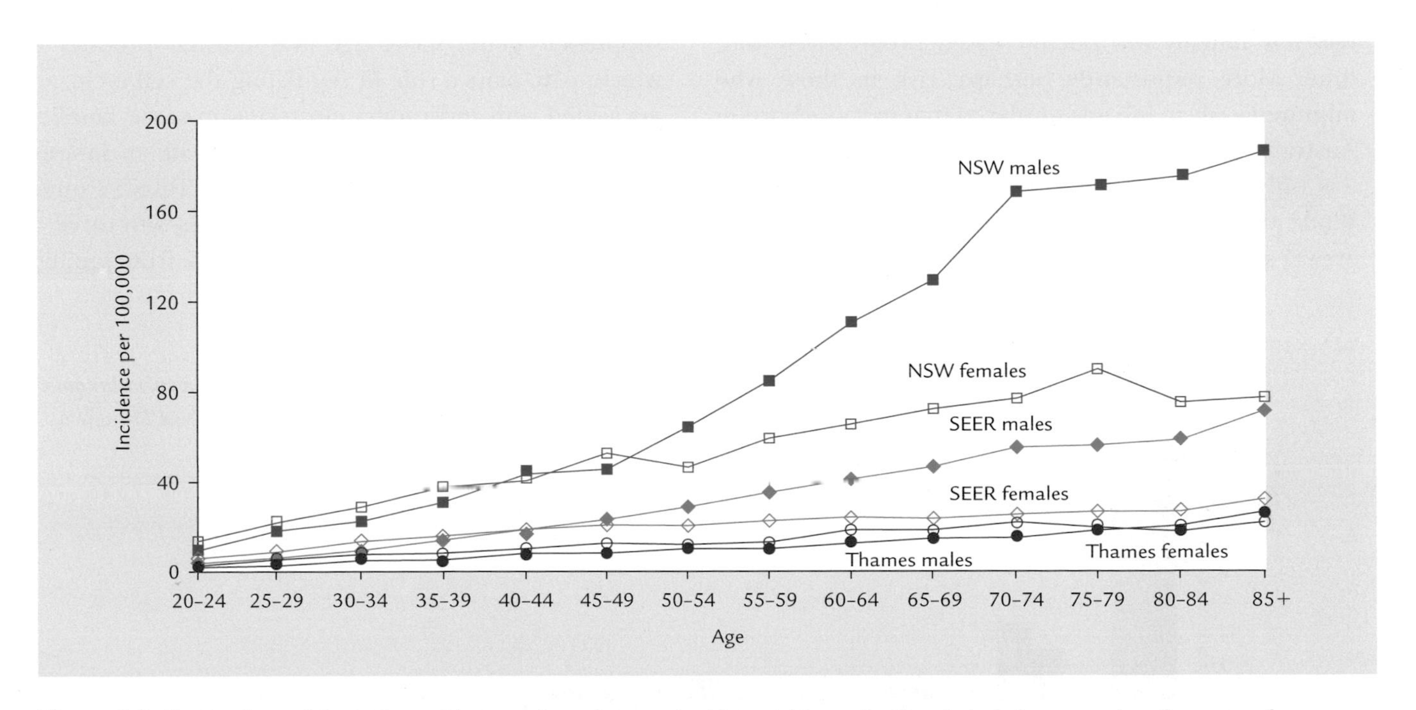

Figure 6.2 *Comparison of the pattern of increase in melanoma incidence with age in three populations covering the range of melanoma incidence – New South Wales, Australia (NSW), the SEER cancer registry populations of the USA, and the South West Thames cancer registry population of England.*[7]

Ethnicity

Ethnic background is an important correlate of melanoma incidence in mixed race populations. For example, in San Francisco, United States, incidence is substantially lower in Hispanic whites than in non-Hispanic whites (Figure 6.3).[7] Similarly and consistent with the international patterns (Figure 6.1), incidence is much less in blacks and those of Asian origin residing in San Francisco than in those of European origin. These patterns in a single environment suggest that ethnic origin itself is a major factor in determining risk of melanoma.

Migration

The effect on melanoma incidence of migration from one environment to another is best examined by studying populations that migrate from a low incidence area to a high incidence area populated by people of a similar ethnic origin. This has been done for populations migrating from Europe to Australia and New Zealand, Jews migrating from other countries to Israel, and people migrating within the USA.[12]

Typical results are shown in Figure 6.4, based on migrants, mainly from Europe, to Australia.[15] Migrants' risk was initially low but increased progressively with time. More importantly perhaps, risk in those who migrated early in life was similar to that in those born in Australia, whereas risk in those who migrated as adults was only about one third of the Australian born risk. While the effects of duration of residence and age at arrival are inevitably entangled, either pattern suggests that risk of melanoma is strongly determined by long residence in a high risk area and long residence is more probable the earlier in life a person migrates.

RELATION OF CONSTITUTIONAL CHARACTERISTICS TO INDIVIDUAL RISK

Family history and major gene mutations

Melanoma has long been known to run in families.[17] A summary analysis of family history of melanoma in eight case–control studies showed a relative risk of 2.24 (95% confidence interval 1.76 to 2.86) with a history of any affected first degree relative. With only one affected, the relative risk was 2.18, based on six of the studies, and with two or more it was 5.56. Other host factors such as naevus count, freckling, and other pigmentary characteristics did not explain this association. However, families at high risk of melanoma have been shown, in comparison with families not at high risk, to have significantly higher proportions of members who tan poorly and have large numbers of naevi.[18]

Segregation analysis suggests that familial clustering of melanoma cannot be explained by a single major gene mutation.[19] However, mutations in the tumour suppressor gene, CDKN2A, the normal product of which, p16, plays a role in regulating the cell cycle, are associated with melanoma clustering in some families. In a study of 131 Australian patients with melanoma and a family history of it, germ-line CDKN2A mutations were present in 15.1% from families with three or more members with melanoma and 1.5% from families

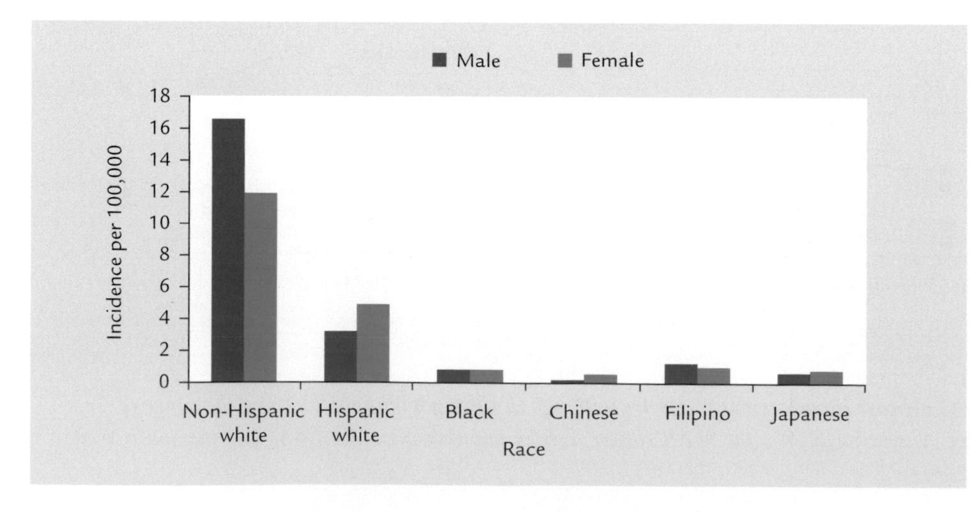

Figure 6.3 *Variation in melanoma incidence by race in San Francisco, USA.*[7]

with only two.[20] The prevalence was even higher, 31.6%, in those from families with three or more members with melanoma one of whom had multiple primary melanomas. In a population based series of 482 patients with melanoma in Queensland (Australia) families at defined risk of melanoma (defined according to the excess of observed cases to expected cases, based on family size, age, sex, and birth years), all nine patients with CDKN2A mutations were among 87 patients from very high risk families (mutation prevalence 10.3%).[21] It could be estimated from this study that 0.2% of patients with melanoma in Queensland had CDKN2A mutations. Thus it seems that even in high risk families, a minority of melanoma patients have germ-line CDKN2A mutations, and these mutations are rare in the general population of people with melanomas.

Number of naevi, atypical naevi, fair complexion, cutaneous sun sensitivity, and sun exposure appear to increase risk of melanoma in people with CDKN2A mutations just as they do in the general population.[22]

A few germ-line mutations in the CDK4 gene have also been observed in patients with melanoma.[23]

Anatomy

Melanomas occur most often on the trunk in males and the lower limbs in females in populations of European origin.[12] Simple proportions or incidences by body site, however, do not correctly represent the propensity of a particular site on the skin to give rise to melanoma because they do not take account of the area of the skin at the site. Density of melanoma per unit surface area is generally highest on the head and neck but also high on the back in both sexes (Figure 6.5[24,25]) and least on the legs in men and the chest and abdomen in women.

Black and Asian populations have a much higher proportion of melanomas on the soles of the feet than

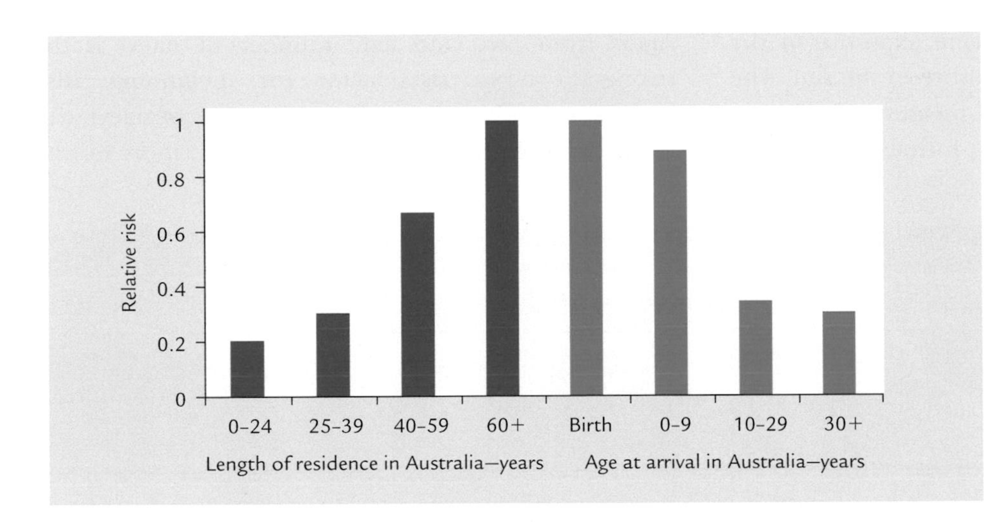

Figure 6.4 *Relative risk of melanoma in migrants to Western Australia by duration of residence and age at arrival.*[16]

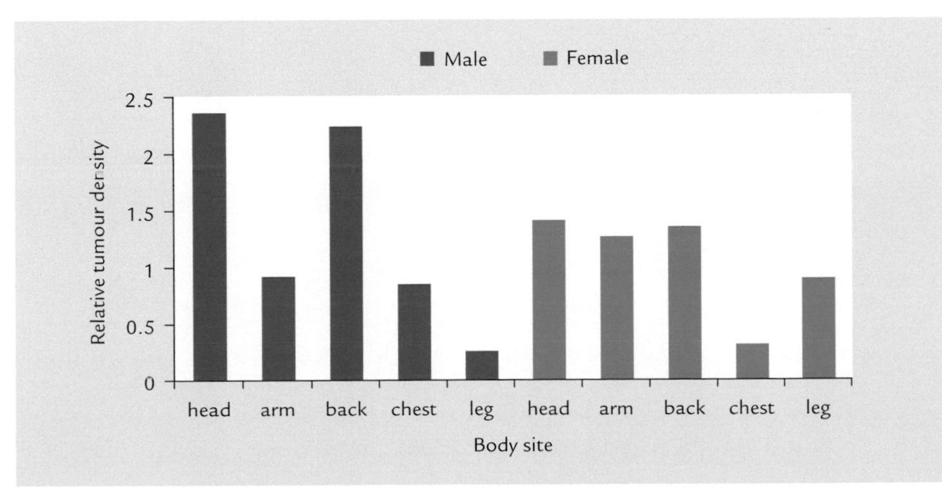

Figure 6.5 *Relative density of melanoma on different body sites (adapted from Elwood and Gallagher 1998*[24]*) (head = face, scalp, ears, and neck; arm = upper arm, forearm and hand; back = back and buttocks; chest = chest and abdomen; legs = hip, thigh, lower leg, foot. Relative density = ratio of observed numbers of melanomas on a body site to the expected number calculated assuming uniform distribution of melanomas in relation to body surface area).*

white populations.[12,26] Available evidence suggests, however, that the absolute incidence of plantar lesions is no higher in these populations than it is in whites.[27,28]

Pigmentary traits and reaction to sunlight

Fair or red hair, blue eyes, pale complexion, and the skin's reaction to sun exposure are well known risk factors for melanoma in populations of European origin. For those with red hair (the highest risk category) relative risk is of the order of 5 with reference to those with black hair (Table 6.1[29]). The risk gradient is less with eye colour and skin colour, the relative risk being around 1.5 for blue eyes with reference to brown and of the order of 2 for darker skin colour with reference to lighter. Difficulties in accurate measurement of skin colour, however, may have biased the association downwards.

The skin's reaction to sun exposure has usually been measured by a questionnaire enquiring about either propensity to burn on acute exposure to the sun or to tan after repeated exposure to the sun. The latter is probably the more valid measure of sun sensitivity because assessment of the former depends on the person's experience of sun exposure sufficient to cause sunburn. While no systematic review has been made of data relating to sun sensitivity, the relative risk in those who do not tan at all, with reference to those who tan easily, has usually been of the order of 2–3.

Freckles

Freckles are associated with increased risk of melanoma (Table 6.1[29]). This risk is attenuated little by adjustment for possible confounding of freckles with naevi. Risk associated with freckles appears to be higher in younger people than older people.

Acquired melanocytic naevi

Naevus remnants have been found in histological contiguity with up to 72% of melanomas.[12]

Number of naevi

Apart from race and age, number of naevi is the strongest known risk factor for melanoma. Risk increases steeply with increasing number of naevi with relative risks typically of the order of 10 or more for the

Table 6.1 *Effect of pigmentary characteristics and freckling on risk of melanoma (summarized from Bliss et al. 1995[29])*

Risk factors and classification categories	Relative risks (95% Confidence intervals)
Adult hair colour (eight studies)	
Black or dark brown	1.00
Light brown	1.49 (1.31 to 1.70)
Blonde or 'fair'	1.84 (1.54 to 2.21)
Red	2.38 (1.90 to 2.97)
Eye colour (10 studies)	
Brown	1.00
Green, grey or hazel	1.34 (1.17 to 1.54)
Blue	1.55 (1.35 to 1.78)
Skin colour (seven studies)	
Various	1.67 to 2.73 for lightest category relative to darkest category
Freckling (seven studies)	
Various	2.25 (2.00 to 2.54) for heaviest category relative to the lightest

highest number category.[16] The number of naevi at a particular site does not appear to predict risk of melanoma at that site any more strongly than does total number of naevi.[30,31]

Atypical naevi

Clinically atypical and histopathologically dysplastic naevi are associated with a high risk of melanoma in some families. Atypical naevi are also associated with a high risk of melanoma without a strong family history (for example relative risk of 12, 95% CI 4.4 to 31, for 10+ atypical naevi) and this association is independent of and stronger than that with number of all naevi >2 mm in diameter (for example relative risk of 3.4, 95% CI 2.0 to 5.7, for 100+ naevi).[32] Number of large (>5 mm) naevi, on the other hand, does not predict risk of melanoma more strongly (relative risk 2.3, CI 1.2 to 4.3, for 10+ large naevi) than number of naevi >2 mm.

RELATION OF ENVIRONMENTAL EXPOSURES TO INDIVIDUAL RISK

Exposure to the sun

The evidence that sun exposure causes melanoma is summarized in Table 6.2.[12,33] Except in the area of personal exposure to the sun, which is bedevilled by difficulties in measuring exposure, this table presents a consistent pattern of positive associations with generally indirect indicators of sun exposure. Although not consistently related to direct measures of total (occupational and non-occupational) sun exposure, melanoma has been quite consistently, and often quite strongly, related to history of recreational sun exposure and of sunburn, which presumably reflects high levels of recreational exposure. A summary analysis of published results for recreational or 'intermittent' sun exposure in 29 case–control studies produced a summary relative risk of 1.87 (95% CI 1.67 to 2.09) for the highest exposure category relative to the lowest.[34]

Melanoma has been associated negatively (inversely) with occupational sun exposure as often as it has been associated positively. In the summary analysis of 29 case–control studies, the estimate of relative risk in the highest category of occupational exposure was 0.76 (95% CI 0.68 to 0.86) – paradoxically slightly protective.[34] More continuous, non-occupational sun exposure also appears to be associated with a lower risk of melanoma.[35]

Some understanding of these paradoxical results for occupational sun exposure is offered by studies that suggest that incidence of melanoma on usually covered body sites is highest in indoor workers and on usually exposed sites is highest in outdoor workers.[36,37] It is worth noting too that the reference exposure category in studies of occupational sun exposure is generally people without occupational exposure, not people without any exposure. Given the evidence of potent effects of recreational sun exposure on melanoma risk, these apparently protective effects of occupational exposure may not be surprising, particularly if occupationally exposed people have less recreational exposure than other people do.

An interesting perspective on the contributions of ambient solar radiation and a recreational pattern of sun exposure to melanoma can be seen in the relation of latitude and longitude to incidence of melanoma in New South Wales, Australia.[4] Incidence of melanoma falls significantly with increasing latitude (falling ambient solar radiation) and falling longitude (increasing distance from the coast) in both males and females (Figure 6.6). Interestingly, latitude explains only 6% to 9% of the variance in melanoma rates, whereas longitude explains 15% in females and 36% in males (27% if a straight line rather than a quadratic curve is fitted). Access to recreational sun exposure opportunities is much greater along the coast of New South Wales than it is inland.

Effect of pattern of exposure

That melanoma shows weak or absent associations with occupational sun exposure, consistent associations with recreational exposure, and moderately high densities on body sites that are only occasionally exposed to the sun have suggested the intermittent exposure hypothesis.[9]

This hypothesis proposes that risk of melanoma is related to pattern as well as amount of sun exposure and is illustrated in Figure 6.7,[38] as it may be now conceived. It proposes that amount and pattern of sun exposure are independently related to melanoma. That is, given a particular pattern of exposure to sunlight, risk of melanoma increases monotonically with increasing amount of exposure and, given a particular amount

Table 6.2 *Summary of evidence that melanoma is caused by sun exposure (adapted from English et al. 1997[31])*

Area of evidence	Nature of evidence	Strength of evidence*
Related to ambient solar radiation		
Population location	In reasonably homogeneous populations of European origin (for example Australia, United States), incidence of melanoma increases with increasing ambient solar radiation	++
Personal residence history	Individual risk of melanoma increases in proportion to duration of residence in areas of high ambient solar radiation	++
Migration	People of European ethnic origin born in a place of low ambient solar radiation who migrate to an area of high ambient solar radiation have a lower risk of melanoma than people of similar ethnic origin born in the area of high solar radiation	++
Related to cutaneous sun sensitivity		
Ethnic origin	Melanoma is most common in fair-skinned people of European origin and least common in darker skinned people of African and Asian origin	++
Colour of unexposed skin	In people of European origin, risk of melanoma decreases with increasing pigmentation of unexposed skin	++
Ability to tan	In people of European origin, risk of melanoma decreases with increasing ability to develop a tan on exposure to the sun	++
Favours body sites exposed to the sun		
When skin surface area is taken into account, density of occurrence of melanoma is greatest on skin usually exposed to the sun, intermediate on skin occasionally exposed to the sun, and least on skin rarely exposed to the sun		++
Related to personal sun exposure		
Total lifetime exposure	Case–control studies have not shown a consistent relation between recalled total lifetime sun exposure and risk of melanoma	0
Recent total exposure	Similarly, they have not shown a consistent relation between recent or present usual frequency of sun exposure and risk of melanoma	0
Occupational exposure	Most relevant case–control studies have not shown a positive relation between estimated lifetime occupational exposure to the sun and risk of melanoma and some have shown an apparent inverse relation	0
Non-occupational exposure	Most relevant case–control studies have shown one or more significant positive associations between sun exposure during outdoor recreation and risk of melanoma	++
Sunburn	Case–control studies have consistently shown significant associations between recalled frequency or severity of sunburn and risk of melanoma	++
Associated with other sun related conditions		
Almost all relevant case–control studies have shown significant positive associations between risk of melanoma and measures of other sun related skin conditions, such as non-melanocytic skin cancers, solar elastosis, solar lentigines, and solar keratoses		++

*Key: ++, strong evidence of causal effect unlikely to be explained by bias or confounding; +, weak evidence, association is present but may be explained by bias or confounding; 0, conflicting evidence or lack of evidence.

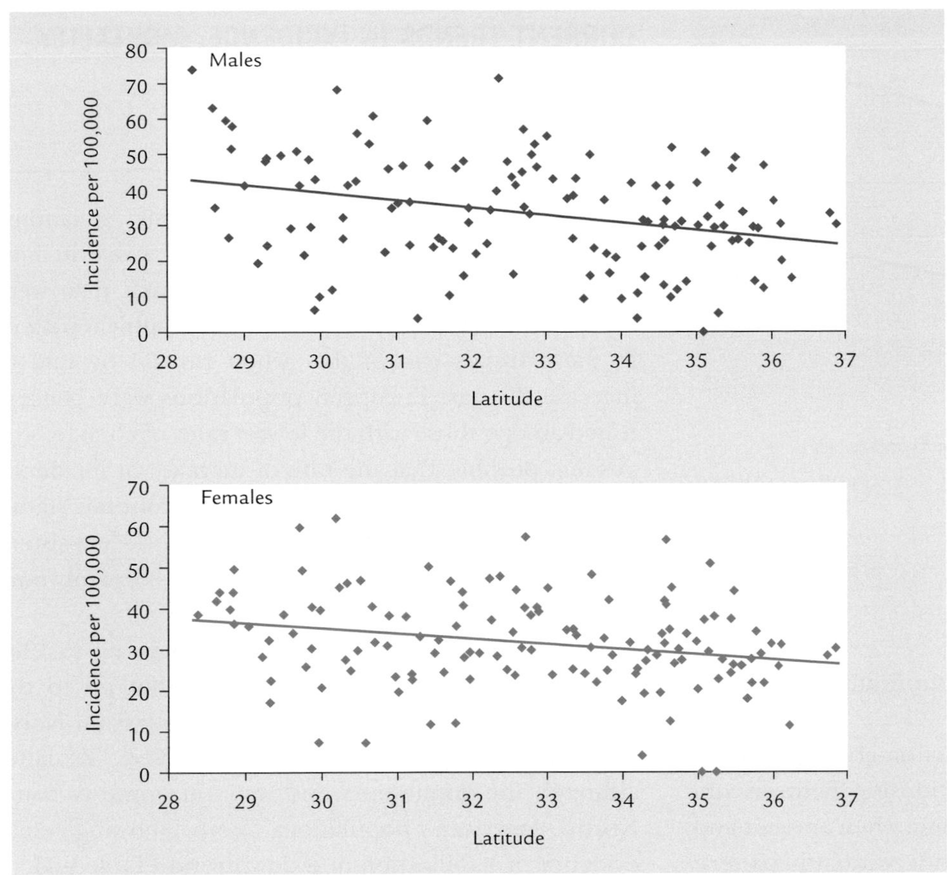

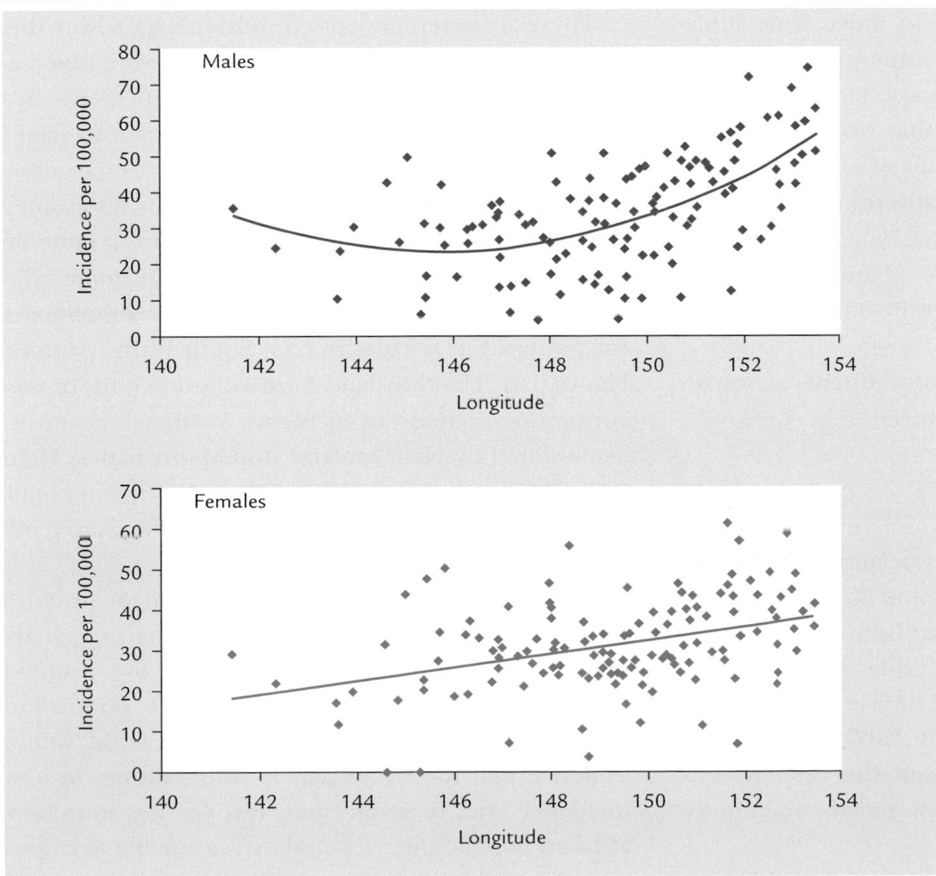

Figure 6.6 *Relation between melanoma incidence and latitude and longitude in New South Wales, Australia.*[4]

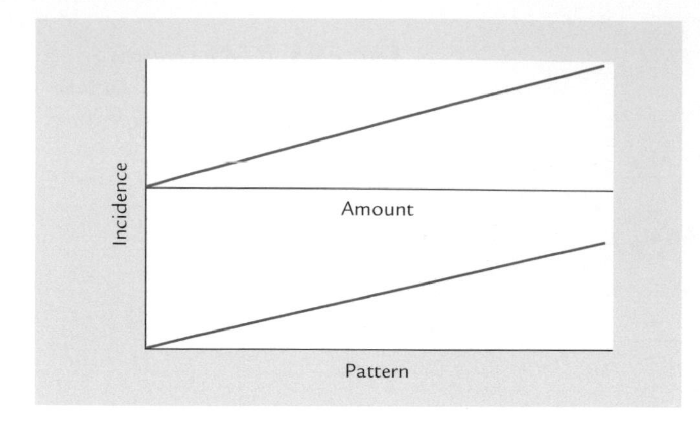

Figure 6.7 *Schematic conception of the hypothesized independence of amount and pattern of sun exposure in causing melanoma.*[37]

of exposure, risk increases monotonically as exposure becomes more intermittent.

This hypothesis makes a prediction about the exposure-response curve for the relationship between sun exposure and melanoma. In real life, when amount and pattern of exposure do not vary independently, pattern of exposure would be expected to move from more intermittent to more continuous as amount of exposure increases. This change would be expected to moderate the increase in melanoma risk that would otherwise follow from the increase in amount of exposure. What few data there are on the exposure-response relation for sun exposure and melanoma suggest that this does indeed occur; i.e. the rate of increase in risk with increasing amount of exposure falls as amount increases.[39]

A biological basis for the intermittent exposure hypothesis has recently been advanced.[40]

Other environmental exposures

Evidence has been obtained of associations of a range of other environmental exposures and lifestyle variables with melanoma, extending from artificial sources of UV radiation to aspects of diet. The evidence for these is generally quite weak. For the sake of brevity, these associations have been summarized in Table 6.3. In most cases Armstrong and English[12] cite the relevant evidence, but some important, more recent, references have been added to the table.

CURRENT TRENDS IN INCIDENCE, MORTALITY, AND SURVIVAL

Time trends in incidence

Between the early 1960s and the late 1980s, melanoma incidences increased by averages of 3–7% a year in most populations of European origin for which data were available.[3] There was little evident geographical pattern in these trends except that when ranked by rate of increase the east European populations were concentrated among those with the lowest rates of change, suggesting, possibly, that the rate of increase in incidence of melanoma has been related to socioeconomic status.

There was, over the same period, little consistent trend, either up or down, in populations of mainly non-European origin.[3]

Data in populations of European origin up to 1992 suggest a more diverse pattern than that up to the late 1980s.[7] In representative populations from North America, Europe, Australia, and New Zealand, although the dominant trend was still upwards, some North American populations were showing clear evidence of stabilization or a downtrend (Table 6.4).

There are heterogeneous trends with age within these populations. Four broad trend patterns were observed. The first, and rarest, was a downtrend in incidence in all age groups. This is exemplified by the pattern seen in Hawaii (Figure 6.8). The second pattern, seen in a number of United States, Canadian, Australian, and some of the higher rate European populations, was a flattening in the uptrend in older age groups and, generally, a downtrend in younger age groups (as exemplified by the pattern for females in New South Wales, Australia; Figure 6.8). The third and most common pattern was a continuing increase in incidence in all age groups (as exemplified by New Zealand non-Maori males; Figure 6.8). This pattern was seen mostly in European populations, New Zealand, and some of the lower rate Australian populations.

Although not argued rigorously here, it would be reasonable to suggest that these patterns suggest that the emerging downtrends in incidence are mainly in more affluent, generally high-incidence populations. Incidence is still increasing, on the other hand, without evidence that the trend may be moderating, in lower incidence and, in some cases, less (or less long term) affluent populations. It would be reasonable to suggest,

Table 6.3 *Summary of associations between environmental and lifestyle variables other than sun exposure that have been associated with melanoma risk*

Exposure	Direction of association	Strength of evidence*	Comments
Artificial sources of UV radiation			
Fluorescent lighting	Causative	0	Some fluorescent tubes emit small amounts of short wavelength UV radiation
Sunbeds or sunlamps	Causative	+[41]	Mainly emit UVB but may also emit some UVA
PUVA (combination of oral psoralen and UVA irradiation of skin)	Causative	+[42,43]	Used to treat psoriasis
Occupational exposures			
Ionizing radiation	Causative	+[44–46]	
Chemicals	Causative	+[44,47]	
Printing industry employment	Causative	+[48]	
Medications			
Oral contraceptives	Causative	+[49]	Risk only evident in long term users and may be present only in current users
Oestrogen replacement	Causative	0	
Immunosuppressive treatment	Causative	+	
Diet			
High intake of polyunsaturated fat	Causative	0[50]	
High alcohol intake	Causative	0	
Antioxidant vitamins	Protective	+	Association is more consistent for vitamin E than for beta-carotene
High selenium intake	Causative	+[51]	
High body weight and height	Causative	+	Evidence is stronger for obesity than high body height
Other			
Use of hair dyes	Causative	0	
Infections causing fever	Protective	0[52]	
Skin trauma	Causative	+[53,54]	Evidence relates mainly to acral melanoma

*Key: ++, strong evidence of causal effect unlikely to be explained by bias or confounding; +, weak evidence, association is present but may be explained by bias or confounding; 0, conflicting evidence or lack of evidence.

Table 6.4 *Percentage changes in age standardized incidence (1983–87 to 1988–92) and patterns of change in age specific incidence (1978–82, 1983–87, 1988–92) of melanoma in large populations of European origin*[7,55,56]

Population	Males		Females	
	% change	Pattern of change	% change	Pattern of change
Canada, British Columbia	+2.1	2	−4.7	2
USA, Hawaii white	−12.2	1	−16.8	1
USA, Los Angeles white	+9.6	2	−2.6	2
USA, San Francisco white	+23.3	3	+9.2	2
USA, Seattle	+11.9	2	+18.9	3
Denmark	+14.3	3	+19.4	3
Finland	+18.2	3	+11.7	2
France, Bas Rhin	+29.4	3	+25.8	3
France, Isere	+46.4	3	+82.4	3
Germany, Saarland	−20.8	3	−27.1	3
Italy, Varese	+30.8	2	+13.6	2
Netherlands, Eindhoven	+33.3	3	+34.4	3
Norway	+34.3	3	+13.3	2
Poland, Warsaw City	+15.2	2	+37.0	3
Slovakia	+22.2	3	+10.0	3
Slovenia	+30.6	3	+35.0	3
Spain, Zaragoza	+0.0	2	+65.0	3
Sweden	+15.8	2	+15.6	3
Switzerland, Zurich	+47.3	3	+9.9	2
UK, England and Wales	+53.3	3	+32.0	3
UK, Scotland	+36.4	3	+18.6	2
Australia, New South Wales	+27.8	2	+8.0	2
Australia, South Australia	+55.3	3	+22.7	2
Australia, Tasmania	+72.8	3	+22.9	3
Australia, Victoria	+36.6	3	+12.8	2
Australia, Western Australia	+29.3	3	+6.4	2
New Zealand, non-Maori	+34.4	3	+29.6	3

Pattern: 1, downtrend in all or nearly all age groups; 2, flattening in uptrend in older age groups and a flattening or downtrend in younger age groups; 3, continuing rise in incidence in all age groups.

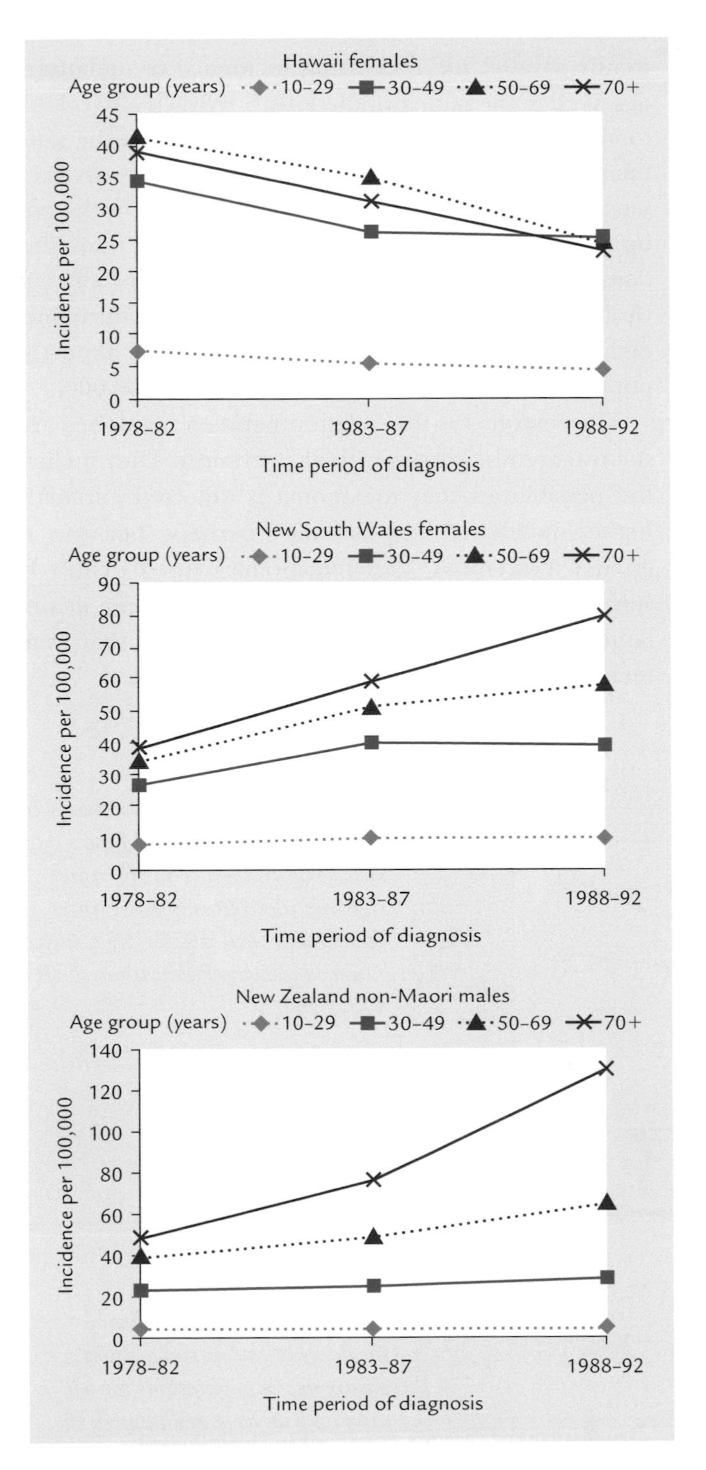

Figure 6.8 *Three different patterns in time trend of age specific incidences of melanoma: downtrend in all or nearly all age groups, illustrated by Hawaii white females; flattening in uptrend in older age groups and a flattening or downtrend in younger age groups, illustrated by New South Wales females; continuing rise in incidence in all age groups, illustrated by New Zealand non-Maori males.*

from one view of melanoma epidemiology, that the ultimate driver behind these patterns is a shift from a mainly occupational to a mainly recreational pattern of sun exposure with increasing affluence. This shift would produce, initially, increasing incidence rates of melanoma, which ultimately stabilize or fall with moderation or cessation of the increase in recreational sun exposure and increasing control of exposure to solar radiation when in the sun.

Time trends in mortality

Melanoma mortality in populations of European origin shows similar patterns to those described above, except that they are more advanced towards eventual or actual downtrends.

La Vecchia et al.[57] described trends in skin cancer mortality (estimated 80–90% melanoma) from 1955 to 1995 in people 20–64 years of age in 18 European countries, the United States, Canada, Australia, and New Zealand. Mortality rose between 1955 and 1984 at 20–44 and 45–64 years of age in men and women with just three exceptions in 88 age, sex, and country specific observations. Whereas between 1985 and 1995, mortality fell in 25 of 44 observations in those 20–44 years of age and in 15 of 44 in those 45–64 years of age.

A more detailed analysis of similar mortality data showed essentially the same three patterns of temporal change in mortality by age as have been described above for incidences.[58] These were:

- increasing rates until generations born around 1930 to 1935 followed by decreasing rates in more recent birth cohorts (Australia, the Nordic countries, and the United States);
- increasing rates until generations born during the second world war, followed by flattening or slightly decreasing rates in more recent birth cohorts (United Kingdom, Canada); and
- a steep, almost linear increase with no major changes in this trend (France, Czechoslovakia, and Italy).

These patterns generally seem more advanced than do those in the incidence trends, thus suggesting that there are factors driving the mortality trends other than the underlying incidence trends. The shift towards thinner lesions with increasing incidence (see below), in part perhaps resulting from better detection, is probably one of these.

Site and thickness of incident melanomas

Increases in incidence in European populations have generally been most pronounced on the trunk, particularly in men, while the incidence of melanoma of the face remained reasonably stable over time.[3] In most, but not all, populations, the relative increases have been seen in the thinnest melanomas, but absolute increases have occurred in thick as well as thin melanomas.[3,59]

Time trends in survival

There is a general trend for relative survival from melanoma after diagnosis to increase with time in populations of European origin as illustrated for the SEER populations of the United States in Figure 6.9. These trends parallel the increasing incidence of melanoma observed in the same populations. Survival is also related to incidence in different populations at about the same time (Figure 6.10). In this case, 5-year relative survival is seen to increase with increasing incidence in both sexes up to about an incidence of 12/100,000 and thereafter does not seem to increase further. Put another way, survival was greater than 80% in all populations with an incidence above 12/100,000 and less than 80% for almost all populations with an incidence less than 5/100,000.

The reasons for this relation between incidence and survival are not known with any certainty. They include the possibilities that melanoma is detected earlier in higher incidence populations (perhaps because of greater awareness), that melanoma caused mainly by sun exposure is less aggressive than melanoma arising largely in the absence of sun exposure, and that treatment is better in high incidence populations.

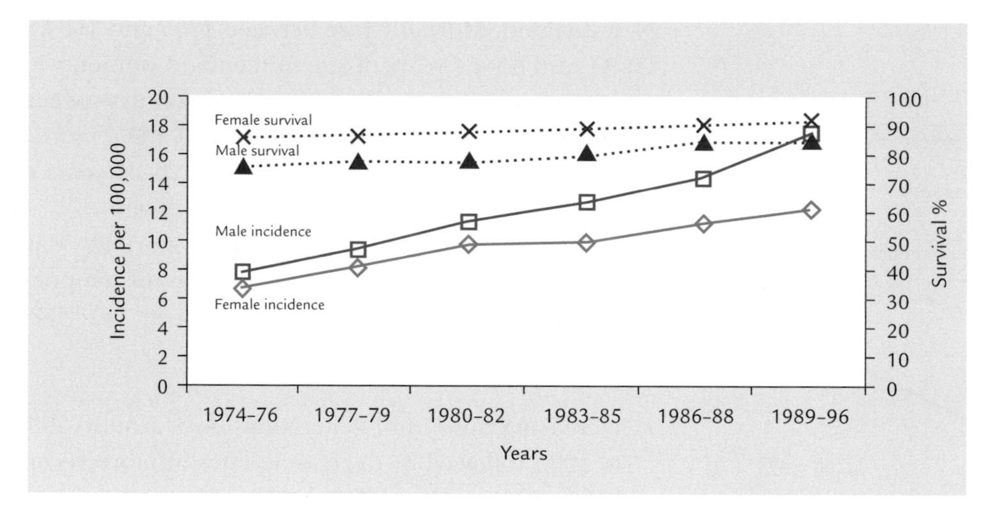

Figure 6.9 *Comparison in trends in incidence of and survival from melanoma in the US SEER cancer registries (data from SEER Cancer Statistics Review, 1973–1997, http://seer.cancer.gov/Publications/CSR1973_1997/).*

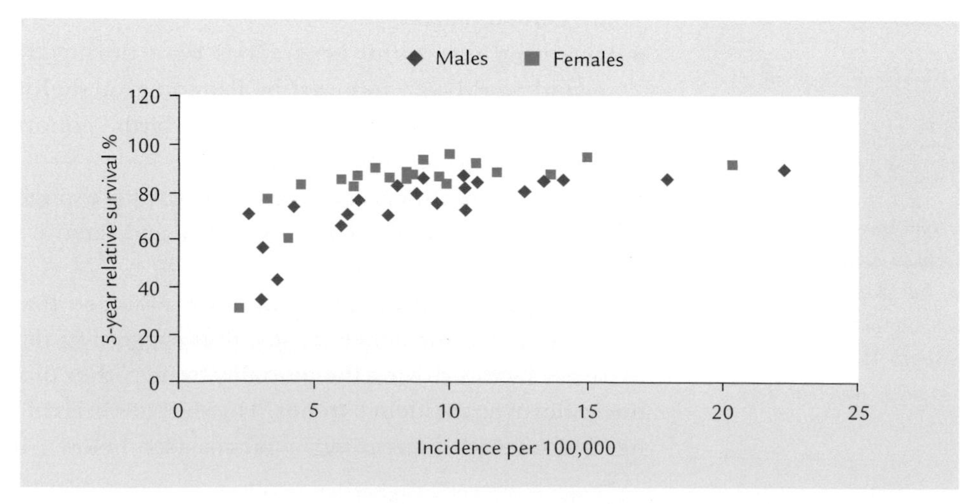

Figure 6.10 *Relation between incidence of and survival from melanoma in populations for which data on both were available in the mid 1980s (Canada Ontario, Quebec and Saskatchewan; USA Atlanta, Connecticut, Detroit, Hawaii, Iowa, New Mexico, San Francisco-Oakland, Seattle, Utah; Denmark, Finland, France Bas Rhin, Italy Latina, Netherlands Eindhoven, Norway, Slovenia, Switzerland Geneva, Sweden; UK North Western England and Scotland; South Australia[7,60]).*

REFERENCES

1. Parkin DM, Pisani P, Ferlay J, Estimates of the worldwide incidence of 25 major cancers in 1990. *Int J Cancer* 1999; 80: 827–41.
2. Pisani P, Parkin DM, Bray F, Ferlay J, Estimates of the worldwide mortality from 25 cancers in 1990. *Int J Cancer* 1999; 83: 18–29.
3. Armstrong BK, Kricker A, Cutaneous melanoma. *Cancer Surv* 1994; 19: 219–40.
4. Nguyen HL, Armstrong B, Coates M, Cutaneous melanoma in NSW in 1983 to 1995. New South Wales: Sydney Cancer Council, 1997.
5. Subramaniam R, Smith D, Coates M, Armstrong B, Survival from cancer in New South Wales in 1980 to 1995. NSW Cancer Council: Sydney, 1999.
6. Armstrong BK, Kricker A, How much melanoma is caused by sun exposure? *Melanoma Res* 1993; 3: 395–401.
7. Parkin DM, Whelan SL, Ferlay J, et al, Cancer incidence in five continents Volume VII. International Agency for Research on Cancer: Lyon, 1997.
8. Australian Institute of Health and Welfare and Australasian Association of Cancer Registries, *Cancer in Australia 1998* (Cancer Series No.17). Canberra: Australian Institute of Health and Welfare, 1998, p42.
9. Armstrong BK, Melanoma of the skin. *Br Med Bull* 1984; 40: 346–350.
10. Holman CD, Mulroney CD, Armstrong BK, Epidemiology of pre-invasive and invasive malignant melanoma in Western Australia. *Int J Cancer* 1980; 25: 317–23.
11. Bulliard JL, Site-specific risk of cutaneous malignant melanoma and pattern of sun exposure in New Zealand. *Int J Cancer* 2000; 85: 627–32.
12. Armstrong BK, English DR, Cutaneous malignant melanoma. In: *Cancer epidemiology and prevention* (eds Schottenfeld D, Fraumeni JF). Oxford University Press: New York, 1996: 1282–312.
13. Harrison RA, Haque AU, Roseman JM, Soong SJ, Socioeconomic characteristics and melanoma incidence. *Ann Epidemiol* 1998; 8: 327–33.
14. Kirkpatrick CS, Lee JA, White E, Melanoma risk by age and socio-economic status, *Int J Cancer* 1990; 46: 1–4.
15. Holman CD, Armstrong BK, Cutaneous malignant melanoma and indicators of total accumulated exposure to the sun: an analysis separating histogenetic types. *J Natl Cancer Inst* 1984; 73: 75–82.
16. Holman CD, Armstrong BK, Pigmentary traits, ethnic origin, benign nevi, and family history as risk factors for cutaneous malignant melanoma. *J Natl Cancer Inst* 1984; 72: 257–66.
17. Cawley EP, Genetic aspects of malignant melanoma. *AMA Arch Dermatol Syphilol* 1952; 65: 440–50.
18. Aitken JF, Duffy DL, Green A, et al, Heterogeneity of melanoma risk in families of melanoma patients, *Am J Epidemiol* 1994; 140: 961–73.
19. Aitken JF, Bailey-Wilson J, Green AC, et al, Segregation analysis of cutaneous melanoma in Queensland. *Genet Epidemiol* 1998; 15: 391–401.
20. Holland EA, Schmid H, Kefford RF, Mann GJ, CDKN2A (P16(INK4a)) and CDK4 mutation analysis in 131 Australian melanoma probands: effect of family history and multiple primary melanomas. *Genes Chromosom Cancer* 1999; 25: 339–48.
21. Aitken J, Welch J, Duffy D, et al, CDKN2A variants in a population-based sample of Queensland families with melanoma. *J Natl Cancer Inst* 1999; 91: 446–52.
22. Goldstein AM, Falk RT, Fraser MC, et al, Sun-related risk factors in melanoma-prone families with CDKN2A mutations. *J Natl Cancer Inst* 1998; 90: 709–11.
23. Soufir N, Avril MF, Chompret A, et al, Prevalence of p16 and CDK4 germline mutations in 48 melanoma-prone families in France. The French Familial Melanoma Study Group. *Hum Mol Genet* 1998; 7: 209–16.
24. Green A, MacLennan R, Youl P, Martin N, Site distribution of cutaneous melanoma in Queensland. *Int J Cancer* 1993; 53: 232–6.
25. Elwood JM, Gallagher RP, Body site distribution of cutaneous malignant melanoma in relationship to patterns of sun exposure. *Int J Cancer* 1998; 78: 276–80.
26. Kukita A, Ishihara K, Clinical features and distribution of malignant melanoma and pigmented nevi on the soles of the feet in Japan, *J Invest Dermatol* 89; 92: 210S–13S.
27. Elwood JM, Epidemiology and control of melanoma in white populations and in Japan. *J Invest Dermatol* 1989; 92: 214S–21S.
28. Stevens NG, Liff JM, Weiss NS, Plantar melanoma: is the incidence of melanoma of the sole of the foot really higher in blacks than whites. *Int J Cancer* 1990; 45: 691–3.
29. Bliss JM, Ford D, Swerdlow AJ, et al, Risk of cutaneous melanoma associated with pigmentation characteristics and freckling: systematic overview of 10 case–control studies. The International Melanoma Analysis Group (IMAGE). *Int J Cancer* 1995; 62: 367–76.
30. Weinstock MA, Colditz GA, Willett WC, et al, Moles and site-specific risk of non-familial cutaneous malignant melanoma in women. *J Natl Cancer Inst* 1989; 81: 948–52.
31. Swerdlow AJ, English J, MacKie RM, et al, Benign melanocytic naevi as a risk factor for malignant melanoma, *BMJ* 1986; 292: 1555–9.
32. Tucker MA, Halpern A, Holly EA, et al, Clinically recognized dysplastic nevi. A central risk factor for cutaneous melanoma. *JAMA* 1997; 277: 1439–44.
33. English DR, Armstrong BK, Kricker A, Fleming C, Sunlight and cancer. *Cancer Causes Control* 1997; 8: 271–83.
34. Elwood JM, Jopson J, Melanoma and sun exposure: an overview of published studies. *Int J Cancer* 1997; 73: 198–203.
35. Walter SD, King WD, Marrett LD, Association of cutaneous malignant melanoma with intermittent exposure to ultraviolet radiation: results of a case–control study in Ontario, Canada. *Int J Epidemiol* 1999; 28: 418–27.
36. Beral V, Robinson N, The relationship of malignant melanoma, basal and squamous skin cancers to indoor and outdoor work. *Br J Cancer* 1981; 44: 886–91.
37. Vagero D, Ringback G, Kiviranta H, Melanoma and other tumors of the skin among office, other indoor and outdoor workers in Sweden 1961–1979. *Br J Cancer* 1986; 53: 507–12.
38. Armstrong BK, Kricker A, English DR, Aetiology and pathogenesis of skin cancer: sun exposure and skin cancer. *Australas J Dermatol* 1997; 58: S1–S6.
39. Elwood JM, Gallagher RP, Hill GB, Pearson JC, Cutaneous melanoma in relation to intermittent and constant sun exposure – the Western Canada Melanoma Study. *Int J Cancer* 1985; 35: 427–33.
40. Gilchrest BA, Eller MS, Geller AC, Yaar M, The pathogenesis of melanoma induced by ultraviolet radiation. *NEJM* 1999; 340: 1341–8.
41. Westerdahl J, Ingvar C, Masback A, et al, Risk of cutaneous malignant melanoma in relation to use of sunbeds: further evidence of UV-A carcinogenicity. *Br J Cancer* 2000; 82: 1593–9.
42. Stern RS, Nichols KT, Vakeva LH, Malignant melanoma in patients treated for psoriasis with methoxsalen (psoralen) and ultraviolet A radiation (PUVA). The PUVA Follow-Up Study, *NEJM* 1997; 336: 1041–5.
43. Lindelof B, Sigurgeirsson B, Tegner E, et al, PUVA and cancer risk: the Swedish follow-up study. *Br J Dermatol* 1999; 141: 108–12.
44. Austin DF, Reynolds P, Investigation of an excess of melanoma among employees of the Lawrence Livermore National Laboratory, *Am J Epidemiol* 1997; 145: 524–31.
45. Ron E, Preston DL, Kishikawa M, et al, Skin tumor risk among atomic-bomb survivors in Japan. *Cancer Causes Control* 1998; 9: 393–401.
46. Gundestrup M, Storm HH, Radiation-induced acute myeloid leukaemia and other cancers in commercial jet cockpit crew: a population-based cohort study. *Lancet* 1999; 354: 2029–31.
47. Moore DH, Patterson HW, Hatch F, et al, Case–control study of malignant melanoma among employees of the Lawrence Livermore National Laboratory, *Am J Ind Med* 1997; 32: 377–91
48. Nielsen H, Henriksen L, Olsen JH, Malignant melanoma among lithographers. *Scand J Work Environ Health* 1996; 22: 108–11.
49. Feskanich D, Hunter DJ, Willett WC, et al, Oral contraceptive use and risk of melanoma in premenopausal women. *Br J Cancer* 1999; 81: 918–23.
50. Veierod MB, Thelle DS, Laake P, Diet and risk of cutaneous malignant melanoma: a prospective study of 50,757 Norwegian men and women, *Int J Cancer* 1997; 71: 600–4.
51. Vinceti M, Rothman KJ, Bergomi M, et al, Excess melanoma incidence in a cohort exposed to high levels of environmental selenium. *Cancer Epidemiol, Biomarkers Prev* 1998; 7: 853–6.
52. Kolmel KF, Pfahlberg A, Mastrangelo G, et al, Infections and melanoma risk: results of a multicentre EORTC case–control study.

European Organization for Research and Treatment of Cancer. *Melanoma Res* 1999; 9: 511–9.

53. Rolon PA, Kramarova E, Rolon HI, et al, Plantar melanoma: a case–control study in Paraguay. *Cancer Causes Control* 1997; 8: 850–6.
54. Green A, McCredie M, MacKie R, et al, A case–control study of melanomas of the soles and palms (Australia and Scotland). *Cancer Causes Control* 1999; 10: 21–5.
55. Muir C, Waterhouse J, Mack T, et al, Cancer incidence in five continents Volume V. International Agency for Research on Cancer: Lyon, 1987.
56. Parkin DM, Muir CS, Whelan SL, et al, Cancer incidence in five continents Volume VI. International Agency for Research on Cancer: Lyon, 1992.
57. La Vecchia C, Lucchini F, Negri E, Levi F, Recent declines in worldwide mortality from cutaneous melanoma in youth and middle age, *Int J Cancer* 1999; 81: 62–6.
58. Severi G, Giles GG, Robertson C, et al, Mortality from cutaneous melanoma: evidence for contrasting trends between populations, *Br J Cancer* 2000; 82: 1887–91.
59. Dennis LK, Analysis of the melanoma epidemic, both apparent and real: data from the 1973 through 1994 surveillance, epidemiology, and end results program registry, *Arch Dermatol* 1999; 135: 275–80.
60. Berrino F, Sant A, Verdecchia R, et al, Survival of cancer patients in Europe: the EUROCARE study. International Agency for Research on Cancer: Lyon, 1995.

7

Prevention strategies, early detection, and results of education programmes

Jason K Rivers, Robert C Burton

INTRODUCTION

In many countries the incidence of malignant melanoma (MM) has increased steadily for several decades.[1–5] Moreover, there is some suggestion that MM may be the most rapidly increasing cancer in white populations.[1] Although there is some concern that the apparent epidemic may be due in part to aggressive screening, there are data to suggest that the increase in both MM incidence and mortality is real.[6,7]

As MM continues to be a public health problem in many countries, there has been an impetus to develop prevention, early detection, and educational programmes that will help to reduce the morbidity and death associated with this disease. This chapter will review some of the issues related to these public health topics.

PREVENTION STRATEGIES

It has been suggested that the burden of MM may be lowered through effective primary and secondary preventive measures. Primary prevention emphasizes the reduction of sun exposure from childhood onwards, whereas secondary prevention strategies focus on early detection of skin cancer.

Armstrong and Kricker have estimated that 80% or more of MM are caused by sun exposure even in white populations resident in areas of low solar flux and with low incidences of MM.[8] Although the mechanism remains unclear, many investigators have concluded that acute, intense exposure to sunlight, especially exposure that causes erythema and inflammation (sunburn) is strongly linked to the development of MM.[9] People who have had MM are twice as likely to have experienced at least one episode of severe sunburn and are more than three times as likely to report several episodes of severe sunburn compared with those with no history of the disease. However, epidemiological data to suggest that sunburns occurring early in life carry a higher risk of MM remain limited.[9,10]

When one thinks of sun protection, sunscreens immediately come to mind. However, recent concern has been voiced that sunscreens may in fact increase the risk of developing MM because the use of high SPF sunscreen promotes extended duration of sun exposure.[11] Although one study showed a protective effect of chemical sunscreen against MM, most previous studies have suggested either no association or a positive correlation between sunscreen use and MM risk.[12–17] The presence of melanocytic naevi (moles) is a strong risk factor for the development of MM.[18] Therefore, the results of a recently published prospective study that demonstrated broad spectrum sunscreens may attenuate the number of moles in white children, especially if they freckle, is encouraging.[19] These findings suggest that sunscreens should still be considered an important part of a comprehensive programme to reduce overall sun exposure. However, it should be emphasized that sunscreens need to be applied liberally and before sun exposure to be effective.[20]

Australia, with the highest incidence of MM worldwide, has taken the lead in public health education.[21]

The ultimate goal of public health campaigns against MM is to reduce the incidence and mortality to the lowest achievable level. There is no strong evidence of a relation between diet, vitamin A, β-carotene, and related compounds in the pathogenesis of MM.[22] Therefore, the main focus of primary prevention programmes is the protection of children and adolescents from excessive sun exposure. Education campaigns have focused on natural protection as the best protection. This includes avoiding the sun when the ultraviolet (UV) radiation is maximal (the two hours around solar noon), use of clothing and hats, and seeking shade while outside. Sunscreens (with a sun protection factor of 15 or higher) are advocated as an adjunct to natural protection, not a replacement for it. In Australia, structural changes have included the development and institution of occupational health and safety guidelines, working with local officials for policies on the provision of shade in public areas, the distribution of effective yet inexpensive sunscreens, and the establishment of standards for testing the sun protective ability of clothing materials. An evaluation of this type of programme indicates that there may in fact be a paradigm shift occurring in Australia.[21] Fewer people are being sunburnt each summer, and the pursuit of the perfect tan is waning. Furthermore, it has been predicted that a comprehensive Australian national skin cancer primary prevention programme would provide excellent 'value for money': a 20-year commitment of A$5m annually (28 cents per person) would avoid 4300 premature deaths and cost only A$1360 per life-year saved.[23]

Other countries such as the United States and Canada have implemented public education campaigns that have effectively reached large sectors of the population by means of a mix of media approaches (television, radio, written brochures, and pamphlets).[24,25] An excellent manual published by the International Union Against Cancer offers guidelines for the implementation of MM control programmes for those who are interested.[26] In the United States, numerous non-profit organizations provide resources for public education on sun education and skin cancer prevention.[27] The internet is fast becoming a major resource source for both public and professional information. For this, the reader is directed to two sites of interest: http://www.aad.org and http://www.nci.nih.gov/info/what.htm.

EARLY DETECTION

Early detection of disease is the second approach to MM control. Melanoma is curable when detected early: the 5-year survival is 95–99% when the tumour has a Breslow thickness of <0.75 mm.[28] Therefore, the goal of secondary prevention (early detection) is to reduce mortality by teaching professionals and lay people alike the clinical features of early MM.

Early detection of MM by the healthcare professional

In order for healthcare professionals to help in the reduction of mortality associated with MM they must be able to accurately assess a pigmented lesion in order to determine the likelihood that it is malignant.

About a decade ago, Curley et al. demonstrated that only half of 116 apparently benign pigmented lesions were diagnosed correctly.[29] Three of these lesions were MM, and all were misdiagnosed by at least one of the three experienced observers. In another study, for 21% of cases of MM at least two months elapsed between physicians' observation of lesions and a definitive diagnosis of MM, while 13% of cases were diagnosed at a minimum of four months after a visit to a physician.[30] However, in another setting, Doherty and Mackie confirmed that delays in diagnosis could be reduced through an education programme directed to the primary care provider.[31] More recent reports continue to emphasize the problem. Stephenson et al. reported that more than 50% of family physicians surveyed stated they lacked confidence in being able to recognize MM.[32] Yet, thin MMs are more likely to be detected by physicians than the patients themselves, suggesting that increased awareness by all physicians may result in greater detection of early MMs.[33] This point is highlighted by the study of Burton et al. that showed that trained general practitioners were notably better than untrained general practitioners at diagnosing as MM suspicious pigmented lesions that subsequently proved to be MM.[34] Therefore, educational programmes directed to general practitioners may help to increase their confidence and ability to diagnose MM at an early stage of disease.

What about skin specialists? The diagnostic accuracy for MM by dermatologists has been reported to range between 31% and 64% depending on their level of experience.[35,36] Grin et al. have shown that, in a series of

265 histologically confirmed MMs, the correct clinical diagnosis of MM was made in almost 85%, indicating a high degree of sensitivity.[37] Gerbert et al. have recently shown that, although dermatologists and resident dermatologists may not accurately diagnose MM clinically 25% of the time, primary care residents fail to do so 40% of the time.[38] Thus, dermatologists can diagnose MM, but there is certainly room for improvement.

The skin lends itself readily to inspection, and this can be performed in a matter of minutes. Rigel et al. have presented data to suggest that patients having complete cutaneous examinations are more likely to have an MM detected than those having a partial skin review, though this has been contested.[39,40] Only 20% of MM arise on skin regularly exposed to the sun. Thus, if examination is to be limited, it is most important to at least examine the difficult to see areas such as the back.

A number of tools have been developed to aid in the diagnosis of early MM. These include telemedicine, photographic techniques, epiluminescence microscopy, and computer based image analysis.

Telemedicine

As we enter the 21st century, telemedicine is becoming established as a way of reaching patients in remote communities or serving as a way to bring the specialist to the community. A pilot study of digital imaging in skin cancer showed that there was almost complete agreement among and between clinical and digital examiners, on differential diagnosis and biopsy recommendations.[41] In another study, three of four MMs were correctly diagnosed by telemedicine suggesting that video conferencing equipment can be used with a reasonable degree of accuracy for the diagnosis of MM.[42] Although the United Kingdom's multicentre teledermatology trial did not include patients with MM, the results indicated that a high proportion of dermatological conditions could be managed successfully by real-time teledermatology.[43] Patients find telemedicine acceptable, which lends further support to more research in this area.[44,45]

Photography

The use of photographs to document new or changing melanocytic naevi is broadly accepted in the literature.[46,47] Photographs provide an objective means by which a physician can tell a patient that a particular lesion has or has not changed with time.

Some feel that total body photography is too labour intensive to perform in a clinical setting. However, once experienced in the technique, a photographer can efficiently perform the series of images involved in total body photography in less than 5 minutes.[48] As changes in naevi may be difficult to detect, a baseline set of photographs may in fact reduce the time for a cutaneous examination, especially if the patient has hundreds of lesions.

In one study, early diagnosis of low risk MMs was possible in 10 of 18 patients followed for atypical naevi as a direct result of changes detected on baseline photographs.[49] In another study, 20 new MM were detected in 16 patients – an incidence of 46 times that of the general Australian population.[46] Eleven were detected because of changes evident in comparison with baseline photographs. Surveillance of this sort was much more cost-effective in preventing life threatening MM than prophylactic excision of atypical naevi.

Polaroid photography of a single suspicious naevus and follow up of the patient to assess whether the naevus had changed or not promises to be an effective aid to the diagnosis of MM in primary health care.[50] In this Australian study, which compared the diagnosis of MM by primary healthcare physicians (general practitioners) in two rural cities, general practitioners who were provided with Polaroid cameras and an algorithm maintained their rate of diagnosis of MM but halved the ratio of naevi to MM which they excised. This aid to the diagnosis of MM is applicable generally and would complement whole body photography in patients with many normal and/or atypical naevi.

It should be borne in mind that an accurate representation of the lesions is key: variable lighting and camera exposure settings will result in inaccurate replication of the image colour and size. Different film developing techniques and even different types of film can modify the final image. Therefore, to compare images accurately over time, photographic techniques should be standardized in terms of ambient light, film type, exposure setting, and distance from a measured reference lesion.[48]

Epiluminescence microscopy

Epiluminescence microscopy (EM) is a non-invasive technique involving skin magnification in conjunction with oil immersion. It is used to examine pigmented lesions of the skin through the enhancement of the subsurface structures that allows for the identification of features not readily appreciated by the naked eye. Hand held EM devices, dermoscopes, have been available to the clinician for the past 14 years. Dermoscopy is a valuable tool for those formerly trained in its use.[51] Steiner et al. found that EM improved diagnostic accuracy by 12–21%.[52] By means of EM, Nachbar et al. conducted a prospective study of 172 melanocytic lesions. In this series, diagnostic accuracy of MM was 80.0% with EM compared with 64.4% using the unaided eye.[53] A complete discussion on EM will be found in Chapter 18 in this book.

Computer image analysis

EM images can be attained for computerized image analysis. Initially, images were digitized from photographic slides with the Heine dermoscopic camera. Later, analog video camera/frame grabber combinations were developed for direct acquisition, display, and processing of digitized images.

The computer automatically subjects the digitized images to an analytic sequence, which begins with lesion segmentation – determination of the boundary separating the lesion from the surrounding normal skin. Surprisingly, this is a difficult issue and has not been completely resolved.[54] Next, feature extraction takes place. That is, diagnostically important features in the image characteristic for either MM or benign lesions are evaluated. For example, Seidenari et al. evaluated lesion area, symmetry, shape, colour distribution, and texture.[55] One hundred per cent sensitivity and 92% specificity were reported for a test set of 365 naevi and 18 thin invasive MMs. Others have also shown sensitivity and specificity ranging between 90–98% and 74–81%, respectively.[56,57]

Most recently, another group has developed multispectral digital microscopy employing a unique version of 'expert system' software designed for automatic image processing from segmentation through feature extraction and classification.[58] For each lesion, the system acquires 10 dermoscopic images, each using light of a different wavelength – ranging over the visible region into the near infrared region. Classification can be determined in less than five minutes. In preliminary studies, 100% sensitivity to MM was achieved, at 85% specificity, when the images of 63 MMs and 183 melanocytic naevi were processed automatically.[59]

Early detection of MM in the community

Ultimately, the responsibility for the early detection of MM rests with the individual. Several reports have documented that patient delay in seeking treatment for MM stems from a lack of knowledge.[59,60] Women are more likely to perform skin self examination and to seek skin cancer screening, at least in some countries.[24,61,62] Furthermore, women are more likely to discover their own lesions as well as those of their spouse.[63] Men are more likely to present with a thick primary tumour.[64] However, in a percentage of patients, poor prognosis can be accounted for by aggressive rapidly growing tumours rather than delays in diagnosis.[65]

In the United States, increases in knowledge and awareness have occurred without major evidence of behavioural change.[25] Miller et al. found that 74% of a sample of white Americans older than 50 years were aware of MM and more than 60% had ever examined their skin for cancer.[66] In other studies, self examination is estimated to range from 20% to 48% and the level is consistently lower in men and those with less education.[67–69]

The ability of patients without MM to document skin findings associated with an increased risk for MM was studied by Gruber et al.[70] Patients identified clinical findings, relative to physician examination as a standard, with sensitivity ranging from 63% to 88% and specificity ranging from 83% to 95% for three cutaneous risk markers. These findings suggest that patients can self select themselves for being at an increased risk to develop MM. More recently in another study,[71] patients' and physicians' counts of atypical naevi were compared directly: 73% of counts agreed within +/− three naevi, but patients tended to overcount naevi on visible body parts, undercount elsewhere and ignore flat naevi. This could have important implications because early MM often appears as a flat cutaneous lesion, and this attribute should be emphasized in public health programmes.

Screening and early detection programmes represent other approaches to secondary prevention. The theoretical and practical aspects of MM screening is the subject of Chapter 9 and has been recently reviewed by Koh et al.[25] In brief, MM is an appealing disease for screening because it is externally visible, it has well known risks factors, and the screening process (visual examination) is acceptable to patients.

Additionally, MM screening fulfils the criteria outlined by Cole and Morrison in that it has serious consequences, is more readily treatable at an early screen detected stage, and has a significant prevalence in the presymptomatic stage.[72] It should be emphasized that screening for MM, whether by self examination or by physician examination, remains controversial. Although some groups advocate its use, others have concluded that there is no rigorous evidence to support its value.[61,73]

Koh et al. have suggested that screening directed to high risk groups would be the most efficient approach to maximize positive predictive value and lower false positives.[25] This could be done at the primary care physician's office as most of the population has seen their doctor in the past two years and, in one sample, 63% of patients diagnosed with MM had seen their doctor in the year before diagnosis.[74]

Optimally, effective screening should be assessed by randomized trials, but logistically this is difficult to accomplish.[73,75] Short term non-randomized studies should be interpreted with caution. Surrogates for decreased mortality such as tumour thickness and improved skin awareness have been suggested as end points for early screening or early detection programmes.

The campaign mounted in Scotland by MacKie et al. best exemplifies the potential impact of an early detection programme.[76] These researchers increased the level of knowledge of skin cancer among general practitioners and established specific pigmented lesion clinics for patient referral. This was followed by mass media education of the general public.

Audit of this programme indicated a significant increase in the proportion of thin MMs diagnosed after the programme was introduced. More important, there was an encouraging fall in the absolute number of thick MM and also of MM related mortality but this was seen only in women. These findings emphasize the need for surveillance of high risk groups such as elderly men, people with an increased number of moles, individuals with clinically atypical naevi, and those with a family history of MM.

It should be noted that a similar campaign caused an appreciable increase in the workload at pigmented lesion clinics, with the greatest increase in referral rate occurring in the three months immediately after the start of the campaign.[77] As well, general practitioners experienced a two- to three-fold increase in workload for pigmented lesions in the weeks immediately after the start of the campaign. The MM to non-MM ratio was 1:33 at the pigmented lesion clinics during the campaign, which compares to the ratio of 1:250 reported at walk-in clinics staffed by dermatologists in the United States.

In the United States, as a response to the increase in MM incidence, primary care providers have been encouraged to increase skin cancer detection efforts. Wender has summarized several of the barriers to effective cancer detection from the perspective of the general practitioner and cites the following: skin cancer is a low priority in primary care; physicians lack the time to perform a complete skin check; practitioners lack the adequate expertise to assess pigmented skin lesions; there is a lack of positive feedback from skin examinations because most primary providers will detect an MM only once or twice per decade; and, there is a perception of inadequate remuneration for time spent on preventive care.[78]

In spite of these concerns, there is evidence, as outlined above, that public health initiatives on the early detection of skin cancer do have a positive impact, especially for high risk populations.

RESULTS OF EDUCATION CAMPAIGNS

The evaluation of MM control programmes in terms of benefits and risks (including costs) is critical for long term policy planning. The ultimate evaluation of a randomized control study would show a sustained decrease in MM mortality in a defined population. However, this type of study would take years to accomplish and would be difficult to implement for logistic reasons. Therefore, researchers have looked for more short term indices to determine whether an educational intervention has had a positive impact on the target group in question. These include (1) improvement in knowledge, attitudes and beliefs about sun protection; (2) decreased rates of deliberate sunbathing, sunburn, and tanning; (3) increased rates of use of sunscreens, hats and protective clothing; (4) decreased use of tanning salons; and (5) evidence of changing societal norms about safe sun behaviour.[25]

Although public education campaigns have been initiated in a number of countries, for most cases, the programmes have focused on educating primary care physicians and the general population regarding the risks of excessive sun exposure and the warning signs of skin cancer.[79–89] The ultimate goal of education programmes in skin cancer prevention is to change people's behaviour so that they will adopt a healthy respect for the sun. Behavioural change, however, must be preceded by knowledge of the hazards associated with sun exposure and a change in attitude. Once a changed behaviour is enacted, it must be sustained for long term effects to be noted.

Knowledge

Investigators have consistently shown that knowledge about MM and safe sun behaviour can be improved through education campaigns.[90–98] In the United States, a nationally representative random digit dial sample of 502 white Americans showed that 74% were aware of MM and the major risk factors were widely known.[90] By contrast, in Australia, over 90% of the population have heard of MM and over 95% of people believe that skin cancer is a serious illness.[85] This difference is probably reflected in the fact that Australia has implemented community wide efforts to reduce sun exposure since the early part of the 1980s.[99]

Attitude

In recent surveys of young American adults roughly two thirds felt healthier and more attractive with a suntan, while 61% stated that people look better with a tan.[25] Australian adolescents' desire for a tan and interest in sunbathing were obstacles to their sun protection on beaches in Victoria.[100] Parents still believe that a tan makes people look better and that children are unlikely to develop skin cancer during their lifetime.[101] More concerning, 54% of a sample of Canadian medical students believed that a tanned appearance was healthy before the implementation of an education curriculum.[97]

However, attitudes can be changed. In Scotland, Fleming et al. reported that parents of school children showed significant improvements in attitude after a 'sun awareness week' campaign.[94] Glanz et al. recently reported on the results of a four week intervention in Hawaii.[95] These investigators developed SunSmart, a skin cancer prevention programme for 6- to 8-year-old children, their parents, and staff at outdoor recreation sites. Positive changes were noted not only in knowledge, but also in readiness to change behaviours. In another study, elementary students from Arizona participated in a 5-week curriculum, Sunny Days, Healthy Ways.[93] The curriculum consisted of five multidisciplinary units and a student workbook. Each unit was about 50 minutes in length and contained lesson material, in class and take home activities, in addition to a student/parent newsletter. Two months after completing the curriculum, students receiving the programme showed less preference for tanning and believed that there were fewer barriers to sunscreen use than did students in the control arm of the study. In France, a prospective, multicentre study evaluated a school based campaign of four weeks duration.[96] Standardized questionnaires were administered eight months before the intervention and again two months after the campaign. Compared with the precampaign answers, more children after the campaign considered that a T-shirt and shade provided better protection than sunscreen, and considered sunlight as a risk factor for skin cancer. Children with fair complexions showed the best improvement in their responses.

Gooderham and Guenther reported first-year medical students in Canada showed a notable change in their attitude to tanning after a one-week dermatology curriculum.[97] However, this was measured at the end of the curriculum so long term changes could not be evaluated. Further interventions aimed at this group of subjects are important because these future physicians will be educating patients through their teaching and behaviour.

Behaviours

In Australia, Girgis et al. implemented an intensive 4-week programme called Skin Safe as part of the school curriculum.[102] Compared with a control group or a group of students that received a standard 30 minute lecture, students who experienced the intervention were more likely to have used a high level of solar protection at both four weeks and eight months follow up. In France, a 4-week programme aimed at primary grade students (aged 9 years) was shown to result in notably less time uncovered in the sun after the intervention.[96] By contrast, Hughes et al. found that, although their intervention (pamphlets, workbooks, and a video) was effective in modifying knowledge and attitudes of secondary school students, the programme had no significant effect on behaviour of the educated group compared with the control group.[92] They concluded that adolescents were a group that is difficult to influence, an observation noted by others.[103] Thus innovative strategies will need to be developed if we are to reach this group of the population, the group most likely to get maximal sun exposure.[104]

Parents of schoolchildren were likely to improve their sun exposure behaviours after a sun awareness media campaign in Scotland. Further, parents who personally take part in sun protection may be more likely to take precautions for their children.[94,105] Thus, programmes that target the entire family may have a greater impact on improved sun safety.

In Australia, population based surveys over the period 1991–98 have shown that the proportion of the population avoiding mid-day weekend sun exposure increased from 50% to 65% and the wearing of hats increased from 40% to 50%; wearing clothes that covered most exposed skin and sunscreen use remained steady at about 45%.[106] The proportion of the population surveyed who reported being sunburnt at weekends halved during this period. Around the world people are using more sunscreen, suggesting that people are modifying their behaviours. Policy change, such as 'no hat, no play', has taken place in Australian schools, and other countries are beginning to follow suit by providing protective clothing and shade provision to outdoor workers.

The ultimate measures of effective prevention and early detection programmes are decreases in MM incidence and mortality. Incidences are levelling off in younger cohorts in some countries, and mortality is now falling in some populations.[1,6,107–109] However, some education programmes have led to transient increases in incidence, which has been attributed to early detection of MM that would have presented at a more advanced stage at a later date, and to the identification of a non-aggressive form of the disease.[3,110] It is hoped that with continued implementation of innovative education programmes that encourage people to both adopt a healthy respect for the sun and perform self screening for MM, these favourable trends in incidence and mortality will continue.

REFERENCES

1. Armstrong BK, Kricker A, Cutaneous melanoma. *Cancer Surveys* 1994; 19: 219–39.
2. Armstrong BK, Epidemiology of malignant melanoma: intermittent or total accumulated exposure to the sun? *J Dermatol Surg Oncol* 1988; 14: 835–49.
3. Burton RC, Coates MS, Hersey P, et al, An analysis of a melanoma epidemic. *Int J Cancer* 1993; 55: 765–70.
4. Franceschi S, La Vecchia C, Lucchini F, Cristofolini M, The epidemiology of cutaneous malignant melanoma: aetiology and European data. *Eur J Cancer Prev* 1991; 1: 9–22.
5. Gloster HM, Brodland DG, The epidemiology of skin cancer. *Dermatol Surg* 1996; 22: 217–26.
6. Hall HI, Miller DR, Rogers JD, et al, Update on the incidence and mortality from melanoma in the United States. *J Am Acad Dermatol* 1999; 40: 35–42.
7. Dennis LK, Analysis of the melanoma epidemic, both apparent and real. Data from the 1973 through 1994 surveillance, epidemiology, and end results programme registry. *Arch Dermatol* 1999; 135: 275–80.
8. Armstrong BK, Kricker A, How much melanoma is caused by sun exposure? *Melanoma Res* 1993; 3: 395–401.
9. Whiteman D, Green A, Melanoma and sunburn. *Cancer Causes Control* 1994; 5: 564–72.
10. Westerdahl J, Olsson H, Ingvar C, At what age do sunburn episodes play a crucial role for the development of malignant melanoma. *Eur J Cancer* 1994; 30A: 1647–54.
11. Autier P, Dore JF, Cattaruzza MS, et al, Sunscreen use and duration of sun exposure: a double-blind, randomized trial. *J Natl Cancer Inst* 1999; 91: 1304–9.
12. Holly EA, Aston DA, Cress RD, et al, Cutaneous melanoma in women, 1: exposure to sunlight, ability to tan, and other risk factors related to ultraviolet light. *Am J Epidemiol* 1995; 141: 923–33.
13. Holman CD, Armstrong BK, Heenan PJ, Relationship of cutaneous malignant melanoma to individual sunlight-exposure habits. *J Natl Cancer Inst* 1986; 76: 403–14.
14. Elwood JM, Gallagher RP, More about: sunscreen use, wearing clothes and a number of nevi in 6- to 7-year-old European children [letter]. *J Natl Cancer Inst* 1999; 91: 1164–6.
15. Autier P, Dore JF, Schifflers E, et al, For the EORTC Melanoma Cooperative Group. Melanoma and use of sunscreens: an EORTC case–control study in Germany, Belgium, and France. *Int J Cancer.* 1995; 61: 749–55.
16. Westerdahl J, Olsson H, Masback A, et al, Is the use of sunscreens a risk factor for malignant melanoma? *Melanoma Res.* 1995; 5: 59–65.
17. Beitner H, Norell SE, Ringborg U, et al, Malignant melanoma: aetiological importance of individual pigmentation and sun exposure. *Br J Dermatol* 1990; 122: 43–51.
18. Evans RD, Kopf AW, Lew RA, et al, Risk factors for development of malignant melanoma I: Review of case control studies. *J Dermatol Surg Oncol* 1988; 14: 383.
19. Gallagher RP, Rivers JK, Lee TK, et al, Broad-spectrum sunscreen use and the development of new nevi in white children. A randomized controlled trial. *JAMA* 2000; 283: 2955–60.
20. Rivers JK, Sunscreens: Is an ounce of prevention worth the hassle? *Dermatol Surg* 2000; 26: 513–14.
21. Marks R, Skin cancer control in Australia. The balance between primary prevention and early detection. *Arch Dermatol* 1995; 131: 474–8.
22. Kirkpatrick CS, Epidemiology of diet and melanoma incidence: a brief review. In: *Epidemiological aspects of cutaneous malignant melanoma.* (eds Gallagher RP, Elwood JM) Boston: Kluwer, 1994: 243–51.
23. Carter R, Marks R, Hill D, Could a national skin cancer primary prevention campaign in Australia be worthwhile? An economic perspective. *Health Prom Int* 1999; 14: 73–82.
24. Rivers JK, Gallagher RP, Public education projects in skin cancer. Experience of the Canadian Dermatology Association. *Cancer* 1995; 75: 661–6.
25. Koh HK, Geller AC, Miller DR, et al, Prevention and early detection strategies for melanoma and skin cancer. Current status. *Arch Dermatol* 1996; 132: 436–43.

26. Marks R, Hill D, *The public health approach to melanoma control: prevention and early detection.* International Union Against Cancer; Geneva: 1992.
27. Robinson, JK, Hornung, RL, Non-profit organizations and public education: a compendium of resources for physicians. *Clin Dermatol* 1998; 16: 461–5.
28. Johnson TM, Smith JW II, Nelson BR, Chang A, Current therapy for cutaneous melanoma. *J Am Acad Dermatol* 1995; 32: 689–707.
29. Curley, RK, Marsden RA, Fallowfield M, Cook MG, Diagnostic accuracy in the clinical evaluation of melanocytic lesions. *Br J Dermatol* 1988; 119(Supp33): 34–5.
30. Cassileth BR, Temoshok L, Frederick BE, et al, Patient and physician delay in melanoma diagnosis. *J Am Acad Dermatol* 1988; 18: 591–8.
31. Doherty VR, Mackie RM, Experience of a public education programme on early detection of cutaneous malignant melanoma. *BMJ* 1988; 287: 388–91.
32. Stephenson A, From L, Cohen A, et al, Family physicians' knowledge of malignant melanoma. *J Am Acad Dermatol* 1997; 37: 953–7.
33. Epstein DS, Lange JR, Gruber SB, et al, Is physician detection associated with thinner melanomas? *JAMA* 1999; 281: 640–3.
34. Burton RC, Howe C, Adamson L, et al, General practitioner screening for melanoma: sensitivity, specificity and effect of training. *J Med Screen* 1998; 5: 156–61.
35. Lindelof A, Hedblad M, Accuracy of clinical diagnosis and patterns of malignant melanoma at a dermatological clinic. *J Dermatol* 1994; 21: 461–4.
36. Perednia DA, Gaines J, Rossum AC, Variability in physician assessment of lesions in cutaneous images and its implications for skin screening and computer-assisted diagnosis. *Arch Dermatol* 1992; 128: 357–64.
37. Grin CM, Kopf AW, Welkovich B, et al, Accuracy in the clinical diagnosis of malignant melanoma. *Arch Dermatol* 1990; 126: 763–6.
38. Gerbert B, Maurer T, Berger T, et al, Primary care physicians as gatekeepers in managed care. *Arch Dermatol* 1996; 132: 1030–8.
39. Rigel DS, Friedman RJ, Kopf AW, et al, Importance of complete cutaneous examination for the detection of malignant melanoma. *J Am Acad Dermatol* 1986; 14: 857–60.
40. De Rooij MJM, Rampen FHJ, Schouten LJ, et al, Total skin examination during screening for malignant melanoma does not increase the detection rate. *Br J Dermatol* 1996; 125: 42–5.
41. Whited JD, Mills BJ, Hall RP, et al, A pilot trial of digital imaging in skin cancer. *J Telemed Telecare* 1998; 4: 108–12.
42. Oakley AMM, Astwood DR, Loane M, et al, Diagnostic accuracy of teledermatology: results of a preliminary study in New Zealand. *NZ Med J* 1997; 110: 51–3.
43. Loane MA, Corbett R, Bloomer MA, et al, Diagnostic accuracy and clinical management by realtime teledermatology. Results from the Northern Ireland arms of the UK Multicentre Teledermatology Trial. *J Telemed Telecare* 1998; 4: 95–100.
44. Loane MA, Bloomer SE, Corbett R, et al, Patient satisfaction with realtime teledermatology in Northern Ireland. *J Telemed Telecare* 1998; 4: 36–40.
45. Oakley AMM, Duffill MB, Reeve P, Practising dermatology via telemedicine. *NZ Med J* 1998; 111: 296–9.
46. Kelly JW, Yeatman JM, Regalia C, et al, A high incidence of melanoma found in patients with multiple dysplastic naevi by photographic surveillance. *Med J Aust* 1997; 167: 191–4.
47. Rhodes AR, Intervention strategy to prevent lethal cutaneous melanoma: Use of dermatologic photography to aid surveillance of high-risk persons. *J Am Acad Dermatol* 1998; 39: 262–7.
48. Slue W, Kopf AW, Rivers JK, Total body photographs of dysplastic nevi. *Arch Dermatol* 1988; 124: 1239–43.
49. Rivers JK, Kopf AW, Vinokur AF, et al, Clinical characteristics of malignant melanomas developing in persons with dysplastic nevi. *Cancer* 1990; 65: 1232–36.
50. Del Mar C, Green AC, Aid to the diagnosis of melanoma in primary health care. *BMJ* 1995; 305: 492–5.
51. Binder M, Schwarz M, Winkler A, et al, Epiluminescence microscopy: A useful tool for the diagnosis of pigmented skin lesions for formerly trained dermatologists. *Arch Dermatol* 1995; 131: 286–91.
52. Steiner A, Pehamberger H, Wolff K, In vivo epiluminescence microscopy of pigmented lesions. II. Diagnosis of small pigmented skin lesions and early detection of malignant melanoma. *J Am Acad Dermatol* 1987; 17: 584–91.
53. Nachbar F, Stolz W, Merkle T, et al, The ABCD rule of dermatoscopy. *J Am Acad Dermatol* 1994; 30: 551–9.
54. Gao J, Zhang, Fleming MG, Pollak I, Gognetta AB, Segmentation of dermatoscopic images by stabilized inverse diffusion equations. *Proceedings of the International Conference on Image Processing 1998.* Vol. 3, , Piscataway, NJ; IEEE, 1998: 823–7.
55. Seidenari S., Pellacani G, Giannetti A, Digital Videomicroscopy and image analysis with automatic classification for detection of these melanomas. *Melanoma Res.* 1999; 9: 163–71.
56. Binder M, Kittler H, Seeber A, et al, Epiluminescence microscopy-based classification of pigmented lesions using computerized image analysis and an artificial neural network. *Melanoma Res* 1998; 8: 261–6.
57. Fleming MG, Image analysis for melanoma diagnosis. *Melanoma Letter* 2000; 18: 1–3.
58. Elbaum M, A unique multispectral digital dermoscope for diagnosis of early melanoma. *Melanoma Letter* 2000; 18: 4–6.
59. Cassileth BR, Clark WH Jr, Heiberger RM, et al, Relationship between patients' early recognition of melanoma and depth of invasion. *Cancer* 1982; 49: 198–200.
60. Temoshok L, DiClemente RJ, Sweet DM, et al, Factors related to patient delay in seeking medical attention for cutaneous malignant melanoma. *Cancer* 1984; 54: 3048–53.
61. Berwick M, Begg CB, Fine JA, et al, Screening of cutaneous melanoma by skin self-examination. *J Natl Cancer Inst* 1996; 88: 17–23.
62. Koh HK, Geller AC, Miller DR, et al. Who is being screened for melanoma/skin cancer? Characteristics of persons screened in Massachusetts. *J Am Acad Dermatol* 1991; 24: 271–7.
63. Brady, MS, Oliveria SA, Christos PJ, et al, Patterns of detection in patients with cutaneous melanoma. Implications for secondary prevention. *Cancer* 2000; 89: 342–7.
64. Hersey P, Sillar RW, Howe CG, et al, Factors related to the presentation of patients with thick primary melanomas. *Med J Aust* 1991; 154: 583–7.
65. Richard MA, Grob JJ, Avril MF, et al, Melanoma and tumor thickness. Challenges of early diagnosis. *Arch Dermatol* 1999; 135: 269–74.
66. Miller DR, Koh HK, Geller AC, Lew RA, National survey of skin cancer awareness and prevention practices in older Americans. In: *Programme and Abstracts of the American Public Health Association Meeting, October 20–24, 1993.* San Francisco, Session 2132.
67. Koh HK, Miller DR, Geller AC, et al, Who discovers melanoma? Patterns from a population-based survey. *J Am Acad Dermatol* 1992; 26: 914–9.
68. Girgis A, Campbell EM, Redman S, Sanson-Fisher RW, Screening for melanoma: a community survey of prevalence and predictors. *Med J Aust* 1991; 154: 338–43.
69. Friedman RJ, Rigel DS, Silverman MK, et al, Malignant melanoma in the 1990s. The continued importance of early detection and the role of physician examination and self examination of the skin. *CA Cancer J Clin* 1991; 41: 201–26.
70. Gruber SB, Roush GC, Barnhill RL, Sensitivity and specificity of self-examination for cutaneous malignant melanoma and risk factors. *Am J Prev Med* 1993; 9: 50–4.
71. Lawson DD, Moore DH II, Schneider JS, et al, Nevus counting as a risk factor from melanoma: comparison of self counts with counts by physicians. *J Am Acad Dermatol* 1994; 31: 438–44.
72. Cole P, Morrison AS, Issues in population screening for skin cancer. *J Natl Cancer Inst* 1980; 64: 1263–72.
73. Elwood JM, Skin self-examination and melanoma. *J Natl Cancer Inst* 1996; 88: 3–15.
74. Geller AC, Koh HK, Miller DR, et al, Use of health services before diagnosis of melanoma: implications for early detection and screening. *J Gen Intern Med* 1992; 7: 154–7.
75. Koh HK, Geller AG, Miller DR, Lew RA, Early detection of melanoma: An ounce of prevention may be a ton of work. *J Am Acad Dermatol* 1993; 28: 645–7.

76. MacKie RM, Hole D, Audit of public education campaign to encourage earlier detection of malignant melanoma. *BMJ* 1992; 304: 1012–15.
77. Melia J, Cooper EJ, Frost T, et al, Cancer Research Campaign health education programme to promote the early detection of cutaneous malignant melanoma. I. Work-load and referral patterns. *Br J Dermatol* 1995; 132: 405–13.
78. Wender RC, Barriers to effective skin cancer detection. *Cancer* 1995; 75: 691–8.
79. Barnes L, Sun education in Ireland. *Clin Dermatol* 1998; 16: 517–18.
80. Brenner S, Wohl Y, Landau M, Sun education in Israel. *Clin Dermatol* 1998; 16: 518–20.
81. George AO, Sun education in Africa: Nigeria and West African subregion. *Clin Dermatol* 1998; 16: 520–1.
82. Goihman-Yahr M, Sun education in Venezuela. *Clin Dermatol* 1998; 16: 522–3.
83. Graham-Brown RAC, Sun education in the United Kingdom. *Clin Dermatol* 1998; 16: 523–5.
84. Katsambas, AD, Katoulis, AC, Varotsos C, Sun education in Greece. *Clin Dermatol* 1998; 16: 525–6.
85. Kim ST, Sun education in Korea. *Clin Dermatol* 1998; 16: 526–7.
86. Marks, R, Sun education in Australia. *Clin Dermatol* 1998; 16: 528–30.
87. Rivers JK, Sun education in Canada. *Clin Dermatol* 1998; 16: 530–1.
88. Schulz EJ, Sun education in South Africa. *Clin Dermatol* 1998; 16: 531–3.
89. Zaitz C, Campbell I, da Rosa Santos OL, Sun education in Brazil. *Clin Dermatol* 1998; 16: 533–4.
90. Koh HK, Geller AC, Miller DR, Lew RA, The current status of melanoma early detection and screening. *Dermatol Clin* 1995; 13: 623–34.
91. Bourke JF, Healsmith MF, Graham-Brown RAC, Melanoma awareness and sun exposure in Leicester. *Br J Dermatol* 1995; 132: 251–6.
92. Hughes BR, Altman DG, Newton JA, Melanoma and skin cancer: evaluation of a health education programme for secondary schools. *Br J Dermatol* 1993; 128: 412–17.
93. Buller DB, Buller MK, Beach B, Ertl G, Sunny Days, Healthy Ways: Evaluation of a skin cancer prevention curriculum for elementary school-aged children. *J Am Acad Dermatol* 1996; 35: 911–2.
94. Fleming C, Newell J, Turner S, Mackie R, A study of the impact of sun awareness week 1995. *Br J Dermatol* 1997; 136: 719–24.
95. Glanz K, Chang L, Song V, et al, Skin cancer prevention for children, parents, and caregivers: A field test of Hawaii's SunSmart programme. *J Am Acad Dermatol* 1998; 38: 413–17.
96. Bastuji-Garin S, Grob JJ, Grognard, C, et al, Melanoma prevention. Evaluation of a health education campaign for primary schools. *Arch Dermatol* 1999; 35: 936–40.
97. Gooderham MJ, Guenther L, Impact of a sun awareness curriculum on medical students' knowledge, attitudes, and behaviour. *J Cutan Med Surg* 1999; 3: 182–7.
98. Gooderham MJ, Guenther L, Sun and the skin: Evaluation of a sun awareness programme for elementary school students. *J Cutan Med Surg* 1999; 3: 230–5.
99. Sinclair C, Borland R, Davidson M, et al, From slip! slap! slop! to sunsmart: A profile of a health education campaign. *Cancer Forum* 1994; 18: 183–7.
100. Pratt K, Borland R, Predictors of sun protection among adolescents at the beach. *Aust Psychol* 1994; 29: 135–9.
101. Buller DB, Borland R, Public education projects in skin cancer prevention: childcare, school, and college-based. *Clin Dermatol* 1998; 16: 447–59.
102. Girgis A, Sanson-Fisher RW, Tripodi DA, et al, Evaluation of interventions to improve solar protection in primary schools. *Health Educ Quart* 1993; 20: 275–87.
103. Koblenzer CS, The psychology of sun-exposure and tanning. *Clin Dermatol* 1998; 16: 421–8.
104. Lovato CY, Shoveller JA, Peters L, Rivers JK, Canadian National Survey on sun exposure and protective behaviours: youth at leisure. *Cancer Prev Control* 1998; 2: 117–22.
105. Zinman R, Schwartz S, Gordan K, et al, Predictors of sunscreen use in childhood. *Arch Pediatr Adolesc Med* 1995; 149: 804–7.
106. Burton R, Malignant melanoma in the year 2000. *CA Cancer J Clin* 2000; 50: 209–13.
107. MacKie RM, Hole D, Hunter JAA, et al, Cutaneous malignant melanoma in Scotland: incidence, survival, and mortality, 1979–94. *BMJ* 1997; 315: 1117–21.
108. Jemal A, Devesa SS, Fears TR, Hartge P, Cancer surveillance series: changing patterns of cutaneous malignant melanoma mortality rates among whites in the United States. *J Natl Cancer Inst* 2000; 92: 811–8.
109. Giles GG, Armstrong BK, Burton RC, et al, Has mortality from melanoma stopped rising in Australia? Analysis of trends between 1931 and 1994. *BMJ* 1996; 312: 1121–5.
110. Burton RC, Armstrong BK, Non-metastasizing melanoma? *J Surg Oncol* 1998; 67: 73–6.

8

The role of sunscreens in melanoma prevention

Philippe Autier, Jean-François Doré

INTRODUCTION

Sun exposure is believed to be the main environmental determinant of skin cancers, and sunburn experience is known to be associated with skin cancer occurrence.[1, 2] Ultraviolet (UV) radiation is deemed to represent that part of the solar spectrum involved in the development of skin cancers, actinic keratoses, and melanocytic naevi. The UV radiation reaching the earth's surface comprises UVB (280–315 nm) and UVA (315–400 nm). The proportion of UVB is highest around noon and decreases with latitude. The carcinogenic properties of the UVB component of the solar spectrum have been known since the 1930s, and it has also been long known that UVB is about one thousand times more erythemogenic than UVA.[1] In the 1980s, the suspicion was raised that UVA might also be involved in the development of skin malignancies.

Sunscreens were primarily formulated for the prevention of sunburn.[3] Besides their ability to delay sunburn occurrence, however, sunscreens can reduce several UV induced skin phenomena. These include the development of non-melanoma skin cancers in rodents, local immunological depression, mutations of the p53 gene in keratinocytes, and the development of actinic keratoses and squamous cell skin cancers in humans.[4–10] As a consequence, sunscreen use has become generally recommended as a sun protection method, and that protection is deemed to increase with increasing sun protection factor (SPF). The SPF value indicates the ability of a sunscreen to delay the skin erythemal reaction induced by solar radiation. In the 1990s, chemical substances specifically designed to block UVA began to be added to sunscreens.

In contrast to laboratory data, retrospective and prospective epidemiological studies have repeatedly shown sunscreen use to be associated with a moderately increased risk for cutaneous melanoma and basal cell skin cancer, and higher numbers of naevi.[11–13] Careful analysis of epidemiological data suggested that the increased risk associated with sunscreen use was not likely to be merely the result of 'indication biases' (sunscreen use would simply be a marker of higher sun exposure or higher natural susceptibility to sunlight).[14–16] However, these studies dealt mainly with earlier types of sunscreens with low SPF ratings, and assessment of past sunscreen use was not accurate. To determine whether findings from epidemiological studies applied to modern high SPF sunscreens, we studied in 1995–96 the determinants of naevus numbers in 631 white European children aged 6–7 years.[17] Sunscreens used by these children had a median SPF value of 17, and most of them contained UVA filters. After adjustment for sun exposure and host characteristics, the number of naevi on the trunk was found to increase steadily with increasing sunscreen use, but to decrease with increasing wearing of clothes (Figure 8.1). The SPF value had no effect on naevus counts, even when the SPF was ≥20. The sharp contrast between results for the wearing of clothes and sunscreen use was also present in the only other epidemiological study that examined the value of clothing in sun protection, in which it was found that

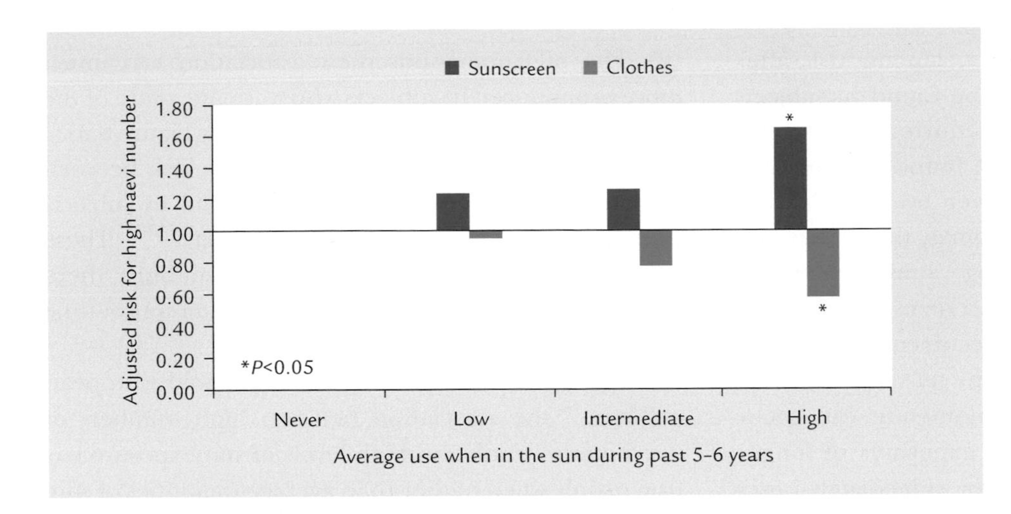

Figure 8.1 *Sunscreen use, wearing clothes, and number of naevi in European children aged 6–7 years (Autier et al., 1998[17]).*

there was a reduced risk of melanoma with increased wearing of clothes.[18]

Most recent data indicate that the sunscreen-melanoma association essentially concerns naevi and melanomas arising on the trunk.[16,17] Since melanoma of the trunk is more common in men than in women, it is not surprising that the association between sunscreen and melanoma has generally been found to be more apparent in men than in women.[16,19]

The apparent contradictions between experimental and observational data raised considerable controversy. Investigation of that puzzling issue was partly hampered by our ignorance about the solar radiations involved in the genesis of melanomas, and partly by the absence of a valid animal model for human melanoma. However, recent epidemiological data suggested that behavioural issues could also be involved in the sunscreen-melanoma association. In the remainder of this chapter, behavioural issues associated with sunscreen use are considered.

EVIDENCE FOR AN ASSOCIATION BETWEEN BEHAVIOURAL ISSUES AND SUNSCREEN USE

If the moderate increase in the risk of developing melanoma and basal cell cancer, and of having a higher number of naevi associated with sunscreen use was true, then what could be the underlying mechanism? How could application onto the skin of products containing organic and inorganic chemical substances able to block UV radiation result in a greater probability of developing a melanoma, a basal cell cancer, or a greater number of naevi?

Epidemiological data were not consistent with a direct carcinogenic effect of any compound incorporated in sunscreens.[13,17] For instance, the association between sunscreen use and melanoma, basal cell cancer and number of naevi was found in different countries at different points in time, and hundreds of sunscreen products of different formulations were used by the individuals who were involved in the epidemiological investigations. The only sunscreen for which a photocarcinogenic effect was suspected was commercialized in France, Belgium, and Greece before 1995, and was prepared with bergamot oil, a natural substance that contains 5-methoxypsoralen (5-MOP). The 5-MOP is a tanning activator and a photocarcinogen. Availability of these 5-MOP sunscreens in France, Belgium, and Greece for use by the general public use was based on laboratory experiments suggesting that 5-MOP sunscreens could be more protective against sun induced DNA damage than regular sunscreens.[20,21] In 1995 epidemiological data providing evidence for a high risk of melanoma associated with the use of 5-MOP sunscreens were published.[14] The risk was particularly great among sun sensitive subjects. In the same year, the European Commission put a ban on these products.[22]

A second possibility was that protection conferred by sunscreens was 'incomplete'.[13] For example, most sunscreens in use before 1990 had a low ability to filter UVA. Therefore, some authors speculated that the melanoma-sunscreen association could be due to UVA that was not stopped by the sunscreen. However, the suggestion of incomplete protection implies that sunscreen use would confer at least some protection.

Following that logic, the highest melanoma risk, after appropriate adjustments, should be found in subjects who have never used sunscreens during intense sun exposure, but this result was not found in most epidemiological studies.[14,16,17] Moreover, even if UVA was involved in the genesis of melanomas, the higher risk of melanoma observed among sunscreen users implies that, although the sunscreens block UVB (and thus delay sunburn occurrence), greater amounts of UVA reach the skin cells than in the absence of sunscreen. This phenomenon can occur only if sunscreen use allows sun exposures of longer duration.[23] The latter consideration immediately raises the matter of behavioural issues.

What is the evidence from observational data for a behavioural problem associated with sunscreen use?

(1) As noted above, invoking the concept of incomplete protection by sunscreens against solar radiation to explain the sunscreen-melanoma association implies that sunscreen use increases the time spent in the sun. Epidemiological data showed a higher risk of melanoma associated with sunbathing when a sunscreen was used than when no sunscreen was used (Figure 8.2).[14] Hence, the induction of extended sun exposure by sunscreen use must be especially marked for intense, brutal sun exposures such as those that occur during sunbathing activities.

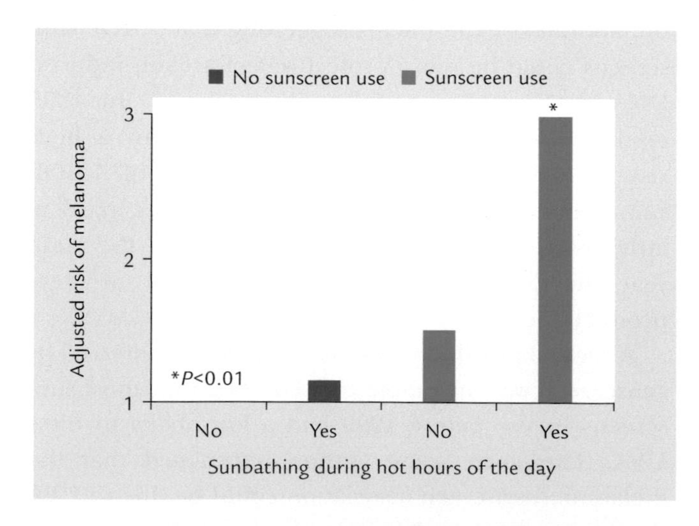

Figure 8.2 *Melanoma risk according to sunbathing activities and sunscreen use in European adults (Autier et al., 1995.[14] Risk adjusted for age, sex, and natural sun sensitivity).*

(2) The melanoma-sunscreen association was much more pronounced in subjects who were not aware of the hazards linked to excessive sun exposure (Figure 8.3).[19]
(3) The largest difference in melanoma risk between sunscreen users and non-users was found in subjects without a history of sunburn in recent years.[14,16,17] These results suggested that in the absence of sunburn, there is virtually no physiological limit to the amount of time spent in the sun.
(4) In the study of naevi in 6- to 7-year-old European children,[17] the association between high numbers of naevi on the trunk and high levels of sun exposure was true mainly when higher than average quantities of sunscreens were used. Taken together, these observations suggested that sunscreen use had a direct influence on the ability to support lengthy exposures of the trunk to intense solar radiation.

STUDIES OF BEHAVIOURAL ISSUES IN RELATION TO SUNSCREEN USE

The most likely hypothesis to explain the sunscreen-melanoma association was that because of their ability to delay sunburn occurrence, sunscreens would encourage sun exposures of greater duration (the 'compensatory hypothesis').

The likelihood of the compensatory hypothesis being correct was supported by the results of a double blind randomized trial conducted in Lyons (France) and in Lausanne (Switzerland) during the summer of 1997.[24] This study of sunscreen use by European

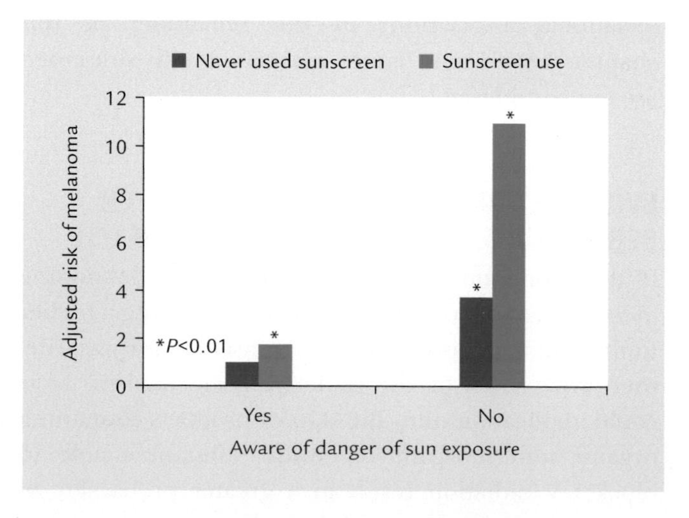

Figure 8.3 *Awareness of dangers of sun exposure and melanoma risk in European adults (Autier et al, 1997[19]).*

students showed that sun exposure was of significantly longer duration ($P<0.01$) when a SPF 30 sunscreen was used compared with when a SPF 10 sunscreen was used. The increase in duration of sun exposure was particularly marked for sunbathing activities. In the first days of holidays, students in both groups started sunbathing at about the same hour (Figure 8.4). However, as holidays progressed, students who used higher SPF products tended to start sunbathing more around noon, when the sunlight is more aggressive (with a greater proportion of UVB radiation), while students who used low SPF sunscreen tended to start sunbathing later in the afternoon. The in study sunburn experience was similar for the two SPF groups. Changes in sun exposure behaviours induced by sunscreens were totally unconscious. During the summer of 1998, the same study was performed in Paris and Thionville (France), and in Brussels (Belgium).[25] A similar difference in daily sunbathing duration was found between the SPF 10 and SPF 30 groups ($P<0.05$), and a similar change in starting hours of sunbathing activities (Figure 8.4).

INTENTIONAL AND NON-INTENTIONAL SUN EXPOSURE

If the compensatory hypothesis is correct, a difficulty arises in the interpretation of results from three human randomized experiments that provided evidence for a protective effect of sunscreen use against the development of actinic keratoses and the number of squamous cell cancers (but not of basal cell cancers).[8–10] Recent data allow a better interpretation of the apparent discrepancies between experimental and observational studies.

Sun exposure is believed to be the main environmental risk factor for the development of naevi, solar keratoses and skin cancers. However the term 'sun exposure' encompasses a wide variety of behaviours. In considering this, a distinction must be made between non-intentional and intentional sun exposure. Non-intentional sun exposure (NISE) is sun exposure occuring as part of normal daily life. During NISE, uncovered body parts are generally the face, the ears, the neck, and the hands. Forearms and legs (especially in women) may also be uncovered, but the trunk is rarely exposed.

Intentional sun exposure (ISE) is essentially motivated by the desire to acquire a tan, or by the wish to go uncovered in the sun. During ISE, significant portions of the trunk and limbs are often exposed. Intentional exposure to ultraviolet light sources other than the sun has also become popular with the increasing availability of artificial tanning devices.

Examples of NISE are outdoor activities such as gardening, but also activities such as skiing, because the primary motive for skiing is not to get a tan. A typical ISE activity is sunbathing. NISE would be more likely to lead to the development of actinic keratoses and squamous cell cancers, while ISE would be more likely to be associated with melanoma development.

ISE, NISE AND THE SUNSCREEN CONTROVERSY

Sun exposure is usually a mix of variable proportions of NISE and ISE. A greater proportion of NISE occurs as chronic sun exposure, and a greater proportion of ISE occurs during holidays in sunny areas (the so called

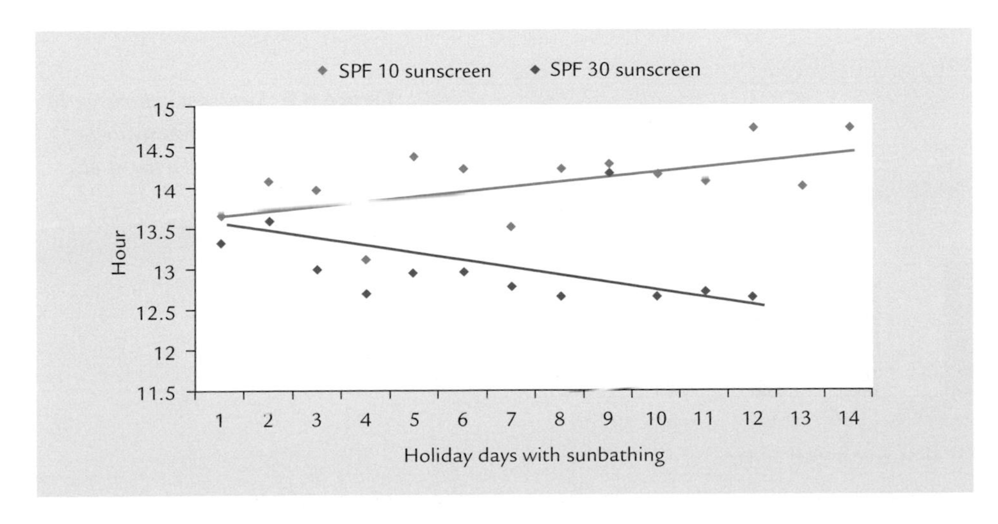

Figure 8.4 *Starting hour of sunbathing during the summer 1998 trial, according to randomization group (Autier et al., 1999[24]).*

intermittent sun exposure pattern). This distinction is relevant to the sunscreen controversy. For example, most observational studies that have suggested a positive association between sunscreen use and melanoma were more concerned about the role of ISE in melanoma occurrence. Sunscreens were primarily designed to prevent sunburn in children and in adults, and most sunburn occurs during ISE.[17,26–28]

The human experiments that demonstrated the ability of sunscreens to prevent the development of actinic keratoses and squamous cell cancers were conducted in NISE situations, with sunscreen (or placebo lotion) applied essentially on the face, ears, neck, and hands. During these trials, subjects either did not experience sunburn, or the number of sunburns was significantly lower in the intervention group.[8,9,29] Also, in the latter trial, there was no evidence of increasing time spent in the sun among subjects allocated to the intervention group.[29] Other studies in NISE situations have provided evidence that sunscreen use can reduce sunburn occurrence.[30]

In contrast, the human experiments that documented longer sun exposure duration with sunscreen use were conducted during ISE situations, among students eager to acquire a tan during their summer holidays.[24,25] In these trials, the sunburn experience was identical for participants using the SPF 10 or the SPF 30 sunscreens.

Several surveys on sunscreen use and sun exposure patterns in ISE situations have yielded data suggesting that sunscreen use (or use of higher SPF products) was associated with longer time spent in the sun, and also with sunburn experience similar to or even worse than if no sunscreen was used.[31–34] For example, in a study among beach attendants in Texas, sun exposure duration increased in parallel with the SPF of the sunscreen used, but use of high SPF sunscreens seemed to be associated with more sunburn episodes (Figures 8.5 and 8.6).[33] Hence, use of a sunscreen during ISE, or use of a higher SPF sunscreen, seem to have little or no impact on sunburn occurrence, a phenomenon most probably attributable to the fact that sun seekers tend to stay in the sun until sunburn modifies their behaviour.

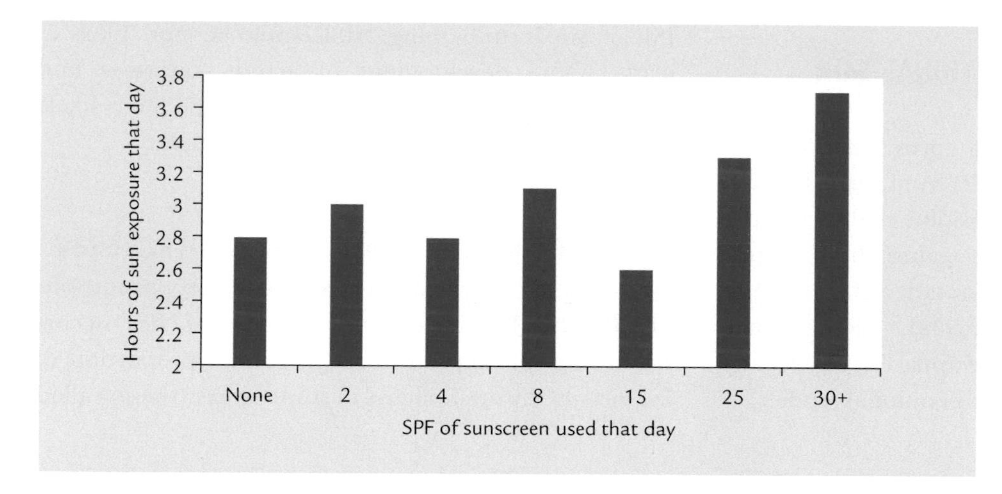

Figure 8.5 *Duration of sun exposure in 55 Texan (US) subjects ready to leave the beach (McCarthy et al., 1999[33]).*

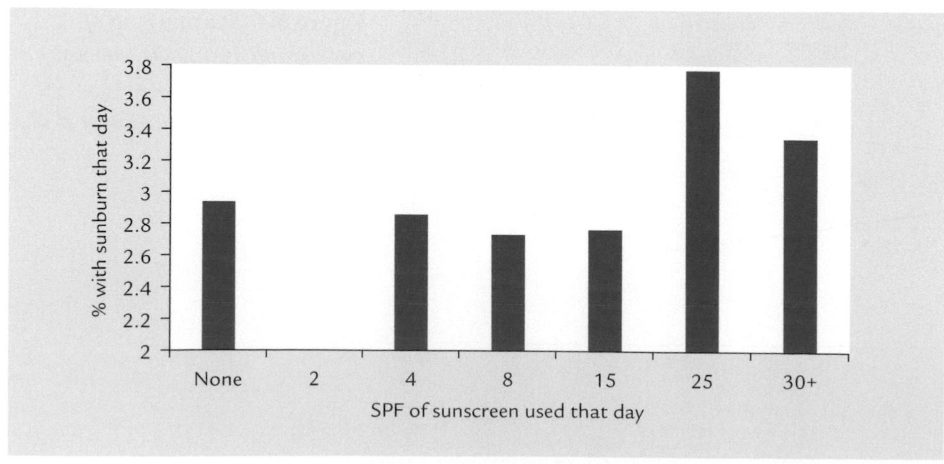

Figure 8.6 *Sunburn experience in 55 Texan (US) subjects ready to leave the beach (McCarthy et al., 1999[33]).*

A case–control study of childhood melanoma in Queensland, Australia (the area with the highest skin cancer incidence in the world) illustrates the importance of distinguishing between ISE and NISE situations.[35] Figure 8.7 shows that control children more frequently used a sunscreen when they were on holiday than when they were at school. Despite the comparatively low numbers of cases and controls, the melanoma risk associated with sunscreen use seemed absent when sunscreen used at school was considered, whereas it tended to increase for sunscreen used during holidays (Figure 8.8).

ISE, NISE, AND SUNSCREEN USE

The changes in tanning fashions and the increasing tendency to take holidays in sunny areas that took place in many industrialized nations after the second world war resulted in a dramatic increase in ISE among sun sensitive populations. Since the late 1980s, many studies have been conducted on patterns of sunscreen use. However, assessment of sunscreen use was often ill defined, making comparisons over time and between study areas difficult.[36] Also, it is not always clear whether sunscreen use was assessed in ISE or NISE situations.

Regardless of the variable quality of survey methods, the various studies clearly indicate that sunscreens are mainly used during ISE. Between 1994 and 1999 in Europe, North America, and New Zealand, sunscreen use was reported by more than 50% of subjects attending beaches or open-air sporting facilities such as swimming pools.[24,37–47] Sunscreen use by European adults or children was directly correlated with time spent in leisure or holiday activities in sunny areas.[14,17] A survey among British adults showed that only 27% had used a sunscreen when at home, but 71% when on holiday abroad.[48]

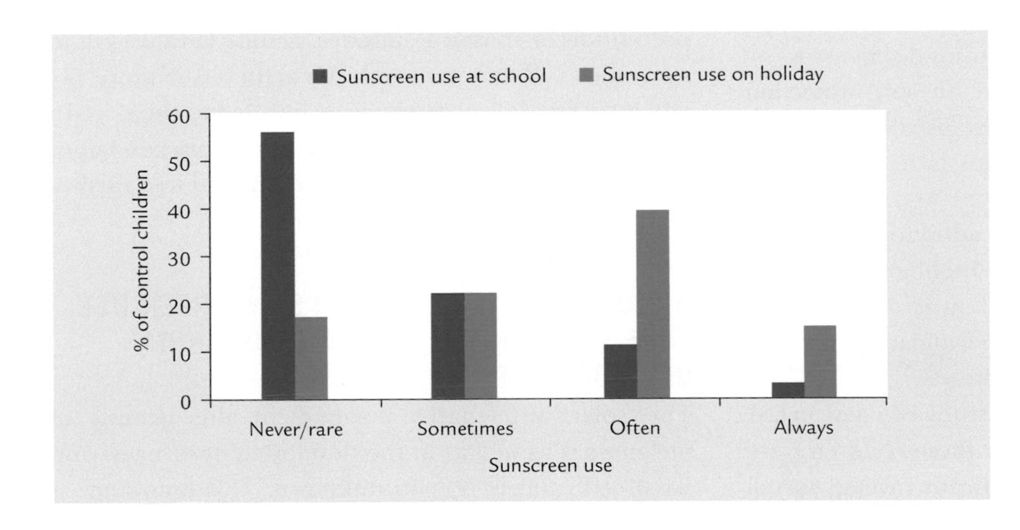

Figure 8.7 *Sunscreen use by children younger than 15 years in Queensland (Whiteman et al., 1997[35]).*

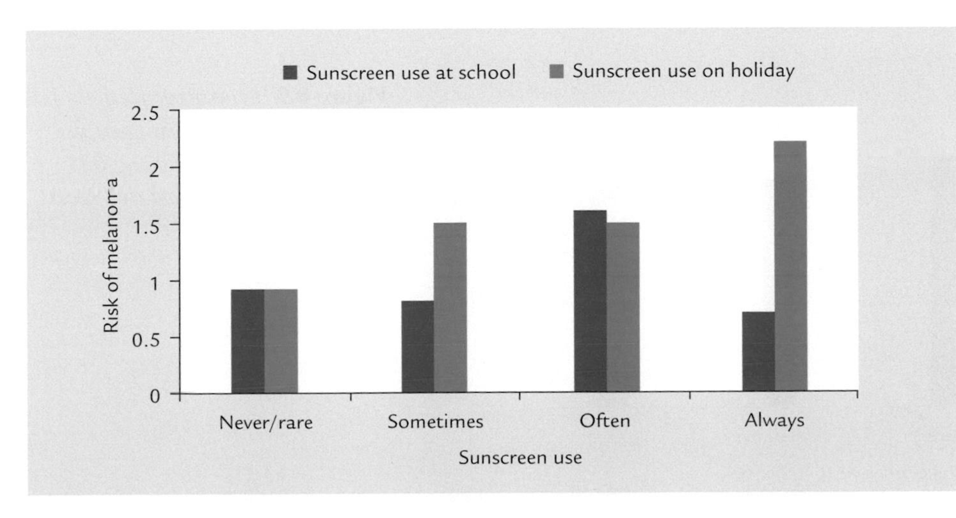

Figure 8.8 *Melanoma risk in children younger than 15 years and sunscreen use in Queensland (Whiteman et al., 1997[35]).*

Although sunscreen use during NISE seems more common in Australia than in North America and in Europe, some studies suggest that sunscreen use in sunny climates is also more usually associated with ISE than with NISE. In northern areas of Australia, 71% of women and 68% of men present on beaches had applied a sunscreen.[49] In contrast, less than 20% of fair-skinned adults attending an outdoor market were found to have applied a sunscreen on uncovered skin areas.[50] In a Queensland study of melanoma in children, 83% of control children used a sunscreen when on holiday, but only 44% when they were at school.[35]

ISE, NISE AND OTHER SUN PROTECTION METHODS

Individual sun protection methods usually recommended are the wearing of appropriate clothes and sunglasses, the avoidance of sunlight whenever possible (searching for shade), the wearing of a hat, and the application of a sunscreen on uncovered skin areas.

Studies that have concentrated on sun protection during daily life (during NISE) have usually found that the wearing of appropriate clothes is more frequent than sunscreen use.[51–55]

Studies that have examined the adoption of sun protection methods during ISE have highlighted the fact that, in both children and adults, sunscreen use is far more frequently reported than sun avoidance measures and the wearing of protective clothes.[17,26,34,37,39,41,56–62]

Figure 8.9 is derived from the study of naevi in 631 European schoolchildren.[17] When these children were engaged in ISE activities, a significant inverse correlation existed between sunscreen use and the wearing of clothes. The difference between sunscreen use and wearing of clothes or sun avoidance may be considerable: for example, in a 1997 United States survey, 53% of parents reported that they protected their children with sunscreens, but only 8% did so with a shirt.[63] Intervention studies promoting sun protection have generally been more effective in increasing sunscreen use than in increasing other sun protection methods.[41,64–67]

QUANTITIES OF SUNSCREEN USED

The SPF of a sunscreen is measured according to internationally agreed standards, using 2 mg/cm^2 of the sunscreen being tested, but it is well known that most people apply only between 0.5 mg and 1 mg of sunscreen per square centimetre of uncovered skin.[3] The argument that people do not use enough sunscreen is often proposed as an explanation for the discrepancy between laboratory and epidemiological data. It is highly probable that in NISE situations, more effective prevention of sunburn episodes, actinic keratoses, and squamous cell cancers would be achieved if more liberal quantities of sunscreen were applied to the skin. In ISE situations, however, it is likely that use of larger quantities of sunscreens would merely lead to a further increase in the time spent in the sun.

BIOLOGICAL LINKS BETWEEN SUNSCREEN USE, TIME SPENT IN THE SUN, AND MELANOMA DEVELOPMENT

The solar wavelengths involved in the genesis of melanomas as well as in the development of naevi and basal cell cancers remain unknown. This ignorance is partly due to the absence of a valid animal model for

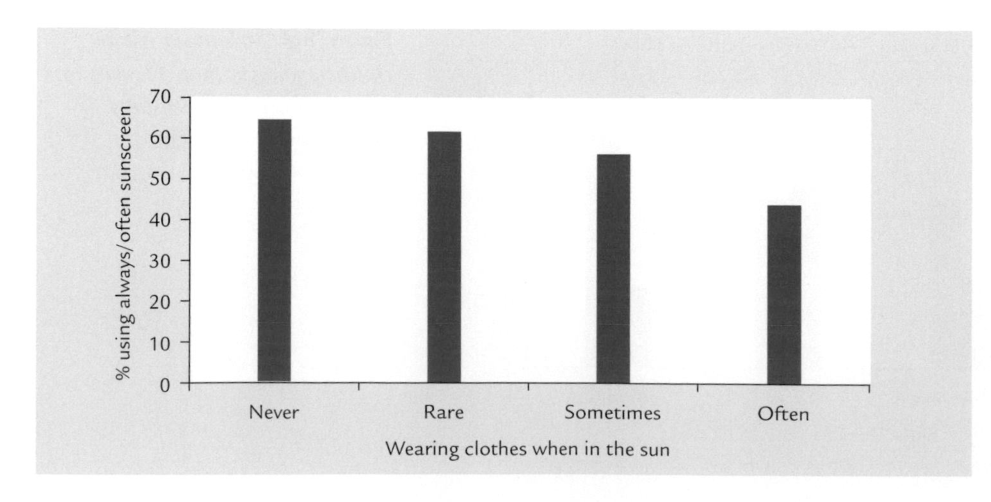

Figure 8.9 *Inverse correlation (P<0.01) between sunscreen use and wearing clothes among 631 European children aged 6–7 years (Autier et al., 1998[17]).*

human melanoma. In contrast, there is now ample evidence from animal and human studies that high doses of UVB (usually leading to sunburn in sun sensitive individuals) are involved in the development of actinic keratoses and squamous cell skin cancers, accompanied by a high frequency of abnormalities (for example, UV signature mutations) in the p53.[68,69]

The reasons why the longer durations of sun exposure related to sunscreen use contribute to an increased risk of cutaneous melanoma development are still speculative. Trial results strongly support the hypothesis that sunscreen use encourages sun exposure, but it is still unclear how the increase in sun exposure time influences the melanoma risk. One possibility would be that longer time spent in the sun while using a sunscreen could lead to larger quantities of UVA reaching the skin. There is also the possibility of dose fractionation and dose attenuation of the UV radiation delivered to the skin. A UV radiation dose (especially of UVB) is more effective for triggering skin cancers in rodents when delivered as a succession of small doses than as a single large dose (dose fractionation).[1,70] A UV radiation dose is also more carcinogenic when delivered over a long period of time than if delivered over a short period of time (dose attenuation). Evidence that sunscreen use may contribute to dose fractionation and dose attenuation of solar UV radiation is supported by several observations. For example, sunscreen use encourages sun exposure around noon, when the proportion of UVB in the solar spectrum is highest.[24,71] Thus it seems that by attenuating the amount of UV radiation reaching the skin, sunscreen use allows intense sun exposures that would not be possible otherwise. However, because more time is spent in the sun when a sunscreen is used, the overall dose of UV radiation delivered to the skin is similar to the dose that would have been delivered if no sunscreen was used, but is delivered to skin cells over a longer period of time. This interpretation is substantiated by the fact that in randomized studies of time spent in the sun according to the SPF of sunscreens,[24] participants had a similar sunburn experience in both high and low SPF groups.

IS THERE A ROLE FOR SUNSCREENS IN SUN PROTECTION?

Table 8.1 summarizes the current state of knowledge about the effects of sunscreen use and the wearing of protective clothing on sunburn and the development of various malignant skin lesions, actinic keratoses and melanocytic naevi, according to the type of sun exposure. Question marks indicate that no data are available about the type of association linking sunscreen use or clothing with a particular skin lesion.

In NISE situations, sunscreen use leads to a decrease in sunburn incidence, and decreases the development of actinic keratoses and squamous cell cancers (SCC). No impact on basal cell cancer (BCC) incidence has yet been shown, but it is probable that an effect would be demonstrated if randomized trials were of longer duration. A protective effect could also be possible as a result of reduced naevus numbers (and thus probably also on melanoma occurrence), but the latter hypothesis remains unproved. Nonetheless, priority should be given to protective clothing, the provision and use of shade, and reduction of sun exposure. Sunscreen use is only an adjunct to a global sun protection strategy, to be applied on skin areas that cannot be protected by other methods.

ISE is a hazardous behaviour that should be discouraged. When used during ISE, sunscreens can involuntarily modify behaviour towards longer durations of sun exposure, and encourage sun exposure in the middle of the day, around noontime (when the sunlight is richest in UVB). The consequence of these behaviour

Table 8.1 *Impact of sunscreen use and clothing on various sun induced skin lesions in humans*

	NISE*	ISE*
SS on SE duration	No effect	Increase
SS on sunburns	Decrease	No effect
SS on actinic keratosis	Decrease	?
SS use on SCC	Decrease	?
SS use on BCC	No effect	Moderate increase
SS use on naevi number	?	Moderate increase
SS use on melanoma	?	Moderate increase
Clothing on naevi number	?	Decrease
Clothing on melanoma	?	Decrease

* NISE: non-intentional sun exposure; ISE: intentional sun exposure (see text for more details on definitions). SS: sunscreen; SCC: squamous cell cancer; BCC: basal cell cancer

patterns is an increased likelihood of developing a melanoma. It is therefore better to avoid recommending use of a sunscreen to sun seekers who cannot refrain from engaging in ISE activities.

In North America and Europe, the general public receives most information about sunscreens through commercial advertising. In most instances, advertising for sunscreens encourages sun exposure and acquisition of a tan, and it often provides a false sense of security to sun enthusiasts.[71] Advertising for sunscreens should instead place emphasis on global sun protection and cease giving the impression that ISE activities are safer when a sunscreen is used. Finally, a possible way to encourage the use of global sun protection would be to advise that a sunscreen should never be applied on the trunk and shoulders.

REFERENCES

1. International Agency for Research on Cancer, *Solar and ultraviolet radiation.* Monographs on the evaluation of the carcinogenic risk of chemicals to humans. Vol 55. IARC: Lyons, 1992: 285–90.
2. Elwood M, Jopson J, Melanoma and sun exposure: An overview of published studies. *Int J Cancer* 1997; 73: 198–203.
3. Diffey B, Has the sun protection factor had its day? *BMJ* 2000; 320: 176–7.
4. Gasparro FP, Mitchnick M, Nash JF, A review of sunscreen safety and efficacy. *Photochem Photobiol* 1998; 68: 243–56.
5. Naylor MF, Farmer KC, The case for sunscreens: A review of their use in preventing actinic skin damage and neoplasia. *Arch Dermatol* 1997; 133: 1146–54.
6. Ananthaswany HN, Loughlin SM, Cox P, et al, Sunlight and skin cancer: inhibition of p53 mutations in UV-irradiated mouse skin by sunscreens. *Nat Med* 1997; 3: 510–14.
7. Damian DL, Halliday GM, Barnetson RS, Broad-spectrum sunscreens provide greater protection against ultraviolet-radiation-induced suppression of contact hypersensitivity to a recall antigen in humans. *J Invest Dermatol* 1997; 109: 146–51.
8. Thompson SC, Jolley D, Marks R, Reduction of solar keratoses by regular sunscreen use. *NEJM* 1993; 329: 1147–51.
9. Naylor MF, Boyd A, Smith DW, et al, High sun protection factor sunscreens in the suppression of actinic neoplasia. *Arch Dermatol* 1995; 131: 170–5
10. Green A, Williams G, Neale R, et al, Daily sunscreen application and betacarotene supplementation in prevention of basal-cell and squamous-cell carcinomas of the skin: a randomised controlled trial. *Lancet* 1999; 354, 723–9.
11. Bigby M, The sunscreen and melanoma controversy. *Arch Dermatol* 1999; 135: 1526–7.
12. Autier P, Sunscreen and melanoma revisited. *Arch Dermatol* 2000; 136: 423.
13. Elwood JM, Gallagher RP, More about: Sunscreen use, wearing clothes, and number of naevi in 6-to7-year-old European children. *J Natl Cancer Inst* 1999; 13: 1164–5.
14. Autier P, Doré JF, Schifflers E, et al, for the EORTC Melanoma Cooperative Group. Melanoma and use of sunscreens: an EORTC case-control study in Germany, Belgium and France. *Int J Cancer* 1995; 61: 749–55.
15. Westerdahl J, Olsson H, Masback A, et al, Is the use of sunscreens a risk factor for malignant melanoma? *Mel Res* 1995; 5: 59–65.
16. Westerdahl J, Ingvar C, Masback A, Olsson H, Risk of Cutaneous malignant melanoma in relation to use of sunbeds: further evidence for UVA carcinogenicity. *Br J Cancer* 2000; 82: 1593–9.
17. Autier P, Doré JF, Cattaruzza MS, et al, for the EORTC Melanoma Group. Sunscreen use, wearing clothes and naevi number in 6- to 7-year-old European children. *J Natl Cancer Inst* 1998; 90: 1873–81.
18. Holman CDJ, Armstrong BK, Heenan P, Relationship of cutaneous malignant melanoma to individual sunlight-exposure habits. *J Natl Cancer Inst* 1986; 76: 403–14.
19. Autier P, Doré JF, Renard F, et al, Melanoma and sunscreen use: Need for studies representative of actual behaviours. *Melanoma Res* 1997; 7 (suppl. 2): S115–20.
20. Young AR, Potten CS, Chadwick CA, et al, Inhibition of UV radiation-induced DNA damage by a 5-methoxypsoralen tan in human skin. *Pigment Cell Res* 1988; 1: 350–4.
21. Young AR, Potten CS, Chadwick CA, et al, Photoprotection and 5-MOP photochemoprotection from UVR-induced DNA damage in humans: the role of skin type. *J Invest Dermatol* 1991; 97: 942–8.
22. Autier P, Doré JF, Césarini JP, Boyle P, Should subjects who used psoralen suntan activators be screened for melanoma? *Ann Oncol* 1997; 8: 435–7.
23. Autier P, Doré JF, Severi G, More about: Sunscreen use, wearing clothes, and number of naevi in 6-to-7-year-old European children. *J Natl Cancer Inst* 1999; 13: 1165–6.
24. Autier P, Doré JF, Négrier S, et al, Sunscreen use and duration of sun exposure: A double blind randomized trial. *J Natl Cancer Inst* 1999; 15: 1304–9.
25. Autier P, Doré JF, Conde Reis A, et al, Sunscreen use and recreational exposure to ultraviolet A and B radiation: A double blind randomized trial using personal dosimeters. *Br J Cancer* 2000; 83: 1243–8.
26. Melia J, Bulman A, Sunburn and tanning in a British population. *J Public Health Med* 1995; 17: 223–9.
27. McGee R, Wiliams S, Glasgow H, Sunburn and sun protection among young children. *J Paediatr Child Health* 1997; 33: 234–7.
28. Hill D, White V, Marks R, et al, Melanoma prevention: behavioral and non behavioral factors in sunburn among an Australian population. *Prev Med* 1992; 21: 654–69.
29. Green A, Williams G, Neale R, Battistutta D, Betacarotene and sunscreen use: author's reply. *Lancet* 1999; 354: 2164.
30. Hill D, White V, Marks R, Borland R, Changes in sun-related attitudes and behaviors, and reduced sunburn prevalence in a population at high risk of melanoma. *Eur J Cancer Prev* 1993; 2: 447–56.
31. Berwick M, Fine JA, Bolognia JL, Sun exposure and sunscreen use following a community skin cancer screening. *Prev Med* 1992; 21: 302–10.
32. Wulf, HC, Stender IM, Lock-Andersen J, Sunscreens used at the beach do not protect against erythema: a new definition of SPF is proposed. *Photodermatol Photoimmunol Photomed* 1997; 13: 129–32.
33. McCarthy E M, Ethridge K P, Wagner R F, Beach holiday sunburn: the sunscreen paradox and gender differences. *Cutis* 1999; 64: 37–42.
34. Robinson JK, Rigell DS, Amonette RA, Summertime sun protection used by adults for their children. *J Am Acad Dermatol* 2000; 42: 746–53.
35. Whiteman DC, Valery P, McWhirter W, Green AC, Risk factors for childhood melanoma in Queensland, Australia. *Int J Cancer*, 1997; 70: 26–31.
36. Buller DB, Borland R, Skin cancer prevention for children: A critical review. *Health Educ Behav* 1999; 26: 317–43.
37. Vergnès C, Daures J P, Sancho-Garnier H, et al, [Sun exposure behavior of children between 3–15 years of age living in Montpellier] [in French]. *Ann Dermatol Venereol* 1999; 126: 505–12.
38. Ross SA, Sanchez JL, Recreational sun exposure in Puerto Rico: trends and cancer risk awareness. *J Am Acad Dermatol* 1990; 23: 1090–2.
39. Zitser BS, Shah AN, Adams ML, St Clair J, A survey of sunbathing practices on three Connecticut State beaches. *Conn Med* 1996; 60: 591–4.
40. Hillhouse JJ, Stair AW, Adler CM, Predictors of sunbathing and sunscreen use in college undergraduates. *J Behav Med* 1996; 19: 543–61.
41. Miller D R, Geller A C, Wood M C, et al, The Falmouth Safe Skin Project: evaluation of a community program to promote sun protection in youth. *Health Educ Behav* 1999; 26: 369–84.
42. Stender I, Lock Andersen J, Wulf HC, Sun exposure and sunscreen

use among sunbathers in Denmark. *Acta Derm Venereol (Stockh)* 1996; 76: 31–3.
43. Jerkegren E, Sandrieser L, Brandberg Y, Rosdahl I, Sun-related behaviour and melanoma awareness among Swedish university students. *Eur J Cancer Prev* 1999; 8: 27–34.
44. Banks BA, Silverman RA, Schwartz RH, Tunnessen WW Jr, Attitudes of teenagers toward sun exposure and sunscreen use. *Pediatrics* 1992; 89: 40–2.
45. Boldeman C, Beitner H, Jansson B, Nilsson B, Ullen H, Sunbed use in relation to phenotype, erythema, sunscreen use and skin disease. A questionnaire survey among Swedish adolescents. *Br J Dermatol* 1996; 135: 712–16.
46. McGee R, Williams S, Cox B, et al, A community survey of sun exposure, sunburn and sun protection. *NZ Med J* 1995; 108: 508–10.
47. Wichstrom L, Predictors of Norwegian adolescents' sunbathing and use of sunscreen. *Health Psychol* 1994; 13: 412–20.
48. Bourke JF, Graham-Brown RA, Protection of children against sunburn: a survey of parental practice in Leicester. *Br J Dermatol* 1995; 133: 264–6.
49. Pincus MW, Rollings PK, Craft AB, Green A, Sunscreen use on Queensland beaches. *Australas J Dermatol* 1989; 32: 21–5.
50. Whiteman DC, Frost CA, Whiteman CA, Green AC, A survey of sunscreen use and sun-protection practices in Darwin. *Aust J Public Health* 1994; 18: 47–50.
51. Hoegh HJ, Davis BD, Manthe AF, Sun avoidance practices among non-Hispanic white Californians. *Health Educ Behav* 1999; 26: 360–8.
52. Rademaker M, Wyllie K, Collins M, Wetton, N, Primary school children's perceptions of the effects of sun on skin. *Australas J Dermatol* 1996; 37: 30–6.
53. Grin CM, Pennoyer JW, Lehrich DA, Grant-Kels JM, Sun exposure of young children while at day care. *Pediatr Dermatol* 1994; 11: 304–9.
54. Fritschi L, Green A, Solomon PJ, Sun exposure in Australian adolescents. *J Am Acad Dermatol* 1992; 27: 25–8.
55. Buller DB, Callister M, Reichert T, Skin cancer prevention by parents of young children: Health information sources, skin cancer knowledge, and sun protection practices. *Oncol Nursing Forum* 1995; 22: 1559–66.
56. Lovato CY, Shoveller JA, Peters L, Rivers JK, Canadian National Survey on Sun Exposure & Protective Behaviours: parents' reports on children. *Cancer Prev Control* 1999; 2: 123–8.
57. Grob JJ, Guglielmina C, Gouvernet J, Zarour H, Noe C, Bonerandi JJ, Study of sunbathing habits in children and adolescents: application to the prevention of melanoma. *Dermatology* 1993; 186: 94–8.
58. Reynolds KD, Blaum JM, Jester PM, et al, Predictors of sun exposure in adolescents in a Southeastern U.S. population. *J Adolesc Health* 1996; 19: 409–15.
59. Martin RH, Relationship between risk factors, knowledge and preventive behaviour relevant to skin cancer in general practice patients in South Australia. *Br J Gen Pract* 1995; 45: 365–7.
60. Goodherham MJ, Guenther L, Sun and the skin: Evaluation of a sun awareness program for elementary school students. *J Cutan Med Surg* 1999; 5: 230–5.
61. Glanz K, Carbone E, Song V, Formative research for developing targeted skin cancer prevention programs for children in multiethnic Hawaii. *Health Educ Res* 1999; 14: 155–66.
62. Cockburn J, Hennrikus D, Scott R, Sanson-Fisher R, (1989) Adolescent use of sun-protection measures. *Med J Aust* 1989; 151: 136–40.
63. Robinson JK, Rigel RS, Amonette RA, Sun-protection behaviors used by adults for their children – United States. *JAMA* 1997; 280: 317–18.
64. Dixon H, Borland R, Hill D, Sun protection and sunburn in primary school children: the influence of age, gender, and coloring. *Prev Med* 1999; 28: 119–30.
65. Bastuji-Garin S, Grob JJ, Grognard C, et al, Melanoma prevention: evaluation of a health education campain for primary schools. *Arch Dermatol* 1999; 135: 936–40.
66. Dietrich AJ, Olson AL, Sox CH et al, A community-based randomized trial encouraging sun protection for children. *Pediatrics* 1998; 102: 1468–9.
67. Cockburn J, Thompson SC, Marks R, et al, Behavioural dynamics of a clinical trial of sunscreens for reducing solar keratoses in Victoria, Australia. *J Epidemiol Community Health* 1997; 51: 716–21.
68. Ziegler AM, Jonason AS, Leffell DJ, et al, Sunburn and p53 in the onset of skin cancer. *Nature* 1994; 372: 773–6.
69. Nataraj AJ, Trent JC, Ananthaswamy HN, p53 gene mutations and photocarcinogenesis. *Photochem Photobiol* 1995; 62: 218–30.
70. Forbes PD, Photocarcinogenesis: An overview. *J Invest Dermatol* 1981; 77: 139–43.
71. George PM, Kuskowski M, Schmidt C, Trends in photoprotection in American fashion magazines, 1983–1993. *J Am Acad Dermatol* 1996; 34: 424–8.

9

Population screening for melanoma: current evidence and a community based randomized trial

Joanne Aitken, Mark Elwood

INTRODUCTION

Regular skin examination should, in principle, lead to earlier diagnosis of melanoma, thinner tumours, and fewer deaths. But, in contrast to the situation for other cancers for which screening is recommended, such as breast or colorectal cancer, there is no evidence from prospective trials that screening actually does reduce deaths. Melanoma is one of the commonest cancers in populations of European origin living in sunny climates, such as Australia, New Zealand, Hawaii and California. In these high incidence countries, the survival rate tends to be higher than in areas where melanoma is less common, and the survival rates have improved over time. This is likely to be due to both increased public awareness of the disease and more effective management, particularly in the initial diagnosis. In most moderate and high incidence countries, over 90% of melanomas are diagnosed before there is regional or distant metastatic spread, so survival depends on the depth of invasion of the primary lesion. In most countries, at least until recently, the trend in mortality rates has been upwards.[1] In Australia and the United States mortality is stabilizing or beginning to fall in younger age groups but continues to increase in older subjects (Figure 9.1).[2,3] In this chapter, the issues relating to skin screening will be discussed, with particular attention to the Australian situation.

THICKNESS DISTRIBUTION OF MELANOMA

Queensland, Australia, has the world's highest recorded incidence of melanoma, with annual age-standardized rates for invasive melanoma in 1999 of 49.5 and 38.7

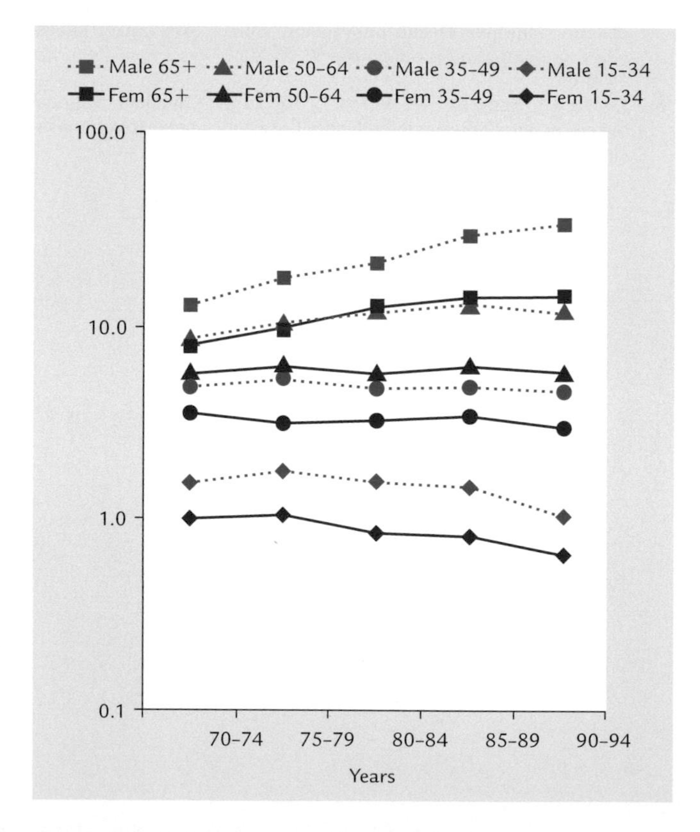

Figure 9.1 *Melanoma mortality trends in Australia: age specific rates per 100,000 per year by 5-year periods 1970–74 to 1990–94.*[2] *Log scale.*

per 100,000 for men and women respectively. Melanoma incidence has increased sharply in Queensland and in other white-skinned populations over the past three decades and, although the pace of increase has now slowed, rates are still rising in this state.[4–7] Age adjusted incidence has increased in Queensland in all thickness categories and the biggest increase, as in other populations, has been for lesions less than 1.5 mm thick (Table 9.1).[4,8,9] This has resulted in a shift in the proportional distribution of melanoma in Queensland towards thinner lesions, particularly in men. In 1979/80, 64% of incident invasive melanomas in men and 79% in women (excluding metastatic disease from an unknown primary and tumours of unknown depth) were recorded as less than 1.5 mm thick. By 1997, this had increased to 79% in men and 83% in women. This comparison probably understates the true improvement, as depth was not recorded for over one quarter of all cases in 1979/80 compared with only 5% of cases in 1997, and most of these are likely to have been thicker lesions.

Public and professional education campaigns about skin cancer and melanoma have been conducted in Queensland since the early 1960s, and the distribution of tumour depth in Queensland today compares favourably with that in other countries where education and detection programmes have been conducted over shorter periods (Table 9.2).[6,10–13] In this high risk and highly aware population, how much of the comparatively greater increase in incidence of thin lesions is explained by overdiagnosis of biologically non-progressive disease is a matter of some debate, as discussed later in this chapter.[7,8,14,15] Nevertheless, it is also likely to be due at least in part to a shift from thick to thin lesions caused by earlier diagnosis of invasive disease.[2,4,8] If so, this should result in a slowdown in the rate of rise in melanoma mortality, as has been observed in Queensland and in other Australian states.[2] Despite these improvements, 20% of incident melanomas of known depth in Queensland in 1997 were thicker than 1.5 mm, and there remains the potential for further improvement in depth distribution, particularly among older patients (Figure 9.2).

Tumour thickness increases with age at diagnosis in most populations. In Queensland, the disparity in thickness distribution between young and old has increased over the past two decades. In Queensland in 1997 11% (in men) and 8% (in women) of invasive

Table 9.1 *Age-standardized rates of invasive melanoma in Queensland, Australia, by tumour thickness for three time periods*

Thickness	1979/80§				1987#				1997‡			
	Male		Female		Male		Female		Male		Female	
	No.	*ASR**	No.	*ASR*	No.	*ASR*	No.	*ASR*	No.	*ASR*	No.	*ASR*
Total invasive	280	*22.6*	317	*25.8*	755	*49.6*	626	*40.4*	1223	*57.7*	889	*42.4*
<0.75 mm	78	*6.6*	148	*12.6*	358	*23.9*	321	*21.5*	665	*32.1*	532	*26.4*
0.75–1.49 mm	48	*4.1*	36	*3.1*	134	*9.0*	148	*9.7*	215	*10.1*	136	*6.8*
1.5–2.24 mm	27	*2.3*	18	*1.5*	45	*3.0*	47	*2.7*	91	*4.2*	62	*2.8*
2.25–2.99 mm	13	*0.99*	9	*0.6*	37	*2.4*	9	*0.5*	40	*1.8*	22	*0.8*
≥3.00 mm	32	*2.5*	21	*1.6*	77	*4.7*	32	*1.9*	107	*4.7*	55	*1.9*
Metastatic	n/r¶		n/r		50	*3.1*	20	*1.2*	51	*2.3*	39	*1.8*
Unkn. thick.†	82	*6.6*	85	*6.6*	54	*3.5*	49	*2.9*	54	*2.5*	43	*2.0*

§From MacLennan et al. (1992).[4]
From Queensland Melanoma Register.
‡ From Queensland Cancer Registry.
* *ASR*: Rate per 100,000 per year age-standardized to world standard population.
¶ n/r: metastatic not recorded for 1979/80.
† Unkn. thick.: thickness not recorded on pathology form.

Table 9.2 *Age-standardized rates of invasive melanoma by tumour thickness in four countries*

Thickness	Queensland‡ 1997				New Zealand¶ 1997				USA# 1996				Scotland§ 1995–1997			
	Male		Female		Male		Female		Male		Female		Male		Female	
	No.	*ASR**	No.	*ASR*	No.	*ASR*	No.	*ASR*	No.	*ASR*	No.	*ASR*	No.	*ASR*	No.	*ASR*
Total invasive	1223	*57.7*	889	*42.4*	769	*33.1*	759	*29.9*	2916	*13.7*	2305	*9.6*	732	*7.3*	1121	*9.8*
<0.75 mm	665	*32.1*	532	*26.4*	333	*14.4*	361	*15.1*	1343	*6.4*	1163	*5.0*	230	*2.4*	458	*4.5*
0.75–1.49 mm	215	*10.1*	136	*6.8*	178	*7.7*	156	*6.3*	518	*2.5*	416	*1.8*	145	*1.4*	232	*2.1*
1.5–2.24 mm	91	*4.2*	62	*2.8*	55	*2.3*	70	*2.6*	233	*1.1*	162	*0.7*	76	*0.7*	122	*1.0*
2.25–2.99 mm	40	*1.8*	22	*0.8*	30	*1.3*	25	*0.8*	88	*0.4*	73	*0.3*	45	*0.5*	56	*0.4*
≥3.00 mm	107	*4.7*	55	*1.9*	103	*4.3*	88	*2.9*	235	*1.1*	147	*0.5*	194	*1.7*	205	*1.4*
Metastatic	51	*2.3*	39	*1.8*	+		+		118	*0.5*	46	*0.2*	39	*0.4*	44	*0.3*
Unkn. thick.†	54	*2.5*	43	*2.0*	70	*3.1*	59	*2.2*	381	*1.8*	298	*1.2*	3	*<0.1*	4	*<0.1*

‡ From Queensland Cancer Registry.
¶ From New Zealand Cancer Registry.
# From Surveillance, Epidemiology, and End Results (SEER) Cancer Incidence Public-Use CD-Rom (1973–1996) National Cancer Institute, DCCPS, Cancer Surveillance Research Programme, Cancer Statistics Branch, released April 1999, based on the August 1998 submission.
§ From the Scottish Melanoma Group.
* ASR: Rate per 100,000 per year age-standardized to world standard population.
+ Not available.
† Unkn. thick.: thickness not recorded on pathology form.

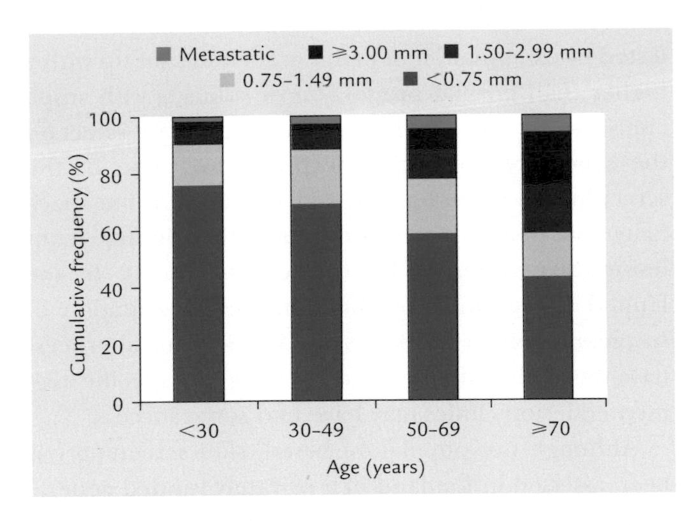

Figure 9.2 *Cumulative distribution of invasive melanoma in Queensland, Australia in 1997 by tumour thickness, for four age groups.*

tumours in patients aged 30 to 49 years were 1.5 mm or thicker, compared with 19% and 15% for men and women aged 50 to 69 years, and 33% and 41% for those 70 years or older. There is a strong correlation between tumour thickness and lower survival, and melanoma mortality is thus also higher in older patients. The reasons may include more biologically aggressive tumours in older patients and also delays in diagnosis owing to failure to recognize early signs of melanoma or to seek timely medical attention.[16–19] This suggests some potential for further improvement through targeted education programmes.

Thus, four decades of increasing publicity and education about skin cancer in Queensland have been accompanied by a shift in melanoma thickness distribution to thinner tumours likely to result at least in part from earlier diagnosis. New strategies, with a particular focus on older people, should now be considered. It would be reasonable to aim to shift the thickness distribution of melanoma in those over 50 years to that seen in younger patients. On the basis of recent Australian figures for melanoma survival according to tumour depth at diagnosis such a shift could be accompanied, at least in theory, by up to a 44% reduction in 10-year melanoma mortality in this group.[20] Mortality gains might be expected with improvements in early diagnosis in all age groups, and the question then is how best to achieve this.

OPTIONS FOR EARLY DIAGNOSIS

Screening is only one method of achieving earlier diagnosis. Other programmes for the early diagnosis of melanoma include media based education to the general public about the early signs of melanoma; open access clinics, offering skin checks or spot checks; and case finding as a component of routine primary care. Although all these include an element of screening, the term screening, as used in other cancer contexts such as for breast or cervical screening, implies a systematic offer of the screening test to an entire defined eligible population.

In Scotland, a programme of public education about the early signs of melanoma was backed by educational support to general practitioners in dealing with pigmented lesions. This was followed by reductions in the incidence of thick melanoma and in melanoma mortality, but only in women; no beneficial trend was seen in men.[6,21,22] Programmes in some other areas have not been followed by any decrease in thick melanoma.[23] Educational campaigns may have substantial effects on the demand for referral services.[24,25] In Queensland, a descriptive analysis by time period in one city looked at the effect of two public education campaigns, showing a 24% increase in the total number of melanocytic skin lesions excised.[26] The authors found no change in the detection rate or the thickness distribution of melanomas, and questioned the effectiveness of such campaigns.

Open access skin checks range from beach patrols and informal skin screening sessions in community halls, to a process by which general practitioners or specialists will open their premises on occasions specifically to offer free skin checks. This approach has been assessed in the United States, the Netherlands, and Western Australia.[27–32] The participation rates on a population basis are usually low, despite the large number of attendees. For example, the US total of some 282,000 subjects screened in 1992–94 translates to only about 2% of the population at risk, if defined as white-skinned adults over the age of 30.[28] The positivity rate is a central issue. Defining this as the proportion of subjects given a label of suspected melanoma or something similar, gives modest positivity rates of between 1% and 4%, and the predictive value – the proportion of such patients who are subsequently found to have melanoma – is substantially higher. The US programme defined 1.6% of participants as having suspected melanoma, and this was confirmed in 8.2%.[28] However, the proportions of subjects who have a positive screening result – in management terms they are recommended to take further action, are much higher, 10–12% in the Netherlands, 31% in an early Massachusetts programme (reduced later), and 17% in Western Australia.[27,29,31,32] Most of the subjects referred were clinically labelled as having suspected basal cell carcinomas, squamous cell carcinomas, or a range of other conditions including dysplastic naevi; all these conditions have such good outcomes in normal clinical practice that any improvement from screening is unlikely. If only those with clinically suspected melanomas were followed up, some melanomas would be missed; more selective referral accepts a reduction in sensitivity for a substantial gain in specificity. In the Geraldton (Australia) survey, six out of 20 melanomas diagnosed were clinically labelled basal cell carcinoma, and would have been missed by a selective referral process.[33]

By case finding, we refer to the process of questioning a patient who visits his or her primary care provider for another reason about recent skin changes; or offering a partial or full skin examination. The essential difference between screening and case finding is that case finding is opportunistic, adding extra questioning or examination, but only for those people who visit the general practitioner for other reasons. In contrast, screening, as it is used in other disease contexts, implies a programme to encourage visits to the general practitioner (or other screener) for that purpose, whether or not the patient is aware of skin changes, signs, or symptoms. The improvements in melanoma survival over time have probably been produced by improved case finding, allied to improved referral decisions and prompt and accurate further management. There are few studies of efforts to improve case finding at primary care level. There is evidence in high risk countries that the level of expertise in general practitioners is high. In a survey of a large representative sample of general practitioners in New Zealand, over 95% described the correct management for three presented scenarios involving early melanoma, and the responses were not greatly different from those of a small sample of specialist dermatologists.[34] Skill levels were higher in younger than in older general practitioners and were increased in those who had dealt personally with at least one melanoma patient. In Australia, the effect of a one day training course for general practitioners on their diagnostic abilities was tested by examination of patients at clinics set up with a higher than normal proportion of subjects with suspicious lesions.[35] The training had no significant effect on the sensitivity, specificity, or predictive value of the screening. In general the sensitivity was high but specificity low, that is many subjects with non-malignant lesions were referred for further assessment. In the United Kingdom, delays both in the presentation of suspicious lesions to doctors and in the referral process have been documented, and setting up specific pigmented lesion clinics may have had some success.[25,36,37]

Although not population based, skin screening has been assessed in England in a privately funded general health screening centre.[38] A complete skin check was carried out by a doctor, usually a general practitioner, and the position and characteristics of any pigmented lesion regarded as suspicious or changing was marked on a skin chart, and assessed by a seven point check list system. All lesions were then photographed using Polaroid cameras and the pictures assessed independently by two consultant dermatologists. Of 39,922 subjects screened, 948 (2.4%) had at least one skin lesion assessed and photographed. Of the 1052 lesions in these subjects, 231 were assessed as requiring follow up, and among these there were 11 melanomas, but follow up was incomplete. The authors concluded that photography greatly reduced the need for specialist referral, but their estimate of sensitivity was only 37%.

The above approaches – public education, open access clinics, and case finding – all have some overlap with screening but lack the systematic population based approach characteristic of a screening programme. Screening for melanoma could be by the active promotion of self screening or by specific invitation based screening in routine primary care supplemented with additional screening services at dedicated skin screening clinics. While any campaign that attempts to educate about the early signs of melanoma must encourage people to be aware of or look at their skin, some initiatives specifically encourage a self screening protocol. This can range from a simple checklist to comprehensive regular screening methods such as those promoted by the American Cancer Society.[39,40]

EFFECTS OF SCREENING

The purpose of screening for melanoma is to reduce mortality and morbidity. This assumes that intervention at an earlier stage in the natural history results in a better outcome for the patient. However, early intervention for a lesion that is not progressive will not be beneficial. There is substantial evidence that a proportion of thin melanomas may not progress or progress only very slowly.[8,15,41,42] There has been a very rapid rise in the incidence of melanomas in Australia in the 1980s (Figure 9.3). This was due mainly to a great increase in lesions classified as invasive, but thin (less than 0.75 mm thickness). In situ lesions also increased. At this time the total number of people having skin lesions removed increased by 14% per year, and a careful analysis of this situation suggested that increased diagnosis of a non-metastasizing form of melanoma could be a major part of the explanation.[8] If this is so, both the incidence and the survival rates of melanoma will be overestimated. A skin screening programme will be likely to lead to increased diagnosis of such lesions, which will add to its cost. The problem cannot be resolved clinically until there are biological markers to distinguish potentially fatal melanomas from those which do not invade. We are conducting a case–control study of melanoma designed to estimate the proportion of melanomas diagnosed after screening which represent non-progressive lesions.

Even if effective, a reduction in mortality would be seen only several years after the introduction of screening. The more immediate effect should be an increase in the proportion of thin lesions, due to an increase in the incidence rate of thin lesions, and within a few years a decrease in the incidence rate of thick lesions. A short term increase in the total incidence of melanoma is likely. If the programme is successful and is continued, this short term increase in incidence should fall away, being replaced by a similar constant incidence rate as before, but with a thinner depth distribution. If, however, more surveillance is causing the diagnosis of non-progressive lesions, then this later stable incidence rate will be higher than that occurring before screening. Thus, although the proportional distribution by thickness is misleading as an indicator of the benefits of screening, the incidence rate of thick melanomas should be a good predictor of the death rate from melanoma.

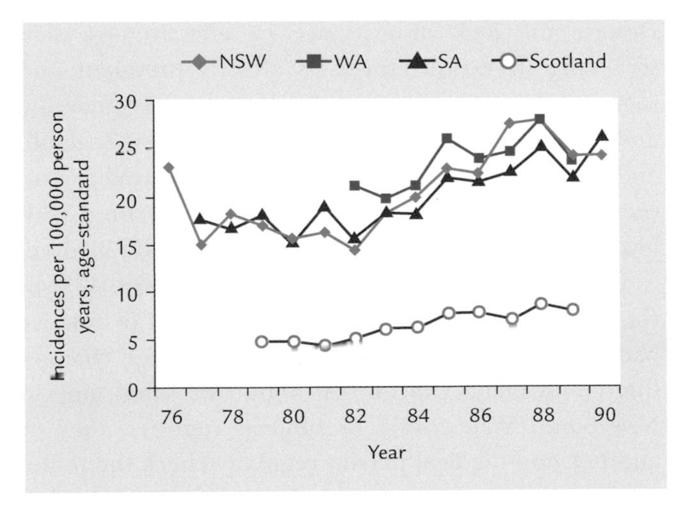

Figure 9.3 *Incidence trends for melanoma in Australia and in Scotland (females).[15] NSW: New South Wales; WA: Western Australia; SA: South Australia.*

Skin surveillance programmes will also lead to the diagnosis of basal cell and squamous cell cancers, lentigo maligna lesions, and a wide range of other skin lesions. Their earlier diagnosis is unlikely to be of great benefit, as these lesions have excellent outcomes even if diagnosed in normal clinical practice.

If screening does give reduced mortality or morbidity from melanoma, the relevant questions then relate to the comparison of these benefits with the costs and detrimental effects (such as false positives) of screening. This comparison will be more favourable in populations with a higher mortality and a higher incidence of deeply invasive melanoma.

EVALUATION OF MELANOMA SCREENING

There are very few studies that assess the effects of screening for melanoma. Self screening has been assessed in Connecticut using a case–control study.[43] From the population based registry, subjects with 'lethal' (fatal or advanced) melanoma were identified and compared to population controls. The key factor assessed, by questionnaire shortly after diagnosis, was the history of self examination, defined as 'a careful, deliberate and purposeful examination of the skin'. The study assessed whether screening was related to a decrease in the risk of lethal melanoma among all melanoma patients, and showed a substantial but non-significant reduction (risk ratio 0.58, 95% confidence interval 0.31 to 1.11), which is consistent with a beneficial effect of screening on postdiagnosis survival. The study however also showed a reduction in total melanoma incidence in people who practiced self screening (risk ratio 0.66, 95% confidence interval 0.44 to 0.99). This is unexpected and difficult to explain. The main mechanism by which incidence could be reduced is by self screening leading to the recognition and removal of precursor lesions, but there is no direct evidence of this from the study.[44] By combining both effects, the authors estimated that self examination may reduce mortality from melanoma by 63% (risk ratio 0.37, 95% CI 0.16 to 0.84). But the reduction in incidence could also indicate observation bias or confounding within the study, raising questions about the validity of the other results. Assessing screening by case–control methods is inherently difficult, and although this is a well performed study, alternative explanations of the results cannot be easily ruled out.

We are not aware of any controlled study that assessed a population based programme of screening other than this single case–control study. This highlights the discrepancy between a substantial body of opinion that assumes that screening is beneficial and the lack of empirical evidence on the issue.

Selective screening of high risk groups is discussed elsewhere in this book. There seem to be no randomized trials of alternative types of follow up surveillance in high risk groups, but careful regular surveillance, based on clinical observation supplemented by photography, has been shown to give an improved thickness distribution of subsequent melanomas.[45–47] The value of screening for less well-defined risk groups, such as subjects with some dysplastic naevi, or a high total naevus count, is less clear.[48–50]

ECONOMIC ISSUES

A cost-effectiveness analysis has been published for the Australian situation which assumes mortality reductions of 15–34% with either two or five yearly screening, starting at age 50.[51] With analytical assumptions including discounting and assuming five yearly screening, 60% sensitivity, 98% specificity, and a 27% reduction in mortality, the estimated costs per year of life saved were A$6800 for men and A$11,100 for women. With a specificity of 90%, costs per life year saved increased to A$9700 (men) and A$15,700 (women). These costs are comparable to those of breast cancer screening. The critical assumption is that screening does produce a substantial reduction in mortality. Another analysis, which assumed 95% sensitivity and 49% specificity, as measured for a random sample of general practitioners in Newcastle, New South Wales, Australia, produced costs per life year saved for men of A$16,800.[35]

The number needed to screen (NNS) per death prevented can be assessed by an approximate calculation (Table 9.3). For Australia, age range 50–69, both sexes, and assuming a 20% reduction in mortality from a screening test every two years, with a positivity rate (the proportion of screenees requiring further investigation) of 5% on the first screen, reducing to 2% on the second screen, to prevent one death would require screening 2500 persons and performing some 25,000 screens. The number of false positives to be investigated would be about 575. As the mortality is higher in men, the NNS (both sexes) is around 1800 for men and 4000 for women in this age group. In contrast, for the much lower mortality rate in the United Kingdom, the NNS is about 7000. This is an approximate calculation only, although this approach gives generally similar results to the full analysis given in the last paragraph, if the same parameters are used.

The cost-benefit of screening will be more favourable in a group with a higher mortality. A screening programme can be easily targeted by age and gender. However, if screening is restricted to some other high risk group – for example, to subjects with a family history or a high risk skin type – it is then important to add in the costs, and the accuracy or otherwise, of whatever method is used to define that group.

EXTENT OF SCREENING AT PRESENT

Despite the lack of evidence of effectiveness, skin screening in various forms is already prevalent and seems to be increasing in populations with moderate and high incidences including Australia, New Zealand, and the United States. Little information is available on the prevalence of skin screening in populations with low melanoma incidence, including the United Kingdom.

In a nationwide survey in Australia in 1988, 47% of respondents reported that they or a friend or relative had ever deliberately checked their skin for changes that could mean cancer.[52] At about the same time in New South Wales, 48% of subjects reported they or another non-medical person regularly check the moles on their body for changes.[53] In Victoria in 1990, 54% of respondents reported they or a friend or relative had ever deliberately checked their skin for changes that could mean skin cancer.[54] In Queensland in 1992–93

Table 9.3 *Approximate calculation of number needed to screen, and costs (ignoring discounting), for melanoma screening applied to populations with different death rates. Cost data from*[51]

Population	Australia 1996, both sexes	Australia 1996, men	Australia 1996, women	UK, both sexes
Assumptions:				
Mortality per 100,000 per year, age 50–69	10.00	13.80	6.40	3.50
Proportional mortality reduction	0.2	0.2	0.2	0.2
Starting age	50	50	50	50
Length of programme (years)	20	20	20	20
Screening interval (years)	2	2	2	2
Cost per screen A$	24	24	24	24
Cost per positive A$	140	140	140	140
Risk of false positive in first screen	5.0%	5.0%	5.0%	2.0%
Risk of false positive in subsequent screens	2.0%	2.0%	2.0%	1.0%
Derived:				
Risk of melanoma death in programme period	0.002	0.00276	0.00128	0.0007
Probability of death averted; d	0.0004	0.000552	0.000256	0.00014
Number of screenings per person; s	10	10	10	10
Cost per person screened A$	240	240	240	240
Risk of a false positive in whole programme; p	23.0%	23.0%	23.0%	11.0%
Cost of false positives in whole programme per person screened	32.2	32.2	32.2	15.4
Total programme cost per person A$ c	272.2	272.2	272.2	255.4
To prevent one death from melanoma:				
Number of subjects in programme = number needed to screen = 1/d	2500	1812	3906	7143
Number of screens = s/d	25,000	18,116	39,063	71,429
Number of false positives = p/d	575	417	898	786
Total cost, A$000 = c/d	681	493	1063	1824

65% of subjects reported that they or another non-medical person currently checked their skin for early signs of skin cancer.[55] More recently in Queensland, we conducted in 1998 a large telephone survey of a random sample of 3110 adults aged 30 or more. A total of 74% of subjects said they or another non-medical person had in the past year deliberately checked the skin on all or parts of their body for early signs of skin cancer, not including checks of particular moles or spots. This is the highest prevalence of self screening yet reported in Australia. Self screening involving a systematic whole body assessment is less common, and historical data are lacking. In the most recent Queensland survey, over one quarter of subjects reported that they or another non-medical person had in the past 12 months deliberately checked the skin on their whole body for early signs of skin cancer, with the additional prompt 'By this I mean, checked all your skin, front and back'. Unlike the previous Queensland study, skin self examination practice did not increase with age and was most commonly reported in men and women aged 30 to 49 years.

In regard to skin screening by a doctor, 17% of subjects in a 1988 survey in New South Wales reported having had a doctor check their moles in the past year, and in Victoria in 1990, 22% reported a doctor had ever systematically examined all or most of their skin for signs of skin cancer.[53,54] In Queensland in 1990, 18% of subjects said they went to their general practitioner or skin specialist to have their whole body checked, although no time frame was specified.[55] In our 1998 survey in Queensland, 39% of subjects reported a doctor had in the past year deliberately checked the skin on all or parts of (the) body for early signs of skin cancer not including checks of particular moles or spots of concern, and 13% of the total sample reported whole body skin examination, down to underwear, by a doctor in the past year. Twenty two per cent had had at least one such examination in the past three years. Although melanoma risk increases markedly with age, whole body screening by a doctor in this most recent survey did not. Like self screening, it was more frequent in people aged 30–49 years than in older subjects.

Screening is similarly widespread in New Zealand where, like Australia, public education campaigns for skin cancer prevention and early detection have been conducted for some decades in response to a high incidence of melanoma. In a survey in the mid 1980s, 44% of subjects reported that they, a family member or friend had checked their skin in the past year, and in 1993/94, 53% of 21-year-olds reported that they themselves had deliberately checked their skin in the past year.[56,57]

In the United States, with a lower incidence of melanoma, the nationwide prevalence of skin self examination seems now to be approaching the level seen in Australia and New Zealand a decade ago. In each of two national telephone surveys in the United States in 1995 and 1996 almost half of the respondents reported that they had closely examined themselves for signs of melanoma or skin cancer in the past year.[58,59] In a survey of 200 residents of Rhode Island in 1997, 59% of subjects reported that they at least sometimes actually looked at all the different areas of the skin deliberately and systematically, although only 9% were regarded as performing thorough skin examination, defined as always or almost always examining at least seven of eight listed areas of the body.[60] The response rate for this survey was quite low (42%) and middle aged and higher income people were overrepresented; nevertheless the proportion reporting skin self examination represents a large increase from a decade before when 24% of subjects in Connecticut reported they or someone other than a physician had ever carefully examined their own skin, that is, checked the surfaces of their skin deliberately and purposefully.[43,61]

Comparisons between surveys conducted at different times and places, in different populations and age groups, and using different definitions of screening and different questionnaire wording, are necessarily limited. Nevertheless, it seems that the practice of skin screening is increasing, presumably as a result of increasing public education and awareness about skin cancer. In Queensland, skin screening by a doctor, although not recommended by the Australian Cancer Society because of the lack of evidence of effectiveness, occurs across most adult age groups at a level now approaching that of breast cancer screening in women over 40.[52] It is clearly time for the benefits, risks, and cost-effectiveness of population based skin screening to be properly evaluated and communicated to doctors and consumers with clear evidence based guidelines for starting ages and screening intervals. Such evidence can come best from a randomized controlled trial.

A RANDOMIZED TRIAL OF SCREENING FOR MELANOMA

In this chapter, we have presented the case for a randomized trial of screening for melanoma. Although primary prevention campaigns may reduce the incidence of melanoma in the long term, the only option currently available to reduce deaths from melanoma in the short term is early diagnosis. Although skin screening has the potential to achieve early diagnosis and improved prognosis, the effectiveness of any form of screening for melanoma has not been established. Despite this, we have shown that informal screening has increased in Australia and other white-skinned populations over the past decade, and interest in screening among the medical profession and the public is likely to grow, with accompanying increases in cutaneous excisions, morbidity, patient anxiety, and cost.[42]

A randomized controlled trial with melanoma mortality as the end point is the definitive means of determining whether screening is effective. It may now be our last opportunity for such a trial to proceed with a reasonable chance of success, before screening becomes an accepted and expensive, although unproven, aspect of health care, and the means of determining its effectiveness become practically, and ethically, impossible.

The pilot phase for a randomized controlled trial of a community based screening programme for melanoma is under way in Queensland.[62] This is one of the few places in the world where such a trial is feasible, given this state's high melanoma incidence. The aim of the trial is to determine the effectiveness of a three-year community based screening programme in reducing mortality from melanoma. The design provides 85% power to detect a 20% reduction in mortality in the 15 years from the beginning of the intervention period. Such a result would represent a significant public health benefit, comparable to the reduction in mortality demonstrated by randomized trials of screening for breast and colorectal cancer.[63–66]

Overview of trial design

The sample comprises a total of 44 eligible Queensland communities with an aggregate population of 559,000 persons aged 30 years or over (Figure 9.4). Communities will be paired according to their size, broad geographic location , and socioeconomic status, based on standard indicators, and randomized within pairs into intervention or control groups.

In intervention communities, the community based melanoma screening programme will be delivered over three years. This will comprise a community education programme to promote self screening, prompt medical attention for suspicious lesions thus detected, and whole body clinical skin examination; an education and support programme for general practitioners; and the provision of supplementary screening services. No programme activities will be conducted in control communities. The target population for the trial will comprise all adults aged 30 years or more resident in the geographical boundaries of the intervention and control communities as defined by the Australian Bureau of Statistics. The inception cohort will comprise all adults aged 30 years or more resident in these communities at the beginning of the intervention period and registered on the Queensland electoral roll.

Deaths from melanoma, deaths from all causes, incident cases of melanoma, and the thickness of melanoma at diagnosis among inception cohort members during the 15 years from the beginning of

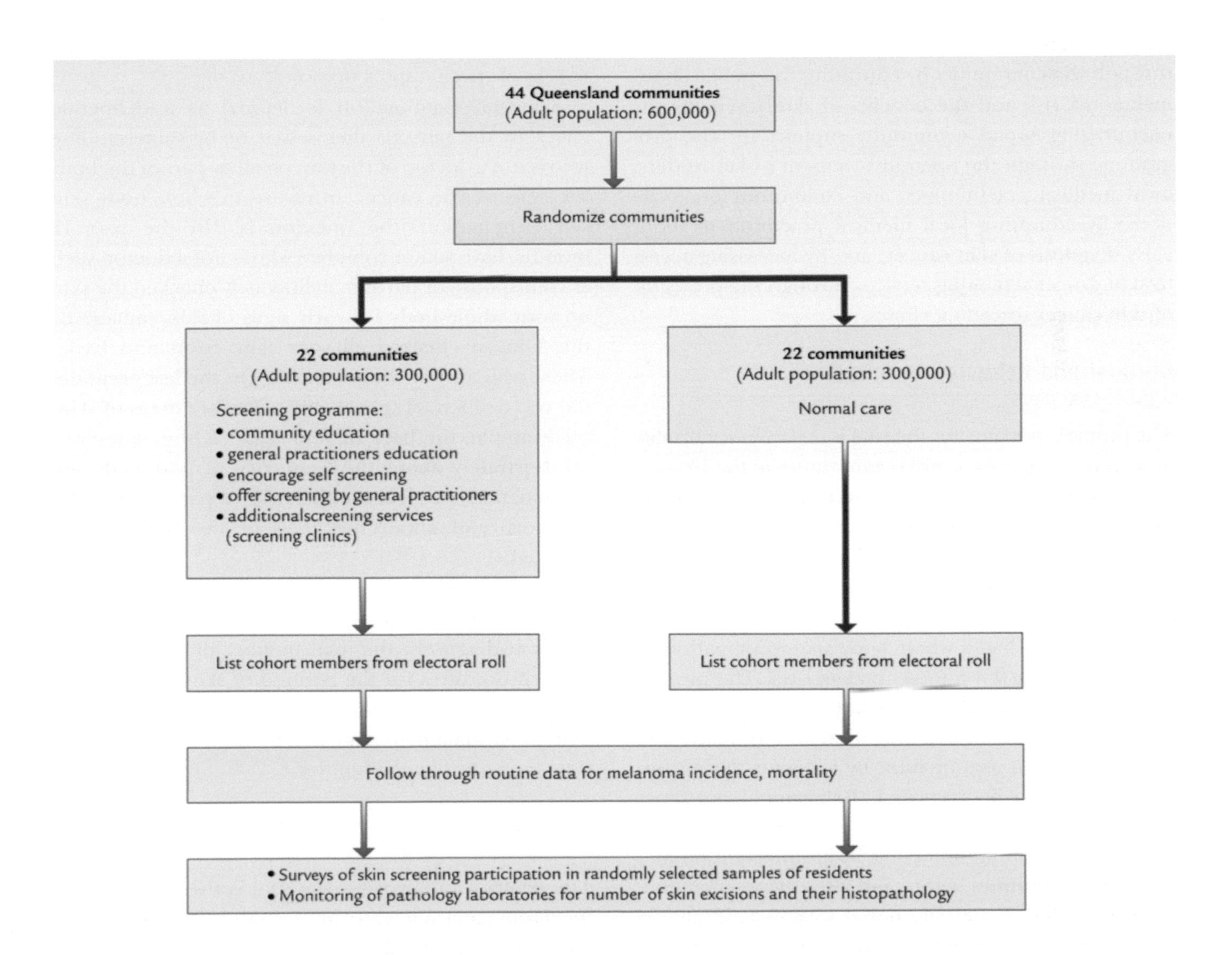

Figure 9.4 *Design of a randomized trial of a community based melanoma screening programme.*[62]

the intervention period will be identified using routine mortality collections and state cancer registry notifications.

The community based melanoma screening programme

The goal of the screening programme is to ensure that during the three-year intervention period, at least 60% of the adult population has at least one whole body skin examination by a general practitioner (an approximate three-fold increase from baseline), and at least 40% has at least two such examinations separated by no less than a year.

The programme is based on established theories of behavioural change.[67,68] The programme is designed to facilitate the uptake of skin screening and its diffusion through the community by educating the public about melanoma risk and the benefits of skin screening; by encouraging broad community support for the programme through the open involvement of key leaders, local medical practitioners, and community organizations; by educating local medical practitioners about early diagnosis of skin cancer; and by increasing access to skin cancer screening services through the provision of skin cancer screening clinics.

Clinical and behavioural outcomes

The primary outcome for the trial is melanoma mortality in intervention and control communities in the 15 years after the introduction of the screening programme, including only those deaths from melanoma that occur among cases diagnosed during this period.

The primary behavioural outcome is the proportion of the population in intervention and control communities who have had a whole body skin examination by a doctor during the intervention period. The proportions of the population who have performed whole and part body skin self examination and who have had a part body skin examination by a doctor during this period will also be recorded. Behavioural outcomes will be measured through cross-sectional community surveys by telephone interview in all intervention and control communities before and after the intervention. In addition, cross-sectional postal surveys at 12 and 24 months after the start of the intervention will be used to monitor the uptake of screening and allow fine tuning of the intervention if required, through the redirection of resources for advertising and skin screening clinics to those communities where uptake may be slow.

Clinical skin examination is defined as a visual examination by a doctor of the skin on all or part of the body for signs of skin cancer. For whole body clinical skin examination, the relevant survey question is: 'In the past 12 months, has a doctor deliberately checked the skin on your whole body? Usually, this would involve taking your clothes off at least down to your underwear (bra and underpants).' For those who answer yes to this, the interviewer asks, 'On the last occasion you had a whole body check, did you take your clothes off at least down to your underwear?' Other questions ask separately about a doctor checking particular parts of the body for early signs of skin cancer, not including checks of specific spots or moles.

Skin self examination is defined as a deliberate check by the persons themselves, or by someone else who is not a doctor, of the skin on all or part of the body for signs of skin cancer. In regard to whole body skin self examination, the question is: 'In the past 12 months, have you or someone who is not a doctor, such as your spouse or partner, deliberately checked the skin on your whole body for early signs of skin cancer? By this I mean checked all your skin, front and back.' Those who answer yes are asked, 'On the last occasion, did you deliberately check difficult to see areas of skin, for example, the back of your legs?' Other questions ask separately about the frequency of part body self examination, not including checks of particular moles or spots, and about the areas of the body usually checked.

Secondary clinical outcomes include the incidence of melanoma during the 15-year period according to depth at diagnosis; the total number of excisions and other procedures for the removal of skin lesions, both melanocytic and non-melanocytic; and the ratio of benign to malignant skin lesions excised in intervention and control communities.

Statistical analysis and study power

The principal analysis for the trial is the difference in melanoma mortality rates between the intervention and control groups during the 15 years of follow up. The mortality rate will be estimated using the method of

Duffy et al. for cluster-randomized designs in which the power of the analysis is improved by using pretrial melanoma mortality rates to estimate variance between towns in melanoma mortality.[69] Assuming 15 years of follow up, versus (the square of the coefficient of variation of cluster specific death rates) of 0.25 as estimated from historical information on the number of melanoma deaths in each community provided by the Queensland Cancer Registry, and using 25 years of antecedent data, the trial has 85% power (95% confidence interval 82% to 88%) to detect a 20% reduction in melanoma mortality between intervention and control groups for a two-sided test where alpha = 0.05. If screening produced a mortality benefit of much less than 20%, the study may not have the power to detect it. However, such a mortality benefit would be unlikely to be sufficient to justify institution of a population screening programme.

Ethical issues

This trial will assess the effectiveness of an increasingly common clinical procedure for which the potential benefits, but also the potential harm and costs, are great. In this circumstance, it is important to complete this trial as quickly as possible so that doctors and patients can make truly informed decisions about skin screening. Those in communities in the control group will not be disadvantaged, as they will continue to receive normal care. Written informed consent will be obtained from all patients presenting to the screening clinics in intervention communities. The pilot phase for the trial has received ethical approval from a duly constituted institutional ethics committee, and separate approval will be obtained for additional surveys and studies done as part of the project.

Screening participation at baseline and changes after 12 months of the pilot phase

During the pilot phase, the melanoma screening programme was launched in nine small communities, beginning in the first community in February 1998 with the other eight communities launched subsequently one at a time at intervals of one month. Surveys of screening participation at baseline and after 12 months of the intervention have been completed in these, and their matched control communities.

Progress to date is promising in terms of early increases in screening participation in intervention communities in the pilot phase. Skin cancer screening clinics were provided from the beginning of the intervention period for three communities in the pilot phase. In these three communities, the prevalence of whole body skin examinations by a doctor in the previous 12 months has increased almost three-fold from 10.8% at baseline to 27.1% one year after the start of the intervention. There has been no significant increase in screening participation in the three matched control communities (10.9% at baseline to 12.1% after 12 months).

In the remaining six intervention communities in the pilot phase, skin clinics were provided from the second year of the intervention to meet the demand for screening generated by the community education campaign. Where it has been completed to date, the second annual survey has measured a similar increase in screening participation as described above for the first three communities, and again, no increase in screening in the matched control communities. The provision of supplementary screening services through skin screening clinics is likely to remain a key component of the programme in all intervention communities.

The pilot phase of this project has demonstrated that a randomized trial of a community based screening programme is feasible within a reasonable budget, and results to date indicate that it is likely to achieve the level of community support and screening participation necessary for the long term success of the project.

RECOMMENDATIONS ON SCREENING POLICY

Given the lack of empirical evidence, it is not surprising that the conclusions of expert groups on skin screening vary considerably.[70–73] Many expert groups who base their findings on an evidence based review of scientific literature do not recommend screening: such groups include the US Preventive Services Task Force, the US National Cancer Institute, the American College of Preventive Medicine, the Canadian Task Force on the Periodic Health Examination, and the International Union against Cancer (UICC).[74–79] The 1999 Australian Clinical Guidelines, which were produced by the Australian Cancer Network and the National Health and Medical Research Council after extensive consultation and review, do not recommend screening for average risk people.[80,81] The Australian and New Zealand cancer societies do not recommend screening.[82,83] Several of these groups do recommend screening of high risk subjects, and advocate awareness and good clinical management of skin lesions. In contrast, many American groups, such as the American Cancer Society, the American Academy of Dermatology and a National Institutes of Health Consensus Conference support regular screening, on its own or linked to a general health check.[40,84–87] The differences in recommendations relate to the relative weight given to empirical evidence of benefit, the professional viewpoints of the groups, whether economic factors are explicitly considered, and perhaps the difference in approach between American and European medical cultures that has been noted in other screening contexts;[88,89] the Australian approach seems closer to the European.

CONCLUSIONS

Screening for cancer on a population basis requires strong evidence. Screening programmes for breast cancer and colorectal cancer are supported by evidence from large scale population based randomized trials; screening for uterine cervical cancer does not have randomized trial evidence but has a large number of strong cohort and case–control studies to support it. In other cancer screening situations, for example, for ovarian cancer, the predominant view is that screening should not be undertaken until the results of current randomized trials become available. In contrast, the evidence base for screening for melanoma is extremely weak. There are no available results from randomized trials or cohort studies, the only analytical study result being the single case–control study. The main argument for the effectiveness of screening is based on the assumption that earlier diagnosis will produce mortality and morbidity benefits, which in turn is based on the large differences in postdiagnosis survival with depth of invasion, for patients diagnosed in normal clinical practice. This assumption may be correct, but without empirical evidence, it remains a hypothesis.

The difficulties of carrying out the ideal evaluation study, a randomized trial, are considerable. One such study has been designed, and the pilot phase has been successfully completed; if funding support is given, this trial should provide important results on the effectiveness of one approach to screening. Other evaluations, in other countries and using different screening methods, could use randomized or non-randomized trials, or well designed cohort, case–control, or time series designs. Until such evidence becomes available, the effects of screening will remain uncertain.

ACKNOWLEDGEMENTS

We thank the following people for their assistance in providing data on international comparisons of melanoma depth distribution: Judy Symmons, Philippa Youl and Anna Chung (Queensland); Jim Fraser (New Zealand); Robert Greenlee (USA) and Rona MacKie, David Hole and Caroline Bray (Scotland). We thank Philippa Youl for calculation of incidence rates and Sue Aspinall for assistance in reviewing the literature.

REFERENCES

1. Rigel DS, Friedman RJ, Kopf AW, The incidence of malignant melanoma in the United States: issues as we approach the 21st century. *J Am Acad Dermatol* 1996; 34: 839–47.
2. Giles GG, Armstrong BK, Burton RC, et al, Has mortality from melanoma stopped rising in Australia? Analysis of trends between 1931 and 1994. *BMJ* 1996; 312.
3. Roush GC, McKay L, Holford TR, A reversal of the long-term increase in deaths attributable to malignant melanoma. *Cancer* 1992; 69: 1714–20.
4. MacLennan R, Green AC, McLeod GRC, Martin NG, Increasing incidence of cutaneous melanoma in Queensland, Australia. *J Natl Cancer Inst* 1992; 84: 1427–32.
5. Cooke K, McNoe B, Hursthouse M, Taylor R, Primary malignant melanoma of skin in four regions of New Zealand. *N Z Med J* 1992; 105: 303–6.
6. MacKie RM, Hole D, Audit of public education campaign to encourage earlier detection of malignant melanoma. *BMJ* 1992; 304: 1012–15.
7. Dennis LK, Analysis of the melanoma epidemic, both apparent and real. Data from 1973 through 1994 surveillance, epidemiology, and end results program registry. *Arch Dermatol* 1999; 135: 275–80.
8. Burton RC, Coates MS, Hersey P, et al, An analysis of a melanoma epidemic. *Int J Cancer* 1993; 55: 765–70.
9. Lipsker DM, Hedelin G, Heid E, et al, Striking increase of thin melanomas contrasts with stable incidence of thick melanomas. *Arch Dermatol* 1999; 135: 1451–6.
10. Davis NC, Herron JJ, Queensland melanoma project: organization and a plea for comparable surveys. *Med J Aust* 1966; 1: 643–4.
11. Smith T, The Queensland melanoma project – an exercise in health education. *BMJ* 1979; 1: 253–4.
12. Woolcock HR, Thearle MJ, *A History of the Queensland Cancer Fund 1961–1991.* Brisbane: Queensland Cancer Fund, 1991.
13. Stanganelli I, Raccagni AA, Baldassari L, et al, Analysis of Breslow tumor thickness distribution of skin melanoma in the Italian region of Romagna, 1986–1991. *Tumori* 1994; 80: 416–21.
14. Swerlick RA, Chen S, The melanoma epidemic. Is increased surveillance the solution or the problem? *Arch Dermatol* 1996; 132: 881–4.
15. Burton RC, Armstrong BK, Current melanoma epidemic: a non-metastasizing form of melanoma?. *World J Surg* 1995; 19: 330–3.

16. Richard MA, Grob JJ, Avril MF, et al, Melanoma and tumour thickness. Challenges of early diagnosis. *Arch Dermatol* 1999; 135: 269–74.
17. MacKie RM, Thickness and delay in diagnosis of melanoma. How far can we go? *Arch Dermatol* 1999; 135: 339–40.
18. Hanrahan PF, Hersey P, D'Este CA, Factors involved in presentation of older people with thick melanoma. *Med J Aust* 1998; 169: 410–14.
19. Hersey P, Sillar R, Howe CG, et al, Factors related to the presentation of patients with thick primary melanomas. *Med J Aust* 1991; 154: 583–7.
20. South Australian Cancer Registry, *Epidemiology of cancer in South Australia: incidence, mortality and survival 1977–1997, incidence and mortality 1997.* Adelaide: Openbook Publishers, 1998.
21. Doherty VR, MacKie RM, Experience of a public education programme on early detection of cutaneous malignant melanoma. *BMJ* 1988; 297: 388–91.
22. MacKie RM, Melanoma prevention and early detection. *Br Med Bull* 1995; 51: 570–83.
23. Melia J, Early detection of cutaneous malignant melanoma in Britain. *Int J Epidemiol* 1995; 24: S39–S44.
24. Graham-Brown RAC, Osborne JE, London SP, et al, The initial effects on workload and outcome of a public education campaign on early diagnosis and treatment of malignant melanoma in Leicestershire. *Br J Dermatol* 1990; 122: 53–9.
25. Whitehead SM, Wroughton MA, Elwood JM, et al, Effects of a health education campaign for the earlier diagnosis of melanoma. *Br J Cancer* 1989; 60: 421–5.
26. Del Mar CB, Green AC, Battistutta D, Do public media campaigns designed to increase skin cancer awareness result in increased skin excision rates? *Aust NZ J Public Health* 1997; 21: 751–3.
27. Koh HK, Caruso A, Gage I, et al, Evaluation of melanoma/skin cancer screening in Massachusetts. *Cancer* 1990; 65: 375–9.
28. Koh HK, Norton LA, Geller AC, et al, Evaluation of the American Academy of Dermatology's national skin cancer early detection and screening program. *J Am Acad Dermatol* 1996; 34: 971–8.
29. Rampen FHJ, van Huystee BEWL, Kiemeney LALM, Melanoma/skin cancer screening clinics: experiences in the Netherlands. *J Am Acad Dermatol* 1991; 25: 776–7.
30. Rampen FH, Casparie-van Velsen JI, van Huystee BE, et al, False-negative findings in skin cancer and melanoma screening. *J Am Acad Dermatol* 1995; 33: 59–63.
31. de Rooij MJ, Rampen FH, Schouten LJ, Neumann HA, Volunteer melanoma screenings. Follow-up, compliance, and outcome. *Dermatol Surg* 1997; 23: 197–201.
32. Katris P, Crock JG, Gray BN, Research note: the Lions Cancer Institute and the Western Australian Society of Plastic Surgeons skin cancer screening programme. *Aust NZ J Surg* 1996; 66: 101–4.
33. Kricker A, English DR, Randell PL, et al, Skin cancer in Geraldton, Western Australia: a survey of incidence and prevalence. *Med J Aust* 1990; 152: 399–407.
34. McGee R, Elwood M, Sneyd MJ, et al, The recognition and management of melanoma and other skin lesions by general practitioners in New Zealand. *NZ Med J* 1994; 107: 287–90.
35. Burton RC, Howe C, Adamson L, et al, General practitioner screening for melanoma: sensitivity, specificity, and effect of training. *J Med Screening* 1998; 5: 156–61.
36. Doherty VR, MacKie RM, Reasons for poor prognosis in British patients with cutaneous malignant melanoma. *BMJ* 1986; 292: 987–9.
37. Kirkpatrick JJ, Taggart I, Rigby HG, Townsend PL, A pigmented lesion clinic: analysis of the first year's 1055 patients. *Br J Plast Surg* 1995; 48: 247–51.
38. Edmondson PC, Curley RK, Marsden RA, et al, Screening for malignant melanoma using instant photography. *J Med Screening* 1999; 6: 42–6.
39. Fitzpatrick TB, Rhodes AR, Sober AJ, Mihm CM Jr, Primary malignant melanoma of the skin: the call for action to identify persons at risk; to discover precursor lesions; to detect early melanomas. In: *Naevi and melanoma: incidence, interrelationships and implications; pigment cell no. 9.* (Elwood JM, ed.) Basel: Karger, 1988: 110–17.
40. Friedman RJ, Rigel DS, Silverman MK, et al, Malignant melanoma in the 1990s: the continued importance of early detection and the role of physician examination and self-examination of the skin. *CA Cancer J Clin* 1991; 41: 201–26.
41. Burton RC, Armstrong BK, Recent incidence trends imply a non-metastasizing form of invasive melanoma. *Melanoma Res* 1994; 4: 107–13.
42. Burton RC, Analysis of public education and the implications with regard to nonprogressive thin melanomas. *Curr Opin Oncol* 1995; 7: 170–4.
43. Berwick M, Begg CB, Fine JA, et al, Screening for cutaneous melanoma by skin self-examination. *J Natl Cancer Inst* 1996; 88: 17–23.
44. Elwood JM, Skin self-examination and melanoma. *J Natl Cancer Inst* 1996; 88: 3–5.
45. Rhodes AR, Intervention strategy to prevent lethal cutaneous melanoma: use of dermatologic photography to aid surveillance of high-risk persons. *J Am Acad Dermatol* 1998; 39: 262–7.
46. Masri GD, Clark WH Jr, Guerry DIV, et al, Screening and surveillance of patients at high risk for malignant melanoma result in detection of earlier disease. *J Am Acad Dermatol* 1990; 22: 1042–8.
47. MacKie RM, McHenry P, Hole D, Accelerated detection with prospective surveillance for cutaneous malignant melanoma in high risk groups. *Lancet* 1993; 341: 1618–20.
48. Tucker MA, Halpern A, Holly EA, et al, Clinically recognized dysplastic nevi. *JAMA* 1997; 277: 1439–44.
49. Jackson A, Wilkinson C, Ranger M, et al, Can primary prevention or selective screening for melanoma be more precisely targeted through general practice? A prospective study to validate a self administered risk score. *BMJ* 1998; 316: 34–8.
50. Grob JJ, Gouvernet J, Aymar D, et al, Count of benign melanocytic nevi as a major indicator of risk for nonfamilial nodular and superficial spreading melanoma. *Cancer* 1990; 66: 387–95.
51. Girgis A, Clarke P, Burton RC, Sanson-Fisher RW, Screening for melanoma by primary health care physicians: a cost-effectiveness analysis. *J Med Screening* 1996; 3: 47–53.
52. Hill D, White V, Borland R, Cockburn J, Cancer-related beliefs and behaviours in Australia. *Aust J Public Health* 1991; 15: 14–23.
53. Girgis A, Campbell EM, Redman S, Sanson-Fisher RW, Screening for melanoma: a community survey of prevalence and predictors. *Med J Aust* 1991; 154: 338–43.
54. Borland R, Meehan JW, Skin examination for signs of cancer. *Aust J Public Health* 1995; 19: 85–8.
55. Balanda KP, Lowe JB, Stanton WR, Gillespie AM, Enhancing the early detection of melanoma within current guidelines. *Aust J Public Health* 1994; 18: 420–3.
56. McGee R, Elwood JM, Social epidemiology of health problems: Cancer. In: *Social dimensions of health and disease: New Zealand perspectives* (Spicer J, Trlin A, Walton JA, eds) Palmerston North: Dunmore Press, 1994: 67–82.
57. Douglass HM, McGee R, Williams S, Are young adults checking their skin for melanoma? *Aust NZ J Public Health* 1998; 22: 562–7.
58. Miller DR, Geller AC, Wyatt SW, et al, Melanoma awareness and self-examination practices: results of a United States survey. *J Am Acad Dermatol* 1996; 34: 962–70.
59. Robinson JK, Rigel DS, Amonette RA, What promotes skin self-examination? *J Am Acad Dermatol* 1998; 39: 752–7.
60. Weinstock MA, Martin RA, Risica PM, et al, Thorough skin examination for the early detection of melanoma. *Am J Prev Med* 1999; 17: 169–75
61. Oliveria SA, Christos PJ, Halpern AC, et al, Evaluation of factors associated with skin self-examination. *J Am Acad Dermatol* 1999; 34: 962–70.
62. Aitken JF, Elwood JM, Lowe JB, Firman DW, Balanda KP, Ring IT, A randomised trial of population screening for melanoma. *J Med Screening* 2002; 9: 33–7.
63. Shapiro S, Venet W, Strax P, Venet L, *Periodic screening for breast cancer: the health insurance plan project and its sequelae, 1963–1986.* Baltimore: Johns Hopkins University Press, 1988.
64. Alexander FE, Anderson TJ, Brown HK, et al, The Edinburgh randomised trial of breast cancer screening: results after 10 years of follow-up. *Br J Cancer* 1994; 70: 542–8.
65. Hardcastle JD, Chamberlain JO, Robinson MHE, et al, Randomised controlled trial of faecal-occult-blood screening for colorectal cancer. *Lancet* 1996; 348: 1472–7.

66. Kronborg O, Fenger C, Olsen J, et al, Randomised study of screening for colorectal cancer with faecal-occult-blood test. *Lancet* 1996; 348: 1467–71.
67. Bandura A, *Social foundations of thought and action.* Englewood Cliffs, NJ: Prentice Hall, 1986.
68. Rogers EM, *Diffusion of innovations.* New York: Free Press, 1983.
69. Duffy SW, South MC, Day NE, Cluster randomization in large public health trials: The importance of antecedent data. *Stat Med* 1992; 11: 307–16.
70. Lipskie TL, A summary of cancer screening guidelines. *Chronic Dis Can* 1998; 19: 112–30.
71. Rampen RH, Mass population skin cancer screening is not worthwhile. *J Cutan Med Surg* 1998; 2: 128–9.
72. Weinstock MA, Mass population skin cancer screening can be worthwhile (if it's done right). *J Cutan Med Surg* 1998; 2: 129–32.
73. Elwood JM, Screening for melanoma and options for its evaluation. *J Med Screening* 1994; 1: 22–38.
74. United States Preventive Services Task Force, Screening for skin cancer: recommendations and rationale. *Am J Prev Med* 2001; 20: 44–6.
75. National Cancer Institute, *PDQ database – detection and prevention.* http://cancernet.nci.nih.govt, 1999.
76. Hill L, Ferrini RL, Skin cancer prevention and screening: summary of the American College of Preventive Medicine's practice policy statements. *CA Cancer J Clin* 1998; 48: 232–5.
77. Canadian Task Force on the Periodic Health Examination, *The Canadian guide to clinical preventive health care.* Ottawa: Health Canada, 1994.
78. Miller AB, Chamberlain J, Day NE, et al, Report on a workshop of the UICC project on evaluation of screening for cancer. *Int J Cancer* 1990; 46: 761–9.
79. International Union Against Cancer (UICC), *Melanoma control manual.* Geneva: UICC, 1992.
80. Marks R, Elwood JM, Screening for skin cancer. In: *Guidelines for preventive interventions in primary health care – cardiovascular disease and cancer.* (Health Advancement Standing Committee, ed.) Canberra: National Health and Medical Research Council (NHMRC): 1996: 100–15.
81. Australian Cancer Network, National Health and Medical Research Council, *Clinical practice guidelines: the management of malignant melanoma.* Commonwealth of Australia: Canberra, 1999.
82. The Cancer Council Australia, National cancer prevention policy 2001–2003. Sydney: The Cancer Council Australia, 2001.
83. Elwood JM, Glasgow H, *The prevention and early detection of melanoma in New Zealand.* Wellington: Cancer Society of New Zealand and Department of Health, 1993.
84. American Cancer Society, Update January 1992: the American Cancer Society guidelines for the cancer-related check-up. *CA Cancer J Clin* 1992; 42: 44–5.
85. McDonald CJ, American Cancer Society perspective on the American College of Preventive Medicine's Policy Statements on Skin Cancer Prevention and Screening. *CA Cancer J Clin* 1998; 48: 229–31.
86. Goldsmith L, Koh HK, Bewerse B, et al, Proceedings from the national conference to develop a national skin cancer agenda. *J Am Acad Dermatol* 1996; 34: 822–3.
87. Hall WH, Goldsmith LA, Askin FB, et al, Diagnosis and treatment of early melanoma. *JAMA* 1992; 268: 1314–19.
88. Jatoi I, Baum M, American and European recommendations for screening mammography in younger women: a cultural divide? *BMJ* 1993; 307: 1481–3.
89. Elwood JM, Breast cancer screening in younger women: evidence and decision making. *J Eval Clin Pract* 1997; 3: 179–86.

10

The histological diagnosis and classification of melanoma

Kerry Crotty, Stanley McCarthy, Martin C Mihm Jr

INTRODUCTION

The histological diagnosis of melanocytic lesions is one of the greatest challenges for pathologists. Although most benign and malignant melanocytic lesions can be diagnosed with certainty, significant numbers of cases are diagnostically difficult and may lead to varied diagnoses even among expert melanopathologists.[1] This difficulty in diagnosis is compounded by the fact that smaller and less classical lesions are being removed because of increasing awareness among clinicians and patients about the need for vigilance concerning melanocytic lesions. The use by clinicians of instruments, both computer aided and hand held, that provide magnification of the macroscopic appearance of lesions has also led to a different pattern of excision of lesions.

PATHOLOGICAL DIAGNOSIS

There is no single histological criterion that definitely separates benign and malignant melanocytic lesions. Every characteristic that has been described in melanoma has also been found in benign naevi. There are several different types of benign melanocytic naevi, including banal junctional, compound, and dermal melanocytic naevi, as well as congenital, dysplastic (atypical), blue, cellular blue, deep penetrating, Spitz (spindle and epithelioid), ancient, desmoplastic, balloon cell, and halo naevi. Each type of benign naevus may simulate malignant melanoma and vice versa.

A further confounding factor in the diagnosis of melanoma is that melanomas are frequently adjacent to or admixed with benign naevi including banal and dysplastic types.

The histological features must be evaluated in conjunction with clinical and macroscopic data. Pathologists should make their histological assessment initially without reference to the clinical context. However, the histological features have to be further assessed in the clinical context. This stresses the importance of the clinician providing all relevant data in the pathology request form including age, sex, site, pregnancy, history of previous melanomas or naevi at the site of the current lesion or elsewhere, and recent change in the lesion. The clinician should also provide their provisional and differential diagnoses to the pathologist. Accurate diagnosis of melanocytic lesions may require a consultation between the clinician and the pathologist, either by telephone, by email, or in person at the microscope.

The histological diagnosis of melanocytic lesions requires assessment of architectural and cytological features. Histological features that are more often present in melanoma than benign naevi include asymmetry, ulceration, cytological atypia, pagetoid involvement of the epidermis, lack of maturation, and dermal mitoses including deep and atypical types.

Asymmetry

Symmetry is assessed by looking at the silhouette of the lesion, and the distribution of its characteristics around a central vertical plane. Benign naevi are usually symmetrical whereas melanomas are often asymmetrical (Figure 10.1). This reflects the disordered growth of melanomas. Features contributing to symmetry and asymmetry include the extent of lateral spread, the pattern of dermal infiltration, the presence of pigmentation and the host response. Benign lesions are usually uniform and monotonous, whereas melanomas are varied and disordered. However, many melanomas, especially those that are small, may be symmetrical and uniform.

Ulceration

The presence of non-traumatic ulceration is an indication that the lesion is probably malignant (Figure 10.2). In addition, ulceration is a poor prognostic feature in melanomas and the greater the extent of ulceration the worse the prognosis.[2]

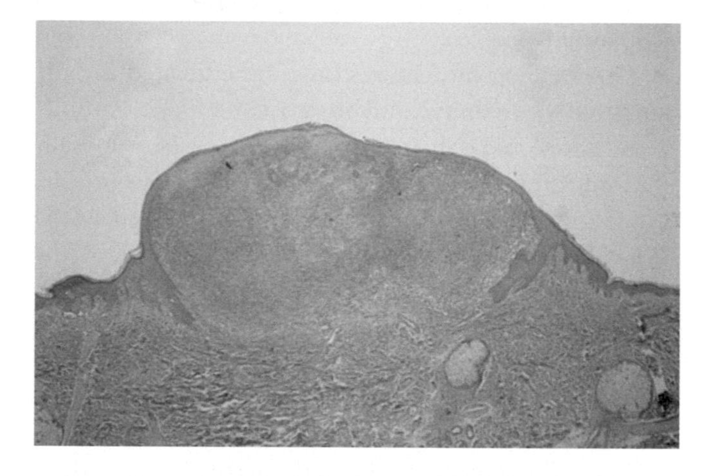

Figure 10.1 *Malignant melanoma exhibiting asymmetry. The two halves of the lesion are not mirror images.*

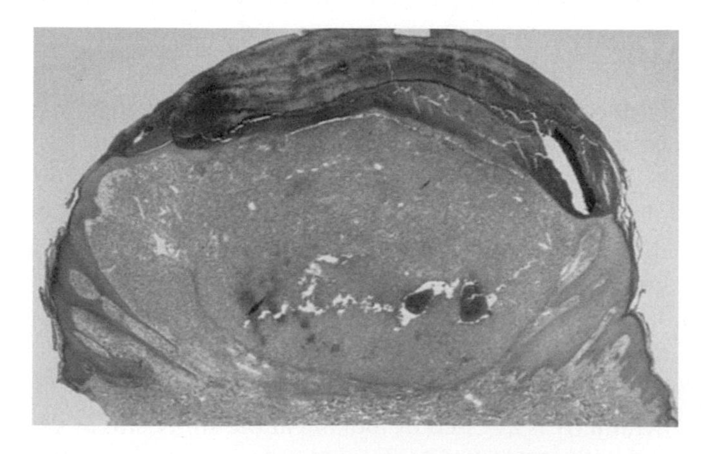

Figure 10.2 *Ulcerated nodular malignant melanoma.*

Cytological atypia

There is great variety in the cells that may be present in melanoma. The cells may vary from very small to very large in size. Their shape may be round, oval, polygonal, spindled, dendritic, or irregular. The cytological features of melanoma are protean, and melanoma may mimic other neoplasms. Cytological atypia is usually present (Figure 10.3) and is assessed mainly by looking at nuclear features. The nuclei often have irregular membranes, coarse chromatin, and hyperchromasia. Nuclear pseudoinclusions may be present. There is also great variety in the cytoplasmic features of melanoma. The cytoplasm may be eosinophilic, basophilic, amphophilic, granular, ground glass, pale, and/or vacuolated.[3] While the cytological features of melanoma are usually atypical, in some cases the melanoma cells can be very bland and resemble a banal naevus, the so called naevoid melanoma. On the other hand, some benign naevi such as Spitz naevi exhibit cytological atypia that may lead to confusion in diagnosis.

Melanin may or may not be present in the cytoplasm of melanoma cells. If no pigment is present the pathologist needs to seek confirmation that the lesion is melanocytic in origin. This confirmation can include the presence of a junctional component or the use of immunohistochemical stains such as S-100 protein or Melan-A. One useful feature that may help in the diagnosis of melanomas is the presence or absence of pigment in the deepest component of the lesion. Naevus cells usually, but not always, lose their pigment with descent into the dermis, whereas melanomas often exhibit melanin in the deep dermal cells.

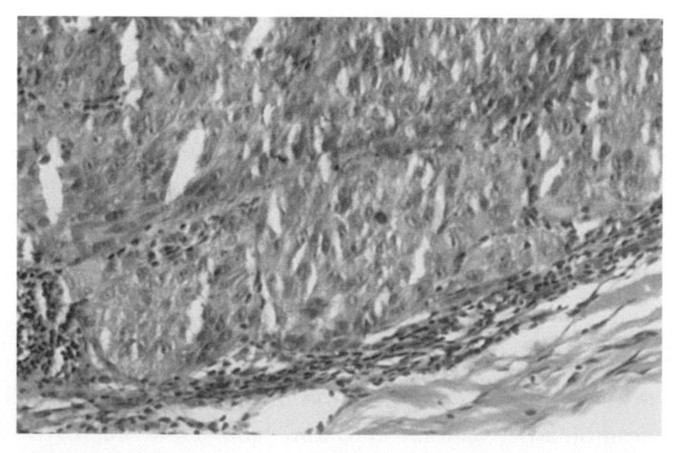

Figure 10.3 *Malignant melanoma showing large atypical cells, lack of maturation, and a deep mitosis.*

Pagetoid involvement of the epidermis

The presence of atypical melanocytes singly and in small groups of two or three cells above the basal layer is a clue to the diagnosis of melanoma, particularly if the melanocytes are present up to and including the granular layer (Figure 10.4). This is termed pagetoid epidermal invasion, because of its similarity to Paget's disease of the nipple. The differential diagnosis of atypical cells in the epidermis includes Bowen's disease, in situ melanoma and Paget's disease.[4] Pagetoid spread may also be seen at times in benign melanocytic lesions including recurrent, Spitz and acral naevi.

Lack of maturation

As the melanocytes of benign naevi descend into the deeper dermis they usually become smaller both in cell and nuclear size compared with the melanocytes present in the superficial zone of the lesion. This is termed maturation. In melanomas there is often poor or no maturation (Figure 10.3), or there may be apparent maturation in which the cells become smaller but still possess significant atypia. It is also important not to mistakenly label as maturation the presence of an associated banal naevus at the base of a melanoma.

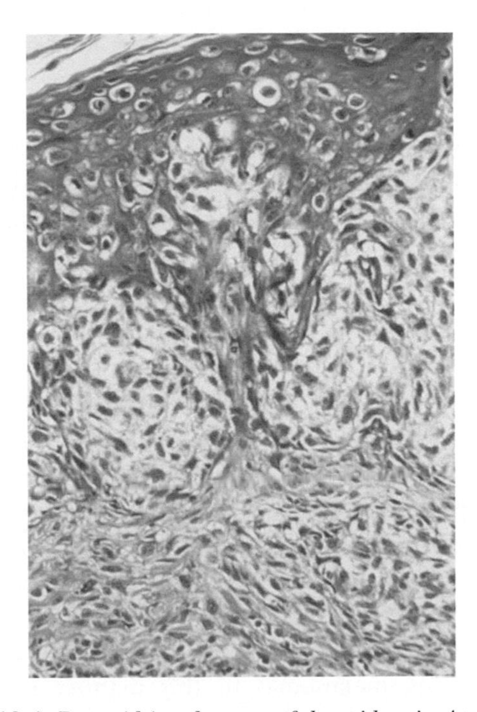

Figure 10.4 *Pagetoid involvement of the epidermis. Atypical melanocytes are present throughout the full thickness of the epidermis.*

Dermal mitoses including deep and atypical types

Mitoses are generally not present in benign naevi. Exceptions include Spitz naevi, traumatized naevi, halo naevi, and naevi in pregnant women. The presence of mitoses in a melanocytic lesion, especially if numerous and particularly if they are deep and/or atypical, should arouse suspicion of malignancy.[5]

Each lesion must be judged in its entirety together with the clinical details, including age, site and history of recent change. Additional special techniques may also be used.

SPECIAL TECHNIQUES

The pathologist may be assisted by ancillary techniques in the diagnosis of melanoma. These techniques include immunohistochemistry, DNA ploidy and morphometry, silver nucleolar organizer regions, proliferation studies, and genetic analysis.

Immunohistochemistry

Immunohistochemistry is standard practice in the diagnosis of melanocytic lesions. All melanocytic lesions stain with antibodies to S-100 protein. It is very sensitive but not very specific as it stains normal components of the skin including nerves, dendritic cells and sweat glands as well as many neoplasms including those of neural origin.[6] Both benign and malignant melanocytic lesions will stain with antibodies to S100 protein so it is of no use in differentiating benignity and malignancy (Figure 10.5). However, it is useful in poorly differentiated tumours to separate epithelial and other tumours from melanoma.

Melan-A (MART-1) is a melanosome associated glycoprotein that is recognized by autologous cytotoxic T cells.[7] It does not stain normal skin components such as nerves and Langerhans cells but it does stain naevus cells and most melanoma cells.[8] It is of no use in distinguishing a benign naevus from malignant melanoma but it is useful in distinguishing melanocytic tumours from non-melanocytic neoplasms. However, there are rare non-melanocytic neoplasms that are positive with Melan-A, including angiomyolipoma, adrenocortical

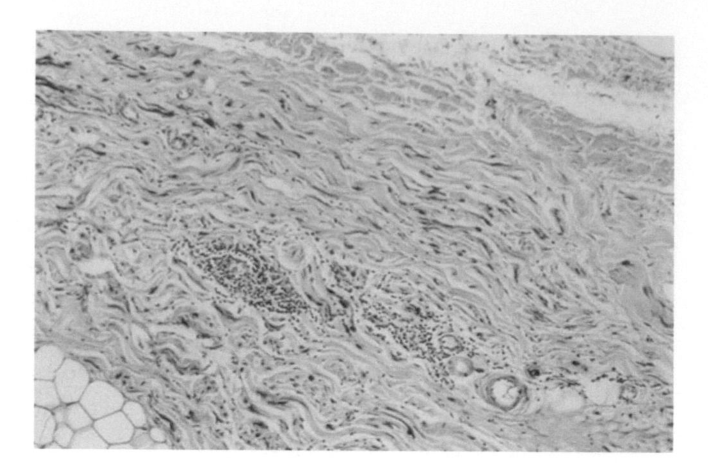

Figure 10.5 *S-100 staining the cells of a desmoplastic melanoma. Note the focal collection of lymphocytes in the centre. The presence of lymphocytes is a clue to the diagnosis of melanoma.*

adenomas and carcinomas, Leydig cell tumours, and Sertoli–Leydig cell tumours.

HMB-45 is a useful marker in the diagnosis of melanocytic lesions. It is rarely positive in benign naevi except in the junctional component and in blue naevi. It is often negative in melanoma, but if a lesion is positive for HMB-45 in the dermal component, especially the deep dermal component, the pathologist must be alerted to the lesion having a high probability of being melanoma.[9]

Proliferation markers such as proliferating cell nuclear antigen and Ki67(MIB-1) may be useful in distinguishing benign and malignant melanocytic lesions. Melanomas usually have a higher proliferation rate than naevi and there may be evidence of proliferation throughout the dermal component whereas evidence of proliferation is usually negative or confined to the superficial dermal component of benign naevi.[10] There is, however, some overlap between Spitz naevi and melanoma.

AgNORs

Nucleolar organizer regions (NORs) are ribosomal DNA that encode ribosome RNA and control the formation of ribosomes and proteins.[11] NORs can be visualized by silver (argyrophilic) staining of NORs associated proteins (AgNORs). AgNORs are considered to act as a marker of rDNA and its level of transcriptional activity. There is some overlap between naevi and melanoma, however, in general, melanoma tends to have a higher AgNORs count and more irregular AgNORs than benign naevi.[12]

DNA microdensitometry and nuclear morphometry

DNA microdensitometry measures the DNA nuclear profile by a technique using transmitted light passing through the specimen on a microscope stage. In general, benign naevi tend to have a normal DNA content, that is, they are diploid, whereas melanomas tend to be aneuploid. However, many melanomas are diploid.[12]

Nuclear morphometry is the measurement of nuclear features such as area, perimeter and length.[13] Morphometry can be a measure of the degree of cytological atypia and can be used to objectively assess the presence of maturation.[12]

CLASSIFICATION OF MELANOMA

Histological interpretation has led to a recognition of two stages in the progression of melanoma.[14,15] These are the radial or horizontal growth phase and the vertical growth phase. Melanomas are believed to begin as a proliferation of melanocytes in the epidermis (melanoma in situ). After a certain period of intraepidermal proliferation, many melanomas invade the papillary dermis as single cells or small nests of cells (microinvasion). Melanomas are then believed to grow and proliferate in the dermis. The intraepidermal and microinvasive phase is termed radial growth phase (RGP). The RGP is considered to have no capacity for metastasis. The proliferative phase is called vertical growth phase (VGP) and is considered to have capacity for metastasis. RGP is recognized by the presence of in situ melanoma with or without invasion of the papillary dermis by single cells or small nests of melanoma cells. Mitoses are absent in the RGP. VGP is recognized by the presence of sheets and/or large nest or nests of melanoma cells in the dermis. Mitoses are often present. There has been widespread acceptance of the RGP and VGP concept. However, there has not been universal adoption by pathologists of the practise of classifying melanomas in this manner in routine pathology reporting. One of the factors that has led to some reluctance to routinely classify melanomas according to growth phase is that it can be difficult to distinguish between microinvasive RGP and VGP. It must also be remembered that pathologists are only looking at a limited number of representative sections, and it is possible that evidence of a VGP may be missed because it is not present in the examined sections. This last caveat must be applied to all parameters assessed in melanocytic lesions.

There is some debate about the need for further subclassification of melanoma but there is no doubt that there are certain groupings of melanoma that can be separated by clinical and pathological features. Large numbers of melanomas do not readily fit into the classical groupings.[16] Classical groupings of melanoma include superficial spreading melanoma, nodular melanoma, lentigo maligna melanoma, and acral lentiginous melanoma.[14] Other rare types include desmoplastic, neurotropic, naevoid, balloon cell, myxoid, melanophagic (animal type), and signet ring cell melanomas.

Superficial spreading melanoma (SSM)

This is the most common subtype of melanoma, representing about two thirds of all melanomas. It can be present at any cutaneous site with the trunk of men and the lower limbs of women being the most common sites. Histologically, SSM is marked by an intraepidermal component that extends laterally more than three rete ridges beyond the dermal component. Pagetoid spread is common (Figure 10.6). The dermal component is variable but is often composed of nests and sheets of epithelioid melanocytes.[3,14]

Nodular melanoma (NM)

These are nodular or polypoid rapidly growing lesions that can occur on any cutaneous site. They are often brown, red, grey, or black but may be amelanotic. NM constitutes about 10% of cutaneous melanoma.[17] Histologically, they are marked by a lack of lateral spread of the epidermal and junctional component beyond the dermal component, that is, they seem to lack a radial growth phase and are classified as vertical growth phase only (Figure 10.2). The epidermal component is often ulcerated. The cells are usually epithelioid.

Lentigo maligna melanoma (LMM)

LMM usually arise on sun exposed sites, particularly head, neck, back, and upper extremities, of middle aged and elderly people. LMM arises in a precursor lesion called lentigo maligna (Hutchinson's melanotic freckle), which is a slow growing, irregularly shaped, pigmented macule. Lentigo maligna shows abnormal melanocytes confined to the epidermis, usually distributed as a continuous lentiginous proliferation in the basal layer of an atrophic epidermis. The melanocytic proliferation usually extends down appendages (Figure 10.7). The development of a pagetoid pattern of intraepidermal proliferation is considered to be a precursor

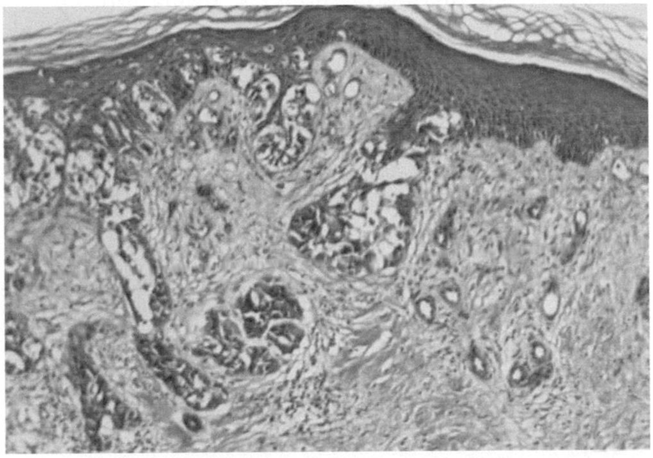

Figure 10.6 *Superficial spreading melanoma with the epidermal component extending beyond the dermal component. There is also pagetoid involvement of the epidermis.*

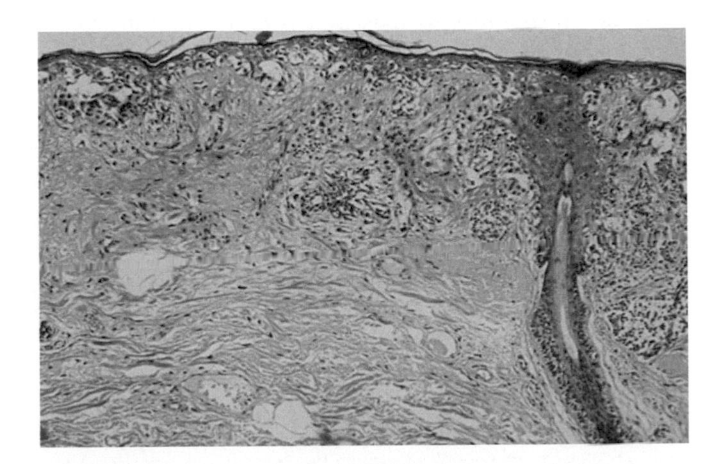

Figure 10.7 *Lentigo maligna showing atypical melanocytes in the basal layer of the atrophic epidermis. The melanocytic proliferation extends down a hair follicle. There is solar elastosis in the dermis.*

to dermal invasion.[18] LMM is often heralded clinically by a change in pigmentation or the development of a palpable nodule within the lentigo maligna. Invasive melanoma occurs in only a small group of lentigo maligna with the lifetime risk said to be about 5%.[19]

Acral lentiginous melanoma (ALM)

ALM arises on palms, soles, and subungual sites. It is the most common form of melanoma in Asian and black populations and accounts for less than 5% of melanomas in white populations. The epidermis is often hyperplastic, with an associated lentiginous proliferation of melanocytes which show varying degrees of atypia (Figure 10.8). The dermal component is often spindled.[3] The lesions often present at an advanced age because they may be mistaken by patients and clinicians as warts, or inflammatory or traumatic conditions.

Desmoplastic melanoma

This rare spindle cell melanoma may occur as a part of one of the more classical subtypes such as SMM, LMM, or ALM or it may arise de novo with only a very slight or no epidermal component. It is marked histologically by spindle cells embedded in a fibrotic stroma (Figure 10.9). A clue to diagnosis is the presence of scattered lymphocyte aggregates (Figure 10.5). This is one of the melanomas that are often misdiagnosed clinically and by the pathologist because it is usually amelanotic and its histological features are not typical of melanoma. It is often misdiagnosed as scar tissue, dermatofibroma, blue naevus, atypical fibroxanthoma, or other spindle cell tumour.[20] The sclerosing blue naevus may be especially problematic. One helpful aspect is the strong decoration of blue naevus cells with HMB-45, whereas desmoplastic melanoma cells almost invariably do not stain for this antibody.

Neurotropic melanoma

These are usually associated with desmoplastic melanoma and show infiltration around or within nerves (Figure 10.10) or neural differentiation.[20]

Naevoid melanoma

This heterogeneous group of melanomas represent one of the greatest challenges for pathologists. The melanoma may resemble a banal compound naevus and be easily misdiagnosed as such if diagnosis relies on low power scanning magnification.[21] It is important to recognize the cytological atypia and lack of maturation. Another naevus that can easily be mistaken for melanoma is Spitz naevus. In approximately 6.6% of melanoma cases referred to one specialist pigmented lesion clinic, review of the histopathology sections resulted in a change of diagnosis from malignant melanoma to a benign naevus.[22] Most of these benign naevi were Spitz naevi. Common features that melanomas and Spitz naevi share include prominent epidermal involvement, large and pleomorphic cells, and numerous mitoses. Features which are more likely in melanoma include asymmetry, ulceration, lack of

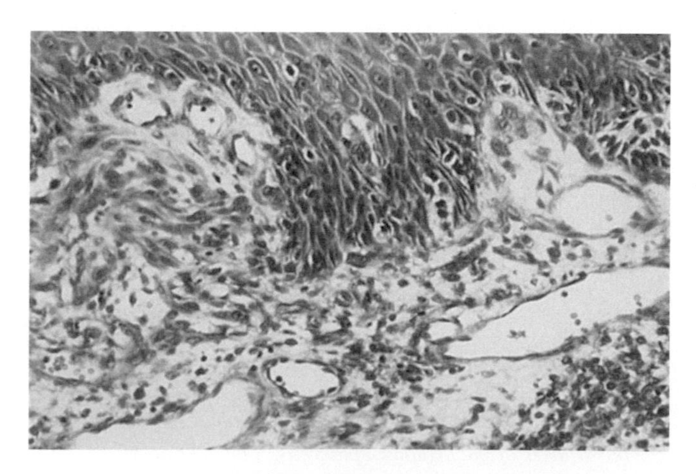

Figure 10.8 *Acral lentiginous melanoma on the toe of a 68-year-old man.*

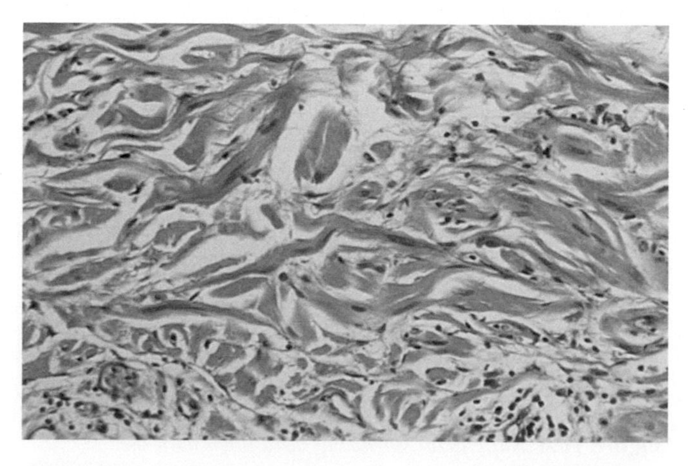

Figure 10.9 *Desmoplastic melanoma showing scattered atypical melanocytes in a fibrotic stroma.*

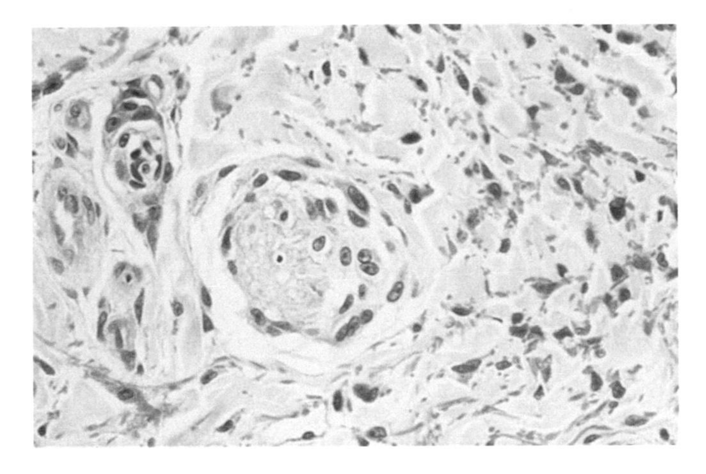

Figure 10.10 *Melanoma exhibiting neurotropism with the melanoma cells infiltrating around the nerve.*

maturation, marked cytological atypia, a brisk mitotic rate, deep mitoses, atypical mitoses, involvement of the subcutis, diameter >6 mm, epidermal thinning, and pagetoid spread. Features that are more likely to be seen in Spitz naevi include diameter <6 mm, diffuse epidermal hyperplasia, prominent hypergranulosis, terminal nests, uniformity of nests from side to side, numerous, and/or confluent Kamino bodies, subepidermal clefts, spindle shaped cells, maturation, and lack of deep and atypical mitoses. Evaluation of these multiple criteria determined that the most useful for distinguishing between melanoma and Spitz naevus were (1) Kamino bodies, (2) symmetry, (3) uniformity of nests from side to side, (4) a brisk mitotic rate, (5) mitoses close to the base of the lesion, (6) abnormal mitoses. The first three features are more helpful in diagnosing Spitz naevus and the latter three features point to a diagnosis of melanoma.[23]

CONCLUSION

Most melanomas can be diagnosed with certainty. However, in a small but significant group of cases the diagnosis is not clear, and it may be difficult to distinguish between a benign and a malignant melanocytic lesion. It may be necessary to give a guarded report describing the lesion and indicating that the biological behaviour of the lesion is uncertain.

REFERENCES

1. Farmer ER, Gonin R, Hanna MP, Discordance in the histopathologic diagnosis of melanoma and melanocytic naevi between expert pathologists. *Hum Pathol* 1996; 27: 528–31.
2. Cochran AJ, Elashoff D, Morton DL, Elashoff R, Individualized prognosis for melanoma patients. *Hum Pathol* 2000; 31: 327–31.
3. Barnhill RL, Mihm MC, The histopathology of cutaneous malignant melanoma. *Semin Diagn Pathol* 1993; 10: 47–75.
4. Kohler S, Rouse RV, Smoller BR, The differential diagnosis of pagetoid cells in the epidermis. *Mod Pathol* 1998; 11: 79–92.
5. Crotty K, McCarthy S, Palmer A, et al, Malignant melanoma in childhood: A clinicopathologic study of 13 cases and comparison with Spitz nevi.' *World J Surg* 1992; 16: 179–85.
6. Ruiter, D, Brocker E, Immunohistochemistry in the evaluation of melanocytic tumors. *Semin Diag Pathol* 1993; 10: 76–91.
7. Busam, K, Chen Y, et al, Expression of melan-A (MART1) in benign melanocytic naevi and primary cutaneous malignant melanoma. *Am J Surg Pathol* 1998; 22: 976–82.
8. Blessing, K, Sanders D, et al, Comparison of immunohistochemical staining of the novel antibody melan-A with S100 protein and HMB-45 in malignant melanoma and melanoma variants. *Histopathology* 1998; 32: 139–46.
9. Prieto, V. Expression of HMB-45 antigen in spindle cell melanoma. *J Cutan Pathol* 1997; 24: 580–1.
10. Li L-XL, Crotty KA, McCarthy SW, et al, A zonal comparison of MIB1–Ki67 immunoreactivity in benign and malignant melanocytic lesions. *Am J Dermatopathol* 2000; 22: 489–95.
11. Crocker J, Nucleolar organizer regions (NORs) in neoplasms. In: *Oxford textbook of pathology. Volume 1. Principles of pathology* (eds McGee JOD, Isaacson PG, and Wright NA) New York: Oxford University Press, 1992: 586–9.
12. Li L, Crotty K, McCarthy S, Palmer A, Krik J, Special laboratory techniques for studying cutaneous melanocytic lesions. *Cancer Forum* 1998: 180–2.
13. Stolz W, Vogt T, Landthaler M, et al, Differentiation between malignant melanomas and benign melanocytic nevi by computerized DNA cytometry of imprint specimens. *J Clin Pathol* 1994; 21: 7–15.
14. Clark WH, Elder DE, Van Horn M, The biological forms of malignant melanoma. *Hum Pathol* 1986; 17: 443–50.
15. Clark WH, Elder DE, Guerry D, IV Model predicting survival in Stage I melanoma based on tumour progression. *J Natl Cancer Inst* 1989; 81: 1893–904.
16. Ackerman AB, David KM, A unifying concept of malignant melanoma: biological aspects. *Hum Pathol* 1986; 17: 438–40.
17. McGovern VJ, Shaw HM, Milton GW, Prognostic significance of a polypoid configuration in melanoma. *Histopathology* 1983; 7: 663–72.
18. Tannous ZS, Lerner LH, Duncan LM, et al, Progression to invasive melanoma from malignant melanoma in situ, lentigo maligna type. *Hum Pathol* 2000; 31: 705–8.
19. Weinstock MA, Sober AJ, The risk of progression of lentigo maligna to lentigo maligna melanoma. *Br J Dermatol* 1987; 116: 303–10.
20. Quinn MJ, Crotty, KA, Thompson, JF, et al, Desmoplastic and desmoplastic neurotropic melanoma: experience with 280 patients. *Cancer* 1998; 83: 1128–35.
21. Wong TY, Duncan LM, Mihm MC Jr, Melanoma mimicking dermal and Spitz's nevus ('nevoid' melanoma) *Sem Surg Oncol* 1993; 9: 188–93.
22. Orchard D, Dowling J, Kelly J, Spitz naevus histologically misdiagnosed as melanoma. Prevalence and clinical profile. *Australas J Dermatol* 1997; 38: 12–14.
23. Walsh N, Crotty KA, Palmer A, McCarthy SW, Spitz nevus versus spitzoid malignant melanoma: an evaluation of the current distinguishing histopathological criteria. *Hum Pathol* 1998; 29: 1105–12.

11

Pathological reporting of cutaneous melanoma

Alistair J Cochran, Kerry Crotty

INTRODUCTION

The pathologist's role in the management of cutaneous melanoma is crucial, not only in determining the diagnosis but also in determining the margins of excision and in providing prognostic indicators. This chapter is based on our previously published comments and the recommendations for the reporting of tissues removed as part of the surgical treatment of cutaneous melanoma presented by the Association of Directors of Anatomic and Surgical Pathology.[1–3]

In the pathological reporting of a primary malignant melanoma, desirable features include: characteristics of the melanoma, including subtype; whether the lesion has been completely excised; and an evaluation of prognostic indicators. This will allow critical decisions regarding extent of surgery and possible use of potentially morbid adjuvant therapy to be made, as well as reducing the chances of local recurrence and removing melanoma cells that could serve as a source of metastases.

EVALUATION OF THE GROSS SPECIMEN

A careful inspection of the submitted biopsy should provide much useful information. The optimal biopsy to determine melanoma characteristics and prognostic parameters is an excision biopsy but pathologists are also called upon to interpret incision, shave and punch biopsies.

Incision biopsies

These are most often derived from lesions that are large or in cosmetically sensitive areas, or in which the diagnosis of a melanocytic lesion is not suspected. An incision biopsy may not be representative of the entire lesion and the diagnosis of melanoma may be missed in a small biopsy. It may not be possible accurately to determine parameters such as Clark level, Breslow thickness, or the presence of regression from such biopsies.

Shave biopsies

This technique is popular with clinicians and patients because it is rapid, inexpensive, and leaves a wound that usually heals with a good cosmetic result. However, shave biopsies are generally unpopular with pathologists because they include little or no surrounding tissue so that it is often not possible to evaluate the radial growth phase of melanomas. Shave biopsies, even 'deep' shave biopsies, seldom completely remove the deeper parts of a tumour. Tissue distortion secondary to pressure and crush artifact is common. These features may make accurate evaluation impossible, and the diagnosis of melanoma may be missed or overcalled. It is rarely possible to assess Clark level or Breslow thickness accurately. It is usually not possible to reconstruct Clark level or Breslow thickness by combining data from the initial shave with the re-excision specimen because of tissue changes that occur during healing after the initial shave and as a result of the effects of haemostatic chemicals such as aluminium chloride or, worse still, diathermy or cautery of the wound. For all these reasons, shave biopsies should not, in general, be performed for any lesion that is clearly melanocytic.

Punch biopsies

These too have little place in the evaluation of pigmented lesions and should be avoided where possible. They may however be of some value in assessing large or heterogeneous pigmented lesions. Punch biopsies are frequently crushed by the forceps used to remove them. Even minor degrees of distortion of nuclei may create an appearance that resembles nuclear atypia, a problem that is also seen with shave biopsies.

EXCISION SPECIMENS

Excision specimens permit the most accurate evaluation of melanocytic lesions. The excision should include normal tissue lateral to and deep to the pigmented lesion. Assessment may be enhanced by pinning out the specimen on cardboard or cork during fixation. Fixation for 24 hours (with one change of formalin) before dissection is desirable but should be for at least 8–12 hours. Surgical margins should be identified and preferably inked, possibly with different coloured inks applied to the various margins. A written description of the gross specimen should include:

(1) Colour, thickness, and texture of the skin.
(2) Extent and quality of hair present.
(3) Measurement of the length, width, and thickness of the tissue.
(4) The presence of orienting features such as stitches, clips, and marker inks applied by the clinician.
(5) The main tumour is described in terms of its:
   - profile elevation or flatness,
   - diameter and height of the dominant lesion,
   - pigmentation – presence, degree, and homogeneity or heterogeneity,
   - ulceration – presence or absence,
   - border – regularity or irregularity.
(6) The skin surrounding the main lesion is examined for any abnormality of pigmentation that may represent a radial growth phase lesion, an area of regression or an associated naevus. A detailed description should be given of each such lesion present, including dimensions.
(7) Describe and measure any scars that are present.
(8) Measure the distance(s) in millimetres between the edge of the main tumour/radial growth phase, other lesions including scars and the nearest surgical margins.

Dissection of gross skin specimens

For most tumours, especially those up to 1 cm in diameter, the surgical ellipse may be sectioned from pole to pole across the long axis of the ellipse (parallel transverse sections). If these blocks are embedded serially, a stereoscopic image of the whole tumour can be obtained. This method is preferred if the transverse sections can include the surgical margins in the blocks (Figure 11.1). Alternatively, if tumour tissue is needed for special studies or research, a section can be taken from pole to pole along the long axis of the ellipse. In the latter case minimum clearance is evaluated by taking sections at right angles to the initial cut in the

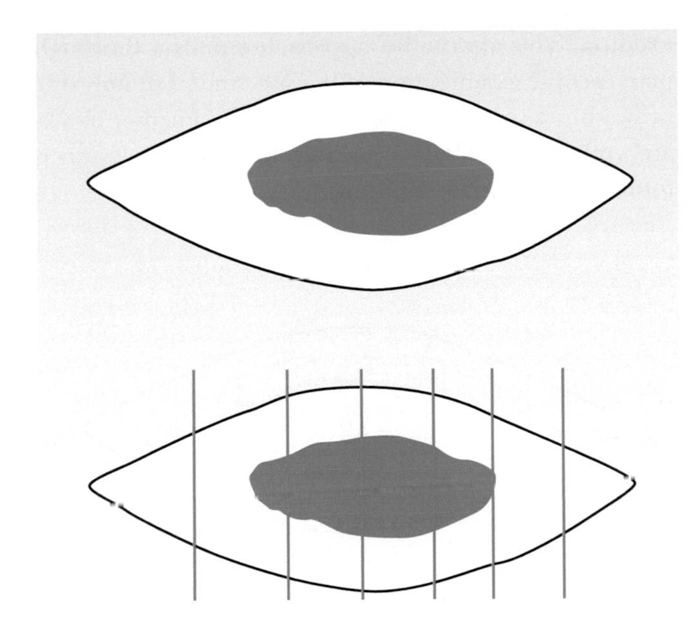

Figure 11.1 *An approach for the evaluation of an ellipse of skin removed to excise a small primary melanoma if the transverse sections can include the surgical margins. The surgical margins are inked. A diagram (or Polaroid photograph) is prepared and the source of the blocks marked on it.*

areas where the tumour, on gross inspection, is closest to the margin.

In larger ellipses it may be necessary to take separate blocks of the surgical margins (Figure 11.2). A comprehensive method of examining all surgical margins is to place the blocks face down in the cassettes and cut sections 'en face' to provide an excellent overview of the true surgical margins. In this method the processing procedure must be explained in detail to the technicians and understood by the clinician. This approach is especially valuable in desmoplastic and neurotropic melanomas.

Re-excision specimens

The scar should be measured, and any residual or satellite lesions, benign melanocytic lesions, or non-melanocytic lesions present in the specimen should be described, measured, and oriented relative to the scar and to the surgical margins. These specimens are often managed similarly to the large specimen shown in Figure 11.1, whether or not residual tumour is present. An alternative approach is used in some laboratories when there is no obvious residual melanocytic lesion and/or when the previous biopsy showed complete excision. This alternative approach entails a thorough macroscopic examination of the specimen but only one or two blocks of the scar are embedded.[4] Further blocks are embedded only if a residual melanocytic lesion is found on microscopic review.

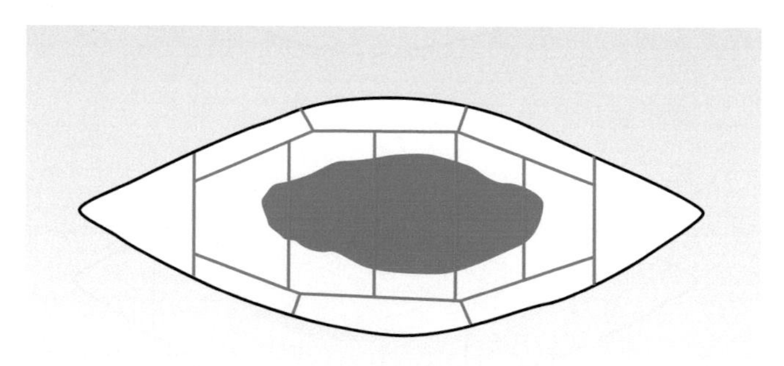

Figure 11.2 *An approach for the evaluation of an ellipse of skin removed to excise a melanoma. The surgical margins are inked. A diagram or Polaroid photograph is prepared and the source of the blocks marked on it. The peripheral marginal blocks, taken separately, are placed inked face down to allow sectioning of the true surgical margin. This approach is useful especially if the tumour shows neurotropism.*

MICROSCOPIC EVALUATION OF PRIMARY LESION

The pathologist must confirm that the lesion is malignant and look for and assess those features associated with different biological behaviours and clinical outcomes (see Chapter 10).

Determination of primary status of melanoma

Distinction between primary and metastatic melanomas is extremely important, since treatments for these two stages of the disease are entirely different. Determination of primary status may be difficult if the tumour shows extensive ulceration or the cells of the junctional component have undergone regressive changes.

Ulceration

If present, the diameter of ulceration should be measured using a micrometer. Ulceration is an independent prognostic factor. Patients with more extended ulceration are more likely to develop metastases and die of their melanoma.[5–7]

Histogenetic subtypes of melanoma

There is considerable debate as to whether there are truly subtypes of melanomas.[8] If possible we consider that it is useful to subtype primary melanomas according to:

(1) Growth phase[9]
  (a) Radial
  (b) Vertical.
(2) Histological subtype
  (a) Superficial spreading
  (b) Acral lentiginous
  (c) Lentigo maligna
  (d) Nodular
  (e) Other.

Micrometer measured thickness[10]

The thickness of the primary tumour is measured from the granular layer to the deepest contiguous melanoma cell or associated satellite tumour, or from the base of an ulcer to the same deeper limits (Figure 11.3). With increasing thickness there is a reduction in survival.

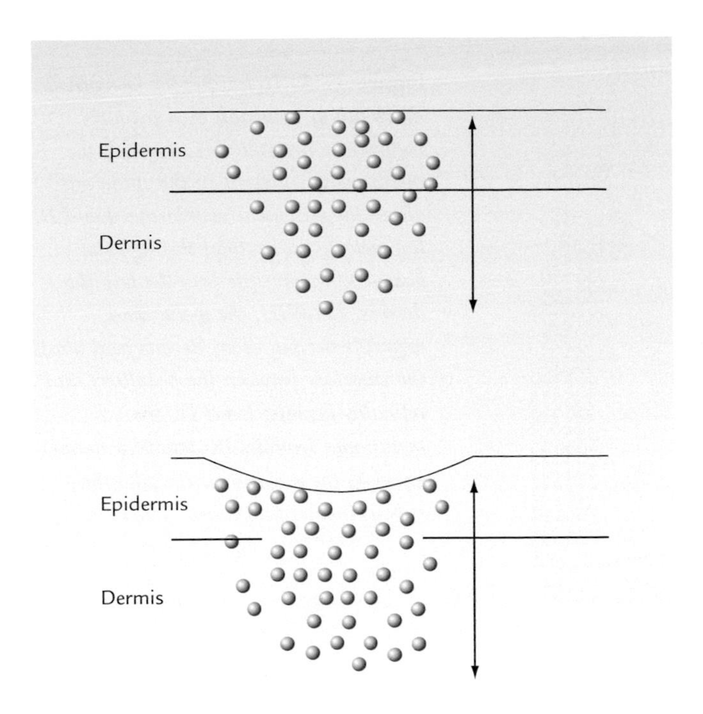

Figure 11.3 *Measurement of tumour thickness by Breslow's technique. An ocular micrometer is used to measure the thickest area of the tumour from the granular layer (or ulcer base) to the deepest contiguous melanoma cells (or satellite base).*

Depth of invasion of the melanoma[11]

This simple technique of determining the depth of invasion of the melanoma related to the standard skin components: epidermis, papillary dermis, reticular dermis and subcutis (Figure 11.4) was developed by the late Wallace Clark. Increasing depth is associated with an increased likelihood of metastasis and reduced survival.

Mitotic rate

The mitotic frequency in a melanoma should be recorded per millimetre square. This is best achieved using a microscopic grid. Assessments of mitoses per high power field is less desirable as different pathologists use different combinations of lenses to achieve a high power magnification. While markers of cells in the proliferation cycle, such as Ki67(MIB-1), have some place in separating benign from malignant lesions, these markers are not routinely used in evaluating the proliferative activity of melanomas.[12]

Assessment of lymphatic/blood vascular invasion

This can be a surprisingly difficult determination to make, even if immunohistochemical markers are used to delineate blood vessels. We record lymphatic/vascular invasion only when we are convinced that we see tumour cells within a vessel bounded by endothelium.

Desmoplasia

Desmoplasia is often seen in melanomas, particularly those where the tumour is comprised of spindle cells and in the melanomas that develop from lentigo maligna.[13,14] Desmoplasia may also be seen in superficial spreading melanomas and acral lentiginous melanomas.[15] Desmoplasia should be recorded, as it provides some indication that this is a class of tumour that may also demonstrate neurotropism. An S100 stain may be useful in delineating the extent of a desmoplastic melanoma and certainly makes it easier to find the cutaneous nerves.

Neurotropism

It is important to identify and record the presence of neurotropism.[13–15] Neurotropic melanomas often require very extensive local surgery to eradicate them. Recurrence is common. It may be necessary to use immunohistochemistry with S100 protein to be sure that all cutaneous nerves have been identified.

Margins of excision

We routinely record the distance from the tumour to the closest lateral margin and the distance from the deepest part of the tumour to the deep margin. Care must be taken in assessing the excision margins of desmoplastic/neurotropic melanomas and it may be necessary to scrutinize the entire margin, using 'en face' sections of the external cut surface of the specimen, similar to the method used in Figure 11.2.

OPTIONAL FEATURES

There are other histological features of considerable interest, but that have not yet been conclusively proved to be directly related to prognosis. We encourage

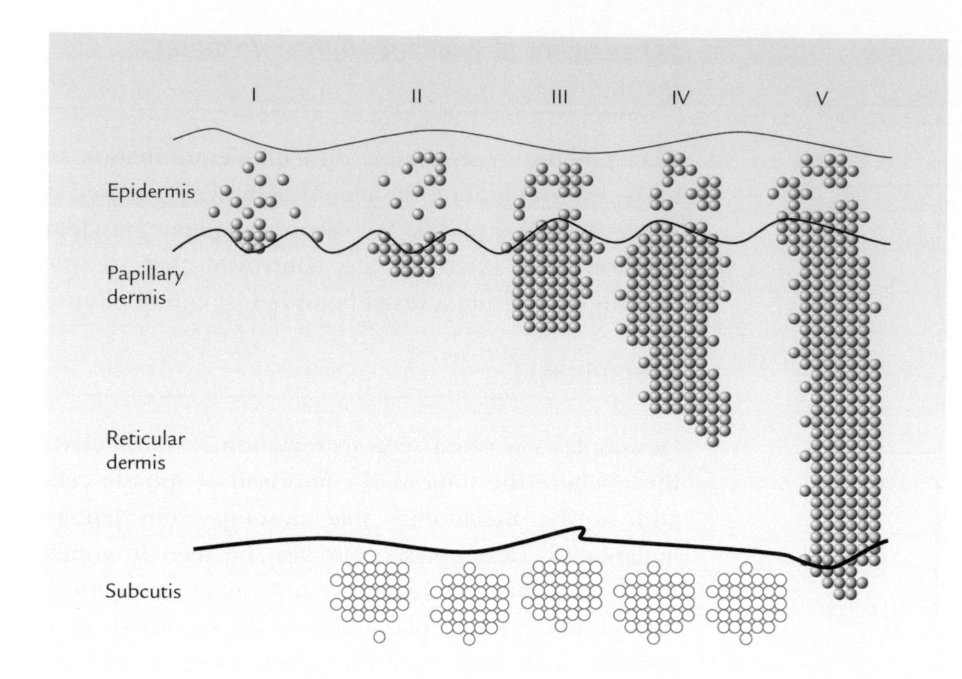

Figure 11.4 *Technique for measuring the depth of invasion by a primary melanoma into the skin. Level I, the melanoma is present in the epidermis above the basement membrane. Level II, the melanoma invades through the basement membrane into the papillary dermis. Level III, the melanoma expands the papillary dermis and abuts the interface between the papillary and reticular dermis. Level IV, the melanoma invades the reticular dermis. Level V, the melanoma invades the subcutaneous fat (Clark, 1967[11]).*

pathologists to record these features and study their relation to outcome. Such features include: regressive changes in relation to the invasive and radial growth components, the distribution and extent of tumour infiltrating lymphocytes (TILs), the dominant cell type, the presence and position of a preexisting naevus, the presence and extent of necrosis, the presence of microsatellites, and the presence of heterologous cytological features.

EVALUATION OF LYMPH NODE SPECIMENS

Therapeutic lymph node dissections

Ideally, the specimen should be palpated before fixation to detect any enlarged lymph nodes that are present. If extranodal tumour extension is suspected, the outside surface of the specimen is inked. The tissues can be partially sectioned at 1 cm intervals to facilitate the penetration of fixative once the ink has dried. Ideally fixative should be changed at least once, after 6–8 hours, but at least overnight fixation should occur.

The specimen should be measured as to length, breadth and thickness, and orientation markers placed by the surgeon should be identified and recorded. The examining pathologist palpates the specimen for nodes and dissects out all nodes. The pathologist records the number of lymph nodes, the size of the largest node or nodes, the presence or absence of grossly apparent tumour, whether or not the nodes are pigmented, the consistency of the node (soft, rubbery, hard), and whether tumour is confined to the node or is present in the extracapsular tissue.[16]

Elective lymph node dissection

These specimens are handled in exactly the same manner as tissues removed at therapeutic lymph node dissection. If possible, the proximal and distal ends of the specimen are identified. Close attention should be paid to the lymph nodes located nearest to the primary tumour, as these are the nodes in which early metastatic melanoma is most likely to be present.[17]

Selective ('sentinel') lymph node removal

This comparatively new technique has rapidly achieved great popularity in recent years despite the absence of evidence that it is therapeutically advantageous.[17] The surgeon identifies the sentinel nodes using blue dye and/or radioisotopes. These are usually the nodes nearest to a primary melanoma on the direct lymphatic drainage route. If specimens containing several lymph nodes are submitted following sentinel node biopsy, any lymph nodes that stain blue and that have relatively high radioactivity should be regarded as sentinel. Because the isotope moves relatively rapidly along the lymphatic chain, not all nodes that are radioactive are sentinel nodes, though sentinel nodes are almost always selectively radioactive. Nodes in such specimens that are not blue stained are 'incidental', non-sentinel nodes. Frozen section evaluation of sentinel nodes should be avoided as it is technically demanding and wasteful of potentially diagnostic material.

Sentinel nodes should be cut into two equal parts along the longest equator of the lymph node and both halves placed face down in the cassette (Figure 11.5). A practical approach to sampling these nodes is as follows. The technician is requested to obtain a full face section as rapidly as possible and then to cut 10 serial sections. Sections 1, 3, 5 and 10 (Figure 11.5) are stained by H&E, section 2 is reacted with an antibody to S100 protein, and section 4 with antibody to HMB-45 (or MART-1). Sections 6 and 7 are negative controls for immunoperoxidase studies, and sections 8 and 9 either can be used as spares to repeat unsuccessful initial studies or can be stained for S100 and HMB-45.[18,19] If material is required for experimental studies (for example, molecular biological approaches), the researchers should be given sections interleaved with the conventionally evaluated sections. We recommend that the arbitrary provision of portions of a node for research purposes be avoided because a diagnostic portion of the node may be lost.

A radioactive marker may be used to identify the sentinel lymph node. This is usually technetium and represents a limited hazard to those handling the tissue. We recommend that these nodes should be stored for 24 hours before being definitively handled. It should be noted that the amount of radioactivity in the skin specimen may be substantially higher and such material should be handled with due caution.[20]

If tumour is found in the sentinel lymph node, surgeons will perform a standard lymphadenectomy providing a 'completion lymphadenectomy' specimen. These specimens are handled in the same way as tissues from a therapeutic lymph node dissection (see above). It is arguable that the nodes from completion lymphadenectomies should also be evaluated by immunohistochemistry such as S100, but the substantial cost of such investigations must be weighed against their expected benefits. There is at present no clear evidence that immunohistochemistry is necessary in the routine evaluation of completion lymphadenectomy specimens.

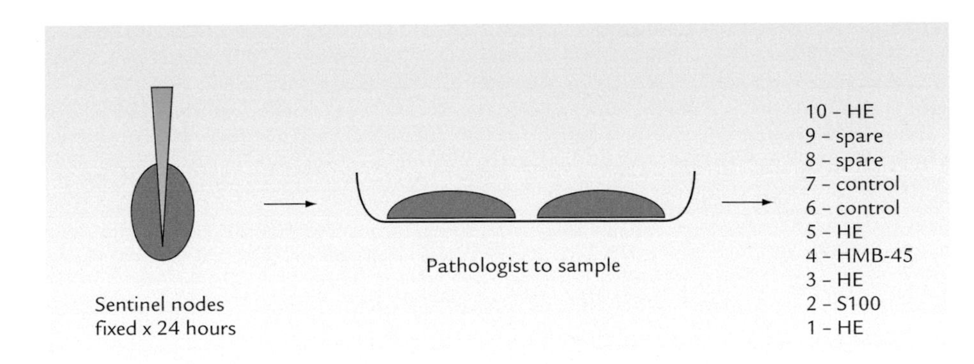

Figure 11.5 *Recommendations for sampling a sentinel node. The node is exactly bisected along the longest circumference and both cut faces are sampled. Serial full face sections are evaluated as indicated.*

REFERENCES

1. Cochran AJ, Bailly C, Cook M, et al, Reporting tissues removed as part of the treatment of cutaneous melanoma. *Path Case Rev* (in press).
2. Cochran AJ, Bailly C, Cook M, et al, Standardized reporting of melanoma as recommended by the Association of Directors of Anatomic and Surgical Pathology. *Hum Pathol* 1997; 28: 1123–5.
3. Cochran AJ, Bailly C, Cook M, et al, Recommendations for the reporting of tissues removed as part of the surgical treatment of cutaneous melanoma. *Virchow's Arch* 1997; 431: 79–81.
4. Martin HM, Birkin AJ, Theaker JM, Malignant melanoma re-excision specimens – how many blocks? *Histopathology* 1998; 32: 362–7.
5. Cochran AJ, Bailly C, Paul E, Remotti F, *Melanocytic tumors: A guide to diagnosis.* Philadelphia and New York: Lippencott-Raven, 1997.
6. Balch CM, Wilkerson JA, Murad TM, et al, The prognostic significance of ulceration of cutaneous melanoma. *Cancer* 1980; 45: 3012–18.
7. Cochran AJ, Elashoff D, Morton DL, Elashoff R, Individualized prognosis for melanoma patients. *Hum Pathol* 2000; 31: 327–31.
8. McGovern VJ, Shaw HM, Milton GW, Farago GA, Is malignant melanoma arising in Hutchinson's melanotic freckle a separate disease entity? *Histopathology* 1980; 4: 235–42.
9. Clark Jr WH, Elder DE, Guerry D, et al, Model predicting survival in stage I melanoma based on tumour progression. *J Natl Cancer Inst* 1989; 81: 1893–904.
10. Breslow A, Thickness, cross-sectional areas and depth of invasion in the prognosis of cutaneous melanoma. *Ann Surg* 1970; 172: 902–8.
11. Clark WH, Jr, A classification of malignant melanoma in man correlated with histogenesis and biologic behavior. In: *Advances in the biology of the skin.* (eds Montagna W, Hu F) New York: Pergamon Press, 1967; 8: 621–47.
12. Li LiL-X, Crotty KA, McCarthy SW, et al, A zonal comparison of MIB1–Ki67 immunoreactivity in benign and malignant melanocytic lesions. *Am J Dermatopath* 2000; 22: 489–95.
13. Conley J, Lattes R, Orr W, Desmoplastic malignant melanoma (a rare variant of spindle cell melanoma). *Cancer* 1971; 28: 914–36.
14. Jain S, Allen PW, Desmoplastic malignant melanoma and its variants. *Am J Surg Pathol* 1989; 13: 358–73.
15. Quinn, MJ, Crotty, KA, Thompson, JF, et al, Desmoplastic and desmoplastic neurotropic melanoma: experience with 280 patients. *Cancer* 1998; 83: 1128–35.
16. Cochran AJ, Robert ME, Wen D-R, Pathology of the lymph nodes in patients with malignant melanoma. *State of the Art Review in Pathology* 1994; 2: 385–400.
17. Morton DL, Wen D-R, Wong JH, et al, Technical details of intraoperative lymphatic mapping for early stage melanoma. *Arch Surg* 1992; 127: 392–9.
18. Cochran AJ, Wen D-R, Herschman JR, Occult melanoma in lymph nodes detected by antiserum to S-100 protein. *Int J Cancer* 1984; 34: 159–63.
19. Cochran AJ, Wen D-R, Morton DL, Occult tumor cells in the lymph nodes of patients with pathological Stage I malignant melanoma: An immunohistological study. *Am J Surg Pathol* 1988; 12: 612–18.
20. Cochran AJ, The pathologist's role in sentinel lymph node evaluation. *Sem Nuclear Med* 2000; 30: 11–17.

12

Immunohistochemistry and special diagnostic techniques

Dirk J Ruiter, Wolter J Mooi, Goos NP van Muijen, Alistair J Cochran

INTRODUCTION

To arrive at a definive pathological diagnosis of melanoma, inspection of routinely H&E-stained sections is generally sufficient. However, in more complex cases ancillary techniques such as histochemistry, (immuno)electronmicroscopy, in situ hybridization, immunohistochemistry, or cytochemistry may be of help. Since in practice immunohistochemistry is the technique most often used, especially to determine the expression of melanocytic markers and/or melanoma associated antigens, we will concentrate on this technique.

Since our previous review of this subject[1] several important aspects of immunohistochemistry and other special diagnostic techniques have changed. New markers have been identified, and special procedures have been developed to enhance antigen detection in fixed tissues. Progress has been made in the application of molecular techniques that are potentially of diagnostic relevance, and recently developed molecular strategies promise the identification of new markers.

We will discuss the classification of melanoma antigens and their important properties, the various immunohistochemical detection methods and techniques to detect genomic changes. After a critical appraisal of the diagnostic application of immunohistochemistry and its role in the prediction of prognosis, likely future developments are outlined.

MELANOMA ASSOCIATED ANTIGENS

This section deals with the classification of melanoma antigens and their important properties.

Classification of melanoma associated antigens

Melanoma associated antigens can be classified on the basis of their functional or structural properties or their clinical application(s). No ideal classification exists, and overlap between the different categories is therefore unavoidable. A working classification, based on a compilation of theoretical and practical aspects of these molecules, was devised at the Lausanne consensus meeting on melanoma antigens in 1992 and will be followed here.[2] Table 12.1 illustrates the rationale for this classification.

Both melanocytic differentiation antigens and melanoma progression antigens are potentially useful as markers for cell biological and therapeutic purposes. Antigens that serve as targets for antibodies and/or cytotoxic T lymphocytes are relevant to attempts at immunotherapy. A majority of the different categories of antigens can be identified and localized by immunocytochemistry and/or immunohistochemistry. Different classes of antigens are discussed separately in the following paragraphs.

Properties of melanoma associated antigens

Melanocytic differentiation antigens

A melanocytic differentiation antigen is a marker for melanocytic cell lineage, including benign (naevus) and malignant tumour cells (melanoma cells) that are melanocyte derived. The ideal marker would have very high sensitivity – it would recognize all stages of melanocyte evolution and of melanocytic tumour progression – and very high specificity – it would not be associated with other non-melanocytic types of cellular differentiation. Such an ideal differentiation marker does not (yet) exist. Based on a review of the literature and our own experience there are two different groups of melanocytic differentiation markers, one with very high sensitivity but limited specificity, and the other with moderate to high sensitivity and a high specificity. Prototypes of the first group are S-100 protein[3–4] and high molecular weight-melanoma associated antigen (HMW-MAA).[5–6] Examples of the second group are gp 100 (HMB-45, NKI-beteb), tyrosinase and MART-1 (syn: Melan-A). Representative expression patterns of various markers are shown in Figures 12.1a and b. The different antigens and the properties of various markers are listed in Table 12.2.[3–14] In diagnostic histopathology most experience currently exists with immunohistochemistry using antibodies recognizing S-100 or gp 100. AntiHMW-MAA antibodies are not broadly applied as they cannot be used with formalin fixed and paraplast/paraffin embedded tissues. For research purposes anti-HMW-MAA is useful for the identification of pericytes, microvascular smooth muscle cells, in frozen tissue sections. Antityrosinase and antiMART-1 (antiMelan-A) are

Table 12.1 *Classification of melanoma associated antigens*[2]

Classification	Rationale/application
Melanocytic differentiation antigens	Marker for melanocytic cell lineage; diagnosis; staging
Melanoma progression antigens	Marker for certain stages of melanocytic tumour progression; prognosis
Melanoma antigens as targets for antibodies	Immunoscintigraphy and immunogenetherapy
Melanoma antigens as targets for cytotoxic T cells	Immunotherapy
Other antigens	Biologically or clinically relevant functions that do not fit in the previous categories

Table 12.2 *Melanocytic differentiation antigens*

Antigen	Properties	Further specification	Antibodies*	References
S-100	Family of acidic calcium binding proteins	Homo or heterodimers of S-100a and S-100b	Rabbit polyclonal (P)	3,4
HMW-MAA	Chondroitin sulphate proteoglycan	Two chains of 420 and 250 KD	225.28S, Mel.14 (F)	5,6
Gp 100	Unknown	Present in melanosomes	HMB-45, NKI-beteb (F and P)	4,7,8
Tyrosinase	Enzyme of melanin biosynthesis	Present in melanosomes	T311 (F and P)	9, 10
MART-1 (Melan-A)	Unknown	Transmembrane protein	A103, M2, 7C10 (F and P)	11, 12
TRP-1 TRP-2	Tyrosinase related proteins gp 75	Regulate the quality of melanin	TMH-1 (F)	13, 14

P = paraplast sections
F = frozen sections
* For further information, see websites http://mol.genes.nig.ac.jp/hlda and http://www.ncbi.nlm.nih.gov./PROW/.[4]
Antibodies mentioned are monoclonal unless specified otherwise.
The antibodies mentioned are examples only.

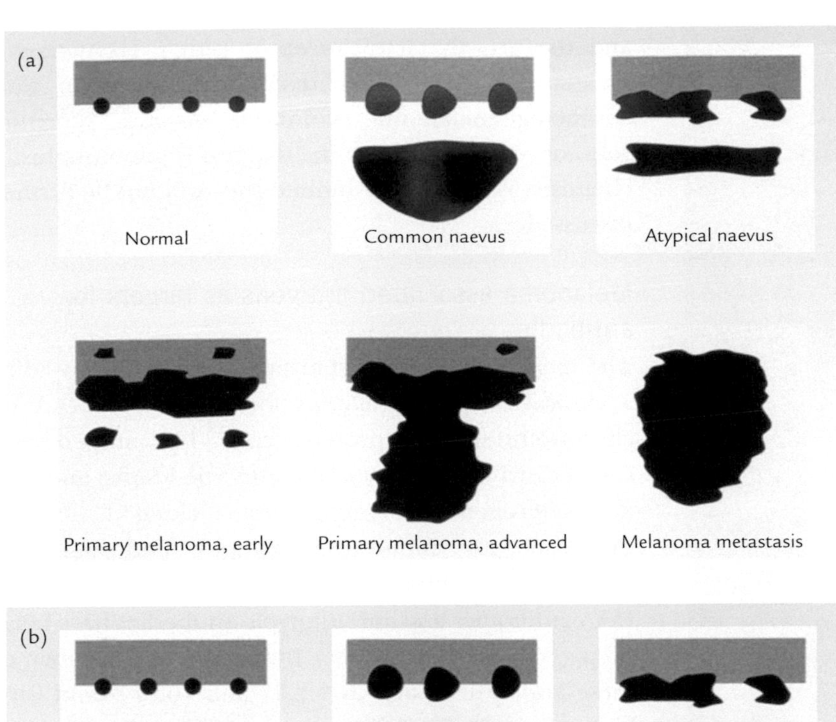

Figure 12.1 *(a) Melanocytic differentiation antigen with a high sensitivity, showing extensive expression in all stages of melanocytic tumor progression. (b) Melanocytic differentiation antigen with a moderate sensitivity due to diminished expression in the advanced tumour lesions.*

recent antibodies that seem to have a tissue distribution that parallels that of anti-gp 100 antibodies.[15] This is not surprising as they nearly all recognize proteins associated with the melanosome, the organelle that is associated with melanin synthesis, and thus a key feature of melanocytic differentiation and function. Recent experience however suggests a higher sensitivity for MART-1 than gp 100.[11,12,15,16] Information on the specificity of the antigens of melanocytic lineage and their application to diagnosis is given below. Representative immunohistochemical images are shown in Figure 12.2.

Melanoma progression antigens

These antigens have a tissue distribution restricted to one or more stages of melanoma progression. On the basis of variable distribution with tumour evolution 'early', 'intermediate', and 'late' progression antigens can be identified.[1] An early antigen is preferentially expressed by common naevocellular naevi and atypical (dysplastic) naevi, an intermediate antigen is associated with melanomas in situ and early primary melanomas, and a late antigen is typical of advanced primary melanomas and melanoma metastases. A representative distribution pattern is illustrated in Figure 12.3. Representative progression antigens and their important properties are listed in Table 12.3.[17–25] Most progression antigens are growth factors, growth factor receptors, proliferation molecules, adhesion molecules, proteases and related components, or immunomodulatory molecules.

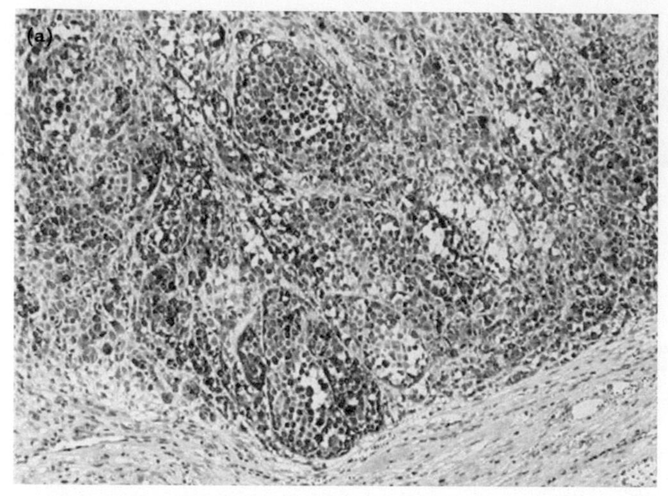

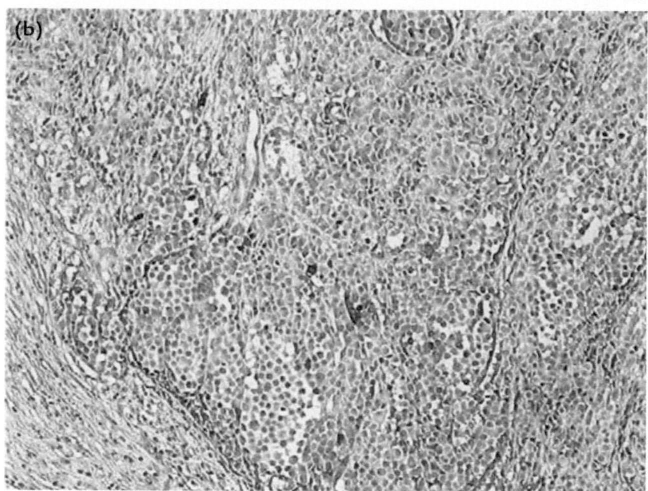

Figure 12.2 *(a) Immunohistochemical staining of a melanoma metastasis using an antiMART-1 antibody. Note extensive expression. APAAP procedure with haematoxylin counterstaining, ×100. (b) As (a), using an anti-gp 100 antibody. Note less extensive expression.*

From the nature of these molecules clear specificity limited to melanocytic cells cannot be expected for progression antigens or markers. The association of expression of such molecules with specific stages in melanoma progression suggests that they subserve a pathogenetic role for one or more steps in the complex process of neoplastic progression.[26] In addition, the so called cancer/testis antigens discussed below are considered progression markers. In addition to antigens that show increased expression with melanoma progression, other antigens have an inverse relationship to tumour progression. Such antigens may represent suppressor gene products: for example certain adhesion molecules (integrin $\alpha4\beta6$) and the growth factor receptor c-kit.[27] HLA class I antigens also may show decreased expression with advancing melanoma evolution.[1] As the potential role of such antigens in diagnostic immunohistochemistry is likely to be limited they will not be further discussed.

Melanoma associated antigens as targets for antibodies

The melanoma associated antigen most widely used as a clinical target for alloantibodies is HMW-MAA or chondroitin sulphate proteoglycan.[28] This antigen has a broad distribution among melanocytic lesions and limited heterogeneity of expression, making it an ideal candidate for immunoscintigraphy and immunotherapy.[5,6] A number of murine and human antiHMW-MAA antibodies and anti-idiotypic antibodies have been prepared, including F(ab′) fragments.[29] A number of these antibodies, such as 9.2.27 and 763.74 bind with high affinity and specificity to the HMW-MAA. There is evidence that certain antigens like HMW-MAA are immunodominant in vitro and probably also in vivo.[28] Preclinical studies of radiolabelled antibodies targeting melanomas growing in nude mice indicate their considerable clinical potential.

Melanoma cells express the ganglioside antigens GM3, GD3, GM2, and GD2 on their surface. These gangliosides can induce specific IgM antibodies, and high concentrations of these antibodies are reported to have a beneficial impact on survival.[30]

Melanoma associated antigens as targets for cytotoxic T lymphocytes

Appreciable progress has been achieved in the identification of melanoma antigens recognized by cytotoxic T lymphocytes.[6,31] These antigens belong to three main groups, i.e. cancer/testis antigens (MAGE, BAGE, GAGE), melanocytic differentiation antigens (gp 100, tyrosinase), and mutated or aberrantly expressed antigens (MUM-1, CDK4).[32] It is quite surprising that HLA class I presented peptides derived from melanocytic differentiation antigens can serve as targets for cytotoxic T cells. The development of a significant immune response to the peptides of differentiation antigens is limited by tolerance to these critical 'self' antigens, restricting the influence of T lymphocytes to antigens with low affinity T cell receptors.[31] Among the melanocytic differentiation antigens listed in Table 12.2 only

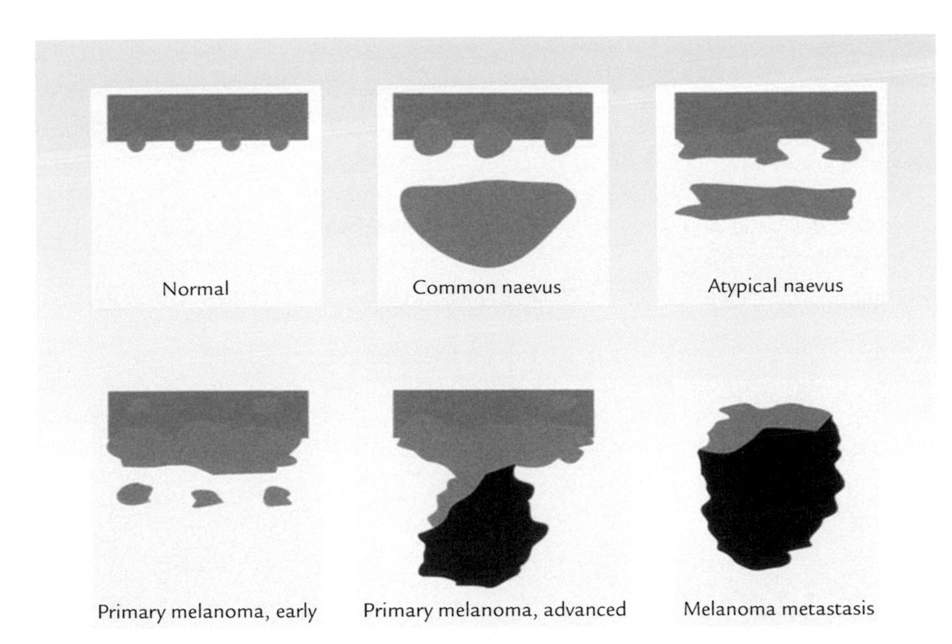

Figure 12.3 *Representative expression pattern of a melanoma progression antigen, that preferentially shows expression in the advanced tumour lesions.*

Table 12.3 *Melanoma progression antigens*

Groups of antigens	Examples	Antibodies*	References
Growth factors/receptors	EGF, EGF-R	2E9, 425, 225	17
Proliferation molecules	Ki67 antigen, PCNA	Ki67(F), MIB-I(P)	4, 18
Adhesion molecules			
Integrins	α_V, β_3	SSA6, SAP	19
Ig-superfamily	ICAM-1, ALCAM	CL 203. 4, clone 16	4, 20
Cadherins	E-cadherin	Clone 13 A9	4, 21
Others	CD44	T2. F4, BU 52	4, 22
Proteases/-related components			
Serine proteases	uPA, uPAR	Rabbit Pab (P),	23
Matrix metalloproteases	MMP2	R2(F)	24
Immunomodulatory molecules	HLA-DR	917D7	4, 25

* For further information see[4] and websites mentioned below Table 12.2.

gp 100 has been shown to be a tumour regression antigen. The cancer/testis specific antigens listed in Table 12.4 are potentially highly immunogenic and contain several HLA class I binding sites.[30–39] In contrast to melanocyte differentiation antigens only a few antibodies recognize cancer/testis specific antigens. Expression of this group of antigens is usually assessed from the mRNA level using reverse transcriptase-polymerase chain reaction (RT-PCR) procedures. To select patients suitable for immunotherapy it is necessary to determine the level of expression of the antigen(s) in tissues representative of the lesions to be treated by immunotherapy. Immunohistochemistry was used to estimate tumour expression of gp 100 and tyrosinase in a trial of vaccination with peptides of these antigens or peptide-loaded antigen presenting cells.[40]

Other antigens

Another melanoma antigen that does not fit into the previous categories is heparin sulfate (HS)/heparin, the most heterogeneous class within the group of

Table 12.4 *Melanoma antigens as targets for cytotoxic T cells*

Antigen	Properties	Antibodies* or target	References
Cancer/testis antigens:			
IMAGE 1–12	No specific function found yet. Located on chromosome X	57 B (P) (MAGE-3) (P)	31–33
MAGE, GAGE	Ibid	Not yet prepared	34
FRAME	Ibid	Not yet prepared	35
NY-ESO-1	Ibid	Autologous	36
SSX 1–2	Ibid	E3AS (P)	37
CTpll	Ibid	Not yet prepared	38
Melanocytic differentiation antigens: see Table 12.1		Peptides	3–14
Mutated or aberrantly expressed antigens:			
MUM-1	Transporter protein	Point mutation	32, 40
CDK4	Cell cycle regulation	Point mutation	32, 40
β catenin	Cell-cell adhesion	Exon 3 mutations	32, 40
Gp 100– in 4	Differentiation antigen	Non-mutated epitope	32, 40
P15	Unknown	Non-mutated epitope	32, 40
N-acetylglucosaminyl-transferase V	Unknown	Splice variant	32, 40

* For further information see[4] and websites mentioned below Table 12.2.

glycosaminoglycans.[41] HS binds, stores, and modulates a variety of growth factors implicated in angiogenesis and metastasis. Highly metastatic human melanoma cell lines express high concentrations of surface associated HS.[41] Antibodies in preparation against the various HS species expressed by melanoma cells will serve as new tools for immunohistochemistry, immunoscintigraphy and immunotherapy. The hyaluronic acid receptor CD44 and its splice variants also deserve to be mentioned. Increase of CD44 and some splice variants were found by immunohistochemistry and PCR to be associated with melanoma progression.[22,26]

Other antigens worth mentioning include cytokeratins 8 and 18, which may be co-expressed with vimentin in cell lines from invasive and metastatic human melanomas.[42]

DETECTION OF MELANOMA ANTIGENS

Immunohistochemistry permits the identification and localization of specific antigens by means of antigen-antibody interactions. The site of binding is identified by applying a visible labelling molecule that is directly bound to the first antibody or by the use of a secondary labelling method.

Immunohistochemical detection methods

Immunohistochemical techniques can be classified into direct and indirect methods. In the direct method a single (primary) antibody that recognizes the target antigen is applied to the section. This antibody is linked with a reporter molecule (fluorochrome or enzyme) that permits visualization of the antigen. As each antibody batch must be labelled individually, and since this technique is comparatively insensitive, this approach is not frequently used in routine pathology. Indirect staining methods are preferred as they greatly amplify the original signal. The most common indirect techniques are: (1) a two or three step incubation with layers of antibodies directed against antigens of differing species specificity, (2) a peroxidase-antiperoxidase (PAP) or alkaline phosphatase anti-alkaline phosphatase (APAAP) technique, and (3) an avidin-biotin complex technique. In immunohistochemistry for melanocytic lesions amino-ethylcarbazole (AEC), which has a red colour, is preferable as a chromogenic substrate for the peroxidase approach, to diethyl-aminobenzidine (DAB). The brown colour of the latter may lead to confusion with the yellow-brown melanin pigment. Another option is to remove melanin by bleaching with potassium permanganate and oxalic acid.[43] This treatment, however, may have an adverse effect on some antigens. A full range of appropriate controls must be stained in parallel.

Antibodies

Immunohistochemistry was initially performed using polyclonal antibodies against often impure antigenic preparations. This resulted in staining patterns that were often not 'specific'. Polyclonal antibodies must be extensively characterized by rigorous immunochemical techniques and preferably be affinity purified. With the advent of monoclonal antibodies, which are absolutely specific for a single epitope, problems of cross reactivity were greatly reduced. Only if an antigenic sequence is shared by more than one type of molecule is cross reactivity a problem. The monospecificity of monoclonal antibodies can be problematic. Multivalent polyclonal antibodies have a strong capacity to detect antigens and are generally more sensitive than monoclonal antibodies. Theoretically the problem of lower sensitivity with monoclonal antibodies can be circumvented by developing a defined polyclonal antiserum by mixing several well defined monoclonal antibodies against different epitopes on the same antigen. In practice this is only rarely done. Another disadvantage of monoclonal antibodies, also due to their monospecificity, is their sensitivity for reagents used for tissue fixation. When antigenic determinants recognized by a monoclonal antibody are changed (or destroyed) by the fixative the antibody can not or only insufficiently bind to its epitope and the staining result will be negative or at least markedly reduced. For this reason most monoclonal antibodies could only successfully be used on frozen sections and not on routinely formalin fixed and paraffin embedded tissues. Nowadays, however, immunoreactivity can often be restored by the use of antigen retrieval techniques.

Antigen retrieval

Antigen retrieval is a technique that re-exposes epitopes and makes them again detectable by immunohistochemistry. Both proteolytic treatment and heat mediated antigen retrieval have been shown to improve immunohistochemical staining with a great number of antibodies. By protease treatment enzymes such as trypsin and pronase break the cross linking bonds caused by the formalin fixation and reveal the antigenic sites. In the early 1990s it was found that antigens previously unreactive, even after protease treatment, could be retrieved by heating sections in a microwave oven or even after boiling in a pressure cooker. Both unmasking by protease treatment and by heat treatment complement each other. Furthermore, it has been shown that successful microwave treatment for various antigens is pH-dependent.[44] Finally, it is important to stress that for each antibody to be used in combination with any antigen retrieval technique an extensive quality controlled study should be performed to avoid misinterpretation due to false negative or false positive staining.[45]

Enhancement

Sometimes there may be reasons for enhancing the intensity of the staining result (detection of small amounts of antigen or need for good conditions for photography). Enhancement of the brown DAB stain can be achieved by intensification during the peroxidase reaction (addition of cobalt or nickel salts or of imidazole) or by postreaction intensification with heavy metal salts (copper sulphate). A recent and very powerful enhancement technique is tyramine signal amplification or CARD.[46] This method may be applied to all chromogens in an avidin-biotin technique. Regarding all enhancement techniques we should realize that the initial reaction (with the primary antibody) should have no background staining since this will also be intensified.

Interpretation

Important aspects regarding the interpretation of the staining results are the sensitivity and specificity of the staining procedure. Sensitivity can be defined as the lowest amount of antigen detectable. From the above it is clear that sensitivity of detection depends on several aspects like fixation of the tissue, immunohistochemical detection method used, and application of enhancement techniques or not. Although a number of antibodies can now be used on formalin fixed tissue, for reliable staining results we recommend the use of an indirect staining technique on frozen tissue sections. Specificity can be defined in relation to its cell or tissue distribution. Expression of differentiation antigens for example should be specific for cells of a certain lineage. Regarding melanocytic differentiation markers we know that some (tyrosinase, MART-1) seem to be melanocytic lineage specific both on the mRNA and protein level, whereas others (gp 100) show some 'illegal' transcription in non-melanocytic cells. Most other antigens described in this chapter have a broader tissue distribution.

Regarding the interpretation of the staining results we have to realize that this markedly depends on the complexity of the expression pattern and the experience of the observer. A reliable and relatively simple scoring system assures accuracy and reproducibility. A scoring system should include specification of type(s) of positive cell(s), the proportion of positive cells, and the intensity of staining. We advise use of a semi-quantitative scoring system for the proportion of positive cells: 0% (absent), 1–5% (sporadic), 6–25% (local), 26–50% (occasional), 51–75% (majority), 76–100% (large majority). Scoring the intensity of staining we neglect faint staining. We score intensity of staining as – (negative), + (dull), 2+ (moderate), and 3+ (marked, strong).[15]

DETECTION OF GENOMIC CHANGES

Regarding the total DNA content of tumour cells, flow cytometric studies have illustrated a correlation between aneuploidy and tumour progression in various types of tumour including melanoma. In addition, Southern blotting and restriction fragment length polymorphism analysis have been used in the study of single genes. Also, cytogenetic studies have shown changes of specific chromosomes in melanoma, namely chromosomes 1, 6, and 7 in late stages of progression. However, karyotyping studies of earlier lesions are very difficult because of their low mitotic index and limited amount of tissue. Therefore it is worth while to study chromosomal changes in cell preparations and tissue sections.

In situ hybridization

In situ hybridization (ISH) techniques enable the visualization of DNA targets in interphase nuclei, a method termed interphase cytogenetics. Numerical chromosomal aberrations in interphase nuclei in tumours have been reliably detected by DNA probes that hybridize to the (peri-) centromeric region of a specific chromosome. The technical procedure on paraplast sections consists of air drying and subsequent heating for 16 hours at 56°C, dewaxing, blocking of endogenous peroxidase activity, and pretreatment with Na SCN, followed by enzyme digestion with pepsine. Biotinylated probe DNA, herring sperm DNA, and baker's yeast RNA are added as hybridization buffer. The reaction is visualized using mouse antibiotin serum, peroxidase labelled rabbit antimouse serum and di-aminobenzidine. Nuclei are counterstained with haematoxylin solution.

Using DNA in situ hybridization on paraplast sections of primary melanoma, De Wit et al.[47] found nuclei with one, two, three, and four spots per nucleus for the chromosome 1 and 7 targets. For chromosome 1 nuclei with five spots were observed as well. The corresponding metastases also showed numerical aberrations on chromosomes 1 and 7. In contrast, in normal skin no nuclei with more than two spots were seen. These results indicate that DNA ISH can be applied to detect targeted repetitive DNA sequences at the single cell level. ISH on tissue sections enables direct comparison to histopathological characteristics (Figure 12.4.).

DIAGNOSTIC APPLICATION

Immunohistochemistry and molecular diagnostic techniques are of practical use in several ways – for example, if, on histology, the lesion is obviously melanocytic but it is difficult to make the distinction between naevus and melanoma; if the lesion is a morphologically undifferentiated tumour that may be melanoma or an undifferentiated carcinoma, sarcoma, or large cell

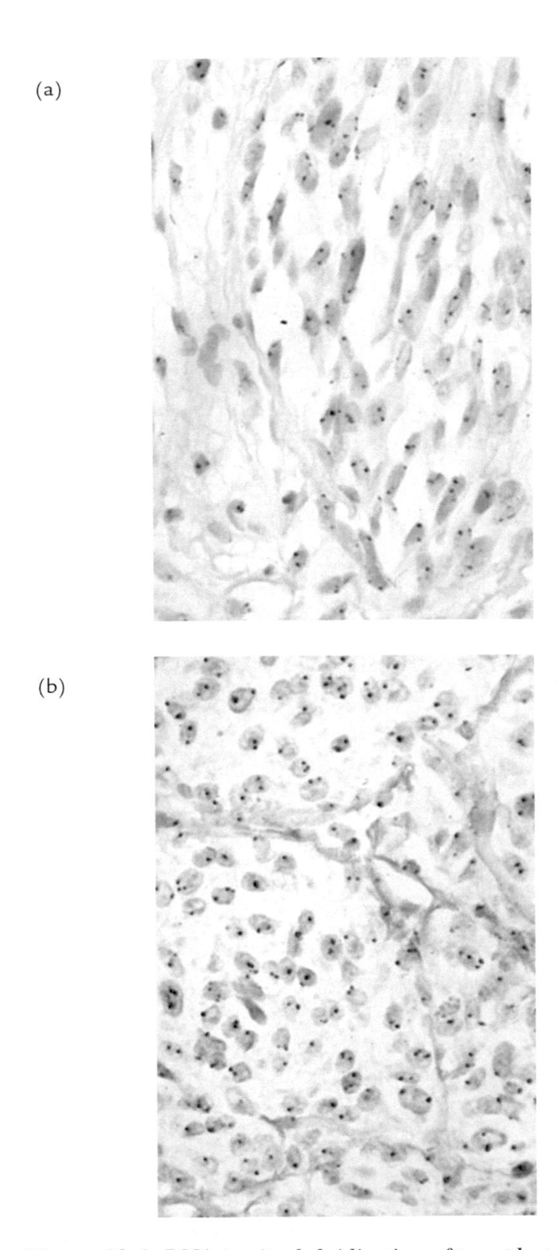

Figure 12.4 *DNA in situ hybridization of paraplast sections of a Spitz naevus (a) and a primary melanoma (b) recognizing a centromere probe for chromosome 1. Note an increased number of nuclear spots in (b) as compared to (a) (× 250, with haematoxylin counterstaining).*

lymphoma; or if very small numbers of melanoma cells are present that are difficult to detect on the basis of cytomorphology alone. In each of these situations, the careful employment of additional techniques may be of significant help.

Immunohistochemistry as an aid in distinguishing between melanocytic naevi and melanoma

The differential diagnosis of naevus versus melanoma can usually be resolved on the basis of histological evaluation. A discussion of the practical aspects of this separation is outside the scope of this chapter; the interested reader is referred to the available texts.[48–50] The expression of markers related to the melanocytic differentiation pathway, such as melanogenesis related enzymes or products of melanin/melanosome synthesis such as tyrosinase, gp 100, and MART-1, do not reliably distinguish between benign and malignant melanocytic tumours, although expression patterns of these molecules can assist in the evaluation of lesional architecture.[51]

Most melanocytic naevi that extend into the dermis exhibit a gradual diminution in the size of naevomelanocytes and their nuclei in the deeper part of the lesion. Cell distribution may be compacted in superficial parts of a naevus, whereas in deeper parts naevocytes are usually arranged in dissociated and ill defined aggregates or are loosely dispersed as single cells. This reduction in naevocyte density is often associated with a switch from a rounded to a more elongated cell morphology, so called neuroid change. Almost all melanocyte derived cells, whether physiological or part of a benign or malignant tumour, express S-100 protein. Thus, S-100 expression per se does not distinguish between benign and malignant melanocytic tumours. S-100 immunostaining does provide a 'one glance' impression of lesional architecture, which may be of help in the diagnosis of problem cases. Suspiciously compact nodules of melanocytic tumour cells, marked variations in cellularity, and other suspicious architectural findings are often highlighted by S-100 immunostaining. It is critically important to accumulate experience of the range of architectures of different melanocytic tumours as indicated by S-100 immunostaining before relying on such appearances in diagnostic practice. To the inexperienced observer, variations in architecture highlighted by S-100 may appear more striking than would be expected from assessment of H&E stained slides, leading to the possibility of overdiagnosis of melanoma. Melanin synthesis in naevi is generally restricted to upper parts of the lesion. gp 100, recognized by monoclonal antibody HMB-45, is a melanosomal protein and (predictably) stains the superficial dermal and intraepidermal naevomelanocytes of common naevi, but not the deep dermal naevocytes.[52,53] Recently Meije et al. found a similar diminution of expression of the melanocytic differentiation-related antigens, pigment associated antigen (PAA) and TRP-1 (tyrosinase-related protein) in deeper melanocytes.[54] Notably in blue naevus and its variants, such as deep penetrating naevus, the capacity for melanogenesis is retained by naevocytes at all levels of the lesion, including the deepest lesional cells.

Immunostaining of inflammatory infiltrates, using a pan-lymphocytic marker such as CD45, may distinguish between halo naevus (Sutton naevus), in which the infiltrate is more or less evenly distributed throughout the dermal component of the lesion, and melanoma, where lymphocyte distribution is generally more irregular. In regressing melanoma irregular inflammatory infiltrates are usually associated with irregularities in distribution of the melanoma cells that are highlighted by S-100 immunostaining.

Deep proliferative activity

Immunostaining for proliferation markers such as MIB-1 promises to be of assistance, although definitive studies of problem cases with adequate follow up are awaited. The widely accepted absence of deep mitotic figures in most naevi (with blue naevus and its variants again being important exceptions to this rule) is paralleled by rarity of MIB-1 positive nuclei in naevi especially in the deeper part of the lesions. This contrasts with melanomas, where MIB-1 positive nuclei are substantially more common and are encountered at all levels of the tumour. MIB-1 positivity in 2% or more of nuclei was observed in 96 % of melanomas but only 6 % of Spitz naevi.[55] A subsequent study confirmed this difference but provided different absolute figures: the average proportion of MIB-1 positive nuclei in Spitz naevus was 3.2% compared with 15.3% in melanomas.[56] In Spitz naevi, a gradual diminution of cyclin Dl immunoreactivity was noted towards the base;[56] probably indicating the gradual disappearance of proliferative activity towards the base.

Other studies have shown that naevi and melanomas differ in the expression of several other markers, but none of these seems of use as an accurate indicator of benignity or malignancy. These include beta 3 integrin, which is expressed in most vertical growth phase melanomas and melanoma metastases, but expressed at low levels or not at all in most naevi, with the notable exceptions of neurotized naevi and Spitz naevi.[19] Immunohistochemical positivity for p53 protein is frequent in melanoma but rare in benign naevi.[51,57] However, the difference seems insufficient for diagnostic use, although a report on application of the approach to problem cases with follow up is awaited. Interestingly, in 20 melanomas apparently derived from contiguous benign naevus the immunoreactivity was increased for p53 and expression of p_{16}^{ink4a} and Bcl-2 decreased. This attests to the probable relevance of dysregulation of these important controllers of cell proliferation and survival in the processes of malignant transformation that result in the development of melanoma.[58]

p53 gene mutations are comparatively rare in melanoma, which may relate to the frequency of mutations of the $p_{16}^{ink4a}/p_{19}^{arf}$ locus. Disruption of p_{19}^{arf} function results in diminished or aborted binding of the p_{19}^{arf} protein to Mdm2, leading in turn to increased Mdm2 mediated degradation of p53 and therefore diminished p53 function despite the absence of p53 mutations.[59] However, p53 mutations are present in some melanocytic tumours, including some benign naevi.[60] Thus, the presence of a p53 mutation clearly does not prove that a melanocytic lesion is malignant. Vascular endothelial growth factor (VEGF) was expressed by almost half of melanomas in a recent series but was not seen in the naevi tested.[61] The practical diagnostic relevance of this observation requires independent confirmation and an analysis of expression patterns in problem cases.

A recently identified antigen designated CTpll, was expressed by seven of 10 melanomas but was absent from melanocytic naevi.[38]

Analyses of the clonality of melanocytic naevi have produced discrepant results, and the role of this approach is unresolved. Using the analysis of X chromosome inactivation in females, one group reported that all informative cases of a series of 20 junctional and compound melanocytic naevi were polyclonal.[62] A second study, using the same approach, found monoclonality in 37 of 47 naevi.[63] It is possible that the patch size of the X chromosome inactivation mosaic of normal tissues may have influenced these disturbing discrepancies. Analysis of clonality cannot at present be recommended as means of distinguishing between naevus and melanoma. Aneuploidy as assessed by DNA image cytometry was detected in 16% of benign naevi, in contrast with 86% of primary melanomas and 83% of metastatic melanomas.[64] Notably, all metastasizing melanomas in the study were aneuploid.[64] In situ hybridization using probes directed to centromeres probes identifies aneusomias and may be able to distinguish between naevi from melanomas in paraffin sections. Using this approach, de Wit et al. found clear differences between Spitz naevi and melanomas in considering the number of nuclei with more than two signals highlighted by a probe for the chromosome 1 centromere.[47] It is important that de Wit et al. specifically addressed a subgroup of problem cases and included follow up data. Although still a laborious technique, comparative genomic hybridization (CGH) may have a diagnostic application. Aberrations of chromosomes 1, 6, 7, 8, 9, and 10 are common in melanoma but were absent from a recent series of 17 Spitz naevi.[65] However, it is of interest that gains of lip and 7q21-ter were found in four of these Spitz naevi.[65] Wettengel et al. recently confirmed the rarity of numerical chromosomal abnormalities in Spitz naevi.[66]

Immunohistochemistry as an aid to identification of melanocytic origin of a morphologically undifferentiated tumour

In the absence of melanin pigment, the distinction between melanoma and other malignancies may be difficult. The problem can usually be resolved by the use of immunohistochemistry. Several antibodies are useful and best used as a small panel of antibodies, including markers specific for the other malignancies that fall within the differential diagnosis. S-100 is perhaps the most widely used marker for melanoma.[3] It is expressed by practically all melanomas, including the challenging group of amelanotic tumours.[50] Levels of expression of S-100 in melanoma generally result in strong and convincing positivity located in the cytoplasm and the nucleus. A wide variety of other benign and malignant tumours that take their origin from cells other than melanocytes also express S-100 protein.[50] Cytology and histology as well as the clinical context in which these non-melanocytic tumours occur generally allow their distinction from melanocytic naevi or melanomas. Myoepithelial tumours and salivary gland tumours are characterized by their special anatomical location, clinical and histological appearance as well as their coexpression of keratins (absent or expressed at low levels in the most melanomas) and sometimes calponin. Malignant peripheral nerve sheath tumours (MPNST) generally exhibit poor and focal S-100 immunoreactivity and may express other neural markers. The MPNST may show a connection with a large nerve at surgery or by careful microscopy. Cellular neurilemmoma is a benign tumour that requires special mention here, since it strongly S-100 immunoreactive and has a densely cellular histological appearance, which may confuse those not familiar with this entity and lead them erroneously to interpret the tumour as a melanoma.[67] Lack of nuclear atypia and very low mitotic activity, both of which contrast with the high cellularity of this S-100 positive spindle cell tumour, are important indicators of the correct diagnosis. Liposarcomas, chondrosarcomas, and Langerhans cell histiocytomas all express S-100 protein, but because these tumours have quite singular histological characteristics this will seldom lead to diagnostic problems. Clear cell sarcoma of tendons and aponeuroses is essentially a melanoma of soft tissues and as such exhibits the immunophenotypic profile that is characteristic of melanoma. Distinction of this quite rare tumour from the much more common cutaneous melanoma is based on histology and the tissue of origin of the tumour. Clear cell sarcoma originates in the deep soft tissues and only secondarily extends to the more superficial tissues, including the skin.

The tissue and tumour distribution pattern of gp 100, the protein harbouring the epitopes recognized by monoclonal antibodies HMB-45 and NKI-beteb, is much more restricted. Apart from melanocytes and melanocytic tumours, gp 100 is expressed by lesions, including tumours, that are believed to derive from the so called perivascular epithelioid cell; these entities include angiomyolipoma, epithelioid angiomyolipoma, lymphangioleiomyomatosis, and 'benign sugar tumour' of the lung.[68] In view of their characteristic appearance on conventional miscroscopy, these lesions rarely pose diagnostic problems, unless they present in an unusual site such as the nasal cavity, or if the lesion is highly cellular, with atypical features.[69] High cellularity and atypia are seen in the recently described cellular/epithelioid angiomyolipoma, which may be made up of epithelioid cells that resemble the tumour cells of some melanomas. Such tumours may present in the liver.[70]

Melan-A is an antibody that recognizes the MART-1 antigen, expressed by melanocytes and their tumours, as well as the HMB-45 reactive perivascular epithelioid cell lesions mentioned above. In addition, Melan-A stains adrenocortical carcinoma, Leydig cell tumours, and other steroid producing cells and tumours.[68,71]

The monoclonal antibody NKI-C_3, raised against melanoma, has had some popularity as a marker of melanoma; but it should not be used to differentiate melanoma from other malignancies because of its lack of specificity. Tyrosinase, a key enzyme in melanogenesis, can be recognized in paraffin sections by monoclonal antibody T311 and serves well as a differentiation marker in that it will distinguish between melanoma and other malignancies.[68,72] Monoclonal antibody KB A. 62, which can be used on paraffin sections, can be employed in panels with other melanocytic markers.[68,73] KB A. 62 is highly sensitive but has the disadvantage that it stains a minority of carcinomas. Microphthalmia transcription factor, Mitf, is a recently developed and highly promising marker of melanocytic differentiation. In a recent consecutive series of 100 melanomas all exhibited nuclear staining with Mitf, while 60 varied non-melanocytic tumours were either negative (58 cases) or had cytoplasmic staining without evident nuclear reaction (two cases).[74]

It is of importance to realize that melanoma cells may express markers that are more characteristic of other types of differentiation, such as keratins, smooth muscle actin and histiocytic markers, including CD68, alpha 1-antitrypsin, and muramidase.[75–77] The problem of the determination that a lesion is of melanocytic origin is not confined to malignant tumours. Unusual types of naevi may simulate non-melanocytic lesions, and immunohistochemistry using markers of melanocytic differentiation may be required to make the separation. These include desmoplastic naevus, intradermal Spitz naevus, and naevus cell aggregates of lymph nodes.[78,79] Immunostaining for S-100 is generally of help, and Melan-A (MART-1) may be an even better marker by virtue of its greater specificity.[80]

ESTIMATION OF PROGNOSIS

Despite the wide range of histopathological appearances that are encountered when evaluating melanomas, the prognostic factors that are assessed by the pathologist have emphasized tumour size and the degree of local extension and spread rather than tumour subtype or grade. This contrasts with many other areas of tumour pathology, where grading has been shown to be of independent prognostic significance and is part of the daily routine of the surgical pathologist. Nonetheless, the need for additional prognostic parameters continues to increase.[81]

When they come to clinical attention, melanomas are often small and thin, and the chance of cure is substantial for the great majority of patients. There is, however, a need specifically to identify the minority of patients with small, apparently early melanomas who have a significant risk of life threatening spread. Treatment that is tailored to variables of tumour aggressiveness rather than just tumour spread, might be more effective. Attempts in this direction have had varying success. Studies of genotypic and phenotypic properties of melanoma provide new insights into the heterogeneity of this disease and may permit rational subdivision into subgroups of varying aggressiveness. In addition, immunohistochemistry and PCR based molecular techniques allow identification of very small numbers of melanoma cells in lymph nodes or other tissues.[3,82,83] When applied appropriately and meticulously, such approaches can increase diagnostic sensitivity without jeopardizing specificity. We first review the detection of minimal melanoma and subsequently the issue of qualitative differences between individual melanomas that are of potential prognostic significance.

DETECTION OF SMALL NUMBERS OF MELANOMA CELLS

Primary tumour site

The pathologist may need immunohistochemistry to identify small numbers of melanoma cells in the primary diagnostic excision specimen or subsequent definitive re-excision. In total or subtotal regression of melanoma there is often a dense inflammatory infiltrate, the mixed lymphohistiocytic infiltrate may obscure scattered single melanoma cells, which are diagnostically important for the confident diagnosis of invasive melanoma. Immunostaining for S-100 protein is of limited help, since histiocytes and Langerhans cells are positive. The combination of large cell size (relative to adjacent leukocytes), epithelioid morphology, large nuclei with prominent eosinophilic nucleoli or nuclear inclusions of cytoplasm, cell distribution (small aggregates) and S-100 immunoreactivity of cytoplasm and nucleus may, however, be sufficient to allow confidence that the cells present are melanoma cells. Immunostaining with other melanocyte markers, especially Melan-A/MART-1 promises to be of additional diagnostic value, but further systematic studies will be necessary.

Small numbers of invasive melanoma cells in the papillary dermis underlying an in situ melanoma (invasive radial growth phase) are more easily identified by immunostained sections. However, dermal histiocytes and Langerhans cells may give an erroneous impression of invasion, especially in lentigo maligna. In case of doubt, we believe that it is better to err on the safe side and conclude that there is no (micro)invasion. Even if truly minimal invasion is present, the chance of metastasis and of local recurrence after surgery with clear margins is minimal. The true extent of spread of spindle cell melanoma may be exceedingly difficult to identify on H&E slides. Immunostaining for S-100 protein is of notable help in this respect.[83] Similarly, the detection of residual disease in a re-excision specimen may be facilitated by S-100 staining. However, it is well to remember that, in scar tissue elongated fusiform S-100 positive cells of uncertain derivation (though some may be nerve related) are often present. After excision of a spindle cell melanoma the mere presence of scattered, often attenuated, fusiform cells that are S-100 positive is not sufficient to determine that residual tumour is present. Perineural or intraneural spread of melanoma may at times be extremely difficult to identify. S-100 immunostaining is of limited benefit here, as many nerve associated cells are normally S-100 positive. Careful comparison of H&E and S-100 stained nerves in sections prepared from contiguous levels is often the only approach to evaluate neurotropism. Most sections will contain normal nerves as well as those suspected of being involved by melanoma and carefully contrasting normal and suspect in the immunostained and conventionally stained sections is often instructive. Desmoplastic melanoma is usually S-100 positive and rarely HMB-45 positive but may exhibit properties not usually associated with melanocytic differentiation, such as marked expression of smooth muscle actin.

Regional lymph nodes

The procedures to be followed in sentinel node detection, biopsy, and diagnostic processing are described in Chapter 27 and our various previous publications on the topic.[84,85] Here, we limit ourselves to a discussion of potential pitfalls in the immunohistochemical detection of small numbers of metastatic melanoma cells.

S-100 positive macrophages and antigen presenting dendritic cells

Macrophages can usually be separated from melanoma cells on the basis of cell size, the comparatively small size, an often reniform shape of the nucleus and the occasional presence of phagocytosed material. If background staining of macrophages is present it will usually affect mainly the cytoplasm of the cells and the prominent nuclear staining seen in melanoma cells will be absent. Macrophages are negative with HMB-45 and Melan-A. In some instances, large numbers of macrophages within sinuses, as in sinus histiocytosis, may be a problem. The absence of compact cell clumps usually points away from melanoma cells, though single melanoma cells may be encountered. Dendritic antigen presenting cells of the paracortex sometimes present a problem.[86] Such cells are smaller that melanoma cells (other than naevocytoid melanoma cells), and are largely confined to the paracortical nodules with maximum concentration at the periphery of the nodules and lack the large nuclei and nucleoli of melanoma cells. They are polydendritic in reactive paracortices and their complex dendrites seem to anastomose or interlace. In inactive (immune suppressed) nodes the dendritic cells have had few or no dendrites. Although strongly S-100 positive, these cells are negative with HMB-45 and Melan-A.

Melanocytic naevus cell aggregates within the lymph node capsule can usually be identified because of their location within the fibrous capsule and trabeculae (rather than the marginal sinus) and by their monomorphic cytologic and nuclear features.[79] Such naevus cell aggregates were detected in 22% of lymphadenectomy specimens from melanoma patients in one large systematic study undertaken during the development of the sentinel node technique.[79] This study combined morphology and immunohistology. Nodal naevi are a serious cause for concern when attempts to detect metastatic melanoma are based on non-morphological techniques such as RT-PCR using primers for tyrosinase or other melanocyte differentiation markers.[87] Naevus cells and possibly Schwann cells and other cell types can cause false positive results with such techniques. Tyrosinase transcripts have been reported to be present in a wide variety of tissues including normal lymph nodes.[88] Techniques that combine the possibility of morphology and the exquisite sensitivity of the PCR approach are very appealing, but present considerable technical problems and are currently unsuited for routine use.[89,90]

Blue naevi of lymph nodes have been reported repeatedly in the literature but in our experience are rare. Blue naevi are characterized by naevomelanocytes, often substantially pigmented and fusiform or partly dendritic, within the lymph node parenchyma. Because of their rarity and the fact that metastatic melanoma also involves the lymph node parenchyma, the alternative diagnosis of metastatic melanoma should always be a very serious consideration. Immunostaining for currently available melanocytic markers cannot help to separate these entities.

Blood and distant tissue sites

PCR based molecular techniques have the power to identify very small numbers of tumour cells in a large population of other cells, as long as they can be based on the detection of a (DNA, RNA) marker that is qualitatively different from non-neoplastic cells, or which is totally absent from the non-neoplastic cells in the sample. These techniques have been employed to detect melanoma micrometastases in regional lymph nodes or distant sites, or within the blood.[91] Very strict negative controls are mandatory in order to prevent false positive results, especially when extensive DNA or cDNA amplification is employed in order to reach very high detection sensitivities. In this respect, the occurrence of small numbers of non-neoplastic melanocytes at sites where their presence is less well known becomes very relevant. Mucous membranes, meninges, thymus, and, possibly, deep tendons and aponeuroses contain non-neoplastic melanocytes, and the so called perivascular epithelioid cells that presumably give rise to HMB-45 and MART-1 positive tumours may result in false positive results if melanoma associated expression markers, rather than specific mutations previously identified in the melanoma under study, are targeted in the PCR based micrometastasis detection.[92] Despite their intrinsic technical appeal, the clinical usefulness of these novel assays needs further critical study before clinical treatment decisions and planning can be based on the results obtained with them. Indeed, in view of the poor correlation of findings with subsequent course of disease, a recent study of RT-PCR based detection of melanoma cells cast doubt on the practical applicability of this technique in the identification of patients with subsequent distant metastasis.[93] Immunocytochemistry of cytospin preparations of bone marrow aspirates, using HMB-45, can be used to detect small numbers of metastatic melanoma cells that escape detection using conventional cytological screening; such cells were detected in 4/20 patients undergoing surgery for lymph node metastases.[94]

In a recent study, RT-PCR based detection of melanocytes in peripheral blood after surgical removal of the primary tumour was associated with increased likelihood of recurrence of tumour.[95] Interestingly, MART-1 positivity within the blood was less likely to be followed by disseminated disease recurrence than tyrosinase positivity, which led the authors of the study to speculate that an antiMART-1 immune response might account for this decreased likelihood of tumour recurrence within the 2-year observation period.

Prognostic relevance of various genotypic and immunophenotypic properties of melanoma

Proliferative activity

In numerous studies, it has been established that high proliferative activity, as evidenced by high mitotic counts, high S-phase fraction, and large numbers of tumour cells positive for proliferation associated proteins are recognized by antibodies such as Ki-67 PCNA, and MIB-1, is correlated with increased likelihood of melanoma recurrence and/or increased pace of tumour progression.[96–106] Variations in variables investigated, techniques used, cut-off points defined, and melanoma series subjected to study preclude more detailed conclusions. The role of proliferative activity assessments in many thin stage I melanomas seems to be limited in view of the marked variations in cellular density of primary melanomas and the comparatively small absolute numbers of tumours cells in any one histological section of such melanomas. Despite the plethora of studies showing significant correlation with prognosis, assessment of proliferative activity and the application of special techniques to investigate it, have not become part of the standard histological evaluation of primary melanoma as it has in, for example, the evaluation of breast carcinoma or soft tissue sarcomas.

Vascularity

Animal models have provided ample evidence that outgrowth of tumours, including melanoma, requires the establishment of a vascularized supportive stroma. In accordance with this, Barnhill et al. found a significantly greater mean number of vessels associated with macrometastases than with micrometastases of melanoma.[107] Lack of such induction of vascular proliferation may account for so called tumour dormancy (persistent presence but lack of outgrowth of tumour for prolonged periods of time). Differences in vascularity of primary melanomas have been related to prognosis in several studies; but the emerging picture is not clear since increased vascularity was linked to unfavourable prognosis, to favourable prognosis, or lack of prognostic impact.[108–111]

Oncogenes and tumour suppressor genes

A variety of oncogenes have been investigated for their possible relevance to melanoma prognosis. Most studies deal with increased expression, as detected by immunohistochemistry, and have focused on oncogenes whose oncogenic mode of action is solely or largely mediated by increased expression. Immunohistochemical positivity of primary melanoma for c-myc was associated with increased thickness, ulceration, and decreased survival in a recent study;[112] within the group of melanomas over 3 mm in thickness, it was an independent prognostic factor. However, in another study of 40 primary melanomas, c-myc immunoreactivity, present in 10 cases, did not correlate with survival, so that the matter remains unresolved.[113]

Immunoreactivity for p53 protein, which is often the result of missense mutations of the p53 gene resulting in an abnormally stable protein with altered biological activities, was the subject of a number of studies; no obvious prognostic influence emerged from these studies since some reported an association with poorer prognosis, whereas others found an improved survival or no significant prognostic influence.[114–117]

Various markers

Interleukin 8 (IL-8) has been shown to act as a significant growth factor for melanoma cells in vitro. Recently, increased IL-8 expression in primary melanoma or in the epidermal keratinocytes overlying the tumour, as detected by in situ hybridization, was associated with decreased time to progression of the melanoma.[118]

NM23, which is associated with decreased metastatic potential of some animal tumour models, can be shown immunohistologically in many melanomas. Some found a favourable prognostic significance of immunopositivity for this marker, but others have not found a relation with tumour recurrence or patient survival.[119–123]

Expression of the activated leukocyte cell adhesion molecule, ALCAM/CD 166, which has been associated with metastatic capacity of melanoma cell lines in an animal model, was recently shown to increase with increasing thickness and Clark level of primary melanomas, being positive in $<10\%$ of melanomas under 1.5 mm and in $>70\%$ of melanomas over 1.5 mm in thickness.[124] Studies of the prognostic significance of ALCAM/CD 166 expression after stratification for thickness and other classical prognostic factors will be needed before the possible usefulness of this biologically interesting marker becomes clear. Expression of $\alpha_v\beta_3$ integrin as well as ICAM-1 is more common on malignant than in benign melanocytic tumours, and in the group of melanomas their expression was associated with increased thickness and their combined expression was associated with a higher frequency of tumour recurrence in a recent study.[125] Expression of p75NGFR, NCAM/CD56 and GAP-43 is common in the intradermal component of melanocytic naevi, possibly as a reflection of a recapitulation of early Schwannian differentiation in dermal naevus cells; but the expression of these markers was significantly lower in melanomas.[126] A transmembrane receptor with tyrosine kinase activity c-kit (CD117) is expressed in normal melanocytes, melanocytic naevi, as well as radial growth phase melanoma, but was there was little or no staining in vertical growth phase melanoma and metastatic melanoma, so that its loss of expression in melanoma seems to be prognostically significant.[127] Accumulation of peanut agglutinin binding glycoconjugates was found in roughly two thirds of melanomas but not in non-neoplastic melanocytes or naevus cells, and in the groups of melanomas, the presence of positive cells was associated with worse outcome in a recent study.[128]

Ploidy assessment of lymph node metastases of melanoma is of potential interest since in a recent study, diploid and aneuploid lymph node melanoma metastases were associated with a 12-month survival of 87% and 41%, respectively.[129]

These studies, many of which await independent confirmation, illustrate that in future, improved prediction of melanoma prognosis will probably be possible, to the benefit of patients.

FUTURE PERSPECTIVES

The past decade has been characterized by the development of molecular biology extending to molecular medicine. In the diagnostics of a number of tumour types such as lymphomas, molecular assays have already been introduced. In this ongoing molecular revolution three phases can be distinguished. The first phase is gene discovery. In this phase genes are identified that were previously unknown. Identification of the whole human genome has been accomplished now. Since several types of changes/mutations in DNA are crucial in tumourigenesis and tumour progression as DNA chips are already available to detect cancer relevant genomic changes/mutations. The second phase is molecular fingerprinting. In this phase the genomic status and the mRNA (cDNA) expression patterns are correlated with functional status of cells and/or tissues. This phase will provide insight into which (new) molecules are functionally important, and this will lead to a more precise diagnosis and targets for a better treatment of cancer patients. To determine specific mRNA expression profiles cDNA chips for various types of tumours including melanoma are available for diagnostic and prognostic purposes.[130] The third phase puts protein information into functional pathways and will result in a functional understanding of the pathophysiology of disease. Simply establishing which genes are transcribed and which proteins are translated in a specific cell type will not provide enough information. Ultimately it is important to know how these proteins interact with each other in networks and pathways in cells and/or tissues in situ.[131] This will reveal the differences between normal function in healthy cells and aberrant function in diseased cells. An understanding of these processes will be the basis for diagnosis and individual therapeutic design.

REFERENCES

1. Ruiter DJ, Broecker E-B, Immunohistochemistry in the evaluation of melanocytic tumors. *Semin Diagn Pathol* 1993; 10: 76–91.
2. Reisfeld RA, Report of the International Consensus Conference on Human Melanoma Antigens, Lausanne, Switzerland, 12–14 November 1992. *Melanoma Res* 1993; 3: 209–17.
3. Cohran AJ, Wen D-R, Herschman HR, Gaynor RB, Detection of S-100 protein as an aid to the identification of melanocytic tumors. *Int J Cancer* 1982; 30: 295–7.
4. Leong A S-Y, Cooper K. Leong FJWM, *Manual of diagnostic antibodies for immunohistology*. London: Greenwich Medical Media, 1999.
5. Graf LH Jr, Ferrone S, Human melanoma-associated antigens. *Immunol Ser* 1989; 43: 643–79.
6. Carrel S, Rimoldi D, Melanoma-associated antigens. *Eur J Cancer* 1993; 29A: 1903–7.
7. Gown AM, Vogel AM, Hoak D, et al, Monoclonal antibodies specific for melanocytic tumor distinguish subpopulations of melanocytes. *Am J Pathol* 1986; 123: 195–203.
8. Vennegoor C, Hageman P, Van Nouhuys H, et al, A monoclonal antibody specific for cells of the melanocyte lineage. *Am J Pathol* 1988; 130: 179–92.
9. Chen YT, Stockert E, Tsang S, et al, Immunophenotyping of melanomas for tyrosinase: implications for vaccine development. *Proc Natl Acad Sci USA* 1995; 92: 8125–9.
10. Hofbauer GF, Kamarashev J, Geertsen R, et al, Tyrosinase immunoreactivity in formalin-fixed, paraffin-embedded primary and metastatic melanoma: frequency and distribution. *J Cutan Pathol* 1998; 25: 204–9.
11. Busam KJ, Jungbluth AA, Melan-A, a new melanocytic differentiation marker. *Adv Anat Pathol* 1999; 6: 12–18.
12. Orosz Z, Melan-A/Mart-1 expression in various melanocytic lesions and in non-melanocytic soft tissue tumours. *Histopathology* 1999; 34: 517–25.
13. Xu Y, Setaluri V, Takechi Y, et al, Sorting and secretion of a melanosome membrane protein, gp 75/TRP1. *J Invest Dermatol* 1997; 109: 788–95.
14. Nishioka E, Funassak Y, Kondoh H, et al, Expression of tyrosinase, TRP-1 and TRP-2 in ultraviolet-irradiated human melanomas and melanocytes. TRP-2 protects melanoma cells from ultraviolet B induced apoptosis. *Melanoma Res* 1999; 9: 433–43.
15. De Vries TJ, Fourkour A, Wobbes T, et al, Heterogeneous expression of immunotherapy candidated proteins gp 100, MART-1, and tyrosinase in human melanoma cell lines and in human melanocytic lesions. *Cancer Res* 1997; 57: 3223–9.
16. Blessing K, Sanders DS, Grant JJ, Comparison of immunohistochemical staining of the novel antibody Melan-A with S-100 protein and HMB-45 in malignant melanoma and melanoma variants. *Histopathology* 1998; 32: 139–46.
17. De Wit PEJ, Moretti S, Koenders PG, et al, Increasing epidermal growth factor receptor expression in human melanocytic tumor progression. *J Invest Dermatol* 1992; 99: 168–78.
18. Niezabitowski A, Czajecki K, Rys J, et al, Prognostic evaluation of cutaneous melanoma: a clinicopathologic and immunohistochemical study. *J Surg Oncol* 1999; 70: 150–60.
19. Van Belle PA, Elenitsas R, Satyamoorthy K, et al, Progression-related expression of beta 3 integrin in melanomas and nevi. *Hum Pathol* 1999; 30: 562–7.
20. Van Kempen LCLT, Van den Oord JJ, Van Muijen GNP, et al, Activated leukocyte cell adhesion molecule/CD 166, a marker of tumor progression in primary malignant melanoma of the skin. *Am J Pathol* 2000; 156: 769–74.
21. Silye R, Karayiannakis AJ, Syrigos KN, et al, E-cadherin/catenin complex in benign and malignant melanocytic lesions. *J Pathol* 1998; 186: 350–5.
22. Manten-Horst E, Danen EH, Smit L, et al, Expression of CD44 splice variants in human cutaneous melanoma and melanoma cell lines is related to tumor progression and metastatic potential. *Int J Cancer* 1995; 64: 182–8.

23. Ferrier CM, Van Geloof WL, De Witte HH, et al, Epitopes of components of the plasminogen activation system are re-exposed in formalin-fixed paraffin sections by different retrieval techniques. *J Histochem Cytochem* 1998; 46: 469–76.
24. Vaisanen A, Kallioinen M, Taskinen PJ, et al, Prognostic value of MMP-2 immunoreactive protein (72 kD type IV collagenase) in primary skin melanoma. *J Pathol* 1998; 186: 51–8.
25. Moretti S, Pinzi C, Berti E, et al, In situ expression of transforming growth factor beta is associated with melanoma progression and correlates with ki67, HLA-DR and beta 3 integrin expression. *Melanoma Res* 1997; 7: 313–21.
26. Ruiter DJ, Van Muijen GNP, Markers of melanocytic tumor progression, Editorial, *J Pathol* 1998; 186: 340–2.
27. Moretti S, Pinzi C, Spallanzani A, et al, Immunohistochemical evidence of cytokine networks during progression of human melanocytic lesions. *Int J Cancer* 1999; 84: 160–8.
28. Desai SA, Wang X, Noronha EJ, et al, Characterization of human anti-high molecular weight-melanoma-associated antigen single-chain Fv fragments isolated from a phage display antibody library. *Cancer Res* 1998; 58: 2417–25.
29. Hamby CV, Chinol M, Palestro CJ, et al, Improved tumor targeting of rhemium-186-labeled anti-human high-m.w. melanoma-associated antigen monoclonal antibody 763. 74 following purification with anti-idiotypic monoclonal antibody MK2-23. *Int J Cancer* 1998; 78: 486–90.
30. Takahaski T, Johnson TD, Nishinaka Y, et al, IgM Anti-ganglioside antibodies induced by melanoma cell vaccine correlate with survival of melanoma patients. *J Invest Dermatol* 1999; 112: 205–9.
31. De Plaen E, Arden K, Traversari C, et al, Structure, chromosomal localization, and expression of 12 genes of the MAGE family. *Immunogenetics* 1994; 40: 360–9.
32. Kirkin AF, Dzhandzyhugazyan K, Zeuthen J, Melanoma-associated antigens recognized by cytotoxic T lymphocytes. *AMPiS* 1998; 106: 665–9.
33. Hofbauer GF, Schaefer C, Noppen C, et al, MAGE-3 immunoreactivity in formalin-fixed, paraffin-embedded primary and metastatic melanoma: frequency and distribution. *Am J Pathol* 1997; 151: 1549–53.
34. Van den Eynde BJ, Boon T, Tumor antigens recognized by T lymphocytes. *Int J Clin Lab Res* 1997; 27: 81–6.
35. Ikeda H, Lethe B, Lehmann F, et al, Characterization of an antigen that is recognized on a melanoma showing partial HLA loss by CTL expressing an NK inhibitory receptor. *Immunity* 1997; 6: 199–208.
36. Chen Yt, Scanlan MJ, Sahin U, et al, A testicular antigen aberrantly expressed in human cancers detected by autologous antibody screening. *Proc Natl Acad Sci USA* 1997; 94: 1914–18.
37. Dos Santos NR, Torensma R, De Vries TJ, et al, Heterogeneous expression of the SSX cancer/testis antigens in human melanoma lesions and cell lines. *Cancer Res* 2000; 60: 1654–62.
38. Zendman AJW, Cornelissen IMHA, Weidle UH, et al, CTpll, a novel member of the family of human cancer/testis antigens. *Cancer Res* 1999; 59: 6223–9.
39. Ohnmacht GA, Marincola FM, Heterogeneity in expression of human leukocyte antigens and melanoma-associated antigens in advanced melanoma. *J Cell Physiol* 2000; 182: 332–8.
40. Castelli C, Rivoltin L, Andreola G, et al, T Cell recognition of melanoma-associated antigens. *J Cell Physiol* 2000; 182: 323–31.
41. Van Muijen GNP, Danen EH, Veerkamp JH, et al, Glycoconjugate profile and CD44 expression in human melanoma cell lines with different metastatic capacity. *Int J Cancer* 1995; 61: 241–8.
42. Zarbo RJ, Gown AM, Nagle RB, et al, Anomalous cytokeratin expression in malignant melanoma: one- and two-dimensional western blot analysis and immunohistochemical survey of 100 melanomas. *Modern Pathol* 1990; 3: 494–501.
43. Orchard GE, Calonje E, The effect of melanin bleaching on immunohistochemical staining in heartily pigmented melanocytic neoplasms. *Am J Dermatopathol* 1998; 20: 357–61.
44. Ferrier CM, Van Geloof WL, de Witte HH, et al, Epitopes of components of the plasminogen activation system are re-exposed in formalin-fixed paraffin sections by different retrieval techniques. *J Histochem Cytochem* 1998; 16: 469–76.
45. Ruiter DJ, Ferrier CM, van Muijen GNP, et al, Quality control of immunohistochemical evaluation of tumor-associated plasminogen activators and related components. *Eur J Cancer* 1998; 34: 1334–40.
46. Kerstens HM, Poddighe PJ, Hanselaar AG, A novel in situ hybridization signal amplification method based on the deposition of biotinylated tyramine. *J Histochem Cytochem* 1995; 43: 347–52.
47. De Wit PE, Kerstens HM, Poddighe PJ, et al, DNA in situ hybridization as a diagnostic tool in the discrimination of melanoma and Spitz naevus. *J Pathol* 1994; 173: 227–33.
48. Elder DE, Murphy GF, Melanocytic tumors of the skin. Atlas of tumor pathology 1. *Armed Forces Institute of Pathology* 1991.
49. Mooi WJ, Krausz T, *Biopsy pathology of melanocytic disorders.* London: Chapman and Hall Medical, 1992.
50. Cochran AJ, Bailly C, Paul E, Remotti F, *Melanocytic tumors: a guide to diagnosis.* Philadelphia: Lippincott-Raven, 1997.
51. Bergman R, Azzam H, Sprecher E, et al, A comparative immunohistochemical study of MART-1 expression in Spitz nevi, ordinary nevi, and malignant melanomas. *J Am Acad Dermatol* 2000; 42: 496–500.
52. Smoller BR, McNutt NS, Hsu A, HMB-45 staining of dysplastic nevi: support for a spectrum of progression toward melanoma. *Am J Surg Pathol* 1989; 13: 680–4.
53. Mirecka J, Korabiowska M, Schauer A, Comparative distribution of S-100 protein and antigen HMB-45 in various types of melanoma and naevi. *Pol J Pathol* 1995; 46: 167–72.
54. Meije CB, Mooi WJ, Le Poole C, et al, Micro-anatomy related antigen expression in melanocytic lesions. *J Pathol* 2000; 190: 572–8.
55. Kanter-Lewensohn L, Hedblad MA, Wejde J, Larsson O, Immunohistochemical markers for distinguishing Spitz nevi from malignant melanoma. *Modern Pathol* 1997; 10: 917–20.
56. Nagasaka T, Lai R, Medeiros LJ, Brynes RK, et al, Cyclin Dl overexpression in Spitz nevi: an immunohistochemical study. *Am J Dermatopathol* 1999; 21: 115–20.
57. Kanoko M, Ueda M, Nagano T, Ichihashi M, Expression of p53 protein in melanoma progression. *J Dermatol Sci* 1996; 12: 97–103.
58. Radhi JM, Malignant melanoma arising from nevi, p53, p16 and Bcl-2 expression in benign versus malignant components. *J Cutan Med Surg* 1999; 3: 293–7.
59. Chin L, Merlino G, DePinho RA, Malignant melanoma: modern black plague and genetic black box. *Genes Dev* 1998; 12: 3467–81.
60. Levin DB, Wilson K, Valdares de Amorim G, et al, Detection of p53 mutations in benign and dysplastic nevi. *Cancer Res* 1995; 55: 4278–82.
61. Bayer-Garner IB, Hough AJ Jr, Smoller BR, Vascular endothelial growth factor expression in malignant melanoma: prognostic versus diagnostic usefulness. *Modern Pathol* 1999; 12: 770–4.
62. Harada M, Suzuki M, Ikeda T, et al, Clonality in nevocellular nevus and melanoma: an expression-based clonality analysis at the X-linked genes by polymerase chain reaction. *J Invest Dermatol* 1997; 109: 656–60.
63. Robinson WA, Lemon M, Elefanty A, et al, Human acquired naevi are clonal. *Melanoma Res* 1998; 8: 499–503.
64. Pilch H, Gunzel S, Schaffer U, et al, Evaluation of DNA ploidy and degree of DNA abnormality in benign and malignant melanocytic lesions of the skin using video imaging. *Cancer* 2000; 15: 1370–7.
65. Bastian BC, Wesselman U, Pinkel D, Leboit PE, Molecular genetic analysis of Spitz nevi shows clear differences to melanoma. *J Invest Dermatol* 1999, 113: 1065–9.
66. Wettengel GV, Draeger J, Kiesewetter F, et al, Differentiation between Spitz nevi and malignant melanomas by interphase fluorescence in situ hybridization. *Int J Oncol* 1999; 14: 1177–83.
67. Fletcher CDM, Davies SE, McKee PH, Cellular schwannoma: a distinct pseudosarcomatous entity. *Histopathology* 1987; 11: 21–35.
68. Busam KJ, Jungbluth AA, Melan-A, a new melanocytic differentiation marker. *Adv Anat Pathol* 1999; 6: 12–18.
69. Watanabe K, Suzuki T, Mucocutaneous angiomyolipoma. A report of 2 cases arising in the nasal cavity. *Arch Pathol Lab Med* 1999; 123: 789–92.
70. Tsui WM, Colombari R, Portmann BC, et al, Hepatic angiomyolipoma: a clinicopathological study of 30 cases and delineation of unusual morphological variants. *Am J Pathol* 1999; 23: 34–48.

71. Kaufmann O, Koch S, Burghardt J, et al, Tyrosinase, melan-A, and KBA62 as markers for the immunohistochemical identification of metastatic amelanotic melanomas on paraffin sections. *Modern Pathol* 1998; 11: 740–6.
72. Hofbauer GF, Kamarashev J, Geertsen R, et al, Tyrosinase immunoreactivity in formalin-fixed, paraffin-embedded primary and metastatic melanoma: frequency and distribution. *J Cutan Pathol* 1998; 25: 204–9.
73. Cohen-Knafo E, al Saati T, Aziza J, et al, Production and characterization of an antimelanoma monoclonal antibody KB A. 62 using a new melanoma cell line reactive on paraffin wax embedded sections. *J Clin Pathol* 1995; 48: 826–31.
74. King R, Weilbaecher KN, McGill G, et al, Microphthalmia transcription factor. A sensitive and specific melanocyte marker for melanoma diagnosis. *Am J Pathol* 1999; 155: 731–8.
75. Miettinen M, Franssila K, Immunohistological spectrum of malignant melanoma. The common presence of keratins. *Lab Invest* 1989; 61: 623–8.
76. Riccioni L, Di Tommaso L, Collina G, Actin-rich desmoplastic malignant melanoma: report of three cases. *Am J Dermatopathol* 1999; 21: 537–41.
77. Pernick NL, DaSilva M, Gangi MD, et al, 'Histiocytic markers' in melanoma. *Modern Pathol* 1999; 12: 1072–7.
78. Harris GR, Shea CR, Horenstein MG, et al, Desmoplastic (sclerotic) nevus: an underrecognized entity that resembles dermatofibroma and desmoplastic melanoma. *Am J Surg Pathol* 1999; 23: 786–94.
79. Carson KF, Wen D-R, Li P-X, et al, Nodal nevi and cutaneous melanomas. *Am J Surg Pathol* 1996; 20: 834–40.
80. Evans MJ, Sanders DS, Grant JH, Blessing K, Expression of Melan-A in Spitz, pigmented spindle cell nevi, and congenital nevi: comparative immunohistochemical study. *Pediatr Dev Pathol* 2000; 3: 36–9.
81. Cochran AJ, Elashoff D, Morton DL, Elashoff R, Individualized prognosis for melanoma patients. *Human Pathol* 2000; 31: 327–31.
82. Cochran AJ, Wen D-R, Morton DL, Occult tumor cells in the lymph nodes of patients with pathological stage I malignant melanoma: an immunohistological study. *Am J Surg Pathol* 1988; 12: 612–18.
83. Eng W, Tschen JA, Comparison of S-100 versus hematoxylin and eosin staining for evaluating dermal invasion and peripheral margins by desmoplastic melanoma. *Am J Dermatopathol* 2000; 22: 26–9.
84. Morton DL, Wen D-R, Wong JH, et al, Technical details of intraoperative lymphatic mapping for early stage melanoma. *Arch Surg* 1992; 127: 392–9.
85. Cohran AJ, Surgical pathology remains pivotal in the evaluation of 'sentinel' lymph nodes. *Am J Surg Pathol* 1999; 23: 1169–72.
86. Van der Velde-Zimmermann D, Schipper ME, et al, Sentinel node biopsies in melanoma patients: a protocol for accurate, efficient, and cost-effective analysis by preselection for immunohistochemistry on the basis of Tyr-PCR. *Ann Surg Oncol* 2000; 7: 51–4.
87. Cohran AJ, Wen D-R, Herschman JR, Occult melanoma in lymph nodes detected by antiserum to S-100 protein. *Int J Cancer* 1984; 34: 159–63.
88. Battyani Z, Xerri L, Hassoun J, et al, Tyrosinase gene expression in human tissues. *Pigment Cell Res* 1993; 6: 400–5.
89. Li P-X, Cheng L, Wen D-R, et al, Demonstration of cytoplasmic tyrosinase mRNA in tissue cultured cells by reverse transcriptase (RT) in situ polymerase chain reaction (PCR) and RT PCR in situ hybridization. *Diagn Mol Pathol* 1997; 6: 26–33.
90. Guo J, Cheng L, Wen D-R, et al, Selection of tyrosinase mRNA in formalin fixed paraffin-embedded archival sections of melanoma, using the reverse transcriptase in situ polymerase chain reaction. *Diagn Mol Pathol* 1998; 7: 10–15.
91. Ghossein RA, Carusone L, Bhattacharya S, Review: polymerase chain reaction detection of micrometastases and circulating tumor cells: application to melanoma, prostate, and thyroid carcinomas. *Diagn Mol Pathol* 1999; 8: 165–75.
92. Parker JR, Ro JY, Ordonez NG, Benign nevus cell aggregates in the thymus: a case report. *Modern Pathol* 1999; 12: 329–32.
93. Hanekom GS, Stubbings HM, Johnson CA, Kidson SH, The detection of circulating melanoma cells correlates with tumor thickness and ulceration but is not predictive of metastasis for patients with primary melanoma. *Melanoma Res* 1999; 9: 465–73.
94. Thybusch-Bernhardt A, Klomp HJ, Maas T, et al, Immunocytological detection of isolated tumor cells in the bone marrow of malignant melanoma patients: a new method for the detection of minimal residual disease. *Eur J Surg Oncol* 1999; 25: 298–502.
95. Curry BJ, Myers K, Hersey P, MART-1 is expressed less frequently on circulating melanoma cells in patients who develop distant compared with locoregional metastases. *J Clin Oncol* 1999; 17: 2562.
96. Sondergaard K, Schou G, Survival with primary cutaneous malignant melanoma, evaluated from 2012 cases. A multivariate regression analysis. *Virchows Arch Pathol Anat Histopathol* 1985; 406: 179–85.
97. McCarthy WH, Shaw HM, McCarthy SW, et al, Cutaneous melanomas that defy conventional prognostic indicators. *Semin Oncol* 1996; 23: 709–13.
98. Spatz A, Shaw HM, Crotty KA, et al, Analysis of histopathological factors associated with prolonged survival of 10 years or more for patients with thick melanomas (>5 mm). *Histopathology* 1998; 33: 406–13.
99. Karlsson M, Boeryd B, Carstensen J, et al, DNA ploidy and S-phase in primary malignant melanoma as prognostic factors for stage III disease. *Br J Cancer* 1993; 67: 134–8.
100. Karjalainen JM, Eskelinen MJ, Nordling S, et al, Mitotic rate and S-phase fraction as prognostic factors in stage I cutaneous malignant melanoma. *Br J Cancer* 1998; 77: 1917–25.
101. Martin G, Halwani F, Sibata H, Meterissian S, Value of DNA ploidy and S-phase fraction as prognostic factors in stage III cutaneous melanoma. *Can J Surg* 2000; 43: 29–34.
102. Soyer HP, Ki 67 immunostaining melanocytic skin tumors. Correlation with histologic parameters. *J Cutan Pathol* 1991; 18: 264–72.
103. Ramsay JA, From L, Iscoe NA, Kahn HJ, MIB-1 proliferative activity is a significant prognostic factor in primary thick cutaneous melanoma. *J Invest Dermatol* 1995; 105: 22–6.
104. Boni R, Doguoglu A, Burg G, Muller B, Dummer R, MIB-1 immunoreactivity correlates with metastatic dissemination in primary cutaneous melanoma. *J Am Acad Dermatol* 1996; 35: 416–18.
105. Sparrow LE, English DR, Taran JM, Heenan PJ, Prognostic significance of MIB-1 proliferative activity in thin melanomas and immunohistochemical analysis of MIB-1 proliferative activity in melanocytic tumors. *Am J Dermatopathol* 1998; 20: 12–16.
106. Vlakova T, Talve L, Hana-Kemppinen M, et al, MIB-1 immunoreactivity correlates with blood vessel density and survival in disseminated malignant melanoma. *Oncology* 1999; 57.
107. Barnhill RL, Piepkorn MW, Cochran AJ, et al, Tumor vascularity, proliferation, and apoptosis in human melanoma micrometastases and macrometastases. *Arch Dermatol* 1998; 134: 991–4.
108. Rongioletti F, Miracco C, Gambini C, et al, Tumor vascularity as a prognostic indicator in intermediate-thickness (0.76–4 mm) cutaneous melanoma: a quantitative assay. *Am J Dermatopathol* 1996; 18: 474–7.
109. Ilmonen S, Kariniemi AL, Vlaykova T, et al, Prognostic value of tumor vascularity in primary melanoma. *Melanoma Res* 1999; 9: 273–8.
110. Barnhill RL, Busam KJ, Berwick M, et al, Tumor vascularity is not a prognostic factor for cutaneous melanoma. *Lancet* 1994; 344: 1237–8.
111. Guffey JM, Chaney JV, Stevens GL, et al, Immunohistochemical assessment of tumor vascularity in recurrent Clark II melanomas using antibody to type IV collagen. *J Cutan Pathol* 1995; 22: 122–7.
112. Ross DA, Wilson GD, Expression of c-myc oncoprotein represents a new prognostic marker in cutaneous melanoma. *Br J Surg* 1998; 85: 46–51.
113. Konstadoulakis MM, Vezeridis M, Hatziyianni E, et al, Molecular oncogene markers and their significance in cutaneous malignant melanoma. *Ann Surg Oncol* 1998; 5: 253–60.
114. Lee CS, Pirdas A, Lee MW, P53 in cutaneous melanoma: immunoreactivity and correlation with prognosis. *Australas J Dermatol* 1995; 36: 192–5.
115. Essner R, Kuo CT, Wang H, et al, Prognostic implications of p53 overexpression in cutaneous melanoma from sun-exposed and non-exposed sites. *Cancer* 1998; 15: 309–16.
116. Weiss J, Heine M, Korner B, Pilch H, Jung EG. Expression of p53 protein in malignant melanoma: clinicopathological and prognostic implications. *Br J Dermatol* 1995; 133: 23–31.

117. Talve L, Kainu J, Collan Y, Ekfors T, Immunohistochemical expression of p53 protein, mitotic index and nuclear morphometry in primary malignant melanoma of the skin. *Pathol Res Pract* 1996; 192: 825–33.
118. Nurnberg W, Tobias D, Otto F, et al, Expression of interleukin-8 detected by in situ hybridization correlates with worse prognosis in primary cutaneous melanoma. *J Pathol* 1999; 189: 546–51.
119. Betke H, Korabiowska M, Brinck U, et al, The role of nm23 in melanoma progression and its prognostic significance. *Pol J Pathol* 1998; 49: 93–6.
120. McDermott NC, Milburn C, Curran B, et al, Immunohistochemical expression of nm23 in primary invasive melanoma is predictive of survival outcome. *J Pathol* 2000; 190: 157–62.
121. Easty DJ, Maung K, Lascu I, et al, Expression of NM23 in human melanoma progression and metastasis. *Br J Cancer* 1996; 74: 109–14.
122. Saitoh K, Takahashi H, Yamamoto M, et al, Expression of metastasis suppressor gene product, nm23 protein, is not inversely correlated with the tumour progression in human malignant melanomas. *Histopathology* 1996; 29: 497–505.
123. Van den Oord JJ, Maes A, Stas M, et al, Prognostic significance of nm23 protein expression in malignant melanoma. An immunohistochemical study. *Melanoma Res* 1997; 7: 121–8.
124. Van Kempen LC, van den Oord JJ, van Muijen GN, et al, Activated leukocyte cell adhesion molecule/CD 166, a marker of tumor progression in primary malignant melanoma of the skin. *Am J Pathol* 2000; 156: 769–74.
125. Natali PG, Hamby CV, Felding-Habermann B, et al, Clinical significance of alpha(v)beta3 integrin and intercellular adhesion molecule-1 expression in cutaneous malignant melanoma lesions. *Cancer Res* 1997; 15: 1554–60.
126. Reed JA, Finnerty B, Albino AP, Divergent cellular differentiation pathways during the invasive stage of cutaneous malignant melanoma progression. *Am J Pathol* 1999; 155: 549–55.
127. Montone KT, Van Belle P, Elenitsas R, Elder DE, Proto-oncogen c-kit expression in malignant melanoma: protein loss with tumor progression. *Modern Pathol* 1997; 10: 939–44.
128. Cochran AJ, Wen DR, Berthier-Vergnes O, et al, Cytoplasmic accumulation of peanut agglutinin-binding glycoconjugates in the cells of primary melanoma correlates with clinical outcome. *Human Pathol* 1999; 30: 556–61.
129. Martin G, Halwani F, Shibata H, Meterissian S, Value of DNA ploidy and S-phase fraction as prognostic factors in stage III cutaneous melanoma. *Can J Surg* 2000; 43: 29–34.
130. Bittner M, Meltzer P, Chen Y, et al, Molecular classification of cutaneous malignant melanoma by gene expression profile. *Nature* 2000; 406: 536–40.
131. Ruiter D, Bogennieder T, Elden D, Hamlyn M, Melanoma–stroma interactions. Structural and functional aspects. *Lancet Oncol* 2002; 3: 35–43.

13

Ultrastaging of melanoma patients: molecular detection of micrometastatic disease

Bret Taback, Dave S B Hoon

INTRODUCTION

There has been an increasing interest in the application of molecular markers, used to detect occult metastasis, to the clinical setting. As a prognostic aid the amplification of tumour specific molecular markers using polymerase chain reaction (PCR) offers the promise of more accurately staging disease over conventional imaging methods. The advantages of early detection are well known and include identification of patients with minimal residual disease who are at increased risk of recurrence and may benefit from additional treatment. Furthermore, tumour specific genetic events may permit the identification of molecular targets to tailor individual treatment and potentially assess response. Biological changes can occur during tumour progression (such as chemotherapy resistance, de-differentiation, and tumour aggressiveness) and molecular markers specific for these events offer the clinician the potential of assessing these events on a subclinical level and intervening accordingly. Finally, because reverse transcriptase (RT)-PCR can be performed easily and rapidly on a variety of tissue and body fluid samples in their entirety, this process can be adopted routinely in a cost-effective manner. The limitations to date are validation and robustness of the assays.

This molecular approach to disease detection and diagnosis, staging, screening, monitoring response to treatment, and surveillance for recurrence provides a new frontier for the field of medicine. Many strategies entail the use of molecular markers as surrogates for subclinical disease presence, as indicators of tumour progression, and as a prognostic factor. There is no doubt that RT-PCR analysis for the detection of metastatic disease in tissues and body fluids is revolutionizing surgical pathology and altering approaches to the diagnosis and management of many tumours.[1–4] The field is constantly growing and adopting innovative technologies that provide additional information to improve patient care. However, we are still in the infancy of this 'new approach'. Molecular diagnosis of haemopoietic cancers is far more advanced and has been very successfully integrated into the routine management of patients.[5,6] Molecular approaches for assessing solid tumours have not yet reached that stage. Among all the solid tumours, melanoma diagnosis by molecular methods is most advanced. This may be related to the aggressive behaviour of melanoma and the extremely poor prognostic implications associated with detecting early metastasis. In the future, integrating each patient's tumour specific molecular marker expression pattern (tumour profiling) into a personal diagnostic and treatment plan offers the opportunity to assess more accurately prognosis and tailor treatment to an individual's unique tumour targets. This customized approach may further maximize benefits while minimizing the adverse risks associated with treatment. Improvements in technology and in our understanding of the genetic events associated with the initiation and progression of tumours will make molecular diagnostics and therapeutics more of a certainty in the care of cancer patients.

PROGNOSTIC SIGNIFICANCE OF LYMPH NODE METASTASIS

Melanoma is a highly unpredictable disease in terms of rate and sites of recurrence.[7] Numerous variables have been investigated to obtain prognostic insight into the disease course.[8,9] These have included clinical characteristics (age, sex, race, lesion size and anatomical location, pregnancy status, etc) and histopathological features (growth pattern, ulceration, pigmentation, lymphovascular invasion, lymphocyte infiltration, regression, etc). In a multivariate analysis of 13 commonly cited risk factors, Balch identified the pathological stage of disease (presence of lymph node metastasis) as the most important prognostic variable for determining survival.[10–12] As a result, lymph node status was considered a hallmark for systemic metastasis, and all patients diagnosed with primary melanoma were subject to a formal lymphadenectomy.[13,14] However, pathological studies have shown that the majority of patients (approximately 75% or more) presenting without clinically suspicious lymph nodes will not have metastasis detected by routine histochemistry.[15–17] Therefore, performing such radical surgery for prognostic purposes, which has long been considered the standard of care, was not warranted in the majority of patients. Furthermore, the added cost of an additional surgical procedure and its potential morbidity (such as lymphoedema, neuropathy, infection) could be avoided. Moreover, any therapeutic benefit an elective or prophylactic lymph node dissection confers in early clinical stage disease is currently controversial.[18–25] In only one subgroup of patients has this method shown a survival advantage, in people under 60 years old with primary melanomas 1–2 mm thick.[26] With evidence suggesting that early intervention with immunotherapy may prolong relapse-free and overall survival in high risk patients, lymph node status remains the most important factor identifying patients who may benefit most from further but potentially toxic treatment.[27,28] Additionally, regional lymph node status imparts valuable prognostic information that provides both the patient and physician with substantive support for any future decision making.

Identifying primary tumour characteristics that correlate with tumour aggressiveness offered a more definitive opportunity to determine those patients who may benefit from the prognostic information obtained from a lymph node dissection. In 1970, Breslow correlated increasing tumour thickness with an increased 5-year rate of disease recurrence.[29] Subsequent studies have shown significant correlation between increasing tumour thickness and the incidence of regional lymph node metastasis.[8,13,16] Tumours <0.76 mm thick were associated with a very low incidence of lymph node metastasis (<3%). In contrast, tumours >4.0 mm in thickness were shown to have a greater than 60% incidence of lymph node metastasis. However, any prognostic information obtained from a lymph node dissection was overshadowed by the overwhelming incidence of systemic micrometastasis (>80%). This systemic disease is clearly present in these patients during their initial presentation and accounts for their dismal course (less than 20% are alive at 5 years).[23] Therefore, it is in those patients with intermediate thickness melanomas (1.0–4.0 mm) where the ratio of benefit to risk of performing a lymphadenectomy, to obtain prognostic information, is of greatest value.

Today, despite many advances in cancer diagnosis and detection, lymph node status remains the single most important prognostic factor predicting survival in patients with melanoma or any epithelial malignancy.[9,30] The histological identification of lymph node metastasis supersedes any other prognostic factor associated with a primary melanoma and upstages disease (American Joint Committee on Cancer, AJCC, stage III) in all cases when present.[31] Once patients are diagnosed with lymph node metastasis, their 5-year survival decreases by 40%.[18] Such a dramatic reduction occurs with no other known prognostic factors aside from the finding of systemic metastasis. It is no wonder that such an aggressive search for detecting lymph node metastasis is undertaken in early stage patients.

HISTOLOGICAL ASSESSMENT OF LYMPH NODES

Haematoxylin and eosin (H&E) has long been considered the standard method for staining tissues submitted for histological examination. It is well known that this method may underestimate the true incidence of lymph node metastasis.[32–35] In an attempt to improve the sensitivity of identifying occult melanoma cells in regional lymph nodes over conventional H&E, which is not specific for tumour cells, Cochran et al. used an antibody to S-100, a protein previously identified from primary and metastatic melanomas.[36–39] They were able to identify 30% more tumour-containing lymph nodes with this technique compared with conventional H&E staining in advanced patients with clinically suspicious lymph nodes.[40] In a follow up study, 100 early-stage melanoma patients without histological evidence of lymph node metastasis had immunohistochemical (IHC) analysis performed. IHC identified 14 patients (14%) with tumour cells in their lymph nodes.[41] Furthermore, almost twice as many patients diagnosed with metastasis by this method died compared with patients in whom no occult tumours cells were identified. Although this difference in outcome fell short of achieving statistical significance, it was nevertheless pioneering in demonstrating the clinical implications of further evaluating surgical specimens for the presence of micrometastasis. One caveat of this study, limited specificity, was the cross reactivity of this antibody to dendritic cells, sinus macrophages and Schwann cells of nerves which may be co-habitants in regional lymph nodes and contain S-100 protein. The two most widely used IHC markers in clinical practice today are antibodies to S-100 and gp100 (HMB-45).[42,43] As noted, antibodies to S-100 protein may lack specificity whereas HMB-45 antibody showed a lack of sensitivity, identifying less than 70% of micrometastases in one study.[44] These findings and others have shown limitations in specificity and sensitivity associated with IHC techniques.[45] Furthermore, serial sectioning and IHC evaluation can be an expensive and cumbersome proposition when performed routinely to assess all lymph nodes from a standard lymphadenectomy specimen dependent on surgery (that contains on average 10–20 lymph nodes).

CELL CULTURE TECHNIQUE

Although IHC has proved to be highly useful for improving the rate of detecting lymph node micrometastases by 10–15% over routine H&E, cell culture techniques have shown that it is possible to grow tumour cells from these histopathologically negative lymph nodes.[15] Heller et al. were able to culture tumour cells from 155 (48%) of 323 lymph nodes from 41 clinically node negative patients with primary tumour thicknesses between 0.76 mm and 4.0 mm. They found 20 lymph nodes (6%) from 12 patients (29%) positive for tumour by IHC, however the cell culture technique identified an additional 74 lymph nodes (23%) from nine patients (22%) with occult metastasis. Three of the nine patients developed a recurrence after a mean follow up of 18 months, in comparison to none of the patients whose lymph nodes were culture negative. These findings suggest that lymph nodes considered negative by both clinical and pathological evaluation may contain submicroscopic tumour cells which may be prognostically significant. However, the feasibility of performing this technique on a routine basis is limited by the stringent requirements of cell culturing. In addition, with this method, culture results often take 4–6 weeks, which is not practical in a clinical setting.

INDICATIONS FOR LYMPH NODE DISSECTION

Melanoma patients succumb to their disease as a result of systemic metastasis that may occur through two routes: lymphatic and haematogenous. Historically, lymph node dissection was performed consistently for either therapeutic or prognostic reasons. Previously, clinical studies have shown an improved long term survival in patients whose tumour-bearing lymph nodes were resected early in the course of their disease.[13,23] These findings supported the role of lymph node dissection as a therapeutic manoeuvre in patients with clinically advanced disease.[46,47] More recently, with an increase in early detection, the incidence of clinically palpable lymph node metastases is declining. So far no studies have shown a consistent survival disadvantage in patients whose lymph nodes were not resected until clinically suspicious regional metastasis had occurred.[16,18,21,22] We believe that the role of lymph node dissection as a therapeutic modality for early stage disease will recede and this procedure will be most valuable as a prognostic tool. Because of this emphasis towards earlier detection, the role of evaluating lymph nodes for the presence of smaller (micro-) metastases may be critical.

Detecting the presence of occult metastases will require a more aggressive and thorough approach. Standard histological processing involves bisecting the lymph node, then sectioning and staining, which provides less than 1% of the submitted material for analysis.[48] Because melanoma micrometastasis tends to occur focally in a lymph node, routine histopathological assessment may miss the presence of occult tumour cells.

RATIONALE FOR SENTINEL NODE EVALUATION

In 1992, Morton described the technique of sentinel node biopsy.[49] A sentinel node was defined as the first node in the regional lymphatic basin that drains the primary tumour. Metastases were detected in the sentinel lymph nodes from 40 of 194 lymph node basins assessed (21%). Their false negative rate was less than 1%, indicating the extremely high accuracy with which the sentinel lymph node can predict the pathological status of the regional drainage basin. The addition of IHC improved the sensitivity for detecting sentinel node micrometastasis by 9% over H&E alone (12%). The low incidence of skip metastases documented in this and other studies confirms a sequential progression of melanoma tumour cells through the regional lymphatics, contributing to this technique's success.[17,50–55] This procedure now allows the pathologist to perform a more focused and cost-effective examination of the small number of lymph nodes most likely to harbour occult metastasis. Therefore, via a minimally invasive procedure, significant prognostic information can be obtained from a small amount of tissue.

Only recently, with adequate long-term follow up, has the clinical significance of these occult metastases become more evident. Gershenwald evaluated the recurrence pattern in 243 patients with negative sentinel lymph nodes by H&E analysis.[56] Twenty seven patients (11%) developed a recurrence. With a median follow up of 35 months, the most common site of first recurrence was in the previously mapped lymph node basin, occurring in 10 patients (4.1%). Upon reevaluation of the sentinel lymph nodes with additional serial sectioning and IHC, occult metastases were identified in eight (80%) of these 10 patients, showing the limited sensitivity associated with routine H&E examination. Of greater concern was the lack of any detectable lymph node metastasis with the addition of IHC in all eight patients (3.3%) who developed distant disease as their primary site of relapse.

In a similar study involving 89 sentinel node negative patients, Gadd identified 11 patients (12%) who developed recurrent disease, at a median follow up of 23 months, with seven (7.9%) occurring first in the regional lymph nodes.[57] Retrospective analysis with serial sectioning and IHC of the sentinel lymph nodes available from four of these patients identified tumour cells in one patient (25%). Two patients (2.3%) developed distant metastasis as their first site of recurrence, and only one patient's sentinel node contained metastatic melanoma on re-examination. From these studies it is evident that the combination of sentinel node biopsy and a more thorough histological examination, with serial sectioning and IHC, can accurately assess the lymph node status and indicate the risk of recurrence in almost 90% of cases. However, even such an aggressive histological evaluation may not be completely adequate for detecting lymph node metastasis in all patients. This may be a consequence of the limitations associated with current technology's sensitivity or practicality and/or the biological behaviour of the disease whereby metastasis may occur through a path, presumably haematogenous, that is not assessed.

RT-PCR ASSAYS FOR THE DETECTION OF METASTATIC MELANOMA

Specificity and sensitivity

RT-PCR is a highly sensitive molecular biology technique that may prove useful for identifying early submicroscopic melanoma metastasis. RT-PCR permits the amplification of a limited number of gene transcripts that can then be analyzed against a constitutively expressed control or 'housekeeping' gene to confirm the integrity of the PCR reaction. RT-PCR allows the amplification of 'desired' mRNA transcripts from cells to levels detectable by solid phase (gel electrophoresis) or solution phase detection systems. The assay specificity and sensitivity will strongly depend on the gene evaluated and the source of the specimen (lymph node or blood). These two factors play a significant part in the validation and utility of the assay and must be considered in experimental design. RT-PCR assays can detect specific gene mRNA concentrations as low as femtograms of total RNA. This depends on amplification techniques and the number of gene transcripts present in the total sample. RT-PCR analysis of serial dilution of tumour cells in normal cells can detect as few as several melanoma cells among 10^7 lymphocytes in in vitro assays. These assessments represent only potential sensitivities and should be considered with caution about the sensitivity of the entire method.

In general, RT-PCR shows superior sensitivity in comparison to conventional H&E staining (which can detect in the range of one melanoma cell in 10^4

lymphocytes) and IHC (which can detect one melanoma cell in 10^5 lymphocytes).[48,58] With the extensive use of PCR in the laboratory, the application of this technique as an adjunct to currently available staging methods can be accomplished quite readily. Pathologists have always established their diagnosis on the basis of visual identification of tumour cells. The use of RT-PCR in surgical pathology has received criticism from sceptics who suggest that if tumour cells cannot be detected by conventional methods they are not present and therefore not pathological. Although conventional histopathology is regarded as the gold standard, it is far from being completely accurate.[42,59] The role of RT-PCR for molecular staging will continue to be the subject of considerable debate until results are validated and marker specificity and sensitivity are confirmed in large scale multicentre studies that adhere to unified guidelines for performing the technique.

RT-PCR is a powerfully sensitive method that can be prone to false positive results, and strict adherence to standard operating procedures and meticulous technique is required.[60,61] Even the most minimal variation can be exploited by the extreme sensitivity of PCR to produce false or inconsistent results. Differing results have been shown to occur between separate laboratories processing the same sample as well as within the same laboratory.[62–64] mRNA integrity and freedom from contamination is critical to avoid misinterpreting results. For example, we determined early in assay development that during blood collection the 'skin plug' obtained upon needle puncture was a source of contamination and this required discarding the first few millilitres of blood. In addition, methods of tissue collection require specific review for attention to detail. Contamination of scalpels and surgical equipment with tumour tissue can produce false positive lymph nodes. Maintaining the fidelity of the mRNA product to be assessed is crucial and can be compromised by improper methods of collection, storage, and processing. A diagram of our method for processing the sentinel lymph node for histopathological examination and RT-PCR assessment is shown in Figure 13.1.

Other factors in the assay that must be considered are the influence of pseudogenes and illegitimate mRNA transcription that can produce false positive results.[65,66] Primer designs and probes are critical in assay specificity and sensitivity. Often investigators use reported primers without carefully evaluating the sequences and specificity. The extraction method, quality and amount of RNA used in the assay will influence results. Often

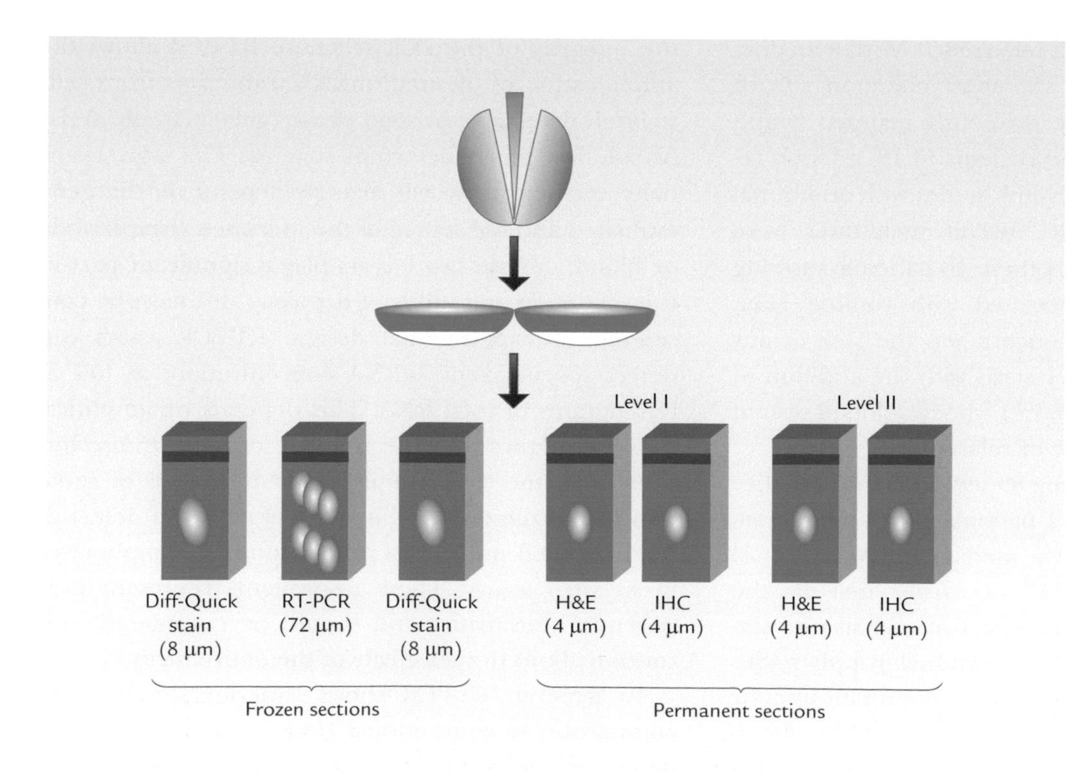

Figure 13.1 *Sentinel node technique. Serial sectioning for analysis bivalving, sectioning and assaying.*

RNA is assessed by ultraviolet spectrophotometry. This may not be consistently reliable and can produce false readings of RNA concentration. DNA and protein contamination will heavily influence specific mRNA detection. The type of thermocycler, number of cycles, and annealing temperatures can significantly affect results.[67] Even individual wells from a single thermocycler can demonstrate differences in conformity. In general, assessing for RT-PCR cDNA products without validation of the products such as with specific probes can result in false interpretations. The most common method reported in literature to date in assessing melanoma RT-PCR cDNA products is by gel electrophoresis and ethidium bromide staining. This approach is highly subjective for detection and varies noticeably from one laboratory to another. If one is searching for micrometastatic disease, the sensitivity of this assay has its limitations. Improvement or validation of these results has been through Southern blotting with specific probes.[68] In general, gel electrophoresis based systems are cumbersome and have limitations with regard to quantitation and sensitivity. More recently, assay methods are being converted to solution phase systems, which allow for a higher throughput, quantitation, standardization, and, most importantly reproducibility among the various laboratories. This has been well documented in viral assay systems.[69] These are just some of the factors that must be considered when designing clinical studies using PCR techniques for tumour staging.

Independent of PCR assay conditions, there exists the problem of tumour heterogeneity for the expression of specific mRNA markers.[70] It is well known that differences may exist among tumours from various patients as well as between the primary tumours and the corresponding metastases within the same patient.[71] Furthermore, changes in gene expression can occur during disease progression and/or in response to treatment (for example, resistance).[2] These inherent tumour cell characteristics are always a significant obstacle in designing a detection assay. We intend to evaluate the role of RT-PCR in ultrastaging melanoma patients based on assessment of individual body compartments: sentinel lymph node, blood, and bone marrow. An emphasis will be on the detection of occult metastasis in the sentinel lymph nodes from patients with early stage melanoma where current results seem more in agreement and demonstrate correlations with known clinical and pathological prognostic variables (tumour thickness and stage).

Lymph nodes

The most common mRNA marker studied in melanoma is the tyrosinase gene transcript. This enzyme is involved in the early steps of melanin biosynthesis, and its expression was shown to occur in 100% of melanoma cell lines and tumour cell cultures, indicating a potentially high specificity of this marker for detecting occult disease.[72] In 1994, Wang et al. showed the presence of tyrosinase mRNA in the lymph nodes of patients at high risk for recurrence (clinically node negative with intermediate thickness lesions).[73] They detected tyrosinase mRNA in the lymph nodes from 19 (66%) of 29 patients assessed, which included all 11 patients with lymph nodes positive by routine histology. No false negative RT-PCR results occurred (RT-PCR negative but histology positive) and nine non-melanoma tumour controls were negative for tyrosinase. Using this technique, Wang et al. were able to upstage eight patients, in this original study. They concluded that RT-PCR was more sensitive than conventional histochemical analysis for the detection of occult lymph node metastasis. In addition, this technique proved highly efficient, allowing the evaluation of an entire lymph node, if necessary, in less time than standard histological processing.

Initially combining these two highly efficient methods (sentinel node biopsy and RT-PCR), one study was able to upstage six of 12 patients with histologically negative sentinel nodes.[74] The authors concluded that RT-PCR assessment of the sentinel node is more sensitive and less labour intensive, thereby providing a cost-effective method for detecting occult metastatic disease, which may have prognostic significance.[75] To address the prognostic value of this approach, two large studies reported results from patients with early clinical stage melanoma who underwent RT-PCR analysis of their sentinel nodes and clinical follow up.[76,77] In 1998, Shivers reported results from a study consisting of 114 patients who underwent sentinel node biopsy and molecular analysis for tyrosinase mRNA. The overall rate of recurrence was 18% (21 patients) during a mean follow up period of 28 months. Fourteen recurrences (61%) had occurred in 23 patients with sentinel lymph nodes positive by histology and RT-PCR, whereas six recurrences

(13%) were noted to occur in the 47 patients with sentinel lymph nodes negative by histology but positive by RT-PCR, and only one recurrence occurred in the 44 patients with sentinel nodes negative by both histology and PCR. In a similar study, Blaheta et al. examined sentinel nodes from 116 patients and identified 36 patients with sentinel nodes positive only by RT-PCR.[77] In this group nine patients (25%) relapsed after a median follow up of 19 months, compared with four patients with sentinel nodes negative by both RT-PCR and histology. These studies show the poorer prognostic implications in patients with occult disease detected by molecular methods and provide convincing evidence for their use in clinical practice. The further finding of a significant correlation between increasing Breslow thickness and RT-PCR lymph node positivity provided a biological explanation for this relation.[78]

Despite an increase in the detection of occult lymph node metastasis with single marker RT-PCR for tyrosinase, ranging from 6–50% (Table 13.1), this method is not infallible, as previously mentioned. We have shown that although a number of melanoma associated antigen (MAA) mRNA markers are expressed in cultured melanocytes and cell lines with 100% frequency, expression levels from a variety of tumour specimens can be significantly less (Table 13.2).[72]

We have subsequently applied this multimarker molecular approach to detect occult melanoma tumour cells in the sentinel lymph nodes of patients who have no clinical evidence of metastasis.[79] From our collection, three mRNA markers were chosen that showed the greatest degree of expression in primary and metastatic tumour tissues: MAGE-A3, MART-1, and tyrosinase. Using this technique we assessed 93 sentinel lymph nodes from 72 patients. No single mRNA marker was found to be exclusively expressed by all sentinel nodes that were considered positive by PCR. MART-1 was the most commonly expressed marker identified in 15 (88%) of 17 patients with sentinel nodes positive by histochemistry (Table 13.3). In contrast, of the 55 patients with sentinel nodes negative by histology, MAGE-A3 was most frequently expressed. Histologically positive sentinel nodes more often expressed two or more mRNA markers (94% patients) compared with histologically negative sentinel nodes (36% of patients). Using multivariate analysis we identified three factors associated with an increased risk for sentinel node metastasis: tumour thickness, age less than 60 and/or sentinel nodes expressing multiple markers. After a mean follow up of 12 months, patients with sentinel nodes expressing two or more markers had a significantly increased risk for early relapse (Figures 13.2 and 13.3). These findings substantiate our hypothesis that combinations of molecular markers to detect occult tumour metastasis may have certain prognostic implications relevant to the clinical setting.

The multimarker approach may also show an advantage in distinguishing true metastases from benign naevus cells, which may reside in regional lymph nodes.[79–81] Multiple markers may allow for the differential identification of these cells, on the basis of varying amounts and types of mRNA transcripts as compared to tumour cells. To date RT-PCR analysis of sentinel nodes has been performed on fresh or frozen tissue or sections because of the instability of RNA at room temperatures and the technical difficulties associated with extraction from paraffin embedded tissues. We have recently had success in detecting metastases in paraffin-embedded nodal tissue sections using multimarker RT-PCR in conjunction with a highly sensitive quantitative technique: electrochemiluminescence (ECL) (Figure 13.4).

Finally the multimarker approach may offer a selective advantage in identifying occult metastasis from different body compartments, whereby variations in microenvironment may select for clones with a unique pattern of gene expression. We have shown varying efficiency for detecting different mRNA markers from selected sites of metastasis.[72] These differences can be due to dilutional effects from non-related mRNA from normal cells, tumour cell heterogeneity, organ microenvironment, and changes in the levels of gene expression during tumour progression.[70,82,83]

Blood

The histological identification of tumour cells in lymph nodes in early clinical stage disease is currently the most widely accepted evidence that metastasis has occurred and its association with a poor patient prognosis is irrefutable. But it must be noted that lymph node analysis provides limited information with regard to disease course. A significant latent period may exist between the initial diagnosis and the development of clinically significant metastasis, whereby the disease course may progress differently in response to each individual's host immune system and/or various therapeutic

Table 13.1 *RT-PCR upstaging of the sentinel node in published series. (Values in brackets are all percentages unless otherwise specified)*

Author	Date	No. of patients	Histology (+)	RT-PCR (+)	Patients upstaged by RT-PCR	Clinical follow up (months)	Incidence of recurrence according to sentinel node status (%)		
							H&E (+) and RT-PCR (+)	H&E (−) and RT-PCR (+)	H&E (−) and RT-PCR (−)
Goydas et al.[81]	1998	50	10 (20)	13 (26)	3 (8)	7 (mean)	N/A	0/3 (0)	N/A
Shivers et al.[76]	1998	114	23 (20)	70 (61)	47 (52)	28 (mean)	14/23 (61)	6/47 (13)	1/44 (2)
Bielgik et al.[80]	1999	26	6 (23)	19 (73)	13 (65)	11.8 (median)	1/6 (17)	0/13 (0)	0/7 (0)
Bostick et al.[79]	1999	72	17 (24)	28 (39)	20 (36)	12 (mean)	5/16 (31)	3/20 (15)	0/35 (0)
Blaheta et al.[77]	2000	116	15 (13)	51 (44)	36 (36)	19 (median)	10/15 (67)	9/36 (25)	4/65 (6)

All studies assessed sentinel lymph nodes for the presence of tyrosinase mRNA by PCR. In addition, Goydas assayed for the presence of MART-1 and Bostick's multimarker assay included MART-1 and MAGE-A3.
+, positive −, negative.
NA = not available.

Table 13.2 *MAA mRNA expression by cell lines, tissues, and blood.* (Values in brackets are all percentages unless otherwise specified)*[72]

RNA Source	MAA mRNA markers expressed			
	Tyr	TRP–1	TRP–2	MART–1
Cultured melanocytes (1)	1 (100)	1 (100)	1 (100)	1 (100)
Cell lines (6)	6 (100)	6 (100)	6 (100)	6 (100)
Tumours (23)	23 (100)	18 (78)	19 (83)	20 (87)
TDLN (28)	26 (93)	18 (64)	20 (71)	24 (86)
Blood (35)	30 (86)	20 (57)	26 (74)	29 (83)

* Results represent MAA RT-PCR plus Southern blotting of various types of tissues and cells. Percentages (in brackets) represent MAA mRNA marker expression per individual specimen source. mRNA markers assessed included Tyr (Tyrosinase), TRP-1 (Tyrosinase-Related-Protein-1), TRP-2 (Tyrosinase-Related-Protein-2), and MART-1/Melan-A. Tumours refer to primary and metastatic (excluding TDLN) melanomas that were assessed by H&E histopathology as involved with melanoma. All TDLNs represent nodes that were pathology positive by H&E staining for melanoma, with one exception. Bloods were from AJCC stage I–IV (I and II, n = 2; III and IV, n = 33) melanoma patients. RNA integrity was confirmed by RT-PCR analysis for β-actin mRNA, which was identified in all specimens. Reproduced from *Cancer Research,*[72] with permission from American Association for Cancer Research © 1997.

Table 13.3 *Correlation of mRNA marker expression and sentinel node histology. (Values in brackets are all percentages unless otherwise specified)*[79]

Sentinel node status	mRNA marker expressed		
	MAGE-A3	MART-1	Tyrosinase
Histology (+) (n = 17)	12 (71)	15 (88)	12 (71)
Histology (−) (n = 55)	24 (44)	20 (36)	16 (29)

+, positive −, negative.

interventions. Lymph node micrometastasis is merely a surrogate marker for risk of distant disease recurrence, and its prognostic value is restricted to the time the biopsy is obtained. This diagnostic procedure does not allow for the continuous monitoring of subclinical disease progression, nor does it identify sites at risk for recurrence. Currently, no assay exists to evaluate treatment response in these early stage patients. Molecular techniques that assess different body compartments (blood, bone marrow, cerebrospinal fluid, drainage fluid from a operative site, etc) may offer the opportunity to more accurately monitor disease presence and/or progression, which can provide invaluable information to the physician and the patient. Studies evaluating recurrences in early stage melanoma patients with histologically negative sentinel lymph nodes have shown that 3% will recur systemically as the first site of relapse (Table 13.4).[56,57,76,77,79] Because distant metastasis can occur through a haematogenous route, and blood is an easily accessible resource to sample that is in constant contact with a tumour, this is considered the most logical site to screen for the presence of subclinical disease progression.

In 1991 Smith et al. first showed the ability to detect circulating tumour cells in the blood from patients with metastatic melanoma using RT-PCR for detection of tyrosinase mRNA.[84] Since then numerous studies have been published showing a wide array of results for detecting circulating tumour cells in patients with advanced stage melanoma (range 0–100%).[63,64,74,85–89] Furthermore, clinical correlations with stage and disease progression are conflicting.[62,87] We believe that

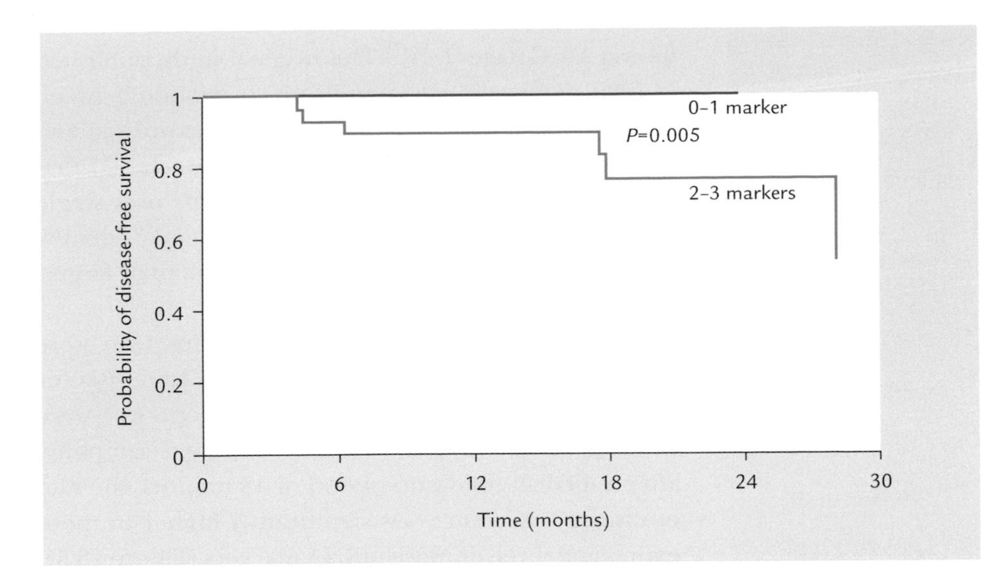

Figure 13.2 *Disease-free survival for RT-PCR marker expression in the sentinel lymph node. Kaplan–Meier curves: 2–3 markers (n = 36); 0–1 marker (n = 36). Reproduced with permission from*[79] *Lippincott Williams & Wilkins ©.*

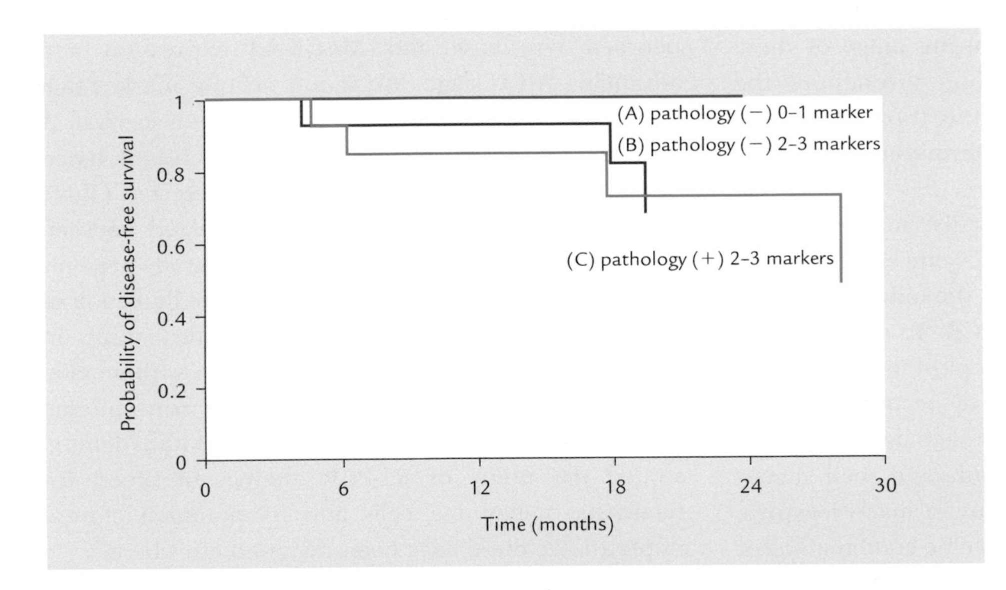

Figure 13.3 *Correlation of sentinel lymph node histopathology and RT-PCR marker expression to disease-free survival. Groups: A, 35 patients; B, 20 patients; C, 16 patients. Group A versus B, P = 0.02; Group C = highest risk of disease relapse (P = 0.01). Reproduced with permission from*[79] *Lippincott Williams & Wilkins ©.*

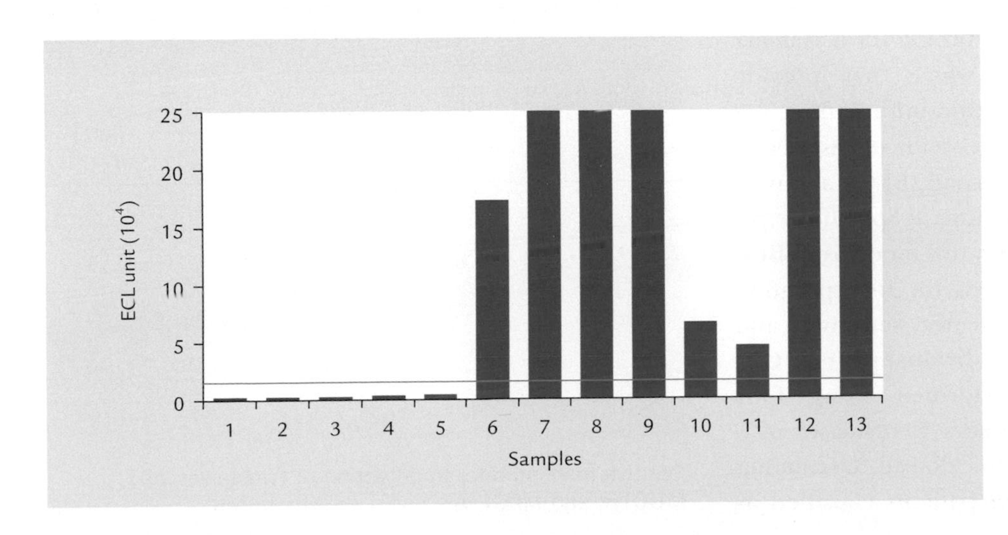

Figure 13.4 *Representative ECL data for RT-PCR study of paraffin embedded tissue. Assessment of melanoma metastasis in tumour-draining lymph nodes; TRP-2 marker assay. Specimens above the ruled line are positive (7350 above controls). Specimens: 1–5, normal lymph nodes; 6–11, micrometastatic lymph nodes; 12–13, melanoma cell lines.*

Table 13.4 *Incidence of distant metastasis as the first site of recurrence in patients with histologically negative sentinel lymph nodes*

Author	Clinical follow up (months)	Patients with distant metastasis/ total patients (%)
Blaheta[77]	19	3/101 (3.0)
Bostick[79]	12	1/55 (1.8)
Gadd[57]	23	2/89 (2.3)
Gershenwald[56]	35	9/243 (3.7)
Shivers[76]	28	3/91 (3.3)
Average	23	3.6/116 (3.1)

using a multimarker approach, PCR sensitivity and specificity can be increased, resolving many of these issues. Additionally, serial sampling throughout the clinical follow up period may identify those patients in whom tumour cells are shed intermittently into the systemic circulation.[88]

This lack of a particular molecular marker, that is 100% tumour specific and tissue specific and expressed under all circumstances, may limit the universal clinical application of single marker RT-PCR. To combat these issues we have proposed the concept of multiple markers for the molecular detection of occult metastasis. Theoretical advantages of this approach include (1) the ability to evaluate multiple tumours and their metastases, which can be heterogeneous in marker expression, (2) the ability to follow a specific combination of tumour markers expressed throughout the disease course, which can vary during tumour progression, (3) the establishment of a molecular profile for a primary tumour and/or its metastasis, which may provide additional prognostic or therapeutic information, (4) improved detection sensitivity for occult metastases in sites highly diluted by normal cells and (5) the ability to anticipate gene transcript regulations at specific organ sites. An additional advantage with this model is its flexibility over single marker methods for incorporating future markers that may increase the sensitivity and specificity of this assay for each individual patient. Our initial investigations were performed using four melanoma associated gene markers (tyrosinase, p97, MUC 18, and MAGE-A3) to detect circulating melanoma cells in the blood of patients classified as having AJCC stages I–IV.[89] This original study, published in 1995, demonstrated a significant correlation between the number of positive RT-PCR markers expressed and advanced AJCC stage (Table 13.5). We concluded that this approach provides improved sensitivity over single marker systems. More importantly, this may identify specific tumour-associated antigens as potential targets for treatment.

We evaluated the prognosis of patients who were clinically disease-free but have an increased risk for developing metastatic disease.[90] In 46 patients who were clinically disease-free at the time of blood sampling, after a median follow up period of 43 months, the rate of disease recurrence was significantly higher in those expressing three or more mRNA markers (Figure 13.5). Of the four markers assessed, tyrosinase, p97, MUC-18, and MAGE-A3, a significant correlation was noted between tyrosinase and MAGE-A3 expression and advancing AJCC stage. We found no one marker that correlated significantly with recurrence or survival. A predictive model for recurrence was established, based on AJCC stage and number of markers detected (Table 13.6), with a significant difference detected between the three risk groups (Figure 13.6). This study presents evidence that multimarker RT-PCR for the detection of minimal residual disease can be of clinical utility in assessing the risk of recurrence in patients without clinical evidence of disease as detected by conventional imaging techniques. Other studies have also demonstrated the utility of RT-PCR analysis of blood for metastatic melanoma cells and its potential clinical implications; these have been reviewed elsewhere.[91]

Table 13.5 *Number of RT-PCR markers correlated to disease stage*[89]

AJCC stage	Number of positive markers					Total patients
	0	1	2	3	4	
I	3	0	1	2	0	6
II	1	6	2	2	0	11
III	5	6	18	7	0	36
IV	3	15	21	20	7	66
Total	12	27	42	31	7	119

Positive markers refer to detection of tyrosinase, p97, MUC18, and MAGE-A3.

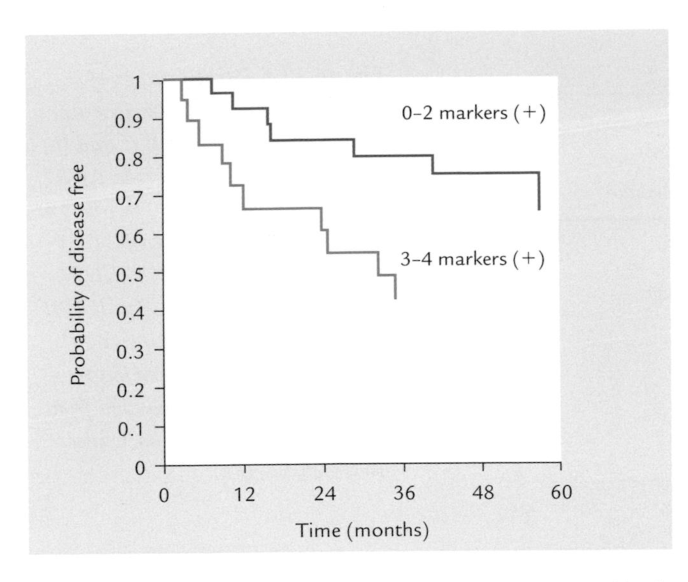

Figure 13.5 *Correlation of number of positive markers in blood to disease recurrence in months (P = 0.024). Reproduced from* Cancer Research,[90] *with permission from American Association for Cancer Research © 2000.*

Bone marrow

Serial RT-PCR assessment of the blood provides an optimal source for routine monitoring of occult tumour progression. This route is the most likely course for the dissemination of early stage micrometastasis, particularly if lymph nodes are negative for tumour cells. Blood is an abundant reservoir, in constant contact with tumours, that can be readily accessed through a minimally invasive procedure. It allows tumour presence and related changes in response to treatment to be monitored. However, blood is a harsh environment for tumour cells to survive, and monitoring potential organ sites for the presence of viable metastases may not only improve yield but also have greater prognostic value.

Recent studies have shown the presence of micrometastases in the bone marrow of patients with an assortment of early stage cancers.[60] In some instances these findings have shown prognostic value.[2,92] Ghossein et al. showed an increased incidence of occult metastasis in the bone marrow, as opposed to blood, of patients with melanoma.[93] In their series of 109 patients, 18 (17%) had bone marrow aspirates positive by RT-PCR for tyrosinase (stage II: 4 of 16 patients (25%), stage III: 11 of 62 patients (18%) and stage IV 3 of 31 patients (10%). In comparison, blood samples from only nine of 73 patients (12%) were positive. There was no correlation between bone marrow or blood RT-PCR positivity and clinical stage of disease, and only positive blood samples from patients with stage II and III disease significantly correlated with a decreased overall survival. These findings show the limited sensitivity associated with single marker RT-PCR for detecting occult tumour cells from various sources.

To evaluate the feasibility and sensitivity of our multimarker approach for assessing the presence of subclinical metastasis, we analyzed rib biopsies obtained from stage IV patients undergoing metastectomy for isolated disease. In 15 of 26 patients (58%) bone marrow biopsies were positive for tyrosinase by RT-PCR. The addition of several markers further improved detection, identifying two additional patients. This

Table 13.6 *Risk factor model for recurrence*[90]

Risk group	Total patients*	Year 1 recurrence	Year 2 recurrence	Year 3 recurrence	Year 4 recurrence
Low	50	0	0	0	0
Medium	25	2	4	6	7
High	16	5	7	9	9
Total	46	7	11	15	16
Log rank test: *P* value		0.081	0.048	0.022	0.034

*Patients were classified as low, medium, or high risk for disease recurrence according to their disease stage and number of positive markers: high risk, if patients had stage III/IV with 3 to 4 positive markers; low risk, if they had stage I/II with 0 to 2 positive markers; and medium risk, if they had stage I/II with 3 to 4 markers and stage III/IV with 0 to 2 markers. For year 1, recurrence occurring after 1 year was considered disease-free, and follow up time longer than 1 year was counted as 1 year. The same approach was applied to all other years' recurrence.

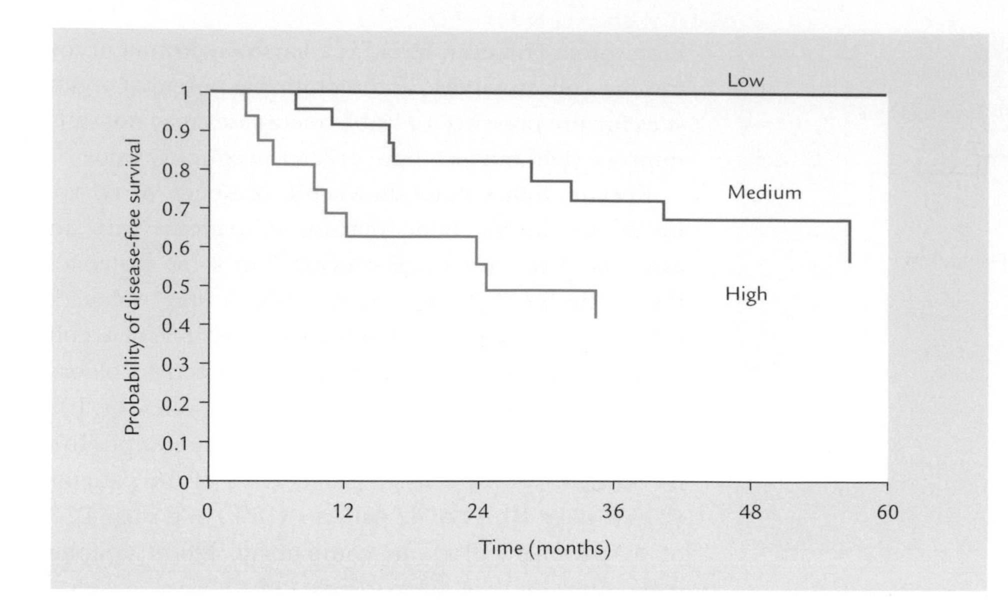

Figure 13.6 *Stratification of disease risk groups for recurrence. Low risk: AJCC Stage I/II and 0–2 (+) markers. Medium risk: AJCC Stage I/II and 3–4 (+) markers or AJCC Stage III/IV and 0–2 (+) markers. High risk: AJCC III/IV and 3–4 (+) markers. Significant differences between groups (*P = *0.037). Reproduced from* Cancer Research,[90] *with permission from American Association for Cancer Research © 2000.*

study shows the feasibility and enhanced sensitivity of performing multimarker RT-PCR and the flexibility afforded by this technique for the incorporation of supplementary markers which may further identify occult tumour cells from various sites and at various stages of disease.

DNA PCR

Advances in tumour genetics have shown that the pathogenesis and progression of tumours follows an accumulation of multiple genetic events. One such alteration involves loss of putative tumour suppressor genes or metastasis suppressor genes. This occurrence can be manifest as loss of heterozygosity (LOH) of DNA microsatellites on specific chromosome arms. LOH has been identified in a variety of tumour types including melanoma. The acquisition of these genetic events seems to be clonal in origin and therefore provides a highly conserved and specific marker to follow subclinical tumour progression. Recently we have shown that DNA microsatellites with tumour specific LOH can be detected in the plasma of patients with melanoma.[94] In our study we evaluated paired tumour biopsies and plasma from 40 patients with melanoma, for LOH at 10 different loci on six different chromosomes. We found LOH in tumour and plasma samples from 34 (85%) and 23 (58%) patients, respectively. In the plasma of 21 of 23 patients (91%), the specific molecular marker demonstrating LOH matched that found in the tumour. A significant correlation was observed between the incidence of LOH microsatellite markers detected in patients' plasma and advanced clinical stage (Table 13.7). We also noted a significant correlation between LOH on microsatellite marker D3S1293 and clinical disease progression. The same finding was noted using the combination of markers: D9S157 and D3S1293; D9S157 and D1S228; and D11S925 and D3S1293. This study shows the concept that tumour specific DNA microsatellite markers can be detected in melanoma patients' plasma with a high degree of accuracy. Advantages of using multimarker assays to assess tumour genetic events include the stability of DNA in comparison to mRNA, a demonstrated clonality of these LOH events in various tumours and their metastases, making this a more ideal marker for recurrence once the LOH profile is established, and the lack of dependence on expression levels for detection. The identification of

Table 13.7 *Correlation of LOH in melanoma patients' plasma to AJCC stage*

AJCC stage	LOH (+)* (%)	LOH (−) (%)	Total number of patients
I	2 (29)	5 (71)	7
II	3 (25)	9 (75)	12
III	16 (53)	14 (47)	30
IV	17 (63)	10 (37)	27

*At least one locus detected has LOH (Reproduced from *Cancer Research* 1999.[94]

these markers in melanoma patients' blood may have significant clinical implications, and serial assessments may provide practical methods of evaluating those genetic events associated with tumour progression and monitoring responses to therapy.

CONCLUSIONS

The role of molecular markers in cancer detection will undoubtedly increase in the future as technical advances continue to occur. Furthermore, as patient and physician awareness of the prognostic importance of early disease detection becomes commonplace, more sensitive methods for detecting micrometastases will be needed. Molecular markers with a high sensitivity and specificity for identifying occult tumour cells offer one such approach. As our understanding of tumour biology improves, molecular techniques that permit the profiling of each patient's tumour will allow for a more improved assessment of an individual's risk and provide a novel method of monitoring subclinical responses to customized therapies.

REFERENCES

1. Raj GV, Moreno JG, Gomella LG, Utilization of polymerase chain reaction technology in the detection of solid tumours. *Cancer* 1998; 82: 1419–42.
2. Braun S, Pantel K, Micrometastatic bone marrow involvement: detection and prognostic significance. *Med Oncol* 1999; 16: 154–65.
3. Pelkey TJ, Frierson HF Jr, Bruns DE, Molecular and immunological detection of circulating tumour cells and micrometastases from solid tumours. *Clin Chem* 1996; 42: 1369–81.
4. Zippelius A, Pantel K, RT-PCR-based detection of occult disseminated tumour cells in peripheral blood and bone marrow of patients with solid tumours. An overview. *Ann NY Acad Sci* 2000; 906: 110–23.
5. Hochhaus A, Weisser A, La Rosee P, et al, Detection and quantification of residual disease in chronic myelogenous leukemia. *Leukemia* 2000; 14: 998–1005.
6. Campana D, Pui C, Detection of minimal residual disease in acute leukemias: methodological advances and clinical significance. *Blood* 1995; 85: 1416–34.
7. Barth A, Wanek LA, Morton DL, Prognostic factors in 1,521 melanoma patients with distant metastases. *J Am Coll Surg* 1995; 181: 193–201.
8. Balch CM, Murad TM, Soong SJ, et al, Tumour thickness as a guide to surgical management of clinical stage I melanoma patients. *Cancer* 1979; 43: 883–8.
9. Balch CM, Soong SJ, Milton GW, et al, A comparison of prognostic factors and surgical results in 1,786 patients with localized (stage I) melanoma treated in Alabama, USA, and New South Wales, Australia. *Ann Surg* 1982; 196: 677–84.
10. Balch CM, Soong SJ, Murad TM, et al, A multifactorial analysis of melanoma. II. Prognostic factors in patients with stage I (localized) melanoma. *Surgery* 1979; 86: 343–51.
11. Balch CM, Soong SJ, Murad TM, et al, A multifactorial analysis of melanoma: III. Prognostic factors in melanoma patients with lymph node metastases (stage II). *Ann Surg* 1981; 193: 377–88.
12. Balch CM, Murad TM, Soong SJ, et al, A multifactorial analysis of melanoma: prognostic histopathological features comparing Clark's and Breslow's staging methods. *Ann Surg* 1978; 188: 732–42.
13. Holmes EC, Moseley HS, Morton DL, et al, A rational approach to the surgical management of melanoma. *Ann Surg* 1977; 186: 481–90.
14. Cohen MH, Ketcham AS, Felix EL, et al, Prognostic factors in patients undergoing lymphadenectomy for malignant melanoma. *Ann Surg* 1977; 186: 635–42.
15. Heller R, Becker J, Wasselle J, et al, Detection of occult lymph node metastases in malignant melanoma. *Ann Plast Surg* 1992; 28: 74–7.
16. Balch CM, The role of elective lymph node dissection in melanoma: rationale, results, and controversies. *J Clin Oncol* 1988; 6: 163–72.
17. Reintgen D, Cruse CW, Wells K, et al, The orderly progression of melanoma nodal metastases. *Ann Surg* 1994; 220: 759–67.
18. Morton DL, Sentinel lymphadenectomy for patients with clinical stage I melanoma. *J Surg Oncol* 1997; 66: 267–9.
19. Sim FH, Taylor WF, Ivins JC, et al, A prospective randomized study of the efficacy of routine elective lymphadenectomy in management of malignant melanoma. Preliminary results. *Cancer* 1978; 41: 948–56.
20. Sim FH, Taylor WF, Pritchard DJ, Soule EH, Lymphadenectomy in the management of stage I malignant melanoma: a prospective randomized study. *Mayo Clin Proc* 1986; 61: 697–705.
21. Veronesi U, Adamus J, Bandiera DC, et al, Delayed regional lymph node dissection in stage I melanoma of the skin of the lower extremities. *Cancer* 1982; 49: 2420–30.
22. Veronesi U, Adamus J, Bandiera DC, et al, Inefficacy of immediate node dissection in stage 1 melanoma of the limbs. *NEJM* 1977; 297: 627–30.
23. Balch C, Surgical management of regional lymph nodes in cutaneous melanoma. *J Am Acad Dermatol* 1980; 3: 511–24.
24. Piepkorn M, Weinstock MA, Barnhill RL, Theoretical and empirical arguments in relation to elective lymph node dissection for melanoma. *Arch Dermatol* 1997; 133: 995–1002.
25. Milton GW, Shaw HM, McCarthy WH, et al, Prophylactic lymph node dissection in clinical stage I cutaneous malignant melanoma: results of surgical treatment in 1319 patients. *Br J Surg* 1982; 69: 108–11.
26. Balch CM, Soong SJ, Bartolucci AA, et al, Efficacy of an elective regional lymph node dissection of 1 to 4 mm thick melanomas for patients 60 years of age and younger. *Ann Surg* 1996; 224: 255–263; discussion 263–6.
27. Kirkwood JM, Strawderman MH, Ernstoff MS, et al, Interferon alfa-2b adjuvant therapy of high-risk resected cutaneous melanoma: the Eastern Cooperative Oncology Group Trial EST 1684. *J Clin Oncol* 1996; 14: 7–17.
28. McMasters KM, Sondak VK, Lotze MT, Ross MI, Recent advances in melanoma staging and therapy. *Ann Surg Oncol* 1999; 6: 467–75.
29. Breslow A, Thickness, cross-sectional areas and depth of invasion in the prognosis of cutaneous melanoma. *Ann Surg* 1970; 172: 902–8.
30. Essner R, The role of lymphoscintigraphy and sentinel node mapping in assessing patient risk in melanoma. *Semin Oncol* 1997; 24(1 Suppl 4): S8–10.
31. Balch CM, Buzaid AC, Atkins MB, et al, A new American Joint Committee on Cancer staging system for cutaneous melanoma. *Cancer* 2000; 88: 1484–91.
32. Prognostic importance of occult axillary lymph node micrometastases from breast cancers. International (Ludwig) Breast Cancer Study Group. *Lancet* 1990; 335: 1565–8.
33. Pickren J, Significance of occult metastasis: a study of breast cancer. *Cancer* 1961, 14: 1266–71.
34. Saphir O, Amromin G, Obscure axillary lymph node metastasis in carcinoma of breast. *Cancer* 1948; 1: 238–41.
35. Reichert CM, Rosenberg SA, Weber BL, Costa J, Malignant melanoma: a search for occult lymph node metastases. *Human Pathol* 1981; 12: 449–51.
36. Cochran AJ, Wen DR, Herschman HR, Gaynor RB, Detection of S-100 protein as an aid to the identification of melanocytic tumours. *Int J Cancer* 1982; 30: 295–97.
37. Gaynor R, Herschman HR, Irie R, et al, S100 protein: a marker for human malignant melanomas? *Lancet* 1981; 1: 869–71.
38. Kindblom LG, Lodding P, Rosengren L, et al, S-100 protein in melanocytic tumours. An immunohistochemical investigation of

benign and malignant melanocytic tumours and metastases of malignant melanoma and a characterization of the antigen in comparison to human brain. *Acta Pathol Microbiol Immunol Scand [A]* 1984; 92: 219–30.

39. Gown AM, Vogel AM, Hoak D, et al, Monoclonal antibodies specific for melanocytic tumours distinguish subpopulations of melanocytes. *Am J Pathol* 1986; 123: 195–203.
40. Cochran AJ, Wen DR, Herschman HR, Occult melanoma in lymph nodes detected by antiserum to S-100 protein. *Int J Cancer* 1984; 34: 159–63.
41. Cochran AJ, Wen DR, Morton DL, Occult tumour cells in the lymph nodes of patients with pathological stage I malignant melanoma. An immunohistological study. *Am J Surg Pathol* 1988; 12: 612–18.
42. Duray PH, Ernstoff MS, Titus-Ernstoff L, Immunohistochemical phenotyping of malignant melanoma. A procedure whose time has come in pathology practice. *Pathol Annu* 1990; 25 Pt 2: 351–77.
43. Walts AE, Said JW, Shintaku IP, Cytodiagnosis of malignant melanoma. Immunoperoxidase staining with HMB-45 antibody as an aid to diagnosis. *Am J Clin Pathol* 1988; 90: 77–80.
44. Yu LL, Flotte TJ, Tanabe KK, et al, Detection of microscopic melanoma metastases in sentinel lymph nodes. *Cancer* 1999; 86: 617–27.
45. Bonetti F, Pea M, Martignoni G, et al, False-positive immunostaining of normal epithelia and carcinomas with ascites fluid preparations of antimelanoma monoclonal antibody HMB45. *Am J Clin Pathol* 1991; 95: 454–9.
46. Morton DL, Wanek L, Nizze JA, et al, Improved long-term survival after lymphadenectomy of melanoma metastatic to regional nodes. Analysis of prognostic factors in 1134 patients from the John Wayne Cancer Clinic. *Ann Surg* 1991; 214: 491–499; discussion 499–501.
47. Callery C, Cochran AJ, Roe DJ, et al, Factors prognostic for survival in patients with malignant melanoma spread to the regional lymph nodes. *Ann Surg* 1982; 196: 69–75.
48. Reintgen D, Balch CM, Kirkwood J, Ross M, Recent advances in the care of the patient with malignant melanoma. *Ann Surg* 1997; 225: 1–14.
49. Morton DL, Wen DR, Wong JH, et al, Technical details of intraoperative lymphatic mapping for early stage melanoma. *Arch Surg* 1992; 127: 392–9.
50. Reintgen D, Albertini J, Berman C, et al, Accurate nodal staging of malignant melanoma. *Cancer Control* 1995; 2: 405–14.
51. Krag DN, Meijer SJ, Weaver DL, et al, Minimal-access surgery for staging of malignant melanoma. *Arch Surg* 1995; 130: 654–658; discussion 659–60.
52. Miliotes G, Albertini J, Berman C, et al, The tumour biology of melanoma nodal metastases. *Am Surg* 1996; 62: 81–8.
53. Messina JL, Glass LF, Pathologic examination of the sentinel lymph node. *J Fla Med Assoc* 1997; 84: 153–6.
54. Reintgen D, Rapaport D, Tanabe KK, Ross M, Lymphatic mapping and sentinel node biopsy in patients with malignant melanoma. *J Fla Med Assoc* 1997; 84: 188–93.
55. Thompson JF, McCarthy WH, Bosch CM, et al, Sentinel lymph node status as an indicator of the presence of metastatic melanoma in regional lymph nodes. *Melanoma Res* 1995; 5: 255–60.
56. Gershenwald JE, Colome MI, Lee JE, et al, Patterns of recurrence following a negative sentinel lymph node biopsy in 243 patients with stage I or II melanoma. *J Clin Oncol* 1998; 16: 2253–60.
57. Gadd MA, Cosimi AB, Yu J, et al, Outcome of patients with melanoma and histologically negative sentinel lymph nodes. *Arch Surg* 1999; 134: 381–7.
58. Li W, Stall A, Shivers SC, Lin J, et al, Clinical relevance of molecular staging for melanoma: comparison of RT-PCR and immunohistochemistry staining in sentinel lymph nodes of patients with melanoma. *Ann Surg* 2000; 231: 795–803.
59. Gibbs JF, Huang PP, Zhang PJ, et al, Accuracy of pathologic techniques for the diagnosis of metastatic melanoma in sentinel lymph nodes. *Ann Surg Oncol* 1999; 6: 699–704.
60. Ghossein R, Bhattacharya S, Rosai J, Molecular detection of micrometastasis and circulating tumour cells in solid tumours. *Clin Cancer Res* 1999; 5: 1950–60.
61. Keilholz U, New prognostic factors in melanoma: mRNA tumour markers. *Eur J Cancer* 1998; 34 Suppl 3: S37–41.
62. Glaser R, Rass K, Seiter S, et al, Detection of circulating melanoma cells by specific amplification of tyrosinase complementary DNA is not a reliable tumour marker in melanoma patients: A clinical two-center study. *J Clin Oncol* 1997; 15: 2818–25.
63. Mellado B, Colomer D, Castel T, et al, Detection of circulating neoplastic cells by reverse-transcriptase polymerase chain reaction in malignant melanoma: Association with clinical stage and prognosis. *J Clin Oncol* 1996; 14: 2091–7.
64. Mellado B, Gutierrez L, Castel T, et al, Prognostic significance of the detection of circulating malignant cells by reverse transcriptase-polymerase chain reaction in long-term clinically disease-free melanoma patients. *Clin Cancer Res* 1999; 5: 1843–8.
65. Lambrechts AC, van't Veer LJ, Rodenhuis S, The detection of minimal numbers of contaminating epithelial tumour cells in blood or bone marrow: use, limitations and future of RNA-based methods. *Ann Oncol* 1998; 9: 1269–76.
66. Kaplan J, Kahn A, Chelly J, Illegitimate transcription: its use in the study of inherited disease. *Hum Mutat* 1992; 1: 357–60.
67. Calogero A, Timmer-Bosscha H, Schraffordt Koops H, et al, Limitations of the nested reverse transcriptase polymerase chain reaction on tyrosinase for the detection of malignant melanoma micrometastases in lymph nodes. *Br J Cancer* 2000; 83: 184–7.
68. Bostick PJ, Chatterjee S, Chi DD, et al, Limitations of specific reverse-transcriptase polymerase chain reaction markers in the detection of metastases in the lymph nodes and blood of breast cancer patients. *J Clin Oncol* 1998; 16: 2632–40.
69. Allain JP. Genomic screening for blood-borne viruses in transfusion settings. *Clin Lab Haematol* 2000; 22: 1–10.
70. Fidler I, Review: biologic heterogeneity of cancer metastasis. *Breast Cancer Res Treatment* 1987; 9: 17–26.
71. Dalerba P, Ricci A, Russo V, et al, High homogeneity of MAGE, BAGE, GAGE, tyrosinase and Melan-A/MART-1 gene expression in clusters of multiple simultaneous metastases of human melanoma: implications for protocol design of therapeutic antigen-specific vaccination strategies. *Int J Cancer* 1998; 77: 200–4.
72. Sarantou T, Chi DD, Garrison DA, et al, Melanoma-associated antigens as messenger RNA detection markers for melanoma. *Cancer Res* 1997; 57: 1371–6.
73. Wang X, Heller R, VanVoorhis N, et al, Detection of submicroscopic lymph node metastases with polymerase chain reaction in patients with malignant melanoma. *Ann Surg* 1994; 220: 768–74.
74. van der Velde-Zimmermann D, Roijers JF, et al, Molecular test for the detection of tumour cells in blood and sentinel nodes of melanoma patients. *Am J Pathol* 1996; 149: 759–64.
75. van der Velde-Zimmermann D, Schipper ME, de Weger RA, et al, Sentinel node biopsies in melanoma patients: a protocol for accurate, efficient, and cost-effective analysis by preselection for immunohistochemistry on the basis of Tyr-PCR. *Ann Surg Oncol* 2000; 7: 51–4.
76. Shivers SC, Wang X, Li W, et al, Molecular staging of malignant melanoma: correlation with clinical outcome. *JAMA* 1998; 280: 1410–5.
77. Blaheta HJ, Ellwanger U, Schittek B, et al, Examination of regional lymph nodes by sentinel node biopsy and molecular analysis provides new staging facilities in primary cutaneous melanoma. *J Invest Dermatol* 2000; 114: 637–42.
78. Blaheta HJ, Schittek B, Breuninger H, et al, Detection of melanoma micrometastasis in sentinel nodes by reverse transcription-polymerase chain reaction correlates with tumour thickness and is predictive of micrometastatic disease in the lymph node basin. *Am J Surg Pathol* 1999; 23: 822–8.
79. Bostick PJ, Morton DL, Turner RR, et al, Prognostic significance of occult metastases detected by sentinel lymphadenectomy and reverse transcriptase-polymerase chain reaction in early-stage melanoma patients. *J Clin Oncol* 1999; 17: 3238–44.
80. Bautista NC, Cohen S, Anders KH, Benign melanocytic naevus cells in axillary lymph nodes. A prospective incidence and immunohistochemical study with literature review. *Am J Clin Pathol* 1994; 102: 102–8.
81. Hara K, Melanocytic lesions in lymph nodes associated with congenital naevus. *Histopathology* 1993; 23: 445–51.
82. Goyodos JS, Ravikumar TS, Germino FJ, et al, Minimally invasive staging of patients with melanoma: sentinel lymphadenectomy and

detention of the melanoma-specific proteins MART-1 and tryosinase by reverse transcriptase polymerase chain reaction. *J Am Coll Surg* 1998; 187: 182–188; discussion 188–90.
83. Orlow S, Hearing H, Sakai C, et al, Changes in expression of putative antigens encoded by pigment genes in mouse melanomas at different stages of malignant progression. *Proc Natl Acad Sci* 1995; 92: 10152–6.
84. Smith B, Selby P, Southgate J, et al, Detection of melanoma cells in peripheral blood by means of reverse transcriptase and polymerase chain reaction. *Lancet* 1991; 338: 1227–9.
85. Farthmann B, Eberle J, Krasagakis K, et al, Reverse transcriptase-polymerase chain reaction for Tyrosinase-mRNA-Postive cells in peripheral blood: Evaluation strategy and correlation with known prognostic markers in 123 melanoma patients. *Invest Dermatol* 1998; 110: 263–7.
86. Foss AJE, Guille MJ, Occleston NL, et al, The detection of melanoma cells in peripheral blood by reverse transcription-polymerase chain reaction. *Br J Cancer* 1995; 72: 155–9.
87. Hanekom GS, Stubbings HM, Johnson CA, Kidson SH, The detection of circulating melanoma cells correlates with tumour thickness and ulceration but is not predictive of metastasis for patients with primary melanoma. *Melanoma Res* 1999; 9: 465–73.
88. Curry BJ, Myers K, Hersey P, Polymerase chain reaction detection of melanoma cells in the circulation: Relation to clinical stage, surgical treatment, and recurrence from melanoma. *J Clin Oncol* 1998; 16: 1760–9.
89. Hoon DS, Wang Y, Dale PS, et al, Detection of occult melanoma cells in blood with a multiple-marker polymerase chain reaction assay. *J Clin Oncol* 1995; 13: 2109–16.
90. Hoon DS, Bostick P, Kuo C, et al, Molecular markers in blood as surrogate prognostic indicators of melanoma recurrence. *Cancer Res* 2000; 60: 2253–7.
91. Taback B, Morton D, O'Day S, Nguyen D-H, Nakayama T, Hoon D. The clinical utility of multimarker RT-PCR in the detection of occult metastasis in patients with melanoma. *Recent Results Cancer Res* 2000; 158: 78–92.
92. Diel I, Kaufmann M, Goerner R, et al, Detection of tumour cells in bone marrow of patients with primary breast cancer: a prognostic factor for distant metastasis. *J Clin Oncol* 1992; 10: 1534–9.
93. Ghossein R, Coit D, Brennan M, et al, Prognostic significance of peripheral blood and bone marrow tyrosinase messenger RNA in malignant melanoma. *Clin Cancer Res* 1998; 4: 419–28.
94. Fujiwara Y, Chi DDJ, Wang H, et al, Plasma DNA microsatellites as tumour-specific markers and indicators of tumour progression in melanoma patients. *Cancer Res* 1999; 59: 1567–71.

14

Staging systems for cutaneous melanoma

Jeffrey E Gershenwald, Merrick I Ross, Antonio C Buzaid

INTRODUCTION

A standardized and uniformly accepted cancer staging system is an essential and fundamental requirement for meaningful comparisons to be made across patient populations. The identification of increasingly powerful prognostic factors has led to sequential modifications of the cutaneous melanoma staging system. Although the current staging system is based on well established prognostic factors, future changes are not only inevitable but also desirable, as more refined prognostic factors are identified that better reflect our understanding of melanoma metastasis.

In order to be useful, a staging system must be simple and practical and must accurately reflect the prognoses of applicable patients. The often capricious biological behaviour of melanoma, however, makes developing a staging system for this disease particularly difficult. This chapter provides a historical perspective, as well as a detailed summary and critical review of the current staging system for cutaneous melanoma. A conceptual framework for proposed changes to the staging system is also presented.

HISTORICAL PERSPECTIVE

Early staging systems

In 1947, Ackerman and Del Regato made one of the earliest attempts to define the clinical stages of cutaneous melanoma.[1] These authors proposed four stages, based on the presence (or absence) of clinically and histologically involved regional nodes and/or distant metastases: group a, distant metastases; group b, clinically detectable and histologically confirmed regional node metastases; group c, clinically negative and histologically positive regional nodes; and group d, clinically and histologically negative regional nodes. These classifications were based on crude death rates, which permitted the authors to identify subsets with the best prognosis (group d) and worst prognosis (group a). In 1949, Sylven described a three stage system in a report on 341 patients with melanoma.[2] Stage I included patients with localized melanoma, including local recurrences or satellite lesions; stage II included patients with regional lymph node (confined to one nodal station only) metastases; and stage III included patients with involvement of two or more nodal groups or distant metastases.

In the early 1960s, the TNM staging system was extended to melanoma after its successful application to breast cancer. Although T definitions (T1 <2 cm, T2 ≥2 and <5 cm, and T3 ≥5 cm), which referred to the maximum diameter of the primary lesion, were soon considered to be inappropriate for melanoma, the unequivocal prognostic differences between patients with localized primary disease and patients with nodal and distant metastases influenced the establishment of a three stage clinicopathological system proposed in 1964 by McNeer and Das Gupta from Memorial Sloan-Kettering Cancer Center (Table 14.1).[3] This system was conceptually quite similar to the three stage system outlined by Sylven 15 years earlier and its simplicity made it very popular among melanoma clinicians.[2]

In the late 1970s, a four stage system was developed at the University of Texas M D Anderson Cancer Center specifically to address the subset of patients with local, in-transit, or satellite recurrences who might be suitable for isolated limb perfusion (Table 14.2).[4] Stage I included patients with primary melanoma only; stage II included patients with local recurrence; stage III included patients with regional disease; and stage IV included patients with distant disease. Like the three stage system popularized by McNeer and Das Gupta, however, this staging system was primarily clinical and failed to microstage patients with primary melanomas.

Development of microstaging

Allen and Spitz provided one of the earliest appraisals of potential prognostic factors, including tumour thickness, when they published their classic paper on the diagnosis and prognosis of melanoma in 1953.[5] Other potential prognostic factors identified in their landmark report included the depth and diameter of the tumour, its anatomical location, the presence of ulceration, the number of mitotic figures, the degree of pleomorphism, and the age and sex of the patient.[5] After validation of this concept in 1955 by Lund and Inhen, Petersen et al. described the first classification system based on microscopic examination of the primary lesion – the progenitor of microstaging.[6,7] The authors proposed 3 groups:

Table 14.1 *The McNeer and Das Gupta three stage system*[3]

Stage	Criteria
I	Localized melanoma without metastases to distant or regional lymph nodes A Primary melanoma untreated or removed by excisional biopsy within 1 month B Locally metastatic and/or recurrent melanoma C Multiple primary melanomas
II	Metastases confined to regional lymph nodes A Primary melanoma present with simultaneous metastases B Primary melanoma controlled with subsequent metastases C Locally recurrent melanoma with metastases D Unknown primary with metastases
III	Disseminated melanoma A Organic and/or multiple lymphatic metastases and/or B Multiple cutaneous and/or subcutaneous metastases

Table 14.2 *Four stage M D Anderson staging system*[4]

Stage	Criteria
I	Localized primary melanoma only
II	Local recurrence or satellites (defined as within 3 cm from the primary lesion)
III	Regional disease A In-transit metastasis B Nodal metastasis C In-transit plus nodal metastasis
IV	Distant metastasis A Cutaneous only B Any visceral site

group I, no invasion of the dermis (carcinoma in situ); group II, invasion of the superficial dermis but without 'tumour' formation; and group III, 'tumour formation' with or without a 'pigmented flare'. The 5-year survival rates for these groups were: group I, 100.0%; group II, 82.3%; group III with a pigmented flare, 51.3%; and group III without a pigmented flare 32.3%.

In 1965, Mehnert and Heard confirmed the concept introduced by Peterson et al. and Lund and Inhen and proposed a system composed of four prognostic groups based on level of invasion:[8] group 0, in situ or preinvasive (100.0% 5-year survival rate); group I, invasion of the papillary dermis (77.6% 5-year survival rate); group II, invasion of the reticular dermis superficial to the base of the deepest sweat gland (38.6% 5-year survival rate); and group III, invasion of the subcutaneous fat (8.0% 5-year survival rate). In 1969, Clark et al. refined the microscopic staging of primary melanomas by classifying malignant melanoma into five categories stratified by level of invasion (analogous to the present day Clark level of invasion).[9] In contrast to the earlier studies, however, melanomas were stratified within the papillary dermis, which identified a subpopulation of patients who not only had a relatively poor outcome but also had tumours that filled the papillary dermis while sparing the reticular dermis. The authors also described three distinct histological forms of melanoma – superficial spreading, nodular, and lentigo maligna melanoma – each with associated prognostic significance. In 1970, McGovern corroborated the prognostic importance of these different histological patterns.[10]

In 1970, Breslow approached microstaging using an entirely different approach.[11] In an attempt to more accurately stage patients with primary melanoma and to explain why lesions that appeared very small had recurred or metastasized, he hypothesized that tumour volume might correlate better with prognosis than superficial tumour diameter. Recognizing that accurate determinations of tumour volume could not easily be made solely from histological analysis, he suggested that by measuring the maximal thickness of the lesions we can calculate the maximal cross-sectional area, which should be roughly proportional to the volume of the tumour. In his landmark paper, Breslow clearly showed the significance of the maximum thickness of primary melanomas as a prognostic criterion. In 1978, Breslow et al. and Balch et al. independently compared Breslow depth and Clark level and showed that Breslow depth was a more powerful and reproducible prognostic factor.[12,13] Strikingly, tumour thickness remains the most important primary tumour prognostic factor three decades following the original report.

American Joint Committee on Cancer staging system

The American Joint Committee on Cancer (AJCC) staging system, published in 1977 and 1978, represented the first formal integration of microstaging into the staging criteria for cutaneous melanoma.[14,15] Although a three stage system was described in 1977, four stages were described the following year. Stage I included patients with primary lesions and was further divided into two subgroups: IA, tumour invading the papillary dermis but not the reticular dermis (levels II and III) and ≤1.5 mm thick; and IB, tumour invading the reticular dermis or subcutaneous tissues (levels IV and V) and >1.5 mm thick. Stage II included patients with regional nodal spread (first station nodes only and not massive or fixed), satellites within 2 cm of the primary lesion, or in-transit metastases. Stage III included patients with massive or fixed metastatic regional lymph nodes or contralateral, bilateral, primary, or secondary echelon nodal involvement. Stage IV included patients with distant metastases. This staging system was poorly accepted, however, partly because of the excessively simplistic division between stage I and stage II disease and the ambiguous distinction between some stage II and stage III melanomas.

In 1983, the melanoma subcommittee of the AJCC again recommended a four stage system that incorporated histological microstaging of primary melanomas.[16] This new system established more meaningful cutoff values for tumour thickness, transferred in-transit disease to stages III and IV, and restratified patients with 'limited' or 'advanced' nodal disease into stage III and stage IV, respectively (Table 14.3). Two additional quantitative measures were further included to distinguish between stage III and stage IV disease: size of the nodal mass and number of in-transit metastases. Although more comprehensive than the 1978 system, this staging system was also quite complex and did not significantly shift support from the more popular three stage system.

In an attempt to develop a more universally accepted staging system for melanoma, the Union Internationale Contre le Cancer (UICC) and the AJCC collaborated to

Table 14.3 *The 1983 American Joint Committee on Cancer staging system*[16]

Stage	Criteria
IA	Localized melanoma $\leq$0.75 mm thick or Clark level II (invasion of papillary dermis) (T1, N0, M0)
IB	Localized melanoma $>$0.75 to 1.50 mm thick or Clark level III (invasion of papillary recticular dermal interface) (T2, N0, M0)
IIA	Localized melanoma $>$1.5 to 4.00 mm thick or Clark level IV (invasion of reticular dermis) (T3, N0, M0)
IIB	Localized melanoma $>$4.00 mm thick, Clark level V (invasion of subcutaneous tissue), or satellite(s) within 2 cm of any primary melanoma (T4, N0, M0)
III	Limited nodal metastases involving only one regional lymph node basin, movable nodes that are $\leq$5 cm in diameter, or negative regional nodes and $<$5 in-transit metastases more than 2 cm from the primary site (any T, N1, M0)
IV	Advanced regional metastases defined as involvement of more than one regional lymph node station, regional nodes $>$5 cm in diameter or fixed, $\geq$5 in-transit metastases or any in-transit metastases more than 2 cm from the primary site with regional node involvement (any T, N2, M0), or any distant metastases (any T, any N, M1 or M2)

generate the 1988 UICC/AJCC staging system. This system used the same tumour thickness cutoff values adopted in the 1983 AJCC staging system but added the following qualifying statement:[17] 'When there is discordance between thickness and level, the measured tumour thickness shall take precedence and be used for pT staging.'* This recommendation was added to reflect the growing body of literature showing that thickness was usually a more powerful and reproducible variable than level of invasion. The nodal size cutoff value was also changed from 5 cm to 3 cm, although no justification for this modification was provided.

In 1992, the AJCC modified the 1988 staging system by stating, 'In case of discrepancy between tumour thickness and level, the pT category is based on the less favourable finding'.[18] No specific justification for this alteration was provided. No other significant changes were adopted.

The 1997 edition of the AJCC Cancer Staging Manual, currently in use throughout the world, did not significantly alter the overall staging system for melanoma described in 1992.[19] As in previous editions, the authors stated that in cases of discrepancy between tumour thickness and level, the pT category should be based on the less favourable finding. One noticeable exclusion from the 1997 edition, however, was the detailed description of specific regional nodal drainage patterns for unilateral tumours and for tumours in 'boundary zones'. Table 14.4 describes the TNM definitions and stage groupings of the 1997 AJCC staging system for cutaneous melanoma. A detailed summary of the salient elements of this version of the staging system follows in the next section.

* Note: The 1988 classification staging system as published by the AJCC/UICC incorrectly omitted this important footnote from the pT classifications.

CLASSIFICATION GUIDELINES: THE 1997 AJCC MANUAL FOR STAGING OF CANCER

Primary lesion

The classification of the primary lesion is based on microscopic assessment of Breslow tumour thickness and Clark level of invasion. Breslow microstaging determines the thickness of the lesion, measured in millimetres, using an ocular micrometer to measure the total vertical height of the melanoma from the granular layer to the area of deepest penetration.[11] Clark microstaging defines levels of invasion according to depth of penetration into the dermis.[9] Evaluation of the entire tumour is always advised to find the thickest and deepest part of the lesion. Measurement techniques have been reviewed elsewhere.[20,21] Table 14.4 describes the TNM definitions and stage groupings of the 1997 AJCC staging system for cutaneous melanoma. In cases of discrepancy

Table 14.4 *The 1997 American Joint Committee on Cancer staging system for cutaneous melanoma*[19]

Primary tumour classifications (pT)†	
pTX	Primary tumour cannot be assessed
pTO	No evidence of primary tumour
pTis	Melanoma in situ (atypical melanocytic hyperplasia, severe melanocytic dysplasia), not an invasive lesion (Clark level I)
pT1	Tumour 0.75 mm or less in thickness and invades the papillary dermis (Clark level II)
pT2	Tumour more than 0.75 mm but not more than 1.5 mm in thickness and/or invades to the papillary reticular-dermal interface (Clark level III)
pT3	Tumour more than 1.5 mm but not more than 4 mm in thickness and/or invades the reticular dermis (Clark level IV) pT3a Tumour more than 1.5 mm but not more than 3 mm in thickness pT3b Tumour more than 3 mm but not more than 4 mm in thickness
pT4	Tumour more than 4 mm in thickness and/or invades the subcutaneous tissue (Clark level V) and/or satellite(s) within 2 cm of the primary tumour pT4a Tumour more than 4 mm in thickness and/or invades the subcutaneous tissue pT4b Satellite(s) within 2 cm of primary tumour
Lymph node involvement (N)	
NX	Regional lymph nodes cannot be assessed
NO	No regional lymph node metastasis
N1	Metastases no larger than 3 cm in greatest dimension in any regional lymph node(s)
N2	Metastases more than 3 cm in greatest dimension in any regional lymph node(s) and/or in-transit metastases N2a Metastases more than 3 cm in greatest dimension in any regional lymph node(s) N2b In-transit metastases N2c Both (N2a and N2b)
Distant metastases (M)	
MX	Presence of distant metastases cannot be assessed
MO	No distant metastases
M1	Distant metastases M1a Metastases in skin or subcutaneous tissue or lymph node(s) beyond the regional lymph nodes M1b Visceral metastases

Stage groupings			
Stage I	pT1 pT2	NO NO	MO MO
Stage II	pT3 pT4#	NO NO	MO MO
Stage III	Any pT Any pT	N1 N2	MO MO
Stage IV	Any pT	Any N	M1

† In case of discrepancy between tumour thickness and level, the pT category is based on the less favourable finding.
# The reader should note that the melanoma stage chart in the 1997 AJCC cancer staging manual identifies a pT4NOMO lesion as stage III. In clinical practice, however, many practitioners categorize such lesions as stage II.

between tumour thickness and Clark level, the pT category is based on the less favourable finding. Shave biopsies of suspected melanomas are never indicated.

Satellite lesions—skin or subcutaneous lesions operationally defined as being within 2 cm of the primary tumour—are currently considered extensions of the primary mass and are categorized as pT4b. On occasion, melanomas yield intraepidermal metastases that cannot be distinguished from multiple new primary tumours by the pathologist. The medical histories of affected patients can sometimes help identify intraepidermal metastases because patients often seem to develop multiple primaries in a very short period of time.[22]

Nodal and in-transit metastases

Regional lymph nodes are the most common site of metastatic involvement in patients with melanoma. What constitutes a regional nodal basin clearly depends on the location of the primary tumour. The AJCC has subsequently simplified its approach and currently states that the specific lymph node chains involved by disease depends on the location of the primary lesion, as tumours are passively borne along with the 'draining' lymphatic fluid, usually (emphasis added by author) to the geographically closest nodes. It is now well understood that the closest draining lymph node chains are not always the 'regional' lymph nodes for a given primary melanoma. This is particularly important in the evaluation of melanomas arising on the trunk or head and neck regions, especially when there is no clinical evidence of nodal disease. In these patients, preoperative lymphoscintigraphy is routinely used to determine which nodal basins are at greatest risk for harbouring occult metastatic disease.[23] (See Chapter 30).

In-transit metastases are defined as skin or subcutaneous metastases more than 2 cm from the primary lesion but not beyond the regional nodal basin; they are coded N2b.

Distant metastases

Unfortunately, melanoma has the potential to metastasize to any organ. Distant melanoma metastases commonly involve skin, subcutaneous tissues, lymph nodes, liver, bone, lungs, brain, and visceral organs. Metastases to the skin, subcutaneous tissue, or lymph nodes beyond the regional nodal basins are categorized as M1a. According to the current staging system, iliac lymph nodes are considered to be distant metastases and are also classified as M1a. Despite therapeutic lymphadenectomy, at least four series reported a 5-year survival rate of less than 10% in patients with pathologically involved iliac lymph nodes.[24–27] However, reports by Karakousis et al., as well as recent reports by Strobbe et al. and Mann and Coit, have documented 24% to 35% 5-year survival rates in these patients and support the need to re-evaluate the prognostic significance of iliac nodal metastatic disease.[28–32] Metastases to other distant sites – often referred to as visceral metastases – are categorized as M1b.

CRITICAL ANALYSIS OF THE 1997 AJCC STAGING SYSTEM

Background

Data from several studies support the proposal that the 1997 AJCC staging system for melanoma should be modified to better conform to recent observations. Among the more controversial areas are:

(a) the prognostic relevance of level of invasion compared with tumour thickness;
(b) the optimal cutoff values for tumour thickness;
(c) the importance of ulceration;
(d) whether satellites should be grouped with in-transit metastases;
(e) whether microsatellites and local recurrences should be included as a separate staging criterion;
(f) whether the number of positive nodes should replace the size of the nodal mass in the current staging system;
(g) the significance of finding nodal metastases in more than one nodal basin; and
(h) the prognostic significance of distant metastases.

A discussion of these controversial areas follows.

Tumour thickness versus level of invasion and optimal cutoff points for tumour thickness

Since the reports by Clark et al. in 1969 and Breslow in 1970, several large series have compared the prognostic value of tumour thickness and level of invasion using modern multivariate statistical analysis techniques.[9,11] Vollmer evaluated a multitude of such analyses using data from 48 papers published before his report in 1989.[33] The vast majority of these studies clearly showed that tumour thickness was a more powerful prognostic factor than level of invasion.

In accordance with this finding, the 1988 AJCC staging system stated that in cases of prognostic discrepancy between tumour thickness and level of invasion, tumour thickness would have precedence. In 1992, however, the AJCC staging system was modified, stating that in case of discrepancy between the two factors, the pT category should be based on the less favourable finding. The decision to implement this modification was probably influenced by the John Wayne Cancer Center series reported by Morton et al. in 1993.[34] In this series, the prognostic values of level of invasion and tumour thickness were examined in 3323 patients. Both level of invasion and tumour thickness were highly statistically significant, indicating that level of invasion provided additional prognostic significance beyond tumour thickness alone. The level of invasion retained its high prognostic value when the same authors analyzed it within two thickness groups ($<$1.5 mm and $\geq$1.5 mm).

Büttner et al. examined the prognostic value of tumour thickness and level of invasion combined in a series of 5093 patients with primary cutaneous melanoma followed between 1970 and 1988 at four university centres in Germany.[35] By multivariate analysis, the combination of tumour thickness and level of invasion was found to be prognostically less significant than tumour thickness alone and did not corroborate the John Wayne Cancer Center experience – level of invasion was statistically significant only for tumour thicknesses $\leq$1 mm. The authors also investigated the relation between tumour thickness and survival probability. The relative risk of death due to melanoma as a function of tumour thickness was nearly linear up to a tumour thickness of 6 mm, and stratification of tumour thickness with cutoff values of 1 mm, 2 mm, and 4 mm resulted in the best fit for these data. They therefore suggested that these cutoff values replace the current tumour thickness cutoff values of 0.75 mm, 1.50 mm, and 4.00 mm since the proposed strata were slightly superior in establishing prognostically distinct groups and were simpler to use.

Buzaid et al. performed an exhaustive evaluation of the published data and a reanalysis of data from the University of Alabama and Sydney Melanoma Unit databases on 4568 prospectively followed patients with primary melanoma.[36] In examining the impact of level of invasion and ulceration on the prognostic value of tumour thickness, they concluded that tumour thickness and ulceration (an additional primary tumour factor noted in AJCC guidelines as 'probably important', but not specifically included in the staging system) were the most powerful prognostic indicators in patients with stage I and stage II disease. In contrast, level of invasion provided statistically significant information only in the subgroup of patients whose tumours were $\leq$1 mm thick, but the absolute 10-year survival differences were small and inconsistent. Furthermore, the best statistical fits for tumour thickness cutoff values were identical to those proposed by Büttner. Accordingly, the authors also recommended that the staging system be modified to incorporate these new tumour thickness groupings *and* that level of invasion be eliminated from the staging system.

In summary, although the controversy regarding tumour thickness and level of invasion continues, recent large series suggest that simpler cutoff values of tumour thickness (1 mm, 2 mm, and 4 mm) provide better prognostic information than the breakpoints currently used. Validation of these findings in studies of other large databases is clearly warranted.

Importance of ulceration

Ulceration is defined as a microscopic interruption of the surface epithelium involved by tumour (Figure 14.1).[13] Vollmer identified ulceration as a significant prognostic factor in seven of 11 studies reviewed by multivariate analysis.[33] More recently, Balch conducted a meta-analysis that included 15,798 patients with localized melanoma.[37] Tumour thickness and ulceration were the dominant pathological factors – the same two factors shown to be the strongest predictors of outcome in virtually all other multivariate analyses using Cox regression. The presence of ulceration, therefore, indicated a strikingly more aggressive type of melanoma, even after accounting for other prognostic features, including tumour thickness. In several centres, tumour ulceration was the single most important feature predicting outcome.[37]

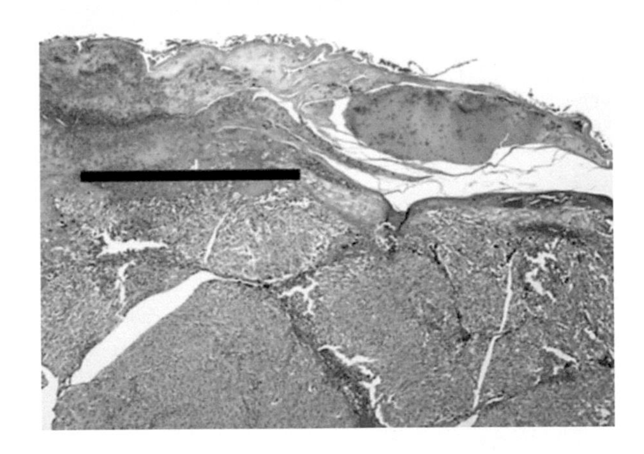

Figure 14.1 *Low power histological image of the cutaneous malignant melanoma. Note the thick pink crust overlying an area lacking epidermis (bar). (Figure courtesy of Victor G Prieto MD, PhD).*

Despite the abundance of data indicating the importance of tumour ulceration as an independent prognostic factor, ulceration is not included in the 1997 AJCC staging system, although the AJCC recommends that it be recorded. Buzaid et al. analyzed the influence of ulceration in four separate tumour thickness groupings (≤1 mm, 1 to 2 mm, 2 to 4 mm, and >4 mm) and demonstrated that the presence of ulceration has a significant adverse effect on survival.[36] The most significant impact was on very thin and very thick lesions. More recently, ulceration has been identified as an important prognostic factor in clinically node negative patients with primary melanoma pathologically staged using the technique of lymphatic mapping and sentinel lymphadenectomy (see Chapter 27).[38,39] On the basis of these and other data, it has been proposed that melanomas with ulceration would be staged higher than melanomas of equivalent thickness without ulceration.

Satellite metastases versus in-transit metastases

In the 1997 staging system, stage II includes both high risk primary tumours (>4 mm) and tumours with satellite nodules (pT4b) – skin involvement within 2 cm of the primary tumour. The system suggests, therefore, that the presence of satellite nodules and high risk primary tumours affect prognosis equally. However, several studies suggest that the presence of satellitosis portends a worse prognosis than that of thick primary tumours and much more similar to the prognosis for patients with in-transit and/or nodal metastases (stage III).[40–44] Moreover, the current definition of satellite metastases is arbitrary and without oncological basis. This contention is well illustrated by Singletary et al. in an analysis of the The University of Texas M D Anderson Cancer Center experience.[45] In a multifactorial analysis of 135 patients with regional cutaneous metastases the authors showed that classifying such lesions as satellite or in-transit metastases on the basis of their distance from the primary tumour had no prognostic significance. Since both satellite and in-transit metastases probably arise secondary to lymphatic dissemination, this observation is not surprising.

Recently, Buzaid et al. employed a graphic overlay technique to compare Kaplan-Meier survival curves of various series from which similar analyses of patients with satellite metastases alone, satellite metastases plus in-transit metastases, and in-transit metastases alone were reported.[36] The survival rates of patients with satellite metastases were similar to those of patients with in-transit or nodal metastases (Figure 14.2). The authors concluded that the melanomas with satellite metastases should, therefore, be classified as stage III and not stage II disease.

Review of the literature also reveals that 10-year survival rates of patients having in-transit and satellite metastases but pathologically negative lymph nodes ranges from 41% to 56%, whereas the survival rates of patients with in-transit and satellite metastases and pathologically positive lymph nodes ranges from 28% to 35%. These data suggest that in patients with satellite and in-transit metastases the pathological status of regional nodes should be included in the staging evaluation.

Microsatellites versus macrosatellites

Another issue that is not specifically addressed in the 1997 staging system pertains to microsatellites. The term 'satellite(s)' as used in the 1997 staging system refers to clinically apparent disease, namely, macrosatellites. Microsatellites, as the name suggests, are defined as discrete nests of melanoma cells that are non-contiguous and clearly separated from the main body of the tumour by normal reticular dermal collagen or subcutaneous fat and are detected histologically.[46] The prognostic significance of microsatellites was

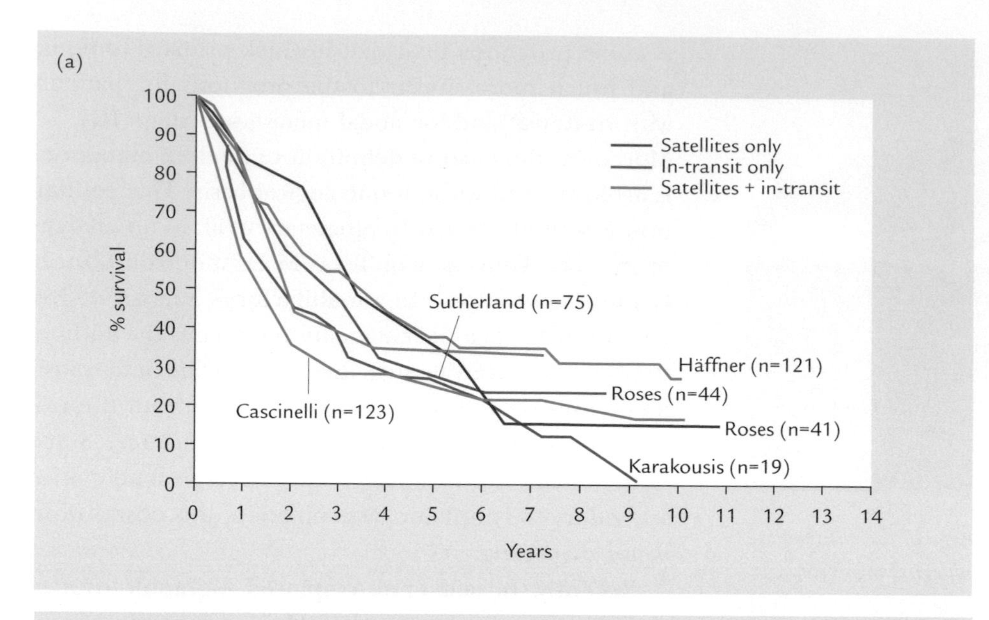

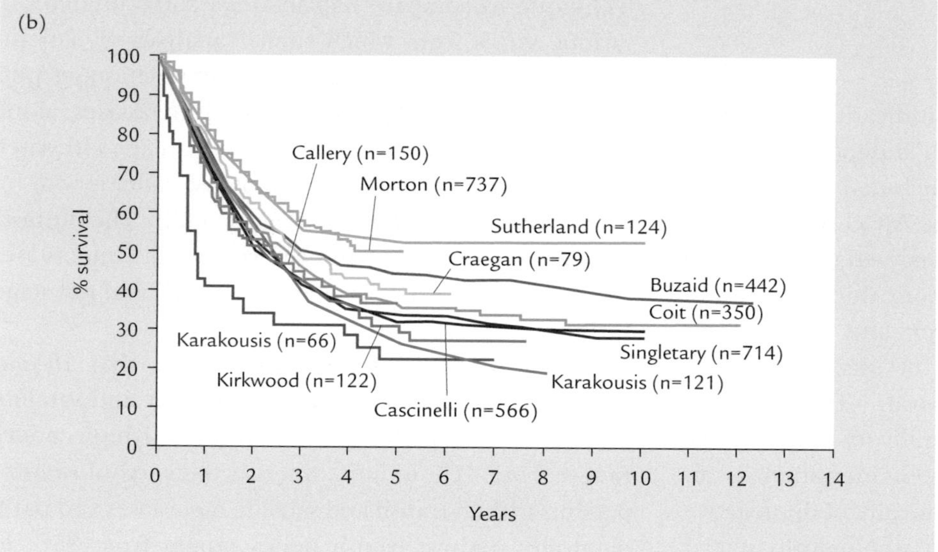

Figure 14.2 *Kaplan-Meier survival curves from (a) various series of patients with satellite, in-transit, or satellite plus in-transit metastases compared with (b) patients with nodal metastases.*[36]

initially reported by Day et al. in 1981.[47] They noted that the 5-year, disease-free survival rate was 36% for patients with microsatellites compared with 89% for patients without microsatellites. A multivariate logistic regression analysis of patients with primary melanoma who underwent elective regional nodal dissection demonstrated that in addition to tumour thickness, the presence of microsatellites was highly associated with occult regional node metastases.[48] More recently, León et al. confirmed the unfavourable prognostic significance of microsatellites in patients with primary melanoma.[46] Compared with matched controls, patients with microsatellites had a significantly decreased 10-year disease-free survival rate (27% versus 60%) and a significantly decreased 10-year overall survival (37% versus 65%). Thus, the prognosis for patients with microsatellites is similar to that for patients with macrosatellites, suggesting that the presence of microsatellites also warrants a stage III classification.

Satellite metastases versus local recurrence

Local recurrence implies the regrowth of neoplastic tissue after an incomplete excision. Most patients with melanoma who develop local recurrences, however, have previously undergone wide local excisions with extensive negative margins. Thus, in these patients, what is normally labelled as local recurrence does not represent true regrowth of the primary tumour but, more likely, growth of tumour that had already spread to surrounding lymphatic channels, namely, a satellite nodule. This contention is strongly supported by the similar outcomes of patients with 'local recurrence' and those with satellite, in-transit, and/or nodal metastases and indicates that these three entities are likely manifestations of the same disease process, namely, lymphatic dissemination (5-year survival rates range from 20% to 40%) (Figure 14.3).[40–45,49–60]

It may be argued that local recurrence should not be included in any staging system because it is not part of the natural progression of the disease; what is usually termed local recurrence is more correctly a form of satellite or in-transit metastasis, since the pathophysiology and prognosis of these entities are comparable. In contrast, the distinction between local recurrence and satellite or in-transit metastases is artificial. However, patients previously misdiagnosed as having a benign naevus after a punch, incisional, or inadequate excisional biopsy who subsequently develop a local recurrence (true regrowth of the tumour) have a significantly better prognosis that is primarily related to the thickness of the recurrence.[61] Thus, these patients' disease should not be classified as stage III.[62]

Prognostic value of lymph node size

The 1983, 1992 and 1997 AJCC staging systems for cutaneous melanoma used nodal size to further stratify patients with regional lymph node metastases. Only five published series have evaluated nodal size as a prognostic factor (Table 14.5).[28,53,63–65] Of these, only a comparatively small series reported by Karakousis et al. showed that size of the nodal mass as determined by physical examination was a significant prognostic factor for survival in patients with axillary nodal metastases.[28] However, size of the nodal mass by physical examination was significant only by univariate analysis, and the cutoffs used for nodal size were different from those used in any of the AJCC staging systems.

The series by Karakousis et al., Coit et al., Bevilacqua et al., and Buzaid et al. were all based on retrospective reviews.[28,53,63,64] To date, only one prospective study, by Drepper et al., has been reported.[65] The authors analyzed the results of the Fachklinik Hornheide study to test the validity of the UICC/AJCC classification for cutaneous melanoma. In this series, however, most patients had primary melanoma without nodal metastases. Of the 103 patients with nodes ≤3 cm by pathological analysis, only 23 patients had palpable nodes; only two patients with nodes >3 cm by both physical examination and pathological analysis had palpable nodes. The authors examined nodal size as a prognostic factor for survival; univariate analysis showed that size was not significant even after stratification according to the cutoff size yielding the greatest apparent separation between the groups.

Several potential prognostic factors have been studied in patients with nodal metastases. The most consistent prognostic factor identified by multivariate analysis is the number of positive nodes.[36] The 10-year survival rates of the reported series according to the number of positive nodes are shown in Table 14.6. The prognostic

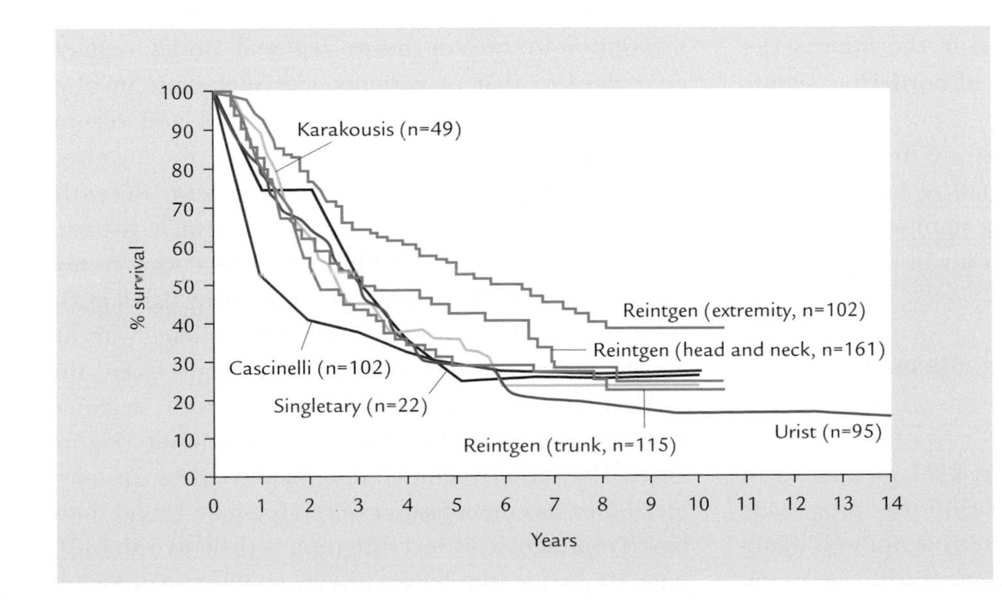

Figure 14.3 *Kaplan-Meier survival curves from various series of patients with local recurrence. Note the similarity of these data compared with data of patients with satellite, in-transit, or nodal metastases shown in Figure 14.2.*[36]

Table 14.5 *Analysis of the prognostic significance of size of the nodal mass*[36]

Study	No. of patients	Size of nodal mass (cm) and method of determination	5-year survival rate (%)	*P* value
Karakousis (1991)[28]	10	<2 (PE)	46	0.0001
	55	2–4 (PE)	22	
	12	>4 (PE)	18	
	9	Large, fixed (PE)	13	
Buzaid (1995)[53]	149	<2 (PE)	51	0.12
	156	2–4 (PE)	47	
	44	>4 (PE)	35	
Bevilacqua (1990)[64]	66	<2 (Path)	37	0.87
	48	2–4 (Path)	42	
	24	>4 (Path)	28	
Buziad (1995)[53]	107	<2 (Path)	50	0.62
	184	2–4 (Path)	44	
	72	>4 (Path)	48	
Coit (1991)[63]	63	<2 (Path)	39	0.15
	44	2–3 (Path)	41	
	25	>3 (Path)	22	
Buzaid (1995)[53]	107	<2 (Path)	50	0.47
	121	2–3 (Path)	44	
	135	>3 (Path)	46	

Path: pathologic analysis; PE: physical examination

significance of the number of positive nodes was evaluated in 20 series. By multivariate analysis, this variable was significant in all but four series.[28,41,54,55,57–59,63–76] In three of these four negative series, the percentage of positive nodes was significant, and in the other series the number of positive nodes was of borderline significance ($P = 0.051$).[57,64,67,70]

In summary, although nodal size was included in the 1997 staging system, only one small series found that size by physical examination was a significant prognostic factor, and this was significant only in the univariate analysis.

Prognostic significance of metastases to more than one lymph node basin

Although many patients are at risk of metastases to more than one lymph node basin, the prognostic significance of this metastatic pattern is not well established. Barth et al. evaluated 21 patients with metastatic melanoma in at least two nodal basins in a review of 175 patients with melanoma who underwent lymphadenectomy at the National Cancer Institute.[77] They concluded that the prognosis of melanoma patients with metastases to two or more regional nodes seemed equivalent to that of patients with metastatic involvement of only one regional nodal basin, and recommended regional lymphadenectomy of the involved lymph node groups with a curative intent. Recently, Dale et al. evaluated factors affecting survival in patients undergoing regional lymph node dissection in two separate basins.[78] In contrast to the study by Barth et al., they determined that compared with patients with an equal tumour burden confined to a single basin, the survival rate of melanoma patients with regional metastases in two lymph node basins is lower (Figure 14.4). They also concluded that patients whose primary melanoma has metastasized to two separate lymph node basins represent a distinct subgroup of patients with AJCC stage III disease who have a less favourable prognosis.

Table 14.6 *10-year survival rates of select series according to the number of positive nodes*[36]

<table>
<tr><th rowspan="2">Series</th><th rowspan="2">No. of patients</th><th rowspan="2">Overall survival rate (%)</th><th colspan="5">Survival rate by no. of positive nodes (%)</th></tr>
<tr><th>1</th><th>2</th><th>3</th><th>4</th><th>≥5</th></tr>
<tr><td>Cohen (1977)[66]</td><td>65</td><td>NS</td><td colspan="3">55</td><td colspan="2">26</td></tr>
<tr><td>Karakousis* (1980)[54]</td><td>125</td><td>27</td><td>41</td><td>30</td><td colspan="3">18</td></tr>
<tr><td>Day* (1981)[67]</td><td>46</td><td>42</td><td colspan="3">48</td><td colspan="2">17</td></tr>
<tr><td>Balch* (1981)[68]</td><td>185</td><td>NS</td><td>58</td><td colspan="3">28</td><td>10</td></tr>
<tr><td>Callery* (1982)[58]</td><td>150</td><td>39</td><td colspan="3">45</td><td colspan="2">21</td></tr>
<tr><td>Cascinelli (1984)[57]</td><td>566</td><td>30</td><td>43</td><td>32</td><td colspan="3">26</td></tr>
<tr><td>Roses# (1985)[69]</td><td>157</td><td>NS</td><td>21</td><td colspan="2">40</td><td colspan="2">31</td></tr>
<tr><td>Koh•# (1986)[70]</td><td>66</td><td>49</td><td colspan="3">53</td><td colspan="2">17</td></tr>
<tr><td>Sutherland (1987)[41]</td><td>124</td><td>53</td><td>72</td><td colspan="2">33†</td><td colspan="2">20†</td></tr>
<tr><td>Kissin* (1987)[71]</td><td>133</td><td>NS</td><td>55</td><td>67</td><td>31</td><td colspan="2">2</td></tr>
<tr><td>Slingluff (1988)[72]</td><td>1273</td><td>NS</td><td>38</td><td colspan="3">31</td><td>18</td></tr>
<tr><td>Calabro (1989)[73]</td><td>1001</td><td>28</td><td>43</td><td colspan="3">32</td><td>18</td></tr>
<tr><td>Bevilacqua (1990)[64]</td><td>176</td><td>NS</td><td>43</td><td colspan="2">37</td><td colspan="2">9</td></tr>
<tr><td>Karakousis* (1990)[55]</td><td>66</td><td>NS</td><td>62</td><td>51</td><td>28</td><td colspan="2">5</td></tr>
<tr><td>Karakousis* (1991)[28]</td><td>105</td><td>NS</td><td>46</td><td colspan="2">32</td><td colspan="2">10</td></tr>
<tr><td>Coit (1991)[63]</td><td>449</td><td>32</td><td>40</td><td colspan="2">40</td><td colspan="2">19</td></tr>
<tr><td>Balch (1992)[74]</td><td>234</td><td>NS</td><td>40</td><td colspan="3">28</td><td>18</td></tr>
<tr><td>Singletary (1992)[75]</td><td>264</td><td>NS</td><td>45</td><td colspan="4">31</td></tr>
<tr><td>Drepper* (1993)[65]</td><td>112</td><td>39</td><td>47</td><td colspan="3">31</td><td>20</td></tr>
<tr><td>Buzaid (1995)[53]</td><td>442</td><td>42</td><td>55</td><td colspan="3">34</td><td>25</td></tr>
</table>

†4-year survival.
*5-year survival.
•7-year survival.
#Only patients with elective node dissection.

Prognostic significance of distant metastasis

Metastases to soft tissue (skin, subcutaneous tissue, or lymph nodes) beyond the regional nodal basins are categorized as M1a, while metastases to other distant sites are categorized as M1b disease. Although patients with iliac nodal metastases are usually managed as if they had regional disease, they usually fare poorly and are therefore currently classified as having M1a disease by the AJCC. This simplistic separation, however, has been questioned recently by investigators who incorporated other parameters into their analyses. For example, Sirott et al. showed that the concentration of lactate dehydrogenase (LDH) was the most powerful prognostic factor in patients with stage IV melanoma.[79] Barth et al. analyzed 1521 patients with stage IV disease

– the largest such series in the literature – and showed that three independent variables predicted survival: initial site of metastases, disease-free interval before distant metastases, and stage of disease before distant metastases were detected. However, LDH concentration was not included in their analysis, so they were unable to corroborate the Sirott findings. In an attempt to reconcile these data, Eton et al. recently reviewed the prognostic significance of site of distant disease, number of disease sites, and LDH concentration in patients with advanced cutaneous melanoma enrolled in clinical trials between 1979 and 1989 at M D Anderson Cancer Center.[81] The authors showed that in univariate and multivariate analyses involving 318 patients with stage IV disease, normal serum concentrations of LDH and albumin, soft tissue and/or single visceral organ metastases (especially lung), and female sex were independent positive predictors for survival. Conversely, the 1997 AJCC criteria did not accurately predict outcome in the multivariate analyses. Additional support for this concept is provided in recently published investigations by Deichmann et al., Franzke et al., and Lagerwaard et al. who independently showed that elevated concentrations of LDH correlated best with disease progression or survival in cohorts of patients with AJCC stage IV melanoma.[82–84]

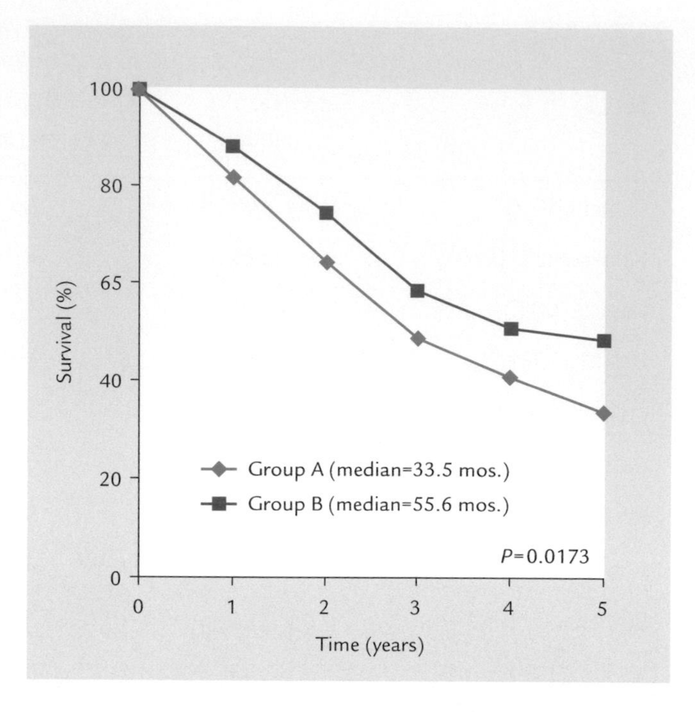

Figure 14.4 *5-year survival in melanoma patients with at least two positive lymph nodes after regional lymphadenectomy stratified by the number of basins containing at least one pathologically positive node. Group A, two pathologically positive basins; group B, one pathologically positive basin.*[78]

PROPOSED CHANGES TO THE AJCC MELANOMA STAGING SYSTEM*

Although the 1997 AJCC staging system was based on well established prognostic factors, several recent reports have identified other prognostic factors not included in the 1997 system, and other studies support the re-evaluation of some of the currently employed staging criteria. Several of these more controversial areas have been discussed. To incorporate these new observations, the staging system is likely to be modified for the 2002–3 AJCC manual for staging cancer.* The Melanoma Task Force of the AJCC has recently summarized its preliminary interpretations of the multitude of studies that examined the prognosis of patients with cutaneous melanoma.[85] A comprehensive analysis of original patient data obtained from many leading cancer centres and cooperative groups throughout the world has also been initiated in an attempt to ensure that proposed staging changes best reflect these recent observations. A brief overview of the conceptual framework for these proposals (awaiting validation) follows below.

With respect to primary melanoma tumour thickness cutoff values, the AJCC has proposed using the breakpoints 1 mm, 2 mm, and 4 mm, since they represent the simplest and best fit between favourable and unfavourable prognoses. Moreover, level of invasion would be largely eliminated as a prognostic factor from the staging system because, although it is predictive, it was found to be less accurate, reproducible, and quantifiable than thickness and ulceration. In contrast, the AJCC has proposed that ulceration be incorporated into the next staging system on the basis of significant data that support its critical prognostic role in patients with primary melanoma; the presence of ulceration would 'upstage' patients compared with those whose melanomas were of equivalent thickness without ulceration.

*Note: These proposed changes were accepted in principle by the AJCC after this chapter had been submitted and is incorporated in the 6th edition of the AJCC staging system (see Balch CM, Buzaid AC, Soon S-J et al., Final version of the American Joint Committee on Cancer staging system for cutaneous melanoma. *J Clin Oncol* 2001; 19: 3635–48). The changes have also been accepted by the UICC. The 2002 AJCC/UICC staging system is summarized in the Appendix (p.180).

With respect to regional lymph node metastases, the AJCC has proposed that size of the nodal mass (determined by physical examination or pathological analysis) be eliminated from the staging system and replaced by number of positive nodes, a more powerful prognostic factor. Since in-transit and satellite metastases can be considered common manifestations of intralymphatic metastases associated with a poor prognosis, the AJCC has also proposed that patients with satellite and/or in-transit metastases be grouped together as having stage III disease to better reflect their cancers' similar biological behaviour. Partly as a result of the widespread use of sentinel lymphadenectomy to accurately stage the regional nodal basins at risk in patients with clinically node negative primary cutaneous melanoma, the AJCC is also contemplating the inclusion of a data element which would identify whether the nodal disease was clinically detectable or occult, that is, identified only after sentinel lymphadenectomy or elective lymph node dissection.

The AJCC Melanoma Task Force recently summarized its initial interpretation of the multitude of studies that examined the prognosis of patients with stage IV melanoma. In all studies analyzing prognosis using a Cox regression analysis, the site(s) of metastases, the number of metastases, and the serum concentrations of LDH were most predictive. Moreover, in all studies evaluated, patients who had distant metastasis in the skin, subcutaneous tissue, or distant lymph nodes had a better prognosis than patients who had metastases in any other anatomical site. In several major studies, patients with metastasis to the lungs and gastrointestinal tract had an 'intermediate' prognosis, whereas metastasis to skin and subcutaneous tissue resulted in a 'better prognosis' and metastasis to all other visceral sites indicated a 'worst prognosis'. In patients with metastasis to multiple organs, the prognosis was dictated by the organ involvement associated with the 'worst' outcome (for example, a patient with lung and liver metastasis would have the 'worst' prognosis because of the presence of disease in the liver). The AJCC melanoma committee has therefore proposed three subgroups for stage IV melanoma based on an outcomes analysis showing anatomical site of metastasis to be the dominant predictor. Additionally, although it is relatively uncommon to include serum factors in an assessment of tumour stage, in all studies where serum LDH concentrations was included in a multivariate analysis, it was among the most predictive of factors, even after accounting for site and number of metastases. To reflect the prognostic significance of serum LDH concentrations, the AJCC has also proposed that patients with stage IV disease who have a raised concentration of serum LDH be classified in the 'worst prognosis' group regardless of the anatomical site of metastasis.

FUTURE DIRECTIONS

Important recent and ongoing developments in molecular biological techniques have enabled investigators to begin to explore the potential prognostic significance of differential gene expression in patients with melanoma. For example, the tyrosinase gene, whose protein product is the rate limiting enzyme in melanin biosynthesis, has been targeted as one of several genes that may serve as possible melanoma markers. It has recently been used in the molecular biological detection of occult regional lymph node metastases by reverse transcriptase-polymerase chain reaction (RT-PCR) after sentinel lymph node biopsy. For a detailed discussion, please see Chapter 13. This technique, therefore, has the potential to identify 'submicroscopic' disease not detected by histological techniques. Although at least two recent reports have validated the concept of identifying tyrosinase gene expression in patients with clinically node negative cutaneous melanoma undergoing sentinel lymphadenectomy (one using tyrosinase alone and the other as part of a multimarker RT-PCR assay, its current role remains investigational, as further studies are required to evaluate the clinical relevance of histologically negative and RT-PCR positive findings.[86,87]

RT-PCR has also been used to detect circulating melanoma cells. In theory, since the tyrosinase gene is not expressed in normal peripheral blood, it could serve as an indicator of the presence of circulating melanoma cells. The initial report by Smith et al. and early subsequent studies showed promising results, with sensitivity rates approaching 100% for patients with stage IV disease.[88–92] Several subsequent studies, however, failed to reproduce this remarkably high detection rate.[93–98] Sensitivity rates were only as high as 50% in one study and, subsequently, less than 30% in two studies evaluating patients with advanced disease.[93,97,98] At present, the value of tyrosinase messenger RNA (mRNA) detection in the peripheral blood by RT-PCR remains controversial and may be of limited value in the staging of patients with melanoma.

Despite current limitations, it is foreseeable that our expanding understanding of the molecular events involved in melanoma metastasis will provide unprecedented opportunities to stage patients with melanoma more accurately in the future.

REFERENCES

1. Ackerman L, Del Regato J, *Cancer diagnosis, treatment and prognosis*, St. Louis: Mosby, MO, 1947: 169–81.
2. Sylven B, Malignant melanoma of the skin. *Acta Radiol* 1948; 32: 33–60.
3. McNeer G, Das Gupta T. Prognosis in malignant melanoma. *Surgery* 1964; 56: 512–18.
4. Smith J. *Histopathology and biological behavior of melanoma, neoplasms of the skin and malignant melanomas.* Chicago: Year Book Medical Publishers, 1976: 293.
5. Allen A, Spitz S. Malignant melanoma. A clinicopathological analysis of the criteria for diagnosis and prognosis. *Cancer* 1953; 6: 1–45.
6. Lund RH, Inhen M, Malignant melanoma: clinical and pathologic analysis of 93 cases. Is prophylactic lymph node dissection indicated? *Surgery* 1955; 38: 652–9.
7. Petersen N, Bodenham D, Lloyd O, Malignant melanomas of the skin. *Br J Plast Surg* 1962; 15: 49–94.
8. Mehnert J, Heard J, Staging of malignant melanoma by depth of invasion. *Am J Surg* 1965; 110: 168–76.
9. Clark W, Jr, From L, Bernardino E, et al, The histogenesis and biologic behavior of primary human malignant melanomas of the skin. *Cancer Res* 1969; 29: 705–26.
10. McGovern V, The classification of melanoma and its relationship with prognosis. *Pathology* 1970; 2: 85–9.
11. Breslow A, Thickness, cross-sectional areas and depth of invasion in the prognosis of cutaneous melanoma. *Ann Surg* 1970; 172: 902–8.
12. Breslow A, Cascinelli N, Van der Esch E, et al, Stage I melanoma of the limbs: assessment of prognosis by levels of invasion and maximum thickness. *Tumouri* 1978; 64: 273–84.
13. Balch C, Murad T, Soong S, et al, A multifactorial analysis of melanoma: prognostic histopathological features comparing Clark's and Breslow's staging methods. *Ann Surg* 1978; 188: 732–42.
14. American Joint Committee for Cancer Staging and End-Results Reporting, Staging of malignant melanoma. In: *Manual for staging of cancer.* Chicago: American Joint Committee, 1977: 131–40.
15. American Joint Committee for Cancer Staging and End-Results Reporting, Staging of malignant melanoma. In: *Manual for staging of cancer.* Chicago: American Joint Committee, 1978: 131–40
16. American Joint Committee on Cancer Melanoma of the skin. In: *Manual for staging of cancer* (eds Beahrs O, Myers M). Philadelphia: J.B. Lippincott, 1983: 117–20.
17. American Joint Committee on Cancer Melanoma of the skin. In: *Manual for staging of cancer* (eds Beahrs O, Henson D, Hutter R, Myers M). Philadelphia: J. B. Lippincott, 1988: 140–2.
18. American Joint Committee on Cancer. Malignant melanoma of the skin. In: *Manual for staging of cancer* (eds Beahrs O, Henson D, Hutter R, Kennedy B). Philadelphia: J. B. Lippincott, 1992: 143–8.
19. American Joint Committee on Cancer, Malignant melanoma of the skin. In: *AJCC Cancer Staging Manual* (eds Fleming I, Cooper J, Henson D, et al). Philadelphia: Lippincott-Raven, 1997: 163–70.
20. Hurt M, Santa Cruz D, Malignant melanoma microstaging: history, premises, methods, problems, and recommendations – a call for standardization. *Pathology Annu* 1994 29: 51–74.
21. Cochran A, Bailly C, Paul F, et al, *Melanocytic tumors: a guide to diagnosis.* Philadelphia: Lippincott-Raven, 1997.
22. Bengoechea-Beeby M, Velasco-Oses A, Fernandez F, et al, Epidermotropic metastatic melanoma: are the current histologic criteria adequate to differentiate primary from metastatic melanoma? *Cancer* 1993; 72: 1909–13.
23. Berger D, Feig B, Podoloff D, et al, Lymphoscintigraphy as a predictor of lymphatic drainage from cutaneous melanoma. *Ann of Surg Oncol* 1997; 4: 247–51.
24. Fortner J, Booher R, Pack G, Results of groin dissection for malignant melanoma in 220 patients. *Surgery* 1964; 55: 485–94.
25. Finck S, Giuliano A, Mann B, et al, Results of ilioinguinal dissection for stage II melanoma. *Ann Surg* 1982; 180–6.
26. McCarthy JG, Haagensen CD, Herter P, The role of groin dissection in the management of melanoma of the lower extremity. *Ann Surg* 1974; 179: 156–9.
27. Coit D, Brennan M, Extent of lymph node dissection in melanoma of the trunk or lower extremity. *Arch Surg* 1989; 124: 162–6.
28. Karakousis C, Goumas W, Rao U, et al, Axillary node dissection in malignant melanoma. *Am J Surg* 1991; 162: 202–7.
29. Karakousis C, Driscoll D, Groin dissection in malignant melanoma. *Br J Surg* 1994; 81: 1771–4.
30. Karakousis CP, Therapeutic node dissections in malignant melanoma. *Ann Surg Oncol* 1993; 5: 473–82.
31. Strobbe L, Jonk A, Hart A, et al, Positive iliac and obturator nodes in melanoma: survival and prognostic factors. *Ann Surg Oncol* 1999; 6: 255–62.
32. Mann G, Coit D, Does the extent of operation influence the prognosis in patients with melanoma metastatic to inguinal nodes? *Ann Surg Oncol* 1999; 6: 263–71.
33. Vollmer R, Malignant melanoma. A multivariate analysis of prognostic factors. *Pathol Annu* 1989; 24: 383–407.
34. Morton D, Davtyan D, Wanek L, et al, Multivariate analysis of the relationship between survival and the microstage of primary melanoma by Clark level and Breslow thickness. *Cancer* 1993; 71: 3737–43.
35. Büttner P, Garbe C, Bertz J, et al, Primary cutaneous melanoma. Optimized cutoff points of tumor thickness and importance of Clark's level for prognostic classification. *Cancer* 1995; 75: 2499–506.
36. Buzaid A, Ross M, Balch C, et al, Critical analysis of the current American Joint Committee on Cancer staging system for cutaneous melanoma and proposal of a new staging system. *J Clin Oncol* 1997; 15: 1039–51.
37. Balch C, Cutaneous melanoma: prognosis and treatment results worldwide. *Semin Surg Oncol* 1992; 8: 400–14.
38. Gershenwald J, Thompson W, Mansfield P, et al, Multi-institutional lymphatic mapping experience: The prognostic value of sentinel lymph node status in 612 stage I or II melanoma patients. *J Clin Oncol* 1999; 17: 976–83.
39. Gershenwald J, Mansfield P, Lee J, et al, The role for lymphatic mapping and sentinel lymph node biopsy in patients with thick (≥4 mm) primary melanoma. *Ann Surg Oncol* 2000; 7: 160–5.
40. Roses D, Karp N, Oratz R, et al, Survival with regional and distant metastases from cutaneous malignant melanoma. *Surg Gynecol Obstet* 1991; 172: 262–8.
41. Sutherland C, Mather F, Krementz E, Factors influencing the survival of patients with regional melanoma of the extremity treated by perfusion. *Surg Gynecol Obstet* 1987; 164: 111–18.
42. Karakousis C, Temple D, Moore R, et al, Prognostic parameters in recurrent malignant melanoma. *Cancer* 1983; 52: 575–9.
43. Häffner A, Garbe C, Burg G, et al, The prognosis of primary and metastasising melanoma. An evaluation of the TNM classification in 2,495 patients. *Br J Cancer* 1992; 66: 856–61.
44. Cascinelli N, Bufalino R, Marolda R, et al, Regional non-nodal metastases of cutaneous melanoma. *Eur J Surg Oncol* 1986; 12: 175–80.
45. Singletary S, Tucker S, Boddie A, Multivariate analysis of prognostic factors in regional cutaneous metastases of extremity melanoma. *Cancer* 1988; 61: 1437–40.
46. León P, Daly J, Synnestvedt M, et al, The prognostic implications of microscopic satellites in patients with clinical stage I melanoma. *Arch Surg* 1991; 126: 1461–8.
47. Day CJ, Harrist T, Gorstein F, et al, Malignant melanoma: prognostic significance of 'microscopic satellites' in the reticular dermis and subcutaneous fat. *Ann Surg* 1981; 194: 108–12.

48. Harrist T, Rigel D, Day C, Jr, et al, 'Microscopic satellites' are more highly associated with regional lymph node metastases than with primary melanoma thickness. *Cancer* 1984; 53: 2183–7.
49. Reintgen D, Vollmer R, Tso C, et al, Prognosis for recurrent stage I malignant melanoma. *Arch Surg* 1987; 122: 1338–42.
50. Urist M, Balch C, Milton G, Surgical management of the primary melanoma. In: *Cutaneous melanoma. Clinical management and treatment results worldwide* (eds Balch C, Milton G). Philadelphia: J.B. Lippincott, 1985: 71.
51. Creagan E, Dalton R, Ahmann D, et al, Randomized, surgical adjuvant clinical trial of recombinant interferon alfa-2a in selected patients with malignant melanoma. *J Clin Oncol* 1995; 13: 2776–83.
52. Coit D, Prognostic factors in patients with melanoma metastatic to regional nodes. *Surg Oncol Clin North Am* 1992; 1: 281–95.
53. Buzaid A, Tinoco L, Jendiroba D, et al, Prognostic value of size of lymph node metastases in patients with cutaneous melanoma. *J Clin Oncol* 1995; 13: 2361–8.
54. Karakousis C, Seddip M, Moore R, Prognostic value of lymph node dissection in malignant melanoma. *Arch Surg* 1980; 115: 719–22.
55. Karakousis C, Hena M, Emrich L, et al, Axillary node dissection in malignant melanoma: results and complications. *Surgery* 1980; 108: 10–17.
56. Kirkwood J, Strawderman M, Ernstoff M, et al, Interferon-alfa-2b adjuvant therapy of high-risk resected cutaneous melanoma: the Eastern Cooperative Oncology Group Trial EST 1684. *J Clin Oncol* 1996; 14: 7–17.
57. Cascinelli N, Vaglini M, Nava M, et al, Prognosis of skin melanoma with regional node metastases (stage II). *Surg Oncol* 1984; 25: 240–7.
58. Callery C, Cochran A, Roe D, et al, Factors prognostic for survival in patients with malignant melanoma spread to the regional lymph nodes. *Ann Surg* 1982; 196: 69–75.
59. Morton D, Wanek L, Nizze L, et al, Improved long-term survival after lymphadenectomy of melanoma metastatic to regional nodes. *Ann Surg* 1991; 214: 491–9.
60. Singletary S, Shallenberger R, Guinee V, et al, Melanoma with metastasis to regional axillary or inguinal lymph nodes: prognostic factors and results of surgical treatment in 714 patients. *South Med J* 1988; 81: 5–9.
61. Brown C, Zitelli J, The prognosis and treatment of true local cutaneous recurrent malignant melanoma. *Dermatol Surg* 1995; 21: 285–90.
62. Drzewiecki K, Andersson A, Local melanoma recurrences in the scar after limited surgery for primary tumor. *World J Surg* 1995; 19: 346–9.
63. Coit D, Rogatko A, Brennan M, Prognostic factors in patients with melanoma metastatic to axillary or inguinal lymph nodes. A multivariate analysis. *Ann Surg* 1991; 214: 627–36.
64. Bevilacqua R, Coit D, Rogatka A, et al, Axillary dissection in melanoma: prognostic variables in node-positive patients. *Ann Surg* 1990; 212: 125–31.
65. Drepper H, Bieß B, Hofherr B, et al, The prognosis of patients with stage III melanoma. *Cancer* 1993; 71: 1239–46.
66. Cohen M, Ketcham A, Felix E, et al, Prognostic factors in patients undergoing lymphadenectomy for malignant melanoma. *Ann Surg* 1977; 186: 635–42.
67. Day CJ, Sober A, Lew R, et al, Malignant melanoma patients with positive nodes and relatively good prognoses: microstaging retains prognostic significance in clinical stage I melanoma patients with metastases to regional nodes. *Cancer* 1981; 47: 955–62.
68. Balch C, Soong S-J, Murad T, et al, A multifactorial analysis of melanoma: III. Prognostic factors in melanoma patients with lymph node metastases (stage II). *Ann Surg* 1981; 193: 377–88.
69. Roses D, Provet J, Harris M, et al, Prognosis of patients with pathologic Stage II cutaneous malignant melanoma. *Ann Surg* 1985; 201: 103–7.
70. Koh H, Sober A, Day CJ, et al, Prognosis of clinical stage I melanoma patients with positive elective regional node dissection. *J Clin Oncol* 1986; 4: 1238–44.
71. Kissin M, Simpson D, Easton D, et al, Prognostic factors related to survival and groin recurrence following therapeutic lymph node dissection for lower limb malignant melanoma. *Br J Surg* 1987; 74: 1023–6.
72. Slingluff CJ, Vollmer R, Seigler H, Stage II malignant melanoma: presentation of a prognostic model and an assessment of specific active immunotherapy in 1,273 patients. *J Surg Oncol* 1988; 39: 139–47.
73. Calabro A, Singletary S, Balch C, Patterns of relapse in 1001 consecutive patients with melanoma nodal metastases. *Arch Surg* 1989; 124: 1051–5.
74. Balch C, Soong S-J, Shaw H, et al, An analysis of prognostic factors in 8500 patients with cutaneous melanoma. In: *Cutaneous melanoma* (eds Balch C, Houghton A, Milton G, et al) 2nd ed. Philadelphia: J.B. Lippincott, 1992: 165–87.
75. Singletary S, Shallenberger R, Guinee V, Surgical management of groin nodal metastases from primary melanoma of the lower extremity. *Surg Gynecol Obstet* 1992; 174: 195–200.
76. Cascinelli N, Bufalino R, Morabito A, et al, Results of adjuvant interferon study in WHO melanoma programme. *Lancet* 1994; 343: 913–14.
77. Barth R Jr, Venzon D, Baker A, The prognosis of melanoma patients with metastases to two or more lymph node areas. *Ann Surg* 1991; 214: 125–30.
78. Dale P, Foshag L, Wanek L, et al, Metastasis of primary melanoma to two separate lymph node basins: prognostic significance. *Ann Surg Oncol* 1997; 4: 13–18.
79. Sirott M, Bajorin D, Wong G, et al, Prognostic factors in patients with metastatic malignant melanoma. A multivariate analysis. *Cancer* 1993; 72: 3091–8.
80. Barth A, Wanek L, Morton D, Prognostic factors in 1,521 melanoma patients with distant metastases. *J Am Coll Surg* 1995; 181: 193–201.
81. Eton O, Legha S, Moon T, et al, Prognostic factors for survival of patients treated sytemically for disseminated melanoma. *J Clin Oncol* 1998; 16: 1103–11.
82. Deichmann M, Benner A, Bock M, et al, S100–beta, melanoma-inhibiting activity, and lactate dehydrogenase discriminate progressive from nonprogressive American Joint Committee on Cancer stage IV melanoma. *J Clin Oncol* 1999; 17: 1891–6.
83. Franzke A, Probst-Kepper M, Buer J, et al, Elevated pretreatment serum levels of soluble vascular cell adhesion molecule 1 and lactate dehydrogenase as predictors of survival in cutaneous metastatic malignant melanoma. *Br J Cancer* 1998; 78: 40–45.
84. Lagerwaard F, Levendag P, Nowak P, et al, Identification of prognostic factors in patients with brain metastases: a review of 1292 patients. *Int J Radiat Oncol Biol Phys* 1999; 43: 795–803.
85. Balch C, Buzaid A, Atkins M, et al, A new American Joint Committee on Cancer staging system for cutaneous melanoma. *Cancer* 2000; 88: 1484–91.
86. Shivers S, Wang X, Li W, et al, Molecular staging of malignant melanoma. *JAMA* 1998; 280: 1410–15.
87. Bostick PJ, Morton DL, Turner RR, et al, Prognostic significance of occult metastases detected by sentinel lymphadenectomy and reverse transcriptase-polymerase chain reaction in early-stage melanoma patients. *J Clin Oncol* 1999; 17: 3238–44.
88. Smith B, Selby P, Southgate J, et al, Detection of melanoma cells in peripheral blood by means of reverse transcriptase and polymerase chain reaction. *Lancet* 1991; 338: 1227–9.
89. Brossart P, Keiholz U, Willhauck M, et al, Hematogenous spread of malignant melanoma cells in different stages of disease. *J Invest Dermatol* 1993; 101: 887–9.
90. Brossart P, Schmier J, Krüger S, et al, A polymerase chain reaction-based semiquantitative assessment of malignant melanoma cells in peripheral blood. *Cancer Res* 1995; 55: 4065–8.
91. Hoon D, Wang Y, Dale P, et al, Detection of occult melanoma cells in blood with a multiple-marker polymerase chain reaction assay. *J Clin Oncol* 1995; 13: 2109–16.
92. Mellado B, Colomer D, Castel T, et al, Detection of circulating neoplastic cells by reverse-transcriptase polymerase chain reaction in malignant melanoma: association with clinical stage and prognosis. *J Clin Oncol* 1996; 14: 2091–7.
93. Battayani Z, Grob J, Xerri L, et al, Polymerase chain reaction detection of circulating melanocytes as a prognostic marker in patients with melanoma. *Arch Dermatol* 1995; 131: 443–7.

94. Foss A, Guille M, Occleston N, et al, The detection of melanoma cells in peripheral blood by reverse transcription-polymerase chain reaction. *Br J Cancer* 1995; 72: 155–9.
95. Kunter U, Buer J, Probst M, et al, Peripheral blood tyrosinase messenger RNA detection and survival in malignant melanoma. *J Natl Cancer Inst* 1996; 88: 590–4.
96. Pittman K, Burchill S, Smith B, et al, Reverse transcriptase-polymerase chain reaction for expression of tyrosinase to identify malignant melanoma cells in peripheral blood. *Ann Oncol* 1996; 7: 297–301.
97. Jung F, Buzaid A, Ross M, et al, Evaluation of tyrosinase mRNA as a tumor marker in the blood of melanoma patients. *J Clin Oncol* 1997; 15: 2826–31.
98. Glaser R, Rass K, Seiter S, et al, Detection of circulating melanoma cells by specific amplification of tyrosinase complementary DNA is not a reliable tumor marker in melanoma patients: a clinical two-centre study. *J Clin Oncol* 1997; 15: 2818–25.

APPENDIX

Summary of the 2002 AJCC/UICC staging system

Skin malignant melanoma	
pT1a	≤1 mm, level II or III, no ulceration
pT1b	≤1 mm, level IV or V, or ulceration
pT2a	>1–2 mm, no ulceration
pT2b	>1–2 mm, ulceration
pT3a	>2–4 mm, no ulceration
pT3b	>2–4 mm, ulceration
pT4a	>4 mm, no ulceration
pT4b	>4 mm, ulceration
N1	1 node
N1a	microscopic
N1b	macroscopic
N2	2–3 nodes or satellites/in-transit without nodes
N2a	2–3 nodes microscopic
N2b	2–3 nodes macroscopic
N2c	satellites or in-transit without nodes
N3	≥4 nodes; matted; satellites/in-transit with nodes

15

The natural history of melanoma and factors predicting outcome

Charles M Balch, Seng-jaw Soong, John F Thompson

INTRODUCTION

Clinical and pathological factors predicting outcome for melanoma patients have been studied for over 30 years. The first multivariate analysis of prognostic factors from a single institution was published in 1978 and the first multivariate analysis of melanoma from a multi-institutional experience in 1981.[1–3] Although a multitude of well designed single institution studies have added to our understanding of prognostic factors in melanoma, few attempts have been made to unify these results into a melanoma staging system to be used in clinical research and clinical practice. Thus, the design and analysis of melanoma clinical trials depends upon the use of relevant predictive or prognostic factors that must be accounted for. Otherwise, treatment differences, or lack thereof, may be influenced more by the mix of the patients' prognostic factors than by the treatment effect being studied. Many melanoma adjuvant therapy trials use such different stratification and patient eligibility criteria that it is difficult, if not impossible, to compare clinical trials conducted by cooperative groups or institutions, or even to reliably compare results of sequential trials conducted by the same investigators.

The Melanoma Staging Committee of the American Joint Committee on Cancer (AJCC) held a series of meetings between 1998 and 2000, to revise the melanoma staging system and to incorporate clinical and pathological factors that more accurately reflected the biology of the disease. The committee recommended a major revision of the melanoma staging system, important elements of which have been recently published.[4–6] The new melanoma staging system better reflects independent prognostic factors that can be used in clinical trials and in reporting the outcomes of various melanoma treatment modalities.

Major changes in the staging system include: (1) melanoma thickness and ulceration but not level of invasion to be used in the T category (except for T1 melanomas); (2) the number of metastatic lymph nodes rather than their gross dimensions and the delineation of clinically occult ('microscopic') versus clinically apparent ('macroscopic') nodal metastases to be used in the N category; (3) the site of distant metastases and the presence of elevated serum lactic dehydrogenase (LDH) to be used in the M category; (4) an upstaging of all patients with stage I, II, and III disease when a primary melanoma is ulcerated; (5) a merging of satellite metastases around a primary melanoma and in-transit metastases into a single staging entity that is grouped into stage III disease; and (6) a new convention for defining clinical and pathological staging so as to take into account the new staging information gained from intraoperative lymphatic mapping and sentinel node biopsy.[4,5]

Members of the melanoma staging committee and additional consultants agreed to an unprecedented collaboration to share prospectively accumulated melanoma outcome data, merged into a single large database for the purpose of validating the proposed revisions to the melanoma staging system. Specifically, the intention was to test: (1) whether the primary determinants of the TNM categories were those most strongly correlated with melanoma specific survival compared with those known independent prognostic factors published previously; and (2) whether the proposed stage groupings partitioned patients into cohorts with similar outcome as measured by melanoma specific survival. The resultant collaborative research project is the largest prognostic factors analysis of melanoma ever conducted. Results of the analysis have been published and are summarized in this chapter, along with a review of other major prognostic factors that were incorporated into the new staging system.[5,7]

THE AJCC MELANOMA STAGING PROJECT

Thirteen institutions and cooperative study groups agreed to contribute prospectively accumulated melanoma patient data. A subcommittee of six experienced clinical statisticians participated in the analysis. The data were merged from 13 prospective databases, all of which has quality control measures in place regarding data entry, pathology and surgery. Details about the data collection, statistical methodologies and results have been published.[7]

The AJCC melanoma database consisted of a total of 30,450 melanoma patients, of which information was available for 17,600 patients (58%) for all of the factors required for the proposed TNM classification and stage grouping. Of the 17,600 patients included in the analysis, 12,837 (73%) had at least 5 years of follow up information, 8633 (49%) had at least 10 years' follow up, and 2485 (14%) had at least 20 years' follow up.

Localized melanoma (stages I and II)

In a multivariate analysis of 13,581 patients with localized melanoma (either clinically or pathologically), the two most powerful independent characteristics of the primary melanoma were tumour thickness and ulceration, among all the prognostic variable analyzed (Table 15.1). These two factors remained the most significant predictors of outcome even after adjustment in the model for the individual centres contributing the data. Other statistically significant prognostic factors were patient age, site of the primary melanoma, level of invasion, and sex (Table 15.1).

When the multivariate analysis was repeated for the cohort of 4750 pathologically staged patients who did not have clinical evidence of nodal metastases preoperatively and who were pathologically staged by sentinel or elective lymphadenectomy, the statistical significance as well as the ranking of factors by χ^2 values was similar to that for the combined group of clinically and pathologically staged patients (Table 15.2). There were two major differences: (1) nodal status (presence or absence of metastases) was the most significant predictor, which could not be accounted for in the clinically staged patients; and (2) level of invasion and patient sex were no longer independent predictors of outcome (Table 15.2).

A non-linear model was fitted to the data to describe the relation between tumour thickness and mortality. Increasing melanoma thickness was highly correlated with 10-year melanoma specific mortality ($P < 0.00001$) (Figure 15.1). This model showed no naturally occurring breakpoints that delineated different biological

Table 15.1 *Cox regression analysis for 13,581 melanoma patients without evidence of nodal or distal metastases. Reproduced with permission from Balch et al.*[7]

Variable	df	χ^2 value (Wald)	*P* value	Risk ratio	95% CI
Thickness	1	244.3	<0.00001	1.558	1.473 to 1.647
Ulceration	1	189.5	<0.00001	1.901	1.735 to 2.083
Age	1	45.6	<0.00001	1.101	1.071 to 1.132
Site	1	41.0	<0.00001	1.338	1.224 to 1.463
Level	1	32.7	<0.00001	1.214	1.136 to 1.297
Sex	1	15.1	0.001	0.836	0.764 to 0.915

Table 15.2 *Cox regression analysis for 4750 melanoma patients without clinical evidence of nodal metastases whose regional lymph nodes were pathologically staged after sentinel or elective lymphadenectomy. Reproduced with permission from Balch et al.*[7]

Variable	df	χ^2 value (Wald)	*P* value	Risk ratio	95% CI
Nodal status	1	100.69	<0.00001	2.239	1.913 to 2.621
Thickness	1	81.85	<0.00001	1.583	1.433 to 1.749
Ulceration	1	78.83	<0.00001	1.938	1.674 to 2.242
Site	1	27.86	<0.00001	1.483	1.281 to 1.716
Age	1	14.25	0.0002	1.095	1.044 to 1.147
Sex	1	1.88	0.1705	0.900	0.774 to 1.046
Level	1	0.01	0.9082	1.007	0.896 to 1.131

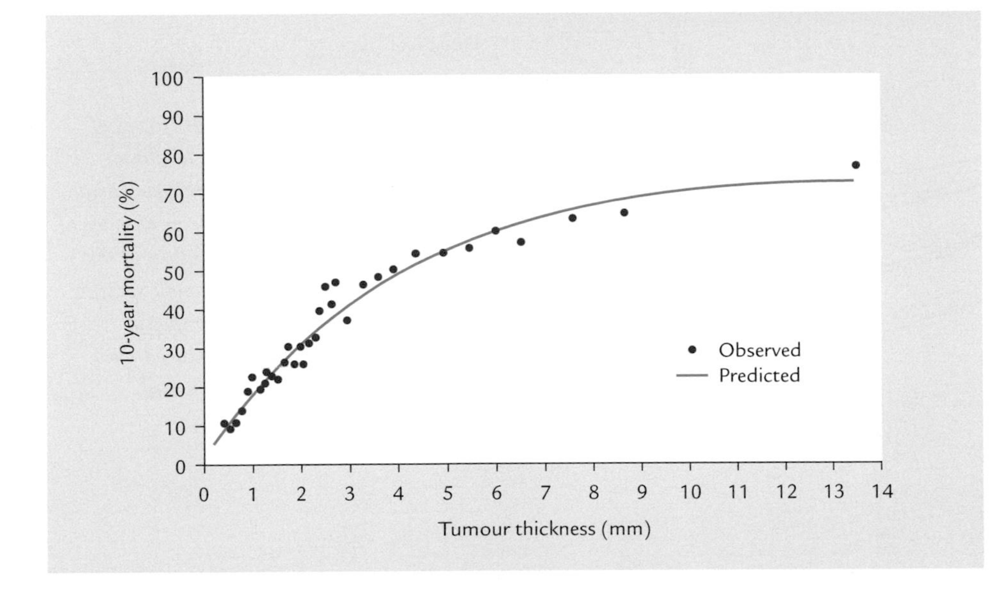

Figure 15.1 *Observed and predicted 10-year mortality of 15,320 patients with clinically localized melanoma based on a mathematical model $f(t) = 1-0.988e^{(-0.211t+0.009\,t^2)}$ derived from the AJCC melanoma database. In the equation, t is the measured tumour thickness (mm) and f(t) is the 10-year melanoma specific mortality rate. The correlation is highly significant (P < 0.0001). There are no naturally occurring breakpoints or thresholds of tumour thickness and mortality. Reproduced with permission from Balch et al.*[7]

risks for melanoma specific mortality. Subsequent analysis of thickness cohorts used the four categories of tumour thickness previously selected by the AJCC melanoma staging committee for clinical convenience and ease of use in the TNM staging system.

The presence or absence of primary tumour ulceration (as documented on histological sections of each melanoma) was the second most powerful predictor of survival, among those independent prognostic factors analyzed. Although this was clearly a predictive feature independent of tumour thickness, the incidence of melanoma ulceration increased with increasing tumour thickness, ranging from 6% for thin (≤1.0 mm) melanomas to 63% for thick (>4.0 mm) lesions (Figure 15.2). It was remarkable that the survival for patients with ulcerated melanomas was diminished to a level equivalent to that for thicker melanomas that were not ulcerated (Figure 15.3). In every instance, the survival rate for ulcerated melanomas was virtually the same as for non-ulcerated melanomas of the next greater thickness category.

To determine the relative predictive strength of these prognostic features within cohorts of tumour thickness, the Cox regression analysis was performed within each of the major thickness subgroups used in the melanoma T categories (Table 15.3). When comparing level of invasion and ulceration within thickness subgroups, there was a hierarchy of relative predictive strength for thin melanoma (≤1.0 mm) that was different from all other thickness groups. Thus, for this

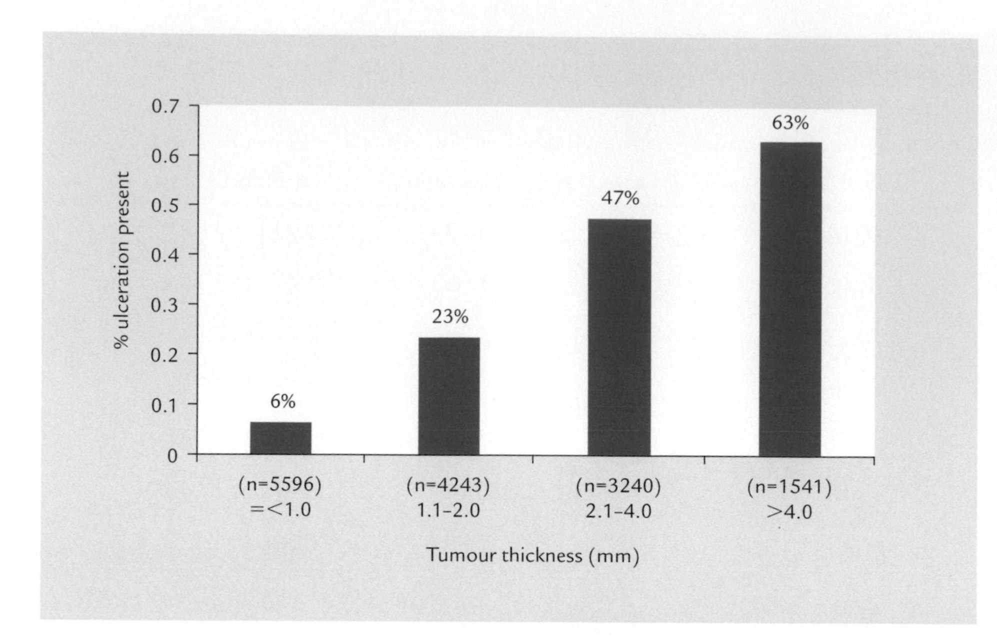

Figure 15.2 *Incidence of melanoma ulceration (determined histopathologically) correlated with tumour thickness for 14,620 patients with localized melanoma. Numbers of patients are shown in parentheses. The correlation is highly significant (P < 0.0001) by χ^2 analysis. Reproduced with permission from Balch et al.*[7]

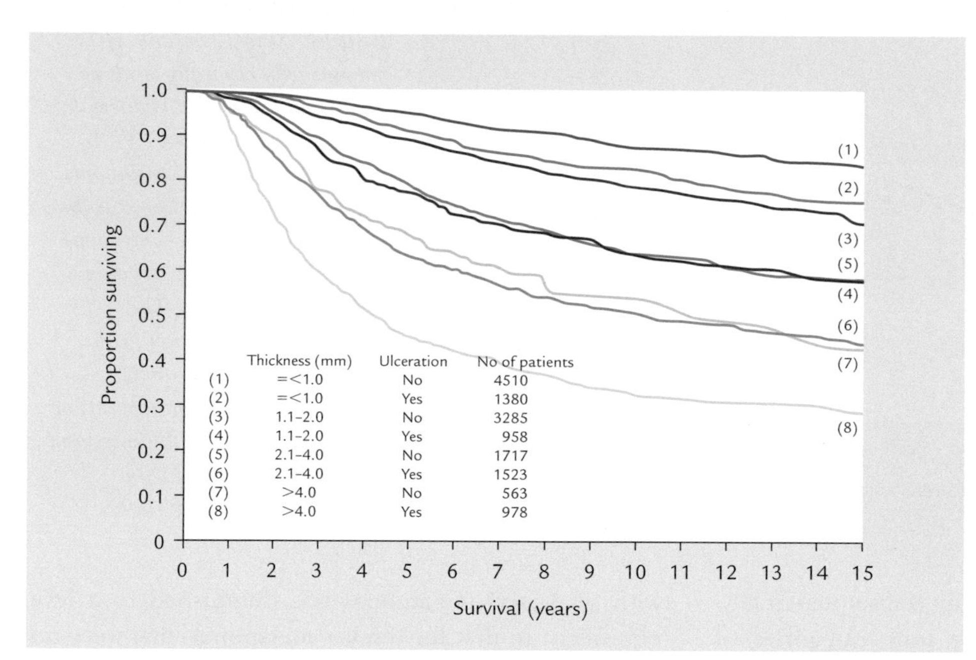

Figure 15.3 *Survival curves of 14,914 patients with localized melanoma stratified by melanoma thickness and presence or absence of ulceration. The correlation of the subgroups with melanoma specific survival is highly significant (P < 0.0001). Reproduced with permission from Balch et al.*[7]

specific subgroup of patients, level of invasion was more predictive of survival outcome than tumour ulceration. The opposite was true for all melanomas thicker than 1.0 mm, where ulceration was clearly the most predictive, and level of invasion ranked below that of patient age and anatomical site of the primary melanoma (Table 15.3).

The incidence of ulceration was quite low overall for patients with thin melanomas (6%) and was slightly greater for deeper levels of invasion (Table 15.4). In this patient series, 10-year survival rates for the 5480 patients with thin melanomas diminished with increasing level of invasion or the presence of ulceration (Table 15.4). Overall, 10-year survival was significantly lower for thin melanomas with ulceration compared to those without ulceration (76% versus 86%, $P < 0.0001$). Only 16% of thin melanomas had level IV invasion (and <0.01% with level V); only 8% of these level IV thin melanomas were ulcerated.

Patient age, sex, and anatomical site of primary melanoma

Increasing patient age was also an independent prognostic factor with respect to overall survival (Tables 15.1

Table 15.3 *Cox regression analysis by tumour thickness category for stages I and II primary melanoma. Reproduced with permission from Balch et al.*[7]

Variable	df	χ^2 value (Wald)	*P* value	Risk ratio	95% CI
		Thickness <1.00 mm (n=5299)			
Level	1	24.778	<0.00001	1.451	1.253 to 1.680
Ulceration	1	17.239	<0.00001	2.073	1.469 to 2.924
Age	1	12.563	0.0004	1.156	1.067 to 1.253
Site	1	6.940	0.0084	1.394	1.089 to 1.784
Sex	1	5.506	0.0189	0.744	0.581 to 0.952
		Thickness 1.01–2.00 mm (n=3943)			
Ulceration	1	57.215	<0.00001	1.965	1.650 to 2.341
Site	1	24.085	<0.00001	1.567	1.310 to 1.876
Age	1	11.613	0.0007	1.101	1.042 to 1.164
Level	1	6.656	0.0099	1.211	1.047 to 1.400
Sex	1	2.668	0.1024	0.861	0.719 to 1.030
		Thickness 2.01–4.00 mm (n=2959)			
Ulceration	1	62.291	<0.00001	1.766	1.634 to 2.034
Age	1	12.529	0.0004	1.087	1.038 to 1.138
Site	1	12.342	0.0004	1.306	1.125 to 1.516
Level	1	4.451	0.0349	1.143	1.010 to 1.294
Sex	1	3.165	0.0752	0.872	0.750 to 1.014
		Thickness >4.00 mm (n=1380)			
Ulceration	1	47.246	<0.00001	1.932	1.601 to 2.331
Age	1	8.745	0.0031	1.087	1.028 to 1.148
Level	1	4.065	0.0438	1.139	1.004 to 1.293
Sex	1	2.875	0.0951	0.858	0.716 to 1.027
Site	1	2.547	0.1106	1.154	0.968 to 1.376

and 15.2) and within each of the thickness subgroups (Table 15.3). There was a significant and consistent stepdown of survival based on increasing decades of life (Table 15.5). In addition to the patient's age, their sex (male patients worse than female ones) as well as the anatomical site (trunk, head and neck site worse than extremities) of their primary melanoma correlated significantly with survival, although their χ^2 values were much lower compared with those for melanoma thickness and ulceration.

Regional metastases (stage III)

Complete clinical and histopathological data were available for 1201 patients with lymph node metastases. A Cox multivariate analysis showed that three factors were

Table 15.4 *10-year survival rate by level and ulceration for thin melanomas (≤1 mm). Reproduced with permission from Balch et al.*[7]

Level of invasion (patient distribution)	Ulceration present (incidence %)	10-year survival	
		Ulceration absent	Ulceration present
All	6	86% ± 0.9% (n = 5174)	76% ± 3.6% (n = 306)
II (45%)	3	88% ± 1.2% (n = 2366)	85% ± 5.6% (n = 76)
III (39%)	7	85% ± 1.8% (n = 1952)	75% ± 5.3% (n = 160)
IV (16%)	8	82% ± 2.3% (n = 789)	70% ± 7.9% (n = 68)

Table 15.5 *5- and 10-year survival rates by age for stage I and II patients. Reproduced with permission from Balch et al.*[7]

Age group	No.	Survival rates	
		5-year % ± S.E.	10-year % ± S.E.
10–19	238	87 ± 2.6	81 ± 3.5
20–29	1400	87 ± 1.1	77 ± 1.6
30–39	2518	86 ± 0.8	77 ± 1.2
40–49	3006	85 ± 0.8	75 ± 1.2
50–59	2945	82 ± 0.9	69 ± 1.3
60–69	2805	78 ± 1.0	63 ± 1.6
70–79	1500	71 ± 1.7	56 ± 2.7
≥80	333	60 ± 5.0	43 ± 7.0

most significant ($P < 0.0001$): (1) the number of metastatic nodes; (2) the tumour burden at the time of staging (microscopic versus macroscopic); and (3) the presence or absence of ulceration of the primary melanoma (Table 15.6). These three factors remained the most significant predictors of outcome even after adjustment in the model for the individual centres contributing the data. The site of the primary melanoma and the patient's age had a somewhat lower, but still statistically significant correlation with survival (Table 15.6).

The actual number of nodal metastases was the most significant predictor of outcome in these patients (Table 15.6). Melanoma specific survival (calculated from the time of primary melanoma diagnosis) decreased significantly with increasing nodal involvement ($P < 0.0001$; Figure 15.4). The best grouping for the number of metastatic nodes that correlated with 5-year survival was 1 versus 2–3 versus ≤4 metastatic nodes. All other statistical groupings, including one combining two to four metastatic nodes, did not produce as significant a difference.

There was a significantly lower survival (calculated from the time of primary melanoma diagnosis) for those patients who presented with macroscopic (palpable) nodal metastases compared with those with microscopic (non-palpable) nodal metastases, even after accounting for lead time bias ($P < 0.0001$; Figure 15.5). Diminishing 5-year survival with increasing tumour burden based upon increasing number of metastatic nodes present was observed for all subgroups ($P < 0.0001$; Table 15.7).

This was true even within each of the stage III subgroups examined, including a two way survival comparison correlating presence or absence of ulceration with

Table 15.6 *Cox regression analysis for 1151 stage III patients with nodal metastases. Reproduced with permission from Balch et al.*[7]

Variable	df	χ^2 value (Wald)	*P* value	Risk ratio	95% CI
No. of metastatic nodes	1	57.616	<0.00001	1.257	1.185 to 1.334
Tumour burden	1	40.301	<0.00001	1.792	1.497 to 2.146
Ulceration	1	23.282	<0.00001	1.582	1.313 to 1.906
Site	1	17.843	0.0001	1.461	1.225 to 1.746
Age	1	13.369	0.0003	1.118	1.053 to 1.187
Thickness	1	1.964	0.1611	1.091	0.966 to 1.233
Level	1	0.219	0.6396	1.033	0.901 to 1.186
Sex	1	0.006	0.9407	1.007	0.836 to 1.213

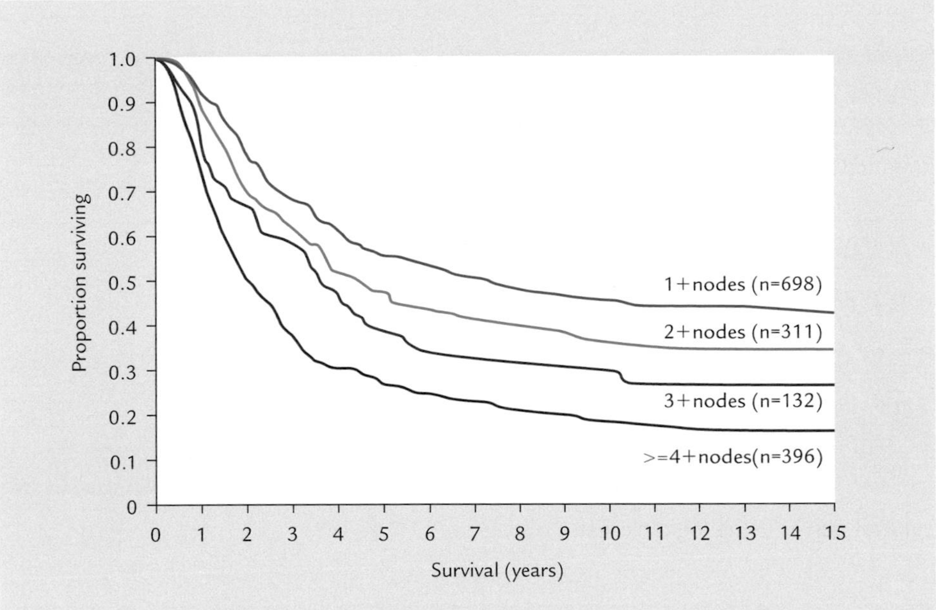

Figure 15.4 *Survival curves of 1528 melanoma patients with lymph node metastases subgrouped by the actual number of metastatic nodes. The correlation is highly significant (P < 0.0001). Reproduced with permission from Balch et al.*[7]

the number of metastatic lymph nodes ($P < 0.0001$; Table 15.8), or a three way comparison that integrated subgroups according to all three of the most important prognostic factors: ulceration of the primary melanoma, nodal tumour burden and the number of metastatic nodes (Table 15.9). Overall, only 49% of all patients with nodal metastases survived 5 years (37% at 10 years), but the range of melanoma specific survival was large, ranging from 13% at 5 years for patients with the highest risk combination of factors, to 69% at 5 years for the lowest risk combination of predictive factors (Table 15.9).

Site of distant metastases (stage IV)

The prognostic influence of different distant metastatic sites was analyzed in 1158 stage IV patients using various combinations of sites of metastases. The most significant differences were noted when visceral versus non-visceral sites (skin, subcutaneous, distant lymph nodes) were compared. Although significant 1-year survival differences were observed when patients with lung metastases were compared with those with metastases in other visceral sites ($P < 0.0001$), no differences were noted when 2-year survival data were compared (Figure 15.6).

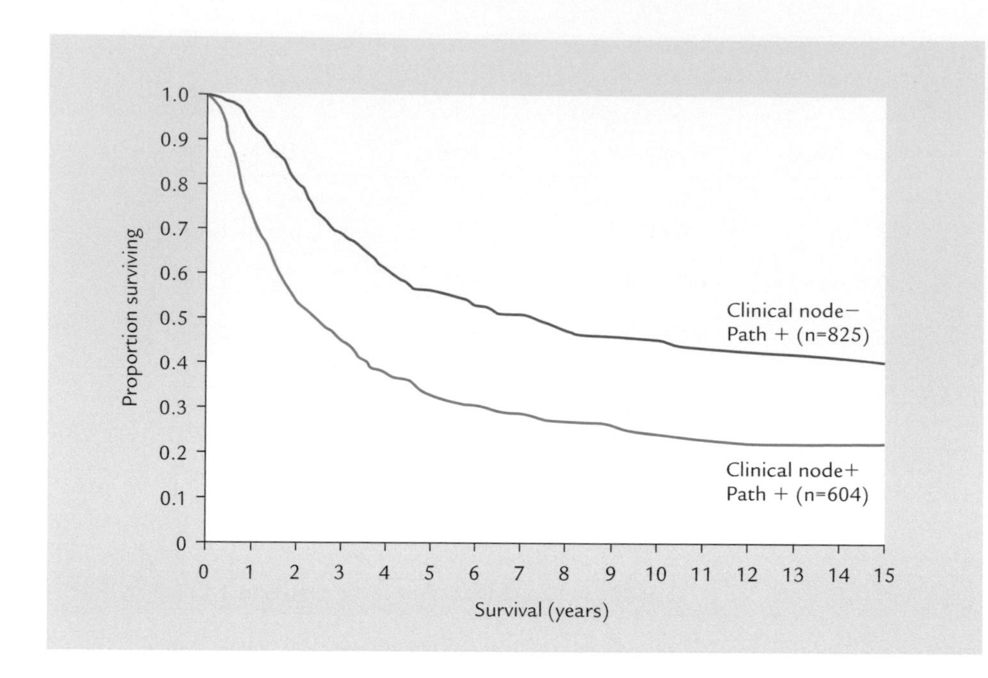

Figure 15.5 *Survival curves of 1429 patients with lymph node metastases subgrouped by their presenting clinical stage. There were 825 patients with clinically occult nodal metastases diagnosed pathologically after either sentinel or elective lymphadenectomy and 604 patients who presented with clinically evident nodal metastases confirmed pathologically after a therapeutic lymphadenectomy. Survival rates were calculated from the time of the primary melanoma diagnosis. The difference in survival rates is highly significant (P < 0.0001). Reproduced with permission from Balch et al.*[7]

Table 15.7 *5-year survival rates for stage III patients with nodal metastases stratified by number of metastatic nodes and tumour burden (microscopic versus macroscopic disease). Reproduced with permission from Balch et al.*[7]

No. of positive nodes	Microscopic + nodes % ± S.E.	Macroscopic + nodes % ± S.E.	*P* value*
1	61 ± 2.8 (n = 469)	46 ± 3.6 (n = 220)	<0.0001
2	56 ± 4.6 (n = 172)	37 ± 4.4 (n = 139)	<0.0001
3	56 ± 8.5 (n = 69)	27 ± 6.0 (n = 63)	<0.001
4	36 ± 8.7 (n = 40)	24 ± 4.4 (n = 106)	0.1034
>4	35 ± 8.7 (n = 73)	24 ± 3.5 (n = 175)	0.0011

**P* value based on the comparison of survival curves using log rank test.

Table 15.8 *5-year survival rates for stage III patients with nodal metastases stratified by number of positive nodes and ulceration. Reproduced with permission from Balch et al.*[7]

No. of positive nodes	Ulcer absent % ± S.E.	Ulcer present % ± S.E.	*P* value*
1	65 ± 3.0 (n = 374)	45 ± 3.3 (n = 315)	<0.0001
2	59 ± 4.6 (n = 153)	30 ± 4.3 (n = 158)	0.0018
3	47 ± 7.7 (n = 70)	32 ± 6.8 (n = 62)	0.0153
4	32 ± 6.7 (n = 63)	17 ± 5.1 (n = 58)	0.0409
>4	26 ± 5.5 (n = 105)	22 ± 4.9 (n = 92)	0.4857

**P* value based on the comparison of survival curves using log rank test.

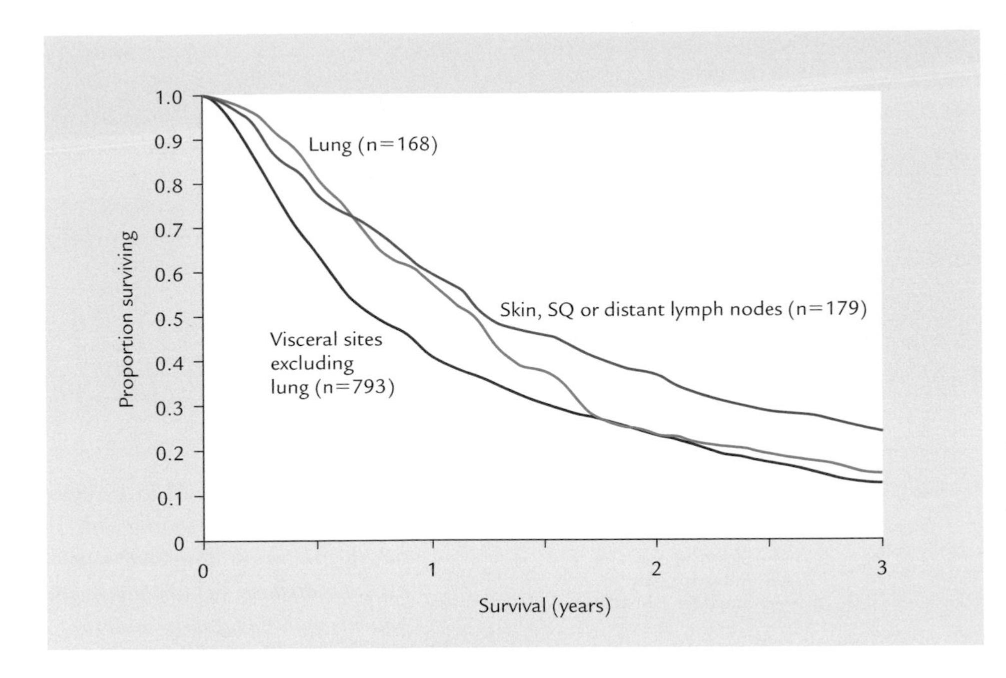

Figure 15.6 *Survival curves of 1158 patients with metastatic melanomas at distant sites subgrouped into three categories or sites: skin, subcutaneous or distant lymph nodes versus lung versus all other visceral sites. The numbers of patients are shown in parentheses. Note that the survival rate for patients with lung metastases is similar to that for non-visceral sites for the first year and then approaches that of other visceral sites after two years. Survival differences are significantly greater for skin, subcutaneous or distant lymph node metastases compared with lung metastases ($P = 0.003$) or other visceral sites of metastases ($P < 0.0001$). Reproduced with permission from Balch et al.*[7]

SUMMARY OF MELANOMA PROGNOSTIC FEATURES

Primary melanoma prognostic features

Melanoma thickness

The use of melanoma thickness was first described by Breslow, who measured the maximum vertical dimension of a melanoma on cross-section using an ocular micrometer.[8–12] In virtually all studies analyzing the prognosis of patients with stage I and II melanoma using a Cox regression analysis, melanoma thickness is the strongest predictor of outcome. This correlation may reflect either the rate and/or the duration of primary melanoma growth. Increasing melanoma thickness correlates with increasing risk for local recurrence, regional metastasis, distant metastasis, and melanoma specific survival. The uniform result of melanoma thickness being the strongest predictor of survival outcome was consistent in multivariate analyses reported from single institutions, from multi-institutional studies and from population based studies that spanned countries in North America, Europe, and Australia.[3,13–46]

Melanoma thickness is a continuous variable for which there are no natural breakpoints.[13,14,17–19,29,47–49] In the previous (1997) version of the melanoma staging system, the threshold of a T1/T2 melanoma was defined as 0.75 mm, a thickness that had been empirically recommended by Breslow in 1970.[8] Subsequently, many melanoma investigators have used a threshold of ≤ 1.0 mm to define a 'thin' or a 'good risk' melanoma. In the new staging version, the T category thresholds of melanoma thickness are defined in even integers (at 1.0 mm, 2.0 mm, and 4.0 mm), both because they represent a statistical 'best fit' and because they are most compatible with current thresholds in clinical decision making and the determination of prognostic groups for 'node negative' (N0) patients.[1,11,18,31,39,50,51]

Melanoma ulceration

Ulcerated melanomas represent a more biologically aggressive form of the disease, associated with a substantially increased risk of metastasis. Indeed, the metastatic capacity of an ulcerated melanoma is similar to that of cancers categorized as 'poorly differentiated' or 'locally advanced' primary tumours. Tumour ulceration is defined as the absence of an intact epidermis overlying a portion of the primary melanoma based upon microscopic examination of the histological sections.[1,50,52,53]

Table 15.9 *5-year survival rates for stage III patients with nodal metastases stratified by number of metastatic nodes, ulceration and tumour burden. Reproduced with permission from Balch et al.[7]*

Melanoma ulceration	Microscopic % ± S.E.			Macroscopic % ± S.E.		
	1 + nodes	2–3 nodes	>3+ nodes	1 + nodes	2–3 nodes	>3+ nodes
Absent	69 ± 3.7 (n = 252)	63 ± 5.6 (n = 130)	27 ± 9.3 (n = 57)	59 ± 4.7 (n = 122)	46 ± 5.5 (n = 93)	27 ± 4.6 (n = 109)
Present	52 ± 4.1 (n = 217)	50 ± 5.7 (n = 111)	37 ± 8.8 (n = 46)	29 ± 5.0 (n = 98)	25 ± 4.4 (n = 109)	13 ± 3.5 (n = 104)

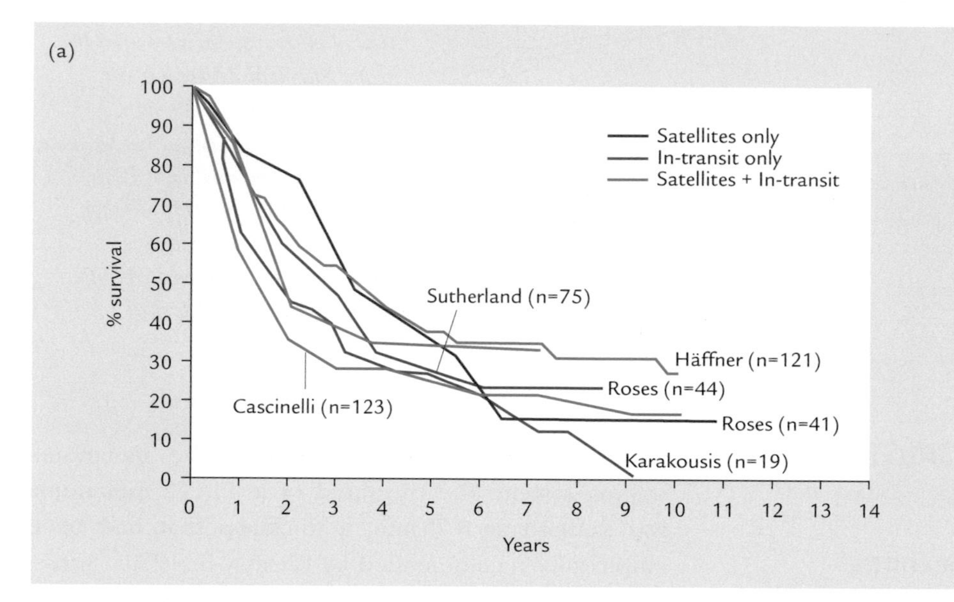

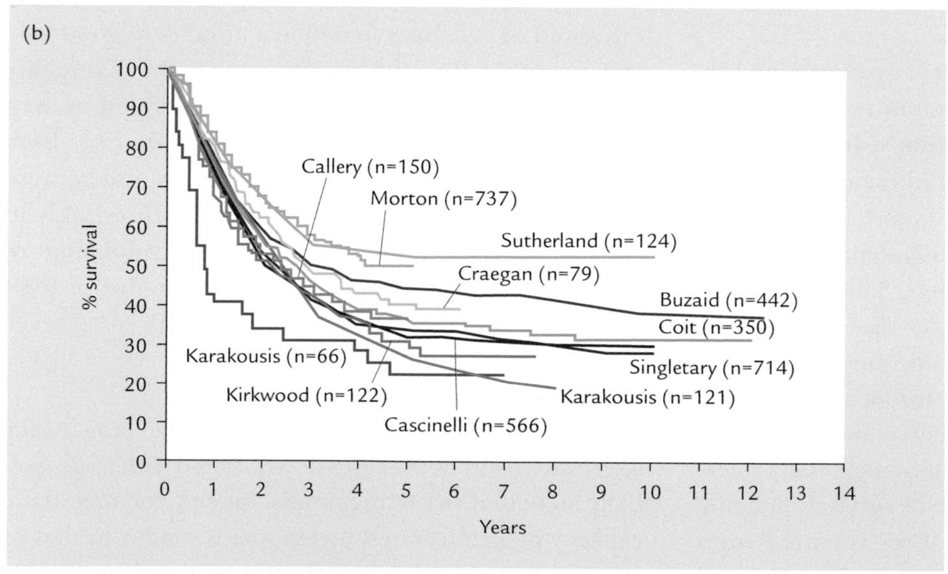

Figure 15.7 *Kaplan-Meier survival curves of patients presenting with satellite, in-transit or satellite + in-transit metastases (a) compared with patients with nodal metastases (b). Reproduced with permission from Buzaid et al.[70]*

It can easily be distinguished from artifactual or traumatic disruption of the epidermis. In fact, the interpretation of melanoma ulceration among pathologists is one of the most reproducible of all the major histopathological features.[54–57] In virtually every Cox regression analysis of prognostic factors that includes ulceration, melanoma ulceration portends a significantly worse prognosis and a higher risk for metastatic disease compared with non-ulcerative melanomas of equivalent thickness.[13,14,16,17,20,22–26,29–31,35,38,42,44,46,53,58–68] The only exception to this observation has been for thin melanomas (≤1.0 mm), where the incidence of ulceration is low overall (6%), even for deeper levels of invasion.

The biological events associated with invasion of a primary melanoma through the overlying epidermis rather than simple upward displacement of it is clearly associated with a greater capacity to metastasize compared with its non-ulcerated counterpart of equivalent thickness. The presence of melanoma ulceration heralds such a high risk for metastasis that its presence 'upstage' the prognosis of all such patients compared with patients with melanomas of equivalent thickness without ulceration. Thus, survival rates for patients with ulcerated melanomas are remarkably similar to those of patients with non-ulcerated melanomas of the next thickness grouping (Figure 15.3). Indeed, the survival rates for thick, ulcerated melanomas (T4b) without nodal metastases are actually worse than for some substages of patients with nodal metastases.[5] Melanoma ulceration correlates with increased mitotic rate within a primary melanoma, further evidence that this factor is associated with increased metastatic behaviour.[29] The presence or absence of ulceration is the only prognostic feature of a primary melanoma that independently predicts outcome in stages I and II as well as in stage III melanoma.[7,38,69,70]

Melanoma level of invasion

The level of invasion has been a gold standard of predictive features of melanoma since it was first defined in the 1960s by Clark.[71] It has been a primary factor in the melanoma TNM staging system and has been widely used as a prognostic factor for decades. However, there are substantial limitations to use of the level of invasion that have gradually caused it to be used less frequently. It requires an interpretation of a tumour's maximum depth (especially for level III and IV), it does not take into account the varying skin thickness of different anatomical parts (for example, skin of the back and the face) and each level is associated with a wide range of melanoma thicknesses. Two studies comparing accuracy of histopathological prognostic factors used by pathologists showed that ulceration and thickness were much more reproducible than level of invasion.[54,72] Moreover, when there is a discrepancy in the prognosis between measured tumour thickness and level of invasion (for example, 'thin' level IV or 'thick' level III), the former is more accurate in predicting survival outcome.[7,18,31,50,51,58,60,70]

Interaction between tumour thickness, level of invasion and ulceration

One of the controversies that was able to be addressed with this large database was the interaction between melanoma thickness, level of invasion, and ulceration. This was particularly important for 'thin' melanomas (≤1.0 mm thickness), where published data had suggested that deeper levels were associated with a worse outcome.[18,66,73–76] Thus, level of invasion does provide additional prognostic discrimination in the specific subgroup of thin (T1) melanomas.[74,77]

The multivariate analysis showed that a deep level of invasion (IV or V) is not a surrogate for ulceration, but an independent factor that eclipses the predictive value of ulceration in this specific subgroup of patients. This relation was not true for all melanomas >1.0 mm, because the level of invasion was no longer a significant predictor of survival outcome, relative to ulceration (presence or absence), increasing age, or the anatomical site of the primary melanoma (trunk; head and neck versus extremity).

Patient age

Even though older patients have thicker melanomas and a higher incidence of ulcerated melanomas, their age is an independent adverse prognostic factor after adjusting for these other factors in a multivariate analysis.[20,34,46,61,78,79] In the AJCC melanoma committee study, there was a consistent and incremental decline in both 5-year and 10-year survival rates with each decade increase of age (Table 15.5). Numerous other studies have shown that older melanoma patients have a lower survival rate, especially those over 60 years of age.[20,33,34,46,61,79–82] This has included a number of multi-institutional clinical trials involving various stages of melanoma, age groups, and treatment effects.[46,61,83–85] Indeed, national cancer statistics in the United States show that melanoma has had the second highest increase in mortality among individuals 65 years of age or older (from 1973 to 1997), especially for men.[86]

Melanoma growth patterns

The data used in the AJCC melanoma prognostic factors analysis, as well as in other studies reported in the literature, were largely based on melanomas with superficial spreading and nodular growth patterns. These two growth patterns, reflecting differences in vertical and radial growth phases, constitute about 90% of melanomas seen in most practices. These two growth patterns are not independent prognostic factors, since their survival rates are almost the same when tumour thickness is accounted for.[1,31,50] There is some evidence that other growth patterns, namely lentigo maligna melanoma, acral lentiginous melanoma, and desmoplastic melanoma, may have a different aetiology and prognosis.[31,37,87–93]

Prognostic features in regional metastases

Stage III melanoma patients include those with regional metastases, either in the regional lymph nodes or as intralymphatic metastases manifesting as satellite or in-transit metastases.

Based on the AJCC analysis and results in the literature, the presence or absence of ulceration is the only prognostic feature of a primary melanoma that independently predicts outcome in stage III melanoma (Table 15.6).[7,38,69,70] Other features of regional metastases are described below.

Number of metastatic lymph nodes

In almost all studies analyzing prognosis using Cox regression analysis, either the number or the percentage of metastatic lymph nodes was the strongest predictor or survival outcome.[17,31,94–106] This was true regardless of whether the patient presentation involved macroscopic or microscopic nodal metastases. Thus, survival correlated best with the number of metastatic nodes even for patients with microscopic (or clinically occult) metastases.

In all studies that have examined prognosis based upon the number of metastatic nodes, patients with one metastatic node did better than those with any combination of two or more metastatic nodes.[17,31,95–101,104] The 'best fit' model for prognosis among patients with nodal metastases was a grouping of 1 metastatic node versus 2–3 metastatic nodes versus 4 or more metastatic nodes (Figure 15.4).

Micrometastases versus macrometastases

A second significant prognostic feature for patients with nodal metastases was the tumour burden of nodal metastases, so designated operationally but not by actual measurements. Tumour burden was defined by whether the nodal metastases were clinically occult (not palpable) and detected by sentinel or elective node dissection (designated operationally as 'micrometastases') or clinically apparent (palpable) metastases and confirmed by therapeutic lymphadenectomy (designated operationally as 'macrometastases'). Thus, those patients without clinical or radiological evidence of lymph node metastases but who have pathologically documented nodal metastases are defined by convention as 'microscopic' or 'clinically occult' nodal metastases. 'Macroscopic' tumour burden refers to clinically evident and pathologically confirmed metastatic deposits. It is recognized that such nodal metastases may vary in dimensions (especially for deepseated nodes or in obese patients), but such a delineation can be identified in the medical record, based upon the preoperative clinical examination and the operative notation about the intent of the lymphadenectomy (whether it was an elective, sentinel, or therapeutic lymphadenectomy). In contrast, melanoma patients with both clinical evidence of nodal metastases and pathological examination documenting the number of nodal metastases (after therapeutic lymphadenectomy) are defined by convention as having 'macroscopic' or 'clinically apparent' nodal metastases. Survival rates for these two patient groups are significantly different.[7,46,107]

Clinical versus pathological nodal staging

Historically, the distinction between clinical staging and pathological staging has not been emphasized because the definitions did not delineate any specific prognostic groups. However, with the widespread use of sentinel lymphadenectomy, it has become apparent that the range of survival rates among various subgroups of pathological stage III patients is enormous (ranging from 13% to 69% 5-year survival and 9% to 63% 10-year survival) because of 'upstaging' based upon directed histopathological examination of sentinel lymph nodes.[7,108]

Our own prognostic factors analysis and those from many other institutions have consistently shown that nodal status is a significant prognostic feature of melanoma.[7,38,106,109] Thus, significant differences were identified when survival rates for melanoma patients who were first staged clinically as having no evidence of nodal metastases and who were subsequently staged pathologically after either sentinel or elective node dissection (Table 15.10). These survival differences were statistically significant among all T substages except for T4b. The differences were most striking in patients with clinical T2bN0M0, T3aN0M0, T3bN0M0 and T4aN0M0 disease, where 5-year survival rates for the clinically node negative patients when staged according to their pathological nodal status varied significantly, with diminished survival ranging from 14% to 30% among clinically versus pathologically staged patients of equivalent T categories (Table 15.10). These results highlight the compelling prognostic value of knowing the nodal status as identified by lymphatic mapping and sentinel lymphadenectomy.

Intralymphatic metastases

The fourth criterion for defining pathological stage III melanoma is the presence or absence of satellites or in-transit metastases, regardless of the number of lesions. The presence of clinical or microscopic satellite metastases around a primary melanoma as well as in-transit metastases between the primary melanoma and the regional lymph nodes represent intralymphatic metastases and portend a poor prognosis.[70,110–113] The available data show no substantial difference in survival outcome for these two anatomically defined entities (Figure 15.7).[70] Furthermore, the available data show that patients with a combination of satellites/in-transit metastases plus nodal metastases have a worse outcome than patients who experience either event alone.[70,95]

Prognostic features of distant metastases

In all studies analyzing prognosis in patients with distant metastases using a Cox regression analysis, the site of metastases, the number of metastatic sites and elevated serum concentration of LDH were most predictive of poor survival.[114–118]

Site of distant metastases

Patients with distant metastases in the skin, subcutaneous tissue or distant lymph nodes have a relatively better prognosis compared with those patients with metastases located in any other anatomical site.[7,31,69,115,118,119] In

Table 15.10 *5- and 10-year survival rates for 5346 patients with clinically negative nodal metastases who were then pathologically staged either by regional lymph node dissection or sentinel lymphadenectomy. Reproduced with permission from Balch et al.*[5]

T stage	Path nodes (N)	5-year survival % ± S.E.	*P* value*
T1a	N− (n = 379) N+ (n = 15)	94 ± 2.0 64 ± 17.7	0.0035
T1b	N− (n = 319) N+ (n = 18)	90 ± 2.5 76 ± 14.9	0.0039
T2a	N− (n = 1480) N+ (n = 150)	94 ± 0.8 73 ± 5.6	<0.0001
T2b	N− (n = 408) N+ (n = 62)	83 ± 2.3 56 ± 8.8	<0.0001
T3a	N− (n = 808) N+ (n = 177)	86 ± 1.6 59 ± 6.0	<0.0001
T3b	N− (n = 639) N+ (n = 176)	72 ± 2.1 49 ± 4.5	<0.0001
T4a	N− (n = 203) N+ (n = 66)	75 ± 3.9 61 ± 7.4	0.0116
T4b	N− (n = 330) N+ (n = 116)	53 ± 3.1 44 ± 5.5	0.2403

**P* value based on the comparison of survival curves using the log rank test.

several studies, patients with metastases in the lung had an 'intermediate' prognosis, compared with those with skin and subcutaneous metastases ('better prognosis') and all other visceral sites ('worse prognosis').[85,114,115]

Number of distant metastases

The number of metastases at distant sites has previously been documented as an important prognostic factor.[31,69,115,118] However, this feature was not incorporated into the staging system because of the significant variability in the deployment of diagnostic tests to comprehensively search for distant metastases. These may range from a chest x ray film only in some centres to PET scanning in others. Until the indications and types of tests used are better standardized, the number of metastases cannot reliably be used for staging purposes.

Elevated serum lactic dehydrogenase

This factor was among the most predictive independent factors of diminished survival in all published studies when it was analyzed in a multivariate analysis, even after accounting for site and number of metastases.[116,117,120–123] Therefore, when the serum concentration of LDH is raised above the upper limits of normal at the time of staging, such patients with distant metastases are designated as M1c regardless of the site of the distant metastases. The use of an elevated serum concentration of LDH should be used only when there are two or more determinations obtained more than 24 hours apart, since an elevated serum concentration of LDH on a single determination can be falsely positive due to haemolysis or other factors unrelated to melanoma metastases.

OVERVIEW AND IMPLICATIONS

The results of these analyses showed: (1) tumour thickness and ulceration were the most powerful predictors of survival in patients with localized melanoma (stage I and II), whereas level of invasion had a significant impact only within the subgroup of thin melanomas; (2) the number of metastatic nodes, the tumour burden ('microscopic' versus 'macroscopic' nodal metastases), the presence or absence of melanoma ulceration and the presence of intralymphatic metastases (satellite or in-transit metastases) were the most powerful predictors of survival in patients with nodal metastases (stage III); and (3) the number and anatomical site of distant metastases and the presence of an elevated serum LDH concentration were the most significant predictors of survival in patients with distant metastases (stage IV).

Patients with metastatic disease in regional lymph nodes should not be considered as a homogeneous group, and recommendations to enter patients into clinical trials should take into account the fact that some stage III patients actually have a reasonably good prognosis. Thus, the integration of major prognostic factors show a marked diversity in the natural history of stage III melanoma. This is demonstrated by more than five-fold differences in 5-year survival rates for defined substages, ranging from 69% for patients with non-ulcerated melanomas (regardless of thickness) who had a single clinically occult nodal metastasis (detected by sentinel or elective lymphadenectomy) to a low of 13% for patients with ulcerated melanomas (regardless of thickness) with four or more clinically apparent nodal metastases (detected by therapeutic lymphadenectomy). It is sometimes assumed that all stage III patients are at particularly high risk for distant metastases, and they may therefore be offered very intensive forms of systemic treatment (biochemotherapy). Understanding these differences in clinical outcome will be important, not only in the design and analysis of melanoma clinical trials, but also in calibrating therapeutic intensity to match metastatic risk.

Once a patient had progressed to stage IV disease, survival rates were measured more in months than in years. There were no prognostic features in this analysis that substantially separated survival rates by more than a few months, and only a minority of stage IV patients survive beyond one year.[85,114,115,117,118,122] In general, the only stage IV patients who live beyond one or two years are those with limited disease who have had a complete surgical resection of their distant metastases.[115,123–129] Whether the long term results reflect a more favourable biology of disease or a therapeutic benefit of surgery (or a combination of the two) is a difficult issue to address in the absence of any randomized trials.

Known prognostic factors should be the primary stratification criteria and end results reporting criteria for melanoma clinical trials. The AJCC melanoma committee recommends that all melanoma patients with clinically negative regional lymph nodes and who may be considered for entry into surgical and adjuvant therapy clinical trials should have pathological staging with sentinel lymphadenectomy to ensure prognostic homogeneity within assigned treatment groups. In this way, investigators will be better able to discern between the natural history impact and the treatment impact being studied in melanoma clinical trials. Moreover, the use of a consistent set of criteria will facilitate the comparability of melanoma clinical trials and thereby accelerate the progress of multidisciplinary melanoma treatment approaches.

It is evident that the next phase of staging melanoma will evolve as new technology allows the clinician to reliably diagnose metastatic melanoma at a level of tumour burden well below that achievable with the light microscope or routine x ray films. This will include molecular diagnostic approaches such as reverse transcriptase-polymerase chain reaction (RT-PCT) to detect relevant gene expression, PET scanning, nuclear magnetic resonance imaging, and use of radiolabelled antimelanoma antibodies, serum markers and genetic/molecular markers that will more accurately detect and stage metastatic melanoma.[120,130–136] Some of these advances in molecular based staging will no doubt supplant those prognostic features of melanoma now determined largely with the light microscope.

APPENDIX

The following institutions, organizations, and cancer cooperative groups generously contributed information from their patient databases for the AJCC prognostic factors study described in this chapter. The clinicians and biostatisticians who were involved in the project are listed in parentheses.

Sydney Melanoma Unit, Royal Prince Alfred Hospital (John F Thompson, MD, Marjorie Colman, BSc)

The University of Texas M D Anderson Cancer Center (Jeffrey E Gershenwald, MD, Merrick I Ross, MD)

Memorial Sloan Kettering Cancer Center (Daniel G Coit, MD)

University of Alabama at Birmingham Cancer Center (Marshall Urist, MD, Seng-Jaw Soong PhD, Rene Desmond, PhD)

University of South Florida/Moffitt Cancer Center (Douglas S Reintgen, MD, Gary Lyman, MD

National Tumour Institute, Milan (Natale Cascinelli, MD, Alberto Morabito, PhD)

University of Washington Cancer Center (David Byrd, MD)

Eastern Cooperative Oncology Group (John M Kirkwood, MD, Michael B Atkins, MD)

Southwest Oncology Group (John A Thompson, MD, Ping-Yu Liu, PhD)

Intergroup Melanoma Surgical Trial (Charles M Balch, MD, Seng-jaw Soong PhD, Renee Desmond, PhD)

World Health Organization Melanoma Program (Natale Cascinelli, MD, Aberto Morabito, PhD)

Sunbelt Melanoma Group (Kelly M McMasters, MD, Patricia B Cerrito, PhD)

REFERENCES

1. Balch CM, Murad TM, Soong SJ, et al, A multifactorial analysis of melanoma: prognostic histopathological features comparing Clark's and Breslow's staging methods. *Ann Surg* 1978; 188: 732–42.
2. Eldh J BB, Peterson LE, Prognostic factors in cutaneous malignant melanoma in Stage I. A clinical, morphological and multivariate analysis. *Scand J Plast Reconstr Surg Hand Surg* 1978; 12: 243–55.
3. Van Der Esch EP, Cancinelli N, Preda F, et al, Stage I melanoma of the skin: evaluation of prognosis according to histologic characteristics. *Cancer* 1981; 48: 1668–73.
4. Balch CM, Buzaid AC, Atkins MB, et al, A new American Joint Committee on Cancer staging system for cutaneous melanoma. *Cancer* 2000; 88: 1484–91.
5. Balch C, Buzaid AC, Soong SJ, et al, Final version of the AJCC staging system for cutaneous melanoma. *J Clin Oncol* 2001; 19: 3635–48.
6. Gershenwald JE, Ross MI, Buzaid AC, Staging systems for cutaneous melanoma, In: *Textbook of Melanoma* (eds Thompson JF, Morton DL, Kroon BBR) London: Martin Dunitz, 2004.
7. Balch C, Soong SJ, Gershenwald JE, et al, Prognostic factors analysis of 17 600 melanoma patients. Validation of the new AJCC melanoma staging system. *J Clin Oncol* 2001; 19: 3622–34.
8. Breslow A, Thickness, cross-sectional areas and depth of invasion in the prognosis of cutaneous melanoma. *Ann Surg* 1970; 172: 902–8.
9. Breslow A, Tumour thickness, level of invasion and node dissection in stage I cutaneous melanoma. *Ann Surg* 1975; 182: 572–5.
10. Breslow A, Problems in the measurement of tumour thickness and level of invasion in cutaneous melanoma. *Human Pathol* 1977; 8: 1–2.
11. Breslow A, Macht SD, Evaluation of prognosis in stage I cutaneous melanoma. *Plast Reconstr Surg* 1978; 61: 342–6.
12. Breslow A, Tumour thickness in evaluating prognosis of cutaneous melanoma [letter]. *Ann Surg* 1978; 187: 440.
13. Balch CM, Murad TM, Soong SJ, et al, A multifactorial analysis of melanoma: prognostic histopathological features comparing Clark's and Breslow's staging methods. *Ann Surg* 1978; 188; 732–42
14. Balch CM, Soong SJ, Murad TM, et al, A multifactorial analysis of melanoma. II. Prognostic factors in patients with stage I (localized) melanoma. *Surgery* 1979; 86: 343–51.
15. Balch CM, Soong SJ, Milton GW, et al, A comparison of prognostic factors and surgical results in 1 786 patients with localized (stage I) melanoma treated in Alabama, USA, and New South Wales, Australia. *Ann Surg* 1982; 196: 677–84.
16. Soong SJ, Shaw HM, Balch CM, et al, Predicting survival and recurrence in localized melanoma: a multivariate approach. *World J Surg* 1992; 16: 191–5.
17. Buzaid AC, Ross MI, Balch CM, et al, Critical analysis of the current American Joint Committee on Cancer staging system for cutaneous melanoma and proposal of a new staging system. *J Clin Oncol* 1997; 15: 1039–51.

18. Buttner P, Garbe C, Bertz J, et al, Primary cutaneous melanoma. Optimized cutoff points of tumour thickness and importance of Clark's level for prognostic classification. *Cancer* 1995; 75: 2499–506.
19. Meyskens FL, Berdeaux DH, Parks B, et al, Cutaneous malignant melanoma (Arizona Cancer Center experience). I. Natural history and prognostic factors influencing survival in patient with I disease. *Cancer* 1988; 62: 1207–14.
20. Averbook BJ, Russo LJ, Mansour EG, A long-term analysis of 620 patients with malignant melanoma at a major referrel centre. *Surgery* 1998; 124: 746–56.
21. Sondergaard K, Depth of invasion and tumour thickness in primary cutaneous malignant melanoma. A study of 2012 cases. *Acta Path Microbiol Immunol Scand A* 1985; 93: 49–55.
22. Urist MM, Balch CM, Soong SJ, et al, Head and neck melanoma in 534 clinical stage I patients. A prognostic factors analysis and results of surgical treatment. *Ann Surg* 1984; 200: 769–75.
23. Gershenwald JE, Thompson W, Mansfield PF, et al, Multi-institutional melanoma lymphatic mapping experience: the prognostic value of sentinel lymph node status in 612 stage I or II melanoma patients. *J Clin Oncol* 1999; 17: 976–83.
24. Thorn M, Ponten F, Bergstrom R, et al, Clinical and histopathologic predictors of survival in patients with malignant melanoma: a population-based study in Sweden. *J Natl Cancer Inst* 1997; 86: 761–9.
25. Kuehnl-Petzoldt C, Wiebelt H, Berger H, Prognostic groups of patients with stage I melanoma. *Arch Dermatol* 1983; 119: 816–19.
26. Essner R, Conforti A, Kelley MC, et al, Efficacy of lymphadenectomy and selective complete lymph node dissection as a therapeutic procedure for early-stage melanoma. *Ann Surg Oncol* 1999; 4: 442–9.
27. Wanebo HJ, Cooper PH, Young DV, et al, Progostic factors in head and neck melanoma. Effect of lesion location. *Cancer* 1988; 62: 831–7.
28. Schuchter L, Schultz DJ, Synnestvedt M, et al, A prognostic model for predicting 10-year survival in patients with primary melanoma. *Ann Intern Med* 1996; 125: 369–75.
29. Ostmeier H, Fuchs B, Otto F, et al, Can immunohistochemical markers and mitotic rate improve prognostic precision in patients with primary melanoma? *Cancer* 1999; 85: 2391–9.
30. Balch CM, Wilkerson JA, Murad TM, et al, The prognostic significance of ulceration of cutaneous melanoma. *Cancer* 1980; 45: 3012–7.
31. Balch CM, Cutaneous melanoma: prognosis and treatment results worldwide. *Semin Surg Oncol* 1992; 8: 400–14.
32. Cascinelli N, Marubini E, Morabito A, et al, Prognostic factors for stage I melanoma of the skin: a review. *Stat Med* 1985; 4: 265–78.
33. Masback A, Westerdahl J, Ingvar C, et al, Cutaneous malignant melanoma in southern Sweden 1965, 1975, and 1985. Prognostic factors and histologic correlations. *Cancer* 1997; 79: 275–83.
34. Sahin S, Rao B, Kopf AW, et al, Predicting ten-year survival of patients with primary cutaneous melanoma: corroboration of a prognostic model. *Cancer* 1997; 80: 1426–31.
35. Shaw HM, Balch CM, Soong SJ, et al, Prognostic histopathological factors in malignant melanoma. *Pathology* 1985; 17: 271–4.
36. Soong SJ, Harrison RA, McCarthy WH, et al, Factors affecting survival following local regional, or distant recurrence from localized melanoma. *J Surg Oncol* 1998; 67: 228–33.
37. Urist MM, Balch CM, Soong SJ, et al, Head and neck melanoma in 534 clinical stage I patients. A prognostic factors analysis and results of surgical treatment. *Ann Surg* 1984; 200: 769–75.
38. Gershenwald JE, Thompson W, Mansfield PF, et al, Multi-institutional melanoma lymphatic mapping experience: the prognostic value of sentinel lymph node status in 612 stage I or II melanoma patients. *J Clin Oncol* 1999; 17: 976–83.
39. Haffner AC, Garbe C, Burg G, et al, The prognosis of primary and metastasising melanoma. An evaluation of the TNM classification in 2495 patients. *Br J Cancer* 1992; 66: 856–61.
40. Haddad FF, Stall A, Messina J, et al, The progression of melanoma nodal metastasis is dependent on tumour thickness of the primary lesion. *Ann Surg Oncol* 1999; 6: 144–9.
41. Day CLJ, Mihm MCJ, Lew RA, et al, Prognostic factors for patients with clinical stage I melanoma of intermediate thickness (1.51–3.39 mm). A conceptual model for tumour growth and metastasis. *Ann Surg* 1982; 195: 35–43.
42. Cascinelli N, Marubini E, Morabito A, et al, Prognostic factors for stage I melanoma of the skin: a review. *Stat Med* 1985; 4: 265–78.
43. McGovern VJ, Shaw HM, Milton GW, et al, Prognostic significance of the histological features of malignant melanoma. *Histopathology* 1979; 3: 385–93.
44. Wagner JD, Gordon MS, Chuang TY, et al, Predicting sentinel and residual lymph node basin disease after sentinel lymph node biopsy for melanoma. *Cancer* 2000; 89: 453–62.
45. Straume O, Akslen LA, Independent prognostic importance of vascular invasion in nodular melanomas. *Cancer* 1996; 78: 1211–19.
46. Balch CM, Soong S-J, Ross MI, et al, Long-term results of a multi-institutional randomized trial comparing prognostic factors and surgical results for intermediate thickness melanomas (1.0 to 4.0 mm). *Ann Surg Oncol* 2000; 7: 87–97.
47. Keefe M, Mackie RM, The relationship between risk of death from clinical stage I cutaneous melanoma and thickness of primary tumour: no evidence for steps in risk. *Br J Cancer* 1991; 64: 598–602.
48. Karakousis CP, Emrich LJ, Rao U, Tumour thickness and prognosis in clinical stage I malignant melanoma. *Cancer* 1989; 64: 1432–6.
49. Day Jr CL, Lew RA, Mihm Jr MC, et al, The natural break points for primary-tumour thickness in clinical stage I melanoma. *NEJM* 1981; 305: 1155.
50. Balch CM, Soong SJ, Murad TM, et al, A multifactorial analysis of melanoma. II. Prognostic factors in patients with stage I (localized) melanoma. *Surgery* 1979; 86: 343–51.
51. Balch CM, Murad TM, Soong SJ, et al, Tumour thickness as a guide to surgical management of clinical stage I melanoma patients. *Cancer* 1979; 43: 883–8.
52. Balch CM, Wilkerson JA, Murad TM, et al, The prognostic significance of ulceration of cutaneous melanoma. *Cancer* 1980; 45: 3012–17.
53. McGovern VJ, Shaw HM, Milton GW, et al, Ulceration and prognosis in cutaneous malignant melanoma. *Histopathology* 1982; 6: 399–407.
54. Lock-Angersen J, Hou-Jensen K, Hansen JP, et al, Observer variation in histological classification of cutaneous malignant melanoma. *Scand J Plast Reconstr Surg Hand Surg* 1995; 29: 141–8.
55. Corona R, Mele A, Amini M, et al, Interobserver variability on the histopathologic diagnosis of cutaneous melanoma and other pigmented skin lesions. *J Clin Oncol* 1996; 14: 1218–23.
56. Larsen TE, Little JH, Orell SR, et al, International pathologists congruence survey on quantitation of malignant melanoma. *Pathology* 1980; 12: 245–53.
57. Heenan PJ, Matz LR, Blackwell JB, et al, Inter-observer variation between pathologists in the classification of cutaneous malignant melanoma in Western Australia. *Histopathology* 1984; 8: 717–29.
58. Vollmer R, Malignant melanoma. A multivariate analysis of prognostic factors. *Pathol Annu* 1989; 24: 383–407.
59. Masback A, Westerdahl J, Ingvar C, et al, Cutaneous malignant melanoma in Southern Sweden 1965, 1975, and 1985. *Cancer* 1997; 79: 275–83.
60. Balch CM, Soong SJ, Milton GW, et al, A comparison of prognostic factors and surgical results in 1,786 patients with localized (stage I) melanomas treated in Alabama, USA, and New South Wales, Australia. *Ann Surg* 1982; 196: 677–84.
61. Balch CM, Soong SJ, Bartolucci AA, et al, Efficacy of an elective regional lymph node dissection of 1 to 4 mm thick melanomas for patients 60 years of age and younger. *Ann Surg* 1996; 224: 255–63; discussion 263–6.
62. Balch CM, Urist MM, Karakousis CP, et al, Efficacy of 2-cm surgical margins for intermediate-thickness melanomas (1 to 4 mm). Results of a multi-institutional randomized surgical trial. *Ann Surg* 1993; 218: 262–7; discussion 267–9.
63. Heaton KM, Sussman JJ, Gershenwald JE, et al, Surgical margins and prognostic factors in patients with thick (>4mm) primary melanoma. *Ann Surg Oncol* 1998; 5: 322–8.
64. Kim SH, Garcia C, Rodriguez J, et al, Prognosis of thick cutaneous melanoma. *J Am Coll Surg* 1999; 188: 241–7.
65. Mraz-Gernhard S, Sagebiel RW, Kashani-Sabet M, et al, Prediction of sentinel lymph node micrometastasis by histological features in primary cutaneous malignant melanoma. *Arch Derm* 1998; 134: 983–7.

66. Marghoob AA, Koenig K, Bittencourt FV, et al, Breslow thickness and clark level in melanoma: support for including level in pathology reports and in American Joint Committee on Cancer Staging. *Cancer* 2000; 88: 589–95.
67. MacKie RM, Aitchison T, Sirel JM, et al, Prognostic models for subgroups of melanoma patients from the Scottish Melanoma Group database 1979–86, and their subsequent validation. *Br J Cancer* 1995; 71: 173–76.
68. Day Jr CL, Lew RA, Harrist TJ, Malignant melanoma prognostic factors 4: Ulceration width. *J Dermatol Surg Oncol* 1984; 10: 23–4.
69. Balch CM, Soong SJ, Murad TM, et al, A multifactorial analysis of melanoma: III. Prognostic factors in melanoma patients with lymph node metastates (stage II). *Ann Surg* 1981; 193: 377–88.
70. Buzaid AC, Ross MI, Balch CM, et al, Critical analysis of the current American Joint Committee on Cancer staging system for cutaneous melanoma and proposal of a new staging system. *J Clin Oncol* 1997; 15: 1039–51.
71. Clark Jr WH, From L, Bernardino EA, Mihm MC, The histogenesis and biological behavior of primary human malignant melanoma of the skin. *Cancer Res* 1969; 29: 705–27.
72. Prade M, Sancho-Garnier H, Cesarini JP, et al, Difficulties encountered in the application of Clark classification and the Breslow thickness measurement in cutaneous malignant melanoma. *Int J Cancer* 1980; 26: 159–63.
73. Mansson-Brahme E, Carstensen J, Erhardt K, et al, Prognostic factors in thin cutaneous malignant melanoma. *Cancer* 1994; 73: 2324–32.
74. Morton DL, Davtyan DG, Wanek LA, et al, Multivariate analysis of the relationship between survival and the microstage of primary melanoma by Clark level and Breslow thickness. *Cancer* 1993; 71: 3737–43.
75. Finley JW, Gibbs JF, Rodriguez LM, et al, Pathologic and clinical features influencing outcome of thin cutaneous melanoma: correlation with newly proposed staging system [In Process Citation]. *Am Surg* 2000; 66: 527–531; discussion 531–2.
76. Salman SM, Rogers GS, Prognostic factors in thin cutaneous malignant melanoma [see comments]. *J Dermatol Surg Oncol* 1990; 16: 413–18.
77. Shaw HM, McCarthy WH, McCarthy SW, et al, Thin malignant melanomas and recurrence potential. *Arch Surg* 1987; 122: 1147–50.
78. Austin PF, Cruse CW, Lyman G, et al, Age as a prognostic factor in the malignant melanoma population. *Ann Surg Oncol* 1994; 1: 487–94.
79. Cohen HJ, Cox E, Manton K, et al, Malignant melanoma in the elderly. *J Clin Oncol* 1987; 5: 100–6.
80. Austin PF, Cruse CW, Lyman G, et al, Age as a prognostic factor in the malignant melanoma population. *Ann Surg Oncol* 1994; 1: 487–94.
81. Loggie B, Ronan SG, Bean J, et al, Invasive cutaneous melanoma in elderly patients. *Arch Dermatol* 1991; 127: 1188–93.
82. Shaw HM, McGovern VJ, Milton GW, et al, The female superiority in survival in clinical stage II cutaneous malignant melanoma. *Cancer* 1982; 49: 1941–4.
83. Kirkwood JM, Ibrahim JG, Sondak VK, et al, High- and low-dose interferon alfa-2b in high-risk melanoma: first analysis of intergroup trial E1690/S9111/C9190. *J Clin Oncol* 2000; 18: 2444–58.
84. Kirkwood JM, Strawderman MH, Ernstoff MS, et al, Interferon alfa-2b adjuvant therapy of high risk resected cutaneous melanoma: the Eastern Cooperative Oncology Group Trial EST 1684. *J Clin Oncol* 1996; 14: 7–17.
85. Manola J, Atkins M, Ibrahim J, et al, Prognostic factors in metastatic melanoma: A pooled analysis of eastern cooperative oncology group trials. *J Clin Oncol* 2000; 18: 3782–93.
86. *NCI Fact Book.* Bethesda, MD: National Cancer Institute, 2000.
87. Cascinelli N, Zurrida S, Galimberti V, et al, Acral lentiginous melanoma. A histological type without prognostic significance. *J Dermatol Surg Oncol* 1994; 20: 817–22.
88. McGovern VJ, Shaw HM, Milton GW, et al, Is malignant melanoma arising in a Hutchinson's melanotic freckle a separate disease entity? *Histopathology* 1980; 4: 235–42.
89. Kuchelmeister C, Schaumburg-Lever G, Garbe C, Acral cutaneous melanoma in caucasians: clinical features, histopathology and prognosis in 112 patients. *Br J Dermatol* 2000; 143: 275–80.
90. Slingluff CL Jr, Vollmer R, Seigler HF, Acral melanoma: a review of 185 patients with dentification of prognostic variables. *J Surg Oncol* 1990; 45: 91–8.
91. Garge CBP, Bertz J, et al, Primary cutaneous melanoma: Prognostic classification of anatomical location. *Cancer* 1995; 75: 2492.
92. Carlson J, Dickersin GR, Sober AJ, et al, Desmoplastic neurotropic melanoma. *Cancer* 1995; 75: 478.
93. Quinn MJ, Crotty KA, Thompson JF, et al, Desmoplastic and desmoplastic neurotropic melanoma: experience with 280 patients. *Cancer* 1998; 83: 1128–35.
94. Balch CM, Soong SJ, Murad TM, et al, A multifactorial analysis of melanoma: III. Prognostic factors in melanoma patients with lymph node metastases (stage II). *Ann Surg* 1981; 193: 377–88.
95. Coit DG, Rogatko A, Brennan MF, Prognostic factors in patients with melanoma metastatic to axillary or inguinal lymph nodes. A multivariate analysis. *Ann Surg* 1991; 214: 627–36.
96. Buzaid AC, Tinoco LA, Jendiroba D, et al, Prognostic value of size of lymph node metastases in patients with cutaneous melanoma. *J Clin Oncol* 1995; 13: 2361–8.
97. Koh HK, Sober AJ, Day Jr CL, et al, Prognosis of clinical stage I melanoma patients with positive elective regional node dissection. *J Clin Oncol* 1986; 4: 1238–44.
98. Drepper H, Biess B, Hofherr B, et al, The prognosis of patients with stage III melanoma. *Cancer* 1993; 71: 1239–46.
99. Cascinelli N, Vaglini M, Nava M, et al, Prognosis of skin melanoma with regional node metastases (stage II). *Surg Oncol* 1984; 25: 240–7.
100. Morton DL, Wanek L, Nizze JA, et al, Improved long-term survival after lymphadenectomy of melanoma metastatic to regional nodes. *Ann Surg* 1991; 214: 491–9.
101. Slingluff Jr CL, Vollmer R, Seigler HF, Stage II malignant melanoma: Presentation of a prognostic model and an assessment of specific active immunotherapy in 1,273 patients. *J Surg Oncol* 1988; 39: 139–47.
102. Karakousis CP, Hena MA, Emrich LJ, et al, Axillary node dissection in malignant melanoma: Results and complications. *Surgery* 1990; 108: 10–17.
103. Kissin MW, Simpson DA, Easton D, et al, Prognostic factors related to survival and groin recurrence following therapeutic lymph node dissection for lower limb malignant melanoma. *Br J Surg* 1987; 74: 1023–6.
104. Roses DF, Provet JA, Harris MN, et al, Prognosis of patients with pathologic stage II cutaneous malignant melanoma. *Ann Surg* 1985; 201: 103–7.
105. Calabro A, Singletary SE, Balch CM, Patterns of relapse in 1001 consecutive patients with melanoma nodal metastases. *Arch Surg* 1989; 124: 1051–5.
106. Gershenwald JE, Prieto V, Colome-Grimmer MI, et al, The prognostic significance of microscopic tumour burden in 925 melanoma patients undergoing sentinel lymph node biopsy. *Proc Am Soc Clin Oncol* 2000; 19: 551a.
107. Cascinelli N, Belli F, Santinami M, et al, Sentinel lymph node biopsy in cutaneous melanoma: the WHO Melanoma Program experience [In Process Citation]. *Ann Surg Oncol* 2000; 7: 469–74.
108. Morton DL, Wanek L, Nizze JA, et al, Improved long-term survival after lymphadenectomy of melanoma metastatic to regional nodes. Analysis of prognostic factors in 1134 patients from the John Wayne Cancer Clinic. *Ann Surg* 1991; 214: 491–9.
109. Grenshenwald JE, Colome MI, Lee JF, et al, Patterns of recurrence following a negative sentinel lymph node biopsy in 243 patients with stage I or II melanoma. *J Clin Oncol* 1998; 16: 2253–60.
110. Cascinelli N, Bufalino R, Marolda R, et al, Regional non-nodal metastases of cutaneous melanoma. *Eur J Surg Oncol* 1986; 12: 175–80.
111. Day CJ, Harrist T, Gorstein F, et al, Malignant melanoma: Prognostic significance of 'microscopic satellites' in the reticular dermis and subcutaneous fat. *Ann Surg* 1981; 194: 108–12.
112. Leon P, Daly JM, Synnestvedt M, et al, The prognostic implications of microscopic satellites in patients with clinical stage I melanoma. *Arch Surg* 1991; 126: 1461–8.
113. Harrist T, Rigel D, Day Jr C, et al, 'Microscopic satellites' are more highly associated with regional lymph node metastases than with primary melanoma thickness. *Cancer* 1984; 53: 2183–7.

114. Balch CM, Soong SJ, Murad TM, et al, A multifactorial analysis of melanoma. IV. Prognostic factors in 200 melanoma patients with distant metastases (stage III). *J Clin Oncol* 1983; 1: 126–34.
115. Barth A, Wanek LA, Morton DL, Prognostic factors in 1,521 melanoma patients with distant metastases. *J Am Coll Surg* 1995; 181: 193–201.
116. Keilholz U, Conradt C, Legha SS, et al, Results of interleukin-2-based treatment in advanced melanoma: A case record-based analysis of 631 patients. *J Clin Oncol* 1998; 16: 2921–9.
117. Eton O, Legha SS, Moon TE, et al, Prognostic factors for survival of patients treated systemically for disseminated melanoma. *J Clin Oncol* 1998; 16: 1103–11.
118. Brand CU, Ellwanger U, Stroebel W, et al, Prolonged survival of 2 years or longer for patients with disseminated melanoma. *Cancer* 1997; 79: 2345–53.
119. Bowen GM, Chang AE, Lowe L, et al, Solitary melanoma confined to the dermal and/or subcutaneous tissue: evidence for revisiting the staging classification. *Arch Dermatol* 2000; 136: 1397–9.
120. Deichmann M, Benner A, Bock M, et al, S100-Beta, melanoma-inhibiting activity, and lactate dehydrogenase discriminate progressive from nonprogressive American Joint Committee on Cancer stage IV melanoma. *J Clin Oncol* 1999; 17: 1891–6.
121. Franzke A, Probst-Kepper M, Buer J, et al, Elevated pretreatment serum levels of soluble vascular cell adhesion molecule 1 and lactate dehydrogenase as predictors of survival in cutaneous metastatic malignant melanoma. *Br J Cancer* 1998; 78: 40–5.
122. Sirott M, Bajorin D, Wong G, et al, Prognostic factors in patients with metastatic malignant malanoma. A multivariate analysis. *Cancer* 1993; 72: 3091.
123. Agrawal S, Yao T-J, Coit DG, Surgery for melanoma metastatic to the gastrointestinal tract. *Ann Surg Oncol* 1999; 6: 336–44.
124. Balch C, Surgical treatment of advanced melanoma, In: *Cutaneous melanoma* (eds Balch C, Houghton AN, Sober AJ, Soong SJ) St Louis, MO: Quality Medical Press, 1998: 373–88.
125. Ollila DW, Hsueh EC, Stern SL, et al, Metastasectomy for recurrent stage IV melanoma. *J Surg Oncol* 1999; 71: 209–13.
126. Wong JH, Skinner KA, Kim KA, et al, The role of surgery in the treatment of nonregionally recurrent melanoma. *Surgery* 1993; 113: 389–94.
127. Eton O, Legha SS, Moon TE, et al, Prognostic factors for survival of patients treated systemically for disseminated melanom. *J Clin Oncol* 1998; 16: 1103–11.
128. Khadra MH, Thompson JF, Milton GM, McCarthy WH, The justification for surgical treatment of metastatic melanoma of the gastrointestinal tract. *Surg Gynecol Obstet* 1990; 171: 413–16.
129. LaHei ER, Thompson JF, McCaughan BC, Ramanaden D, Is resection of pulmonary metastases from malignant melanoma worthwhile? *Melanoma Res* 1993; 3: 102.
130. Bostick PJ, Morton DL, Turner RR, et al, Prognostic significance of occult metastases detected by sentinel lymphadenectomy and reverse transcriptase-polymerase chain reaction in early-stage melanoma patients. *J Clin Oncol* 1999; 17: 3238–44.
131. Curry BJ, Farrelly M, Hersey P, Evaluation of S-100beta assays for the prediction of recurrence and prognosis in patients with AJCC stage I-III melanoma. *Melanoma Res* 1999; 9: 556–67.
132. Kelley MC, Ollila DW, Morton DL, Lymphatic mapping and sentinel lymphadenectomy for melanoma. *Semin Surg Oncol* 1998; 14: 283–90.
133. van der Velde-Zimmermann D, Schipper ME, de Weger RA, et al, Sentinel node biopsies in melanoma patients: a protocol for accurate, efficient, and cost-effective analysis by preselection for immunohistochemistry on the basis of Tyr-PCR. *Ann Surg Oncol* 2000; 7: 51–4.
134. van der Velde-Zimmermann D, Roijers JF, Bouwens-Rombouts A, et al, Molecular test for the detection of tumour cells in blood and sentinel nodes of melanom patients. *Am J Pathol* 1996; 149: 759–64.
135. von Schoultz E, Hansson LO, Djureen E, et al, Prognostic value of serum analyses of S-100 beta protein in malignant melanoma. *Melanoma Res* 1996: 6: 133–7.
136. Shivers SC, Wang X, Li W, et al, Molecular staging of malignant melanoma: correlation with clinical outcome. *JAMA* 1998; 280: 1410–15.

16

Melanoma precursor lesions: recognition and management

Richard GB Langley, Seaver Soon, Jason K Rivers

Cutaneous melanoma may arise de novo in previously normal skin, or it may develop in a pre-existing lesion. Such a pre-existing lesion is understood to be a precursor, which implies a temporal and spatial relation, (occurring prior to the malignancy).[1] Certain lesions, such as clinically atypical naevi (dysplastic naevi, Clark's naevi), may be both precursors and markers of an increased risk of melanoma. Recognition of these lesions is of importance in identifying patients at risk of developing melanoma, for surveillance to facilitate the early diagnosis of melanoma, and in certain cases so that prophylactic removal of high risk lesions can be performed. The importance of early diagnosis is well recognized, as thickness of the primary tumour is the most important prognostic indicator in primary cutaneous melanoma.[2–4] Early recognition of melanoma can lead to the detection and excision of highly curable lesions. This chapter will review the clinical features of these precursor lesions and current management guidelines.

CLINICALLY ATYPICAL NAEVI (DYSPLASTIC MELANOCYTIC NAEVI, CLARK'S NAEVI)

Definition

Dysplastic naevi (DN) are acquired, clinically atypical appearing, melanocytic lesions characterized by atypical melanocytes arranged in a lentiginous pattern, with fibroplasia and dermal lymphocytic infiltration. International cohort and case–control studies have provided compelling evidence for the role of DN as a potential precursor to melanoma and as a marker for increased melanoma risk in affected individuals. DN may occur in the context of familial cutaneous melanoma or, more commonly, as a sporadic entity.

International epidemiological studies reveal a relatively high prevalence of DN in white populations. In the United States, 1.8% to 4.9% of adults have been reported to have DN.[5,6] Reported prevalences worldwide vary considerably, ranging from less than 1% to 20% in different populations.[7–13] The observed variation in international prevalence probably reflects differences in the diagnostic criteria used to identify DN.[14]

Clinical features

Considerable controversy and debate in dermatology and dermatopathology has centred on issues of nomenclature, diagnostic features, and the significance of DN. No reliable clinical criteria exist to allow precise distinction between 'normal' naevi, those with degrees of 'atypia' and melanoma. The absence of definite clinical variables, however, highlights the concept that DN probably represents a spectrum of lesions with varying degrees of atypia, rather than a distinct clinical entity.[1]

In general, considerations such as size, colour, symmetry, and border distinguish DN from the common melanocytic naevus, which classically exhibits moderate size (usually <5 mm), uniformity in colour, symmetry and a well demarcated border (Figure 16.1). DN

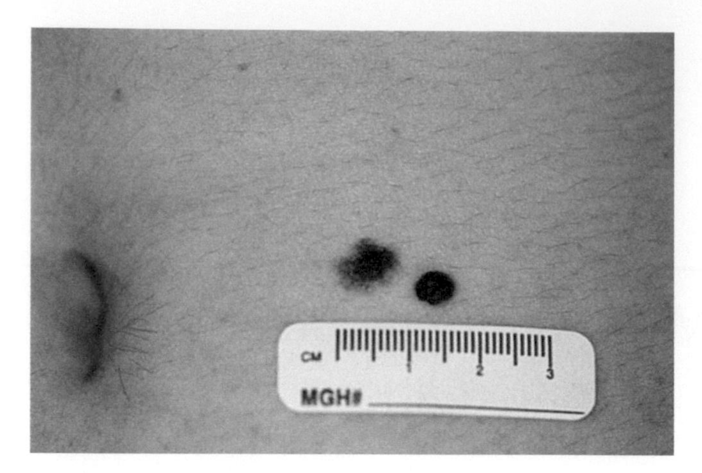

Figure 16.1 *Dysplastic naevus (left) and compound naevus (right). Compare the compound naevus on the right, well circumscribed, uniformly pigmented papule, with the dysplastic naevus on the left, which has minimal colour variation and a border fading into the surrounding skin, Reproduced with permission from Langley RG et al., Clinical presentation: melanoma. In:* American Cancer Society atlas of clinical oncology *(eds Haluska F, Sober AJ). Hamilton: BC Decker, 2001: 49–59.*[93]

denotes a melanocytic lesion 5 mm or greater in diameter with a macular morphology by definition (or the presence of a macular component).[15] The lesions may be round, oval, or asymmetrical, and may show variegation in colour, with shades of brown, tan, and pink within the same lesion (Figure 16.2). Pink coloration may be related to a relative excess of red pheomelanin compared with brown eumelanin pigment in DN, in addition to dermal inflammation.[16] Foci of black pigmentation are comparatively rare. The border in DN may be irregular, poorly demarcated, or 'fuzzy' around the whole or part of its circumference. The border may blend imperceptibly with adjacent normal skin in clinically atypical naevi, whereas the border often has an abrupt, sharp cut off in melanoma. Some DN may exhibit a so-called fried egg or target shaped appearance, where the central naevus is one colour and the peripheral component is another shade. A papular component, if present, is usually located in the centre of an ovoid macule. Outside the familial cutaneous melanoma syndrome, one study reported an average of 10 DN per person, although affected individuals may have just one or several hundred lesions (Figure 16.3).[17] DN are located more often on sun exposed areas such as the back and chest, but may also occur in typically sun protected areas such as the scalp, buttocks, and the female breast. No definite clinical parameters exist to

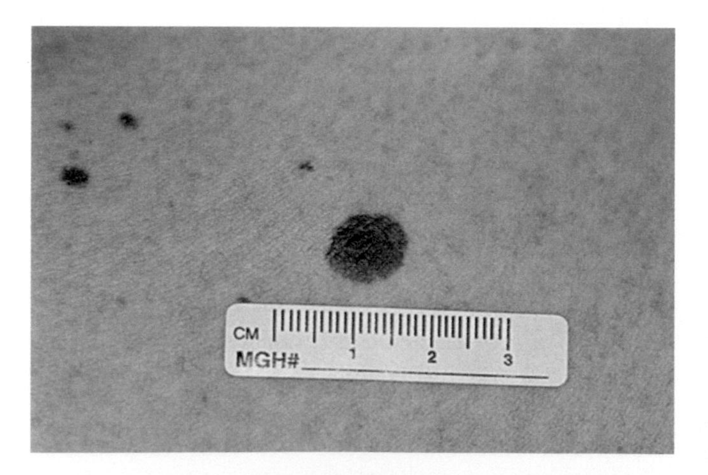

Figure 16.2 *Dysplastic naevus. This lesion has a target-like appearance with darker brown pigmentation centrally and lighter tan brown pigmentation peripherally.*

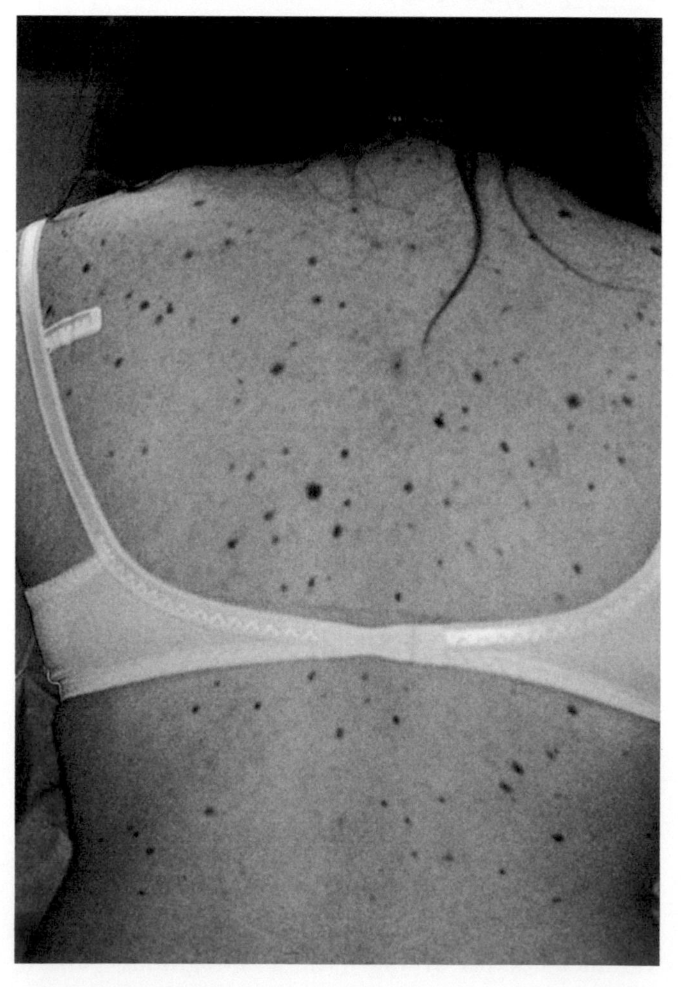

Figure 16.3 *Multiple atypical naevi on the back.*

reliably predict histological atypia; however, total number of naevi, the presence of a macular component, size greater than 4 mm, the presence of irregular or ill defined borders, and pink colour are all associated with varying degrees of histological dysplasia.[18]

DN can undergo dynamic evolution over time. In one cohort study, 153 people with DN were followed for an average of 89 months.[19] Fifty one per cent (297 of 593) of DN showed clinical signs of change during the follow up period: 15% became more atypical, whereas 35% became less atypical. Appearance of new naevi in adulthood was notably more common than previously thought, with 20% of patients over age 50 developing new lesions. Conversely, 38 naevi disappeared in 28 patients.[19] In melanoma prone families, DN usually appear by age 20 years in individuals with ongoing development of new moles over time.[20]

The issue of reliable histological criteria for the diagnosis of DN mirrors its clinical counterpart as a topic of controversy.[21,22] In an attempt to determine reliable histological criteria for DN, the World Health Organization (WHO) Melanoma Program convened a consensus conference to define histological criteria that would yield a high concordance among dermatopathologists' interpretation of melanocytic lesions.[14] Two major and four minor criteria were established that led to a mean concordance of 88% for DN. The major criteria were: (1) basilar proliferation of atypical naevomelanocytes extending at least three rete ridges beyond any dermal naevocellular component (if a dermal component is present) and (2) organization of this intraepidermal proliferation in a lentiginous or an epithelioid cell pattern. Minor criteria were (1) the presence of lamellar fibroplasia or concentric eosinophilic fibrosis, (2) neovascularization, (3) dermal inflammatory response, and (4) fusion of rete ridges. Diagnosis of DN requires the presence of both major criteria and at least two minor criteria.[14] No distinguishing histopathological features of DN were evident based on the presence or absence of a family history of cutaneous melanoma.

A variety of cutaneous lesions may simulate the clinical features of DN. Considerations in the differential diagnosis of DN include: in situ melanoma, seborrhoeic keratosis, pigmented basal cell carcinoma, pigmented spindle cell and/or epithelioid cell naevus, blue naevus, combined naevi (Spitz naevus) and darkly pigmented solar lentigo.[11]

Genetics

Formal genetic analysis suggests an autosomal dominant mode of inheritance for DN, although the precise role of melanoma susceptibility genes in the development of DN remains uncertain. One case–control study drawn from a large private dermatology practice matched 25 patients with DN to 28 controls without DN.[23] Examination for DN of all consenting first degree relatives of both cases and controls revealed atypical naevi in 80% of relatives of cases and in only 4% of relatives of controls. The relative risk of possessing DN if one or more relatives had DN was 7.2. Formal genetic analysis performed on this study group for a hypothetical DN gene yielded an estimated segregation ratio of 0.52. This finding was consistent with an autosomal dominant mode of inheritance.[24]

The evidence for a relation between the putative melanoma susceptibility gene, CDKN2A, and the development of DN is, however, less well defined. A melanoma susceptibility gene on chromosome 9p21 has been confirmed, and the cell cycle regulator CDKN2A, which codes for the protein p16, has been proposed as the candidate gene for this locus.[25–27] Germline mutations in this gene have been identified in about 20% of melanoma prone families.[28] Analysis of various melanoma cell lines showed homozygous deletion of CDKN2A in 61% of various melanoma cell lines.[29] Inclusion of DN in the linkage analysis for 9p, however, produces mixed results. In the Dutch series of melanoma families, lod scores for linkage to 9p were strengthened when DN were included in the model.[30] In the National Cancer Institute series, however, evidence for 9p linkage was weakened by including DN in the analytic model.[31] Microdissection studies nevertheless suggest that CDKN2A mutations may be an important early genetic event in the evolution of sporadic DN.[32] Additional work is necessary in this area to better delineate the relation between DN and melanoma susceptibility genes. In summary, although evidence suggests an autosomal dominant mode of inheritance of DN, the relation of DN to melanoma susceptibility genes remains to be established.

Dysplastic naevus as a marker and precursor for melanoma

DN are markers and potential precursors for cutaneous melanoma. This evidence derives principally from two study methods: (1) case–control studies that show an excess prevalence of DN in melanoma cases relative to controls and (2) cohort studies that show an excess in melanoma incidence in familial melanoma and sporadic DN cohorts relative to the general population.

Numerous case–control studies have established DN as one of the most important markers of increased melanoma risk.[33–47] Table 16.1 summarizes the results of these studies. Methodologically, these studies compare the prevalence of DN or atypical naevi in patients with melanoma (cases) with the prevalence of DN in demographically matched patients (controls). Although most of these studies define and count DN/atypical naevi in different ways, they have in common that all diagnoses of DN were established clinically. Thus, the debate concerning reliable histological criteria for DN diagnosis becomes less relevant to the predominant conclusion that the presence of clinically determined DN represents one of the most important markers of melanoma risk.[28] The prevalence of DN among case–control studies shows that 33% of patients with melanoma possess DN, compared with only 11% of matched controls.[28] The relative risk for melanoma conferred by the presence of DN in case–control studies ranges from 1.0 to 10.4 (median 5.4).[27] The increased risk associated with DN persists after adjustment for potentially confounding melanoma risk factors, such as total number of naevi, hair and eye colour, complexion type, tendency to freckle, history of sun exposure, and family history. Of interest, a number of these studies further report a dose-response relation whereby melanoma risk increases as the total number of DN increases (Table 16.1).[28,33,36,40,43,46,47] One large rigorous case–control study compared 716 melanoma patients with 1014 controls to investigate the relation between number and type of naevi (small naevi: <5 mm, large non-DN: >5 mm and DN) and the development of melanoma.[33] Risk for melanoma was significantly related to increased number of small naevi, large non-DN, and clinically DN ($P<0.001$). However, the degree of risk was substantially higher for DN relative to other types of naevi. The presence of even one DN was associated with a relative risk for melanoma of 2.3, while 10 or more DN conferred a relative risk of 12. By comparison, an increased number of small naevi was associated with a twofold risk, and increased numbers of both small and large non-DN was associated with a fourfold risk. When the results of case–control studies are viewed in aggregate, the increased percentage of melanoma cases and the elevated relative risk profiles associated with DN provide compelling evidence for the central role of DN as a marker for increased melanoma risk.

The status of DN as potent markers of melanoma risk has been further substantiated by cohort studies, which have prospectively documented an excess incidence of melanoma in both familial melanoma kindred[13,20,49–54] and in patients with sporadic DN.[51,52,54–59] Table 16.2 summarizes study results for familial melanoma cohorts, and Table 16.3 summarizes results for nonfamilial DN cohorts. Altogether, cohort studies consistently report three characteristics of melanoma prone kindred that strengthen the relation between DN and melanoma: (1) new melanoma occurs almost exclusively in family members with DN; (2) family members with DN, and especially those with a melanoma diagnosis before study entry, have significantly increased relative risks for melanoma; and (3) close surveillance of melanoma prone kindred leads to higher detection rates of early lesions (35% of all prospectively diagnosed melanomas were identified at an in situ stage).[28] An important cohort study of melanoma prone families evaluated 23 families (14 kindred in Greene et al.[20] with an addition of nine in Tucker et al.[49]) registered in the National Cancer Institute family studies section because the presence of two or more melanomas in their kindred indicated that all 23 kindred had DN in addition to melanoma. In total, 470 family members from 23 melanoma kindred were followed for up to 1591 person-years, during which 47 newly diagnosed melanomas occurred. All incident melanomas occurred in family members with DN. The cumulative risk of melanoma by age 50 years among kindred with DN was 48.9% +/– 4.2%, and rose to 81.6% +/– 6.7% by age 72 years. The relative risk of a prospective melanoma for family members with DN (but no personal history of melanoma) was 85. By comparison, the relative risk of a prospective melanoma among family members with DN and a previous melanoma was 229. There was no excess risk in family members with no DN and no personal melanoma history. Close surveillance was integral to the study design and was associated with a decrease in lesion thickness: 86% of prospective melanomas were less than 0.76 mm compared with 59% previously, and 76% of prospective melanomas were Clark level II or less compared with a previous rate of 52%.

Table 16.1 ***Relative risk of melanoma in case–control studies***

Study	Definition of DN	Number of DN	Relative risk
Nordlund et al.[35]	Atypical naevi	—	7.4
Cristofolini et al.[48]	Dysplastic naevi	—	1.4
Swerdlow et al.[36]	Large naevi	— 0 1–4 5+	3.9 1.0 5.2 5.7
Roush et al.[37]	Dysplastic naevi	—	7.6
Kelly et al.[38]	Dysplastic naevi	— 0 1–5 6+	6.0 1.0 3.8 6.3
Grob et al.[39]	Clinically atypical naevi	—	1.9
Halpern et al.[40]	Dysplastic naevi	—	6.8
Stierner et al.[41]	Dysplastic naevi	—	5.4
Newton et al.[34]	Atypical mole syndrome	—	7.5
Garbe et al.[42]	Clinically atypical naevi	— 0 1–4 5+	2.8 1.0 1.6 6.1
Holly et al.[43]	Large naevi	0 1–3 4–7 8+	1.0 4.5 6.1 16.7
Bataille et al.[46]	Atypical mole syndrome	— 0 1 2–3 4+	10.4 1.0 3.5 5.4 23.7
Grulich et al.[47]	Atypical naevi	0 1–2 3–4 5+	1.0 1.6 3.7 9.0
Tucker et al.[33]	Dysplastic naevi	0 1 2–4 5–9 10+	1.0 2.3 7.3 4.9 12.0

DN, dysplastic naevi.
Adapted from: Greene MH, *Cancer* 1999; 86:2464–77.[28]

Table 16.2 *Prospective melanoma diagnosis in familial dysplastic naevi*

Study	No. of families	No. of prospective cutaneous melanoma	Relative risk for cutaneous melanoma
Greene et al.[20]	14	Series updated in Tucker et al., see below[49]	
Vasen et al.[50]	9	20	NA
Rigel et al.[51]	NA	11	167
Masri et al.[13]	264	28	NA
MacKie et al.[52]	6	8	444
Tucker et al.[49]	23	77	DN 85, DN/CMM 229
Carey et al.[53]	311	40	DN 116, DN/CMM 964
Tiersten et al.[54]	NA	3	53

NA, not available; DN, dysplastic naevus patients; DN/CMM, dysplastic naevus patients with melanoma diagnosed before entry into study.
Adapted from: Greene MH, *Cancer* 1999; 86:2464–77.[28] © 1999 American Cancer Society. Reprinted by permission of Wiley-Liss, Inc., a subsidiary of John Wiley & Sons, Inc.

Table 16.3 *Prospective melanoma diagnosis in non-familial (sporadic) dysplastic naevi*

Study	Prior cutaneous melanoma	No. of subjects	No. of prospective cutaneous melanoma	Relative risk for cutaneous melanoma
Rigel et al.[51]	No Yes	281 66	4 3	16 36
Tiersten et al.[54]	No Yes	157 95	4 4	53 74
Halpern et al.[55]	No	89	2	154/100,000/year
MacKie et al.[52]	No Yes	85 24	9 3	93 91
Kang et al.[56]	No	84	2	NA
Marghoob et al.[57]	No Yes	124 163	10	63 90
Schneider et al.[58]	No	267	5	47
Kelly et al.[59]	No Yes	215 63	9 7	46

Adapted from: Greene MH, *Cancer* 1999; 86:2464–77.[28] © 1999 American Cancer Society. Reprinted by permission of Wiley-Liss, Inc., a subsidiary of John Wiley & Sons, Inc.

Findings of cohort studies in non-familial DN patients mirror those observed in patients with familial DN – except that relative risks for melanoma are lower (Table 16.3). A prospective cohort study by Kelly et al. involved 279 adults, each with five or more clinically DN.[59] The cohort was followed for a mean period of 42 months, and 20 new melanomas were diagnosed prospectively in 16 patients. The melanoma incidence in this cohort of sporadic DN was 46 times the incidence in the general population. A dose-response relation between number of DN and melanoma risk was observed: 5–10 DN was associated with a crude melanoma incidence of 807 whereas 21–50 DN was associated with a crude incidence of 3336. The study by Kelly et al. indicates that clinical photography may be valuable in the follow up of DN patients: 11 of 20 prospectively diagnosed melanomas were identified because of changes evident by comparison to baseline photographs. In summary, findings of numerous case–control and cohort studies of DN, both within and without the familial melanoma context, show that DN constitutes a strong and independent risk factor for melanoma.

Beyond its status as a melanoma risk marker, evidence from anatomical and histological studies suggests a potential role for DN as a precursor to melanoma. In the familial DN setting, one anatomical study correlated DN number and body site distribution in 45 patients with melanoma with body site distribution in a second group of 43 patients from the same DN kindred.[60] Similar sites of predilection for DN and melanoma were observed, providing preliminary evidence for a potential precursor relationship uniting these entities. Histological studies provide additional support for this putative connection by showing melanoma in-contiguity with DN, although the frequency of this histological picture varies between studies. In one large cohort study, Tucker et al. observed 199 melanomas in 23 familial melanoma families.[49] Histological review of these lesions showed 51% (101 of 199) to be associated with DN.[50] In a series of 225 melanoma cases, 'atypical melanocytic hyperplasia' (AMH) associated with lamellar fibrosis and lymphocytic infiltrates was observed in 21.8% of lesions.[61] In one retrospective review of 1101 melanoma cases, 23.3% were associated with melanocytic naevi. Histological classification of these naevi showed 37.7% to be dysplastic, 56.5% to be common acquired, and 5.8% to be congenital.[62] Finally, one population based study of 511 melanomas showed only 7% of melanomas to be contiguous with DN.[63] Overall, histological studies documenting DN in-contiguity with melanoma suggest a potential precursor role for DN in melanoma tumorigenesis, although the majority of melanoma lesions probably arise without an associated precursor. Public education efforts should thus emphasize surveillance for clinical features suggestive of melanoma in clinically normal skin, in addition to those occurring in pre-existing naevi.[62]

Management

Surgical excision of clinically suspicious lesions, regular follow up examinations, and sun protection form the cornerstones of management of DN. In surgical treatment, the challenge is to remove lesions with sufficient cytologic atypia while minimizing surgical morbidity. While seemingly uncomplicated, the frequent lack of correlation between the gross and microscopic appearance of a lesion may confound the assessment of its malignant potential. One study investigated the clinicopathological correlation for 1000 histological specimens submitted with the clinical diagnosis of DN, and found that only 54.7% of submitted lesions showed definitive features of DN.[64] Further, theoretical considerations by Seykora and Elder suggest that very few DN actually progress to become melanomas;[12] they estimate progression rates in the United States at only about one in 3000 sporadic DN. These considerations, and the fact that melanoma frequently arises on clinically normal skin, suggest that DN should not be managed as high risk precursor lesions. It is not practical or necessary to attempt to remove all clinically atypical lesions from patients presenting with numerous DN. In the light of evidence that only a fraction of these naevi will progress to melanoma and that melanoma often arises de novo on normal skin in patients with DN, adopting such a practice may prove clinically injudicious as it may create a false sense of security in patients that may impede follow up care.[1,59] Rather, DN should be understood and managed in the context of evidence relating to their status as a marker of increased melanoma risk requiring regular clinical examination to detect early cutaneous melanoma.

Evaluation of persons for pigmented lesions requires examination of the entire cutaneous surface area. Dermoscopy (dermatoscopy, epiluminescence microscopy) is a non-invasive clinical technique that may be a useful adjunct to clinical examination by enabling the clinician to visualize features not discernible to the naked eye.[65] It has been shown in experienced hands to improve the clinical diagnosis of melanoma and facilitate the differentiation of other benign and malignant pigmented skin lesions.[65,66] Computerized image analysis has also been developed to enhance the discrimination of melanoma from other benign pigmented skin lesions such as dysplastic naevi. Such methods offer the potential advantage of providing objective, reproducible results and avoiding the potential of subjectivity introduced with human interpretation of subtle clinical dermoscopic features.[67]

Baseline total body photographs or selective lesional photographs may also be used to detect new or changing naevi.[59] Lesions suggestive of melanoma must be removed promptly and subjected to histopathological assessment. DN located in difficult to monitor areas, such as the scalp and the perianal area, should be strongly considered for prophylactic removal.[11] The recommended method of removal of pigmented lesions is by excisional biopsy with narrow margins. Surgical excision of suspicious naevi must be followed by regular follow up surveillance for a lifetime in the form of both physician assessment and patient self examination. In addition to formal medical follow up, patients must be instructed in proper skin self examination. This practice should be performed every 1–2 months, with use of a handheld and full length mirror to facilitate visualization of the entire cutaneous surface, including areas that are difficult to assess. Family members should be encouraged to assist in monitoring, particularly of sites such as the scalp and back. Any change in size, pigmentation pattern, elevation, border characteristics, or any new lesion requires immediate attention. A recent population based case–control study suggests that skin self examination may reduce melanoma related mortality through earlier detection.[68] Finally, patients should be instructed in the principles of photoprotection. In particular, patients should be advised to avoid times of peak solar exposure (10 am–3 pm) and sunburns, to use appropriate clothing (such as broad brimmed hats and long sleeved shirts and pants), and sunscreens with a skin protection factor of at least 15 with broad spectrum coverage to protect against ultraviolet A and B.

CONGENITAL MELANOCYTIC NAEVI

Definition

Congenital melanocytic naevi (CMN) are melanocytic naevi present at birth. The naevomelanocytes may be present in an intraepidermal location, a dermal location, or both. Naevomelanocytes can extend deeply into the subcutis and can surround skin appendages, nerves, and vasculature.[69] Congenital naevi, by definition, should be present at birth; however, a rare variant, 'tardive naevi', has been described in which the naevus may not be apparent at birth, but presents up to 2 years of age (Figures 16.4–16.7).

Congential naevi can be classified by the size of the lesion. An arbitrary classification has generally been used which separates congenital naevi into three main groups, by size: small (<1.5 cm); intermediate (≥1.5 but <20 cm); and large (≥20 cm).[70] Large congenital melanocytic naevi (LCMN) have also been defined practically by the ease of surgical excision (inability to close the surgical defect primarily and requiring a skin flap or graft). This definition, although practical, is ambiguous in that certain anatomical sites may not be amenable to primary closure and require tissue movement or grafting based on location rather than absolute

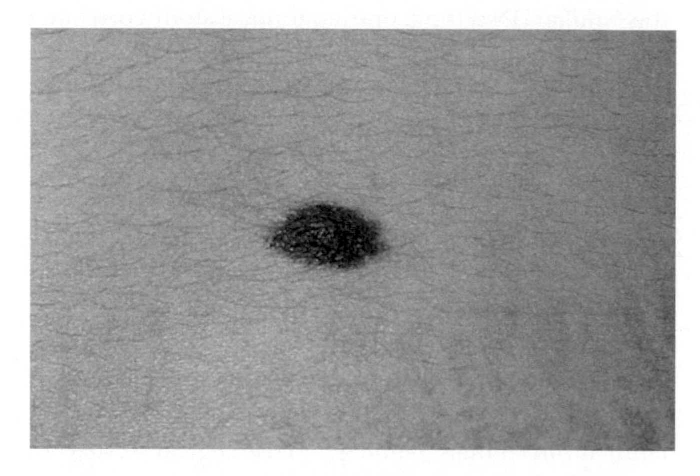

Figure 16.4 *Small congenital naevus. Courtesy of Dr Jennifer Klotz.*

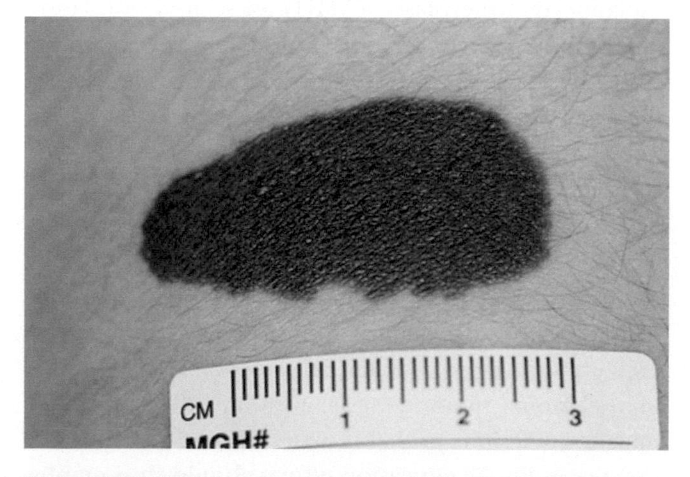

Figure 16.5 *This is an intermediate sized congenital naevus, which by definition was larger than 1.5 cm but extending less than 20 cm. Note the slight irregularity of the border and homogeneous pigmentation.*

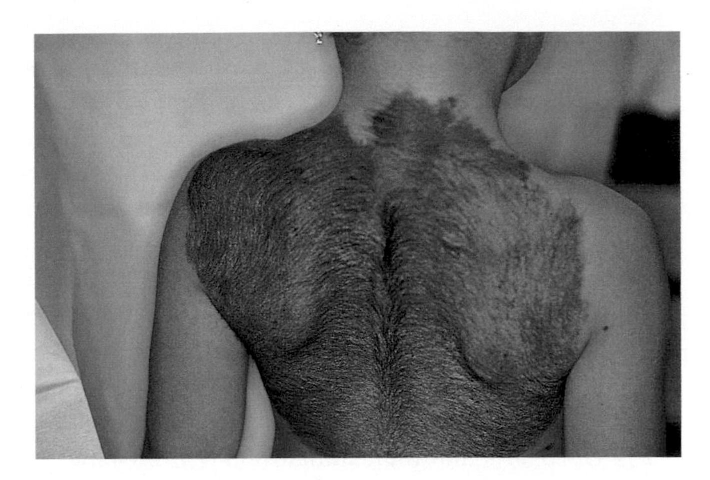

Figure 16.6 *This is a patient with a giant congenital naevus covering a large portion of the back resembling a garment distribution.*

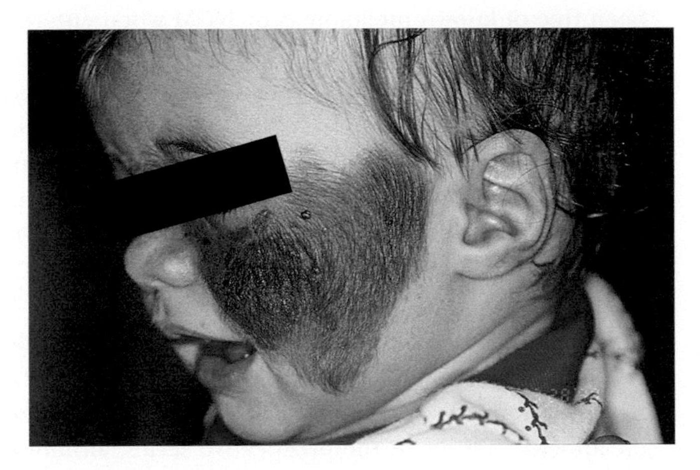

Figure 16.7 *This congenital naevus involved a notable portion of this child's cheek with prominent hypertrichosis evident, and different shades of brown. This lesion is highly disfiguring and was the cause of considerable concern to the parents, and was excised.*

size (i.e. lesions on the nose may be small in diameter, yet require a flap for closure for aesthetic or functional purposes). Large congenital naevi are also known by a number of descriptive synonyms: giant (hairy) naevi; garment naevi; or bathing suit naevi.[11]

Clinical features

Congenital melanocytic naevi may differ in clinical appearance from common naevi by size alone. Small and intermediate sized congenital naevi are typically symmetrical in shape, and round or oval in appearance (Figures 16.4 and 16.5). Large or giant congenital naevi may involve an entire anatomical segment of the trunk (garment or bathing suit distribution), the head and neck, or the extremities (Figure 16.6 and 16.7). There may be associated satellite congenital naevi. Pigmentation can be uniform or may be varied, with different shades of tan to brown colour. Black colour is less frequent and may indicate atypical histopathological features in lightly pigmented patients.[11] Congenital naevi may be hair bearing, often with dark coarse terminal hairs present. The surface of congenital naevi can have a varied appearance, and may be smooth, verrucous, or cerebriform (Figure 16.8). Giant congenital naevi may appear lobular, and may develop nodules within them. These nodules need to be assessed for the presence of malignancy, although they may simply represent benign cellular proliferative lesions.[71]

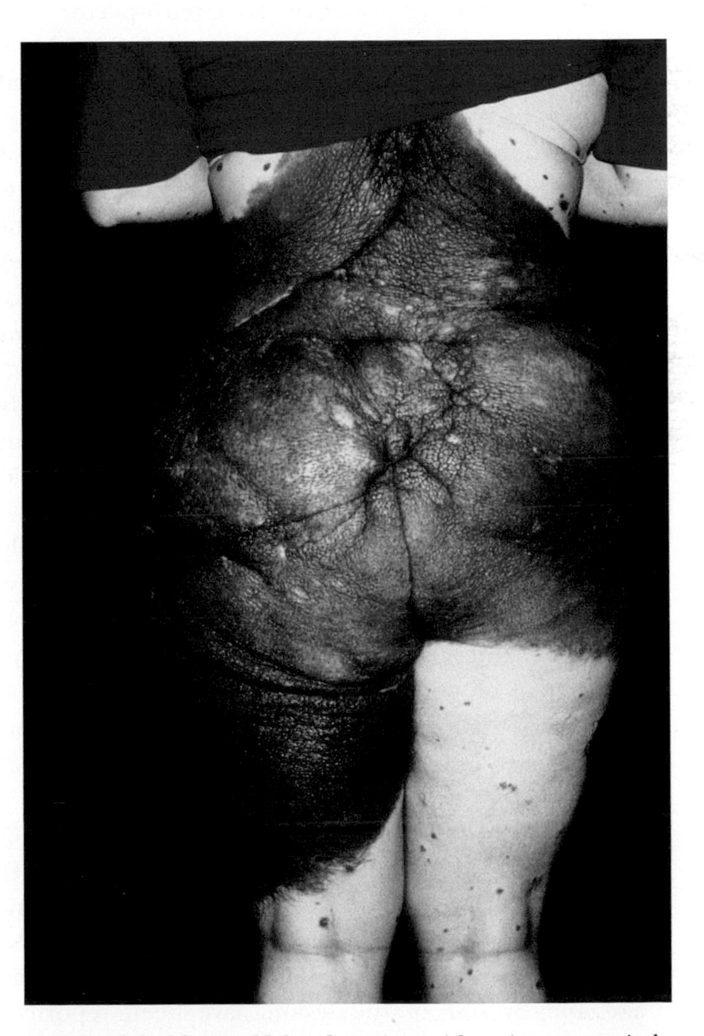

Figure 16.8 *38-year-old female patient with a giant congenital melanocytic naevus. Note the lobular appearance of this lesion. Lobular and nodular areas can develop in these lesions and can be benign, as in this case. Courtesy of Dr Robert Miller.*

Patients with a congenital melanocytic naevus may have associated meningeal involvement, particularly when the naevus overlies the midline. Location and size of the naevus are important: in patients with LCMN present in a posterior axial location there is a greater risk for the development of neurocutaneous melanosis, particularly when associated with 'satellite' melanocytic naevi, compared with patients with LCMN limited to the extremities or those who lack satellite naevi.[72]

Congenital naevi as precursors

Congenital naevi are recognized potential precursors of melanoma, although the degree of risk is contentious depending on the size of the lesion.[73–81] Specifically, there is convincing evidence from retrospective and prospective case–control studies that a substantial risk exists for malignant transformation of large congenital melanocytic naevi.

In general, precise determination of the risk of melanoma developing within a congenital naevus is problematic in that there have been a number of methodological shortcomings in many of the studies reported thus far.[82] Based on existing data from retrospective and more recent prospective series, the current estimates are in the order of 5–42%. A 6% risk of malignant degeneration is widely quoted, based on a study that estimated the risk from a questionnaire follow up of patients from a Danish registry with congenital naevi.[79,83]

Neurocutaneous melanosis is a rare but potentially serious occurrence in patients with congenital naevi and is characterized by benign or malignant proliferation of melanocytes in the central nervous system. The occurrence of neurocutaneous melanosis in patients with congenital naevi is believed to be higher in patients with lesions on the head, paravertebral area, and posterior neck.[84–87]

A review of the world literature and reporting of a prospective study from the New York University (NYU) registry of LCMN,[80,81] identified 34 patients with primary cutaneous melanoma in 289 cases of LCMN. Differences in the risk of development of melanoma by age and by size of the lesion have been reported. Primary cutaneous melanoma developed in 50% of patients (17 of 34) before 5 years of age in the NYU series, and 62% (21 of 34) died from the disease at a median age of 7.1 years. In general, about half of the melanomas developing in giant naevi reportedly do so in the first 3–5 years of life versus malignant transformation after puberty for smaller naevi.[73,84] In addition to the 34 patients in whom melanoma developed within LCMN, 21 patients had primary melanomas in the central nervous system, and 10 had primary cutaneous melanomas outside the LCMN. In the NYU series 92 patients were followed prospectively for an average of 5.4 years, with melanomas developing in extracutaneous sites in 3% (3 of 92).[81] The adjusted relative risk (standardized morbidity ratio) was calculated to be 239 ($P<0.001$) and the cumulative 5-year life-table risk for developing melanoma was 4.5% (not significant).

The NYU series has been recently updated and expanded to include 160 patients with LCMN who had been free of known melanomas or NCM when entered into the registry.[84] Three extracutaneous melanomas developed among 160 patients who were followed prospectively for an average of 5.5 years. Two of the extracutaneous melanomas were in the central nervous system, and one was retroperitoneal. The 5-year cumulative life-table risk for developing melanoma was 2.3% (95% CI 0.8–6.6) and the relative risk was 101 (95% CI 21–296). Four patients developed manifest NCM, 2 with CNS melanomas. The 5-year cumulative life-table risk for developing NCM was 2.5% (95% CI 0.8–7.2). No melanoma occurred within a large congenital melanocytic naevus in the prospective series, although five additional patients in the NYU-LCMN registry, identified retrospectively, had developed melanomas (three in LCMN, one in normal skin, and one in an unknown primary site).

Management

The management of congenital naevi is controversial and ranges from observation only to excision of the entire lesion. The salient considerations in the treatment of congenital naevi include cosmetic and functional outcomes, and the risk of malignant degeneration. Involvement of a visible location can have a significant emotional impact on patients and is an important consideration in the management of these lesions. In patients with atypical congenital naevi where there is a concern about malignancy, prompt removal and histopathological assessment are important.

The decision about whether to observe or prophylactically remove a stable congenital naevus is controversial.

In the NYU prospective series of LCMN, 12% (20/160) were completely excised, 46% (73/160) were partly excised, 41% (66/160) were observed, and in one patient the treatment was not known.[84] If a decision is made to observe the lesion, accurate documentation is important, and photographs can be very useful in detecting changes. Magnetic resonance imaging scans may be useful for patients with LCMN, particularly those at highest risk of NCM, with involvement of the paravertebral, posterior cervical, and/or cephalic areas.[84] Focal darkening, extension of a naevus into adjacent normal skin, and discrete areas that become elevated or develop palpable nodules should prompt evaluation and incisional or, if feasible, excisional biopsy. Prophylactic removal of a large congenital naevus cannot generally eliminate the risk of malignancy since naevus cells may penetrate deeply and involve the meninges. If removal is performed, serial excisions and closure with skin grafting or flap procedures may be required. Tissue expansion may allow excision of the expanded tissue directly.[88,89] Advances in skin grafting with allogeneic split thickness and full thickness skin, autografts, and artificial skin are promising.[90,91]

LENTIGO MALIGNA

Definition

Lentigo maligna (LM) is a type of melanoma in situ, that may eventually become an invasive melanoma and accounts for approximately 4–15% of all melanomas, and up to 26% of all head and neck melanomas.[92] When lentigo maligna becomes invasive, it is referred to as lentigo maligna melanoma (LMM).

Clinical features

Lentigo maligna can present with clinical features similar to those of other subtypes of melanoma, with asymmetry, variegation in colour, and irregularity of border. The lesion typically grows slowly over many years, expanding gradually in diameter. It may initially present as a freckle-like macule and is often likened to a stain on the skin. The lesion has an irregular shape, with differing shades of brown, black, red/pink, or white throughout (Figures 16.9 and 16.10).[93] Amelanotic lentigo maligna is well recognized and may resemble

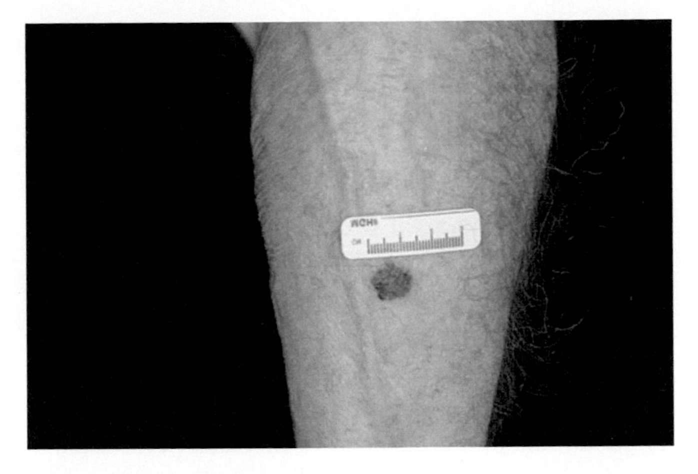

Figure 16.9 *Lentigo maligna. This is a flat lesion on the forearm with prominent focal colour variation.*

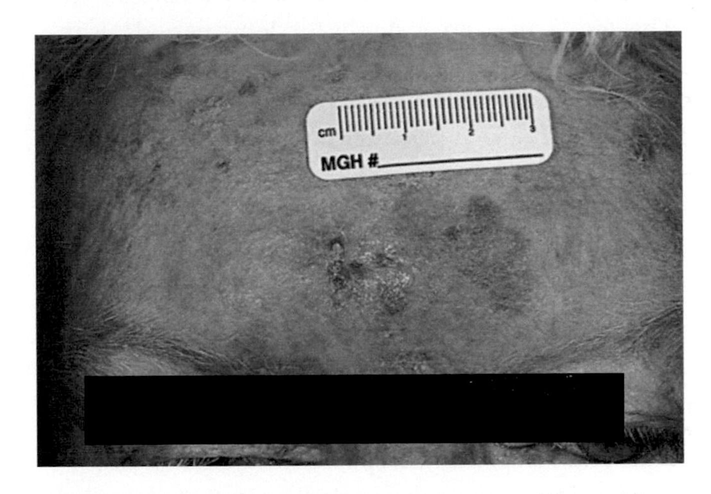

Figure 16.10 *Lentigo maligna melanoma in an 80-year-old female patient. This patient presented with a slowly enlarging lesion with asymmetry and tan brown and dark brown colours.*

eczema, Bowen's disease, or an actinic keratosis.[94–102] Lentigo maligna invariably occurs on sun exposed surfaces, most often in elderly patients on sun damaged atrophic skin in the head and neck region, although it can also present in other locations (Figure 16.10). Irregular mottling or flecking may appear as the lesion enlarges. LM grows by radial spread, increasing in size and assuming a variety of irregular shapes.

It is believed that cumulative exposure to ultraviolet radiation is central to the development of lentigo maligna.[103–105] The anatomical predilection of lentigo maligna for chronically sun exposed areas of the head and neck is in support of the role of solar exposure in the genesis of lentigo maligna. Epidemiological evidence further supporting the role of cumulative sun exposure includes increased risk with: increasing cumulative solar exposure; coexisting actinic damage and basal cell carcinoma; light skin phenotypes; and a history of sunburns.

Lentigo maligna as a precursor

Lentigo maligna can be considered to be precursor lesion in that it may eventually become invasive melanoma. However, it is considered by most authors to be a type of melanoma in situ rather than a precursor to melanoma or a precancer.[92] The exact percentage of LM that progress to LMM is unknown. The lifetime risk of LMM developing from LM has been estimated to be 4.7% at 45 years of age and 2.2% for a 65-year-old.[106] The lesion may grow slowly for long periods, with a latency of approximately 5–15 years in the precursor form before invasion occurs. LM has a prolonged radial growth, but once it becomes invasive it can be fatal.[107]

Management

The only standard treatment for primary cutaneous melanoma is complete surgical excision of the primary lesion (See Chapter 21).[108] For invasive melanomas, prospective randomized surgical trials have helped clearly to define surgical margins for melanomas less than 4 mm thickness except for melanoma in situ.[109,110] Prospective randomized trials have not evaluated the optimal excision margin for in situ melanomas. A National Institutes of Health consensus conference recommended 0.5 cm margins for melanoma in situ.[111] In practice, it is often difficult to define the margin of lentigo maligna, as atypical cells may extend to the clinically defined visible margin, making definitive removal problematic. Mohs micrographic surgery has been utilized to provide frozen section guidance of surgical margins for lentigo maligna. The use of Mohs surgery in this way remains controversial, however, in that the frozen sections can be very difficult to interpret, and the use of rush permanent sections and immunohistochemistry to improve the recognition of clear margins with the procedure have yet to be widely accepted.[67,112,113]

A number of alternative non-surgical treatments have been used for lentigo maligna with variable success when surgery is not an option, and are outlined in Table 16.4. The main disadvantages of non-surgical treatments include the absence of a surgical specimen for confirmation of clearance margins, and the failure to treat deep periappendageal melanocytes.[114]

Table 16.4 *Treatment of lentigo maligna*

Treatment
Surgical
Excision[115]
Mohs micrographic surgery[116–119]
Non-surgical
Cryotherapy[120–123]
Radiation[124–128]
Lasers
-CO_2[129]
-Q switched ruby laser[130]
-Argon[131,132]
Azelaic acid[133]
Imiquimod[134]
5 fluorouracil[135]

REFERENCES

1. Tsao H, Pehamberger H, Sober AJ, Precursor lesions and markers of increased risk for melanoma. In: *Cutaneous melanoma*, 3rd edn. (eds Balch CM, Houghton AN, Sober AJ, Soong SJ), St Louis: Quality Medical Publishing, 1998: 66–79.
2. Balch CM, Soong SJ, Gershenwald JE, et al, Prognostic factor analysis of 17,600 melanoma patients: validation of the American Joint Committee on cancer melanoma staging system. *J Clin Oncol* 2001; 19: 3622–34.
3. Clark WH Jr, From L, Bernardino EA, et al, The histogenesis and biologic behavior of primary human malignant melanomas of the skin. *Cancer Res* 1969; 29: 705–27.
4. Breslow A, Thickness, cross-sectional areas and depth of invasion in the prognosis of cutaneous melanoma. *Ann Surg* 1970; 172: 902–8.
5. Rhodes AR, Sober AJ, Mihm MC, et al, Possible risk factors for primary cutaneous malignant melanoma. *Clin Res* 1980; 28: 252A.
6. Crutcher WA, Sagebiel RW, Prevalence of dysplastic naevi in a community practice. *Lancet* 1984; 1: 729.
7. Scheibner A, Milton GW, McCarthy WH, et al, Prognosis and incidence of multiple primary malignant melanoma[abstract]. *Aust NZ J Surg* 1981; 51: 386.
8. Hernandez-Gill A, Vincente V, Ochotorena MM, et al, Incidence of melanocytic dysplasia in common nevi. First Meeting of the ESPCR, Sorrento/Italy Pigmentary Cell Research, 1988[abstract].
9. Peter RU, Worret WI, Nickolay-Kiesthardt J, Prevalence of dysplastic nevi in healthy young men. *Int J Dermatol* 1992; 31: 327–31.
10. Augustsson A, Stierner U, Suurkula M, et al, Prevalence of common and dysplastic nevi in a Swedish population. *Br J Dermatol* 1991; 124: 152–6.
11. Rhodes AR, Benign neoplasias and hyperplasias of melanocytes. In: *Fitzpatrick's dermatology in general medicine*, 5th edn. (eds Freedberg IM, Eisen AZ, Wolff K, et al), New York: McGraw Hill, 1999: 1018–59.
12. Seykora J, Elder D, Dysplastic nevi and other risk markers for melanoma. *Semin Oncol* 1996; 23: 682–7.
13. Masri GD, Clark WH Jr, Guerry D IV, et al, Screening and surveillance of patients at high risk for malignant melanoma result in detection of earlier disease. *J Am Acad Dermatol* 1990; 22: 1042–8.
14. Clemente C, Cochran AJ, Elder DE, et al, Histopathologic diagnosis of dysplastic nevi: concordance among pathologists convened by the World Health Organization Melanoma Program. *Hum Pathol* 1991; 22: 313–9.
15. Consensus conference: Precursors to malignant melanoma. *JAMA* 1984; 251: 1864–6.

16. Salopek TG, Yamada K, Ito S, et al, Dysplastic melanocytic nevi contain high levels of pheomelanin: quantitative comparison of pheomelanin/eumelanin levels between normal skin, common nevi, and dysplastic nevi. *Pigment Cell Res* 1991; 4: 172–9.
17. Kraemer KH, Greene MH, Tarone R, et al, Dysplastic naevi and cutaneous melanoma risk. *Lancet* 1983; 2: 1076–7.
18. Barnhill RL, Rousch GC, Correlation of clinical and histopathologic features in clinically atypical melanocytic nevi. *Cancer* 1991; 67: 3157.
19. Halpern AC, Guerry D IV, Elder, DE et al, Natural history of dysplastic nevi. *J Am Acad Dermatol* 1993; 29: 51–7.
20. Greene MH, Clark WH Jr, Tucker MA, et al, High risk of malignant melanoma in melanoma-prone families with dysplastic nevi. *Ann Intern Med* 1985; 102: 458–65.
21. Ackerman AB, What nevus is dysplastic, a syndrome and the commonest precursor to malignant melanoma? A riddle and an answer. *Histopathology* 1988; 13: 241–6.
22. Giannotti B, Mihm MC Jr, Review of the proceedings of the consensus workshop on the terminology of melanoma in melanocytic lesions. In: *Cutaneous melanoma,* (eds Veronesi U, Caseinelli N, Santinami M, et al) Academic Press: London, 1987: 517–19.
23. Tucker MA, Crutcher WA, Hartge P, et al, Familial and cutaneous features of dysplastic nevi: a case–control study. *J Am Acad Dermatol* 1993; 28: 558–64.
24. Goldstein AM, Tucker MA, Crutcher WA, et al, The inheritance pattern of dysplastic naevi in families of dysplastic nevus patients. *Melanoma Res* 1993; 3: 15–22.
25. Nancarrow DJ, Mann GJ, Holland EA, et al, Confirmation of chromosome 9p linkage in familial melanoma. *Am J Hum Genet* 1993; 53: 936–42.
26. Nobori T, Miura K, Wu DJ, Lois A, et al, Deletions of the cyclin-dependent kinase-4 inhibitor gene in multiple human cancers. *Nature* 1994; 368: 753–6.
27. Kamb A, Gruis NA, Weaver-Feldhaus J, et al, A cell cycle regulator potentially involved in genesis of many tumour types. *Science* 1994; 264: 436–40.
28. Greene MH, The genetics of hereditary melanoma and nevi: 1998 update. *Cancer* 1999; 86: 2464–77.
29. Haluska FG, Housman DE, Recent advances in the molecular genetics of malignant melanoma. *Cancer Surv* 1995; 25: 277–92.
30. Bergman W, Gruis NA, Sandkuijl LA, et al, Genetics of seven Dutch familial atypical multiple mole-melanoma syndrome families: a review of linkage results including chromosomes 1 and 9. *J Invest Dermatol* 1994; 103 (suppl 5): 122S–5S.
31. Hussussian CJ, Struewig JP, Goldstein AM, et al, Germline p16 mutations in familial melanoma. *Nat Genet* 1994; 8: 15–21.
32. Park WS, Vortmeyer AO, Pack S, et al, Allelic deletion at chromosome 9p21 (p16) and 17p13 (p53) in microdissected sporadic dysplastic nevus. *Hum Pathol* 1998; 29: 127–30.
33. Tucker MA, Halpern A, Holly EA, et al, Clinically recognized dysplastic nevi—a central risk factor for cutaneous melanoma. *JAMA* 1997; 225: 1439–44.
34. Newton JA, Bataille V, Griffiths K, et al, How common is the atypical mole syndrome phenotype in apparently sporadic melanoma? *J Am Acad Dermatol* 1993; 29: 989–96.
35. Nordlund JJ, Kirkwood J, Forget BM, et al, Demographic study of clinically atypical (dysplastic) nevi in patients with melanoma and comparison subjects. *Cancer Res* 1985; 45: 1855–61.
36. Swerdlow AJ, English J, Mackie RM, et al, Benign melanocytic naevi as a risk factor for malignant melanoma. *BMJ* 1986; 292: 1555–9.
37. Roush GC, Nordlund JJ, Forget B, et al, Independence of dysplastic nevi from total nevi in determining risk for nonfamilial melanoma. *Prev Med* 1988; 17: 273–9.
38. Kelly JW, Holly EA, Shpall SN, et al, The distribution of melanocytic naevi in melanoma patients and control subjects. *Australas J Dermatol* 1989; 30: 1–8.
39. Grob JJ, Gouvernet J, Aymar D, et al, Count of benign melanocytic nevi as a major indicator of risk of nonfamilial nodular and superficial spreading melanoma. *Cancer* 1990; 66: 387–95.
40. Halpern AC, Guerry D IV, Elder DE, et al, Dysplastic nevi as risk markers of sporadic (nonfamilial) melanoma. A case–control study. *Arch Dermatol* 1991; 127: 995–9.
41. Stierner U, Augustsson A, Rosdahl I, et al, Regional distribution of common and dysplastic nevi in relation to melanoma site and sun exposure. A case–control study. *Melanoma Res* 1992; 1: 367–75.
42. Garbe C, Buttner P, Weiss J, et al, Risk factors for developing cutaneous melanoma and criteria for identifying persons at risk: multicentre case–control study of the central malignant melanoma registry of the German Dermatological Society. *J Invest Dermatol* 1994; 102: 695–9.
43. Holly EA, Kelly JW, Shpall SN, et al, Number of melanocytic nevi as a major risk factor for malignant melanoma. *J Am Acad Dermatol* 1987; 17: 459–68.
44. Holly EA, Aston DA, Cress RD, et al, Cutaneous melanoma in women. II. Phenotypic characteristics and other host-related factors. *Am J Epidemiol* 1995; 141: 934–42.
45. Swerdlow AJ, English J, MacKie RM, et al, Benign naevi associated with high risk of melanoma (letter). *Lancet* 1984; 2: 168.
46. Bataille V, Newton-Bishop JA, Sasieni P, et al, Risk of cutaneous melanoma in relation to the numbers, types, and sites of naevi. *Br J Cancer* 1996; 73: 1605–11.
47. Grulich A, Bataille V, Swerdlow A, et al, A case–control study of melanoma in New South Wales Australia. *Int J Cancer* 1996; 67: 485–91.
48. Cristofolini M, Franceschi S, Tasin L, et al, Risk factors for cutaneous malignant melanoma in a northern Italian population. *Int J Cancer* 1987; 39: 150–4.
49. Tucker MA, Fraser MC, Goldstein AM, et al, Risk of melanoma and other cancers in melanoma-prone families. *J Invest Dermatol* 1993; 100: 350S–5S.
50. Vasen HFA, Bergman W, Van Haeringen A, et al, The familial dysplastic nevus syndrome: natural history and the impact of screening on prognosis. A study of nine families in the Netherlands. *Eur J Cancer Clin Oncol* 1989; 25: 337–41.
51. Rigel DS, Rivers JK, Kopf AW, et al, Dysplastic nevi. Markers for increased risk for melanoma. *Cancer* 1989; 63: 386–39.
52. MacKie RM, McHenry P, Hole D, Accelerated detection with prospective surveillance for cutaneous malignant melanoma in high risk groups. *Lancet* 1993; 341: 1618–20.
53. Carey WP Jr, Thompson CJ, Synnestvedt M, et al, Dysplastic nevi as a melanoma risk factor in patients with familial melanoma. *Cancer* 1994; 74: 3118–25.
54. Tiersten AD, Grin CM, Kopf AW, et al, Prospective follow-up for malignant melanoma in patients with atypical-mole (dysplastic-nevus) syndrome). *J Dermatol Surg Oncol* 1991; 17: 44–8.
55. Halpern AC, Guerry D IV, Elder DE, et al, A cohort study of melanoma in patients with dysplastic nevi. *J Invest Dermatol* 1993; 100: 346S–9S.
56. Kang S, Barnhill RL, Mihm MC Jr, et al, Melanoma risk in individuals with clinically atypical nevi. *Arch Dermatol* 1994; 130: 999–1001.
57. Marghoob AA, Kopf AW, Rigel DS, et al, Risk of cutaneous malignant melanoma in patients with 'classic' atypical-mole syndrome. A case–control study. *Arch Dermatol* 1994; 130: 993–8.
58. Schneider JS, Moore DH II, Sagebiel RW, Risk factors for melanoma incidence in prospective follow-up. The importance of atypical (dysplastic) nevi. *Arch Dermatol* 1994; 130: 1002–7.
59. Kelly JW, Yeatman JM, Regalia C, et al, A high incidence of melanoma found in patients with multiple dysplastic nevi by photographic surveillance. *Med J Aust* 1997; 167: 191–4.
60. Crijns MB, Bergman W, Berger MJ, et al, On naevi and melanomas in dysplastic nevus syndrome. *Clin Exp Dermatol* 1993; 18: 248–52.
61. Rhodes AR, Harrist TJ, Day CL, et al Dysplastic melanocytic nevi in histological association with 234 primary cutaneous melanoma. *J Am Acad Dermatol* 1983; 9: 563–74.
62. Marks R, Dorevitch AP, Mason G, Do all melanomas come from 'moles'? A study of the histologicalal association between melanocytic naevi and melanoma. *Australas J Dermatol* 1990; 31: 77–80.
63. Hastrup N, Osterlind A, Drzewiecki KT, et al, The presence of dysplastic nevus remnants in malignant melanomas. A population-based study of 551 malignant melanomas. *Am J Dermatopathol* 1991; 13: 378–85.
64. Black VC, Hunt WC, Histological correlations with the clinical diagnosis of dysplastic nevus. *Am J Surg Pathol* 1990; 14: 44–52.

65. Steiner A, Pehamberger H, Wolff K, In vivo epiluminescence microscopy of pigmented lesions. II. Diagnosis of small pigmented skin lesions and early detection of malignant melanoma. *J Am Acad Dermatol* 1987; 17: 584–91.
66. Binder M, Schwarz M, Winkler A, et al, Epiluminescence microscopy. A useful tool for the diagnosis of pigmented skin lesions for formally trained dermatologists. *Arch Dermatol* 1995; 131: 286–91.
67. Elbaum M, Kopf AW, Rabinovitz HS, et al, Automatic differentiation of melanoma from melanocytic nevi with multispectral digital dermoscopy: a feasibility study. *J Am Acad Dermatol* 2001; 44: 207–18.
68. Berwick M, Begg CB, Fine JA, et al, Screening for cutaneous melanoma by skin self-examination. *J Natl Cancer Inst* 1996; 88: 17–23.
69. Mark GJ, Mihm MC, Litteplo MG et al. Congenital melanocytic nevi of the small and garment type. *Hum Pathol* 1973; 4: 395–418.
70. Kopf AW, Bart RS, Hennessey P, Congenital nevocytic nevi and malignanct melanomas. *J Am Acad Dermatol* 1979; 1: 123.
71. Elder DE, Murphy GF, Benign melanocytic tumors (nevi).In: *Atlas of tumor pathology. Melanocytic tumors of the skin.* Washington DC: Armed Forces Institute of Pathology, 1991: 5–101.
72. DeDavid M, Orlow SJ, Provost N, et al, Neurocutaneous melanosis: clinical features of large congenital melanocytic nevi in patients with manifest central nervous system melanosis. *J Am Acad Dermatol* 1996; 35: 529–38.
73. Trozak DJ, Rowland WD, Hu F, Metastatic malignant melanoma in prepubertal children. *Pediatrics* 1975, 55: 191–204.
74. Kaplan EN, The risk of malignancy in large congenital nevi. *Plast Reconstr Surg* 1974; 53: 421–8.
75. Sober AJ, Burstien JM, Precursors to skin cancer. *Cancer* 1995; 75: 645.
76. Hendrickson MR, Ross JC, Neoplasms arising in congenital giant nevi: morphological study of seven cases and a review of the literature. *Am J Surg Pathol* 1981; 5: 109–135.
77. Rhodes AR, Wood WC, Sober AJ, et al, Nonepidermal origin of malignant melanoma associated with a giant congenital nevocellular nevus. *Plast Reconstr Surg* 1981; 67: 782–90.
78. Pers M, Naevus Pigmentosus giganticus: Indikationer for operativ Behandling. *Ugeskr Laeger* 1963; 125: 613.
79. Lorentzen M, Pers M, Bretteville-Jensen G, The incidence of malignant transformation in giant pigmented nevi. *Scand J Plast Reconstr Surg* 1977; 11: 163–7.
80. DeDavid M, Orlow SJ, Provost N, et al, A study of large congenital melanocytic nevi and associated malignant melanomas: review of cases in the New York University Registry and the world literature. *J Am Acad Dermatol* 1997; 36: 409.
81. Marghoob AA, Schoenbach SP, Kopf AW, et al, Large congenital melanocytic nevi and the risk for the development of malignant melanoma: A prospective study. *Arch Dermatol* 1996; 132: 170–5.
82. Swerdlow AJ, English JS, Qiao Z, The risk of melanoma in patients with congenital nevi: A cohort study. *J Am Acad Dermatol* 1995; 32: 595–9.
83. Rhodes AR, Weinstock MA, Fitzpatrick TB et al, Risk factors for cutaneous melanoma. A practical method of recognizing predisposed individuals. *JAMA* 1987; 258: 3146–54.
84. Bittencourt FV, Marghoob AA, Kopf AW, et al, Large congenital melanocytic nevi and the risk for development of malignant melanoma and neurocutaneous melanocytosis. *Pediatrics* 2000; 106: 736.
85. DeDavid M, Orlow SJ, Provost N, et al, Neurocutaneous melanosis: clinical features of large congenital melanocytic nevi in patients with manifest central nervous system melanosis. *J Am Acad Dermatol* 1996; 35: 529–38.
86. Sandsmark M, Eskelan G, Skullerud K, et al, Neurocutaneous melanosis. *Scand J Plast Reconstr Hand Surg* 1994; 28: 151–4.
87. Kadonaga JN, Friden IJ, Neurocutaneous melanosis: definition and review of the literature. *J Am Acad Dermatol* 1991; 24: 747–55.
88. M Argenta LC, Controlled tissue expansion in reconstructive surgery. *Br J Plast Surg* 1984; 37: 520–9.
89. Bauer BS, Vicari FA, An approach to excision of congenital giant pigmentation nevi in infancy and early childhood. *Plast Reconstr Surg* 1988; 82: 1012–21.
90. Soejima K, Nozaki M, Sasaki K, et al, Treatment of giant pigmented nevus using Artificial dermis and a secondary skin graft from the scalp. *Ann Plast Surg* 1997; 39: 489–94.
91. Thomas WO, Rayburn S, LeBlanc RT, et al, Artificial skin in the treatment of a large congenital nevus. *South Med J* 2001; 94: 325–8.
92. Cohen LM, Lentigo maligna and lentigo maligna melanoma. *J Am Acad Dermatol* 1995; 33: 923–36.
93. Langley RG, Mihm MC, Sober AJ, Clinical presentatation: melanoma. In: *American Cancer Society atlas of clinical oncology: skin cancer.* (eds Sober AJ, Haluska F), Hamilton BC: Decker, 2001: 49–59.
94. Su WPD, Bradley RR, Amelanotic lentigo maligna. *Arch Dermatol* 1980; 116: 82–3.
95. Borkovic SP, Schwartz RA, Amelanotic lentigo maligna melanoma manifesting as a dermatitis like plaque. *Arch Dermatol* 1983; 119: 423–5.
96. Lewis JE, Lentigo maligna presenting as an eczematous lesion. *Cutis* 1987; 40: 357–9.
97. Kaufmann R, Nikelski K, Weber L, et al, Amelanotic lentigo maligna melanoma. *J Am Acad Dermatol* 1995; 32: 339–42.
98. Huvos AG, Shah JP, Goldsmith HS, A clinicopathological study of amelanotic melanoma. *Surg Gynaecol Obstet* 1972; 135: 917–20.
99. Burket JM, Amelanotic lentigo maligna. *Arch Dermatol* 1979; 115: 496–7.
100. Lewis JE, Lentigo maligna presenting as an eczematous lesion. *Cutis* 1987; 40: 357–9.
101. Irwin MS, Mercer DM, Walker NPJ, Amelanotic lentigo maligna: a case report and review of the literature. *Br J Plast Surg* 1991; 44: 312–14.
102. Tschen JA, Fordice DB, Reddick M, et al, Amelanotic melanoma presenting as inflammatory plaques. *J Am Acad Dermatol* 1992; 27: 464–5.
103. Holman CDJ, Armstrong BK, Heenan PG, A theory of the etiology and pathogenesis of human cutaneous malignant melanoma. *J Natl Cancer Inst* 1983; 71: 651–6.
104. Holman CDJ, Armstrong BK, Cutaneous malignant melanoma and indicators of total accumulated exposure to the sun: an analysis separating histogenetic types. *J Natl Cancer Inst* 1984; 73: 75–82.
105. Ellwood JM, Gallagher RP, Worth AJ, et al, Etiological differences between subtypes of cutaneous malignant melanoma: Western Canada melanoma study. *J Natl Cancer Inst* 1987; 78: 37–44.
106. Weinstock MA, Sober AJ, The risk of progression of lentigo maligna to lentigo maligna malanoma. *Br J Dermatol* 1987; 116: 303–10.
107. Albert LS, Fewkes J, Sober AJ, Metastatic lentigo maligna melanoma. *J Dermatol Surg Oncol* 1990; 16: 56–8.
108. Langley RGB, Barnhill RL, Mihm MC Jr, et al, Cutaneous melanoma. In: *Fitzpatrick's dermatology in general medicine,* 5th edn. (eds Freedberg IM, Eisen AZ, Wolff K, et al), New York: McGraw-Hill, 1999: 1080–16.
109. Veronesi U, Cascinelli N, Adamus J, Thin stage I primary cutaneous malignant melanoma. *N Engl J Med* 1988; 318: 1159–62.
110. Balch CM, Urist MM, Karakousis CP, et al, Efficacy of 2 cm surgical margins for intermediate-thickness melanomas (1 to 4 mm). *Ann Surg* 1993; 218: 262–7.
111. NIH Consensus Conference. Diagnosis and treatment of early melanoma. *JAMA* 1992; 268: 1314–19.
112. Dhawan SS, Wolf DJ, Rabinovitz HS, et al, Lentigo maligna. The use of rush permanent sections in therapy. *Arch Dermatol* 1990; 126: 928–30.
113. Robinson JK, Margin control for lentigo maligna. *J Am Acad Dermatol* 1994; 31: 79–85.
114. Cohen LM, *What's new in lentigo maligna? Advances in dermatology.* St Louis: CV Mosby, 1999: 203–30.
115. Pitman GH, Kopf AW, Bart RS, et al, Treatment of lentigo maligna and lentigo maligna melanoma. *J Dermatol Surg Oncol* 1979; 31: 758.
116. De Berker D, Lentigo maligna and Mohs. *Arch Dermatol* 1991; 127: 421.
117. Zitelli JA, Moy RL, Abell E, The reliability of frozen sections in the evaluation of surgical margins for melanoma. *J Am Acad Dermatol* 1991; 24: 102–6.
118. Cohen LM, McCall MW, Zax RH, Mohs micrographic surgery for lentigo maligna and lentigo maligna melanoma: A follow up study. *Dermatol Surg* 1998; 24: 673–7.
119. Zitelli JA, Mohs FE, Larson P, et al, Mohs micrographic surgery for melanoma. *Dermatol Clin* 1989; 7: 833–43.

120. Collins P, Rodgers S, Goggin M, et al, Cryotherapy for lentigo maligna. *Clin Exper Dermatol* 1991; 16: 433–5.
121. Zacarian SA, Cryosurgical treatment of lentigo maligna. *Arch Dermatol* 1982; 118: 89–92.
122. Dawber RPR, Wilkinson JD, Melanotic freckle of Hutchinson: treatment of macular and nodular phases with cryotherapy. *Br J Dermatol* 1979; 101: 47–9.
123. Kuflik EG, Gage AA, Cryosurgery for lentigo maligna. *J Am Acad Dermatol* 1994; 31: 758.
124. Tsang RW, Liu F-F, Wells W, et al, Lentigo maligna of the head and neck. Results of treatment by radiotherapy. *Arch Dermatol* 1994; 130: 1008–12.
125. Kopf AW, Bart RS, Gladstein AH, Treatment of melanotic freckle with x-rays. *Arch Dermatol* 1976; 112: 801–7.
126. Harwood AR, Conventional fractionated radiotherapy for 51 patients with lentigo maligna and lentigo maligna melanoma. *Int J Radiation Oncol Biol Phys* 1983; 9: 1019–21.
127. Harwood AR, Conventional radiotherapy in the treatment of lentigo maligna and lentigo maligna melanoma. *J Am Acad Dermatol* 1982; 6: 310–16.
128. Dancuart F, Harwood AR, Fitzpatrick PJ, The radiotherpay of lentigo maligna and lentigo maligna melanoma of the head and neck. *Cancer* 1980; 45: 2279–83.
129. Kopera D, Treatment of lentigo maligna with the carbon dioxide laser. *Arch Dermatol* 1995; 131: 735–6.
130. Lee PK, Rosenberg, CN, Tsao H, et al, Failure of Q-switched ruby laser to eradicate atypical-appearing solar lentigo: Report of two cases. *J Am Acad Dermatol* 1998; 38: 314–17.
131. Arndt KA, Argon laser treatment of lentigo maligna. *J Am Acad Dermatol* 1984; 10: 953–7.
132. Arndt KA, New pigmented macule appearing 4 years after aragon laser treatment of lentigo maligna. *J Am Acad Dermatol* 1986; 14: 1092.
133. Prieto MAR, Lopez PM, Gonzalez IR, et al, Treatment of lentigo maligna with azelaic acid. *Int J Dermatol* 1993; 32: 363: 364.
134. Ahmed I, Berth-Jones J, Imiquimod: a novel treatment for lentigo maligna. *Br J Dermatol* 2000; 143: 843–5.
135. Litwin MS, Krementz ET, Mansell PW, et al, Topical chemotherapy of lentigo maligna with 5-fluorouracil. *Reed RJ* 1975; 35(3): 721–33.

17

Primary cutaneous melanoma: clinical diagnosis

William H McCarthy, Gerald W Milton

With training and experience, around 90% of melanomas can be accurately diagnosed by the taking of a good history, by careful examination of the lesion with a good light and magnification, and by surface microscopy. The remaining 10% of lesions will probably be removed because of patient concern, ill defined suspicion by the attending physician, or cosmetic considerations. The most difficult of clinical diagnoses is the amelanotic melanoma.

Traditionally, clinical melanoma is classified into four main types:

(1) superficial spreading melanoma;
(2) nodular melanoma;
(3) acral lentiginous melanoma; and
(4) lentigo maligna melanoma (melanoma arising in a Hutchinson's melanotic freckle).

In recent years, a fifth type of melanoma has been suggested for inclusion in the classification list – desmoplastic melanoma with or without neural sheath invasion (neurotropism). Clinically, desmoplastic melanoma is currently most commonly classified as one of the more usual variants, including amelanotic melanoma.

This, an essentially morphological classification system, has lost some credence over time because the biological behaviour of these lesions is essentially unrelated to the morphological name applied to the lesion, and prognosis is now related to Breslow tumour thickness rather than the traditional classification system. Prognosis and treatment protocols are now based on the TNM (primary Tumour, lymph Nodes, Metastases) system applied to most other tumours. Some features, such as ulceration and the presence of satellitosis, may influence management, but for the large majority of tumours, only Breslow thickness needs to be considered in determining appropriate initial therapy. The new American Joint Committee for Cancer (AJCC)/UICC classification system for melanoma is summarized in Table 17.1.

In the new system, ulceration is assessed so each of the T classifications is subdivided into tumours (a) with ulceration and (b) without ulceration. The AJCC/UICC staging system is considered in more detail in Chapter 14.

CLINICAL DIAGNOSIS

The important steps in diagnosing pigmented skin lesions are the taking of a careful history, a comparison of the suspect lesion with any other pigmented lesions the patient may have, palpation of the draining lymph node fields, and, in some cases, skin surface microscopy (see Chapter 18).

Table 17.1 ***New AJCC/UICC classification system for melanoma***

• (pTis) Melanoma in situ (no invasion)	
• (pT1) Melanoma ≤1.0 mm	
• (pT2) Melanoma 1.01–2.0 mm	
• (pT3) Melanoma 2.01–4.0 mm	(a) Ulceration
• (pT4) Melanoma >4.0 mm	(b) No ulceration

HISTORY

The history presented by the patient is usually that of a 'sign' rather than a symptom. Almost the only common symptom caused by melanoma is perilesional itch. The itch is characteristically mild, repetitive, and around the mole rather than in the lesion itself. It occurs in approximately 20% of patients, but of itself is not diagnostic, as itch is much more prevalent in common skin lesions, particularly seborrhoeic keratosis. Itching only becomes important when associated with other clinical features.

In evaluating the signs that accompany melanoma, it is desirable to conduct the interview and clinical examination of the patient in the presence of the patient's partner, who in approximately 20% of cases will be the person who first noticed a change in the skin lesion. It is notable that women are more likely to recognize the early changes of melanoma both on themselves and on their partners.[1,2]

It is important to assess the duration of the change in the lesion. The timing of the observed change is relevant to the diagnosis in that a change that has occurred in a skin lesion over a few days or a few weeks is more likely to be inflammation due to such things as infection or irritation from friction, for example pyogenic granuloma. A change observed over years indicates that it is likely to be a benign lesion, especially if it occurs during the teenage years. A melanoma will typically have a history of change over a period of three to 12 months. There is, however, much variability in the duration of changes reported by patients with melanoma.[3]

The features classically observed in a developing melanoma by the patient or their partner are:

(1) a change in colour;
(2) a change in shape;
(3) elevation of part or all of the lesion; and
(4) bleeding as a result of minor trauma.

Pain is rare in early melanoma but may sometimes occur in well advanced melanomas where there is ulceration and infection.

Melanoma may arise from a pre-existing naevus or in unblemished skin. The proportion of melanomas arising in normal skin has been estimated to be from 30% to 70%.[4] It has been suggested that melanomas arising in normal looking skin are usually nodular melanomas and represent isolated malignant change in a single cell, while melanomas arising in pre-existing naevi are usually superficial spreading melanomas (SMM) initially, and may represent a field defect in the pre-existing lesion. However, there is little evidence in support of these conjectures. Over time SSM will develop a nodule, and the lesion is then classified as nodular melanoma.

The diagnosis of amelanotic melanoma is particularly difficult, even with the assistance of surface microscopy. A history of a relatively rapidly expanding pale nodule on the skin is common. On clinical examination it is often featureless, and a diagnosis of basal cell carcinoma (BCC) is often made. Occasionally small areas of brown pigmentation can be seen clinically and more easily with the surface microscope (dermatoscope, episcope) (Figure 17.1). In a recent study of surface microscopy of biopsy proved melanomas, 8% of these lesions had no diagnostic features.[5]

The 'ABCDE' diagnostic system (Rigel et al.), provides a helpful method of evaluating cutaneous pigmented lesions:[6,7]

A = Asymmetry;
B = Border;
C = Colour;
D = Diameter; and
E = Elevation.

These features are considered below.

CLINICAL EXAMINATION

In examining pigmented skin tumours a good even light and magnification are very helpful. A suitable

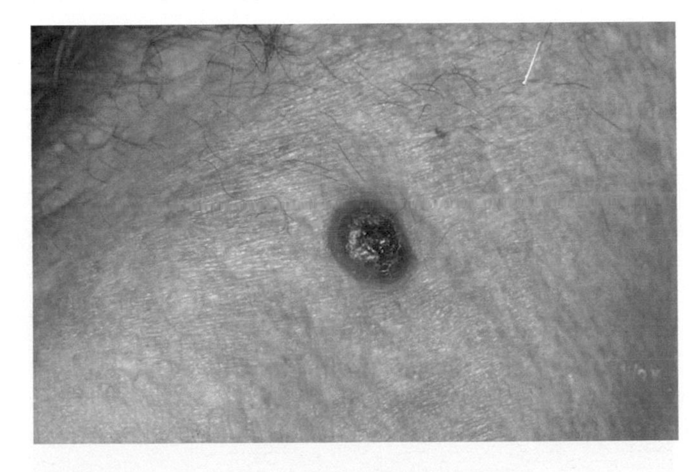

Figure 17.1 *Melanoma with no blue black colour – some pigment is seen at the edge of the lesion.*

handheld fluorescent light incorporating magnification is shown in Figure 17.2.

Asymmetry means asymmetry of pattern and asymmetry of shape (Figure 17.3). Asymmetry of both pattern and shape is usually apparent when using a bright light and magnification. However, asymmetry is easier to assess with surface microscopy (see Chapter 18).

The border of most melanomas becomes irregular because of uneven growth within the lesion. The border is characterized as 'coastline', with bays and promontories as on a map of a country or island (Figure 17.4). The border of a melanoma is often sharply demarcated, at least in some parts of its extent (Figure 17.5). This compares with a dysplastic naevus, where the border is typically ill defined, fading into the adjacent skin (Figure 17.6).

Colour change is often the most dramatic of the features noted in melanoma. The characteristic colours are blue/black (Figure 17.7) but many early melanomas do not contain these characteristic colours (Figure 17.8). Irregularity of colour is more important than the finding of blue/brown/black pigment, and many colours are visible both clinically and with the surface microscope (Figure 17.9). These include brown, tan, red, grey, white, blue, and black. Although irregularity is particularly evident with the surface microscope, it is important to note that small nodular melanomas are often uniformly black in colour and develop a glossy surface, which the patient often describes as looking like a blood blister (Figure 17.10). A grey or white appearance in a melanoma indicates 'regression'(Figure 17.11) and represents an area of the lesion where melanin production ceases and the

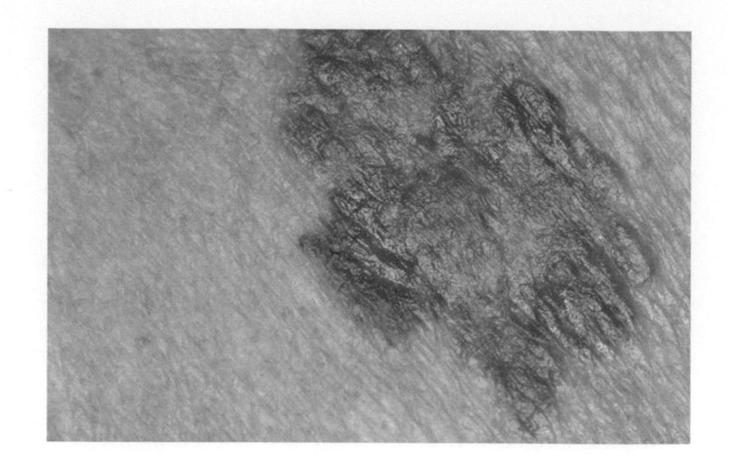

Figure 17.3 *Asymmetry of pattern and shape.*

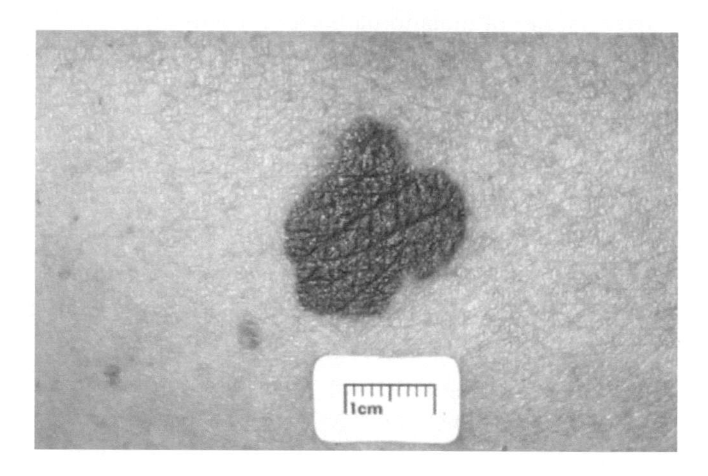

Figure 17.4 *Coastline border.*

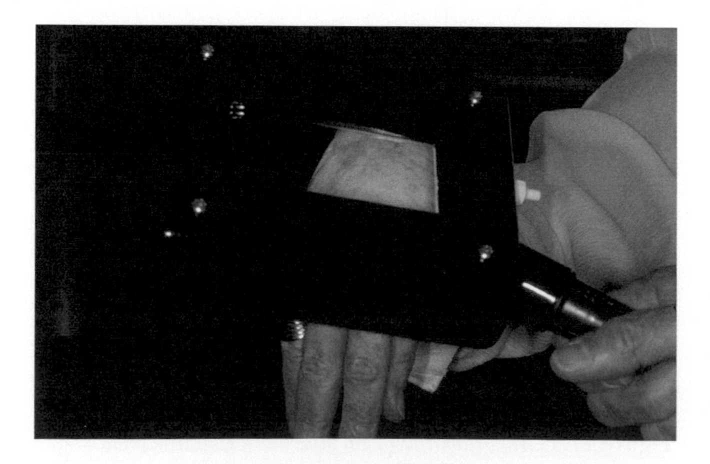

Figure 17.2 *Handheld magnifying lamp.*

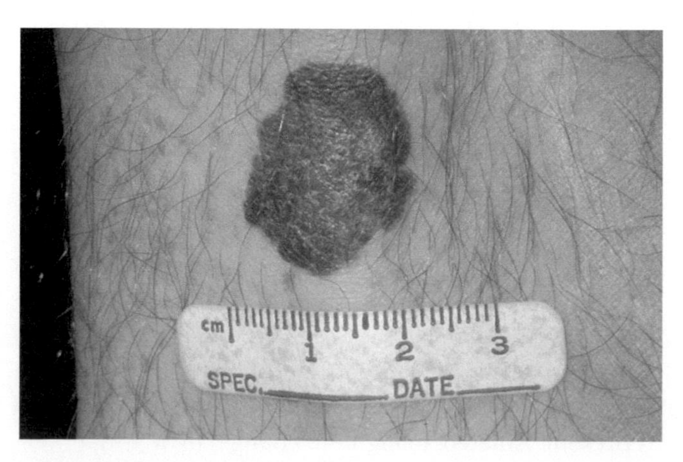

Figure 17.5 *Sharply defined border.*

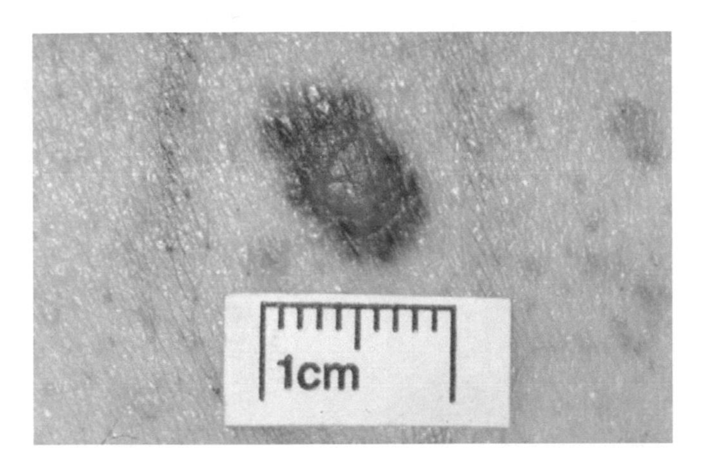

Figure 17.6 *Dysplastic naevus with poorly defined border.*

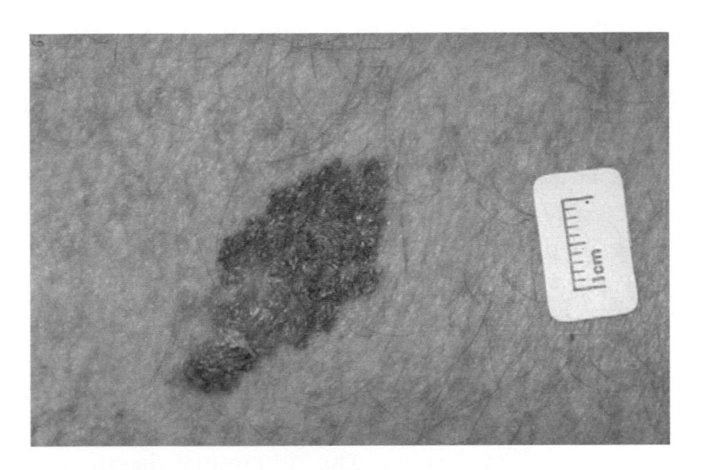

Figure 17.7 *Characteristic blue black colour.*

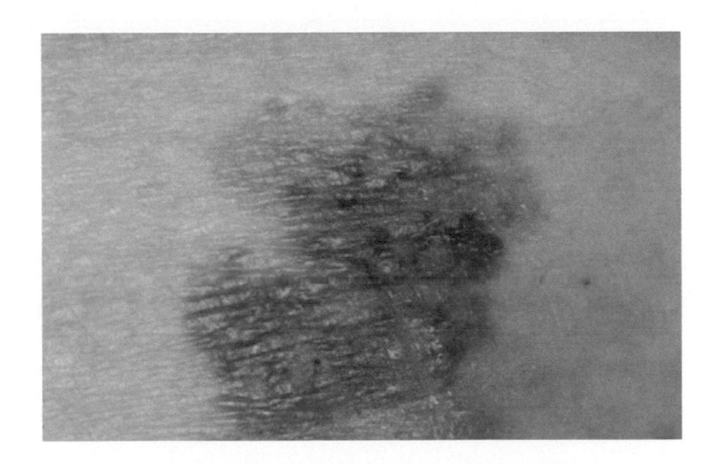

Figure 17.8 *Melanoma with no blue black colour.*

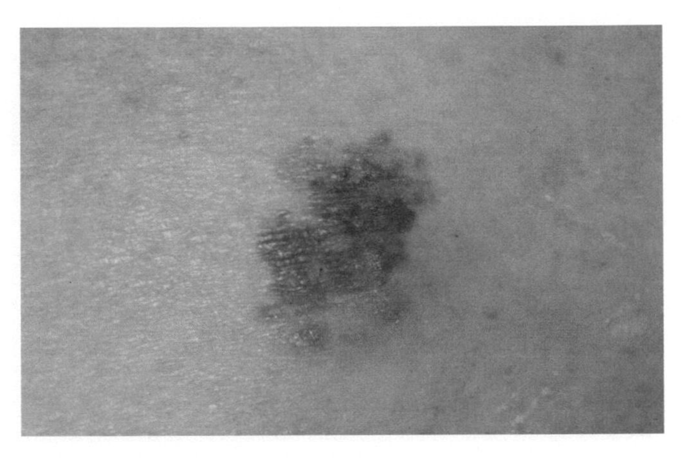

Figure 17.9 *Irregularity of colour.*

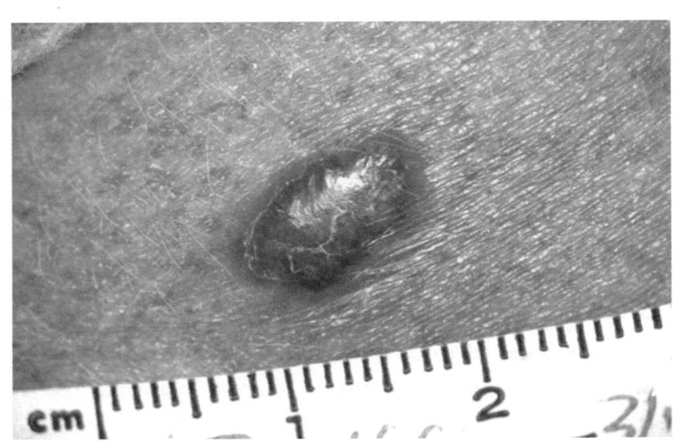

Figure 17.10 *Blood blister appearance.*

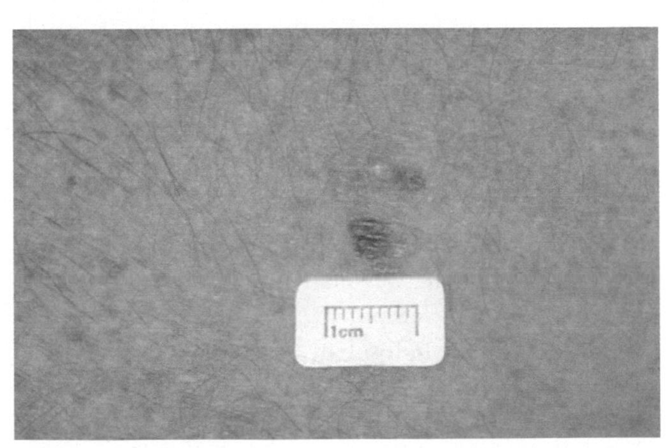

Figure 17.11 *Regression in an early melanoma.*

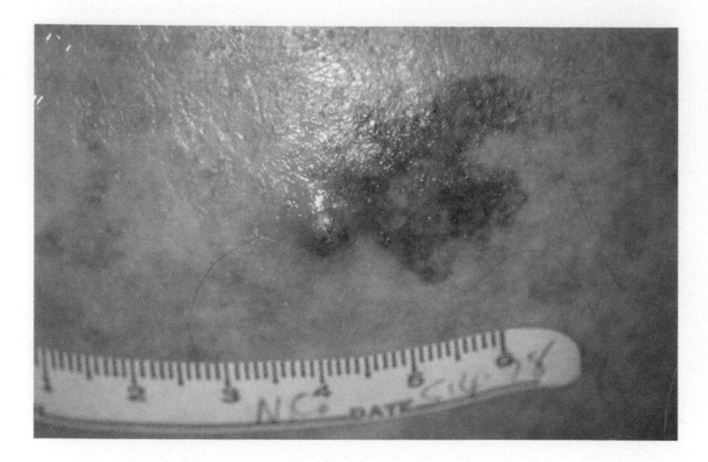

Figure 17.12 *Amelanotic nodule at lower edge.*

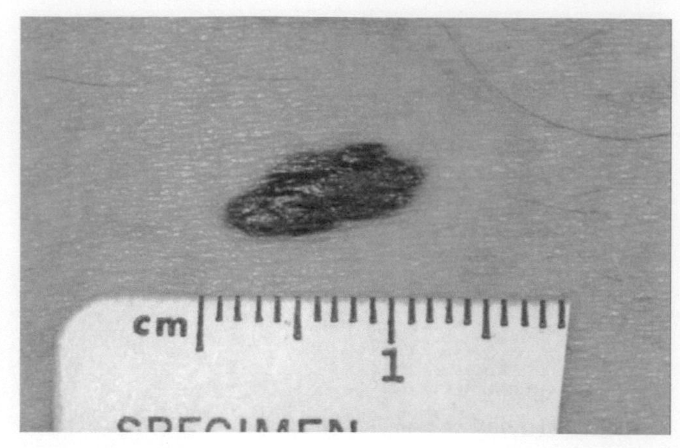

Figure 17.13 *Development of glossy surface.*

melanoma cells may disappear leaving a pale scar-like area. Regression does occur in dysplastic naevi but is much more common in melanoma.

The development of an amelanotic nodule in a lesion thought to be possibly an early melanoma is virtually diagnostic of malignancy in the lesion (Figure 17.12). It should be looked for carefully, with both magnification and the surface microscope.

The diameter of the lesion exceeding 6 mm is not particularly helpful in establishing a diagnosis because many benign lesions, including dysplastic naevi, are 6 mm in diameter or greater. In one Australian study 30% of melanomas at diagnosis were <6 mm in size.[8] However, melanomas developing in dysplastic naevi are usually 6 mm or more in diameter.

Elevation is not useful in the early diagnosis of melanoma. Curable melanomas are flat or only marginally raised above the skin. Elevation represents the development of the vertical growth phase and therefore a more advanced lesion. For this reason, the 'E' could be better used to encourage the clinician to 'Examine' the patient's other naevi. Melanoma is always different from the patient's other naevi. The comparison with existing naevi is thus very useful in determining if the suspect lesion is malignant. Recent elevation is nevertheless important in the history of the lesion, clearly indicating a change, but many benign lesions become elevated during development.

Other features helpful in reaching a diagnosis of melanoma are the development of a glossy, amorphous appearance of part of the lesion where normal skin lines are destroyed by the advancing tumour cells (Figure 17.13). Occasionally, small flakes of keratin become visible on the surface of the lesion (Figure 17.14), although frank keratinization is rare in melanoma, particular in the very early stages. Many early melanomas will retain hairs within the structure of the lesion, and on hair bearing areas such as the scalp, even advanced nodular melanomas may contain hair (Figure 17.15). However, as the tumour progresses and destroys the hair follicles, the melanoma will become hairless.

The clinical diagnosis of melanoma is usually not difficult, but in cases of doubt the clinician may arrive at the diagnosis by exclusion of the other pigmented tumours of the skin, most of which have features not present in a melanoma. The differential diagnosis of melanoma includes dysplastic naevus, Spitz naevus, seborrhoeic keratosis, haemangioma, pigmented BCC,

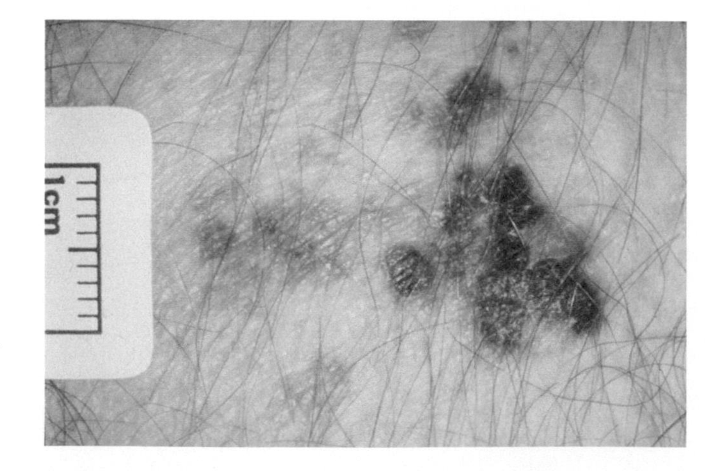

Figure 17.14 *Small flakes of keratin on the surface.*

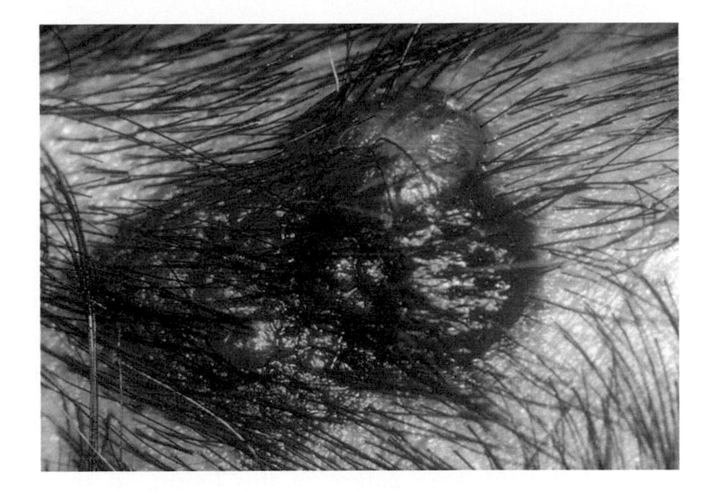

Figure 17.15 *Melanoma on scalp with hair.*

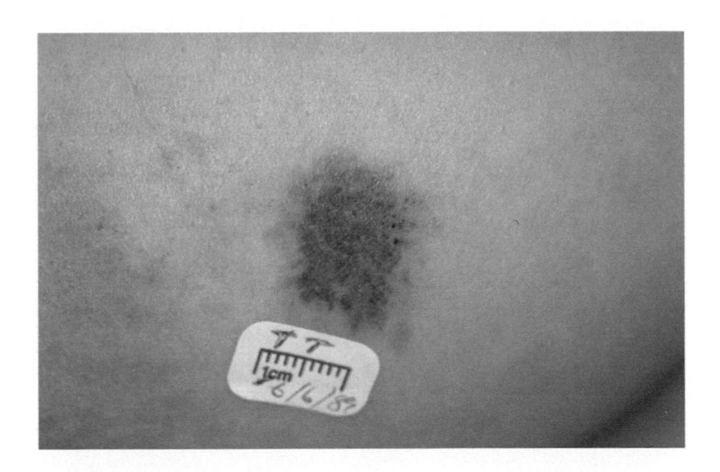

Figure 17.16 *Dysplastic naevus.*

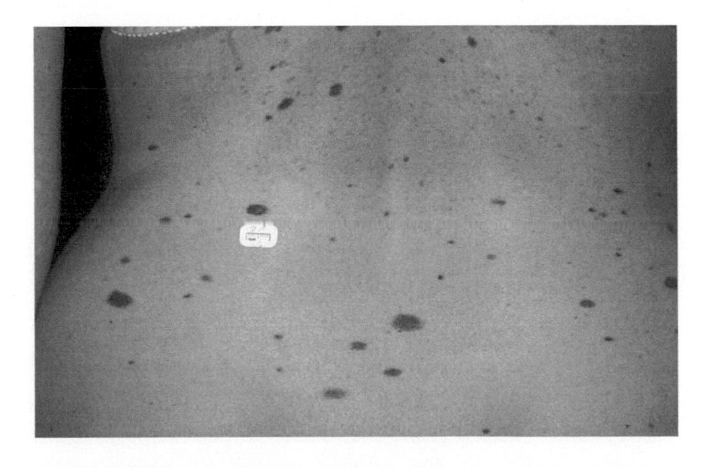

Figure 17.17 *The dysplastic naevus syndrome (DNS/AMS).*

blue naevus, pigmented actinic keratosis, and some rare skin adnexal tumours. Each of these lesions has some characteristic features, enabling it to be distinguished from a primary melanoma.

Dysplastic naevi

Dysplastic naevi (Figure 17.16) provide the greatest challenge to the clinician in distinguishing benign pigmented lesions from early melanoma. A clear linkage exists between dysplastic naevi, melanoma in situ, and invasive melanoma, i.e. multiple dysplastic naevi are markers for malignancy and in some cases precursors of melanoma. However, it is important to note that only rarely do dysplastic naevi evolve into melanoma. The National Institutes for Health consensus conference on dysplastic naevi in 1992 made the strong statement that the single dysplastic naevus has no malignant potential while multiple dysplastic naevi are markers for malignancy.[9]

It is important to note that clinically dysplastic naevi are a common occurrence, suggesting that most people with naevi have at least one clinically dysplastic naevus and that this is not a significant finding.[10,11] It is also important to note that the presence of multiple dysplastic naevi, i.e. the 'dysplastic naevus' or 'atypical mole' syndrome, is associated with an increased risk for melanoma. In these patients, a significant proportion of the melanomas arise in normal skin and not from a clinically dysplastic naevus.[12] Between 17% and 85% of cutaneous melanomas are stated to arise in association with clinically or histologically diagnosed dysplastic naevi.[11]

Multiple dysplastic or atypical naevi are classified into two main syndromes, the dysplastic naevus syndrome (DNS), also known as the atypical mole syndrome (AMS), and the familial DNS also known as FAMS (familial atypical mole syndrome) (Figure 17.17). In the sporadic variant there is no clear family history of a similar distribution of naevi. DNS (AMS) is a clinically defined syndrome in which the patient has at least 50 atypical naevi which vary in shape, size, and colour. The atypical naevi are found in areas not usually sun exposed, e.g. the lower back, under the arms and in the scalp.

Dysplastic naevi when diagnosed clinically are usually greater than 6 mm in diameter. They have an irregular border that fades out into the surrounding tissues ('a shoulder') and variability in colour, with various hues of brown, but sometimes red coloration. Sometimes small areas of the dysplastic naevi tend to become hypopigmented, suggesting clinical regression (Figure 17.18).

Dysplastic naevi tend to be flat or barely palpable and have considerably greater breadth than height, with the raised portion generally being in the centre of the lesion. This appearance, with a central nodule and a surrounding darker pigmentation, is described as a target or 'bulls eye' naevus (Figure 17.6).

In assessing for the presence of the DNS or AMS, it is important to note the great variability in colour, shape and size of the patient's naevi (Figure 17.17).

Spitz naevi (juvenile melanomas)

The Spitz naevus (Figures 17.19 and 17.20) is a variant of a compound naevus occurring predominantly in children but occasionally in adults. Clinically, the lesion usually presents as a rapidly growing, raised, red papular lesion, and is common on the face. It grows rapidly over a period of months, reaching approximately 1 cm in diameter and then remains unchanged for several years. A variant, which produces much pigment, is more difficult to diagnose, as it appears to be uniformly black or brown. It is necessary to excise these heavily pigmented Spitz naevi to determine the diagnosis, as melanoma does occur in children (see Chapter 33).

A form of multiple or agminate Spitz naevus has also been described, and it is thought to be due to local bloodborne spread of naevus cells with the ability to proliferate in the immediate area of the original lesion but not beyond that area.[12]

Spindle cell naevus of Reed

This is an unusual variant of a compound naevus first identified by Reed in 1975.[13] The spindle cell naevus (Figure 17.21) is more common in women on the thigh area. It presents as a densely pigmented, blue/black palpable lesion, usually less than 1 cm in diameter. It can be difficult to diagnose by clinical examination alone, and surface microscopy may be very helpful in determining the true nature of this lesion. In some instances, biopsy is necessary to exclude melanoma.

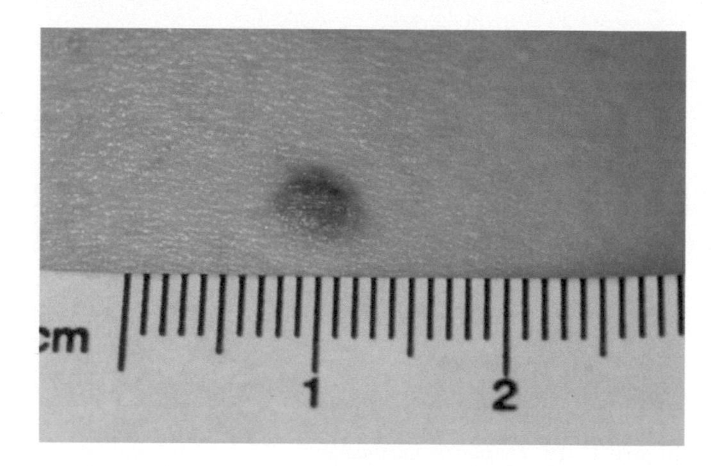

Figure 17.19 *Spitz naevus – non-pigmented.*

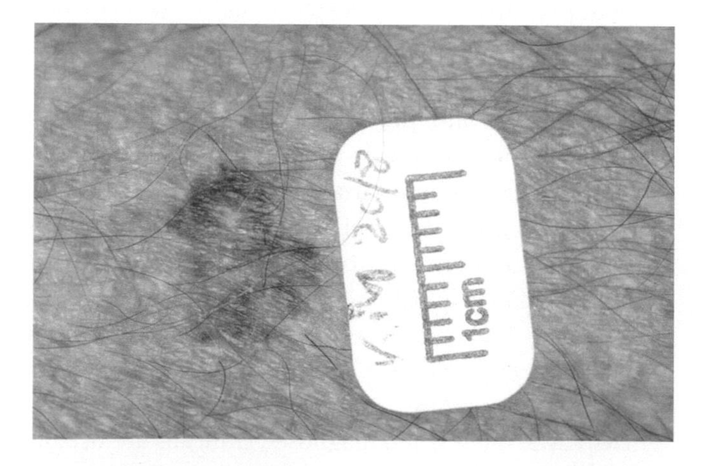

Figure 17.18 *Dysplastic naevus with regression – biopsy is needed to exclude melanoma.*

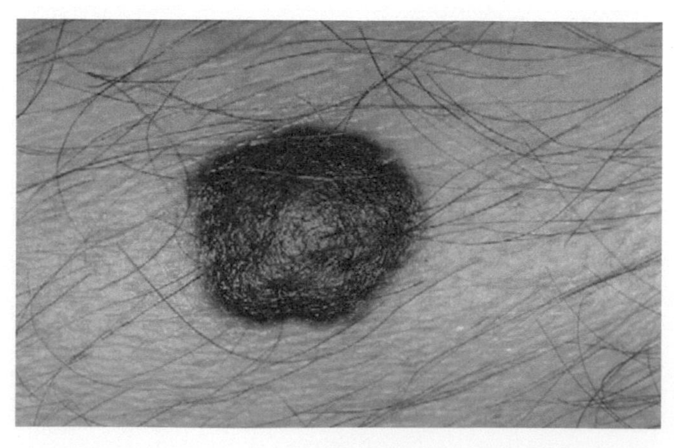

Figure 17.20 *Spitz naevus – pigmented.*

Seborrhoeic keratoses

A seborrhoeic keratosis (Figure 17.22) should not be difficult to diagnose in the majority of cases. The lesions are usually multiple, they seem to be 'stuck on the skin', they have a slightly greasy feel to their surface, and excessive keratinization is characteristic of them. However, in some cases the lesions can be very darkly pigmented and not keratotic. In these cases the pigmentation is usually brown to dark brown and evenly distributed through the tumour. A well circumscribed edge and a superficial 'stuck on' appearance of these lesions distinguishes them from melanomas. Surface microscopy is particularly helpful in diagnosing clinically difficult seborrhoeic keratoses.

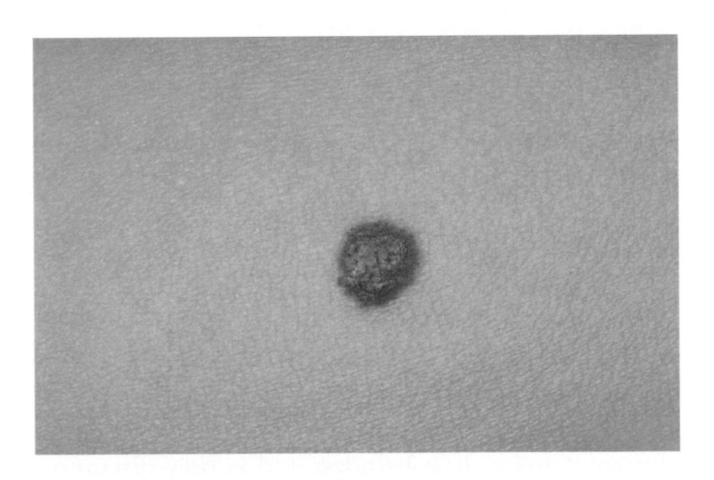

Figure 17.21 *Spindle cell naevus of Reed.*

Haemangiomas

The diagnosis of haemangioma (Figure 17.23) is usually not difficult. It is a well demarcated, discrete, red to violet papule with a smooth lobulated surface. A key feature of these lesions is that they blanch when pressure is applied to the surface by the finger or with a glass slide. Blood is forced out causing the blanching, with colour quickly returning when the glass slide or finger is removed. However, sometimes the draining vessels are small or thrombosed, and definite blanching cannot be achieved. In these situations surface microscopy is particularly helpful in distinguishing haemangiomas. An important finding in some haemangiomas is the presence of a darker pigmentation in the skin around the lesion that the patient has noted to occur quickly (Figure 17.24). This is due to haemorrhage into the dermis from the haemangioma and is characteristic of this particular lesion. Melanoma does not rapidly leak pigment into the surrounding tissues, and this haemosiderin discoloration around the tumour is often helpful in making the clinical diagnosis.

Sclerosing haemangiomas

Sclerosing haemangioma (dermatofibroma) can be mistaken for melanoma if the diagnosis is not considered by the clinician. These lesions are common, particularly on the legs of women, and may be multiple. The history is slow development of a violatious, blue/brown tinged papule (Figure 17.25) that is often itchy. A good clue to the diagnosis of this lesion is the

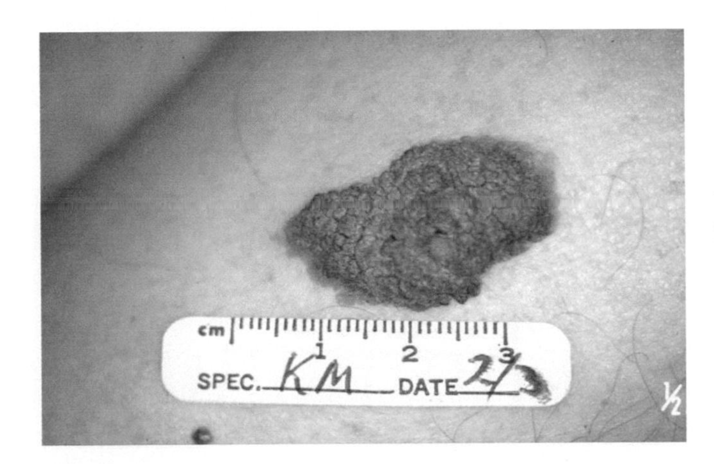

Figure 17.22 *Seborrhoeic keratosis.*

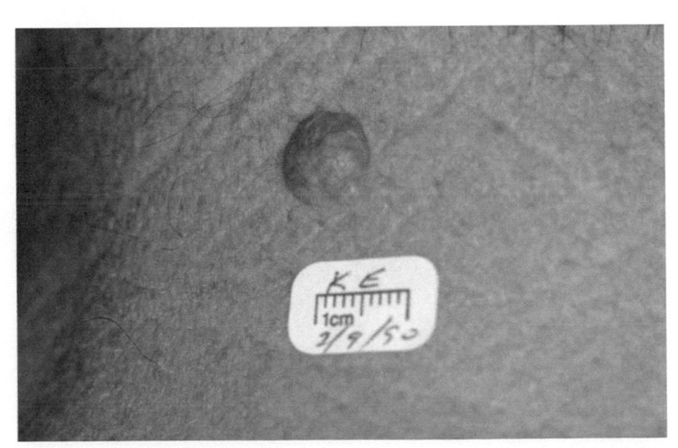

Figure 17.23 *Haemangioma.*

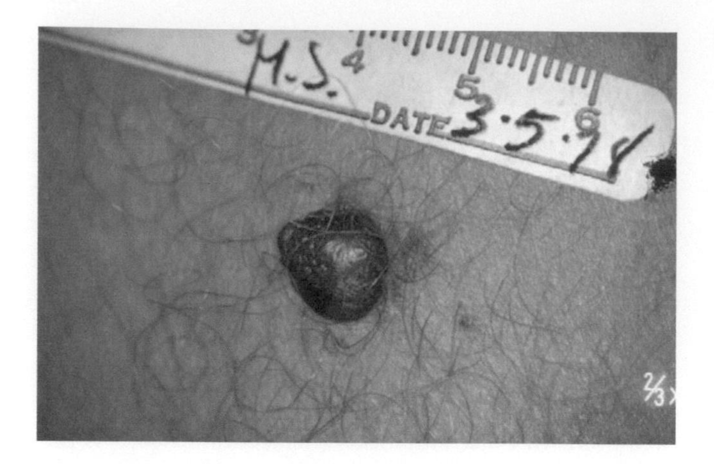

Figure 17.24 *Haemangioma with haemosiderin staining of adjacent skin.*

'dimple' sign, i.e. a dimpling or depression of the centre of the lesion when the margins of the dermatofibroma are pinched between two fingers. This results from a tethering of the epidermis to a deeper fibrous portion of the tissues. The bulk tissue in the dermis is also a helpful sign of sclerosing haemangioma. Most other pigmented lesions do not extend into the dermis with such palpable nodularity.

Blue naevi

The blue naevus (Figure 17.26) should not be difficult to diagnose. The lesion is almost always oval or round, with uniform bluish pigmentation evenly distributed through the tumour. It is characteristically small, less than 5 mm in size, and hairs are often present within a nodule, particularly if the lesion is in hair bearing skin. The history is that of a longstanding lesion, and, again, the surface microscopy appearance can be very helpful.

Pigmented basal cell carcinomas

Pigmented basal cell carcinoma (Figure 17.27) presents as a well defined papular nodule with a translucent pearly quality and overlying telangiectasia in some part of the lesion. There is a long history of a slowly growing lesion, and the pigment is unevenly distributed throughout the tumour, blending imperceptibly with the normal appearance of basal cell carcinoma, i.e. a pearly grey colour and minor telangiectasia on the surface. Pigmented basal cell carcinomas may ulcerate early. The ulcer has the usual characteristics of a rodent ulcer with an incomplete border, a healing base, and border telangiectasia.

Pigmented actinic keratoses

These lesions (Figure 17.28) are characterized by excessive keratinization of the surface and are almost always multiple.

Talon noir

A rare but often misdiagnosed lesion of the sole of the foot is 'talon noir' (black heel). It is haemorrhage into the stratum corneum of the heel and occurs commonly on the feet of athletes and walkers, as a result of trauma during exercise. It is harmless and is only discovered some time after the exercise period (Figure 17.29).

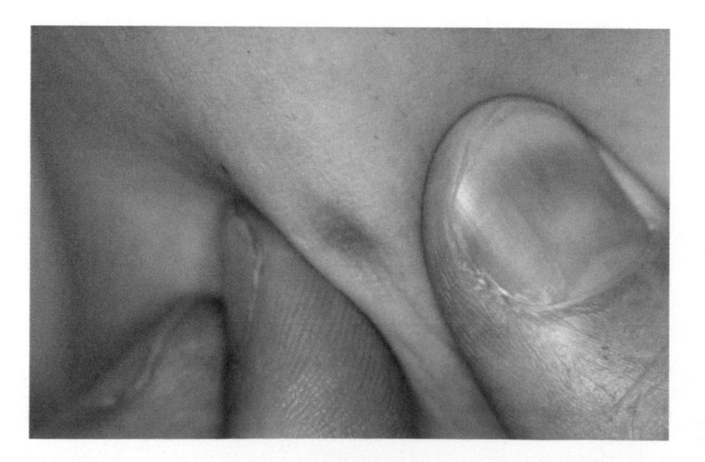

Figure 17.25 *Sclerosing haemangioma – the 'dimple' sign.*

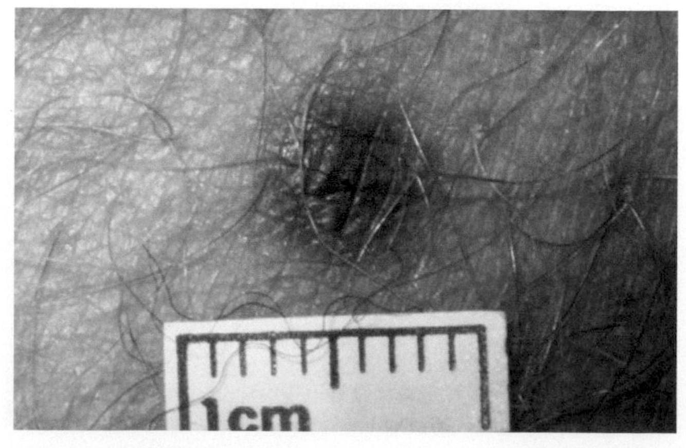

Figure 17.26 *Blue naevus.*

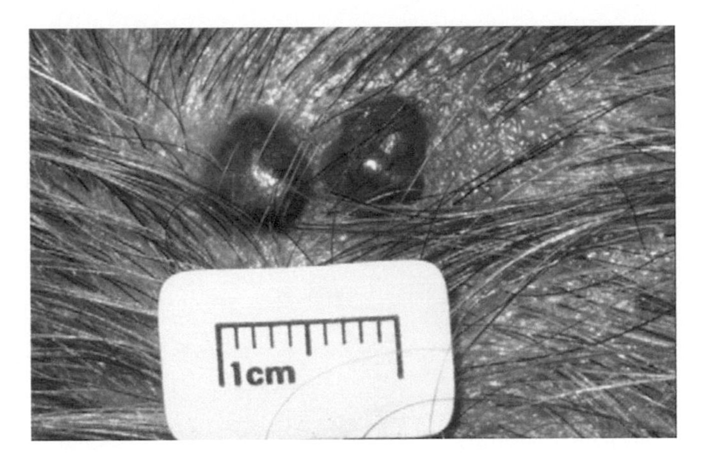

Figure 17.27 *Two pigmented BCCs on the scalp.*

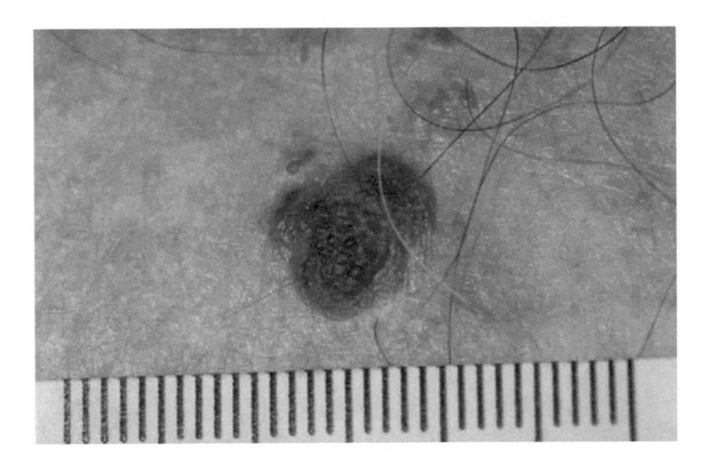

Figure 17.28 *Pigmented actinic keratosis.*

Rare adnexal tumours

It is not possible clinically to diagnose these rare adnexal tumours. A history of relatively slow growth may be helpful, but in most instances only biopsy will provide the definitive diagnosis (Figure 17.30).

CONCLUSION

With a careful history, appropriate clinical examination, pattern recognition using the ABCDE system, consideration and exclusion of the alternative diagnoses, and the assistance of surface microscopy, 92% of pigmented lesions of the skin will be accurately diagnosed. However, it is important to reiterate that for all lesions where a clinical diagnosis cannot be established within two months of observation, excision biopsy is mandatory.

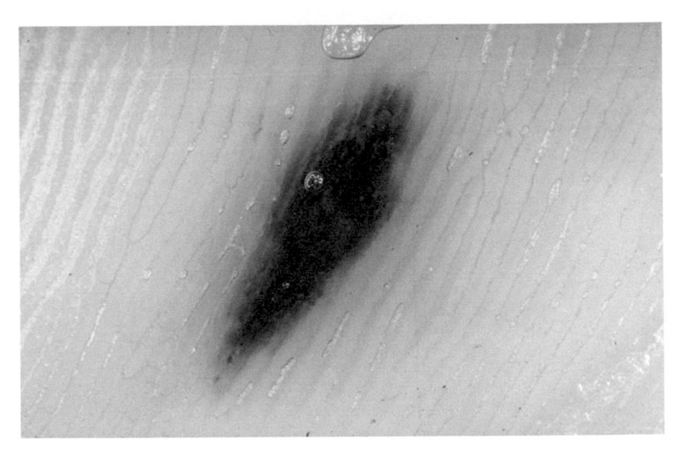

Figure 17.29 *Talon noir.*

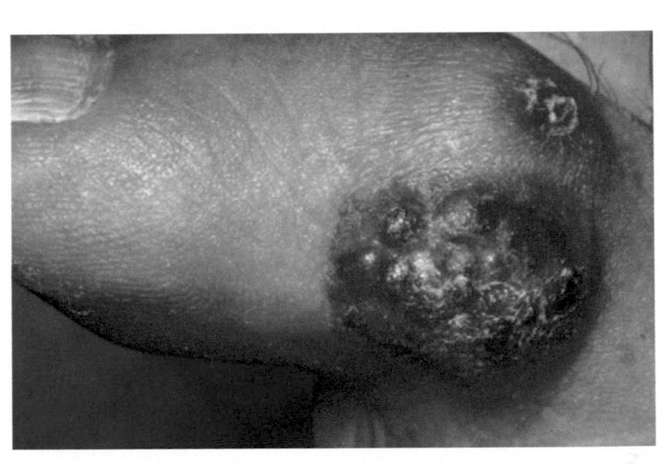

Figure 17.30 *Pigmented adnexal tumour – clinically resembles nodular melanoma.*

REFERENCES

1. Milton GW, Clinical diagnosis of malignant melanoma. *Br J Surgery* 1968; 55: 755–7.
2. Koh HK, Miller DR, Geller AC, et al, Who discovers melanoma? Patterns from a population-based survey. *J Am Acad Dermatol* 1992; 26: 914–19.
3. Fitzpatrick TB, Milton GW, Balch CM, et al, Clinical characteristics. In: *Cutaneous melanoma* 2nd edn. (eds, Balch CM, Houghton AN, Milton GW, et al). Philadelphia: Lippincott, 1992: 223–33.
4. Milton GW, Lewis CWD, The presentation of malignant melanoma (melanoblastoma), *Med J Austr* 1963; 1: 239–42.
5. Menzies S, Ingvar C, Crotty K, McCarthy W, Frequency of morphologic characteristics of invasive melanomas lacking specific surface microscopic features. *Arch Dermatol* 1996; 132: 1178–82.
6. Shaw HM, McCarthy WH. Small-diameter malignant melanoma: a common diagnosis in New South Wales, Australia. *J Am Acad of Dermatol* 1992; 27: 679–82.
7. Anonymous. National Institutes for Health Consensus Conference. 'Diagnosis and Treatment of Early Melanoma' *JAMA* 1992; 268: 1314–19.
8. Elder DE, Goldman LI, Goldman SC, et al, Dysplastic nevus syndrome: a phenotypic association of sporadic cutaneous melanoma. *Cancer* 1980; 46: 1787–94.

9. Albert LS, Sober AJ, The dysplastic nevus as precursor and maker of increased risk for melanoma. In: *Cutaneous melanoma.* 2nd edn. (eds, Balch CM, Houghton AN, Milton GW, et al). Philadelphia: Lippincott, 1992: 60–9.
10. Kopf AW, Goldman RJ, Rivers JK, et al, Skin types in dysplastic nevus syndrome. *J Dermatol Surg Oncol* 1988; 14: 827–30.
11. MacKie, RM. Benign melanocytic lesions. In: *Skin cancer.* 2nd edn. (ed. MacKie RM). London: Martin Dunitz. 1996: 157–81.
12. Brownstein WE, Multiple agriminate juvenile melanoma. *Arch Dermatol* 1975; 106: 89–81.
13. Reed RJ, Ichinose H, Clark WH Jr, Mihm MC Jr, Common and uncommon melanocytic nevi and borderline melanomas. *Semin Oncol* 1975; 2: 119–47.

18

Surface microscopy features of melanoma

Scott Menzies, Wilhelm Stolz

THE TECHNIQUE

In vivo skin surface microscopy, dermatoscopy, dermoscopy, and epiluminescence microscopy are terms that all describe the same process of examination of cutaneous lesions with an incident light magnification system with oil or another fluid, e.g. disinfectant fluid at the skin microscope interface.[1] Fluid application removes the normal scattering of light at the skin surface which results in a translucent non-pigmented epidermis. This, in combination with magnification, permits a detailed examination of the pigmented structures of the epidermis and dermis. As a consequence, a multitude of morphological features not visible with the naked eye can be seen when examining pigmented skin lesions using surface microscopy (Figure 18.1).[2–4] The most commonly used surface microscopes are inexpensive handheld instruments (e.g. Episcope, Welch Allyn Inc, Skaneateles Falls, NY, USA; Dermatoscope, Heine Ltd, Herrsching, Germany; Dermogenius, Rodenstock Ltd, Munich, Germany) which allow a fixed magnification of ×10 (Figure 18.2).

History of surface microscopy

The history of surface microscopy has been reviewed by Stolz.[3] As a general principle, skin surface microscopy was first used to visualize nailfold vessels in 1663, with the use of oil to reduce scattering of light being reported by Unna in the late 19th century.[5,6] The first detailed description of surface microscopy was by Johann Saphier in 1921.[7–10] While Saphier did not use

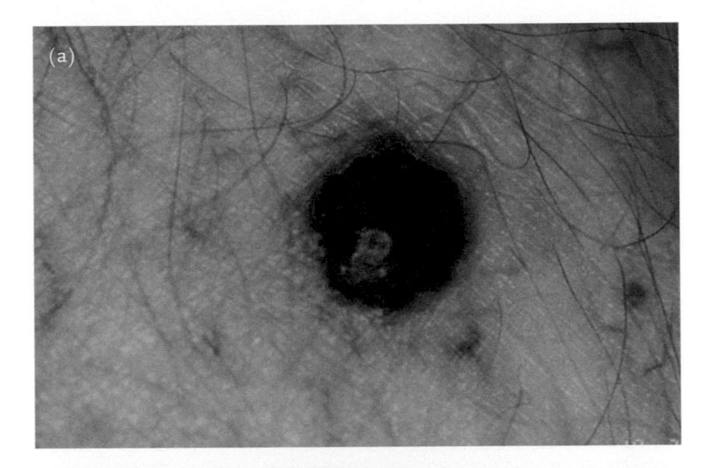

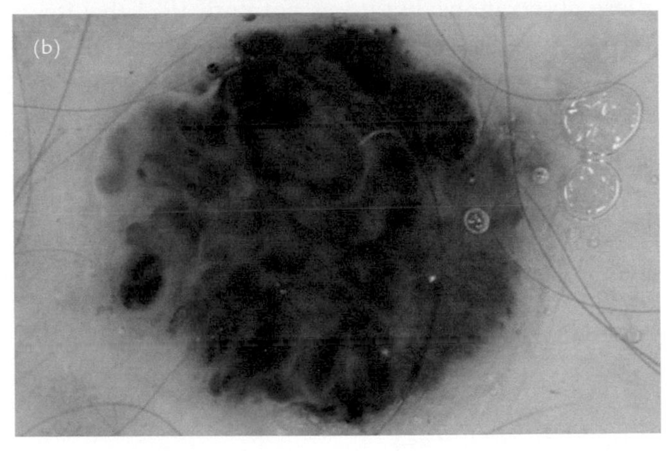

Figure 18.1 *(a) Clinical view of a 2.5 mm Breslow thickness nodular melanoma. (b) Surface microscopy view. The application of oil (which removes scattering of light from the surface of the skin) in combination with magnification results in the appearance of many morphological features not seen on standard clinical examination.*

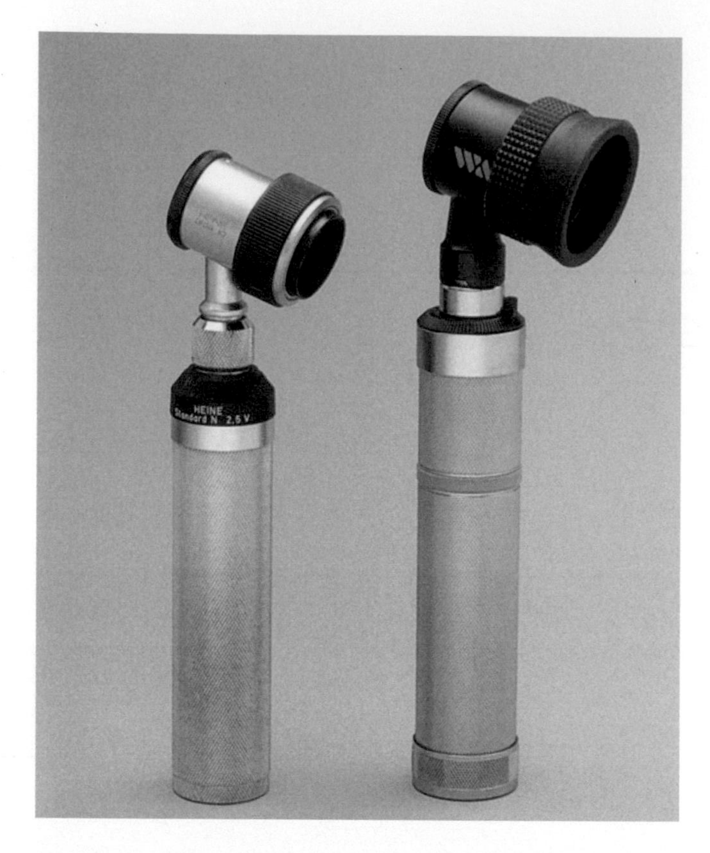

Figure 18.2 *Handheld surface microscopes with × 10 magnification.*

the technique to differentiate benign from malignant pigmented lesions he did describe some features of melanocytic naevi. In the 1950s Goldman extended these observations, but it was not until 1971 that it was recognized that surface microscopy improved the diagnosis of melanocytic lesions.[11,12] During this time and throughout the 1980s surface microscopy techniques used cumbersome and expensive binocular stereomicroscopes. It was the introduction of an inexpensive handheld surface microscope for routine clinical use in 1989 that resulted in a dramatic increase in investigations of the role of surface microscopy in the diagnosis of pigmented skin lesions.[13]

The effect of surface microscopy on melanoma diagnostic accuracy

In most studies skin surface microscopy has been shown to increase the diagnostic accuracy of melanoma.[14–23] Two studies found no significant difference in melanoma diagnosis.[24,25] In one of these studies limitations with the diagnostic model (such as the need for a pigment network to make the diagnosis of melanoma) make the results difficult to interpret.[24] In the other negative study the melanoma median Breslow thickness was greater than 0.75 mm, indicating more advanced lesions.[25] This was reflected in a higher than normal clinical diagnostic sensitivity of 94%. Finally, one study showed an improved sensitivity for melanoma with surface microscopy but a corresponding decrease in specificity.[26] All of these studies have been in an expert setting.

In a study by Binder, dermatologists relatively unfamiliar with the technique showed a significant loss of diagnostic accuracy in comparison with their standard 'clinical' diagnosis.[17] However, after a short training programme, surface microscopy diagnosis was superior to clinical diagnosis.[20] Recently, an education intervention on surface microscopy was designed in order to assess its potential role in the diagnosis of melanoma by the general practitioner (primary care physician).[23] In this study the sensitivity for melanoma diagnosis improved significantly from a clinical baseline pretest of 54.6% to a post-training surface microscopy diagnosis of 75.9%. Such a marked improvement with surface microscopy was seen without a decrease in specificity for melanoma diagnosis, indicating that the effect should occur without increasing the number of needless excisions. Furthermore, as experience with the technique increases, the diagnostic accuracy (which includes specificity) should also increase.[27] It was concluded in this study that all primary care physicians in countries where melanoma leads to significant mortality should be formally trained in skin surface microscopy.[23]

Surface microscopy methods for melanoma diagnosis

The following methods have been formally tested and shown to improve melanoma diagnostic accuracy. Formal comparisons of each method on the same set of pigmented lesions by experts in each method are lacking. Therefore confident comparisons between the diagnostic accuracy of each method are impossible. Rather, the particular method chosen by a clinician may depend upon his or her experience and confidence in using that method. The first two methods are treated in more depth, and the last two methods reviewed briefly.

ABCD rule of dermatoscopy

The ABCD rule of dermatoscopy was the first precisely defined surface microscopy method to diagnose benign from malignant melanocytic lesions.[3,18,28] Using an independent test set of 69 invasive melanomas (median Breslow thickness 1.1 mm) and a benign set of 103 naevi (18% dysplastic), the method gave a 93% sensitivity and 90% specificity for the diagnosis of melanoma. The method also improved the diagnostic accuracy for melanoma, showing 80% with the ABCD rule compared with 64% with the naked eye.

The method is outlined in Table 18.1 and Figures 18.3–18.8. Individual criteria are scored, multiplied by a weighting factor and added to give a total lesion score. A score of greater than 5.45 indicates a high probability of melanoma. A detailed atlas allowing inexperienced clinicians to use the method is available.[3]

The method of Menzies

Following a sensitivity and specificity analysis of the surface microscopy features of invasive melanoma a simple diagnostic method was developed that obtained a sensitivity of 92% and specificity of 71% on both training (62 melanomas and 159 atypical pigmented non-melanomas) and independent test sets (45 melanomas and 119 atypical non-melanomas).[29,30] Importantly, most non-melanomas analysed were considered atypical enough to warrant excision. Therefore the specificity of the method would be much higher in practice. In addition, the non-melanoma set included non-melanocytic lesions such as seborrhoeic keratoses, dermatofibromas, haemangiomas and pigmented basal cell carcinomas. Hence the method is useful for distinguishing all pigmented lesions from melanoma.

The method is described in Table 18.2. For melanoma to be diagnosed a lesion must have neither of both morphological negative features and one or more of the

Table 18.1 *ABCD rule of dermatoscopy*

Criterion	Possible points	Weight factor	Score (min–max)
Asymmetry	0–2	1.3	0–2.6
Border (abrupt)	0–8	0.1	0–0.8
Colours[a]	1–6	0.5	0.5–3.0
Dermatoscopic structures[b]	1–5	0.5	0.5–2.5
TOTAL			1.0–8.9

Each criterion is scored (Figures 18.3–18.8) and multiplied by its weight factor. The total lesion score is the addition of the individual criterion scores. A total score of <4.75 indicates a benign melanocytic lesion, 4.8–5.45 indicates a suspicious lesion suitable for close follow up or excision and >5.45 indicates melanoma.

[a] Colours scored are white, red, light brown, dark brown, slate blue, and black. White is chosen only if it is lighter than surrounding skin.

[b] The different structures scored are network, structureless areas, dots, globules, and streaks.

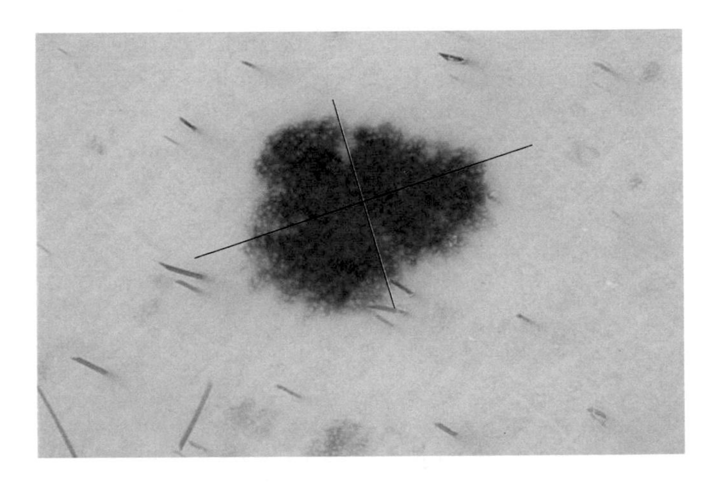

Figure 18.3 ***ABCD method.*** *Asymmetry. This is determined by putting two perpendicular lines in such a way that the lowest score is achieved for mirror symmetry of both shape and pattern. Here symmetry is achieved along the long axis but not the short axis (score 1).*

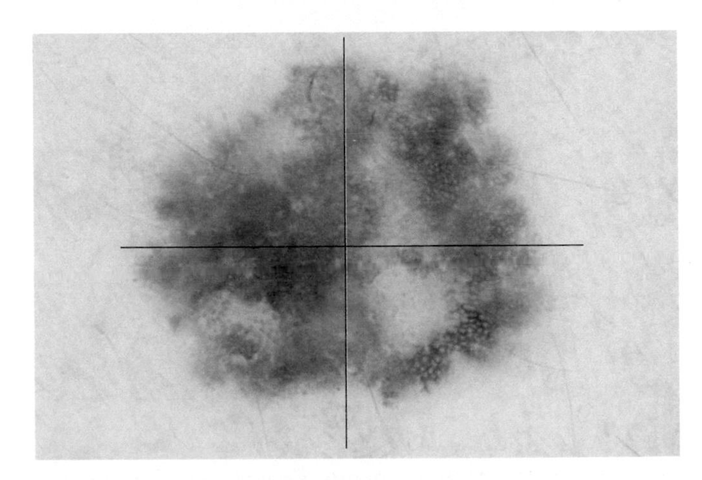

Figure 18.4 ***ABCD method.*** *Asymmetry. Here this 0.4 mm Breslow thickness melanoma has asymmetry of pattern over both axes of symmetry (score 2).*

nine positive features. Lesions illustrating these features and the method are shown in Figures 18.9–18.15. A detailed colour atlas allowing inexperienced clinicians to use the method has been published.[2] This atlas formed the basis of the education intervention that significantly improved the diagnosis of melanoma by primary care physicians (see above).[23] The method is also described in some depth on CD-ROM.[31]

Table 18.2 *Method of diagnosis of invasive melanoma (Menzies)*

Negative features (Both cannot be found)
Symmetry of pattern [a]
Presence of a single colour [b]
Positive features (At least one feature found)
Blue-white veil
Multiple brown dots
Pseudopods
Radial streaming
Scar-like depigmentation
Peripheral black dots/globules
Multiple (5–6) colours [b]
Multiple blue/grey dots
Broadened network

For melanoma to be diagnosed a lesion must have neither of the negative features but have one or more of the nine positive features. Refer to Figures 18.9–18.15 for descriptions of the features.

[a] Symmetry of pattern does not require shape symmetry (see Figure 18.9).

[b] The colours scored are black, grey, blue, dark brown, tan, and red. White is not scored as a colour.

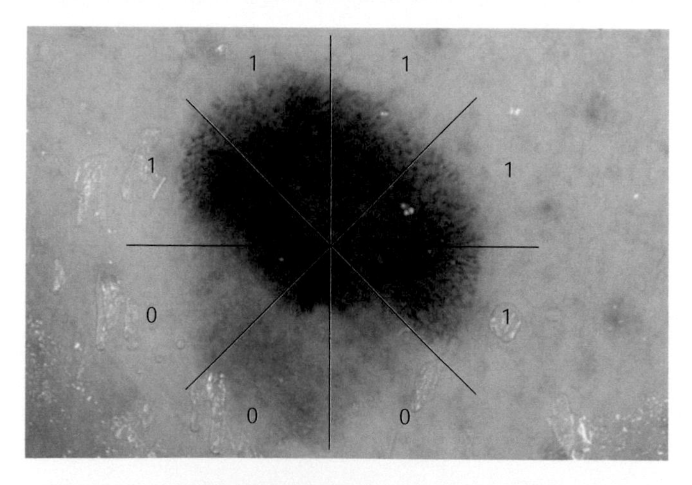

Figure 18.5 ***ABCD method***. *Border. For border scoring the lesion is divided into eight segments. Each segment is scored as 0 if the border graduates (fades) into normal skin and 1 if it ends abruptly. Here this 0.4 mm Breslow thick melanoma has a border score of 5.*

The method of Argenziano – seven-point checklist

A study by Argenziano et al.[32] describes a method using seven diagnostic features, three that are scored as

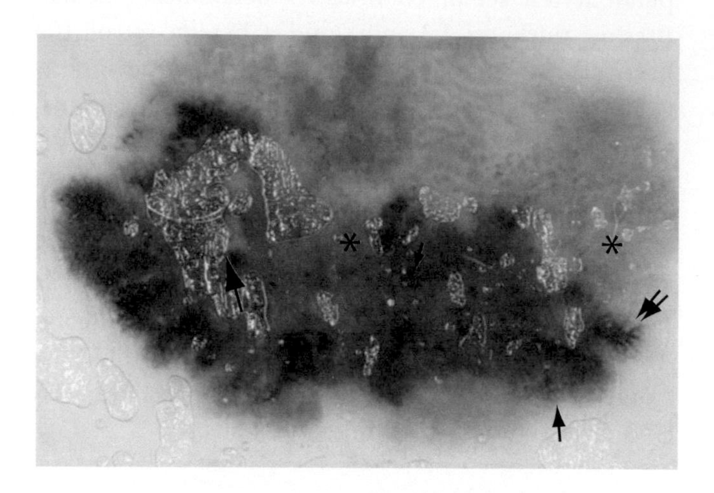

Figure 18.6 ***ABCD method***. *Different structures. Each of the five different structures are given a score of 1. Structureless areas can be of any colour but must occupy more than 10% of the lesion (*). Dots (small arrow) and globules (large arrow) are distinguished by their size and can be of any colour. Dots are scored only if more than one is present. Branched streaks (double arrow) are seen as a result of an aberrant network and are scored only if more than one is present. They can be within or at the edge of a lesion. Pigment network (medium arrow) is scored as a separate feature. Diagnosis: 0.8 mm Breslow thick melanoma.*

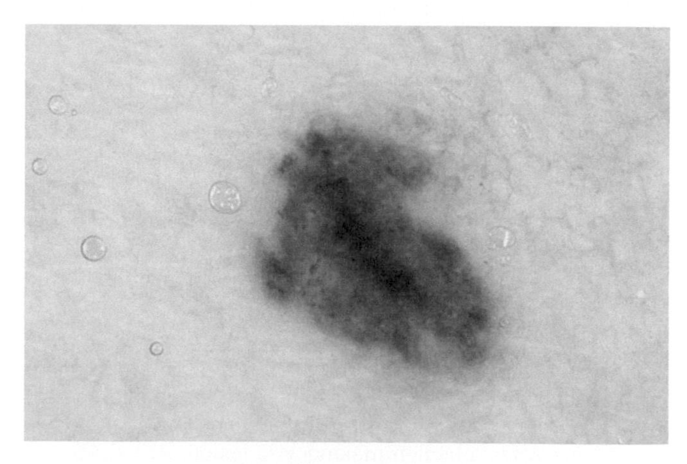

Figure 18.7 ***ABCD method***. *The lesion is scored as follows: Asymmetry 2 (weighted total 2.6), Border 0 (weighted total 0), Colours (light brown, dark brown, slate grey) 3 (weighted total 1.5), Different structures (Structureless areas and globules) 2 (weighted total 1.0). Total lesion score 5.1. Diagnosis: dysplastic compound naevus.*

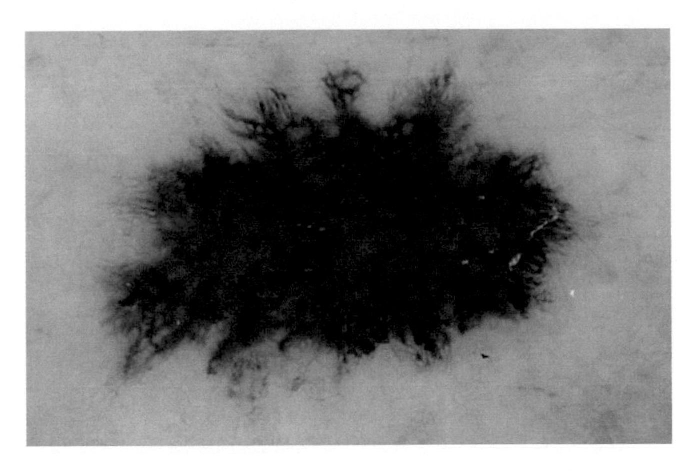

Figure 18.8 ***ABCD method***. *The lesion is scored as follows: Asymmetry 2 (weighted total 2.6), Border 5 (weighted total 0.5), Colours 4 (light brown, dark brown, slate grey, black) (weighted total 2.0), Different structures 5 (Structureless areas, dots, globules, branched streaks and network) (weighted total 2.5). Total lesion score 7.6. Diagnosis: 0.6 mm Breslow thick superficial spreading melanoma.*

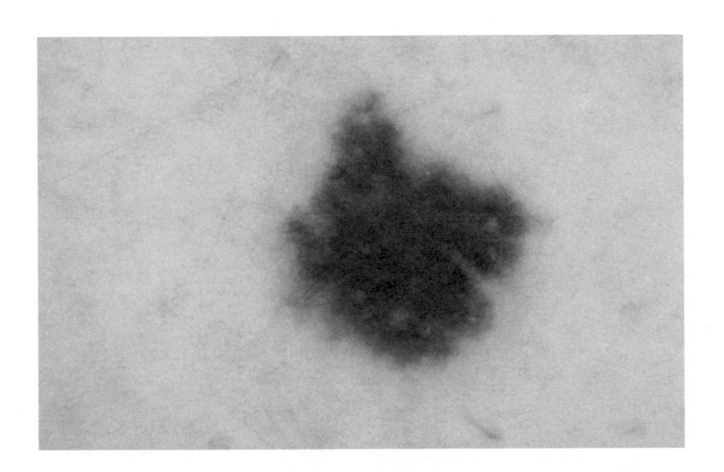

Figure 18.9 ***Method of Menzies.*** *Symmetry of pattern is defined as mirror symmetry of pattern (not shape) over all axes through the centre of the lesion. This dysplastic naevus shows symmetry of pattern despite being asymmetrical in shape. Because it has one of the negative features of melanoma (Table 18.2) it is diagnosed as non-melanoma. Reproduced with permission from Menzies SW et al,* An atlas of surface microscopy of pigmented skin lesions. *Sydney. McGraw-Hill Book Company, 1996.*[2]

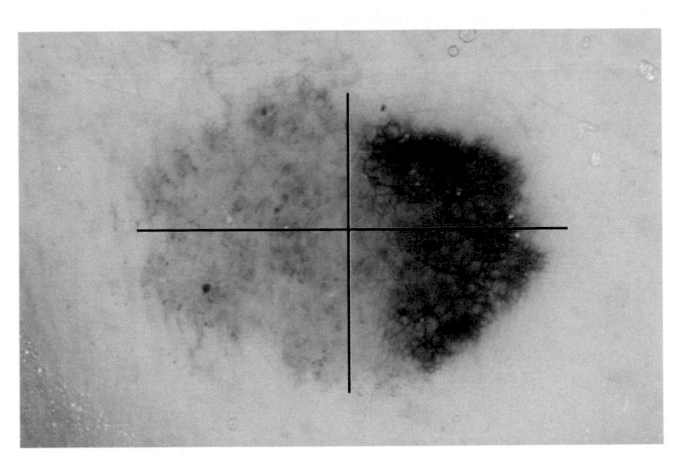

Figure 18.10 ***Method of Menzies.*** *While this lesion has symmetry of pattern over its long axis, it is asymmetrical over its short axis. It is therefore considered as asymmetrical. While this compound naevus has neither of the two negative features it also has none of the nine positive features of melanoma, and therefore is diagnosed as non-melanoma (Table 18.2).*

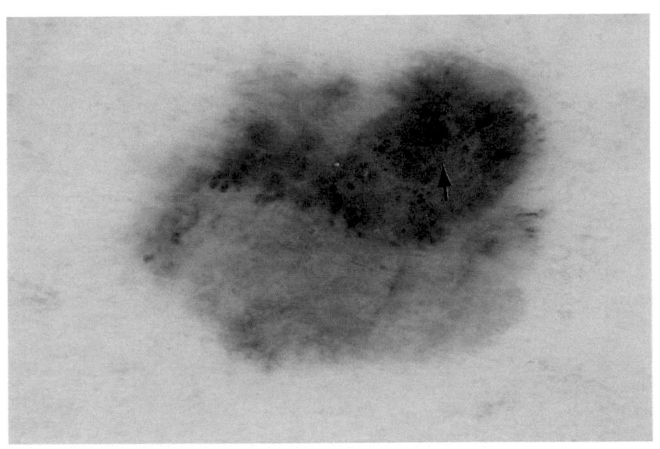

Figure 18.11 ***Method of Menzies.*** *This lesion has neither of the two negative features, and has two positive features of melanoma. Multiple brown dots (arrow) are irregularly distributed focal areas of multiple brown (usually dark brown) dots (not globules). Blue-white veil is seen here as an area of irregular, structureless, confluent blue pigmentation with an overlying white 'ground glass' haze. It can never occupy the entire lesion. Diagnosis. 0.7 mm Breslow thick superficial spreading melanoma.*

major and four as minor (Table 18.3). This was developed from a training set of 57 melanomas and 139 atypical melanocytic derived non-melanomas and tested on an independent set of 60 melanomas and 86 atypical melanocytic non-melanomas. Non-melanocytic derived lesions were not examined. From the total combined sets the method gave a sensitivity of 95% and specificity of 75% for the diagnosis of melanoma. A different method using similar principles has recently been published by others.[33]

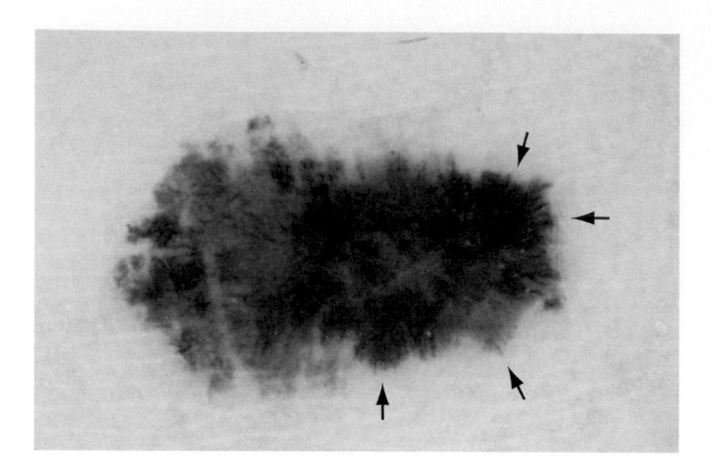

Figure 18.12 ***Method of Menzies.*** *This lesion has neither of the two negative features and has one positive feature of melanoma. Radial streaming (arrows) are finger-like extensions at the edge of a lesion which are never distributed regularly or symmetrically around the lesion. Diagnosis: 0.35 mm Breslow thick superficial spreading melanoma.*

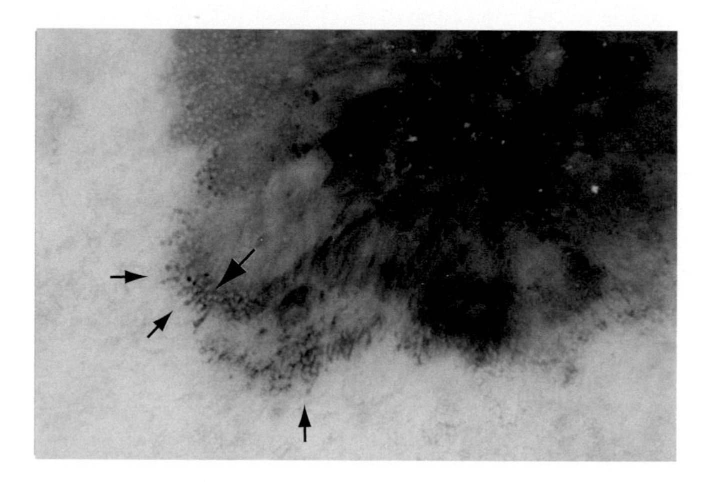

Figure 18.13 ***Method of Menzies.*** *This lesion has neither of the two negative features, and has four positive features of melanoma. The lesion has multiple (5–6) colours. The colours scored are black, grey, blue, dark brown, tan, and red. White is not scored as a colour. Pseudopods (small arrows) are bulbous and often kinked projections that are found at the edge of a lesion either directly connected to the tumour body or pigmented network. They can never be seen distributed regularly or symmetrically around the lesion. A broadened network (large arrow) is a network made up of focally irregular thicker 'cords' of the net. Multiple blue-grey dots are foci of multiple blue or grey dots (not globules) often described as 'pepper-like' in pattern. Here they are seen at bottom left corner of the lesion. Blue-white veil is also seen near the centre of the figure. Diagnosis: 0.9 mm Breslow thick superficial spreading melanoma.*

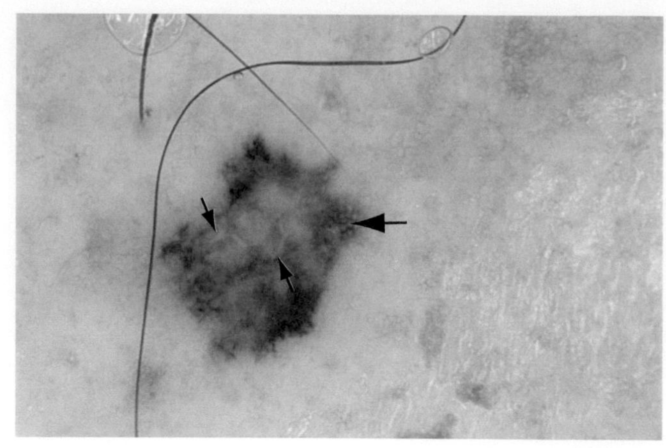

Figure 18.14 ***Method of Menzies.*** *This lesion has neither of the two negative features, and has three positive features of melanoma. Scar-like depigmentation (small arrows) are areas of white distinct irregular extensions (true scarring), which should not be confused with hypo- or depigmentation due to simple loss of melanin. Multiple blue-grey dots are seen scattered throughout the centre of the lesion. A focus of broadened network is also seen (large arrow). Diagnosis: 0.6 mm Breslow thick superficial spreading melanoma.*

Table 18.3 ***Seven-point checklist method of melanoma diagnosis***

Features scored	7-point score
Major criteria	
Atypical pigment network	2
Grey-blue areas	2
Atypical vascular pattern	2
Minor criteria	
Streaks (radial streaming or pseudopods)	1
Blotches	1
Irregular dots and globules	1
Regression pattern (scar-like depigmentation or multiple blue-grey dots)	1

For melanoma to be diagnosed the addition of the scores must be ≥ 3. Atypical pigment network refers to a prominent (hyperpigmented or broadened) and irregular network. Atypical vascular pattern refers to linear, dotted, or globular red structures irregularly distributed outside areas of regression and associated with other melanocytic pigment patterns. Blotches are brown, grey, and black areas of diffuse pigmentation with irregular shape or distribution and abrupt end. Irregular dots and globules are black, brown, or blue round structures irregularly distributed within the lesion.

Pattern analysis

Investigators at the University of Vienna described various 'patterns' used to distinguish melanoma from benign pigmented skin lesions.[16] Others have also described similar specific patterns of pigmented lesions.[2–4] In the Vienna group's work, eight surface microscopy criteria distinguish the various benign and malignant pigmented lesions, with a broad summary shown in Table 18.4. Of the four methods described in this chapter, pattern analysis requires the most experience to be fully utilized. Nevertheless, in experienced hands it improves the diagnosis of most pigmented skin lesions.[16,17,20]

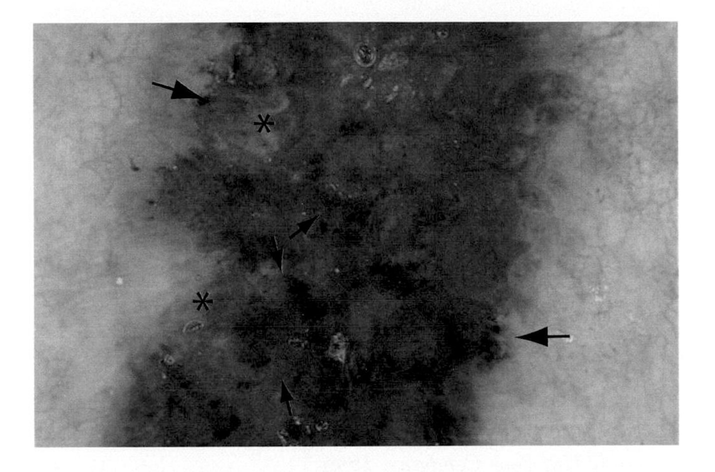

Figure 18.15 ***Method of Menzies.*** *This lesion has neither of the two negative features, and has five positive features of melanoma. Peripheral black dots/globules are black dots or globules found at or near the edge of the lesion (large arrow). Multiple brown dots (small arrows), blue-white veil (*), multiple (5–6) colours and scar-like depigmentation is also seen. Diagnosis: 1.4 mm Breslow thick superficial spreading melanoma.*

Surface microscopy of pigmented non-melanocytic lesions

Surface microscopy can improve the diagnosis of pigmented non-melanocytic lesions. In particular, common lesions that are in the clinical differential diagnosis of melanoma such as pigmented basal cell carcinomas, haemangiomas, and seborrhoeic keratoses have distinct surface microscopy morphological patterns (Figures 18.16–18.18).[2–4,16,34]

Table 18.4 *Summary of pattern analysis for pigmented skin lesions*[16]

Surface microscopy criteria	Benign pigmented skin lesion (PSL)	Melanoma
Pigment network	Regular, delicate, narrow, gradually thins at periphery	Irregular, prominent, wide, abruptly ends at periphery
Diffuse pigmentation	Regular, homogeneous, gradually thins at periphery	Irregular, inhomogeneous, abruptly ends at periphery
Depigmentation	Regular centre	Irregular centre and periphery
Brown globules	Uniform in size and shape, regularly distributed	Varied in size and shape, irregularly distributed
Black dots	Uniform in size and shape, regularly distributed, central position	Varied in size and shape, irregularly distributed, peripheral position
Radial streaming[a]	Absent	Present
Pseudopods	Absent	Present
Grey-blue veil	Absent	Present

For individual pattern analysis profiles of pigmented lesion subtypes refer to Pehamberger et al.[16]
[a] Except within a pigmented Spitz's naevus (starburst lesion); rarely present in dysplastic naevus.

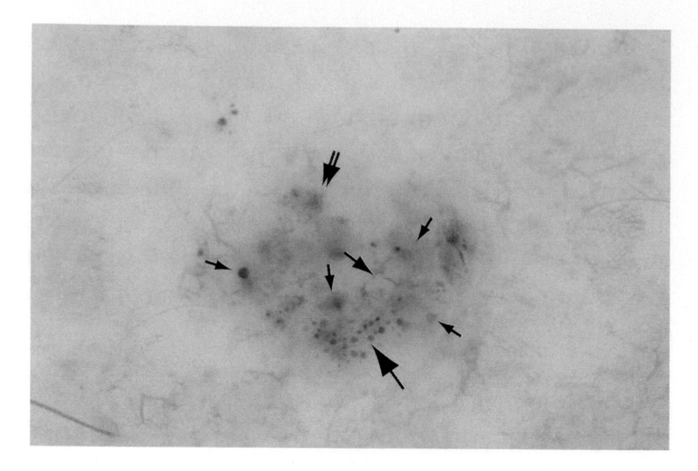

Figure 18.16 ***Surface microscopy of pigmented basal cell carcinoma.*** *Pigmented BCCs can be diagnosed with a sensitivity of 93% and specificity of 89% (invasive melanoma) and 92% (benign pigmented skin lesions) using the following method.*[35] *To be diagnosed they must have no pigment network and one or more of the following positive features; large blue-grey ovoid nests (small arrow), multiple blue-grey globules (large arrow), arborizing (tree-like) telangiectasia (medium arrow), spoke wheel areas (double arrow), maple leaf like areas, and ulceration.*

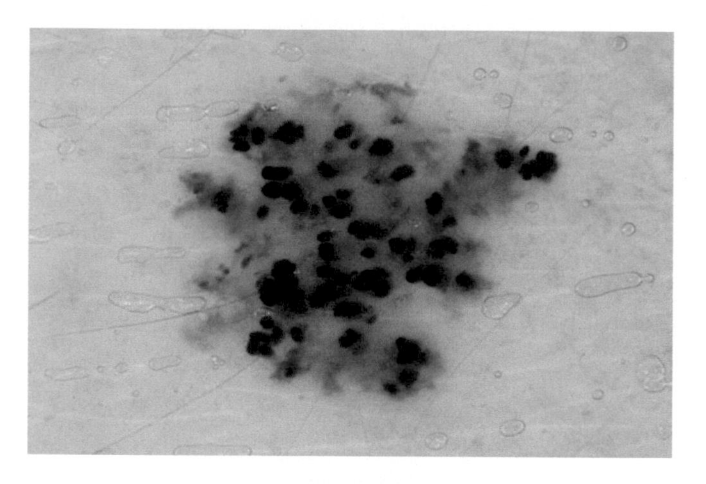

Figure 18.17 ***Surface microscopy of haemangioma.*** *A consistent feature of the surface microscopy of haemangioma is the presence of a single colour of red or red-blue. This pigmentation is often found in lacunae (as seen here). Reproduced with permission from Menzies SW et al,* An atlas of surface microscopy of pigmented skin lesions. *Sydney: McGraw-Hill Book Company, 1996.*[2]

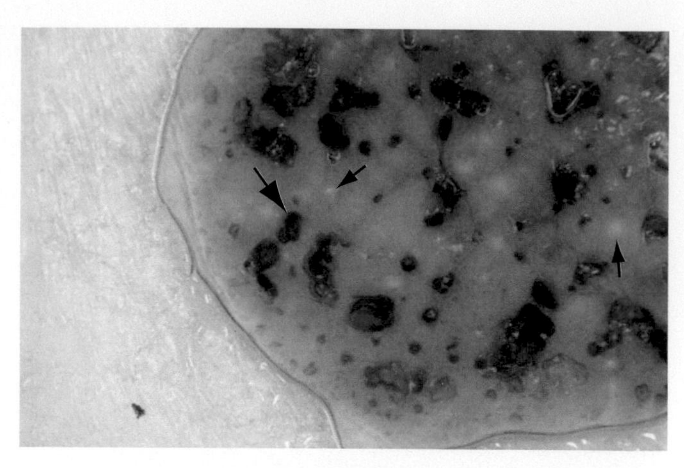

Figure 18.18 ***Surface microscopy of seborrhoeic keratoses.*** *The main features of this common lesion are an absent pigment network, and one or more of the following: multiple milia-like cysts (small arrow), multiple crypts (large arrow) or fissures. Reproduced with permission from Menzies SW et al,* An atlas of surface microscopy of pigmented skin lesions. *Sydney: McGraw-Hill Book Company, 1996.*[2]

REFERENCES

1. Cohen D, Sangueza O, Fass E, Stiller M, In vivo cutaneous surface microscopy: revised nomenclature. *Int J Dermatol* 1993; 32: 257–258.
2. Menzies SW, Crotty, KA, Ingvar C, McCarthy WH, *An atlas of surface microscopy of pigmented skin lesions.* Sydney, Australia: McGraw-Hill International Book Company, 1996.
3. Stolz W, Braun-Falco O, Bilek P, et al, *Colour atlas of dermatoscopy*, 2nd edn. Oxford: Blackwell Science, 2002.
4. Kreusch J, Rassner G, *Auflichtmikroskopie pigmentierter Hauttumoren—Ein Bildatlas.* Stuttgart: Georg Thieme Verlag, 1991.
5. Gilje O, O'Leary P, Baldes E, Capillary microscopic examination of skin disease. *Arch Dermatol* 1958; 68: 136–45.
6. Unna P, Die Diaskopie der Hautkrankheiten. *Berlin Klinische Wochenschrift* 1893; 42: 1016–21.
7. Saphier J, Die Dermatoskopie. I. Mitteilung. *Arch Dermatol Syphilol* 1921; 128: 1–19.
8. Saphier J, Die Dermatoskopie. II. Mitteilung. *Arch Dermatol Syphilol* 1921; 132: 69–86.
9. Saphier J, Die Dermatoskopie. III. Mitteilung. *Arch Dermatol Syphilol* 1921; 134: 314–22.
10. Saphier J, Die Dermatoskopie. IV. Mitteilung. *Arch of Dermatol Syphilol* 1921; 136: 149–58.
11. Goldman L, Some investigative studies of pigmented nevi with cutaneous microscopy. *J Investig Dermatol* 1951; 16: 407–27.
12. MacKie R, An aid to the preoperative assessment of pigmented lesions of the skin. *Br J Dermatol* 1971; 85: 232–8.
13. Stolz W, Bilek P, Landthaler M, Merkle T, Braun-Falco O, Skin surface microscopy. *Lancet* 1989; II: 864–5.
14. Krähn G, Gottlober P, Sander C, Peter RU, Dermatoscopy and high frequency sonography: two useful non-invasive methods to increase preoperative diagnostic accuracy in pigmented skin lesions. *Pigment Cell Research* 1998; 11: 151–4.
15. Steiner A, Pehamberger H, Wolff K, In vivo epiluminescence microscopy of pigmented skin lesions. II. Diagnosis of small pigmented skin lesions and early detection of malignant melanoma. *J Am Acad Dermatol* 1987; 17: 584–91.
16. Pehamberger H, Binder M, Steiner A, Wolff K, In vivo epiluminescence microscopy: improvement of early diagnosis of melanoma. *J Investig Dermatol.* 1993; 100: 356S–62S.
17. Binder M, Schwarz M, Winkler A, et al, Epiluminescence microscopy: a useful tool for the diagnosis of pigmented skin lesions for formally trained dermatologists. *Arch Dermatol.* 1995; 131: 286–91.
18. Nachbar F, Stolz W, Merkle T, et al, The ABCD rule of dermatoscopy: high prospective value in the diagnosis of doubtful melanocytic skin lesions. *J Am Acad Dermatol.* 1994; 30: 551–9.

19. Pazzini C, Pozzi M, Betti R, et al, Improvement of diagnostic accuracy in the clinical diagnosis of pigmented skin lesions by epiluminescence microscopy. *Skin Cancer* 1996; 11: 159–61.
20. Binder M, Puespoeck-Schwarz M, Steiner A, et al, Epiluminescence microscopy of small pigmented skin lesions: short-term formal training improves the diagnostic performance of dermatologists. *J Am Acad Dermatol* 1997; 36: 197–202.
21. Carli P, De Giorgi V, Naldi L, Dosi G, Reliability and inter-observer agreement of dermoscopic diagnosis of melanoma and melanocytic naevi. *Eur J Cancer Prev* 1998; 7: 397–402.
22. Stanganelli I, Serafini M, Cainelli T, et al, Accuracy of epiluminescence microscopy among practical dermatologists: a study from the Emilia-Romagna region of Italy. *Tumori* 1998; 84: 701–5.
23. Westerhoff K, McCarthy W, Menzies S, Increase in the sensitivity for melanoma diagnosis by primary care physicians using skin surface microscopy. *Br J Dermatol* 2000; 143: 1016–20.
24. Cristofolini M, Zumiani G, Bauer P et al, Dermatoscopy: usefulness in the differential diagnosis of cutaneous pigmentary lesions. *Melanoma Res* 1994; 4: 391–4.
25. Soyer HP, Smolle J, Leitinger G, et al, Diagnostic reliability of dermoscopic criteria for detecting malignant melanoma. *Dermatology* 1995; 190: 25–30.
26. Rao BK, Marghoob AA, Stolz W, et al, Can early malignant melanoma be differentiated from atypical melanocytic nevi by in vivo techniques? *Skin Res Technol* 1997; 3: 8–14.
27. Binder M, Kittler H, Steiner A, et al, Reevaluation of the ABCD rule for epiluminescence microscopy. *J Am Acad Dermatol.* 1999; 40: 171–6.
28. Stolz W, Riemann A, Cognetta A, et al, ABCD rule of dermatoscopy: a new practical method for early recognition of malignant melanoma. *Eur J Dermatol* 1994; 4: 521–7.
29. Menzies S, Ingvar C, McCarthy W, A sensitivity and specificity analysis of the surface microscopy features of invasive melanoma. *Melanoma Res* 1996; 6: 55–62.
30. Menzies S, Ingvar C, Crotty K, McCarthy W, Frequency and morphologic characteristics of invasive melanomas lacking specific surface microscopic features. *Arch Dermatol.* 1996; 132: 1178–82.
31. Rabinovitz H, Kopf A, Katz B, Dermoscopy. A practical guide. 1999. (CD-ROM)
32. Argenziano G, Fabbrocini G, Carli P, et al, Epiluminescence microscopy for the diagnosis of doubtful melanocytic skin lesions: comparison of the ABCD rule of dermatoscopy and a new 7-point checklist based on pattern analysis. *Arch Dermatol* 1998; 134: 1563–70.
33. Dal Pozzo V, Benelli C, Roscetti E, The seven features for melanoma: a new dermoscopic algorithm for the diagnosis of malignant melanoma. *Eur J Dermatol* 1999; 9: 303–38.
34. Menzies S, Westerhoff K, Rabinovitz H, et al, The surface microscopy of pigmented basal cell carcinoma. *Arch Dermatol* 2000; 136: 1012–16.

19

Computer aided instrumentation for the diagnosis of primary melanoma

Michael Binder, Scott Menzies

INTRODUCTION: THE NEED FOR INSTRUMENTATION

Efforts to develop automated instrumentation for the diagnosis of melanoma have been increasing in parallel with the worldwide increase in melanoma incidence, while appreciating that the confidence of non-expert clinicians in diagnosing melanoma is not high.[1–3] Conventional clinical examination even in an expert environment achieves suboptimal diagnostic accuracy.[4] The need for automated diagnostic instruments is further underlined by knowledge that screening for melanoma may be cost-effective in areas of high incidence, such as Australia.[5] Such cost-effectiveness depends on the screener being a non-expert primary care physician.

TECHNOLOGICAL APPROACHES

Image analysis

As described in Chapter 18, the technique of surface microscopy (epiluminescence microscopy, dermatoscopy, dermoscopy) increases the morphological detail seen in pigmented lesions and enhances the clinical diagnosis of melanoma. For this reason a general trend is for groups to investigate image analysis of surface microscopy (Figure 19.1) rather than conventional clinical photographic images.[6–9] Such an approach has recently been reviewed.[10]

Initial studies have described image analysis of digitized 35 mm transparencies taken with surface microscopy cameras. Schindewolf et al. examined such images of 194 melanomas and 126 melanocytic naevi.[11] The median melanoma Breslow thickness or number of dysplastic naevi was not stated. A cross-validated model gave a correct classification rate of 78%. The sensitivity and specificity rates were not given. Their surface microscopy image analysis model was not superior to a model of the same lesions analyzed with digitized conventional photographic slides. Menzies et al. examined images of 75 invasive melanomas (median Breslow thickness 0.7 mm) and 95 atypical pigmented non-melanomas, which included 42 dysplastic naevi and a variety of non-melanocytic lesions.[12] Cross-validated analysis gave a 93% sensitivity and 67% specificity for melanoma. Finally, Binder et al. analyzed 37 melanomas (median Breslow thickness 0.72 mm) and 75 melanocytic naevi (including 42 dysplastic naevi).[13] On a small independent test set a model with 90% sensitivity and 74% specificity was obtained.

The encouraging results seen in the above pilot studies of image analysis of digitized surface microscopy photographic slides led to the development of charge coupled device (CCD) video based real time surface microscopy image acquisition devices that could be used to develop automated diagnostic systems (reviewed in[10]). Menzies et al. described a 3 CCD video instrument (Mk1 Skin Polarprobe), which was designed to improve their pilot results by increasing the field of view and allowing control for non-uniformity of illumination and colour calibration.[12,14] Analysis of 45 invasive melanomas (median Breslow thickness 0.62 mm) and 176 atypical

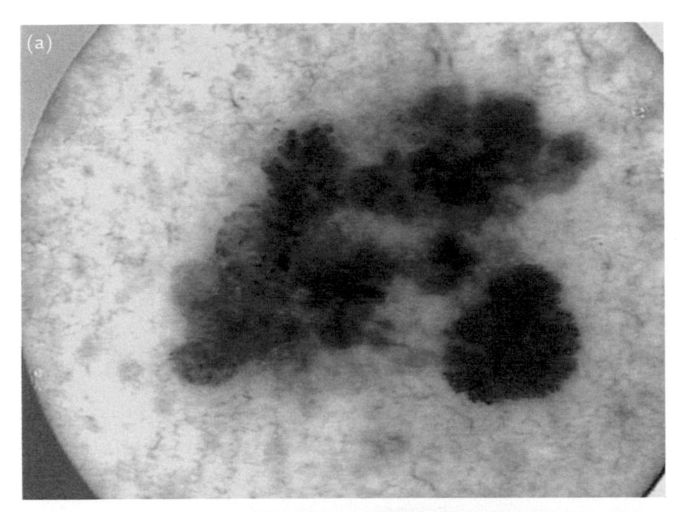

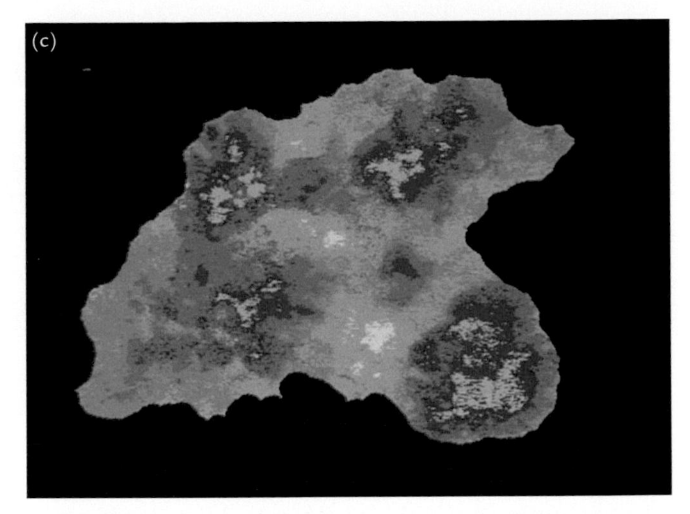

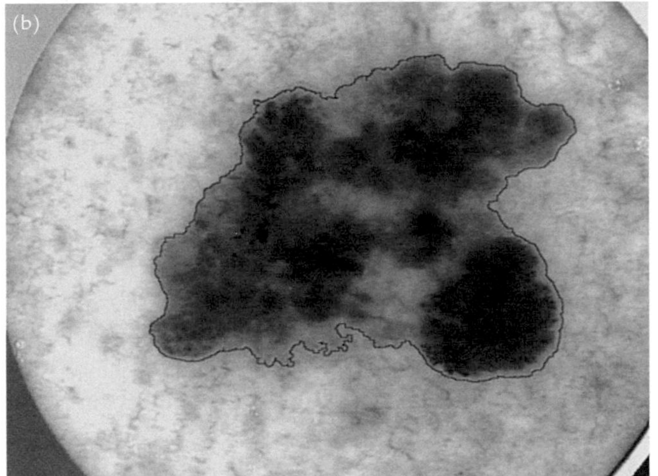

Figure 19.1 *Image analysis of surface microscopy (oil epiluminescence microscopy) digitized pigmented lesions.*
(a) Digitization of surface microscopy images with corner targets allows computerized colour calibration of lesions. This is a fundamental advantage of image analysis when compared with simple visualization by clinicians.
(b) Automated boundary detection algorithms allow isolation of the lesion from the skin.
(c) Automated image analysis such as detailed colour analysis of lesions can be obtained because of colour calibration procedures. These images are from the Mk2 Skin Polarprobe (Polartechnics Ltd, Sydney, Australia).

pigmented non-melanomas (including 73 dysplastic naevi and a variety of non-melanocytic lesions) gave a cross-validated model with a sensitivity of 89% and specificity of 80%. A number of instruments were then designed (Mk2 Skin Polarprobe) and are currently collecting data for model development suitable for a multicentre clinical trial (Figure 19.1).

Analyzing digitized images from a polarizing 1 CCD surface microscopy video instrument using the image analysis software DB-Dermo-MIPS written by the Burroni-Dell'Eva Biomedical Engineering Group (Sienna, Italy), Seidenari et al., created a model from 31 melanomas (mean Breslow thickness 0.73 mm) and 59 naevi.[15] The number of dysplastic naevi was not given. They achieved a 93% sensitivity and 95% specificity for melanoma diagnosis. Details on any cross-validation procedure were not given. Importantly, the model had a greater diagnostic accuracy for melanoma compared with both inexperienced and experienced clinicians (the latter group obtaining a sensitivity of 81% and a specificity of 95% for the same set). Recently this group analyzed another model using the same system on an independent test set of 18 melanomas (Breslow thickness <0.75 mm) and 365 naevi.[16] Again a description of the atypia of the naevi was not given. Although the sample size of melanomas was small, a sensitivity of 100% and specificity of 92% for melanoma were achieved.

More recently, Andreassi et al. described a 3 CCD video image analysis system developed by the Burroni-Dell'Eva Biomedical Engineering Group.[17] In this study, 57 early melanomas (32 in situ and 25 invasive with a Breslow thickness <0.5 mm) and 90 naevi (including 42 dysplastic naevi) were analyzed. A multivariate analysis with cross-validation created a model with a sensitivity of 81% and a specificity of 88% for the diagnosis of melanoma.

The Diagnostic and Neuronal Analysis of Skin Cancer (DANAOS) Consortium (Zentrum für Neuroinformatik, Bochum, Germany) has 13 collection centres within Europe. It collects standardized data sets of lesions, which include calibrated 3 CCD digitized surface microscopy images.[18] The VIDKO system (Regensburg, Germany) supports the classification of pigmented skin lesions by employing bayesian belief networks. Preliminary data indicated a correct classification of pigmented skin lesion (PSL) by the VIDKO system in more than 90%.[19] The increasing number of commercially available 1 CCD video instruments such as MoleMax (Derma Instruments, Vienna, Austria) and FotoFinder Derma (Teach Screen, Griesbach, Germany) that were designed for monitoring pigmented lesions using digitized surface microscopy imaging are also being investigated with a view to producing automated diagnostic instruments. Most recently, Dreiseitl et al. described the classification results of a study using a dataset of 518 digital images (207 benign naevi, 195 atypical naevi and 116 early melanomas) acquired by the MoleMax device.[20] The digital images were automatically segmented, and 45 morphometric parameters were extracted, based on shape, texture, and colour properties of the lesion. In addition, seven clinical parameters based on the patient's history were used as an additional source of information. Artificial neural networks were used as multivariate classifiers. 260 randomly chosen lesions were used as a training set, the remainder of images served as the test set. Using two-way receiver operating characteristics analysis for measuring the performance of classification, common naevi versus dysplastic naevi and dysplastic naevi versus melanoma achieved an area under the curve of 0.895 and 0.929, respectively. The authors also found that adding clinical information to the data set enhanced the performance significantly.

Spectrophotometric analysis

In contrast to regular image analysis, telespectrophotometry (TS) uses an electronic camera that is provided with a set of interference filters. Images are scanned at selected narrow banded wavelengths usually ranging from 420 nm to 1040 nm. The acquired spectral images are stored in a personal computer. Intensity levels and dimensions from the image picture elements from each of the spectral channels are then analyzed and provide several descriptors related to the colour and shape of the imaged lesion. Calibration using reflectance standards and a geometric reference frame allows objective analysis of the images based on quantifying reflectance.

Marchesini et al. focused in a series of studies on the technological background of TS and on the clinical application in pigmented skin lesions.[21,22] In a study of 31 melanomas and 31 benign pigmented skin lesions, applying stepwise discriminant analysis to the data, a sensitivity of 90.3% and a specificity of 77.4% were achieved.[23] In a relatively small study (18 melanomas, 17 common melanocytic naevi and 8 dysplastic naevi) published by Bono et al., a total of 33 (76.7%) lesions were correctly diagnosed by TS, compared with 35 (81.4%) correct clinical diagnoses.[24] Tomatis et al. achieved similar results.[25] Their study included 18 melanomas and 33 benign naevi. An overall sensitivity and specificity of 89% and 88% respectively, was achieved. By introducing morphometric parameters of asymmetry, border features, colour and dimension (ABCD), this approach has been recently extended by Bono et al., who examined 53 melanomas and 142 non-melanoma lesions by the combination of TS and morphometry.[26] By using a multivariate logistic regression model the TS derived parameter of mean reflectance in the infrared spectrum and size as a morphometric parameter were independently associated with melanoma. The Melafind System (EOS Inc, Irvington, NY) uses the TS approach and is currently under clinical investigation. Promising pilot studies have shown both high sensitivity and high specificity of diagnosis.[27]

In vivo confocal microscopy

Confocal microscopy provides higher resolution images with better rejection of out of focus information than conventional light microscopy (reviewed in[28]). Furthermore, the ability of confocal microscopy to obtain optical sections within the depth of intact tissue has made this technique ideally suited to the study of tissue in living animals. Such in vivo confocal microscopy (IVCM) has been shown to be of diagnostic importance in ophthalmology. More recently, high resolution imaging of epidermis and upper dermis has been achieved, particularly with near infrared IVCM.[29–32] While the literature is scant, evidence suggests that with near infrared IVCM (shown at wavelengths of 800 nm and 830 nm) melanin provides a strong contrast by increased backscattering of light. Morphological detail such as cellular and nuclear size of pigmented cells in vivo has been achieved (Figure 19.2).[29,30] It remains to be seen whether such instrumentation will lead to automated diagnosis of primary melanoma in vivo.

Magnetic resonance imaging

Magnetic resonance imaging (MRI) has been considered for supporting the diagnosis of relatively small skin lesions. In the late 1980s the development of surface coils and high field scanners improved the signal-to-noise ratio substantially to meet the requirements for this specialized task.[33] Using MRI melanin is detected as a paramagnetic substance which typically shortens both T1 and T2 relaxation times. Melanocytic tumours therefore show characteristic high signal intensity on MR images.[34] Takahashi found that benign lesions exhibited a more homogeneous signal in T2 weighted scans.[35,36] Melanomas, however, displayed a higher signal in T2 weighted scans compared with tumour-free subcutis. In his studies the negative tumour-to-subcutis contrast was significantly different from the ratios of benign pigmented skin lesions. Maeurer et al. compared 27 melanocytic naevi versus 18 melanomas by high resolution MRI.[34] Their sophisticated approach included sequences with and without contrast enhancement and suppression of the water and fat phase of the sequences. Statistical significance was shown for T2 weighted and fat suppressed, unenhanced, and contrast enhanced sequences. However, because of substantial overlap they concluded that MRI was of limited usefulness for clinical application.

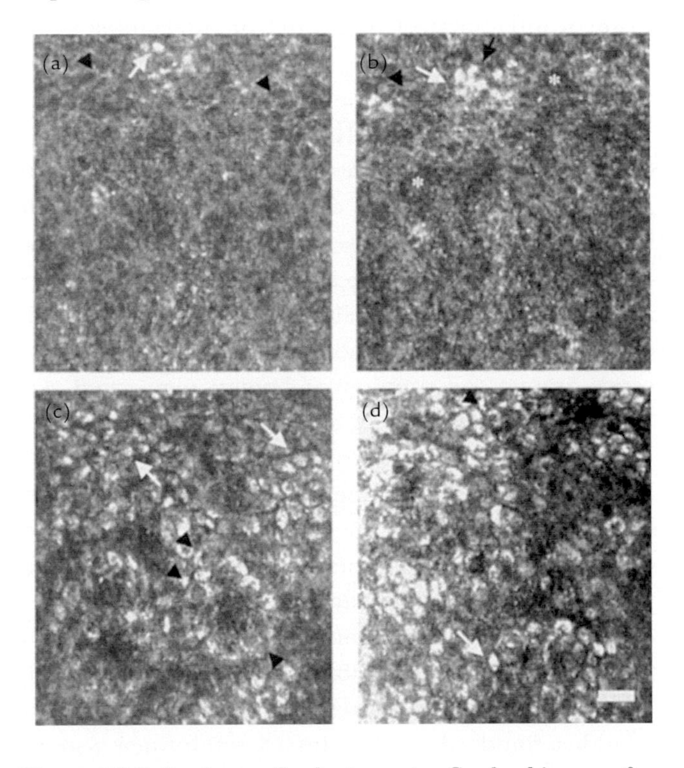

Figure 19.2 *In vivo confocal microscopy. Confocal images of a benign melanocytic lesion (junctional naevus) and surrounding normal skin. (a) and (b) show a transverse section at the dermoepidermal level of inner forearm normal skin. Basal keratinocytes (arrows) are brighter than surrounding spinous keratinocytes (arrowheads) and papillary dermis (*). (c) and (d) correspond to en face sections of a junctional naevus showing a uniform pattern of bright monomorphic cells, naevomelanocytes (arrows) and pigmented basal keratinocytes (arrowheads). (Courtesy of Salvador Gonzalez and Milind Rajadhaksha, Wellman Laboratories of Photomedicine, Department of Dermatology, Massachusetts General Hospital, Boston, MA; Imaging Parameters: VivaScope 1000 – Lucid Inc, Henrietta, NY, 830 nm diode laser, 30×, 0.9 numerical aperture water immersion objective lens; illumination power 5–25 milliwatts at the skin; scale bar 30 μm).*

High frequency ultrasound

Measurements of skin in vivo by high frequency ultrasound B scanning (20 MHz) allows a lateral resolution of 100–500 μm and axial resolution of 20–100 μm. Primary melanoma tumour appears as a hypoechogenic zone (Figure 19.3). Sonography of primary melanomas using such instruments has been shown to correlate highly with histological Breslow thickness measurements.[37–40] However, in a large series of 259 melanomas, sonography measurements showed a mean difference of 0.39 mm (28%) when comparing histological thicknesses.[40] Such differences have been confirmed by others.[38] These differences not only reflect shrinkage of fixed histological tissue but also the inability of sonography to distinguish melanoma cells from other low echo dense structures such as naevus tissue and inflammatory infiltrate. These limitations are such that no automated diagnostic system to distinguish melanoma from naevi can be envisaged with current sonography techniques.

Optical coherence tomography

Optical coherence tomography (OCT) was introduced in the medical domain as a non-invasive method for examining the human eye.[41] Adaptations of the technology for human skin were published in the early 1990s. The underlying principle of OCT is relatively complex and is based on interferometry.[42] Briefly,

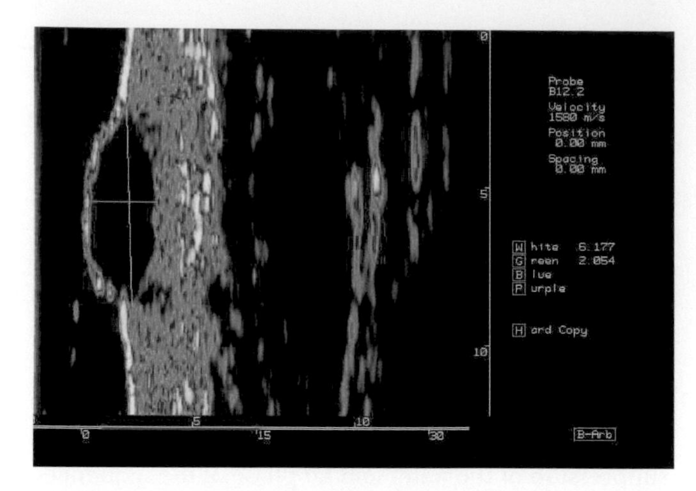

Figure 19.3 *High frequency ultrasound. High frequency (20 Mhz) image of a primary nodular melanoma on the forearm. The thickness of invasion is 1.3 mm. Echogenicity is translated by a look-up table into a spectrum of colours ranging from red to blue. The melanoma itself exhibits almost no echogenicity and is therefore entirely black without reflections from inner structures. Equipment: Dermascan C, 20 Mhz probe (Cortex Technology Inc, Denmark).*

coherent, monochromatic light from an infrared diode (830 nm) is coupled into an optical fibre interferometer. The distribution of the optical path length of the sample beam is measured by interference modulation of a reference beam. Interference occurs only when the propagation distance of both beams matches within the coherence length of the light source. Usually the coherence length determines the depth resolution of the system. The amplitudes of the interference modulation are measured, assigned coordinates, and converted to a logarithmic grey scale for visualization. Lateral scanning of the procedure results in two dimensional cross-sectional images. Resulting images can be compared with B mode ultrasound images. However, OCT measures optical inhomogeneities in the tissue and not the acoustic elastic properties. The penetration depth of OCT range from 0.5 mm to 1.5 mm and allow the visualization of structures of the stratum corneum, the living epidermis, and the papillary dermis. So far studies are focusing on the usefulness of OCT as an adjunct in dermatological diagnosis. Welzel examined healthy skin from different anatomical regions, as well as experimental subepidermal blisters, nail plates, and lentigo maligna melanomas, and compared the results with H&E stained histological slides.[43,44] OCT allowed distinction of the stratum corneum from epidermis and papillary dermis. The axial resolution of 15 μm allowed the visualization of spiral sweat gland ducts and tumour cell formations in lentigo maligna melanomas. However, single cells or subcellular structures were not visible. In conclusion, OCT has a higher resolution than high frequency ultrasound and displays the optical rather than the acoustic properties of the tissue. In comparison to confocal microscopy, OCT has a lower resolution but a substantially higher detection depth. OCT may therefore show some value as intermediate between both methods. However, like ultrasound, OCT with current techniques is unable to distinguish naevus tissue or inflammatory infiltrate from melanoma.

FUTURE IMPROVEMENTS

Despite the promising results from numerous technologies, computer aided diagnosis of pigmented skin lesions has not yet crossed the line that will allow its routine clinical application. Regardless of which approach has been used, almost all studies exhibit substantial weaknesses. Melanoma is a relatively rare occurrence among the number of benign pigmented skin lesions. Sample sizes in published studies are generally too small and pretest probabilities are too high to meet requirements for a representative sample. Up to now, standards for reporting the performance characteristics of classifiers have not been established and mostly do not allow objective comparisons to be drawn between different systems. Using modern communication technology, huge image databases could easily be established and accessed by research groups in order to provide a standardized benchmark test for new systems.

THE REQUIRED DIAGNOSTIC ACCURACY OF AUTOMATED SYSTEMS

As noted previously, the minimal diagnostic accuracy required for a useful clinical automated instrument for diagnosing melanoma is unclear.[12] The most accurate reflection of expert diagnostic ability using conventional non-instrumental aids showed a diagnostic accuracy of 64% and a sensitivity of 84.5% for melanoma.[4] While the specificity was high (99.2%), those correctly classified non-melanomas were still biopsied, presumably in most cases to confirm their non-malignant status. Likewise, while 15.5% of melanomas were misclassified, they were also biopsied. Therefore, if one was to consider the clinician's decision to biopsy as equivalent to the decision of an automated instrument to classify a lesion as melanoma, expert clinical sensitivity will be higher (here the true incidence of misdiagnosed melanomas, i.e. those misdiagnosed and not biopsied, is unknown) but specificity would be considerably lower. A better indicator of expert diagnostic ability may be reflected in the benign:melanoma ratio of all pigmented lesions excised. In a large series, Marks et al. reported a benign:melanoma ratio of 12 for dermatologists in selected areas of Australia compared with 30 for primary care physicians.[45] Del-Mar et al. also reported that only 3% of melanocytic lesions excised by primary care physicians in Australia were invasive melanoma.[46] It could therefore be argued that for an automated instrument to be useful in an expert setting it should achieve a high sensitivity (exceeding 90%) and have a benign:melanoma ratio lower than 12. Data in the non-expert setting of primary care physicians would indicate that such an instrument would have a significant impact on early detection of primary melanomas while decreasing excision rates for benign lesions.

Finally, it should be emphasized that for a significant number of early invasive and in situ melanomas, moderately dysplastic naevi, and adult Spitz naevi, histological diagnostic disagreement is such that a very high diagnostic accuracy will never be obtainable with any automated instrument. The instrument's ability will always be restricted by the histological diagnostic concordance rate.[10]

REFERENCES

1. Weinstock MA, Goldstein MG, Dube CE, et al, Basic skin cancer triage for teaching melanoma detection. *J Am Acad Dermatol* 1996; 34: 1063–6.
2. Lowe JB, Balanda KP, Del Mar CB, et al, General practitioner and patient response during a public education program to encourage skin examinations. *Med J Austr* 1994; 161: 195–8.
3. Paine SL, Cockburn J, Noy SM, Marks R, Early detection of skin cancer. Knowledge, perceptions and practices of general practitioners in Victoria. *Med J Austr* 1994; 161: 188–5,
4. Grin CM, Kopf AW, Welkovich B, et al, Accuracy in the clinical diagnosis of malignant melanoma. *Arch Dermatol* 1990; 126: 763–6.
5. Girgis A, Clarke P, Burton RC, Sanson-Fisher RW, Screening for melanoma by primary health care physicians: a cost-effectiveness analysis. *J Med Screening* 1996; 3: 47–53.
6. Cascinelli N, Ferrario M, Bufalino R, et al, Results obtained by using a computerised image analysis system designed as an aid to diagnosis of cutaneous melanoma. *Melanoma Res* 1992; 2: 163–70.
7. Sober A, Burstein J, Computerised digital image analysis: an aid for melanoma diagnosis. *J Dermatol* 1994; 21: 885–90.
8. Green A, Martin N, Pfitzner J, et al, Computer image analysis in the diagnosis of melanoma. *J Am Acad Dermatol* 1994; 31: 958–64.
9. Hall P, Claridge E, Morris Smith J, Computer screening for early detection of melanoma – is there a future? *Br J Dermatol* 1995; 132: 325–38.
10. Menzies SW, Automated epiluminescence microscopy: human vs machine in the diagnosis of melanoma. *Arch Dermatol* 1999; 135: 1538–40.
11. Schindewolf T, Stolz W, Albert R, Harms H, Comparison of classification rates for conventional and dermatoscopic images form malignant and benign melanocytic lesions using computerised colour image analysis. *Eur J Dermatol* 1993; 3: 299–303.
12. Menzies SW, Bischof L, Peden G, et al, Automated instrumentation for the diagnosis of invasive melanoma: image analysis of oil epiluminescence microscopy. In: *Skin cancer and UV radiation.* (eds Caltmeyer P, Hoffman K, Stucker M). Berlin: Springer-Verlag, 1997.
13. Binder M, Kittler H, Seeber A, et al, Epiluminescence microscopy-based classification of pigmented skin lesions using computerised image analysis and an artificial neural network. *Melanoma Res* 1998; 8: 261–6.
14. Menzies SW, Crook B, McCarthy W, et al, Automated instrumentation for the diagnosis of invasive melanoma. *Skin Res Technol* 1997; 3: 200.
15. Seidenari S, Pellacani G, Pepe P, Digital videomicroscopy improves diagnostic accuracy for melanoma. *J Am Acad Dermatol* 1998; 39: 175–81.
16. Seidenari S, Pellacani G, Giannetti A, Digital videomicroscopy and image analysis with automatic classification for detection of thin melanomas. *Melanoma Res* 1999; 9: 163–71.
17. Andreassi L, Perotti R, Rubegni P, et al, Digital dermoscopy analysis for the differentiation of atypical naevi and early melanoma: a new quantitative semiology. *Arch Dermatol* 1999; 135: 1459–65.
18. Hoffmann K, Husemann R, Toelg S, et al, DANAOS – a European multi-centre study on automated diagnosis of skin cancer. *Melanoma Res* 1997; 7: 19 (Abstract).
19. Stolz W, Schiffner R, Horsch A, et al, The advantage of image analysis for diagnosing and following-up melanocytic lesions. *Melanoma Res* 1997; 7 Suppl 1:20 (Abstract).
20. Dreiseitl S, Ohno-Machado L, Binder M, Comparing three-class diagnostic tests by three way ROC analysis. *Med Decision Making 2000*; 20: 323–31.
21. Marchesini R, Brambilla M, Clemente C, et al, In vivo spectrophotometric evaluation of neoplastic and non-neoplastic skin pigmented lesions – I. Reflectance measurements. *Photochem Photobiol* 1991; 53: 77–84.
22. Marchesini R, Cascinelli N, Brambilla M, et al, In vivo spectrophotometric evaluation of neoplastic and non-neoplastic skin pigmented lesions. II: Discriminant analysis between naevus and melanoma. *Photochem Photobiol* 1992; 55: 515–22.
23. Marchesini R, Tomatis S, Bartoli C, et al, In vivo spectrophotometric evaluation of neoplastic and non-neoplastic skin pigmented lesions. III. CCD camera-based reflectance imaging. *Photochem Photobiol* 1995; 62: 151–4.
24. Bono A, Tomatis S, Bartoli C, et al, The invisible colours of melanoma. A telespectrophotometric diagnostic approach on pigmented skin lesions. *Eur J Cancer* 1996; 32A: 727–9.
25. Tomatis S, Bartoli C, Bono A, et al, Spectrophotometric imaging of cutaneous pigmented lesions: discriminant analysis, optical properties and histological characteristics. *J Photochem Photobiol B* 1998; 42: 32–9.
26. Bono A, Tomatis S, Bartoli C, et al, The ABCD system of melanoma detection: a spectrophotometric analysis of the asymmetry, border, color, and dimension. *Cancer* 1999; 85: 72–7.
27. Elbaum M, Bogdan A, Greenebaum M, et al, Objective detection of early malignant melanoma through multi-resolution representation of multispectral dermoscopic images. *Melanoma Res* 1997; 7 Suppl 1: 19 (Abstract).
28. Petroll WM, Jester JV, Cavanagh HD, In vivo confocal imaging. *Int Rev Exper Pathol* 1996; 36: 93–129.
29. Rajadhyaksha M, Gonzalez S, Zavislan JM, et al, In vivo confocal scanning laser microscopy of human skin II: advances in instrumentation and comparison with histology. *J Investig Dermatol* 1999; 113: 293–303.

30. Rajadhyaksha M, Grossman M, Esterowitz D, et al, In vivo confocal scanning laser microscopy of human skin: melanin provides strong contrast. *J Investig Dermatol* 1995; 104: 946–52.
31. Masters BR, Gonnord G, Corcuff P, Three-dimensional microscopic biopsy of in vivo human skin: a new technique based on a flexible confocal microscope. *J Microscopy* 1997; 185: 329–38.
32. Bertrand C, Corcuff P, In vivo spatio-temporal visualisation of the human skin by real-time confocal microscopy. *Scanning* 1994; 16: 150–4.
33. Zemtsov A, Lorig R, Ng TC, et al, Magnetic resonance imaging of cutaneous neoplasms: clinicopathologic correlation. *J Dermatol Surg Oncol* 1991; 17: 416–22.
34. Maurer J, Knollmann FD, Schlums D, et al, Role of high-resolution magnetic resonance imaging for differentiating melanin-containing skin tumours. *Investig Radiol* 1995; 30: 638–43.
35. Takahashi M, Kohda H, Diagnostic utility of magnetic resonance imaging in malignant melanoma [published erratum appears in *J Am Acad Dermatol* 1993; 28: 513–515] [see comments]. *J Am Acad Dermatol* 1992; 27: 51–4.
36. Takahashi M, Diagnostic utility of magnetic resonance imaging in malignant melanoma. *J Am Acad Dermatol* 1993; 28: 513–15.
37. Lassau N, Spatz A, Avril MF, et al, Value of high-frequency US for preoperative assessment of skin tumours. *Radiographics* 1997; 17: 1559–65.
38. Partsch B, Binder M, Puspok-Schwarz M, et al, Limitations of high frequency ultrasound in determining the invasiveness of cutaneous malignant melanoma. *Melanoma Res* 1996; 6: 395–8.
39. Hoffmann K, Jung J, el Gammal S, Altmeyer P, Malignant melanoma in 20-MHz B scan sonography (published erratum appears in *Dermatology* 1992; 185: 160). *Dermatology* 1992; 185: 49–55.
40. Tacke J, Haagen G, Hornstein OP, et al, Clinical relevance of sonometry-derived tumour thickness in malignant melanoma – a statistical analysis. *Br J Dermatol* 1995; 132: 209–14.
41. Fercher AF, Hitzenberger CK, Drexler W, et al, In vivo optical coherence tomography letter. *Am J Ophthalmology* 1993; 116: 113–14.
42. Huang D, Swanson EA, Lin CP, et al, Optical coherence tomography. *Science* 1991; 254: 1178–81.
43. Welzel J, Lankenau E, Birngruber R, Engelhardt R. Optical coherence tomography of the human skin. *J Am Acad Dermatol* 1997; 37: 958–63.
44. Welzel J, Lankenau E, Birngruber R, Engelhardt R, Optical coherence tomography of the skin. *Curr Probl Dermatol* 1998; 26: 27–37.
45. Marks R, Jolley D, McCormack C, Dorevitch AP, Who removes pigmented skin lesions? *J Am Acad Dermatol* 1997; 36: 721–6.
46. Del Mar C, Green A, Cooney T, et al, Melanocytic lesions excised from the skin: what percentage are malignant? *Austr J Public Health* 1994; 18: 221–3.

20

Initial staging investigations for melanoma

Antonio C Buzaid, Jeffrey E Gershenwald, Merrick I Ross

INTRODUCTION

In general, laboratory tests and imaging studies are of great value in staging patients with cancer. However, it has become increasingly apparent that the cancer staging evaluations performed both at the time of initial diagnosis and during follow up are often excessive. Attempts at justifying these evaluations are based on the tenet that they should be as comprehensive as possible to avoid overlooking any cases of metastatic disease. Although physicians have become more disciplined in the staging evaluation of cancer, prompted largely by the increasingly cost conscious clinical environment, significant room for improvement remains. To help improve staging evaluations, this chapter will review the data and provide practical stage specific guidelines for the initial evaluation of patients with melanoma.

PRIMARY MELANOMA (CLINICAL STAGES I AND II)

At the time of diagnosis, most melanoma patients have disease confined to the skin, i.e. clinical stage I or II disease. Prompted by patient anxiety combined with the average practising physician's limited clinical exposure to the patient with melanoma, the vast majority of these patients still undergo extensive radiological evaluations to exclude distant metastases. However, in an asymptomatic patient with a recently diagnosed primary melanoma, most of these imaging studies are clearly not indicated because the rate of detection of distant metastases in such patients is extremely low. Moreover, the false positive rate, defined here as an abnormal imaging study in the absence of metastatic melanoma, is high (10–20%) and often contributes to additional patient anxiety. For example, at the time of diagnosis of a primary melanoma, the detection rate of distant metastases using chest radiography is virtually 0%.[1–5] In the largest series reported to date, distant metastasis was found in only one of 876 patients (0.1%).[6] However, false positives were identified in approximately 15% of the cases.[6] Similar results were observed for bone scans and other nuclear medicine scans, including liver/spleen and brain scans.[1–3,5,7–10]

The value of computed tomography (CT) has been extensively evaluated in patients having primary melanoma, and it has also been associated with a very low sensitivity. For example, Buzaid et al.[4] systematically analyzed 151 primary melanoma patients using CT scans of the chest and abdomen. In addition, patients having primary tumours of the head or neck had a CT scan of the neck, and those having primary tumours below the waist had a CT scan of the pelvis. Interestingly, 29 of the 151 patients had suspicious CT scans: in 24 (15.8%) of the patients, the abnormalities were ultimately determined to be benign (false positive); in three (2.0%) patients, second primary tumours were discovered (non-Hodgkin's lymphoma, Hodgkin's disease, and renal cell carcinoma); and in the remaining two (1.3%) patients, melanoma metastases were identified (true positive).[4] CT scanning of the brain was also evaluated in several series; no metastases were identified in any of the hundreds of patients studied.[1,3,5,11]

Examples of a false positive CT scan and second primary malignancy identified by extensive radiological examinations are shown in Figures 20.1 and 20.2, respectively.

Another imaging method, positron emission tomography (PET) is currently being evaluated in patients with primary melanoma.[12,13] In one series of 52 melanoma patients whose primary tumour had a Breslow depth >1.5 mm and who had no clinical evidence of lymphadenopathy, PET scanning (done within 4 weeks after wide excision of the primary melanoma) correctly detected nine regional lymph node metastases in four patients.[13] In all four patients, no nodal metastasis was identified by using conventional imaging methods, including high resolution ultrasonography. However, three additional 'lesions' found by using PET were incorrectly identified as metastases (false positives).[13] Although similar results were observed in another smaller study, PET was not useful in at least one study that examined the use of it in imaging lymph node basins in clinically node negative melanoma patients undergoing sentinel node biopsy.[12,14] Thus, the value of PET in patients having stage I or II disease remains unclear, although it seems to be more sensitive than other types of imaging.

In summary, CT scans are clearly not indicated in patients having stage I or II disease because the yield is extremely low (~1%) and the false positive rate is unacceptably high (10–20%). Furthermore, the high false positive rate leads to further patient anxiety and, not infrequently, unnecessary and expensive invasive procedures. Therefore, for these patients, we recommend a staging evaluation consisting of a physical exam (skin and nodal basin survey), chest x-ray, and determination of the lactate dehydrogenase (LDH) and alkaline phosphatase levels (Table 20.1). Although the results of these tests are likely to be normal, they may be useful as baseline examinations for future comparison with subsequent studies during post-treatment surveillance.[15] It is worth emphasizing that when extensive radiological imaging studies have already been performed and are considered suspicious for metastases, the radiological abnormalities are more likely to be benign processes or second primary malignancies. It should therefore never be concluded that metastatic disease is present in a patient with a recently diagnosed primary melanoma solely on the basis of an abnormal imaging study. Pathological confirmation by biopsy is essential before treatment is started.

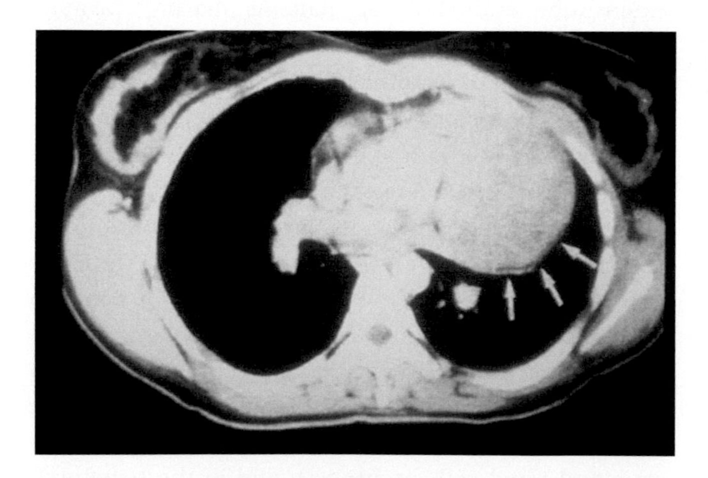

Figure 20.1 *Computed tomography scan of a large mediastinal mass originally seen on the chest x-ray film of a 30-year-old white woman who presented with a 1.7 mm primary melanoma on the right shoulder. A biopsy was performed and showed the mass to be Hodgkin's disease.*

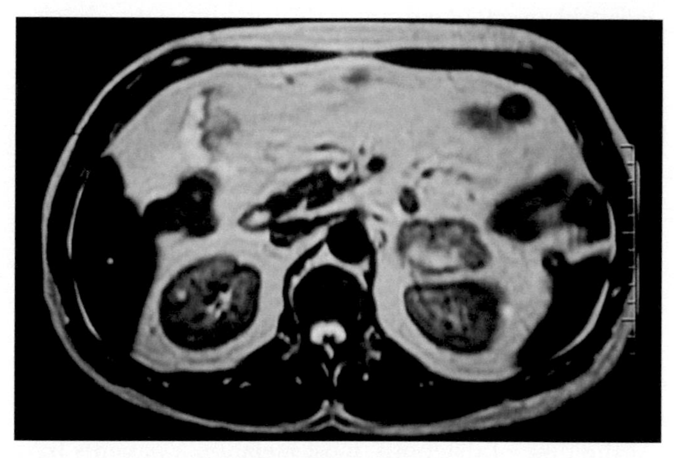

Figure 20.2 *Magnetic resonance imaging (MRI) scan of a large mass anterior to the left kidney in a 50-year-old man who presented with a 0.9 mm Clark level III primary melanoma in the interscapular region. The patient was very anxious during presentation and at his insistence, the attending physician ordered the MRI scan of the abdomen. The left adrenal was normal. Screening for pheochromocytoma was negative. The findings of a fine needle aspiration biopsy of the mass were consistent with those of paraganglioma. The patient underwent resection of the mass, which confirmed the diagnosis of paraganglioma.*

Table 20.1 *Practical recommendations for staging evaluation based on stage at presentation*

Primary tumour (no clinical evidence of regional nodal disease)
- Physical examination
- Chest x-ray film
- Measurement of lactate dehydrogenase (LDH) concentration
- Sentinel lymphadenectomy (see text for inclusion criteria)

Local regional disease
- Physical examination
- Chest x-ray film
- Complete blood count
- Measurement of LDH concentration
- Consideration of sentinel lymphadenectomy concomitant with therapeutic lymph node dissection if definitive wide excision of the primary site has not yet been performed and at least one regional nodal basin is clinically uninvolved by metastatic tumour
- Abdominal computed tomography (CT) scan
- Chest CT scan
- Pelvic CT scan if disease below the waist
- Neck CT scan if disease in the head and neck region
- Consideration of magnetic resonance imaging (MRI) scan of brain
- Additional studies should be done only if clinically indicated or based on symptoms (e.g. bone scan, gastrointestinal series)

Distant metastases
- Physical examination
- Chest x-ray film
- Complete blood count
- Measurement of LDH concentration
- Abdominal CT scan
- Chest CT scan
- Pelvic CT scan if disease below the waist
- Neck CT scan if disease in the head and neck region
- MRI scan of the brain
- Additional studies should be done only if clinically indicated or based on symptoms (e.g. bone scan, gastrointestinal series)

Lymphatic mapping and sentinel lymphadenectomy

While imaging studies are not very useful in staging primary melanoma, a rational alternative to elective lymph node dissection in patients having clinically negative regional lymph node basins has emerged over the past decade that has already notably altered the surgical approach to primary melanoma in most large cancer centres. Initially described by Morton et al., this approach, termed sentinel lymphadenectomy, includes lymphatic mapping and sentinel lymph node biopsy.[16] It is a highly accurate, minimally invasive method of identifying those primary melanoma patients who may have clinically occult nodal metastases. The technique is based on the now well supported hypothesis that lymphatic metastases of melanoma follow an orderly progression through afferent lymphatic channels to sentinel lymph nodes before spreading into other regional, non-sentinel lymph nodes.[17] Several groups have confirmed the accuracy and sensitivity of this technique.[16–26] Although initially sentinel lymph nodes were identified in approximately 80% of the patients who underwent the procedure, current rates approach 100% because of improvements in preoperative lymphoscintigraphy and intraoperative mapping techniques, including combined modality intraoperative sentinel lymph node localization, which uses both dye and radiolabelled colloid.[17–19,22,25,26]

The pathological status of the regional nodal basin in patients having clinically negative lymph nodes provides important prognostic information. For example, Coit et al. reported on 129 patients having tumours ≥4 mm thick or reaching Clark level V who underwent elective lymph node dissection:[27] 63 patients were found to have pathological evidence of nodal metastases, whereas the remaining patients had negative nodes. The overall 5 year survival rate for the 129 patients was 47%, but the rates for node positive and negative patients were 32% and 71%, respectively (P=0.0001 for pathologically positive versus negative nodes). In a recent update of this study, Kim et al. noted that the overall 5 year survival rate was 64%, whereas the rates for patients who initially had stage III and II disease were 48% and 70% respectively.[28] Other investigators observed similar results.[29] Recently, it was shown that the pathological sentinel lymph node status in 612 primary melanoma patients having clinically negative nodes was the most important prognostic factor for recurrence and disease specific survival using multivariate analyses.[26]

On the basis of these observations the authors suggest that, when available, lymphatic mapping and sentinel lymphadenectomy be performed in patients having American Joint Committee on Cancer (AJCC) clinical stage I or II melanoma if their primary tumour is at least 1 mm thick, Clark level IV or V, or ulcerated. Sentinel node biopsy can potentially provide even more accurate staging information than that achievable by elective lymph node dissection because the limited pathological specimen permits more complete assessment of these select lymph nodes, which are most likely to contain metastases using more specialized pathological techniques.[30] Importantly, the AJCC intends to formally incorporate pathological information based on sentinel lymphadenectomy into the new staging system for melanoma.

LOCAL REGIONAL DISEASE (LOCAL, SATELLITE, IN-TRANSIT, AND/OR REGIONAL LYMPH NODE RECURRENCE)

Patients having local regional metastases, including local, satellite, in-transit, or regional nodal disease, have a risk of systemic recurrence that usually exceeds 50%.[31] In other words, at the time of diagnosis of local regional disease, at least 50% of these patients harbour occult distant metastases that will eventually become clinically apparent and are likely to contribute to the patients' untimely death. Despite this high risk of systemic recurrence, staging evaluations that include imaging studies such as CT scans of the brain, chest, abdomen, and pelvis have a relatively low yield in detecting distant metastases at the time of local regional disease diagnosis in asymptomatic patients. However, select imaging studies are warranted in this patient population because the likelihood of identifying metastatic disease is higher than it is in patients with primary disease.

The results of CT scans performed as part of the staging work-up for asymptomatic patients with documented local regional metastases and normal chest x-ray film and serum LDH concentration are summarized in Table 20.2.[32–34] Studies at both the University of Texas MD Anderson Cancer Center and Memorial Sloan-Kettering Cancer Center (MSKCC) documented a true positive rate of approximately 5–6%.[32,34] In contrast, investigators at the University of Michigan noted a true positive rate of 16%.[33] The most striking difference among the studies was in the rate of detection of brain metastases: while no brain metastases were identified in the MD Anderson Cancer Center or MSKCC studies, which collectively totalled almost 200 patients, brain metastases were identified in 6% of the patients in the University of Michigan series (Table 20.3). Additionally, the MD Anderson Cancer Center and MSKCC series showed that CT scanning of the pelvis was beneficial only in patients having inguinal recurrence.[32,34] Other imaging studies such as bone scan have also been evaluated and found to have no clinical value in the evaluation of asymptomatic patients having local regional metastases.[2,3,7,9]

On the basis of the studies described above and our personal experience, we recommend the following staging work-up for patients who present with or develop a local regional recurrence: a complete blood count; liver function tests, including measurement of the alkaline phosphatase and LDH concentrations; a chest x-ray film; and CT scans of the chest and abdomen (Table 20.1). Although the likelihood is low that these tests, particularly the CT scans of the chest and abdomen, will detect distant metastases in asymptomatic patients, they often identify false positive abnormalities and function as an important baseline for future studies in this high risk patient population. For patients whose recurrence is below the waist, we also recommend a CT scan of the pelvis; for those whose recurrence is in the head and neck region, we recommend a CT scan of the neck. Although we do not recommend CT scanning of the brain for all patients with stage III disease, we consider

Table 20.2 *Results of CT scanning of the chest, abdomen, and pelvis in asymptomatic patients with stage III melanoma*

Institution	No. of patients	True positive (%)	False positive (%)	New primary malignancy (%)
MDACC	89	6.7	22.4	0.0
MSKCC	136	4.4	8.4	1.4
Univ. of Michigan	127	16.0	12.0	0.7

Abbreviations: MDACC, The University of Texas MD Anderson Cancer Center; MSKCC, Memorial Sloan-Kettering Cancer Center.

Table 20.3 *Results of computed tomography scanning of the brain in asymptomatic patients with stage III melanoma*

Institution	No. of patients	True positive (%)	False positive (%)
MDACC	82	1.2*	0.0
MSKCC	104	0.0	3.8
Univ. of Michigan	99	6.0	12.0

*This single true positive patient had bone involvement without evidence of brain metastasis.
Abbreviations: MDACC, The University of Texas MD Anderson Cancer Center; MSKCC, Memorial Sloan-Kettering Cancer Center.

it optional on the basis of the experiences at the University of Michigan.[33] Additional studies such as bone scans should be performed only if clinically indicated.

It is important to emphasize that the recommended guidelines for imaging studies were designed for patients who present with or experience their first local regional recurrence. Patients who present with or experience two or more local regional recurrences are at higher risk and should undergo staging evaluations as if they had distant metastases (as described below) until information to the contrary becomes available.

DISTANT METASTASES (STAGE IV)

Unlike patients with primary or local regional disease, those who have known systemic metastases require comprehensive evaluation because the likelihood of detecting other, asymptomatic metastases is significant. Accordingly, we recommend that, as a minimum, these patients should undergo staging consisting of CT or magnetic resonance imaging of the brain and CT scans of the chest and abdomen (Table 20.1). Patients should have a CT scan of the pelvis if they have a history of primary tumour below the waist or if symptoms justify it. All other imaging studies should be done on the basis of specific indications only, e.g. a bone scan for patients with bone pain, a small bowel series for patients with iron deficiency anaemia, etc.

The preliminary experience using PET in patients who have stage IV melanoma suggests that it is more sensitive than CT. For example, in the Sydney Melanoma Unit experience of 100 patients with stage IV disease who underwent both PET and CT scans, a total of 415 metastatic lesions were evaluated.[35] Of these, 388 (93%) were detected by PET scanning. Also, in 20 patients, PET scanning detected 24 metastases up to 6 months earlier than did conventional imaging studies or physical examination. Furthermore, the selection of treatment was influenced by PET findings in 22 patients. In another series of 68 patients, PET scanning detected fewer pulmonary, hepatic, and brain metastases but more lymph node and bone metastases than did conventional CT scanning.[36] These data suggest that PET may be more sensitive than conventional imaging studies in certain regions of the body but less sensitive in others. Therefore, at the present time, PET scanning may more appropriately complement routine imaging studies than completely replace them.

REFERENCES

1. Zartman G, Thomas M, Robinson W, Metastatic disease in patients with newly diagnosed malignant melanoma. *J Surg Oncol* 1987; 35: 163–4.
2. Ardizzoni A, Grimaldi A, Repetto L, et al, Stage I–II melanoma: the value of metastatic work-up. *Oncology* 1987; 44: 87–9.
3. Khansur T, Sanders J, Das S, Evaluation of staging work-up in malignant melanoma. *Arch Surg* 1989; 124: 847–9.
4. Buzaid A, Sandler A, Mani S, et al, Role of computed tomography in the staging of primary melanoma. *J Clin Oncol* 1993; 11: 638–43.
5. Iscoe N, Eisenhauer E, Bodurtha A, Phase II study of trimetrexate in malignant melanoma: a National Cancer Institute of Canada Clinical Trials Group study. *Invest New Drugs* 1990; 8: 121–3.
6. Terhune MH, Swanson N, Johnson TM, Use of chest radiography in the initial evaluation of patients with localized melanoma. *Arch Dermatol* 1998; 80: 233–7.
7. Roth J, Eilber F, Bennett L, Morton D, Radionuclide photoscanning. Usefulness in preoperative evaluation of melanoma patients. *Arch Surg* 1975; 110: 1211–12.
8. Meyer J, Stolbach L, Pretreatment radiographic evaluation of patients with malignant melanoma. *Cancer* 1978; 42: 125–6.
9. Thomas J, Panaussopoulos D, Liesmann G, et al, Scintiscans in the evaluation of patients with malignant melanoma. *Surg Gynecol Obstet* 1979; 149: 574–6.
10. Au F, Maier W, Malmud L, et al, Preoperative nuclear scans in patients with melanoma. *Cancer* 1984; 53: 2095–7.
11. Basseres N, Grob JJ, Richard MA, et al, Cost-effectiveness of surveillance of stage I melanoma. A retrospective appraisal on a 10-year experience in a dermatology department in France. *Dermatology* 1995; 191: 199–203.
12. Macfarlane DJ, Sondak V, Johnson T, Wahl RL, Prospective evaluation of 2-[18F]-2-deoxy-D-glucose positron emission tomography in staging of regional lymph nodes in patients with cutaneous malignant melanoma. *J Clin Oncol* 1998; 16: 1770–6.
13. Rinne D, Baum RP, Hor G, Kaufmann R, Primary staging and follow-up of high risk melanoma patients with whole-body 18F-fluorodeoxyglucose positron emission tomography: results of a prospective study of 100 patients. *Cancer* 1998; 82: 1664–71.
14. Wagner JD, Schauwecker D, Davidson D, et al, Prospective study of fluorodeoxyglucose-positron emission tomography imaging of lymph node basins in melanoma patients undergoing sentinel node biopsy. *J Clin Oncol* 1999; 17: 1508–15.
15. Gershenwald J, Buzaid A, Ross M, Classification and staging of melanoma. *Hematol Oncol Clin North Am* 1998; 12: 737–65.

16. Morton D, Wen D, Wong J, et al, Technical details of intraoperative lymphatic mapping for early stage melanoma. *Arch Surg* 1992; 127: 392–9.
17. Reintgen D, Cruse C, Wells K, et al, The orderly progression of melanoma nodal metastases. *Ann Surg* 1994; 220: 759–67.
18. Albertini J, Cruse C, Rapaport D, et al, Intraoperative radiolymphoscintigraphy improves sentinel lymph node identification for patients with melanoma. *Ann Surg* 1996; 223: 217–24.
19. Thompson JF, McCarthy WH, Bosch C, et al, Sentinel lymph node status as an indicator of the presence of metastatic melanoma in regional lymph nodes. *Melanoma Res* 1995; 5: 255–60.
20. Thompson W, Gershenwald J, Lee J, et al, *Sentinel lymph node identification in melanoma patients using two techniques: Dye vs. dye + radiolabeled colloid.* Atlanta, GA: 49th Annual Meeting of The Society of Surgical Oncology, 1996.
21. Gershenwald J, Thompson W, Mansfield P, et al, *Patterns of failure in melanoma patients after successful lymphatic mapping and negative sentinel node biopsy.* Atlanta, GA: 49th Annual Meeting of The Society of Surgical Oncology, 1996.
22. Krag D, Meijer S, Weaver D, et al, Minimal-access surgery for staging of malignant melanoma. *Arch Surg* 1995; 130: 654–8.
23. Uren R, Howman-Giles R, Thompson J, et al, Lymphoscintigraphy to identify sentinel lymph nodes in patients with melanoma. *Melanoma Res* 1994; 4: 395–9.
24. Reintgen D, Balch C, Kirkwood J, Ross M, Recent advances in the care of the patient with malignant melanoma. *Ann Surg* 1997; 225: 1–14.
25. Gershenwald J, Tseng Ch, Thompson W, et al, Improved sentinel lymph node localization in primary melanoma patients with the use of radiolabeled colloid. *Surgery* 1998; 124: 203–10.
26. Gershenwald J, Thompson W, Mansfield P, et al, Multi-institutional lymphatic mapping experience: the prognostic value of sentinel lymph node status in 612 stage I or II melanoma patients. *J Clinical Oncol* 1999; 17: 976–83.
27. Coit D, Sauven P, Brennan M, Prognosis of thick cutaneous melanoma of the trunk and extremity. *Arch Surg* 1990; 125: 322–326.
28. Kim S, Garcia C, Rodriguez J, Coit D, Prognosis of thick cutaneous melanoma. *J Am Coll Surg* 1999; 188: 241–7.
29. Crowley N, Seigler H, The role of elective lymph node dissection in the management of patients with thick cutaneous melanoma. *Cancer* 1990; 66: 2522–7.
30. Gershenwald J, Thompson W, Mansfield P, et al, Patterns of recurrence following a negative sentinel lymph node biopsy in 243 patients with stage I or II melanoma. *J Clin Oncol* 1998; 16: 2253–60.
31. Buzaid A, Ross M, Balch C, et al, Critical analysis of the current American Joint Committee on Cancer staging system for cutaneous melanoma and proposal of a new staging system. *J Clin Oncol* 1997; 15: 1039–51.
32. Buzaid A, Tinoco L, Ross M, et al, The role of computed tomography in the staging of patients with local-regional metastases of melanoma. *J Clin Oncol* 1995; 13: 2104–8.
33. Johnson T, Fader D, Chang A, et al, Computed tomography in staging of patients with melanoma metastatic to the regional nodes. *Ann Surg Oncol* 1997; 4: 396–402.
34. Kuvshinoff B, Kurtz C, Coit D, Computed tomography in evaluation of patients with stage III melanoma. *Ann Surg Oncol* 1997; 4: 252–8.
35. Damian D, Fulham M, Thompson E, Thompson J, Positron emission tomography in the detection and management of metastatic melanoma. *Melanoma Res* 1997; 6: 325–9.
36. Dietlein M, Krug B, Groth W, et al, Positron emission tomography using 18F-fluorodeoxyglucose in advanced stages of malignant melanoma: a comparison of ultrasonographic and radiological methods of diagnosis. *Nucl Med Commun* 1999; 20: 255–61.

21

Surgical management of primary melanoma: excision biopsy and wide local excision

T Michael D Hughes, Mario Santinami, Leonardo Lenisa, Natale Cascinelli

THE DIAGNOSTIC BIOPSY

An accurate diagnosis of melanoma should be made by excision biopsy before definitive management is contemplated. The histopathological characteristics of the primary melanoma will then be known and can be used to aid decision making concerning the extent of local treatment and whether sentinel lymph node biopsy should be considered. Furthermore, the risk of performing inappropriate radical surgery for benign lesions and non-melanoma skin cancers will then be avoided. In many parts of the body a suspicious lesion can be widely excised without causing any significant cosmetic problem, making a second procedure unnecessary. Unfortunately, however, extensive resection of the primary melanoma site can cause significant alterations in local lymphatic drainage, and sentinel lymph node mapping may then be unreliable.[1,2] The role of sentinel node biopsy is discussed in Chapters 27–28.

Excision biopsy of the primary lesion with a narrow margin of 2–3 mm is the preferred diagnostic technique as it allows examination of the entire lesion. For benign pigmented lesions, including dysplastic naevi and most non-melanoma skin cancers, the procedure will also be therapeutic. There is some anecdotal evidence that the milieu of the healing wound after incomplete excision of naevi, especially dysplastic naevi, may promote transformation to melanoma. The other likely explanation for the observed development of melanoma in previously biopsied naevi is that the original diagnosis was incorrect. Incision biopsy of melanomas has not consistently been shown to affect outcome in terms of survival and local control, but there are no well controlled studies to confirm these observations.[3,4] A study by Rampen et al. of 76 patients showed a significantly worse prognosis in patients treated with incision biopsy compared with those having an excision biopsy.[5] Apart from a potentially adverse effect on prognosis, incision biopsy has the major disadvantage that it might prevent accurate microstaging.[6] Griffiths and Briggs reported that histological specimens were unassessable in over 30% of incision biopsies compared with only 5% of excision biopsies and 0.5% of primary wide excisions.[7] Incision biopsy however is appropriate in circumstances where complete excision will involve disfigurement or the need for a complicated repair of the resulting defect. This is often the case for lesions located on the face or distal extremity. Incision biopsy can be performed by removal of a representative ellipse of full thickness skin using a scalpel or by obtaining a punch biopsy. With both techniques it is imperative that an adequate specimen is obtained. Incision biopsies have the potential to be inaccurate, because the area sampled may not be truly representative of the entire lesion. Furthermore, the specimens can be inappropriately sectioned as a result of difficulties with orientation of the tissue obtained. Shave biopsies do not have any place in the diagnosis of melanoma.

Careful planning must start at the time of excision biopsy. Consideration should be given to the orientation of a subsequent wider excision. Inappropriately orientated biopsy wounds can lead to the need for skin grafting or flap closure of a defect that might otherwise have been managed easily with primary closure. If doubt exists, then the biopsy should be performed by the surgeon who will be performing the wide excision. Meticulous surgical technique and wound care are essential. Poor healing and wound infection can cause delays in treatment and compromise the results of the wide excision.

DEFINITIVE SURGICAL MANAGEMENT – WIDTH OF EXCISION

Introduction

The management plan for an individual patient diagnosed with melanoma must be the result of careful consideration of the aims of treatment, the patient's age and general health, the site and histological characteristics of the primary lesion, and the predicted outcome from a particular strategy based on the evidence available.

The primary aim of adequate local treatment is to prevent systemic disease relapse and death from melanoma by removing all tumour cells from the local region. The second goal of local treatment is to attain good local disease control irrespective of what effect this might have on survival.

The patient should be central to any decisions made about their treatment. Consideration should be given to their age and life expectancy, to comorbidities that will affect anaesthetic risk and wound healing, and to the cosmetic and functional results of any proposed intervention.

The relevance of the characteristics of a primary melanoma in determining definitive management is discussed in detail in the review of the available evidence below. In every case a clinician should take note of the site of the primary, the thickness and diameter of the tumour, the presence or absence of lymphovascular invasion, the presence of microsatellites, and the histological subtype. Desmoplastic and neurotropic melanomas require special consideration, and are discussed in Chapter 34.

The question of how much surrounding skin and subcutaneous fat should be excised for the appropriate treatment of primary cutaneous melanoma has been a matter of great controversy and debate for more than a century and has been only partially addressed in the past two decades. The following paragraphs briefly review the history of surgical management of primary melanoma and the development of the body of evidence on which current recommendations are based.

History

The tradition of taking a wide margin of normal skin around the primary tumour is attributed to Sir William Sampson Handley. His advice was based on the prevailing principles of surgery for breast cancer at the turn of the 19th century and on observations of a single postmortem examination on a patient with metastatic disease from a primary lesion on the heel. As the primary had already been excised Handley admitted: 'No opportunity of investigating the spread of permeation around the primary focus of melanotic growth has fallen to me.'[8] Handley never specified exact margins, but in the second of his Hunterian lectures in 1907 he recommended making an incision 'about an inch' from the edge of the tumour, raising skin flaps 'about two inches in all directions round the skin'.[9]

Different authors recommended a variety of other excision margins over the next few decades. The unifying factor was that the outcomes after radical local surgery were universally disappointing. Pack reported a 5-year overall survival rate of 50% in 189 patients following excision with an 8 cm margin.[10] Lund and Inhem[11] had a 5-year survival rate of 44% with similar margins. Petersen et al. reported the use of 15 cm margins in some cases, once again with disappointing results.[12] Wilson[13] and Lehman et al.[14] obtained a 41% 5-year survival rate for patients treated with wide excision margins or amputations compared with 24% for patients treated with excision biopsy only. These poor results are presumably related to the late presentation or treatment of melanoma in these series.[6,15] Olsen found similar local recurrence rates regardless of margin width, but found a higher metastatic rate for patients treated with narrow margins, concluding that a wide excision might not be necessary in all cases.[16]

Standard treatment remained wide excision with 5 cm margins for many years. The presumed basis for the continued use of these wide margins was the description of the abnormal appearance and distribution of melanocytes in the vicinity of a melanoma, suggesting a field change surrounding tumours with a radial growth phase.[17,18] This concept was supported by Wong, who identified bizarre melanocytes in normal skin 5 cm from the primary.[19] According to Fallowfield and Cook these changes simply represent those of chronic sun damage.[20] A second reason put forward for very wide margins was the observation that microsatellites sometimes arose adjacent to, but not continuous with, the main tumour mass.[21]

The significance of local recurrence

The mechanism by which residual tumour might be related to systemic dissemination has not been well explained. A reasonable argument would be that residual tumour rests may be a persistent source of cells with metastatic potential. Furthermore the regrowth of residual melanoma could attain a depth of penetration into the dermis greater than the original primary. On the basis of the prognostic importance of the depth of penetration, such local recurrences might theoretically affect survival.

The detrimental prognostic significance of local recurrence due to inadequate initial resection remains unclear. The major factor contributing to the lack of clarity is the definition of local recurrence. The traditional definition has been the reappearance of melanoma within 5 cm of the excisional scar or graft and therefore includes the many cases where local failure is in the form of dermal or subcutaneous satellites from lymphatic spread.[4,22–26] These cases in reality represent a localized form of in-transit disease. This contention is strongly supported by the observation that the outcome of patients with local recurrence is similar to that of patients with in-transit metastases.[27] The 10-year survival of patients with local recurrences ranges from 10% to 40%, which is similar to the outcome for patients with in-transit metastases and nodal metastases.[28–37] True local recurrences which occur in spite of wide clearance are most likely to be due to retained, but histologically unrecognized, lateral spread of the melanoma. The significance of the distinction between the two types of local recurrence has been highlighted by Brown and Zitelli.[38] They reported an overall 5-year survival rate of 89% for patients with local recurrence due to inadequate excision, compared with systemic failure rates of 70–90% for patients with satellitosis and in-transit disease.[23] In the former group, prognosis was shown to be related to the depth of either the original primary or the recurrence, depending on which was greater.[38]

The extent of local surgery seems to have little impact on patients with satellitosis in terms of survival, but local control does become an important issue for them, especially in areas not amenable to isolated regional perfusion with high dose chemotherapy.

The past two decades: current practice based on the available evidence

In the last three decades of the twentieth century the long established dogma of 5 cm excision margins and often deforming surgery was challenged. This came about through a combination of events. Firstly, a better understanding of prognostic factors and the subsequent stratification of patients into risk categories according to microstaging identified patients at very low risk of recurrence. Secondly, an increased public awareness of melanoma, with an absolute increase in incidence and a greater proportion of patients presenting with early stage disease, led to the need for well defined surgical guidelines.

Numerous retrospective studies assessing the appropriate width of excision were published in the 1980s. All were confounded by the inherent biases of retrospective, poorly controlled or uncontrolled studies. Nevertheless, a review of their findings provides some insights into the disease itself. Aitken et al. analyzed survival data for 118 patients with localized melanoma and found that excision margins of <2 cm were associated with a worse prognosis than wider margins, if tumours were over 2 mm thick or 1 cm in diameter.[39] Excision margins greater than 3 cm did not appear to influence survival.

Most studies found that surgical excision of primary melanomas with narrower margins did not adversely affect survival, but did increase local recurrence rates when used for thicker melanomas.[40–47]

Schmoeckel et al. found no correlation between the rate of metastasis over 5 years and the width of excision margins in 577 patients who had undergone excision with a variety of excision margins.[48] Breslow reviewed 62 patients with melanomas less than 0.76 mm thick who had been followed for at least 5 years.[40] None developed distant recurrence, including 14 with margins less than 5 mm. Cosimi et al. reported a series of 136 patients who were treated by excision of as much skin as would allow primary closure.[41] Excision margins ranged from 0.7 cm to 4.0 cm. No local recurrences were reported, even though residual melanocytic hyperplasia was present in 12 cases and residual invasive tumour in two. This study showed that wider excision after excision biopsy using less radical margins was quite effective in preventing local recurrence.

Cascinelli et al.[45] reviewed data on 593 patients collected by the collaborating centres of the World Health Organization (WHO) Melanoma Program. The local relapse rate was 9% (9/96) for margins <2 cm and 3% (16/497) for margins >2 cm. The difference in relapse rates disappeared when patients were stratified on the basis of primary tumour thickness <2 mm or >2 mm.

Bagley et al. reviewed the records of 147 patients treated at the Lahey Clinic up to 1979.[4] The rate of local relapse in cases where excision margins had been <1 cm was 12% compared with only 2% in those where margins were wider. Kelly et al. reported on 346 patients with primaries <1 mm;[21] 7.8% of the 51 patients with margins of excision <1 cm had local recurrences. This compared with a rate of 3% in the 295 patients having wider margins. Further studies by O'Rourke et al. and Welvaart et al. have corroborated findings by others that wider margins of excision have little impact on local recurrence rates.[47,49]

The most extensive and well documented experience of outcome after resection of primary melanoma has come from the Sydney Melanoma Unit (SMU). Urist et al. reported on the combined experience of the SMU (936 patients) and the University of Alabama (115 patients) with excision of primary melanomas <1 mm in thickness.[24] Only one local recurrence occurred after a minimum follow up of 5 years. 62% of the patients had margins less than 2 cm. Milton et al. in the same year published the results of treatment of 1839 patients treated at the SMU with 5 years of follow up.[50] This study highlighted the significance of primary tumour thickness in determining the risk of local recurrence. For thick tumours (>3 mm) the local recurrence rate was 21% when margins <2 cm were employed and 9% when wider margins were used. For thin tumours (0.1–0.7 mm) the recurrence rates were 2% and <1%, respectively.

All these studies suggested that there was a minimum safe margin of excision that depended on the depth of invasion of the tumour. The problem at that time was that there was considerable disagreement about the appropriate width of excision for a particular depth of invasion. In 1979 the WHO Melanoma Program designed a randomized prospective clinical trial to address this problem.[51,52] In this trial 612 patients with primary melanomas less than or equal to 2 mm in thickness were randomized to excision margins of either 1 cm or 3 cm. By 1987 the first results were published, with a mean follow up of 55 months. Disease free and overall survival rates were similar, as were the incidence of distant, regional and in-transit metastases in both groups. Local recurrence developed in only six patients (0.9%). This was isolated in three patients, all of whom had primaries >1 mm excised with narrow margins.

The results were updated in 1991, with a mean follow up of 90 months.[52] Once again no significant difference was found in any outcome measure. By 1993 there had been five isolated local recurrences in the narrow margin group and one in the wide margin group. In all cases the primary was >1 mm thick.[6] As a result of this important trial it can be definitively stated that melanomas less than 1mm thick are adequately treated with 1 cm margins. Some have argued that the trial did not resolve the question for melanomas 1–2 mm thick and have suggested that a 2 cm margin might be a reasonable compromise to improve local control.[6,53]

The Intergroup Melanoma Committee conducted a randomized trial for patients with intermediate thickness melanomas (1–4 mm). Margins of 2 cm and 4 cm were compared.[54] The study population consisted of 486 patients with melanoma of the trunk and proximal extremities. When the results were reported the median follow up was 6 years. Distant and in-transit relapse rates were similar for both groups (2 cm – 10.9% distant, 2.5% in-transit; 4 cm – 8.5% distant, 2.1% in-transit). The overall 5-year survival rates were 79.5% for 2 cm margins and 83.7% for 4 cm margins (P=NS). Interestingly the local recurrence rate was higher in the wider excision group (4 versus 2 cases, P=NS). The treatment morbidity and hospital lengths of stay were significantly less in the narrower margin group. This was attributed to the higher rate of skin grafting required in the wide excision group (46% versus 11%). The high morbidity of skin grafts compared with primary closures has been corroborated by O'Rourke and Altmann,[47] who found complications in 31% of patients having skin grafts compared with 6% in those having primary closure.[47]

In the United Kingdom the Melanoma Study Group and British Association of Plastic Surgeons are currently conducting a randomized trial comparing 1 cm with

3 cm margins for patients with primary melanomas 2 mm or more in thickness on the limbs or trunk.

Heaton et al. attempted to clarify the situation for thick primary melanomas (>4 mm) where the risks of local recurrence and systemic recurrence are high (12% and 60%, respectively).[55–57] In a study of 278 patients with a mean follow up of 28 months there was no increase in local recurrence and no decrease in survival for patients treated with narrower margins (2 cm or less) compared with those treated with wider margins.

The evidence presented above does give some guidance to clinical decision making. Melanomas less than 1 mm thick on the trunk or proximal extremities can be managed with 1 cm excision margins. Melanomas thicker than 1 mm on the trunk or proximal extremities do not require excision margins greater than 2 cm. However, there are no data to provide guidelines for the treatment of melanomas on the head, neck and distal extremities. Furthermore, it is clear that 2 cm margins for intermediate and thick melanomas confer only a very slight benefit that has not been shown to be statistically significant and relates only to local recurrence rates. Ross and Balch have sensibly recommended that the 2 cm margin can reasonably be compromised when the risk of disfigurement and surgical morbidity is high.[53]

Micrographic surgery and melanoma

Zitelli et al. have approached the problem of determining appropriate excision margins in a novel way using micrographic surgical techniques.[58] This has not been discussed in earlier reviews of the subject. Micrographic surgery for cutaneous neoplasms was first described by Fredrick Moh. The principle of the technique, and the multitude of technical variations that have since evolved, is to perform microscopic examination of the entire margin of the surgical specimen. Micrographic surgery has principally been used for basal cell carcinoma and squamous cell carcinoma.[59,60] It has also been reported in the treatment of a variety of other skin tumours including dermatofibrosarcoma protuberans, sebaceous carcinoma, Merkel cell carcinoma, and microcystic adnexal carcinoma.[61–64] Further excision is performed at points where the tumour is seen at the margin or closely approaching it. The re-excised margin is then also subjected to examination of its entire margin. The intended result is to have complete tumour resection with minimal risk of local recurrence and at the same time limited excision of normal skin. A number of techniques for tissue preparation and sectioning have been described, including in situ chemical fixation, frozen section assessment, and paraffin embedding to produce permanent sections. The use of this technique for the management of melanoma has been questioned because of doubts about the ability of frozen section examination to detect melanoma reliably and doubts as to whether margins narrow enough to excise the primary lesion alone are adequate.[65]

Micrographic surgery for melanoma has most commonly been described in the management of lentigo maligna (LM) and lentigo maligna melanoma (LMM).[66–70] LM and LMM have lent themselves to this technique because of the characteristic and unpredictable wider extensions of these tumours, which often are not macroscopically apparent. LM and LMM most commonly occur on the face and can reach a considerable size before presentation. Surgical excision using standard margins would result in very large defects. In many cases narrower margins have been used because of anatomical and cosmetic constraints.[71] This has often resulted in positive margins of atypical junctional melanocytic hyperplasia.[72] Left untreated, recurrence can occur in the form of invasive melanoma.[72] Complete surgical resection remains the treatment of choice.[68,73,74] Destructive modalities for the treatment of LM are felt to be suboptimal because of potential failure to treat deep periadnexal melanocytes, inability to detect and treat subclinical disease extension and failure to provide a specimen for detection of invasive melanoma.[74]

Zitelli prospectively collected a series of 535 patients with 553 primary melanomas.[58] All melanomas were excised with a 6 mm margin. The entire margin was then examined by laying out the whole outer circumference and sectioning this in the long axis. Further 3 mm excisions of the circumference were performed where margins were involved. Most cases studied were either in situ or thin melanomas (393/553). Only 67 were greater than 1.5 mm. The final margins of excision were calculated for subgroups based on tumour diameter, location, and thickness. It was found that a margin of 1.2 cm excised 97% of all lesions. In general, wider margins were required on the head and neck compared with the trunk and extremities to achieve clearance rates of 97% (15 mm versus 9 mm). Primary tumour thickness had no bearing on the margins required. Thick primaries did not require wide margins, and in situ disease would have been inadequately removed in many cases by using the recommended 5 mm margin. Tumour diameter >2 cm was a significant predictor of the need for a wider margin. The technique's ability to get clearance has been validated by a local recurrence rate of only 0.5% at a minimum follow up of 5 years. Although micrographic surgery is very time consuming and therefore quite impractical for the majority of patients, Zitelli's work has contributed significantly to our understanding of local recurrence.

Conclusion

Current guidelines for the appropriate margins of excision for primary melanomas should be viewed as such, i.e. as guidelines. Margins of 1 cm for melanomas less than 1 mm thick can be strongly supported. The roles of wider margins for thicker lesions and narrower margins for in situ disease are less clear. Potential benefits of a wider margin must be weighed against the potential cost to the patient in terms of disfigurement, surgical complexity, need for a general anaesthetic, hospital length of stay, and possible morbidity. For lesions thicker than 1 mm consideration should be given to the role of sentinel node biopsy before any operation is performed.

DEFINITIVE SURGICAL MANAGEMENT – BASIC SURGICAL TECHNIQUES

Wide excision of a melanoma biopsy site with appropriate margins can be performed with the expectation of achieving primary closure of the wound in most cases. An elliptical excision is the simplest approach. Dissection should be directly down to the surface of the deep investing fascia. This not only ensures good tumour clearance but also aids closure of the resulting defect. It has been recommended by some that the subcutis should be more widely excised than the skin, in the hope of including any lymphatic tumour emboli. There is no evidence to support this concept, and it potentially increases the risk of wound related problems. Undermining wound edges to aid wound closure is generally unnecessary and usually makes little difference. Closure of wounds can be achieved by any standard technique. A layer of interrupted buried absorbable sutures in the deep dermis can greatly facilitate wound closure and help prevent wound dehiscence. Superficial sutures or staples can then be placed with little difficulty. The wounds are often under some tension and therefore prone to infection and breakdown. Meticulous attention to detail, including haemostasis and careful handling of the skin edges, can minimize the risk of this occurrence. Patients should be advised to restrict activity of the affected area to prevent movement of the opposing wound surfaces.

Larger defects on the trunk and proximal limbs can be closed with the use of a variety of simple local flaps. Rotation flaps are quite satisfactory to close planned V shaped defects. The length of the flap can be increased by excising a triangle of skin at or close to the fixed end. These are known eponymously as Burow's triangles. The use of this flap on both sides of the defect will provide more coverage. The use of small transposition flaps in these regions is to be discouraged as they are usually quite unnecessary. Skin closure could have been achieved primarily in most cases when these flaps have been used.

A split skin graft (SSG) may be necessary at more distal sites and for some large defects at proximal locations. The lower leg and distal limb have little elasticity in the skin, making primary closure impossible in many cases. A SSG has been the usual alternative. Double V-Y advancement flaps can be used and usually provide good clearance, with adequate healing and cosmesis. The scalp also lacks elasticity, but SSGs can be applied with a good outcome. Some controversy exists regarding the appropriate donor site when grafting to the leg. Traditionally, SSGs have been taken from the contralateral limb because of concern that an ipsilateral donor site might be complicated by in-transit metastases. Flook et al. reviewed 186 patients having skin grafts. Skin was obtained from an ipsilateral thigh in 25% of the patients.[75] One patient developed a donor site recurrence, and this was well outside the lymphatic drainage of the primary. Ipsilateral donor sites have the advantage of limiting pain and immobility to one leg. In addition the donor site will be in the field of regional chemotherapy, should in-transit disease occur.

Closure of defects on areas such as the face, distal limbs, hands, and feet often require special reconstructive techniques, and these are outlined in Chapter 22.

REFERENCES

1. Morton DL, Introduction: sentinel lymphadenectomy for patients with clinical stage I melanoma. *J Surg Oncol* 1997; 66: 267–9.
2. Lenisa L, Santinami M, Belli F, et al, Sentinel node biopsy and selective lymph node dissection in cutaneous melanoma patients. *J Exp Clin Cancer Res* 1999; 18: 69–74.
3. Epstein E, Bragg K, Linden G, Biopsy and prognosis of malignant melanoma. *JAMA* 1969; 208: 1369–71.
4. Bagley FH, Cady B, Lee A, Legg MA, Changes in clinical presentation and management of malignant melanoma. *Cancer* 1981; 47: 2126–34.
5. Rampen FHJ, Van Houton WA, Hop WCJ, Incisional procedures and prognosis in malignant melanoma. *Clin Exp Dermatol* 1980; 5: 313–420.
6. Ball AS, Thomas JM, Surgical management of malignant melanoma. *Brit Med Bull* 1995; 51: 584–608.
7. Griffiths RW, Briggs JC, Biopsy procedures, primary wide excisional surgery and long-term prognosis in primary clinical stage I invasive cutaneous malignant melanoma. *Ann R Coll Surg Eng* 1985; 67: 75–8.
8. Handley WS, The pathology of melanotic growths in relation to their operative treatment. Lecture I. *Lancet* 1907; i: 927–33.
9. Handley WS, The pathology of melanotic growths in relation to their operative treatment. Lecture II. *Lancet* 1907; i: 996–1003.
10. Pack GT, End results in the treatment of malignant melanoma: a later report. *Surgery* 1959; 46: 447–60.
11. Lund RH, Inhem H, Malignant melanoma: clinical and pathological analysis of 93 cases. *Surgery* 1955; 38: 611.
12. Petersen NC, Bodenham DC, Lloyd OC, Malignant melanomas of the skin: a study of the origin, development, aetiology, spread, treatment and prognosis. *Br J Plast Surg* 1969; 15: 49–94.
13. Wilson R, Malignant melanoma. A follow up study. West J Surg. 1958; 29.
14. Lehman JA, Cross FS, Richey DW, Clinical study of forty-nine patients with malignant melanoma. *Cancer* 1966; 19: 611.
15. Timmons MJ, Thomas JM, The width of excision of cutaneous melanoma. *Eur J Surg Oncol* 1993; 19: 313–15.
16. Olsen G, Some views in the treatment of melanomas of the skin. *Arch Chir Neerl* 1970; 22: 80–90.
17. Cochran AJ, Studies of the melanocytes of the epidermis adjacent to tumours. *J Invest Dermatol* 1971; 57: 38.
18. Olsen G, The malignant melanoma of the skin: new theories based on a study of 500 cases. *Acta Chir Scand* 1966; 365(suppl): 1128–36.
19. Wong CK, A study of melanocytes in the normal skin surrounding malignant melanomata. *Dermatologica* 1970; 141: 215–25.
20. Fallowfield ME, Cook MG, Epidermal melanocytes adjacent to melanoma and the field effect. *Histopathology* 1990; 17: 397–400.
21. Kelly JW, Sagebiel RW, Calderon W, et al, The frequency of local recurrence and microsatellites as a guide to reexcision margins for cutaneous malignant melanoma. *Ann Surg* 1984; 20: 759–64.
22. MiltonGW, Shaw HM, Farago GA, McCarthy WH, Tumour thickness and the site and time of first recurrence in cutaneous malignant melanoma(stage I). *Br J Surg* 1980; 67: 543–6.
23. Roses DF, Harris MN, Rigel D, et al, Local and in-transit metastases following definitive excision for primary cutaneous malignant melanoma. *Ann Surg* 1983; 198: 65–9.
24. Urist MM, Balch CM, Soong S-J, et al, The influence of surgical margins and prognostic factors predicting the risk of local recurrence in 3445 patients with primary cutaneous melanoma. *Cancer* 1985; 55: 1398–402.
25. Aitken DR, James AG, Carey LC, Local cutaneous recurrence after conservative excision of malignant melanoma. *Arch Surg* 1984; 119: 643–6.
26. Taylor BA, Hughes LE, A policy of selective excision for primary cutaneous malignant melanoma. *Eur J Surg Oncol* 1985; 11: 7–13.
27. Buzaid AC, Ross MI, Balch CM, et al, Critical analysis of the current American Joint Committee on Cancer staging system for cutaneous melanoma and proposal of a new staging system. *J Clin Oncol* 1997; 15: 1039–51.
28. Singletary S, Tucker S, Boddie A, A multivariate analysis of prognostic factors in regional cutaneous metastases of extremity melanoma. *Cancer* 1988; 61: 1437–40.
29. Karakousis C, Temple D, Moore R, et al, Prognostic parameters in recurrent malignant melanoma. *Cancer* 1983; 52: 575–9.
30. Cascinelli N, Bufalino R, Marolda R, et al, Regional non-nodal metastases of cutaneous melanoma. *Eur J Surg Oncol* 1986; 12: 175–80.
31. Reintgen D, Vollmer R, Tso C, et al, Prognosis for recurrent stage I melanoma. *Arch Surg* 1987; 122: 1338–42.
32. Roses D, Karp N, Oratz R, et al, Survival with regional and distant metastases from cutaneous malignant melanoma. *Surg Gynecol Obstet* 1991; 172: 262–8.
33. Coit DG, Rogatko A, Brennan MF, Prognostic factors in patients with melanoma metastatic to axillary or inguinal lymph nodes. A multivariate analysis. *Ann Surg* 1991; 214: 627–36.
34. Calabro A, Singletary SE, Balch CM, Patterns of relapse in 1001 consecutive patients with melanoma nodal metastases. *Arch Surg* 1989; 124: 1051–5.
35. Roses DF, Provet JA, Harris MN, et al, Prognosis of patients with pathological stage II cutaneous malignant melanoma. *Ann Surg* 1985; 201: 103–7.
36. Hughes TMD, Thomas JM, Combined inguinal and pelvic lymph node dissection for stage III melanoma. *Br J Surg* 1999; 86: 1493–8.
37. Hughes TMD, A'Hern RP, Thomas JM, Prognosis and management of patients with palpable inguinal lymph node metastases from melanoma. *Br J Surg* 2000; 87: 892–901.
38. Brown CD, Zitelli JA, The prognosis and treatment of true local cutaneous recurrent malignant melanoma. *Dermatol Surg* 1995; 21: 285–90.
39. Aitken DR, Clausen K, Klein JP, James AG, The extent of primary melanoma excision. *Ann Surg* 1983; 198: 634–41.
40. Breslow A, Macht SD, Optimal size of resection margin for thin cutaneous melanoma. *Surg Gynecol Obstet* 1977; 145: 691–2.
41. Cosimi AB, Sober AJ, Mihm MC, Fitzpatrick TB, Conservative surgical management of superficially invasive cutaneous melanoma. *Cancer* 1984; 53: 1256–9.
42. Balch CM, Murad TM, Soong S-J, et al, Tumor thickness as a guide to surgical management of clinical stage I melanoma patients. *Cancer* 1979; 43: 883–8.
43. Elder DE, Guerry D 4th, Heiberger RM, et al, Optimal resection margin for cutaneous malignant melanoma. *Plast Reconstr Surg* 1983; 71: 66–72.
44. Goldman LI, Byrd R, Narrowing resection margins for patients with low risk melanoma. *Am J Surg* 1988; 155: 242–4.
45. Cascinelli N, van der Esch EP, Breslow A, et al, Stage I melanoma of the skin: the problem of resection margins. *Eur J Cancer* 1980; 16: 1079–85.
46. Day CL, Mihm MC, Sober AJ, et al, Narrower margins for clinical stage I malignant melanoma. *N Engl J Med* 1982; 306: 479–81.
47. O'Rourke MG, Altmann CR, Melanoma recurrence after excision. Is a wide margin justified? *Ann Surg* 1993; 217: 2–5.
48. Schmoeckel C, Bockelbrink A, Bockelbrink H, et al, Low and high-risk melanoma III: Prognostic significance of the resection margin. *Eur J Cancer Clin Oncol* 1983; 19: 245–9.
49. Welvaart K, Hermans J, Zwaveling A, Ruiter DJ, Prognosis and surgical treatment of of patients with stage I melanomas of the skin: a retrospective analysis of 211 patients. *J Surg Oncol* 1986; 31: 79–86.
50. Milton GW, Shaw HM, McCarthy WJ, Resection margins of melanoma. *Aust NZ J Surg* 1985; 55: 225–31.
51. Veronesi U, Cascinelli N, Adamus, et al, Thin stage primary cutaneous malignant melanoma: Comparison of excision with margins of 1 or 3 cm. *N Engl J Med* 1988; 318: 1159–62.
52. Veronesi U, Cascinelli N, Narrow excision (1 cm): A safe procedure for thin cutaneous melanoma. *Arch Surg* 1991; 126: 438–41.
53. Ross MI, Balch CM, Surgical treatment of primary melanoma. In: *Cutaneous melanoma.* (eds Balch CM, Houghton AN, Sober AJ, Soong SJ). St Louis: Quality Medical Publishing, 1998: 141–53.
54. Balch CM, Urist MM, Karakousis CP, et al, Efficacy of 2 cm surgical margins for intermediate-thickness melanomas (1–4 mm): results of a multi-institutional randomized surgical trial. *Ann Surg* 1993; 218: 262–9.
55. Heaton K, Sussman J, Gershenwald J, et al, Surgical margins and prognostic factors in thick(>4mm) primary melanoma patients. *Ann Surg Oncol* 1998; 5: 322–8.

56. Schneebaum S, Briele HA, Walker MJ, et al, Cutaneous thick melanoma: prognosis and treatment. *Arch Surg* 1987; 122: 707–11.
57. Spellman JE, Driscoll D, Velez A Karakousis CP, Thick cutaneous melanoma of the trunk and extremities: An institutional review. *Surg Oncol* 1994: 3: 335–43.
58. Zitelli JA, Brown CD, Hanusa BH, Surgical margins for excision of primary cutaneous melanoma. *J Am Acad Dermatol* 1997; 37: 422–9.
59. Rowe DE, Carroll RJ, Day CL, Long term recurrence rates in previously untreated (primary) basal cell carcinoma: implications for patient follow-up. *J Dermatol Surg Oncol* 1989; 15: 315–36.
60. Mohs FE, *Chemosurgery: microscopically controlled surgery for skin cancer.* Springfield, IL: Charles C Thomas, 1978, 1–356.
61. Parker TL, Zitelli JA, Surgical margins for excision of dermatofibrosarcoma protuberans. *J Am Acad Dermatol* 1995; 32: 233–6.
62. Ratz JL, Duong SL, Kulwin DR, Sebaceous carcinoma of the eyelid treated with Mohs surgery. *J Am Acad Dermatol* 1986; 14: 668–73.
63. Johnson TM, Smith JW, Nelson BR, et al, Current therapy for cutaneous melanoma. *J Am Acad Dermatol* 1995; 32: 689–707.
64. Fleischmann HE, Roth RJ, Wood C, et al, Microcystic adnexal carcinoma treated by microscopically controlled excision. J *Dermatol Surg Oncol* 1984; 10: 873–5.
65. Braun M, Unreliability of frozen section in the histological evaluation of malignant melanoma [abstract]. *J Dermatol Surg Oncol* 1986; 12: 641.
66. Robinson JK, Margin control for lentigo maligna. *J Am Acad Dermatol* 1994; 31: 79–85.
67. Cohen LM, Mc Call MW, Hodge SJ, et al. Successful treatment of lentigo maligna with Moh's micrographic surgery and rush permanent sections. *Cancer* 1994; 73: 2964–70.
68. Coleman WP, Davis RS, Ree RJ, Krementz ET, Treatment of lentigo maligna and lentigo maligna melanoma. *J Dermatol Surg Oncol* 1980; 6: 476–9.
69. Grande DJ, Koranda TC, Whitaker DC, Surgery of extensive, subclinical lentigo maligna. *J Dermatol Surg Oncol* 1982; 5: 493–6.
70. Cohen LM, McCall MW, Zax RH, Mohs micrographic surgery for lentigo maligna and lentigo maligna melanoma. A follow-up study. *Dermatol Surg* 1998; 24: 673–7.
71. Hill DC, Gramp AA, Surgical treatment of lentigo maligna and lentigo maligna melanoma. *Australas J Dermatol* 1999; 40: 25–30.
72. Dhawan SS, Wolf DJ, Rabinovitz HS, Poulos E, Lentigo maligna. The use of rush permanent sections in therapy. *Arch Dermatol* 1990; 126: 928–30.
73. Cohen LM, Lentigo maligna and lentigo maligna melanoma. *J Am Acad Dermatol* 1995; 33: 923–36.
74. Mohs FE, The width and depth of sprad of malignant melanomas as observed by a chemosurgeon. *Am J Dermatopathol* 1984; 6(suppl 1): 123–6.
75. Flook D, Horgan K, Taylor BA, Hughes LE. Surgery for malignant melanoma: from which limb should the graft be taken? *Br J Surg* 1988; 73: 793–5.

22

Surgical management of primary melanoma: reconstruction techniques after wide excision

Michael Quinn, John F Thompson

INTRODUCTION

When considering reconstruction in melanoma management, two important points need to be kept in mind. First, recommended excision margins have decreased in recent years, as discussed in Chapter 21. For melanomas under 1 mm in thickness, a 1 cm margin is now considered adequate, and for melanomas under 4 mm in thickness a 2 cm margin.[1,2] A retrospective study of 278 patients with melanomas greater than 4 mm in thickness found no advantage in terms of recurrence or survival associated with margins of excision greater than 2 cm.[3] In the trunk and proximal limbs, most wide excisions can therefore be repaired by primary closure. Balch showed that with a 4 cm margin, 46% of patients required a skin graft, but with a 2 cm margin only 11% of patients required a skin graft (P=0.001).[2] This study did not, however, include the face. In general, therefore, it is only at specific sites on the distal limbs, face, scalp, and perineum that reconstruction techniques after wide excision for primary melanoma need to be considered. In this chapter these sites will be discussed individually.

The second point is that the thickness of melanomas at the time of diagnosis has decreased in recent years. In most countries some 80% of melanomas will now be less than 1 mm in thickness and thus require only a 1 cm clearance margin (the median thickness at presentation in New South Wales, Australia, for example, is currently 0.7 mm). Except for the body sites mentioned above, the situation can therefore be dealt with in most cases by primary closure of a simple elliptical excision.

PSYCHOLOGICAL ASPECTS

The psychological impact of the surgery undertaken to treat a melanoma also needs to be considered. Cassileth et al. studied this in 176 melanoma patients, and found that accurate prediction of the size of the scar was associated with significantly less distress than if the scar was larger than expected (P< 0.0001).[4] It is noteworthy that two thirds of the patients stated that their scar was larger than expected. Overall, women were more distressed by their scars than were men (P< 0.001). Interestingly, men were more distressed by scars ordinarily covered by clothing, whereas women were more distressed by scars on exposed parts of the body.

These findings imply that when informed consent is obtained preoperatively, not only should the prognosis and the possible risks of surgery be communicated to the patient, but the likely postoperative appearance should also be explained.

PRINCIPLES OF RECONSTRUCTION

In selecting the most appropriate method of reconstruction for a patient after wide excision of a melanoma, the concept of the 'reconstructive ladder' (Figure 22.1) can be utilized, whereby the simplest yet most reliable method is employed as a one stage procedure.[5]

Primary closure

The lowest rung of the reconstructive ladder is primary closure. This is the simplest and most basic method of

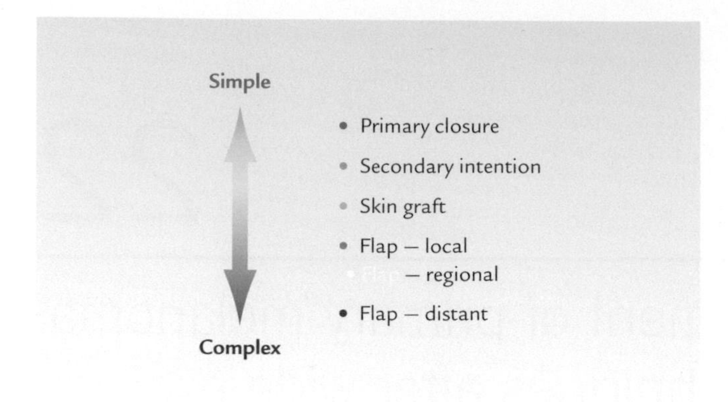

Figure 22.1 *The reconstructive ladder.*

repair of a wide excision defect. It is classically illustrated by the reconstruction of a mid-cheek defect in a young female, where primary closure allows the wound to resemble a traumatic injury, whereas a complex local flap implies that the patient has undergone a surgical operation with its associated stigma.

The use of long term, absorbable sutures in the deep dermis minimizes wound stretch and allows early removal of cutaneous non-absorbable sutures to avoid cross-hatching. However, patients should always be warned of the possibility of wound stretch in high movement areas such as the upper back. Abnormal postoperative scarring can be managed by application of a silicone gel patch, with the addition of pressure when possible. The effect on hypertrophic scarring is probably due both to the occlusive effect and to increased hydration of the superficial scar layers.[6,7]

With recent advances in lymphoscintigraphy showing that lymph does not necessarily drain via the most direct route to regional lymph node fields, thereby negating the concept of 'incontinuity' dissection, elliptical excisions can be orientated in the classic 'lines of resting skin tension', allowing less tension in closure and a more satisfactory wound.[8] An incorrectly oriented biopsy scar can be converted to a more acceptable orientation by excising a 'lazy S' ellipse.[9] In the distal forearm and calf, elliptical excision can result in significant contour deformities, about which the patient should be warned. This is especially significant in the lower limb of females, which is their most common primary melanoma site.

Melanoma of the skin of the female breast can also be treated by wide excision with primary closure, and a mastectomy is not required.[9]

Secondary intention

This implies macrophage initiated wound contraction, starting at about day 10 postoperatively, and epithelial migration, with loss of contact inhibition. It is a process that should have little part to play in melanoma surgery or any reconstructive surgery. Allowing granulation tissue, which is essentially scar tissue, to form, and thereby delaying wound healing, decreases the mobility of surrounding structures and impedes the patient's rehabilitation. Epithelial migration produces a fragile wound closure that, without dermal support, is subject to breakdown with minimal trauma. Wound contraction distorts adjacent structures, and in cosmetically important areas, leads to disfigurement.

On some occasions, however, dressings may still be required, for example in the management of an infected wound producing copious exudate. Over the past 20 years a myriad of new dressings has become available, yet none can be considered a perfect dressing. Wounds can be broadly classified according to their colour: black (eschar), yellow (slough) and red (granulation). Dressings are then indicated by treatment algorithms depending on the wound colour, with each dressing used for a specific purpose. Hydrocolloids are currently the workhorse dressing, whilst alginates are widely used for situations such as that described above.[10]

Recent developments with vacuum assisted wound healing devices[11] have made it possible to close some of the problem wounds occasionally encountered in melanoma surgery, even if they have been previously irradiated.[11,12] When blood vessels are exposed, these devices should of course be used with great caution.

Skin grafts

Split skin grafts are used in distal limbs and the scalp. In the opinion of the authors, all grafts are best perforated with a mesh dermatome. Stapling grafts into position with foam compression inlay moulds is effective and decreases operative time. This technique also allows early postoperative mobilization after excision and split skin grafting for lower limb melanomas. Areas of delayed healing, where granulation tissue is allowed to form, may mimic local recurrence, and should be carefully documented. When minimizing postoperative scarring is particularly important, hidden donor sites should be considered, such as the hair bearing scalp or the pubic triangle in women.

Full thickness grafts are normally used only in the face,[9] harvested from the opposite upper lid for periorbital reconstruction, or from the postauricular and supraclavicular areas for other facial sites.

Flaps

Historically, flap reconstruction after excision of a melanoma was discouraged because of theoretical concerns that local recurrence might be concealed and its detection delayed, with negative prognostic consequences.[13] Clinically, however, flap reconstruction does not seem to worsen either the local recurrence rate or the disease-free survival rate, and detection of local recurrence is not usually a problem.[14]

Local flaps are used mainly in facial reconstruction. They are rarely indicated in the trunk and proximal limbs, given the current guidelines for melanoma excision margins. Regional flaps are used for reconstruction in regional lymph node fields and are of the myocutaneous variety. The inclusion of muscle in these flaps is important, given the greater ability of a muscle flap to resist wound contamination compared to a flap of skin and subcutaneous tissue only.[15]

The final rung of the reconstructive ladder is the free composite graft with microvascular anastomoses. This can be considered as an alternative to a regional flap.

SPECIFIC SITES

Face

Principles

The face is divided into major 'facial units' of forehead, nose, eyelids, cheeks, lips, and chin, and each of these is further divided into site subunits.[16] The central facial units of nose, lips and eyelids are seen in primary gaze and suboptimal reconstruction is readily apparent. The peripheral facial units of the lateral cheeks and forehead are relatively featureless and reconstruction is less demanding. Local flaps, when used, make use of excess skin in the jowl, preauricular, nasolabial, lateral orbital, crow's feet, and glabellar areas.[17]

Balch has proposed that 1 cm is an acceptable excision margin for melanomas of the face.[18] Hudson et al. looked specifically at narrow excision margins in 106 patients with melanomas of the face; of these, 30 had margins of less than 1 cm and 64 had margins of between 1 cm and 2 cm.[19] Mean tumour thickness was 2.2 mm. In the seven patients who developed local recurrence, there was no correlation with surgical margins. Primary closure was achieved in 25% of the patients, and flap closure was achieved in a further 50%.

The Clark level of invasion may be an independent prognostic variable for thin melanomas and for those that arise in thin skin such as the eyelid and ear.[20–22] The Clark level should therefore be considered when determining the appropriate width and depth of excision in these areas.

Periorbital region

The authors of the largest reported series of periorbital melanomas, comprising 40 patients, recommended wide excision according to standard guidelines and provided a treatment algorithm.[23] Melanoma in situ was found in 17 of the patients. The lower eyelid was the commonest site (14 patients), and a melanoma on the upper eyelid was recorded in only one patient. Adjacent facial regions were involved in 31 patients (75%), and this was especially true for melanomas arising at the next commonest site, the lateral canthus (9 patients). The most common method of reconstruction was with a full thickness graft from the opposite upper lid for partial thickness defects of greater than 50% (9 patients). A further six patients had composite grafts with cheek advancement for full thickness defects of greater than 75%. Cervicofacial flaps (Figure 22.2) were used in 19 patients where melanoma extended onto the cheek. Eight patients had an ancillary lateral canthoplasty to maintain lower lid position and avoid postoperative ectropion. An alternative was the use of a laterally based myocutaneous flap from the upper lid which, as the flap contracted, was also protective against ectropion. The average thickness for invasive lesions was 1.47 mm, and there was no local recurrence.

The previous largest series of 24 patients had involvement of contiguous structures in a similar 50% of patients.[24] A review by Zoltie and O'Neill, including the

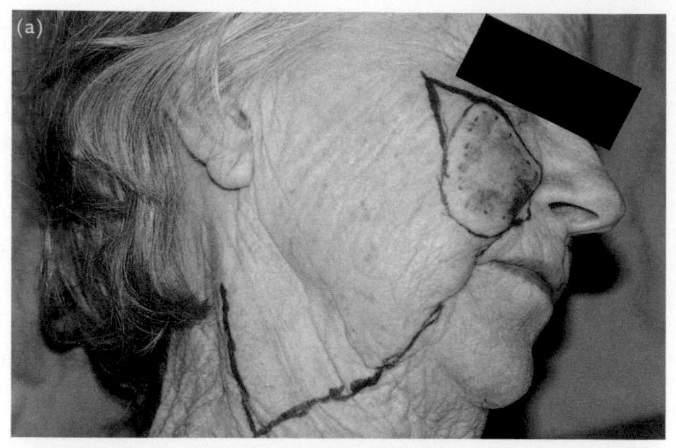

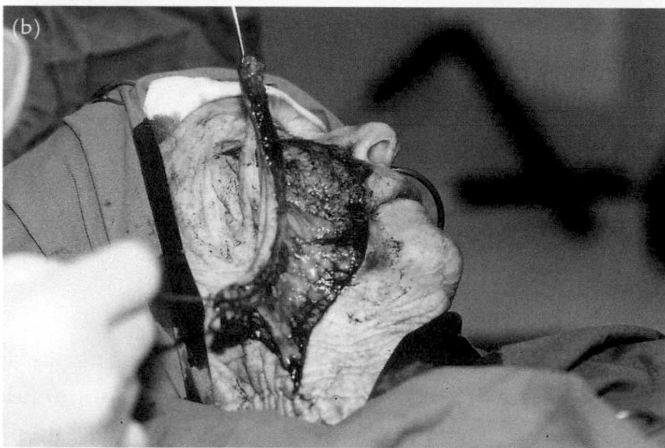

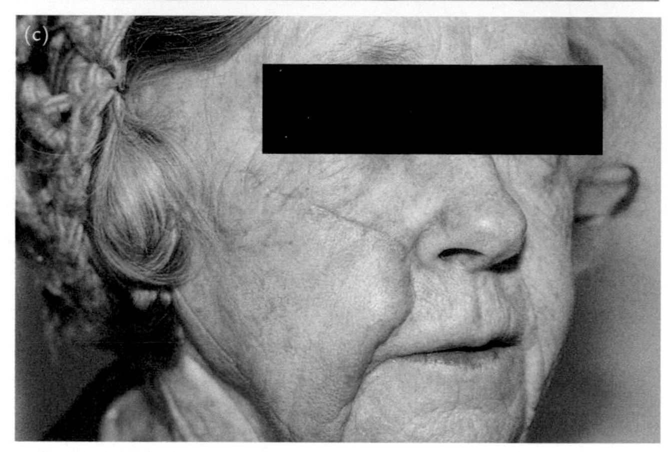

Figure 22.2 *Cervicofacial flap*
(a) Lentigo maligna melanoma of the cheek
(b) Laterally based cervicofacial flap
(c) Postoperative appearance.

latter series, noted that, of the seven accumulated cases of melanoma involving the lid margin, four developed local recurrence and one developed metastatic disease.[25] Melanomas at this site thus require full thickness excision with margins that leave a defect of greater than 75% of the lid. However, the review also notes that no local recurrence occurred when the melanoma did not involve the lid margin, and the authors suggest that more conservative margins can therefore be used when the melanoma does not involve the lid margin.

The review by Zoltie et al. also noted that eyelid skin is the thinnest in the body, often less than 1 mm in total thickness, thus all but the most superficial invasive melanomas will involve the subcutis. However, none of these papers make recommendations on depth of excision for invasive melanomas in the periorbital region. Once again it would seem that a more conservative approach could be adopted, with excision only down to the underlying orbicularis muscle, unless there is obvious involvement of the deep margin.

The adjacent temple area is suitable for reconstruction with a full thickness graft, a double-Z rhombic (DZR) flap, or a Limberg flap, with the flap based on the crow's feet wrinkles.[26,27] McGregor considered this area the best use of the Limberg flap.[17]

Where orbital exenteration is required for extensive local recurrence in the area, the standard reconstruction is with a temporalis muscle flap passed through a lateral orbital rim resection.[28] A split skin graft onto the well vascularized muscle flap can withstand adjuvant radiotherapy.

Cheek

It is now considered that flap reconstruction is best selected according to whether the defect is located in the medial or lateral cheek region. These zones are divided by a line drawn vertically from the lateral canthus. Large defects in the medial cheek are treated by inferolaterally based flaps, and defects in the lateral cheek by medially based flaps avoiding incisions in the medial zone. Incisions in the medial zone are difficult to conceal, as they are apparent on frontal view. Dog ears should not be left as they will not resolve, a principle that is particularly important in the jowl area. Obese patients tend to be difficult as there is little laxity of their facial skin to provide mobility in flap closure.

In a retrospective review of 35 patients who underwent flap reconstruction for head and neck melanomas, the commonest site was the cheek (31%). The preferred local flaps for reconstructing the cheek were cervicofacial and cheek advancement flaps.[29]

Defects in the suborbital and perioral medial cheek skin can often be closed primarily with the scar orientated parallel to the nasolabial fold. Scars are more prominent as the nasal sidewall is approached. A V-Y advancement flap can be used in this area, making use of excess jowl skin, but should not be used to reconstruct the thin periorbital skin.[30] The V-Y advancement flap can also result in problems with ectropion, as can any flap that involves superior advancement. Alternatively a cervicofacial flap can be used, making use of excess jowl and neck skin.[31] This flap, dissected in the deep plane, minimizes scarring because incisions are made within facial subunits.

The mid-cheek area is often able to be closed primarily, making use of excess jowl and nasolabial fold skin, or with a DZR flap, making use of excess nasolabial fold and preauricular skin.

Small defects in the lateral cheek area can be treated by direct excision with either anterior undermining in the subcutaneous facelift plane or making use of excess preauricular skin. A DZR flap is an alternative for larger defects. Larger defects can also be treated by standard cervicofacial flaps based anteriorly.

Overlying the zygomatic body, lentigo maligna melanomas are common, and full thickness graft reconstruction is an option in elderly patients. However, a combination of a V-Y advancement flap for cheek skin and a laterally based upper lid myocutaneous flap for periorbital skin is most often used. The lentigo maligna pigmentation is best delineated with an ultraviolet light.[32] Where lentigo maligna or atypical melanocytic hyperplasia is present at excision margins, in an orientated specimen, these margins should be re-excised until clear. Local recurrence of invasive melanoma has been documented in this situation.[33]

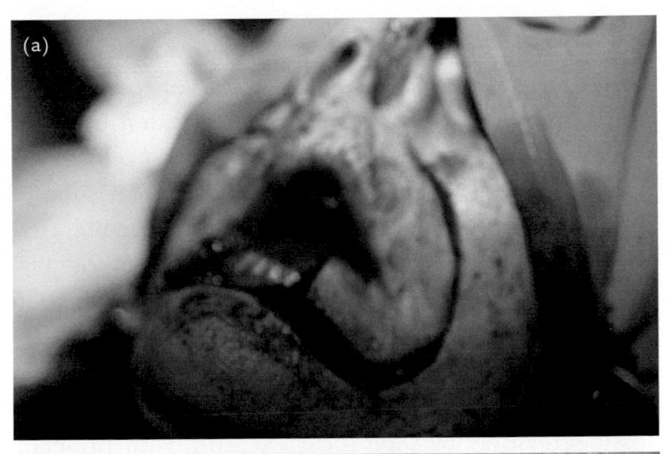

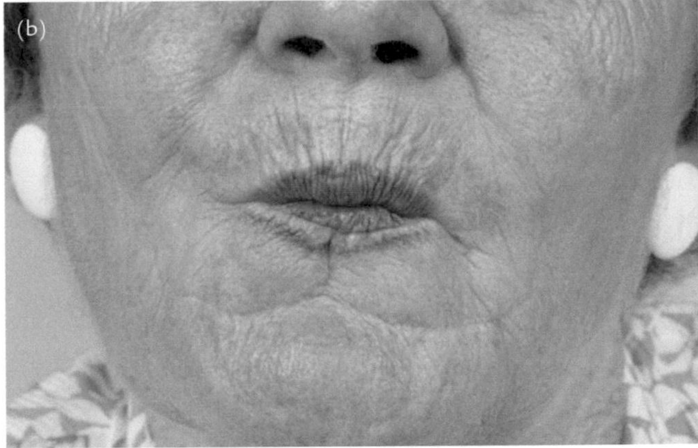

Figure 22.3 *Karapandzic flap*
(a) Defect and Karapandzic flap
(b) Postoperative motor function.

Lip

This is a rare site for melanoma, despite its potential for sun exposure.[34] Such melanomas require wedge excision to attain a 1 cm clearance margin, especially if neurotropism is present, when an even wider margin is desirable.[35] Of the 30 patients in the Sydney Melanoma Unit (SMU) database who had melanomas of the lip, 21 (70%) had neurotropism present. These melanomas require at least a 1 cm clearance.[35] The commonest flap used for reconstruction is the Karapandzic flap (Figure 22.3).[29,36] This allows for both sensory and motor function, but microstomia is an occasional problem, especially for patients with dentures. The upper lip is also amenable to flap reconstruction, although this is more difficult given the increased fixation of the upper lip compared to the lower lip. Only five of the 30 patients on the SMU database with melanomas of the lip had their tumours on the upper lip (17%).

Other innervated composite flaps have also been described, based on the depressor angularis muscle for the lower lip and the levator angularis muscle for the upper lip. These transposed flaps may avoid the problem of microstomia.[37]

Ear

Retrospective reviews of melanomas of the ear at specific institutions suggested that this site was associated with a worse prognosis than other head and neck melanomas, and therefore required aggressive local treatment by wedge excision or partial amputation.[9,38,39] However, other series, including one from the SMU, did not indicate a worse prognosis for this site.[40,41]

The helix is the most common site for melanoma of the ear, being involved in 60% of patients.[29,42] Melanoma of the helical rim can be treated by a rim resection with primary closure, which produces an acceptable rim irregularity.[43] This is particularly useful for superficial spreading melanoma along the rim. Alternatively a wedge excision, or the more complex chondrocutaneous flap reconstruction, can be used. In one series only a single recurrence occurred in 21 patients when this method was employed.[42]

A recent retrospective review of 31 patients treated less aggressively by wide local excision, with preservation of the underlying perichondrium and then skin grafting, showed no local recurrence and no reduction in survival outcome.[40]

The lobule, which is involved in 20% of patients, can be treated by amputation, with the result difficult to detect. Subtotal amputation of the entire external ear is reserved for locally advanced or recurrent melanoma. The root of the helix should be preserved, if possible, to allow the wearing of spectacles.[44]

Scalp

In a review of 998 head and neck melanomas at the SMU, the scalp did appear to be a site of worse prognosis.[41] Taking a 1 cm margin on the scalp usually requires reconstruction in the form of a split skin graft. When pericranium is included in the excision for tumour clearance, or if adjuvant radiotherapy is likely to be required, local flaps are used, employing transposition or rotation designs. Dog ears can be left to settle on the convex surface of the scalp.

Late reconstruction of grafted defects can be achieved with tissue expansion using rectangular or croissant shaped expanders.[45] Incisions are placed radial to the expansion for initial insertion.[46] The circumference of the expanded skin equals the base diameter of the expander plus the diameter of the defect, increased by one third to compensate for skin shrinkage after removal of the expander. The double backcut flap makes best use of the expanded skin.[47] Skull erosion can be a temporary problem in scalp expansion.[48]

Nose

An initial report based on 34 patients from the SMU has shown that this is a rare site for melanoma, involving only 0.4% of patients on the SMU database.[49] Reconstruction is carried out with reference to the nasal subunit principle, with the use of multiple flaps when more than one unit is involved.[50] If more than 50% of a subunit is excised to achieve tumour clearance, the rest of the subunit should also be excised. Although local nasal flaps and full thickness forehead grafts can be used for reconstruction of smaller defects resulting from the far more common non-melanocytic skin cancers, two stage nasolabial and forehead flaps are usually required for melanoma excision defects.[51,52] Alternatively, full thickness grafts can be used. Cartilage is excised only if there is obvious involvement of it, and defects following resection for primary melanomas are rarely full thickness.[53]

The nasal dorsum and sidewall can be reconstructed with full thickness skin grafts harvested from the usual donor sites. Defects following excision of neurotropic melanomas should undergo flap reconstruction to allow adjuvant radiotherapy.

Forehead

Primary closure can occasionally be used in the forehead, with the excision defect oriented horizontally, in line with the forehead wrinkles. This tends to be mainly effective laterally when brow ptosis is present. The patient should be warned about the possibility of eyebrow elevation, which tends to be more of a problem medially. Alternatively, the vertical wrinkle lines present laterally can be used by vertical ellipse orientation to avoid this problem. Dog ears can often be left to settle on the convex surface of the forehead.

When primary closure is not possible, the DZR flap is quite useful in this area. Full thickness grafts are an alternative, especially for larger defects, and the supraclavicular area is a good donor site. A forehead defect is more apparent if the frontalis muscle is included in the excision and patients should be warned of a contour deformity. Where a hemi-forehead defect is present, a forehead scalp flap can be employed.[53]

Distal limb

Extremity melanomas generally have a better prognosis than those on the head, neck, and trunk. However distal lower extremity melanomas (of the distal 1/3 of the leg, the ankle, and the foot) have a prognosis similar to that of trunk melanoma.[54]

Foot

Melanoma is the most common malignant tumour affecting the foot.[55] The plantar surface is the commonest site, and melanomas here tend to be thicker than elsewhere.[56,57] The foot and ankle region is a site associated with a poor prognosis, confirmed by a very large study of 282 patients.[56,58]

Excision of a melanoma on the dorsum of the foot normally requires reconstruction with a split skin graft.[56] The junctional area between the glaborous plantar skin, which is relatively fixed to underlying structures by fibrous septa, and the mobile dorsal skin is a possible site with an increased incidence of melanoma and also a site where dysplastic naevi can be found. Primary closure with the scar crossing perpendicular to the junction between plantar and dorsal skin wherever possible is satisfactory, but grafts can be troublesome in this area.

Adequate excision of a melanoma on the sole of the foot produces a defect that cannot usually be closed primarily.[44]

Split skin grafting of the sole including the weight bearing surfaces is generally recommended, and Woltering et al. reported on the long term results of 11 patients treated in this way.[56,59] Complications were limited to hyperkeratosis around the graft and fissuring of the graft itself. However, a study using the pressure sensitive Harris mat showed an avoidance type gait pattern, with a shift of weight to uninvolved areas of the foot.

Small defects of both the weight bearing and the non-weight bearing plantar surfaces can be reconstructed with a glaborous split skin graft harvested from the instep of the opposite foot. A very thick dermatome setting is used to harvest the skin, which should appear opaque if an adequate thickness of dermis has been obtained. Tie-over and quilting sutures are usually used. These grafts tend to have fewer problems with adjacent hyperkeratosis.

The weight bearing heel can be reconstructed with a medial plantar flap, (Figure 22.4) great care being taken in individuals with peripheral vascular disease.[60] The distal weight bearing forefoot can also be reconstructed with a distally based medial plantar flap, although the dissection is difficult.[61]

The most common site for subungual melanoma of the foot is beneath the nail of the great toe (this was the case in 23 of 25 patients in the SMU series).[62] Amputation of the great toe should attempt to leave the metatarsal head intact to allow more even distribution of weight bearing and better balance as a consequence. This necessitates creating a volar skin flap.[57]

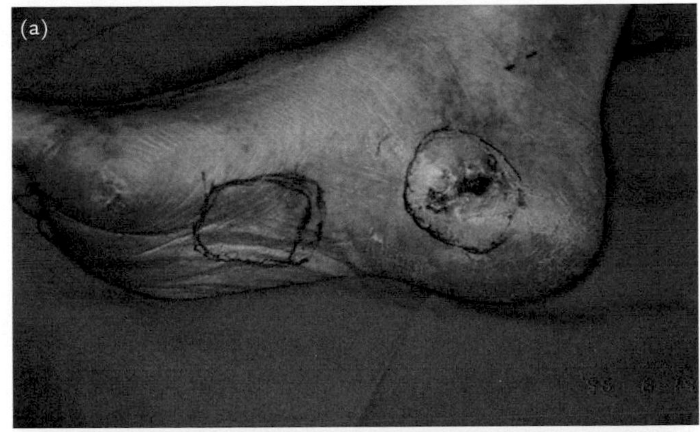

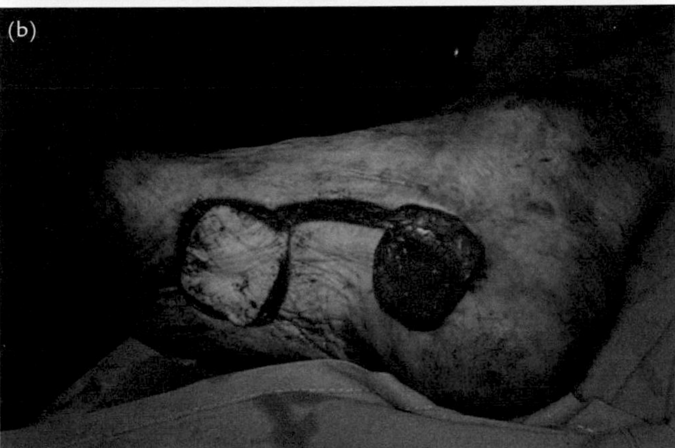

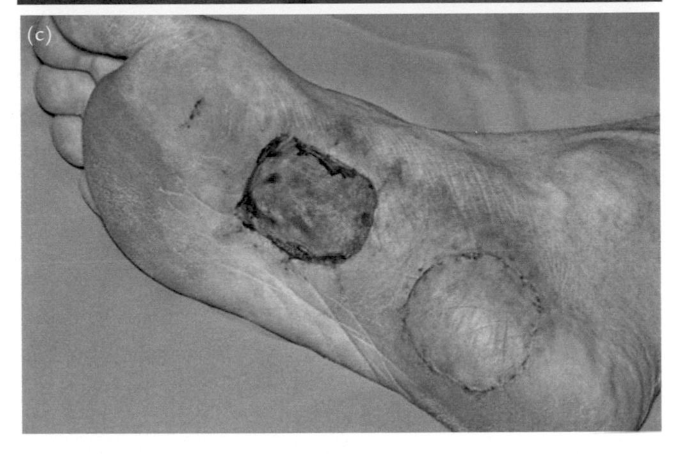

Figure 22.4 *Medial plantar flap*
(a) Acral melanoma on heel
(b) Medial plantar flap
(c) Postoperative appearance with split skin graft on donor site.

Hand

Subungual melanoma can be treated by distal rather than proximal amputation, without increased local recurrence risk.[63] In the thumb, amputation is carried out through the neck of the proximal phalanx. This may be combined with a first web space deepening procedure to allow increased mobility. In a finger, amputation at the level of the midshaft of the middle phalanx allows preservation of the flexor digitorum superficialis tendon insertion and the central slip of the extensor apparatus, thereby preserving movement at the proximal interphalangeal joint. For in situ melanoma, consideration may be given to amputation distal to the profundus insertion with removal of the nail bed. Melanoma of the volar surface is rare (with only two such patients on the SMU database). Melanoma on the dorsum of the hand usually requires reconstruction with a split skin graft. Web space lesions of the hands or feet usually can be excised with adequate margins with flap or graft reconstructions. Double digit ray amputation is usually not indicated.[44]

Mucosal melanomas

Mucosal melanomas generally have a poor prognosis.[64] They represent approximately 1% of melanomas. Most are of the acral lentiginous histogenetic type. Although the equivalent Clark level architecture is not present, thickness and ulceration are known prognostic indicators. Genital and head and neck lesions tend to recur locally, whereas anorectal primaries are more likely to recur systemically.[65]

Head and neck

The head and neck is the most common site for mucosal melanoma. In this region the nasal mucosa is the most frequent site, followed by the oral cavity.[66] However, in Japanese studies of mucosal melanoma, the latter site is more common. The hard palate, which is in turn the commonest site for oral cavity melanoma, can be reconstructed with a split skin inlay graft onto bare bone, which will usually take well (Figure 22.5).[17]

Female genital tract

The labia minora of the vulva is the commonest site for melanomas of the female genital tract, representing 80% of 400 cases in a collected series.[67] This differs from the more common squamous cell carcinoma, which is usually located on the labia majora. Vaginal melanoma is less common, with only 150 cases reported. It has a poor prognosis, with a 5-year survival

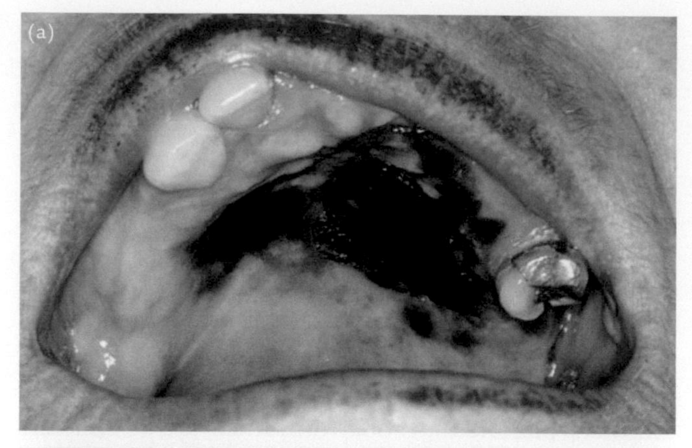

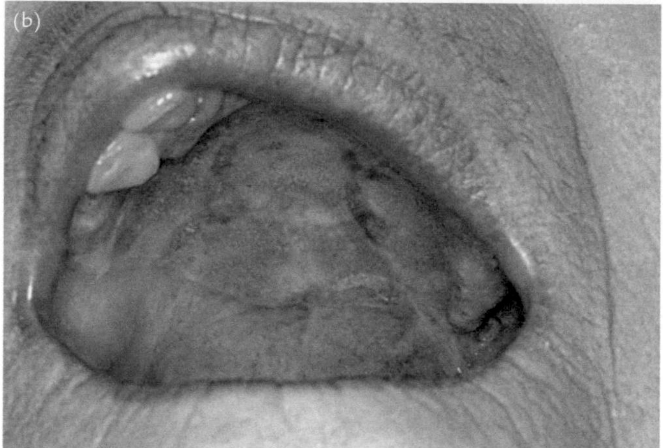

Figure 22.5 *(a) Melanoma of the hard palate (b) Post inlay skin graft reconstruction.*

rate of only 5%.[68] More recently, labia minora melanomas have been excised with primary closure, rather than resorting to radical vulvectomy, but reconstruction with split skin grafts can also be used. Vaginal melanoma can be reconstructed with a split skin graft on a stent, or alternatively fasciocutaneous flaps based on the pudendal arteries and harvested from the groin crease can be employed, with primary closure of the donor site.[69]

Male genital tract

The cutaneous surface of the penis is the commonest site for melanoma of the male genital tract. On the glans penis a simple flap repair is possible in the uncircumcised patient, harvested from the skin of the prepuce.[70]

Anus and lower rectum

Anorectal melanomas have a 90% mortality, many patients presenting with distant metastases.[71,72]

Treatment should consist of wide excision, with preservation of the sphincter mechanism. Abdominoperineal resection does not appear to confer a survival advantage.[71,73]

REFERENCES

1. Veronesi U, Cascinelli N, Narrow excision (1cm): a safe procedure for thin cutaneous melanoma. *Arch Surg* 1991; 126: 438–41.
2. Balch CM, Urist MM, Karakousis CP, et al, Efficacy of 2 cm surgical margins for intermediate-thickness melanomas(1–4mm): results of a multi-institutional randomized surgical trial. *Ann Surg* 1993; 218: 262–9.
3. Heaton KM, Sussman JJ, Gershenwald JE, et al, Surgical margins and prognostic factors in patients with thick (>4mm) primary melanoma. *Ann Surg Oncol* 1998; 5: 322–8.
4. Cassileth BR, Lush EJ, Tenaglia BS, Patients perceptions of the cosmetic impact of melanoma resection. *Plastic Reconstr Surg* 1983; 71: 73–8.
5. Place MJ, Herber SC, Hardesty RA, Basic techniques and principles in plastic surgery. In: *Grabb and Smith's plastic surgery.* 5th ed. (ed. Aston SJ et al.), Philadelphia: Lippincott-Raven, 1997: 13–26.
6. Fulton JE, Silicone gel sheeting for the prevention and management of evolving hypertrophic and keloid scars. *Dermatol Surg* 1995; 21: 947–51.
7. Sawada Y, Sone K, Hydration and occlusion treatment of hypertrophic scars and keloids. 1992; 45: 559–600.
8. Borges AF, *Elective incisions and scar revision.* Boston: Little Brown, 1973.
9. Lee JE, Balch CM, Melanoma. In: *Reconstructive plastic surgery for cancer.* (ed. Kroll SS), St Louis: Mosby, 1996: 64.
10. Ladin DA, Understanding dressings. *Clin Plast Surg* 1998; 25: 433–41.
11. Mullner T, Mrkonjic L, Kwasny O, Vecsei V, The use of negative pressure to promote the healing of tissue defects: a clinical trial using the vacuum sealing technique. *Br J Plast Surg* 1997; 50: 194–9.
12. Argenta LC, Morykwas M, Vacuum-assisted closure: a new method for wound control and treatment. Clinical experience. *Ann Plast Surg* 1997; 38: 563–76.
13. Polk HC, Malignant melanoma: current perspectives with emphasis upon treatment according to prognosis. *J Ky Med Assoc* 1978; 76: 593–8.
14. Lent WM, Ariyan S, Flap reconstruction following wide local excision for primary malignant melanoma of the head and neck region. *Ann Plast Surg* 1994; 33: 23–7.
15. Chang N, Mathes SJ, Comparison of the effect of bacterial innoculation in musculocutaneous and random-pattern flaps. *Plast Reconstr Surg* 1982; 70: 1–9.
16. Menick FJ, Artistry in aesthetic surgery: aesthetic perceptions and the subunit principle. *Clin Plast Surg* 1987; 14: 723–35.
17. McGregor IA, McGregor FM, Reconstructive techniques. In: *Cancer of the face and mouth: pathology and management for surgeons.* (ed. McGregor IA), Edinburgh: Churchill Livingstone, 1986: 22.
18. Balch CM, Excising melanomas: How wide is enough? And how to reconstruct? *J Surg Oncol* 1990; 44: 135–7.
19. Hudson DA, Krige JEJ, Grobbelaar AO, et al, Melanoma of the face: the safety of narrow excision margins. *Scand J Plast Reconstr Hand Surg* 1998; 32: 97–104.
20. Balch CM, Soong S-J, Gershenwald JE, et al, Prognostic factors analysis of 17,600 melanoma patients: validation of the American Joint Committee on Cancer melanoma staging system. *J Clin Oncol* 2001; 19: 3622–34.
21. Pontikes LA, Temple WJ, Cassar SL, et al, Influence of level and depth on recurrence rate in thin melanomas. *Am J Surg* 1993; 165: 225–8.
22. Mansson-Brahme E, Carstensen J, Erhardt K, et al, Prognostic factors in thin cutaneous malignant melanoma. *Cancer* 1994; 73: 2324–32.
23. Glatt PM, Longaker MT, Jelks EB, et al, Periorbital melanocytic lesions: excision and reconstruction in 40 patients. *Plast Reconstr Surg* 1998; 102: 19–27.
24. Garner A, Koorneef L, Levene A, et al, Malignant melanoma of the eyelid skin: histopathology and behaviour. *Br J Ophthalmol* 1985; 63: 180–6.
25. Zoltie N, O'Neill TJ, Malignant melanomas of eyelid skin. *Plast Reconst Surg* 1989; 83: 994–6.
26. Gahhos FN, Cuono CB, Double-Z rhombic technique for reconstruction of facial wounds. *Plast Reconstr Surg* 1990; 85: 869–77.
27. Limberg AA, Design of local flaps. In: *Modern trends of plastic surgery.* 2nd ed. (ed. Gibson T), London: Butterworth, 1996.
28. Webster JP, Temporalis muscle transplants for defects following orbital exenteration. In: *Transactions of the first congress of the International Society of Plastic Surgeons.* Baltimore: Williams and Wilkins, 1957: 291.
29. Bogle M, Kelly P, Shenaq J, et al, The role of soft tissue reconstruction after melanoma resection in the head and neck. *Head Neck* 2001; 23: 8–15.
30. Emmett AJ, The closure of defects by using adjacent triangular flaps with subcutaneous pedicles. *Plast Reconstr Surg* 1977; 59: 45–52.
31. Al-Shunnar B, Manson PN, Cheek reconstruction with laterally based flaps. *Clin Plast Surg* 2001; 28: 283–95.
32. Gilchrest BA, Fitzpatrick TB, Anderson RR, et al, Localization of melanin pigmentation in the skin with Wood's lamp. *Br J Dermatol* 1977; 96: 245–8.
33. AH Johnson TM, Smith JW II, Nelson BR, et al, Current therapy for cutaneous melanoma. *J Am Acad Dermatol* 1995; 32: 689–707.
34. Papadopoulos T, Thompson JF, Quinn MJ, McCarthy WH, Melanoma of the lip. *Aust NZ J Surg* 1996; 66: 327–30.
35. Quinn MJ, Thompson JF, Coates AS, et al, Desmoplastic and desmoplastic neurotropic melanoma—experience with 280 patients. *Cancer* 1998; 83: 1128–35.
36. Karapandzic M, Reconstruction of lip defects by local arterial flaps. *Br J Plast Surg* 1974; 27: 93–7.
37. Tobin GR, O'Daniel TG, Lip reconstruction with motor and sensory innervated composite flaps. *Clin Plast Surg* 1990; 17: 623–32.
38. Hudson DA, Krige JEJ, Strover RM, King HS, Malignant melanoma of the external ear. *Brit J Plast Surg* 1990; 43, 608–11.
39. Byers RM, Smith JL, Russell N, Malignant melanoma of the external ear. *Am J Surg* 1980; 14: 518–21.
40. Cole BJ, MacKay GJ, Walker BF, et al, Melanoma of the external ear. *J Surg Oncol* 1992; 50: 110.
41. O'Brien CJ, Coates AS, Peterson-Schaefer K, et al, Experience with 998 cutaneous melanomas of the head and neck over 30 years. *Am J Surg* 1991; 162: 310–14.
42. Narayan D, Ariyan S, Surgical considerations in the management of malignant melanoma of the ear. *Plast Reconstr Surg* 2001; 107: 20–24.
43. Cohen BJ, Melisi J, Cohen MH, Ear preservation in the treatment of auricular melanoma. *Head Neck* 1990; 12: 346–51.
44. Wagner JD, Gordon MS, Chuang T, Coleman SS, Current therapy of cutaneous melanoma. *Plast Reconstr Surg* 2000; 105: 1744–99.
45. Manders EK, Graham WP III, Schenden MS, et al, Skin expansion to eliminate large scalp defects. *Ann Plast Surg* 1984; 12: 305–12.
46. Matton GE, Tonnard PL, Monstrey SJ, et al, A universal incision for tissue expander insertion. *Brit J Plast Surg* 1995; 48: 172–6.
47. Chao JJ, Longaker MT, Zide BM, Expanding horizons in head and neck expansion. *Oper Techn Plast Reconstr Surg* 1998; 5: 2–11.
48. Penoff J, Skin expansion: a sword that 'stretches' two ways: scalp expansion and bone erosion. *J Craniofac Surg* 1990; 1: 103–5.
49. Papadopoulos T, Rasiah K, Thompson JF, Quinn MJ, Melanoma of the nose. *Br J Surg* 1997; 84: 986–9.
50. Burget GC, Menick FJ, The subunit principle in nasal reconstruction. *Plast Reconstr Surg* 1985; 78: 145–57.
51. Menick FJ, The two stage nasolabial flap for subunit reconstruction of the ala. *Oper Techn Plastic Reconstr Surg* 1998; 5: 59–64.
52. Tardy ME, Sykes J, Kron T, The precise midline forehead flap in reconstruction of the nose. *Clin Plast Surg* 1985; 12: 481–94.
53. Eshima I, The role of plastic surgery in the treatment of malignant melanoma. *Surg Clin North Am* 1996; 76: 1331–42.

54. Menick FJ, Principles of subunit reconstruction of the forehead. *Oper Techn Plastic Reconstr Surg* 1998; 5: 13–15.
55. Hsueh EC, Lucci A, Qi K, Morton DL, Survival of patients with melanoma of the lower extremity decreases with distance from the trunk. *Cancer* 1999; 85: 383–8.
56. Fortin PT, Freiberg AA, Rees R, et al, Malignant melanoma of the foot and ankle. *J Bone Joint Surg Am* 1995; 77: 1396–403.
57. Cowles RA, Johnson TM, Chang AE, Useful techniques for the resection of foot melanomas. *J Surg Oncol* 1999; 70: 255–60.
58. Barnes BC, Seigler HF, Sarby TS, et al, Melanoma of the foot. *J Bone Joint Surg* 1994; 76: 892–8.
59. Woltering EA, Thorpe WP, Reed JK, et al, Split thickness skin grafting of the plantar surface of the foot after wide excision of neoplasms of the skin. *Surg Gynecol Obstet* 1979; 149: 229–32.
60. Morrison WA, Crabb DJM, O'Brien B McC, Jenkins A, The instep of the foot as a fasciocutaneous island and as a free flap for heel defects. *Plast Reconstr Surg* 1983; 72: 56–63.
61. Amarante J, Martins A, Reis J, A distally based median plantar flap. *Ann Plast Surg* 1988: 20: 468–70.
62. Hayes IM, Thompson JF, Quinn MJ, Malignant melanoma of the toenail apparatus. *J Am Coll Surg* 1995; 180: 583–8.
63. II Quinn MJ, Thompson JF, Crotty K, et al, Subungal melanoma of the hand. *J Hand Surg (Am)* 1996; 21: 506–11.
64. DeMatos P, Tyler DS, Seigler HF, Malignant melanoma of the mucous membranes: a review of 119 cases. *Ann Surg Oncol* 1998; 5: 733–42.
65. BX DeMatos P, Tyler DS, Seigler HF, Malignant melanoma of the mucous membranes: a review of 119 cases. *Ann Surg Oncol* 1998; 5: 733–42.
66. SJ, Guillanodegui O, Mucosal melanoma of the head and neck. *Head Neck Surg* 1991; 13: 22–37.
67. Ariel IM, Malignant melanoma of the female genital system: a report of 48 patients and review of the literature. *J Surg Oncol* 1981; 16: 125–43.
68. Brand E, Fu YS, Lagasse LD, et al, Vulvovaginal melanoma: report of seven cases and literature review. *Gynecol Oncol* 1989; 33: 54–60.
69. Wee JTK, Joseph VT, A new technique of vaginal reconstruction using neurovascular pudendal thigh flaps: a preliminary report. *Plast Reconstr Surg* 1989: 83: 701–9.
70. NN Ubrig B, Waldner M, Fallahi M, Roth S, Preputial flap for primary closure after excision of tumors on the glans penis. *Urology* 2001; 58: 274–6.
71. AE Cooper PH, Mills SE, Allens MS Jr, Malignant melanoma of the anus: report of 12 patients and analysis of 255 additional cases. *Dis Colon Rectum* 1982; 25: 693–703.
72. AF Brady MS, Kavolius JP, Quan SH, Anorectal melanoma: a 64 year experience at Memorial Sloan-Kettering Cancer Center. *Dis Colon Rectum* 1995; 38: 146–51.
73. AG Siegal B, Cohen D, Jacob ET, Surgical treatment of anorectal melanomas. *Am J Surg* 1983; 146: 336–8.

23

Elective regional lymph node dissection for melanoma

Natale Cascinelli, Filiberto Belli, William H McCarthy, Helen M Shaw

INTRODUCTION

Despite more than 30 years of debate it is still not possible to state categorically whether elective regional lymph node dissection (ERLND) is indicated for any patients with primary malignant melanoma. Although it is generally agreed that there is no case for ERLND in most patients, the two most recent controlled clinical trials (Intergroup Melanoma Surgical Trial[1] and WHO Melanoma Group Trial #14[2] have continued to show an overall non-statistically significant trend in favour of elective lymph node dissection and have identified a subgroup of patients with intermediate thickness melanomas on the trunk who do seem to have a survival advantage after ERLND.

ELECTIVE REGIONAL LYMPH NODE DISSECTION – THE CASE AGAINST

The main arguments for refraining from ERLND are:

(1) the rationale for performing ERLND is based on the assumption that melanoma metastasizes sequentially, first to regional lymph nodes and later to distant sites by haematogenous dissemination. However, there is much evidence that metastatic spread does not always traverse the regional lymph nodes. In the WHO Melanoma Program Register, only 51% of recurring cases developed their first recurrence in regional lymph nodes, whereas 22% relapsed first at a distant site, and 31% had simultaneous regional node and distant metastases;

(2) in the experience at the National Cancer Institute in Milan, all the main prognostic factors (sex, maximal tumour thickness, site of primary tumour, and ulceration) help identify patients at risk for metastases but fail to predict the site of first recurrence (nodal or distant sites);

(3) only a minority of stage I and II patients submitted to ERLND show evidence of nodal involvement on histological examination;

(4) postoperative morbidity and functional consequences, e.g. lymphoedema, cellulitis, and significant scarring, are factors to be considered in this type of surgery (Table 23.1);

(5) no effective schemes of adjuvant chemotherapy or immunotherapy are currently available for melanoma patients;[3] and

(6) there is no convincing evidence that the survival rate of ERLND patients is improved.

Much of the enthusiasm for advocating ERLND is based on retrospective studies that may have been subject to selection bias.[4–7]

The question of ERLND cannot be resolved on the basis of heterogeneous experiences at different centres around the world, and only controlled and randomized clinical trials can provide an objective answer. In the past 30 years four major randomized trials have been completed, the WHO Melanoma Group Trial #1, the Mayo Clinic Surgical Trial, the WHO Melanoma Group #14, and the Intergroup Melanoma Surgical Trial.[1,2,8–11] These are now briefly considered.

Table 23.1 *Potential complications of regional nodal dissection*

Dissection type	Types of complication
Groin dissection (a) Early complications:	• Persistent seroma*
	• Local infections
	• Skin flap necrosis
(b) Late complications:	• Limb oedema
	• Tight scar
	• Adominal wall hernia
	• Major neurological deficits
Axillary dissection	• Persistent seroma
	• Limb oedema
	• Local infections
Head and neck dissection	• Local scar
	• Major neurological deficits
	• Thoracic duct injury (left side)
	• Persistent seroma*

*More than 10 days.

WHO Melanoma Group Trial #1

This study accrued 553 patients with stage I and II primary melanomas in the distal two thirds of the limbs. Of these patients, 286 (52%) were randomized to receive wide excision of the primary melanoma followed by delayed lymph node dissection (DLND) only if regional nodes became clinically detectable, and 267 (48%) were randomized to receive wide excision plus ERLND. The two groups were matched according to the known major prognostic criteria. However, it should be noted that some currently important prognostic criteria (i.e. ulceration, thickness, and node site identified by lymphoscintigraphy) were not prospectively stratified. No differences in survival were noted between the two groups (Figure 23.1).

Because subgroups of patients may have benefited from ERLND, survival was re-evaluated according to the more recently accepted prognostic criteria: sex, tumour thickness, invasion levels, and ulceration. No significant survival differences were noted in any of these subgroups. When ERLND was re-evaluated on a specific subgroup of 185 melanoma patients with primary tumours of intermediate thickness (between 1.5 mm and 4.0 mm), the overall survival rates were practically identical (Figure 23.2). Ulceration of the melanoma, as defined by histological rather than clinical evaluation, was the only factor associated with survival, including the initial surgical treatment (wide local excision with or without ERLND), sex, age, and maximal tumour diameter.

Mayo Clinic Surgical Trial

Similar results were reported by another randomized study performed at the Mayo Clinic between 1971 and 1976. In this trial, 171 stage I and II patients were randomized to receive (a) observation, (b) ERLND, and (c) delayed lymph node dissection (DLND). The results of this study are indicated in Figure 23.3. No significant differences in survival (P=0.9 and 0.8 respectively; log rank test) were observed even with prolonged follow up.[6,11] However, this study was not stratified according to the current criteria of ulceration and nodal status determined by lymphoscintigraphy.

WHO Melanoma Program Trial #14

A further randomized evaluation of the efficacy of ERLND was conducted by the WHO Melanoma Group from 1982 to 1989, including only patients with a trunk primary lesion 1.5 mm or more in thickness. After wide excision of their primary melanoma, patients were randomized to either immediate regional node dissection or a DLND.

In this trial, ERLND did not affect overall survival rate. The 5-year survival observed in patients who had a DLND was 51.3% (95% confidence interval 41.7 to 60.1) compared with 61.7% (95% CI 52.0 to 70.1) of patients who had an immediate node dissection (P=0.09) (Figure 23.4).

Table 23.2 shows the results of multivariate analysis of survival, taking into consideration sex, Breslow thickness as a continuous variable, patient age, and type of treatment. Age had no impact on survival, Breslow thickness and sex were relevant for prognosis, and the timing of node dissection did not significantly influence survival (P=0.04).

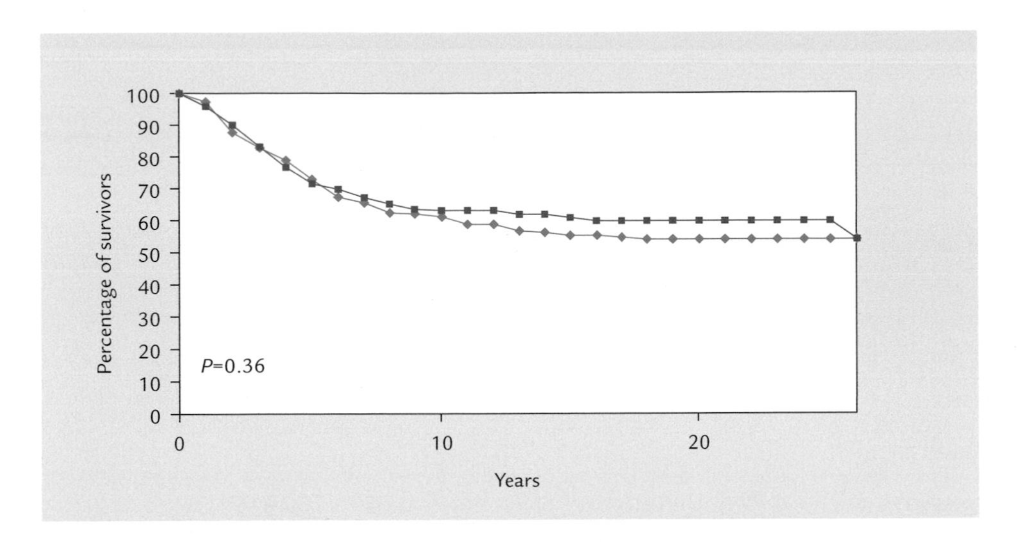

Figure 23.1 *Overall survival of 553 stage I patients, according to treatment. Diamonds depict patients who underwent wide excision followed by delayed lymph node dissection (n=286); squares denote patients who underwent wide excision plus elective lymph node dissection (n=267). Reproduced with permission from Cascinelli et al., The case for minimal margins and delayed regional node dissection for high risk cutaneous melanoma. In: Daky M (ed.),* Current opinion in general surgery *1993, Current Science, 310–15.*

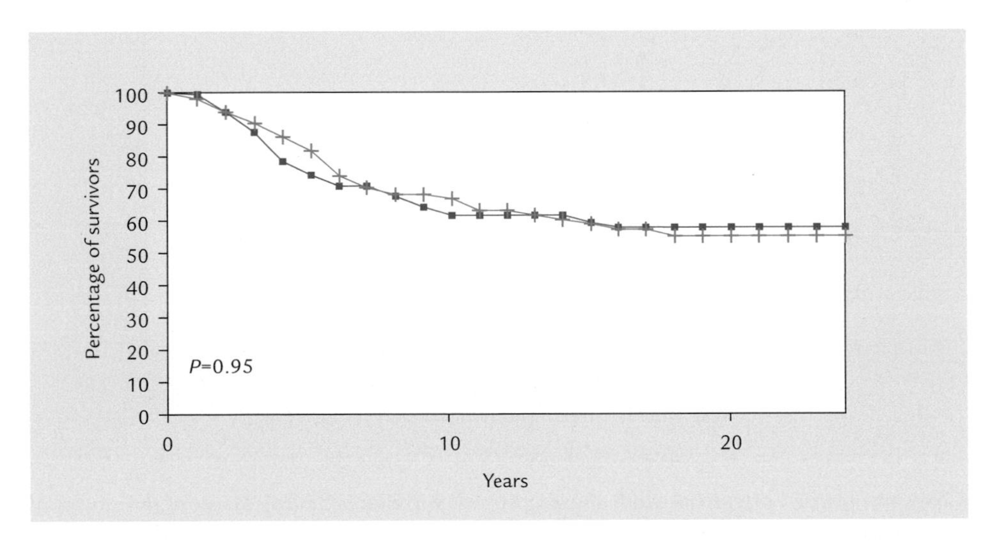

Figure 23.2 *Survival of 185 stage I patients with primary tumour 1.5 to 4 mm thick, according to treatment. Crosses indicate patients who underwent wide excision and delayed lymph node dissection (n=93); squares denote patients who underwent wide excision and elective lymph node dissection (n=92). Reproduced with permission from Cascinelli et al., The case for minimal margins and delayed regional mode dissection for high risk cutaneous melanoma. In: Daky M (ed.),* Current opinion in general surgery *1993, Current Science, 310–15.*

Despite these generally negative results, this trial is now showing one interesting feature. A recent re-analysis of this study evaluated the nodal status of entered patients. Node metastases as the first evidence of dissemination were found in 63 (26%) patients. Twenty-seven (22%) of the 122 patients who had immediate node dissection were found to have occult node metastases (N0+) and 36 (30.5%) of 118 patients who received wide excision only as primary treatment, developed regional node metastases as first recurrence of the disease (N1+) during follow up.

The important finding of this analysis according to nodal status, was that survival rates of patients who never developed node metastases (N0) when primary

Table 23.2 *Multivariate analysis of survival (Cox's model) of 240 evaluable patients: timing of dissection*

Criterion		Hazard ratio	SE	z	*P*>z	95% CI	Likelihood ratio test df	χ^2	*P*
Sex	Male patients	1							
	Female patients	0.49	0.11	−3.26	0.001	0.32 to 0.75	1	12.32	0.0004
Thickness (mm)*		1.11	0.05	2.40	0.02	1.01 to 1.20	1	4.89	0.03
Age	≤60 years	1							
	>60 years	0.92	0.23	−0.35	0.73	0.56 to 1.50	1	0.14	0.71
Wide excision (delayed group)		1							
Wide excision + elective dissection ('immediate' group)		0.72	0.13	−1.77	0.07	0.49 to 1.04	1	4.13	0.04

Log likelihood = −600.26 χ^2(4 df) = 19.71 Prob (χ^2) = 0.0006
*Considered as continuous variable.

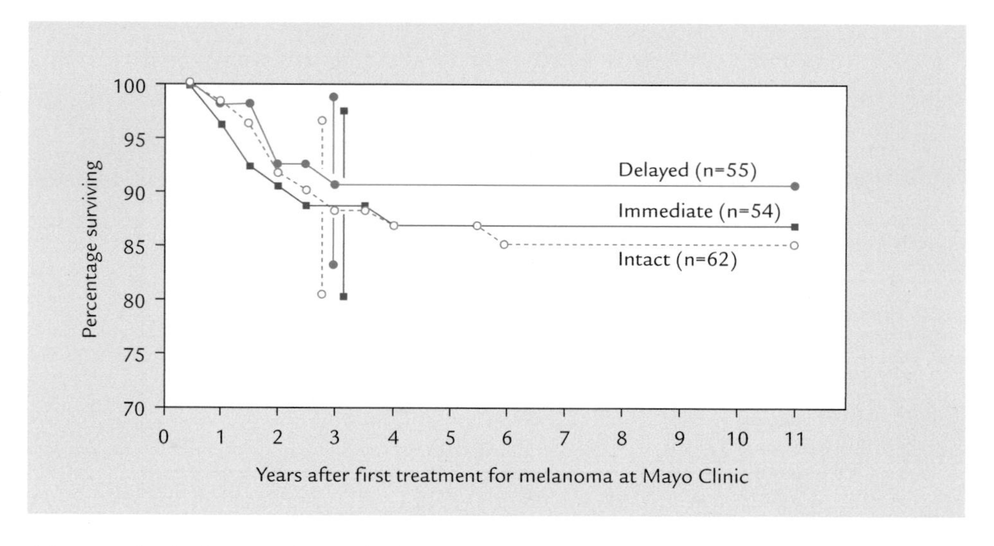

Figure 23.3 *Mayo Clinic randomized prospective study showing overall survival according to one of three surgical treatment arms: immediate lymph node dissection (n=54), elective node dissection delayed until 6 weeks after primary excision (n=55), or nodes intact (n=62). Reproduced with permission from Balch CM, Cascinelli N, Sim FH, et al., Elective lymph node dissection: results of prospective randomized surgical trials. In:* Cutaneous melanoma, *3rd edn, Balch CM, Houghton A, Sober AJ, Soong SJ, (eds), St. Louis: Quality Medical Publishing Inc., 1998, 209–25.*

treatment was wide excision only, and that of patients who were found to have no metastatic deposits in the electively dissected regional nodes (N0−), were similar (*P*=0.63). Survival of patients who were found to have occult node metastases at ERLND (N0+) and that of patients who developed regional node metastases during follow up, and who had DLND (N1), are shown in Figure 23.5. The differences between these two groups were significant (*P*=0.007).

Table 23.3 shows a multivariate analysis of survival when the status of regional nodes was taken into consideration instead of the timing of regional node dissection. Sex maintained its importance, the relevance of Breslow thickness became borderline, and the status of regional nodes had a significant impact on survival (*P*=0.007), as also reported recently by long term results from the Intergroup Melanoma Surgical Trial.[12]

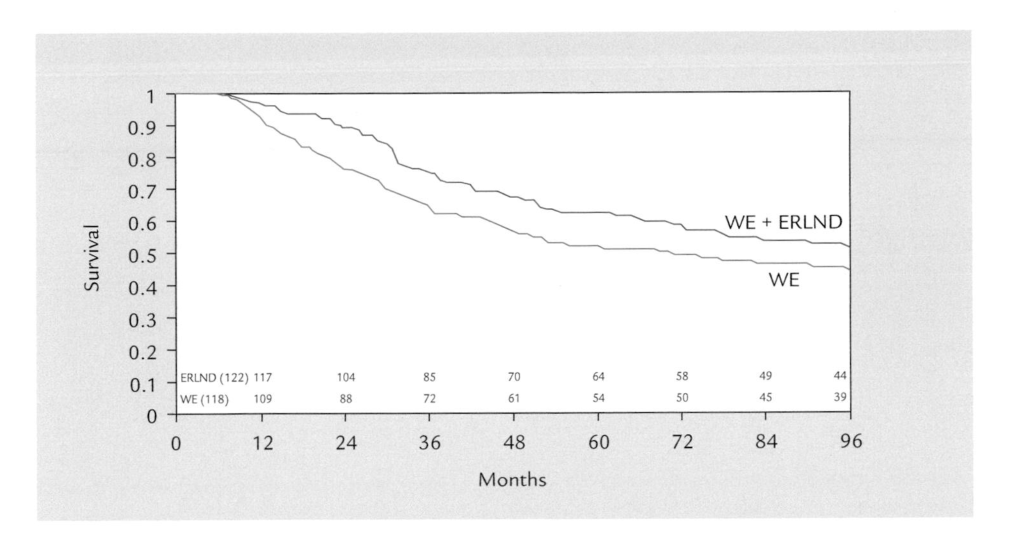

Figure 23.4 *Survival of patients with primary melanoma of trunk (1.5 mm or thicker) according to time of node dissection. ERLND, wide excision and elective regional node dissection (n=122); WE, wide excision and node dissection delayed until time of clinically detectable node metastases (n=118). Reproduced with permission from Cascinelli et al.,* Lancet *1998; 351:793–6.*

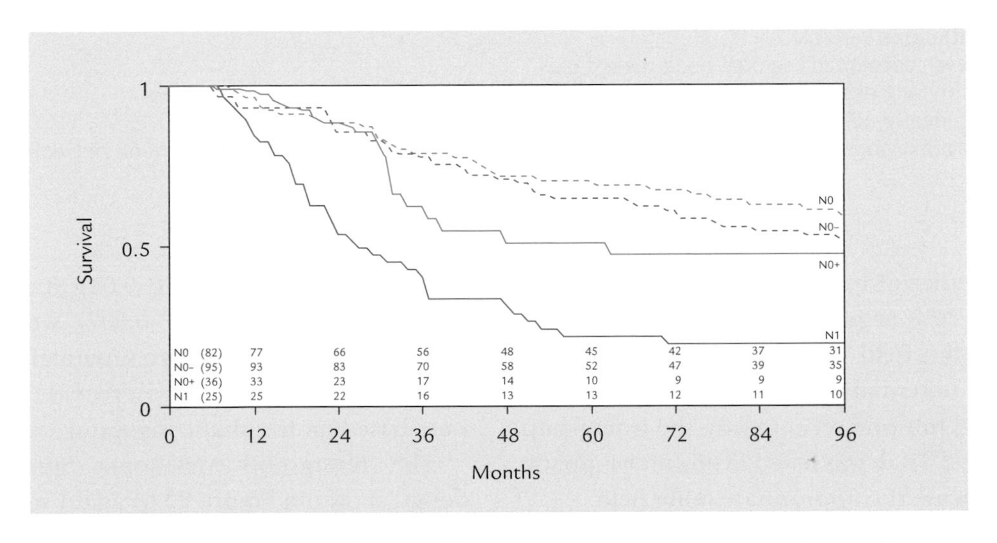

Figure 23.5 *Survival according to status of regional nodes. N0 indicates patients who never developed node metastases after wide excision of primary. N0– depicts patients with clinically negative and histologically negative nodes at elective node dissection. N0+ denotes patients with clinically negative and histologically positive nodes at elective lymph node dissection. N1 indicates patients who developed node metastases during follow up and underwent delayed regional node dissection. Reproduced with permission from Cascinelli et al.,* Lancet *1998 351:793–6.*

ELECTIVE NODE DISSECTION – THE CASE FOR

Many retrospective, non-randomized studies involving over 4000 patients have revealed significant benefits for ERLND, with 10-year survival rates as much as 40% higher for patients with intermediate thickness melanomas. The results of these studies were reviewed in 1992, when a detailed debate on the value of ERLND was published in the *World Journal of Surgery*.[13]

The case against ERLND is based largely on the four studies reviewed above. However, each of these studies has been subject to criticism on the basis of methodological issues such as sex bias, sample size, limited tumour thickness range, lack of assessment of tumour ulceration, and in particular the lack of certainty that the correct node field was dissected (because lymphatic mapping was not generally available at the time of the

Table 23.3 *Multivariate analysis of survival (Cox's model) of 240 evaluable patients: node status*

Criterion		Hazard ratio	SE	z	*P*>z	95% CI	Likelihood ratio test df	χ^2	*P*
Sex	Male patients	1							
	Female patients	0.52	0.11	−2.96	0.003	0.34 to 0.80	1	10.42	0.002
Thickness (mm)*		1.08	0.05	1.77	0.08	0.99 to 1.18	1	2.84	0.09
Age	≤60 years	1							
	>60 years	0.97	0.25	−0.12	0.91	0.59 to 1.59	1	0.03	0.87
N0 (1)		1							
N0− (2)		0.85	0.19	−0.69	0.49	0.54 to 1.34			
N0+ (3)		1.25	0.39	0.71	0.47	0.67 to 2.34	3	12.16	0.007
N1 (4)		2.11	0.56	2.8	0.005	1.25 to 3.57			

Log likelihood = −559.46 χ^2(6 df) = 27.74 Prob (χ^2) = 0.0001
*Considered as continuous variable.
(1) Patients who never developed regional node metastases.
(2) Patients with clinically negative and histologically negative nodes at elective node dissection.
(3) Patients with clinically negative and histologically positive nodes at elective node dissection.
(4) Patients who develop node metastases during follow up and submitted to delayed regional node dissection.

trials). Recent studies of lymphatic pathways have indicated that up to 20% of patients may have had an inappropriate node field dissection when clinical assessment of the potential spread was used to select the dissection field.[14] Only one recent study, the Intergroup Melanoma Surgical Trial, was based firmly on lymphatic mapping to delineate the appropriate node field.

In the WHO Melanoma Group Trial #14, the overall 5-year survival of patients with DLND was 51.3%, compared with 61.7% for those with immediate node dissection. This difference was not statistically significant. However, multifactoral analysis did show a significant benefit for immediate dissection (*P*=0.04). When patients with occult nodal metastases were compared with those developing nodal metastases later, the benefit was statistically significant, confirming that the occult group, if identified, does benefit from early dissection.

The first analysis of WHO Melanoma Group Trial #14 suggested a possible benefit of ERLND for trunk melanoma. That trial was continued to allow a greater entry of patients with truncal melanoma. Overall analysis of the trial showed a 10% advantage for ERLND, but multifactoral analysis revealed a significant advantage for immediate dissection (*P*=0.04) (Table 23.2) and also a significant outcome (*P*=0.007) when patients with occult node metastasis were separately analyzed (Table 23.3). However, only the most recent data from this trial were based on lymphatic mapping.

The Intergroup Melanoma Surgical Trial (trial design shown in Figure 23.6) again suggested a benefit for ERLND for a selected patient group. The trial was based on lymphatic mapping. Although there was no difference in overall 5-year survival between patients whose initial treatment was ERLND (n=379) and those whose lymph nodes were observed (n=361) (Figure 23.7), significant differences were shown between subgroups. The most interesting differences were observed in patients subgrouped as 60 years of age and younger versus older than 60 years. Overall 5-year survival rates of 552 patients under 60 years of age (which was 75% of the total patients) were better with ERLND compared with observation, at 88% versus 81% (*P*=0.04) respectively (Figure 23.8). Patients older than 60 years (n=188) had a lower 5-year survival rate when the treatment was ERLND, being 74% versus 86% (Figure 23.9) for those patients whose lymph nodes were observed.

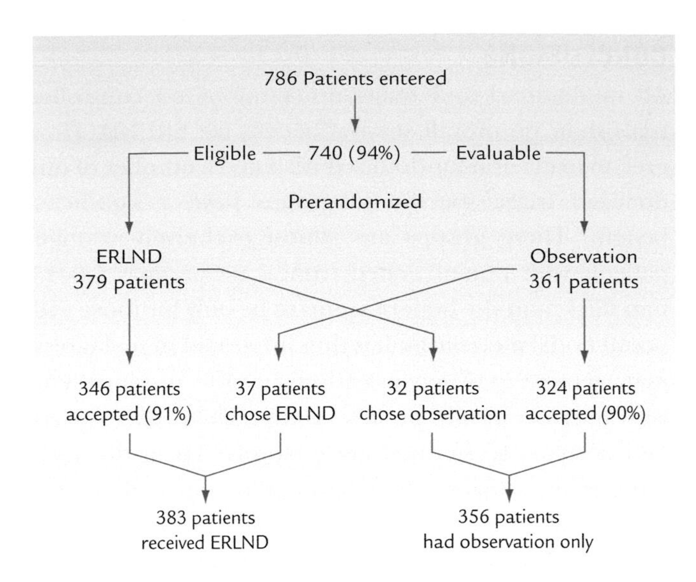

Figure 23.6 *Intergroup Melanoma Surgical Trial.*

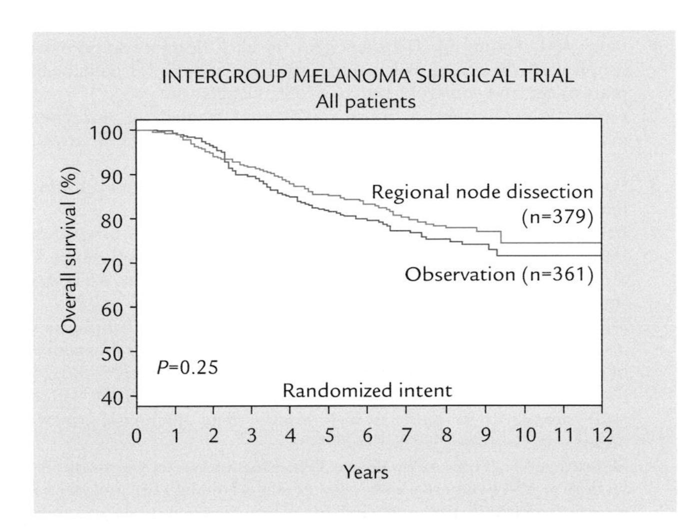

Figure 23.7 *Survival rates for patients undergoing ERLND versus observation. There was no difference in overall survival based on randomized intent or actual treatment received (data not shown). Taken from Balch CM, Cascinelli N, Sim FH, et al. Elective lymph node dissection: results of prospective randomized surgical trials. In: Cutaneous Melanoma 3rd edn (eds Balch CM, Houghton A, Sober AJ, Soong SJ). St Louis: Quality Medical Publishing Inc, 1998: 209–25.*

The patients 60 years of age or younger were further analyzed by subgroups according to tumour thickness and ulceration. In the 403 patients without tumour ulceration, there was a significant increase in 5-year survival when ERLND was performed (95% versus 84% (P=0.01)). In the 284 younger patients with melanomas 1–2 mm thick and no tumour ulceration, there was also an improved 5-year survival rate for ERLND (97% versus 87% (P=0.005)). It is not clear from the literature if the benefits of ERLND, shown by this study, have been

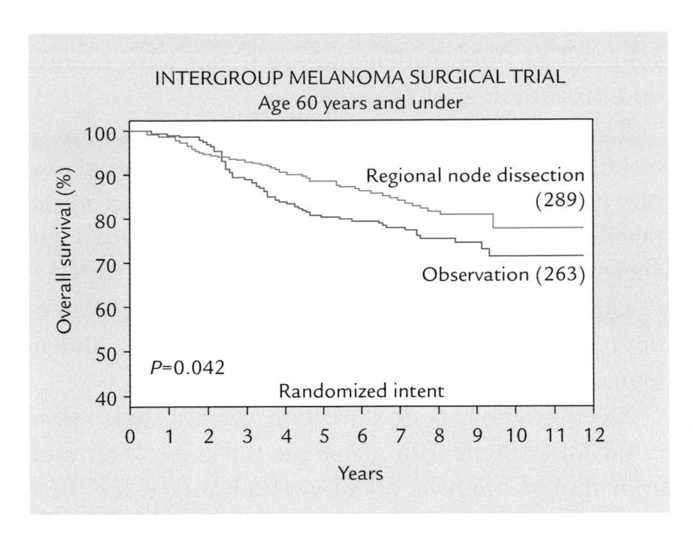

Figure 23.8 *Survival rates by age group based on randomized intent. Patients 60 years of age and younger had higher overall survival rates if they underwent a regional node dissection. Taken from Balch CM, Cascinelli N, Sim FH, et al. Elective lymph node dissection: results of prospective randomized surgical trials. In: Cutaneous Melanoma 3rd edn (eds Balch CM, Houghton A, Sober AJ, Soong SJ). St Louis: Quality Medical Publishing Inc, 1998: 209–25.*

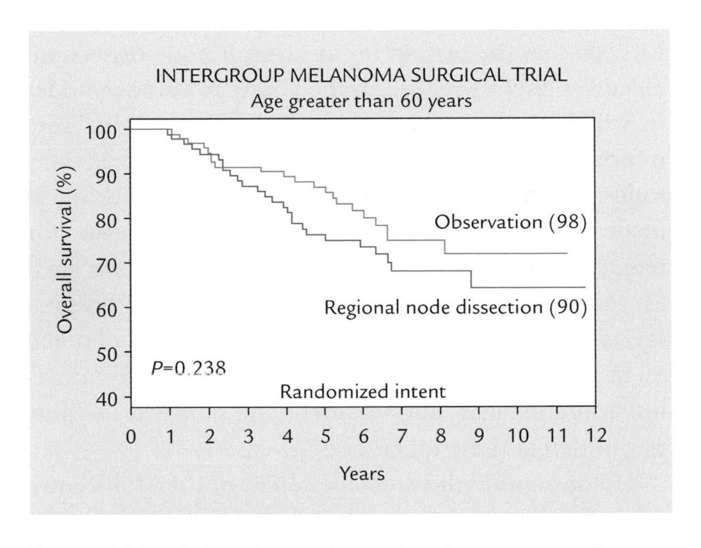

Figure 23.9 *No benefit was observed in the group of patients over 60 years of age receiving a regional node dissection. Taken from Balch CM, Cascinelli N, Sim FH, et al. Elective lymph node dissection: results of prospective randomized surgical trials. In: Cutaneous Melanoma 3rd edn (eds Balch CM, Houghton A, Sober AJ, Soong SJ). St Louis: Quality Medical Publishing Inc, 1998: 209–25.*

confined to those patients whose nodes were positive on histopathological examination.

The degree of lymph node involvement is known to be important in predicting survival. The number of positive lymph nodes has a high degree of relevance to the possibility of survival, as confirmed by a recent large analysis.[15] The number of involved nodes in ERLND is usually one, while therapeutic dissection specimens often contain more than one involved node, and in many cases three or more involved nodes.

Elective lymph node dissection has also been advocated for patients with a tumour thickness >4.0 mm, even though there is no survival advantage for these patients. It is recommended as a form of 'anticipatory palliative surgery', since over 50% of these patients will develop positive nodes during their follow up programme. The operation is thus performed to complete the treatment of the primary lesion and the nodal metastases at one operation. Additionally, ERLND in this group may be of value to detect those patients with positive nodes who can be entered into adjuvant therapy protocols.

Thus it is essentially agreed by the proponents of ERLND that the benefit for any lymph node dissection, elective or selective, lies in the ability to remove nodes in which the tumour burden is microscopic or very minor. With the advent of the selective lymphadenectomy technique, early identification of subclinical involvement of lymph nodes without the necessity for major nodal surgery with concomitant problems such as lymphoedema, infection, and prolonged hospital stay is now possible. Non-surgical identification of nodal metastatic disease may become possible in the future, but at the present time sentinel node biopsy is the only way to detect these metastases.

However, until the outcome report of the Multicenter Selective Lymphadenectomy Trial is available, it is not possible to state whether there is any survival benefit or if there are any negative outcomes after selective lymphadenectomy. It is possible that selective lymphadenectomy may be associated with a higher risk of recurrence in the dissected field because of lymphatic leakage, and that the small group of patients in whom the sentinel node was incorrectly identified, or not removed, may fare worse than patients who had a dissection. Additionally, because of the sentinel node biopsy, delays in diagnosis due to incorrect interpretation of post-biopsy masses in the node field may occur.

CONCLUSIONS

All randomized and many non-randomized controlled trials show no overall survival benefit for ERLND. However, in many non-randomized trials and a number of randomized trials, specific subgroups have a significant benefit. These groups are almost exclusively younger patients with non-ulcerated truncal melanomas 1.0–4.0 mm thick, and the benefit seems to be only for those with occult nodal metastases. It is thus important in melanoma management to dissect as early as possible those patients with microscopically positive nodes. These patients are best detected by sentinel node biopsy,[14] but if this technique is not available, the subgroups identified above may be considered for ERLND or managed by careful follow up and evaluation of the lymph nodes on a regular basis by clinical examination and ultrasonography.

REFERENCES

1. Balch CM, Soong S-J, Bartolucci AA, et al, Efficacy of an elective lymph node dissection of 1 to 4 mm thick melanomas for patients 60 years of age and younger. *Ann Surg* 1996; 224:255–66.
2. Cascinelli N, Morabito A, Santinami M, et al, Immediate or delayed dissection of regional nodes in patients with melanoma of the trunk: a randomised trial. *Lancet* 1998; 351:793–6.
3. Coates AS, Systemic chemotherapy for malignant melanoma. *World J Surg* 1992; 16:277–81.
4. Balch CM, Soong SJ, Milton GW, et al, A comparison of prognostic factors and surgical results in 1786 patients with localized (stage I) melanoma treated in Alabama, USA and New South Wales, Australia. *Ann Surg* 1982; 196:677–84.
5. Milton GW, Shaw HM, McCarthy WH, et al, Prophylactic lymph node dissection in clinical stage I cutaneous malignant melanoma: results of surgical treatment in 1319 patients. *Br J Surg* 1982; 69:108–11.
6. Reintgen DS, Cox EB, McCarty KS, et al, Efficacy of elective lymph node dissection in patients with intermediate thickness primary melanoma. *Ann Surg* 1983; 198:379–83.
7. McCarthy WH, Shaw HM, Milton GW, Efficacy of elective node dissection in 2347 patients with clinical stage I malignant melanoma. *Surg Gynecol Obstetr* 1985; 161:575–80.
8. Veronesi V, Adamus J, Bandiera DC, et al, Inefficacy of immediate node dissection in stage I melanoma of the limbs. *New Engl J Med* 1977; 297:627–30.
9. Veronesi V, Adamus J, Bandiera DC, et al, Delayed regional lymph node dissection in stage I melanoma of the skin of the lower extremities. *Cancer* 1982; 49:2420–30.
10. Sim FH, Taylor WF, Ivins JC, et al, A prospective randomised study of the efficacy of routine elective lymphadenectomy in management of malignant melanoma. *Cancer* 1978; 41:948–56.
11. Sim FH, Taylor WF, Ivins JC, et al, Lymphadenectomy in the management of stage I malignant melanoma: a prospective randomized study. *Mayo Clin Proc* 1986; 61:697–705.
12. Balch CM, Soong S-J, Ross MI, et al, Long-term results of a multi-institutional randomized trial comparing prognostic factors and surgical results for intermediate thickness melanomas (1.0 to 4.0 mm). *Ann Surg Oncol* 2000; 7:87–97.
13. McCarthy WH, Shaw HM, Cascinelli N, Santinami M, Elective lymph node dissection for melanoma: two perspectives. *World J Surg* 1992; 16:203–13.
14. Thompson JF, Uren RF, Shaw HM, et al, Location of sentinel nodes in patients with cutaneous melanoma: new insights into lymphatic anatomy. *J Am Coll Surg* 1999; 189:195–206.
15. Balch CM, Buzaid AC, Atkins MB, et al, A new American Joint Committee on Cancer Staging System for cutaneous melanoma. *Cancer* 2000; 88:1484–91.

24

Therapeutic axillary lymph node dissection for metastatic melanoma

David W Ollila, William H McCarthy, Erin A Felger

INTRODUCTION

The management of the regional lymphatic basin in patients with cutaneous melanoma and no palpable lymphadenopathy has long been a controversial topic. Several non-randomized trials suggested an improved survival for patients undergoing elective complete lymph node dissection (ELND) of the regional node basin at greatest risk for metastatic disease.[1,2] However, no prospective randomized trial has shown an overall survival benefit for those patients undergoing routine ELND (see Chapter 23).[3–6]

With the emergence of sentinel node technology and no randomized trial data supporting the use of routine ELND, melanoma patients can be staged histopathologically using lymphatic mapping and selective lymphadenectomy, and spared the morbidity associated with ELND. Patients whose sentinel nodes are tumour-free require no additional lymph node dissection. For patients whose sentinel nodes contain metastatic melanoma, however, a complete regional lymph node dissection is necessary. This then becomes a therapeutic lymph node dissection.

For patients who present with palpable lymphadenopathy, metastatic disease is best confirmed by fine needle aspiration cytology. Confirmation by needle biopsy in this way minimizes the risk of tumour cell spillage and the disruption of tissue planes which occurs with open surgical biopsy. Sometimes this procedure is non-diagnostic and an incisional or excisional lymph node biopsy is required. However, no comparison of the two biopsy techniques has shown any difference in survival rates.[7]

ANAESTHESIA

There are several anaesthetic options for patients undergoing axillary lymph node dissection, but general anaesthesia is the standard method. An alternative option for patients who wish to avoid general anaesthesia is a paravertebral block combined with intravenous sedation, usually a benzodiazepine and a narcotic.[8,9] A good paravertebral block can achieve up to 23 hours of analgesia in the axillary region, allowing the surgeon sufficient time to perform the axillary dissection and also providing more effective acute pain control.[8,10] Although patients avoid the side effects associated with general anaesthesia, there are potential complications associated with a paravertebral block. Intermittent hypotension occurs in 4% of patients, pleural puncture occurs in 1%, and a pneumothorax develops in 0.5%. These pneumothoraces have been successfully managed without tube thoracostomy.[10,11]

Regional anaesthesia combined with intravenous sedation is possible but not recommended.[8,9] Local anaesthetic in conjunction with intravenous sedation is rarely used because it is very difficult to adequately anaesthetize the axilla with local infiltration of anaesthetic.[12]

ANTIBIOTICS

Perioperative antibiotic treatment has been a source of controversy in many surgical fields, and the arguments apply to axillary lymph node dissection as well. Platt's meta-analysis of perioperative antibiotic studies concluded that antibiotic prophylaxis significantly decreased the risk of postoperative wound infection.[13] A first generation cephalosporin was used in 86% of the cases studied, with a 38% reduction in the incidence of wound infections.[13]

TECHNIQUES OF AXILLARY LYMPH NODE DISSECTION

Descriptions of two techniques of axillary dissection follow. Considerable differences are apparent in the Sydney Melanoma Unit and the John Wayne Cancer Center techniques.

The Sydney Melanoma Unit technique

The general principles for performing an axillary dissection pertain to all other node dissections and to cancer surgery in general. The objective of node dissection is the complete removal of all lymph nodes in the field without lymph leakage or tumour spillage during the procedure. In the axilla this involves removal of all lymph nodes and lymphatic vessels from the edge of the subclavius tendon superiorly to the insertion of the nerve to latissimus dorsi inferiorly. It includes the nodes and lymphatics anterior, superior, inferior, and posterior to the axillary vessels, the central axillary nodes in the main axillary compartment between pectoralis major and latissimus dorsi, the interpectoral nodes between pectoralis major and minor, the anterior (pectoral) nodes along the lateral edge of pectoralis major, and the posterior nodes accompanying the subscapular neurovascular bundle, including an important node in the tissue immediately adjacent and lateral to the origin of the subscapular leash from the axillary vessels. It is important to note that the axillary node field is completely encompassed by a fascial sheath, thus the nodes and associated lymphatics can be removed without lymphatic leak, dividing lymphatic channels only at the apex and the base of the axilla.

The axillary dissection technique described here was developed after demonstration of the axillary lymphatics with blue dye to determine that the procedure could be performed without leakage of blue stained lymph into the field during the dissection. The key principle of this dissection is 'in-continuity' removal of the lymph nodes and lymphatics within their fascial sheath after ligation of the lymphatics at the apex of the axilla. The second general cancer surgery principle is the 'distal to proximal' approach, starting with the division of the lymphatics and fascial tissue as far away as possible from the involved nodes, i.e. commencing at the apex of the axilla.

The important technical aspects of the dissection include sharp dissection with knife or diathermy (rather than with scissors), careful haemostasis, particularly along the axillary vein, avoidance of damage to the nerves to serratus anterior (long thoracic nerve of Bell) and latissimus dorsi (thoracodorsal nerve), and removal of the pectoralis minor in-continuity with the dissection specimen to ensure removal of nodes between the pectoral muscles (the interpectoral or Rotter's nodes) and the nodes immediately behind the upper third of the pectoralis minor.

When bulky disease is present in the axilla, it is imperative that wide exposure is achieved by appropriately placed incisions and, where necessary, division of the pectoralis major near its insertion into the humerus, to ensure easy access to the apical nodes. Excessive traction or pressure on bulky involved nodes is likely to lead to rupture of these nodes and spillage of tumour cells into the operative field.

At the Sydney Melanoma Unit, a 'T'-shaped incision in the axilla is often used (Figure 24.1), commencing over the front of the pectoralis major and extending back to the anterior edge of the latissimus dorsi. The

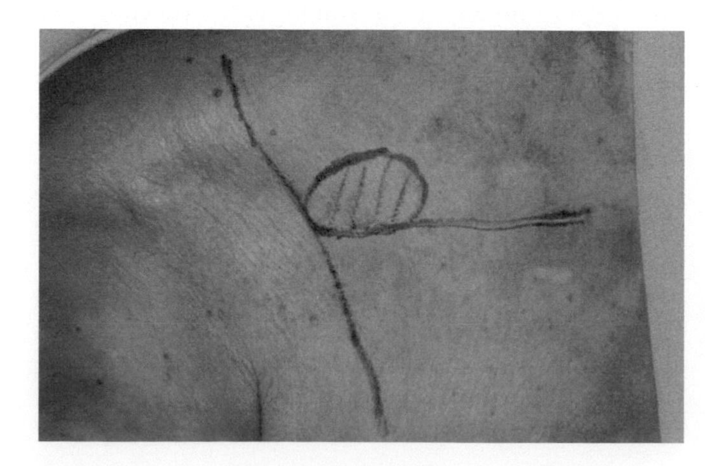

Figure 24.1 *The T incision – Sydney Melanoma Unit.*

vertical arm of the 'T' runs down behind the lateral edge of the pectoralis major. In this way 'barn door' exposure (Figure 24.2) can be achieved by elevation of the three flaps, completely exposing the axillary contents before the actual dissection commences. It is important to note that there is sometimes a superficial node in the central fat of the axilla, and thus it is important that these flaps do not include this very superficial node. However, very thin flaps are not necessary, and the thickness of the flap will necessarily reflect the amount of fat in the axilla. The flaps begin very superficially in the fat along the line of excision and then thicken as the latissimus dorsi and pectoralis major are approached. In this way the blood supply to the flaps is not compromised, and there should be no problems with healing of this wound.

With the axilla fully opened, dissection starts along the front of the pectoralis major 2–3 cm above its edge (Figure 24.3). The pectoral fascia is reflected downwards from the muscle surface and carried down over the edge of the muscle, immediately enclosing the axillary nodes within the pectoral fascia. The dissection then proceeds upwards and medially under the muscle, across the anterior surface of the pectoralis minor to the acromiothoracic vessels and superomedially to the fascia overlying the brachial plexus (Figure 24.4).

At this stage the fat and fascia lateral to the pectoralis minor muscle is gently divided at the coracoid process and swept downwards to allow visualization of the lateral edge of the pectoralis minor. It is helpful at this point to elevate the arm and move it medially to remove tension from the pectoralis major and minor, allowing easy access to the origin of the pectoralis minor from the coracoid process.

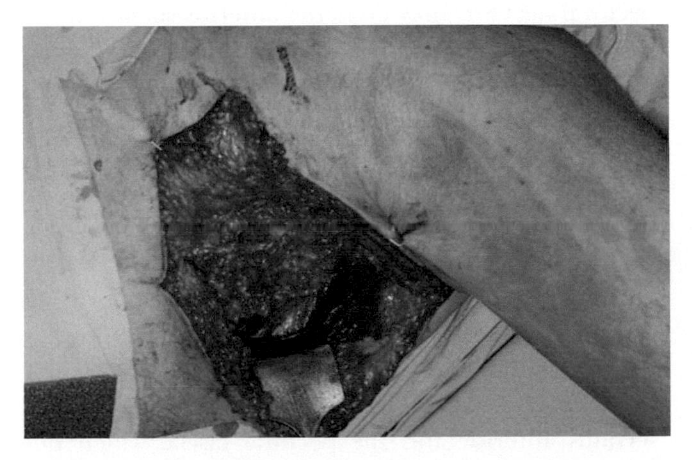

Figure 24.2 *The operative field after elevation of the flaps. The flaps are stapled to the chest wall to maintain exposure during the dissection.*

With both edges of the pectoralis minor insertion now visible, the fascia of the medial edge of the muscle is opened and a finger is inserted under the pectoralis minor to free it from the underlying vessels (Figure 24.5), retaining the underlying nodes within the fascial sheath already delineated by the operation. With a finger behind the pectoralis minor, the insertion is divided with diathermy, to allow the muscle to retract downwards and medially, completely exposing the axillary vein and its tributaries still behind the fascial layer (Figure 24.6). The medial edge of the pectoralis minor is gently dissected free of its underlying fascia, and the muscle is then divided close to its attachment to the chest wall, allowing the whole muscle bulk to remain within the fascial sheath (Figure 24.7). Very lit-

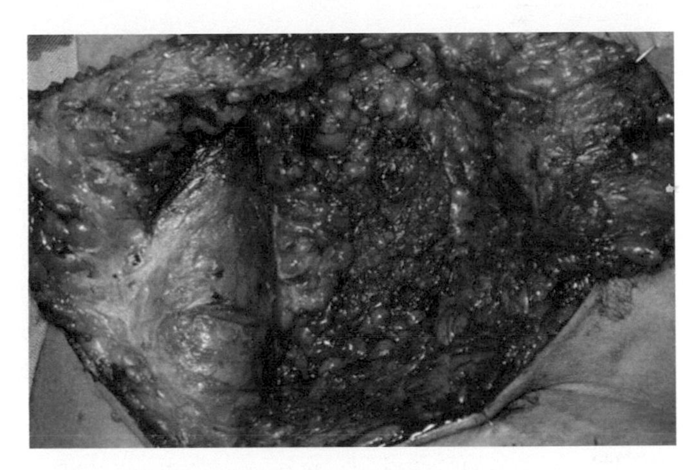

Figure 24.3 *The pectoral fascia is dissected off the pectoralis major edge to retain the nodes in a fascial compartment.*

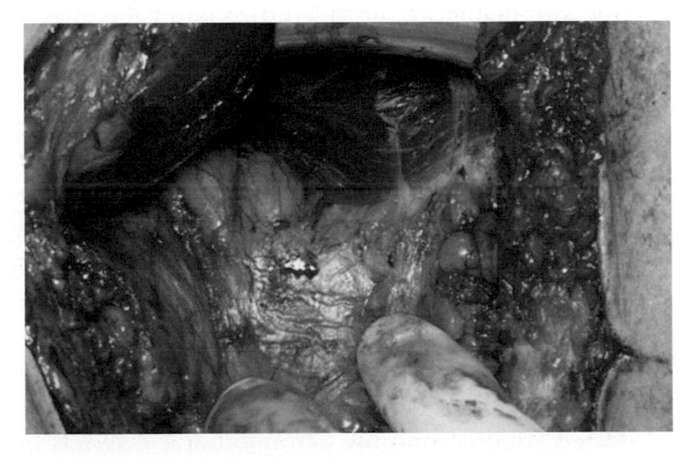

Figure 24.4 *Pectoral fascia dissected from under the surface of pectoral muscles maintaining the closed fascial compartment.*

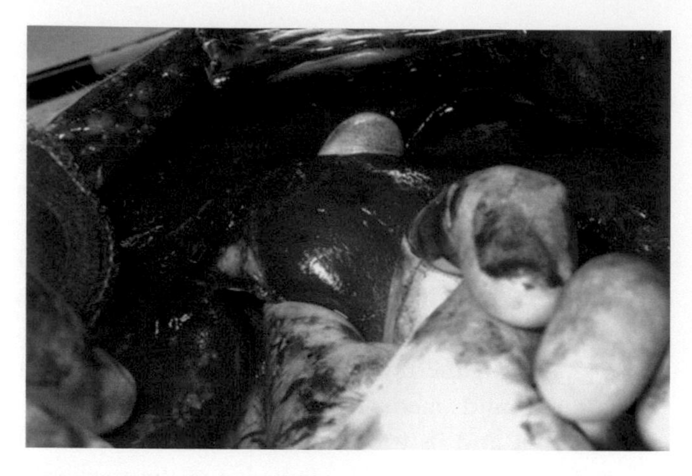

Figure 24.5 *A finger is placed under the pectoralis minor to protect the vessels and the fascial compartment while the muscle is divided.*

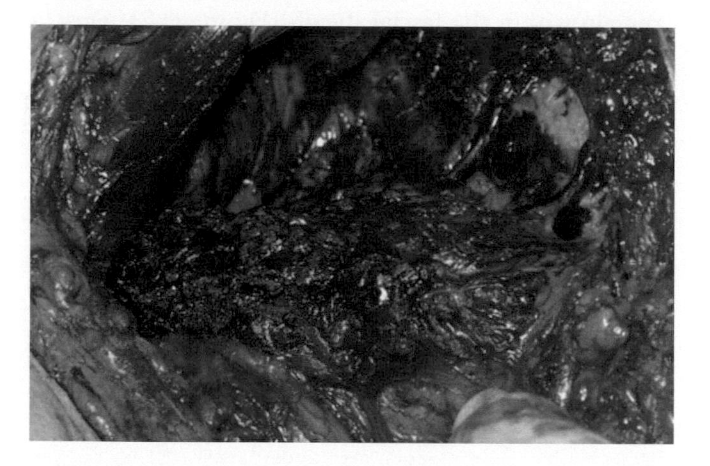

Figure 24.6 *Pectoralis minor has retracted to show underlying tissues.*

tle bleeding eventuates from division of the pectoralis minor with diathermy, provided division of the muscle is undertaken carefully so as not to break through the underlying layer of fascia over the serratus anterior, behind which are small vessels which will bleed if the fascia is penetrated. However, simple diathermy of these bleeding vessels quickly restores a bloodless field. The entire axilla is now exposed, with all the nodes and lymphatics protected by an unbroken layer of pectoral fascia. The fascia overlying the brachial plexus is then gently divided with the scalpel, to allow the fascia to be swept down over the front of the axillary vessels, reaching the acromiothoracic vessels medially. The fascia is dissected from around the acromiothoracic vessels to the lower edge of the subclavius muscle.

It is now important to gain proximal control of the

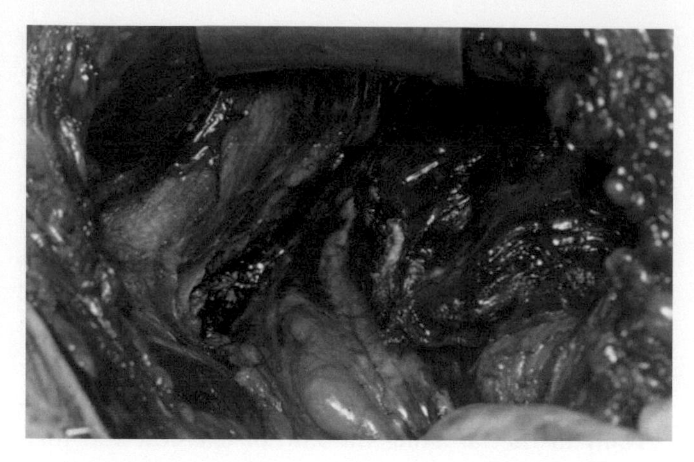

Figure 24.7 *Pectoralis minor is divided at its origin to become part of the operation specimen.*

lymphatics. This is done by dividing the fascial layer on each side of the apical lymphatic channels, close to the subclavius muscle (Figure 24.8), and with right angled forceps, encircling the apical channels, still enclosed in fascia, with two ligatures, the upper one immediately adjacent to the subclavius and the other 1 cm further distally. The apical lymphatics are then divided between the ligatures with diathermy, thus ensuring enclosure of the lymphatics and vessels within the fascial sheath already developed, and achieving proximal control of lymph leakage (Figure 24.9). The proximal ligature is left long to enable the pathologist to identify the apex of the axillary lymphatic leash.

Gentle dissection along the inferior border of the axillary vein is now performed, ligating veins in-continuity and dividing the two branches of the medial pectoral nerve as they cross the anterior surface of the axillary vein (Figure 24.10). As the vessel ligation proceeds laterally, the subscapular vessels will be reached but not ligated. It is important to dissect to the edge of the latissimus dorsi to ensure that an important node, lying laterally in the junction of the subscapular vein and the axillary vein, is included in the dissection (Figure 24.11).

At this stage, dissection along the axillary vein is interrupted to allow dissection medially down the chest wall to identify and preserve the nerve to the serratus anterior. A plane exists between the fascia over the serratus anterior and the pectoral fascia, which now encircles the lymphatics and lymph nodes of the specimen. The divided pectoralis minor and the fascial compartment is gently pulled laterally, and dissection

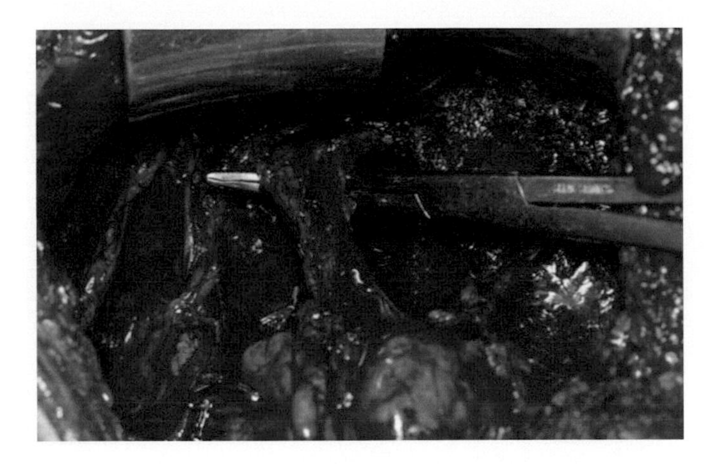

Figure 24.8 *The apical channels have been cleared for division.*

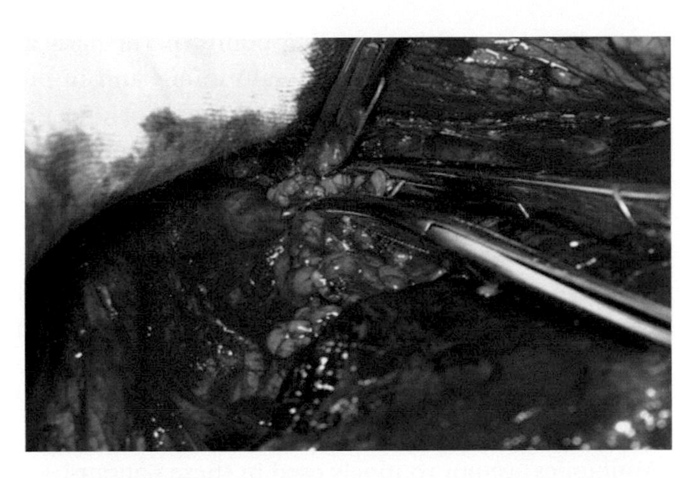

Figure 24.9 *The apical channels are divided between ligatures to prevent lymph leakage.*

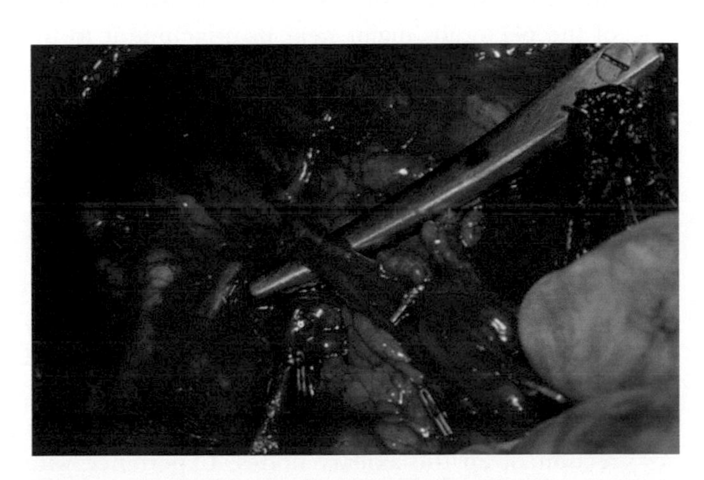

Figure 24.10 *The medial pectoral nerve is divided as it crosses the axillary vein.*

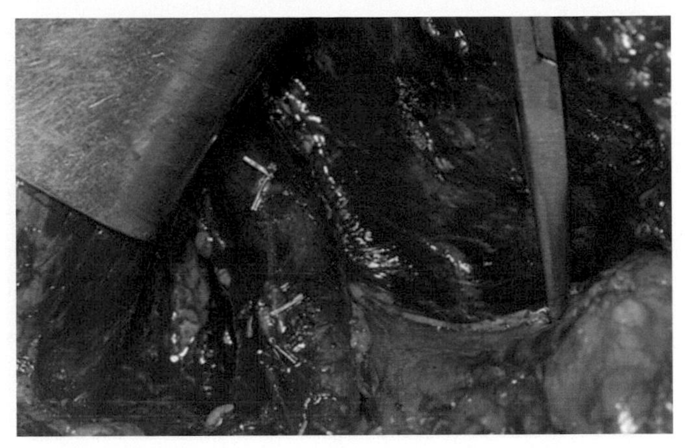

Figure 24.11 *The often important node between the axillary vein and thoracodorsal nerve is identified.*

down the chest wall will display the nerve to serratus anterior (Figure 24.12). It is important to remember that the nerve may be pulled laterally with the fascial sheath and dissection can progress behind the nerve unless it is carefully approached and identified. A scalpel incision along the lateral side of the nerve will allow a finger to be inserted between the nerve and the main specimen. The nerve and its fascia can now be swept medially by moving a finger along the lateral side of the nerve.

Having identified and preserved the nerve to serratus anterior, the operator returns to the dissection along the axillary vein. The objective now is to identify the nerve to latissimus dorsi, which is easily found in the fascia between the axillary vein and the subscapular vessels (Figure 24.10). Gentle dissection in this area will identify the nerve running obliquely across this fascia forming a triangle between the axillary vein and the subscapular vessels (Figure 24.13). Having identified the nerve to latissimus dorsi, the next step is to remove the fascia and possible lymphatics in the tissue between the two nerves. With gentle upward retraction of the axillary vein, the apex of the triangle between the two nerves is dissected downwards and laterally, bringing this tissue into continuity with the main specimen. By gentle knife or diathermy dissection along the chest wall, the fascial compartment containing all the lymphatics and nodes can be swept laterally across the front of the subscapular vessels and the nerve to latissimus dorsi, because of the embryological plane between the subscapular vessels and the pectoral fascia. Some small vessels running laterally from the subscapular vein will

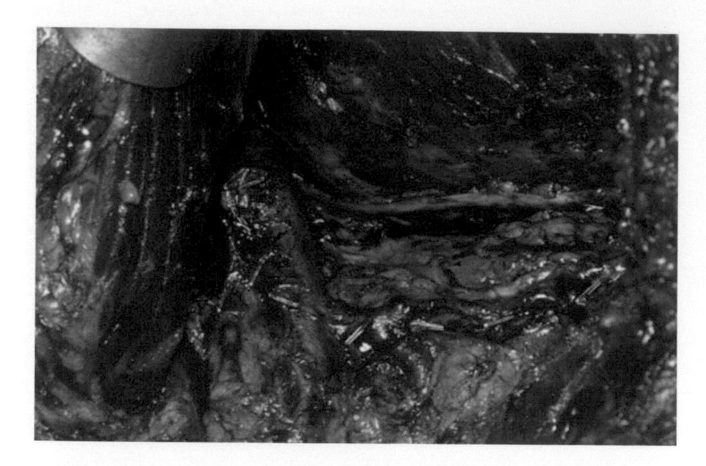

Figure 24.12 *The long thoracic nerve is identified and dissected free from the pectoral fascia.*

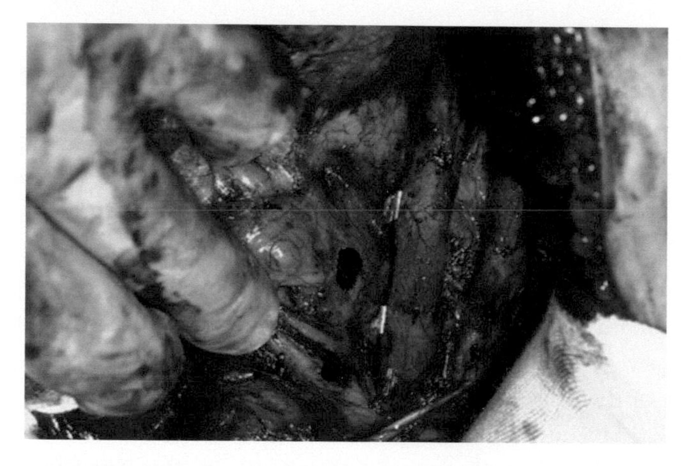

Figure 24.13 *The subscapular leash with the thoracodorsal nerve is cleared of its fascial sheath.*

need to be tied off and divided as the specimen is swept downwards and laterally.

Before completing the sweep across the front of the subscapular leash, the operator moves back to the axillary vein and clears the tissue lateral to the subscapular vessels and below the axillary vein, thus incorporating into the dissection specimen a single lymph node which is usually present in this triangular space (Figure 24.11). This node, with its fascia, is dissected downwards to include it in the main specimen, which is being swept across the front of the subscapular vessels. The dissection is completed by carrying all of the tissue downwards and laterally to the insertion of the nerve to latissimus dorsi. The base of the specimen is divided between ligatures to allow complete removal of all lymphatics and lymph nodes of the axilla, still contained within a fascial sheath (Figure 24.14).

After the specimen has been removed, the axilla is

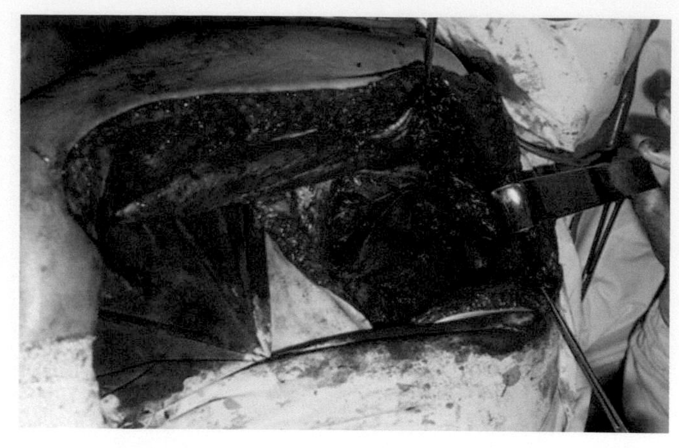

Figure 24.14 *The completed dissection – in this patient pectoralis major muscle has been divided and retracted for more complete exposure.*

carefully inspected for bleeding points, particularly at the site of division of the pectoralis minor and in the space between the nerve to serratus anterior and the nerve to latissimus dorsi. At the Sydney Melanoma Unit the operation is completed with a cytotoxic washout using three solutions sequentially – cetrimide, hydrogen peroxide, and saline. One or two suction drains are placed in the axilla by trocar insertion through normal skin below one of the vertical access incisions and secured with appropriate sutures. The wounds are closed in two layers, using an absorbable suture for the subcutaneous layers and staples for the skin closure. Antibiotics are not routinely used in these patients.

Notes

(1) When the axillary nodes are bulky and heavily involved with tumour, division of the sternal head of the pectoralis major near its attachment to the humerus will allow better vision and thus easier dissection of the entire field without undue retraction or pulling of the affected nodes, which may cause rupture and tumour cell spillage. The muscle is repaired at the close of the dissection and usually heals well, with no significant deficit.

(2) At the Sydney Melanoma Unit a dissection lateral to and below the pectoralis minor, which is commonly performed for breast surgery, (i.e. a level I and II dissection), is not recommended for melanoma. Removal of the pectoralis minor allows a full dissection of all the axillary nodes. Experience with recurrent melanoma in the axilla has indicated that the nodes most commonly found are in three

areas: near the apex of the axilla, behind the pectoralis minor near its insertion, and immediately lateral to the junction of the axillary and subscapular vessels.

The John Wayne Cancer Center technique

The preferred incision for an ELND is a 'modified U' incision. The apex of the U is just inferior to the hair bearing region of the axilla, with a curvilinear medial extension towards the lateral border of the pectoralis muscle and lateral extension towards the lateral border of latissimus dorsi (Figure 24.15). In most patients, this incision gives excellent exposure to all three levels of the axilla and a very good cosmetic result. While the 'modified U' is our preferred incision, the surgeon must be prepared to use other options depending on the location of any previous sentinel node surgery incisions. Other alternatives are a transverse incision made just inferior to the hair bearing region of the axilla extending onto the lateral border of pectoralis major and the lateral border of the latissimus dorsi muscle. We find that this incision provides similar exposure to the 'modified U', but because of the extension onto the skin over pectoralis it is cosmetically inferior. Another alternative is the 'lazy S' incision (Figure 24.16); it is made with a longitudinal incision along the lateral border of pectoralis major turning posterior with a transverse extension across the inferior hair bearing region of the axilla and then again turning longitudinally caudad along the lateral border of the latissimus dorsi muscle. Although this incision gives excellent exposure to the axilla, it is not as cosmetically appealing as the 'modified U' shaped incision. A final alternative is a longitudinal incision along the lateral border of pectoralis major in the anterior axillary line. This incision allows extension up over the coracoid process and allows exposure of the level III nodes. However, lateral exposure of the axillary vein and latissimus dorsi can be difficult, and we find this incision cosmetically inferior to our preferred 'modified U'.

When the therapeutic lymph node dissection is being performed after a sentinel node procedure, the sentinel node biopsy incision site is routinely excised. If the patient is presenting with palpable axillary adenopathy, we then choose the appropriate incision to gain access to all of the palpable adenopathy.

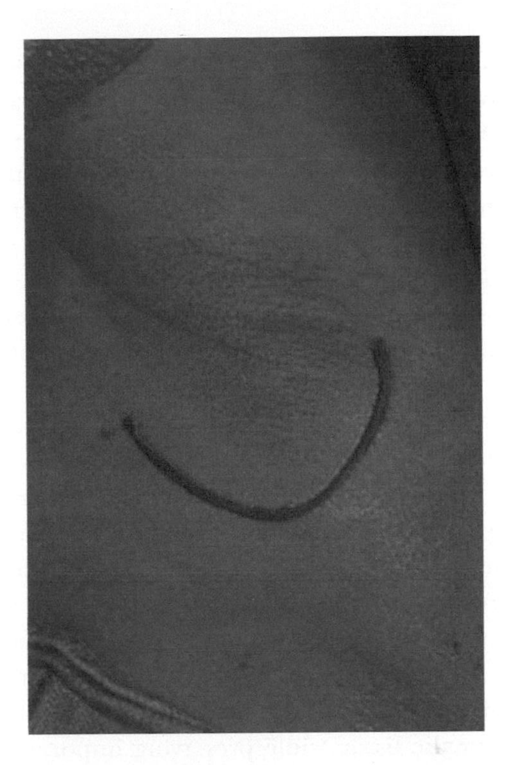

Figure 24.15 *'Modified U' incision.*

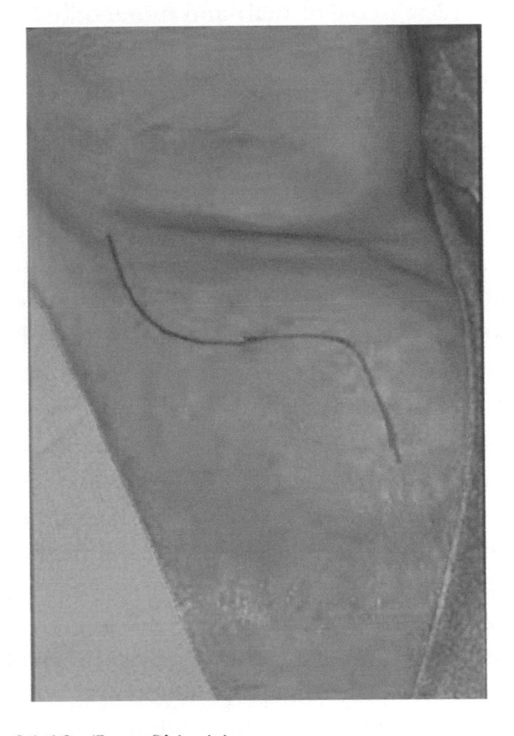

Figure 24.16 *'Lazy S' incision.*

Raising skin flaps

Once the incision has been chosen, the skin is incised with a knife. Cephalad and caudad skin flaps are then raised using electrocautery at the dermal subcutaneous junction. These flaps are created in a uniform thickness of approximately 0.5 cm. To raise the flaps, the assistant holds the skin edge with skin hooks while the surgeon provides countertraction with one hand over the axillary contents. The skin flaps are raised superiorly to the fascia overlying the pectoralis major muscle near its insertion onto the humerus, medially to the lateral border of pectoralis major, inferiorly to the level of the sixth rib and laterally to the lateral edge of latissimus dorsi.

Once the skin flaps have been raised, dissection of the nodal tissue begins. Although most surgeons have a preference, proceeding either from medial to lateral or lateral to medial, we find it most useful to be able to work in either direction. Sometimes the patient's anatomy and previous sentinel node procedure will allow a medial to lateral dissection to proceed with greater ease than a lateral to medial dissection, or vice versa. The most important part of the dissection is to remove all of the lymphatic tissue while preserving important structures, such as the axillary vein, nerve to serratus anterior (long thoracic nerve of Bell) and thoracodorsal nerve.

Dissection of the level I and II axillary lymph nodes

Beginning medially, we identify the lateral border of pectoralis major, which is delineated using electrocautery. The lateral pectoral nerve and pectoral branches of the thoracoacromial artery and vein entering and leaving the pectoralis major muscle are identified and preserved. The lateral pectoral nerve innervates the clavicular portion of the pectoralis major muscle. Gently retracting the pectoralis major medially, the interpectoral nodes and adipose tissue are mobilized to the lateral edge of pectoralis minor and are included with the specimen. The lateral border of pectoralis minor is delineated by incising the deep axillary fascia. The medial pectoral neurovascular complex is preserved as it enters pectoralis minor. Several branches of the medial pectoral nerve innervate pectoralis minor, while others penetrate the muscle to innervate the sternocostal and abdominal portions of pectoralis major (Figure 24.17). Pectoralis minor can now be easily retracted medially and the axilla proper, which contains the majority of the nodal tissue, can be entered.

A handheld retractor is used to retract pectoralis major and pectoralis minor towards the midline. To achieve adequate exposure of the axillary contents, the intercostobrachial nerves are divided sharply as they emerge from the intercostal spaces. Superiorly, the axillary vein is identified and skeletonized distally to the level of latissimus dorsi muscle using sharp dissection along its inferior border; there is often an unnamed superficial tributary of the axillary vein. This tributary can be recognized because there is no accompanying artery or nerve. We prefer to suture ligate this vessel at its junction with the axillary vein. Once the vein has been skeletonized, we then identify the long thoracic nerve of Bell in its usual location along the chest wall just superficial to the investing fascia of the serratus anterior muscle. The nerve is skeletonized proximally from the axillary vein to its insertion onto the anterior surface of serratus anterior muscle. Near this caudad portion of the nerve are one or two crossing veins, which must be ligated. Moving laterally, the thoracodorsal neurovascular complex is identified and preserved, with the vein usually anterolateral to the artery. The thoracodorsal complex is followed to its insertions, into both the latissimus dorsi muscle and the chest wall. Once both nerves are clearly identified, then the intervening nodal tissue between these two nerves is skeletonized down to the posterior extent of the dissection, which is subscapularis muscle. Once this dissection is accomplished, we then reflect the axillary contents from medial to lateral. The lateral perforating branches of the thoracodorsal vascular complex are controlled using small clips. Careful attention is paid to the lymphatic tissue lateral to the thoracodorsal neurovascular complex. This is an area where recurrences occur if the nodal tissue is not completely dissected to the level of latissimus dorsi muscle. The remaining attachments to the lateral border of latissimus dorsi are divided, and the specimen is properly oriented for subsequent pathological examination.

Dissection of the level III axillary lymph nodes

Adequate exposure of level III nodes requires that the area beneath the clavicle including the subclavius muscle can be skeletonized to the costoclavicular ligament. There are several approaches to the level III axillary nodes. These include: (1) adducting the arm over the chest with retraction of the pectoralis muscles anteromedially, (2) detaching the pectoralis minor muscle at or near its attachment to the coracoid process, and (3) making a second incision just inferior to the clavicle.

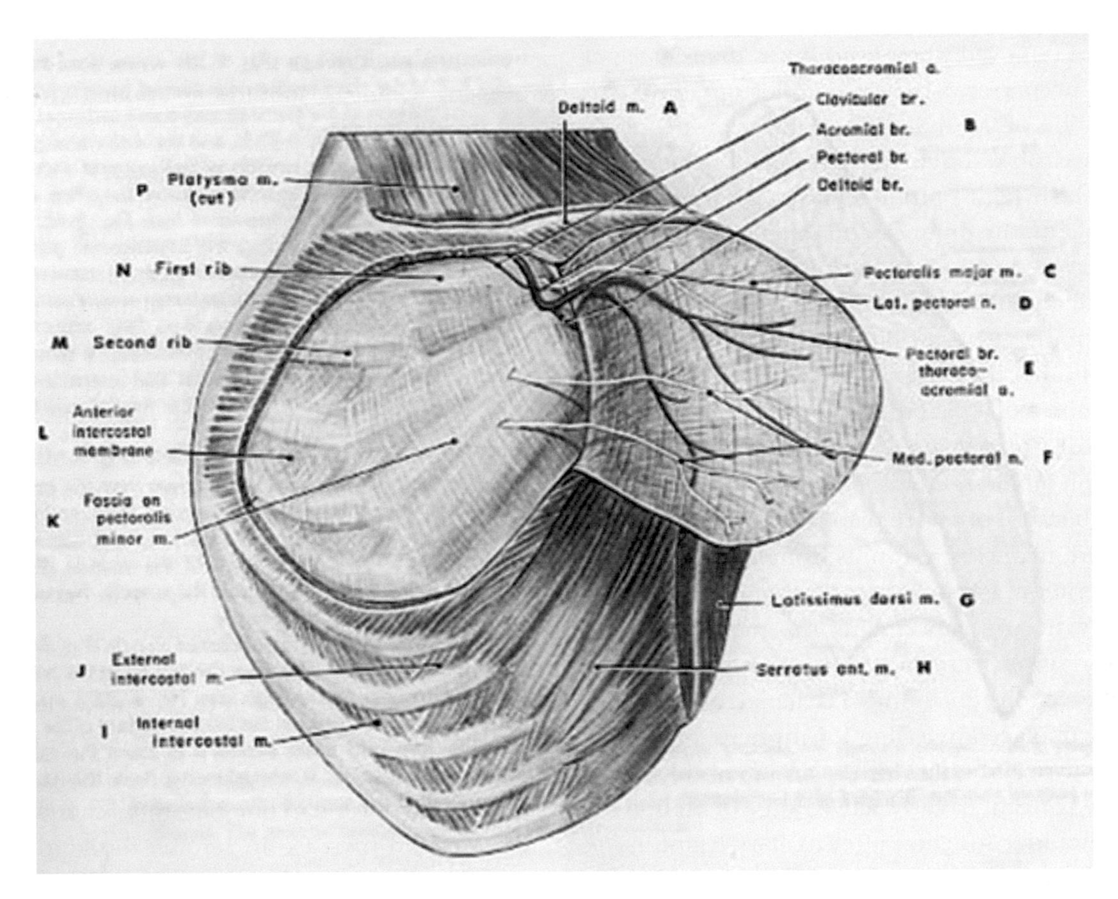

Figure 24.17 *Innervation of pectoralis major. (Reproduced from Crafts RC. A Textbook of human anatomy, 1985 #39: 787).*

Our preferred approach to the level III axillary nodes is with complete muscle paralysis. A retractor is then placed beneath the pectoralis major and pectoralis minor muscles to retract these muscles anteromedially. The arm is adducted across of the chest by the assistant. For most patients, this manoeuvre sufficiently opens up access to the level III nodes so that all nodal tissue can be removed and the axillary vein can be skeletonized as it courses out of the thoracic inlet.

If exposure of the apex of the axilla is inadequate using paralytics and retraction, then the pectoralis minor muscle can be detached sharply off the coracoid process and its origin on the chest wall allowing much better exposure of the level III nodes.[14] This method is particularly useful for patients who have well developed musculature or grossly involved nodal tissue.[15] After the level III nodes have been resected, we reattach the pectoralis minor tendon to the coracoid process.

In some instances, a better approach to the level III lymph nodes may be an infraclavicular approach. This technique may be helpful when the patient has had a previous axillary dissection, and there is recurrent disease in the level III nodes. It also may be of use when there is possible extension into the low cervical chain. A transverse incision is made approximately 1 cm caudad to the inferior border of the clavicle. The pectoralis major muscle is divided from its attachments to the inferior border of the clavicle. The pectoralis minor muscle will be seen crossing the axillary vessels and may be either retracted inferolaterally or divided. Dissection proceeds usually from medial to lateral. Care must be taken to preserve all bundles of the brachial plexus.

POSTOPERATIVE CARE

As with all operations, early ambulation and patient mobilization are the keys to success. Patients undergoing axillary dissection should be ambulatory and on a regular diet by the first postoperative day. Patients should be taught drain care and general care of the involved arm. We encourage limited movement no greater than 90 degrees in any given direction of the affected arm after the operation and before drain removal.[16,17]

Drains are removed when fluid is less than 30 cc per day, which occurs anywhere from postoperative day 5–10. Retention of the drain until flow is low decreases the incidence of seromas and lymphoedema in the affected limb. If high output remains after 10 days of drain placement, the drain can be retained longer if no infection occurs or removed because it may become a nidus for infection. Subsequent aspirations of fluid are carried out in the office.[18,19] If the patient has continued reaccumulation of the seroma, a closed suction drain is replaced in the axilla. Sclerotherapy of the axilla using tetracycline or fibrin sealant to close the space left following lymph node removal has not gained general acceptance because of severe pain from the tetracycline insertion and inconclusive results from fibrin usage.[20,21]

After operation, limited arm and shoulder motion is advocated, with arm movements no greater than 90 degrees in a given direction.[16,17] Patients with more extensive resections including claviculectomy should have their arm placed in a sling for three to four weeks before any physical therapy for the arm. Several studies promote the concept of early active range of motion for improved shoulder function after axillary lymph node dissection; but these patients develop more seromas and wound infections.[22,23] For straightforward dissections, active physical therapy for the arm should begin once the drain has been removed; as arm activity increases, lymphatic drainage increases leading to decreased incidence of lymphoedema.[16] A balanced physical therapy programme includes exercises for shoulder flexion, abduction, internal and external rotation, as well as for functional activity of the arm.[24] To help prevent the development of lymphoedema postoperatively, compression garments, massage therapy, and elevation of the arm in addition to physical therapy must be a part of the patient's postoperative regimen.[17] A fully functional arm with minimal or no oedema is the goal for patients who have undergone an axillary lymph node dissection.[17]

COMPLICATIONS

Wound infections occur in up to 10% of patients who have undergone an axillary node dissection. In patients who develop cellulitis without abscess formation, oral antibiotics are used for treatment. If the infection does not improve or worsens, the patient is placed on intravenous antibiotics.[18,25] When pus is suspected, the incision should be opened and drained, and wet to dry dressing changes should be applied to the wound. Antibiotic coverage is determined from wound cultures, although most of these infections result from skin flora such as staphylococcus or streptococcus.[13]

A lymphocoele or seroma occurs in 2–21% of patients, depending on the type of drain placed and when it is removed.[14,26] The incidence can be decreased by inserting closed suction drains at the time of the operation and leaving them in place until the drainage is less than 30–50 cc per day.[16] Seroma formation is directly related to the length of time the drain is left in place.[25,27] Kopelman et al. compared routine drain removal on postoperative day 3 regardless of output to drain removal only once the output was less than 35 cc per day.[26] Twenty-one per cent of patients who had their drains removed on postoperative day 3 regardless of output developed seromas, whereas only 4% of patients who had drains in place until output was less than 35 cc per day developed seromas ($P = 0.02$).[26] In contrast, others have suggested that drains should be removed on postoperative day one before discharge home, and reported no increase in seroma formation or wound infection and decreased number of office visits to manage the axilla.[25] Most commonly, drains are left in place until the output is less than 30 cc per day or it has been seven to 10 days after the operation. If the drains are removed and a seroma develops, it can easily be aspirated in the office. If the seroma does not resolve with repeated aspiration, a closed suction drain should be placed until the drainage slows significantly.

Lymphoedema after axillary node dissection for melanoma is rare, but no studies of the actual evidence are yet available. It occurs in 4–5% of patients with axillary node dissection for breast cancer but appears to be considerably less common after dissection for melanoma.[28] Conservative treatment options for lymphoedema improve symptoms in most of these patients. Initial management involves arm elevation to decrease intravascular hydrostatic pressure and to increase drainage. Manual lymph drainage, exercises, and massage are also important aspects of management. Skin care is necessary to prevent infection in the affected limb, and compression garments are used to maintain arm size once the oedema has plateaued. For extremely severe cases of chronic lymphoedema that fail to respond to conservative treatment, surgery is the last option. This involves excising excess tissue in the axilla or creating grafts between lymphatic vessels and the venous system to give unobstructed lymphatic drainage, but the outcomes of these procedures have not been impressive. Fortunately, most patients have improved cosmesis and increased function of the arm with conservative measures.[25]

A decreased range of motion in the involved arm sometimes develops when physical therapy has not been started in an appropriate timeframe. Limited arm movements are encouraged immediately after the operation, with active exercises beginning only after the drains are removed; mobilization of the arm is necessary for maintaining its function.[17,18] Massage techniques are also introduced to the patient after the operation to help prevent formation of oedema in the extremity.[24]

Neurapraxia after node dissection is now very rare (less than 0.5%) and even less common if the Patey technique involving placement of the arm above the head for the entire operation is used. This complication is usually temporary and rarely results in a permanent functional deficit.[16,18] Winged scapula secondary to a long thoracic nerve injury is another complication that is of concern in this operation. Injury to this nerve is uncommon because it is visualized and protected throughout the entire procedure.[27]

Haematoma formation is a potential complication for any operation, including axillary node dissection. Meticulous haemostasis during the surgery and a thorough search for small arterial bleeders prior to closure help to lower the rate of this complication. Another rare but important problem that can occur is axillary vein thrombosis due to extensive dissection around this vessel.

SUMMARY

Meticulous surgical technique to remove all of the lymphatic tissue without tumour cell spillage, with preservation of the axillary vein, the long thoracic nerve of Bell, and the thoracodorsal nerve, maximizes the therapeutic benefit to the patient while minimizing long term consequences.

REFERENCES

1. Balch CM, Soong SJ, Milton GW, et al, A comparison of prognostic factors and surgical results in 1,786 patients with localized (stage I) melanoma treated in Alabama, USA, and New South Wales, Australia. *Ann Surg* 1982; 196: 677–84.
2. Milton GW, Shaw HM, McCarthy WH, et al, Prophylactic lymph node dissection in clinical stage I cutaneous malignant melanoma: results of surgical treatment in 1319 patients. *Br J Surg* 1982; 69: 108–11.
3. Veronesi U, Adamus J, Bandiera DC, et al, Inefficacy of immediate node dissection in stage 1 melanoma of the limbs. *New Engl J Med* 1977; 297: 627–30.
4. Veronesi U, Adamus J, Bandiera DC, et al, Delayed regional lymph node dissection in stage I melanoma of the skin of the lower extremities. *Cancer* 1982; 49: 2420–30.
5. Sim FH, Taylor WF, Ivins JC, et al, A prospective randomized study of the efficacy of routine elective lymphadenectomy in management of malignant melanoma. Preliminary results. *Cancer* 1978; 41: 948–56.
6. Balch CM, Soong SJ, Bartolucci AA, et al, Efficacy of an elective regional lymph node dissection of 1 to 4 mm thick melanomas for patients 60 years of age and younger. *Ann Surg* 1996; 224: 255–63.
7. Kelemen PR, Wanek LA, Morton DL, Lymph node biopsy does not impair survival after therapeutic dissection for palpable melanoma metastases. *Ann Surg Oncol* 1999; 6: 139–43.
8. Coveney E, Weltz CR, Greengrass R, et al, Use of paravertebral block anesthesia in the surgical management of breast cancer: experience in 156 cases. *Ann Surg* 1998; 227: 496–501.
9. Richardson J, Lonnqvist P, Thoracic paravertebral block. *Br J Anaesth* 1998; 81: 230–8.
10. Pusch F, Freitag H, Weinstabl C, et al, Single-injection paravertebral block compared to general anaesthesia in breast surgery. *Acta Anaesthesiol Scand* 1999; 4: 770–4.
11. Greengrass R, O'Brien F, Lyerly K, et al, Paravertebral block for breast cancer surgery. *Can J Anaesthesia* 1996; 43: 858–61.
12. Miller R, *Anesthesia*. 5th ed. Philadephia: Churchill Livingston, 2000.
13. Platt R, Zucker JR, Zaleznik DF, et al, Perioperative antibiotic prophylaxis and wound infection following breast surgery. *J Antimicrob Chemother* 1993; 31 (suppl B): 43–8.
14. Karakousis CP, Bland KI, Surgery of the primary lesion and nodal dissections in malignant melanoma. In: *Atlas of surgical oncology*. (eds, Bland KI, Karakousis CP, Copeland EM). Philadelphia: WB Saunders, 1995: 93–128.
15. Harris M, Gumport S, Maiwandi H, Axillary lymph node dissection for melanoma. *Surg Gynecol Obstet* 1972; 135: 936.
16. Karakousis C, Therapeutic node dissections in malignant melanoma. *Sem Surg Oncol* 1998; 14: 291–301.
17. Brennan M, Miller L, Overview of treatment options and review of the current role and use of compression garments, intermittent pumps, and exercise in the managment of lymphedema. *Cancer* 1998; 83: 2821–7.
18. Karakousis C, Goumas W, Rao U, Driscoll D, Axillary node dissection in malignant melanoma. *Am J Surg* 1991; 162: 202–7.
19. Karakousis C, Hena M, Emrich L, Driscoll D, Axillary node dissection in malignant melanoma: results and complications. *Surgery* 1990; 108: 10–17.
20. Moore M, Nguyen D, Spotnitz W, Fibrin sealant reduces serous drainage and allows for earlier drain removal after axillary dissection: a randomized prospective trial. *Am Surg* 1997; 63: 97–102.
21. McCarthy PM, Martin JK Jr, Wells DC, et al, An aborted, prospective, randomized trial of sclerotherapy for prolonged drainage after mastectomy. *Surg Gynecol Obstetr* 1986; 162: 418–20.
22. Petrek JA, Peters MM, Nori S, et al, Axillary lymphadenectomy. A prospective, randomized trial of 13 factors influencing drainage, including early or delayed arm mobilization. *Arch Surg* 1990; 125: 378–82.
23. Jansen RF, van Geel AN, de Groot HG, et al, Immediate versus delayed shoulder exercises after axillary lymph node dissection. *Am J Surg* 1990; 160: 481–4.
24. Na YM, Lee JS, Park JS, et al, Early rehabilitation program in postmastectomy patients: a prospective clinical trial. *Yonsei Med J* 1999; 40: 1–8.

25. Liu C, McFaddend D, Overnight closed suction drainage after axillary lymphadenectomy for breast cancer. *Am Surg* 1997; 63: 868–70.
26. Kopelman D, Klemm O, Bahous H, et al, Postoperative suction drainage of the axilla: for how long? Prospective randomised trial. *Eur J Surgery* 1999; 165: 117–20 (discussion 121–2).
27. Roses DF, Brooks AD, Harris MN, et al, Complications of level I and II axillary dissection in the treatment of carcinoma of the breast. *Ann Surg* 1999; 230: 194–201.
28. Horan D, McMullen M, Assessment and management of the woman with lymphedema after breast cancer. *J Am Acad Nurse Prac* 1998; 10: 155–9.

25

Groin and pelvic dissection for melanoma

Constantine P Karakousis, John F Thompson

INTRODUCTION

Lymph drains to each groin from the skin of the ipsilateral lower extremity and the ipsilateral lower quadrant of the abdomen, the buttock and the perineum. There are normally 10–15 'superficial' inguinal nodes below the level of the inguinal ligament, and 6–8 'deep' nodes, i.e. iliac and obturator nodes, in the pelvis. For patients with palpable, histologically positive nodes in the groin, groin dissection is certainly indicated. The extent of this, however, i.e. whether or not it involves dissection of the pelvic lymph nodes, is dependent on certain criteria advanced by several authors. The positivity of a palpable node is best confirmed by fine needle aspiration cytology. Palpable nodes that contain metastatic melanoma tend to be spherical and firm, whereas hyperplastic nodes retain their fusiform shape and are flat and soft.

With the advent of the technique of sentinel node biopsy, it is no longer considered appropriate to perform elective node dissection in patients with clinically negative inguinal nodes. In most published series, there is a very high rate of identification of the sentinel node in the groin, approaching 100%.[1,2] For patients with a positive sentinel node in the groin, a complete subinguinal ('superficial') groin dissection is indicated, since about 20% of these patients will be found to have additional positive lymph nodes in the same nodal basin.[1]

OPERATIVE TECHNIQUE

A variety of incisions have been employed in carrying out groin dissections. Thus, a transverse incision, or two transverse incisions, or a lazy 'S' incision have been used on the assumption that a vertical incision crossing the inguinal crease might lead to increased morbidity. However, given the layout of the lymph nodes along the femoral vessels in the femoral triangle, it becomes clear that a longitudinal or slightly oblique incision along the course of the femoral vessels provides the best exposure for dissection of the inguinal nodes and accommodates the needs for an in-continuity dissection of the deep nodes should this be indicated. Considering the longitudinal course of the subcutaneous lymphatics in the skin of the femoral triangle, it is also more likely to preserve some of the superficial subcutaneous lymphatics in the flaps that are constructed than a transverse incision in the groin, which cuts across the course of lymphatics and interrupts all of them in the subcutaneous tissue for the length of the incision.

The femoral triangle is bounded superiorly by the inguinal ligament, laterally by the sartorius muscle, and medially by the anterior border of gracilis muscle. The base of this triangle is the inguinal ligament, and the apex of the triangle is the point where the sartorius muscle crosses the superficial femoral vessels. An incision is made about two fingerbreadths superomedial to the anterior superior iliac spine and is carried slightly obliquely, but essentially in a vertical longitudinal fashion, over the centre of the inguinal ligament to the apex of the femoral triangle (Figure 25.1).[3,4] When the intention is to perform a superficial groin dissection only, this incision does not have to be carried above the level of the anterior superior iliac spine, but when the

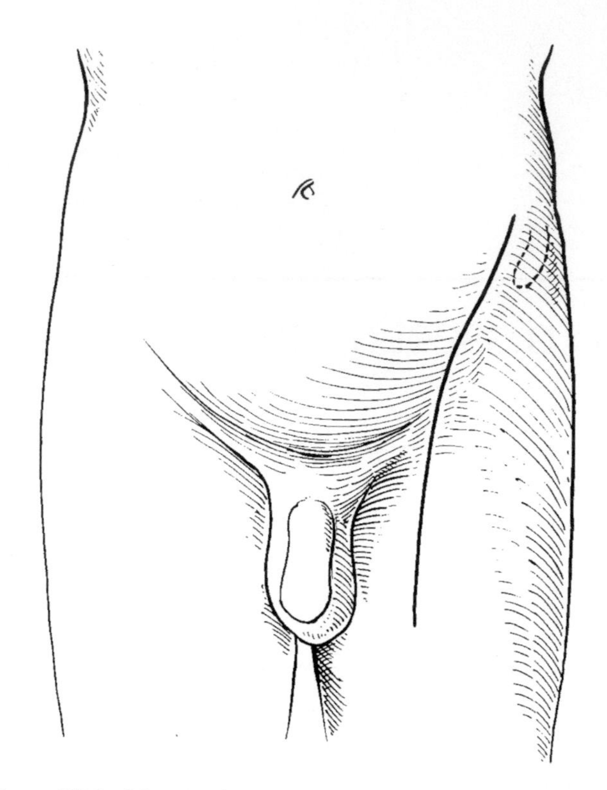

Figure 25.1 *A longitudinal, nearly vertical incision is made from above the anterior superior iliac spine to the apex of the femoral triangle. Reproduced from*[4] *with permission of WB Saunders Co.*

intention is to perform a radical (ilio-inguinal) groin dissection, the incision is commenced two to three fingerbreadths above the level of the anterior superior iliac spine in order to provide proximal exposure for the deep part of the groin dissection.

Flaps are made that are 3–4 mm thick initially, and then as the dissection proceeds toward the base of the flap on each side, the flap is made progressively thicker. Medially, the flap is carried to the pubic tubercle superiorly and inferiorly to the fascia covering the adductor muscles, which is incised along the anterior border of gracilis or the medial edge of adductor longus. Above the level of the pubic tubercle, the dissection is carried out fairly rapidly to the surface of the external oblique aponeurosis and then the adipose tissue, with any lymph nodes above the level of the inguinal ligament and is mobilized to the level of this ligament, skimming over the surface of the spermatic cord in male patients. Below the level of the pubic tubercle, the dissection is continued on the surface of adductor longus first, and then the pectineus, lifting the fascia toward what is to become the specimen. In the inferior part of the dissection of the medial flap, the great saphenous vein is encountered, and is ligated and divided. At the apex of the triangle, the medial border of the sartorius muscle is exposed. The dissection continues on the surface of the adductors until the medial wall of the femoral vein is seen. Some of the tributaries to the femoral vein have to be ligated and divided in order to approach the medial wall of the vein. However, tributaries that are issuing directly from the adductor muscles to the posterior wall of the femoral vein can be preserved. Once the medial wall of the vein is seen, the sheath of the vein is entered and incised longitudinally. The anterior half of the sheath covering the superficial and common femoral vein is lifted off the vein, to be removed en bloc with the rest of the specimen.

About 3–4 cm below the inguinal ligament, the great saphenous vein is visualized as it enters the femoral vein deep to the foramen ovalis (Figure 25.2). The great saphenous vein is clamped deep to the foramen ovalis and divided with a scalpel. The proximal stump of the vein close to the femoral vein is ligated with 2.0 silk and suture-ligated with 3.0 silk or 4.0 prolene, while the distal stump of the great saphenous vein, extremely short, is suture-ligated with 3.0 or 2.0 silk 'U' suture, to prevent slippage of the tie and retraction of this stump superficial to the level of the foramen ovalis, in which case bleeding occurs requiring further suturing. When only a superficial groin dissection is intended, the adipose tissue with lymphatic channels coursing medial to the vein is divided beneath the inguinal ligament at the lower end of the femoral canal. This facilitates lifting of the specimen and further dissection on the femoral vein and more laterally on the superficial and common femoral arteries. When an in-continuity dissection is planned of the inguinal nodes together with the 'deep' iliac and obturator nodes, then this connecting bridge of lymphatic tissue coursing behind the inguinal ligament into the femoral canal is left intact in order to remove en bloc the specimens of the superficial and deep nodes.

The lateral flap is raised in a similar fashion, starting with a thin flap of 3–4 mm over the underlying lymph nodes, and making it progressively thicker as the base of the flap is approached. The base of the flap should be at the lateral border of the sartorius muscle, which is revealed by incising the fascia covering this muscle. Under the proximal portion of the fascia covering the sartorius, about 3–4 cm below the level of the anterior superior iliac spine, the lateral femoral cutaneous nerve

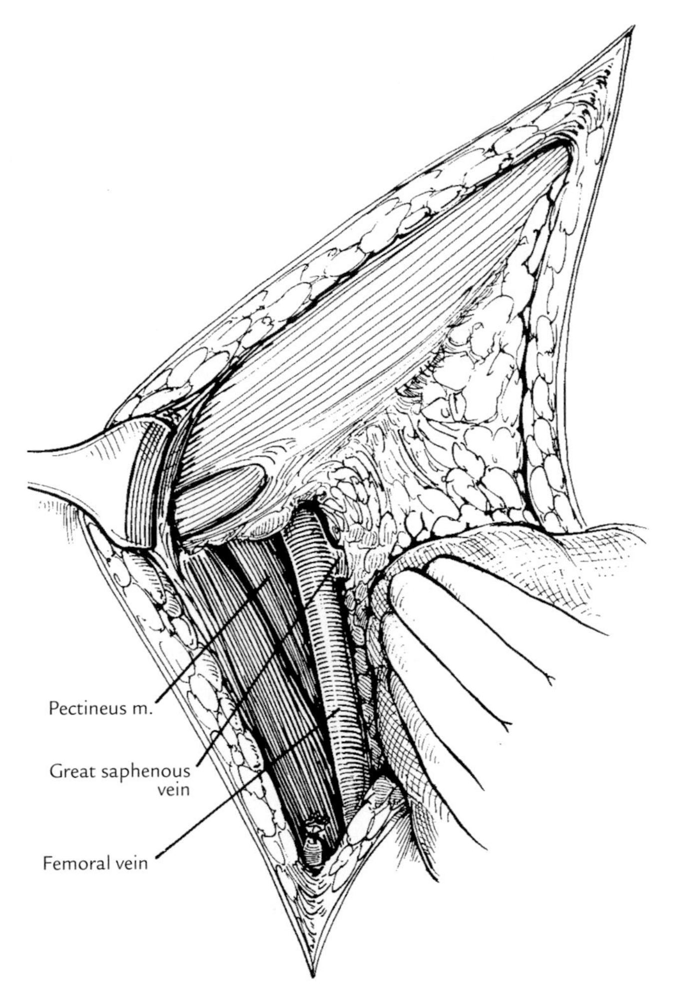

Figure 25.2 *The medial flap has been dissected and the specimen has been mobilized off the adductor longus and pectineus, exposing the femoral vein and the entry of the great saphenous vein into the common femoral vein. Reproduced from*[4] *with permission of WB Saunders Co.*

can be seen directly underneath the fascia as it courses, from its exit point from the retroperitoneal area underneath the lateral end of the inguinal ligament, over the sartorius muscle in an inferolateral direction en route to supplying the skin of the lateral aspect of the thigh. As the fascia covering sartorius is lifted with forceps or Adair clamps, the lateral aspect of the femoral artery is approached, the sheath covering the artery is incised and entered, and small branches issuing from the common and superficial femoral arteries toward the specimen are ligated with fine sutures and divided.

Between the femoral artery and sartorius muscle, the branches of the femoral nerve are exposed. They are branches to the sartorius and some are branches en route to supplying the skin of the anterior and medial aspect of the lower thigh. There is no problem dividing the branches to sartorius. The branch to vastus medialis follows a straight vertical course, while the leash of branches to rectus femoris, vastus intermedius, and vastus lateralis deviate in a lateral direction a few centimetres below the inguinal ligament, between the rectus femoris and vastus intermedius, along with the branches of the lateral femoral circumflex vessels. These motor branches, however, are in a deeper plane and not usually exposed in a typical groin dissection.

As the specimen is mobilized off the front of the femoral vessels, small sensory branches of the femoral nerve coursing in the direction of the specimen have to be sacrificed. The procedure of groin dissection is inevitably associated with numbness around the incision in the area of the flaps, caused by the division of tiny and normally invisible terminal endings of sensory branches in the course of developing the flaps, but the numbness also extends inferiorly almost to the knee as a result of proximal division of the small sensory branches of the femoral nerve issuing below the inguinal ligament and following a short course to enter the specimen en route to supplying the anteromedial aspects of the thigh. After the lateral flap has been developed in the cephalad part of the dissection, the adipose tissue and lymph nodes above the level of the inguinal ligament are dissected off the external oblique aponeurosis to the level of the inguinal ligament, and then the specimen is further mobilized off the femoral artery and femoral vein towards the area of the femoral canal.

As mentioned above, if the intention is to perform only a superficial groin dissection, the specimen should be divided at the level of the femoral canal opening. At this point, if one wishes to use the criterion of the so called node of Cloquet, which is the node normally encountered at the lower end of the femoral canal, this node may be removed and sent for frozen section examination. If it is negative, according to some authors,[5] this is an indication to stop the procedure and perform only a superficial groin dissection. If there is no palpable node at or immediately below the femoral canal, as is often the case, rather than dissect into the apex of the specimen trying to find the highest node to be sent for frozen section, a better option is to detach the inguinal ligament from the pubic tubercle and the adjacent rectus sheath from the pubic crest and thus mobilize and remove the adipose tissue and nodes of the femoral canal. In the opinion of the authors, however, biopsy of Cloquet's node is not a sufficiently sensitive or reliable criterion to justify cutting the lymphatics around a potentially positive node in order to subject it to pathological evaluation, potentially causing wound contamination with tumour cells.

Whenever it is decided that a complete 'radical' (ilio-inguinal) node dissection is to be performed, the specimen should preferably be left in-continuity with the lymphatics in the femoral canal area in order to be removed en bloc with the deep nodes (Figure 25.3). Of course, this is the case whenever one divides the inguinal ligament and performs an in-continuity dissection of the superficial and deep nodes. An alternative technique is to use a separate oblique incision through the lower abdominal musculature above the level of the inguinal ligament and enter the retroperitoneal space through that incision, removing the deep nodes separately from the superficial inguinal group. Either technique, i.e. the in-continuity dissection or separate removal of the superficial and deep nodes, may be satisfactory for most cases. However, the in-continuity dissection has the following practical and theoretical advantages: (1) an improved exposure by dividing the inguinal ligament; (2) removal of possibly involved nodes that could be missed behind an intact inguinal ligament; and (3) avoidance of cutting through potentially contaminated lymphatics in the area of the femoral canal.

In order to perform an in-continuity dissection, the external oblique aponeurosis is incised from a point two to three fingerbreadths or higher superomedial to the anterior superior iliac spine down to a point 1–2 cm lateral to the femoral artery. This is the point at which the inguinal ligament fuses in its lateral third over the iliacus muscle with the iliac fascia. After the external oblique aponeurosis is incised, the internal oblique and transversus abdominis muscles are divided, usually with cautery. The transversalis fascia is then incised, and the retroperitoneal space is entered. The inguinal ligament is divided 1–2 cm lateral to the femoral artery and with blunt and sharp dissection the peritoneum is separated off the external iliac lymph nodes. Superiorly, the peritoneum is separated off the common iliac vessels and the ureter is identified and left on the surface of the peritoneum. The inferior epigastric artery is ligated and divided at its origin (Figure 25.4), as the inguinal ligament is pulled forward, and then the inferior epigastric vein is also ligated and divided close to its point of entry

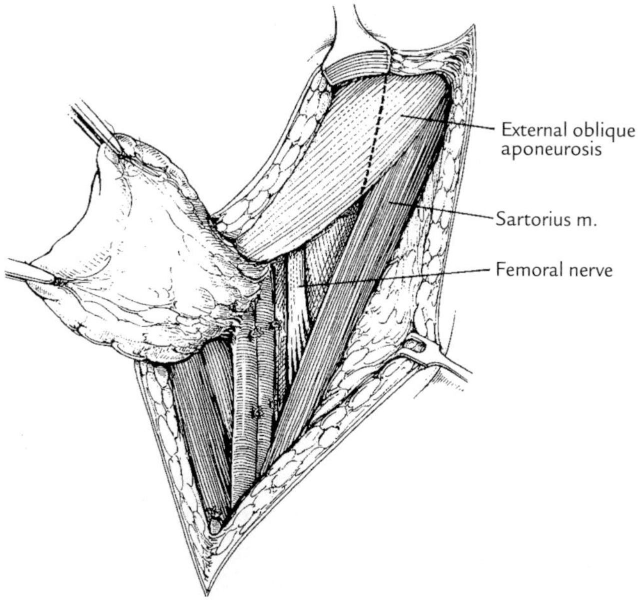

Figure 25.3 *The superficial groin dissection is nearly completed. The specimen is just attached to the femoral canal area for an in-continuity dissection of the deep nodes. The incision over the external oblique aponeurosis for retroperitoneal exposure is outlined. Reproduced from[4] with permission of WB Saunders Co.*

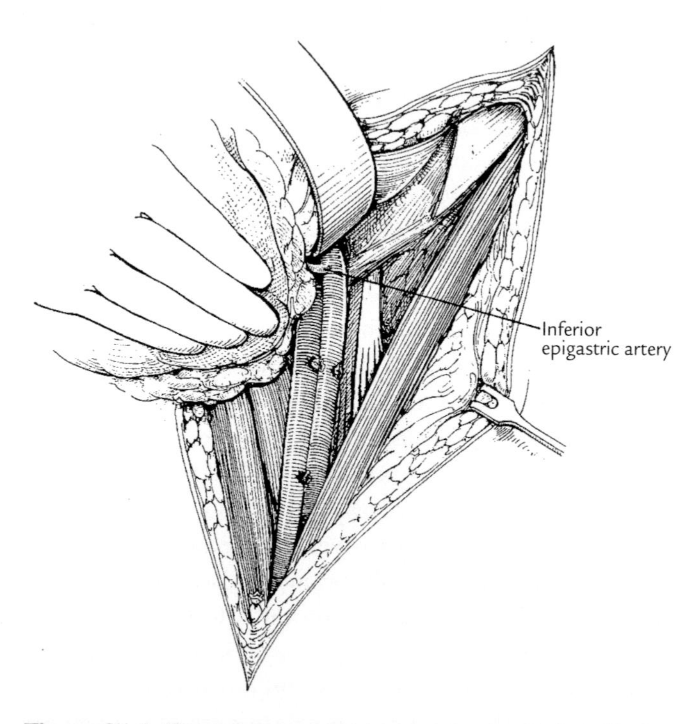

Figure 25.4 *The inferior epigastric artery is exposed in order to ligate and divide it. Reproduced from[4] with permission of WB Saunders Co.*

into the external iliac vein. This allows for the mobilization of the anterior abdominal wall and peritoneum more superiorly from the surface of the external iliac and obturator nodes.

As the blunt dissection of the peritoneum proceeds in an inferomedial direction, the inferior epigastric vessels are encountered anteriorly, are ligated and divided again at a point immediately lateral to the ipsilateral rectus abdominis as they are en route to assuming a position behind that muscle. Thus, a segment of the inferior epigastric vessels between the external iliac vessels and the lateral edge of the rectus abdominis coursing over the deep nodes is removed en bloc with the latter. The bladder is then dissected off the medial aspect of the obturator nodes, the internal iliac artery is visualized, and, if necessary, the superior vesical branch of the internal iliac artery is ligated and divided for greater exposure. Of course, the ureter is always kept under close watch to avoid incidental injury.

In the presence of lymph nodes which appear to be grossly normal, the dissection may start at the bifurcation of the common iliac artery and proceed in a caudal direction, dissecting these lymph nodes off the surface of the external iliac artery and external iliac vein. The area of the obturator nodes is bounded anteriorly by the external iliac vein, posteriorly by the obturator nerve, and inferiorly by the obturator foramen. Superiorly, the boundary is the internal iliac artery. Dissection therefore starts from the internal iliac artery and proceeds to clear these nodes en bloc with the external iliac nodes from the surface of the obturator fascia. This is the fascia covering the obturator internus muscle. Posteriorly, the obturator nerve is visualized and preserved (Figure 25.5). Posterior to the obturator nerve, the obturator vessels are coursing. These vessels issue branches immediately above (cephalad to) the obturator foramen toward the area of Cooper's ligament. These branches need to be ligated and divided. With a dissection that proceeds alternatively from a medial, cephalad, lateral, and caudal point as the facility for exposure dictates, the dissection of the obturator nodes is completed en bloc with the external iliac nodes and the superficial inguinal group of nodes.

In the presence of enlarged nodes in the external iliac or obturator area, it is best to start from the common iliac group of nodes and proceed in a caudal direction. In these cases, in order to obtain greater exposure, the lateral border of the ipsilateral rectus

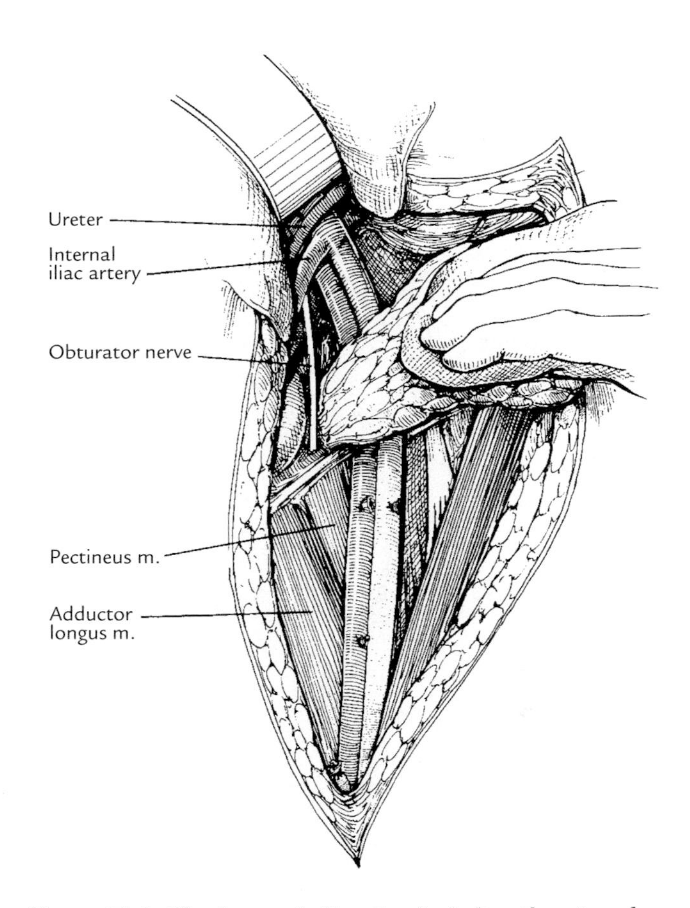

Figure 25.5 *The deep node dissection including the external iliac and obturator nodes is about to be completed. The obturator nodes have been dissected off the obturator nerve at this point. Reproduced from[4] with permission of WB Saunders Co.*

abdominis, as well as the anterior rectus sheath, may be divided off the pubic crest, as necessary, to achieve improved exposure. This completes the dissection of the superficial and deep nodes.

Reconstruction is performed by approximating the transversus abdominis and internal oblique muscles with absorbable continuous sutures, while the external oblique aponeurosis is approximated with a nonabsorbable monofilament running suture all the way to the inguinal ligament (Figure 25.6). Non-absorbable interrupted sutures are then used to approximate the inguinal ligament to Cooper's ligament medial to the vessels and to the iliac fascia lateral to the vessels. The sutures are placed first and then serially tied. The iliac fascia is fairly sturdy at it descends on the iliacus muscle to the level of the inguinal ligament, but then it attenuates below this level. It is exposed by dissecting the fibrofatty tissue and exposing the femoral nerve. The fascia is directly anterior to the femoral nerve, and, with the

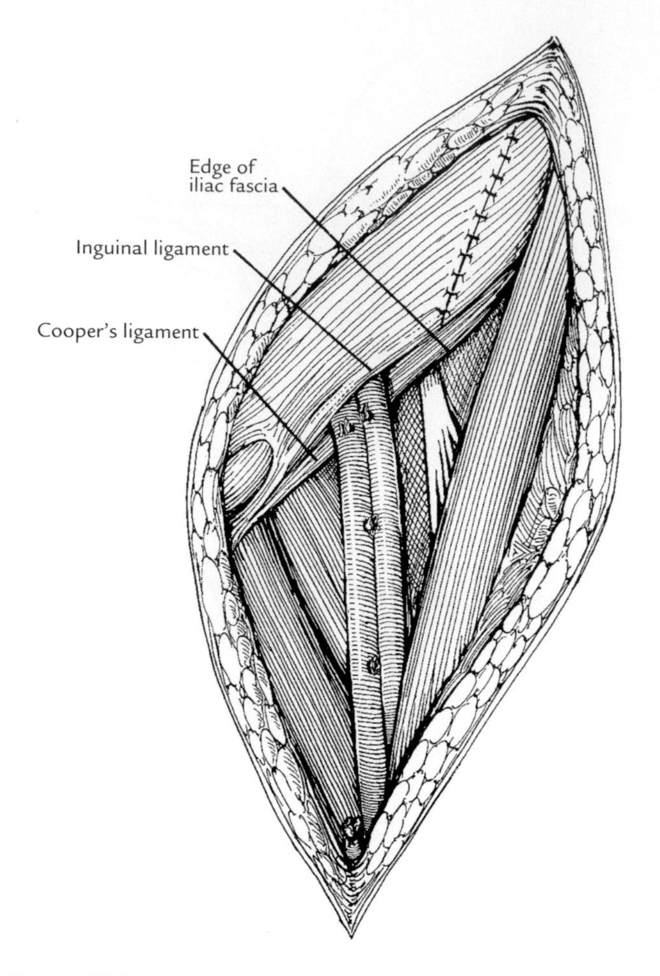

Figure 25.6 *External oblique, internal oblique and transversus abdominis muscles have been approximated. Reproduced from*[4] *with permission of WB Saunders Co.*

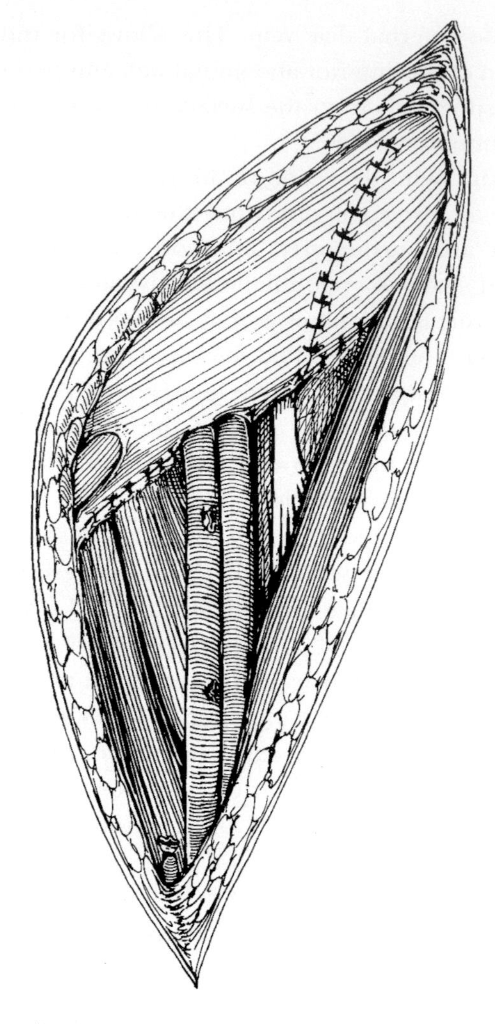

Figure 25.7 *Reconstruction is completed by approximating the medial portion of the inguinal ligament to Cooper's ligament and the lateral portion to the iliac fascia. Reproduced from*[4] *with permission of WB Saunders Co.*

nerve exposed, the sutures can be placed safely between the iliac fascia and the lateral part of the inguinal ligament. This repair, essentially a Cooper's ligament repair, effectively closes the space and prevents the occurrence of an incisional inguinal hernia (Figure 25.7).

To provide vascularized cover for the femoral vessels in the event of wound breakdown, some surgeons advocate routine transposition of the sartorius muscle. This is accomplished by dividing the muscle at its origin from the anterior superior iliac spine. It is dissected along its medial and lateral borders and pulled under the lateral femoral cutaneous nerve when the latter can be preserved. As its proximal to distal dissection proceeds the sartorius muscle is periodically transposed, and an assessment made as to whether it is sufficiently mobilized to cover the femoral vessels adequately. This is done to avoid extensive dissection of the muscle all the way to the apex of the femoral triangle because such dissection may devascularize the proximal part of the muscle and set up a nidus of deep wound infection. The muscle may simply be shifted medially to cover the femoral vessels, preserving its orientation in terms of its anterior and posterior surfaces, or may be reversed if the latter manoeuvre seems to require less mobilization (as it often does), the objective being to minimize the risk of devascularization of the proximal muscle. Once the muscle has been transposed to cover the vessels, it is secured at its proximal end to the inguinal ligament using interrupted figure of eight absorbable sutures. A few additional absorbable sutures are used in a figure of eight manner to approximate the medial border of the muscle to the subjacent adductor muscles and thus effectively cover the femoral vessels (Figure 25.8).

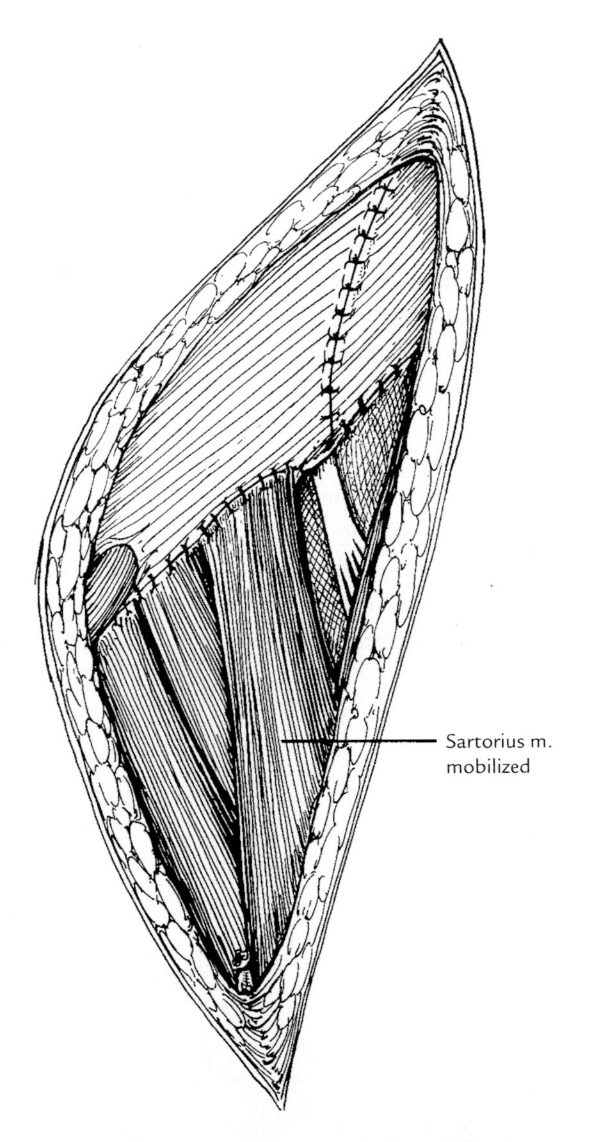

Figure 25.8 *The sartorius muscle has been mobilized to cover the vessels. Reproduced from*[4] *with permission of WB Saunders Co.*

Usually, two suction drains are employed, inserted through small incisions on each side of the lower end of the incision at the apex of the femoral triangle. At this stage a thorough lavage of the entire wound with warm sterile water or cetrimide solution is useful, not only to rinse out clot and fatty debris but also in the hope of lysing any free tumour cells. The subcutaneous tissues are approximated with a running absorbable suture and the skin closed carefully and gently with staples or other suitable material. Staples or a subcuticular suture may have less tendency to interfere with the blood supply of the edges. A dressing is applied, and the tape is usually placed transversely across the incision in order to relieve any tension on the flaps.

Before approximating the edges of the flaps, the viability of each flap is checked and if there is any question about a flap being ischaemic, its edge is trimmed. A 1 cm strip of skin from the central portion on each side can usually be removed without causing undue tension in approximating the flaps. The occurrence of some bleeding from the trimmed edge provides reassurance about the viability of the flap. If only one flap seems to be somewhat ischaemic, then only that particular flap is trimmed before the edges of the flaps are approximated. This is an important step in completing the operation as it may avert the occurrence of flap edge necrosis.

MODIFICATIONS OF THE TECHNIQUE OF GROIN DISSECTION

In the case of large palpable nodes coming close to the skin surface, to avoid an unacceptably close dissection between the skin and these nodes, an ellipse of the skin may be excised at the beginning of the operation so that the skin overlying these lymph nodes is removed en bloc with the nodes. If a large amount of skin needs to be removed in this fashion, then at the end of the procedure one may have to use a skin graft, placed directly on the surface of sartorius muscle. In cases where the sartorius muscle needs to be removed en bloc with the adjacent lymph nodes, which is likely to happen in cases of local recurrence in the groin after a previous groin dissection, one may transpose the rectus femoris to cover the femoral vessels. This is done by dividing the origin of rectus femoris from the anterior inferior iliac spine and shifting the muscle medially to cover the vessels.

If there are grossly enlarged pelvic nodes, the usual technique of ilioinguinal groin dissection may not provide sufficient exposure, and in these cases an abdominoinguinal incision becomes the incision of choice.[6,7] This incision also can provide proximal exposure to the infrarenal aorta and inferior vena cava for a more proximal dissection of potentially involved lymph nodes. In the past, dissection of involved lymph nodes above the level of the inguinal group, i.e. the external iliac and obturator lymph nodes (even more so of the common iliac, preaortic or precaval nodes), was considered inappropriate on the assumption that all these patients had distant occult disease. However, with the current development of adjuvant immunological modalities such as tumour vaccines requiring resection of all of the gross tumour whenever feasible, even in haematogenous stage IV disease, this extensive node dissection may acquire a new rationale and legitimacy.

The abdominoinguinal incision is started just above the level of the umbilicus and carried around the umbilicus and downwards in the midline to the pubic symphysis. The peritoneal cavity is entered for an initial exploration and assessment. The incision is then carried transversely from the pubic symphysis to the mid-inguinal point on the side of involvement and then vertically for a few centimetres to the apex of the femoral triangle (Figure 25.9).

From the vertical part of the incision below the inguinal ligament, flaps are developed medially and laterally, as described for the groin dissection, whereas in the transverse part of the incision a lesser flap is required to remove the adipose tissue and any lymph nodes above the inguinal ligament (Figure 25.10). The ipsilateral anterior rectus sheath and rectus abdominis muscle are divided from the pubic crest, the inguinal ligament is divided from the pubic tubercle, and then the inferior epigastric vein and artery are ligated and divided. More laterally, the lateral third of the inguinal ligament is dissected off the iliac fascia. This provides ample exposure in carrying out manoeuvres needed to dissect large masses of lymph nodes in the pelvic area (Figure 25.11). The transverse part of the incision crosses the spermatic cord in the male. The spermatic cord can be preserved if it is not involved by tumour by opening the floor of the inguinal canal from within and mobilizing the cord and its continuation to vas deferens medially. The internal spermatic vessels may be ligated above the level of the internal ring, if necessary, the testicle normally retaining its viability through scrotal collateral supply.

Reconstruction of the abdominoinguinal incision at the completion of the procedure is fairly simple, by approximating the linea alba with non-absorbable sutures in the abdominal part of the incision, then the anterior rectus sheath and muscle to the pubic crest,

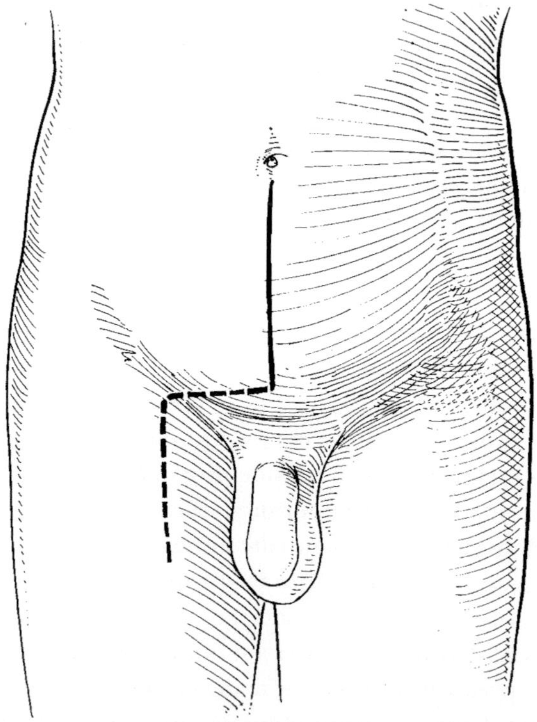

Figure 25.9 *Outline of a right abdominoinguinal incision. Reproduced from[4] with permission of WB Saunders Co.*

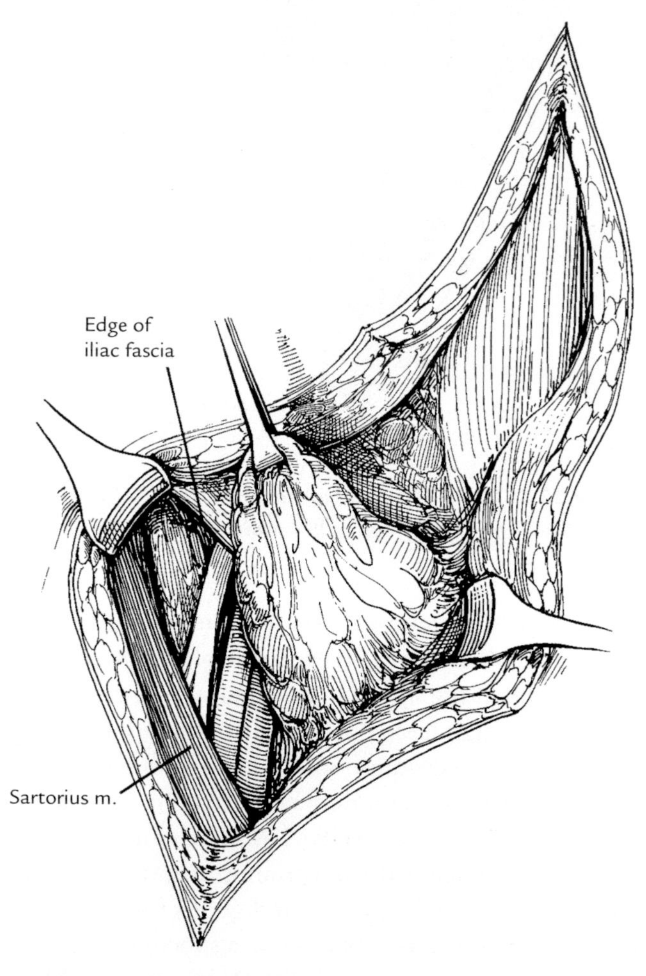

Figure 25.10 *In the area of the femoral triangle, flaps are developed as per groin dissection and the femoral vessels are exposed, as well as the femoral nerve. Reproduced from[4] with permission of WB Saunders Co.*

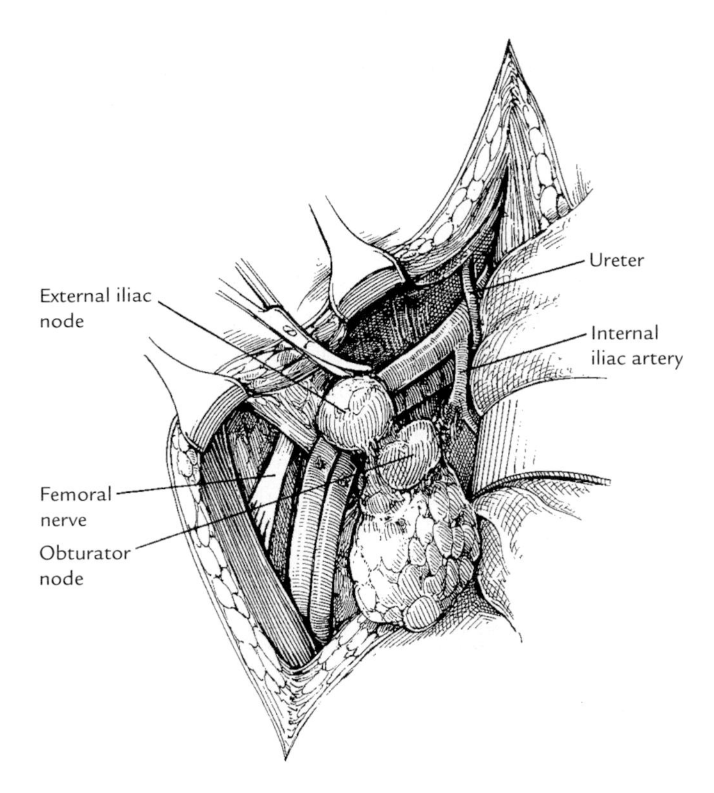

Figure 25.11 *The inferior epigastric vessels have been ligated and divided. Exposure of the retroperitoneal area and the iliac and femoral vessels in-continuity is provided. Reproduced from*[4] *with permission of WB Saunders Co.*

the part of the inguinal ligament medial to the iliofemoral vessels to Cooper's ligament, and the part of the ligament lateral to the vessels to the iliac fascia.

Common technical points between the ilioinguinal and abdominoinguinal procedures are the ligation and division of the inferior epigastric vessels and the provision of a continuous uninterrupted field between the iliac and femoral vessels with their accompanying lymph nodes. The abdominoinguinal incision, in concept a derivative of the ilioinguinal technique, provides improved exposure in the iliac obturator node area and in-continuity exposure of the precaval–preaortic area.

An alternative to the abdominoinguinal approach described above, preferred by some, is a technique that involves extension of the upper part of a slightly oblique but mainly vertically oriented inguinal incision through the skin and subcutaneous tissue upwards and laterally, above the anterior superior iliac spine and well out into the flank. The abdominal musculature can then be split and cut from the lateral edge of the rectus muscle medially to a point well lateral in the flank, allowing satisfactory extraperitoneal exposure not only of the external iliac and obturator regions, but also of the common iliac vessels and nodes, up to the level of the aortic bifurcation and even above this. This involves firm upwards and medial retraction of the intact peritoneum and contents, as well as the ureter, which is carefully identified and preserved, as it runs downwards attached to the peritoneum. Sound repair of the abdominal musculature is readily accomplished when the node clearance has been performed, using continuous nylon in layers, after extraperitoneal placement of a large closed suction drain.

DISCUSSION

Groin dissection for melanoma has in recent years been required only for patients with demonstrable disease in the groin, either in the form of a positive sentinel node or a palpable node which on fine needle aspiration cytology is positive for metastatic melanoma. Nodes involved by metastatic melanoma tend to be spherical and very firm, rather than flat and soft. Inflammatory lymph nodes tend to retain their normal fusiform elliptical shape and are flat and typically quite soft in consistency.

Sentinel node biopsy showing a microscopically positive node should be followed by a superficial groin dissection, since about 20% of these patients may have additional positive groin nodes. In the experience of one of the authors (CPK) with elective ilioinguinal dissection, the incidence of positivity of the deep nodes was 18% for patients with microscopically involved but not clinically palpable subinguinal nodes, perhaps justifying clearance of the pelvic nodes in this clinical situation.[8] With a positive sentinel node, however, the diagnosis of microscopic disease in the groin is likely to be made much earlier and superficial groin dissection should suffice. In the presence of palpable inguinal nodes involved by melanoma, the incidence of involvement of the deep nodes is around 40%, and this, in the opinion of the authors, is certainly at a level that justifies the performance of an ilioinguinal groin dissection.[9] Others, however, have taken a more conservative view towards performing the deep part of a groin dissection and do so only in cases of either a positive Cloquet's node or positivity of a certain number of inguinal nodes.[10] If one performs a superficial groin dissection for microscopically or clinically involved lymph nodes in the groin, computed tomography of the pelvis with attention to the deep iliac and obturator nodes should be part of the follow up.

COMPLICATIONS OF GROIN DISSECTION

The principal short term local complications of groin dissection are wound infection, skin edge necrosis, and seroma formation. Wound infection can be treated by removal of two or three skin sutures or staples, to provide drainage, and the institution of appropriate antibiotic therapy, according to sensitivities. It is not normally necessary to open widely the entire incision. In the case of skin edge necrosis, if it concerns only 2–3 mm on either side of the edge of the flap, it is not usually necessary to perform formal debridement. The skin sutures or staples are simply left for a longer period of time until the eschar that is formed separates naturally, leaving behind healthy granulation tissue. Ambulation may be started on the first postoperative day, although some surgeons believe that maintaining strict bed rest until suction drains are removed reduces the incidence of lymphocoele/seroma formation. If a lymphatic collection does occur after drain removal, it can usually be managed by repeated aspiration, but sometimes formal re-exploration with reinsertion of a suction drain is necessary. The limb should in any case be elevated as much as possible in the immediate postoperative period, and for a period of two to three months postoperatively, especially at night and at periodic intervals during the day, to allow for collateral development of the lymphatic circulation and minimize lymphoedema. In patients with a tendency to develop oedema in the legs, a custom fitted elastic stocking should be prescribed.

The most troublesome long term complication of groin dissection is lymphoedema of the lower extremity, which occurs in 20–30% of patients.[11] The lymphoedema can be alleviated and largely controlled through a regular programme of leg elevation at night and use of elastic graduated compression stockings. This lymphoedema rate of about 20–30% concerns oedema below the level of the knee because nearly all patients with a groin dissection have a localized oedema of the anteromedial aspect of the thigh down to the level of the knee.[12] It is clear that some patients develop sufficient collateral lymphatic circulation via the posterior and lateral aspects of the thigh and then alongside the gluteal and internal iliac vessels. The existence of localized lymphoedema in the anteromedial thigh while the leg below the knee is free of oedema in many of these patients is testament to the existence of such collateral lymphatic circulation. In most series, the rate of lymphoedema is slightly higher after an ilioinguinal dissection than after a superficial groin dissection. The way the surgical procedure is performed may also influence the development of lymphoedema, and, in the opinion of the authors, the incidence of lymphoedema may depend largely on technical factors. A longitudinal incision, for example, is less likely to be followed by lymphoedema compared with a transverse incision across the groin. Fashioning flaps that are not too thin may also help avoid the occurrence of lymphoedema.

SURVIVAL RATES AFTER GROIN DISSECTION

The survival rate after groin dissection varies, as in other nodal areas, according to the number of positive lymph nodes and the thickness of the primary tumour. In patients with clinically negative regional lymph nodes the histological status of the sentinel node is the most important prognostic parameter.[13] In some series, 5-year survival rates after resection of deep positive nodes have been depressingly low, ranging from 0% to 9%.[14–17] However, in other series, 5-year survivals in the range of 35–40% and 10-year survivals in the range of 25–30% have been observed after dissection of positive deep nodes.[18,19] The differences between the reported 5-year survival rates may be partly explained by the selection of patients, since in one of the latter series,[18] a good number of the patients had enlarged, clinically involved nodes in the deep nodal area: this may represent a form of the disease that is not intrinsically aggressive since patients with enlarged lymph nodes in the pelvic area, particularly after superficial groin dissection, without evidence of other systemic disease, may represent biologically less aggressive forms of this particular neoplasm because patients with enlarged pelvic nodes and demonstrable distant disease are selected out.

The status of Cloquet's node may be a useful criterion when deciding on the desirable extent of the node dissection. It is the authors' opinion that patients with a palpable positive node or nodes in the groin should have an ilioinguinal dissection, since the incidence of involvement of the deep nodes is appreciable and the difference in morbidity between a superficial and a radical groin dissection is only slight. In a report by Sterne et al. there was no significant difference in the complication rates for inguinal and ilioinguinal dissections.[20] In this study, there was a substantial rate of iliac or obturator node involvement (>50%) even in patients with a single mobile subinguinal lymph node clinically and no clinical or computed tomographic evidence of deep node involvement. The incidence of groin relapse was lower after ilioinguinal dissection. In a report by Strobbe et al., including 71 patients with positive iliac and/or obturator nodes, the 5- and 10-year survival rates were 24% and 20%, respectively, thus justifying the additional deep lymph node dissections.[21]

In a report by Mann and Coit, the 5-year survival for patients with positive deep nodes was 35%.[22] The extent of surgery in this report was not associated with differential survival since there were other prognostic factors from the nodal basin (e.g. number and size of involved lymph nodes, presence of extranodal spread) and the primary site (e.g. ulceration) that determined metastatic spread. It is obvious, however, that in patients who have positive deep nodes, for the approximately one third of them who do not have distant metastatic disease at the time of diagnosis, the performance of a complete ilioinguinal dissection is of crucial importance. A comprehensive review of the literature on combined inguinal and pelvic lymph node dissection for stage III melanoma was undertaken by Hughes and Thomas.[23]

In conclusion, the indications for groin dissection in patients with melanoma at the present time are a microscopically positive sentinel node (superficial groin dissection probably adequate) or a clinically palpable, histologically positive node or nodes (ilio inguinal dissection desirable).

REFERENCES

1. Balch C, Soong SJ, Gershenwald JE, et al, Prognostic factors analysis of 17,600 melanoma patients: validation of the new AJCC melanoma staging system. *J Clin Oncol* 2001; 19: 3635–48.
2. Karakousis CP, Grigoropoulos P, Sentinel node biopsy before and after wide excision of the primary melanoma. *Ann Surg Oncol* 1999; 6: 785–9.
3. Karakousis CP, Ilio-inguinal lymph node dissection. *Am J Surg* 1981; 141: 299–303.
4. Karakousis CP, Bland KI, Surgery of the primary lesion and nodal dissections in malignant melanoma. In: *Atlas of Surgical Oncology* (eds. Bland KI, Karakousis CP, Copeland EM), Philadelphia: WB Saunders, 1995: 93–128.
5. Coit DG, Extent of groin dissection for melanoma. *Surg Oncol Clin North Am* 1992; 1: 271.
6. Karakousis CP, The abdominoinguinal incision in limb salvage and resection of pelvic tumors. *Cancer* 1984; 54: 2543–8.
7. Karakousis CP, Abdominoinguinal incision in resection of pelvic tumors with lateral fixation. *Am J Surg* 1992; 164: 366–71.
8. Karakousis CP, Emrich LJ, Driscoll DL, et al, Survival after groin dissection for malignant melanoma. *Surgery* 1991; 109: 119–26.
9. Karakousis CP, Emrich LJ, Rao U, Groin dissection in malignant melanoma. *Am J Surg* 1986; 152: 491–5.
10. Coit DG, Brennan MF, Extent of lymph node dissection in melanoma of the trunk or lower extremity. *Arch Surg* 1989; 124: 161–6.
11. Karakousis CP, Heiser MA, Moore RH, Lymphoedema after groin dissection. *Am J Surg* 1983; 145: 205–8.
12. Karakousis CP, Driscoll DL, Groin dissection in malignant melanoma. *Br J Surg* 1994; 81: 1771–4.
13. Gershenwald JR, Thompson W, Mansfield PF, et al, Multi-institutional melanoma lymphatic mapping experience: the prognostic value of sentinel lymph node status in 612 stage I or II melanoma patients. *J Clin Oncol* 1999; 17: 976–83.
14. McCarthy JG, Haagensen CKD, Herter FP, The role of groin dissection in the management of melanoma of the lower extremity. *Ann Surg* 1974; 179: 156–9.
15. Finck SJ, Giuliano AE, Mann BD, et al, Results of ilio-inguinal dissection for stage II melanoma. *Ann Surg* 1982; 196: 180–6.
16. Fortner JG, Booher RJ, Pack GT, Results of groin dissection for malignant melanoma in 220 patients. *Surgery* 1964; 55: 485–95.
17. Coit DG, Extent of groin dissection for melanoma. *Surg Oncol Clin North Am* 1992; 1: 271–80.
18. Karakousis CA, Driscoll DL, Positive deep nodes in the groin and survival in malignant melanoma. *Am J Surg* 1996; 171: 411–22.
19. Morton DL, Wanek L, Nizzie JA, et al, Improved long-term survival after lymphadenectomy of melanoma metastatic to regional lymph nodes. *Ann Surg* 1991; 214: 419.
20. Sterne GD, Murray DS, Grimley RP, Ilio-inguinal block dissection for malignant melanoma. *Br J Surg* 1995; 82: 1057–9.
21. Strobbe LJ, Jonk A, Hart AA, et al, Positive iliac and obturator nodes in melanoma: survival and prognostic factors. *Ann Surg Oncol* 1999; 6: 255–62.
22. Mann GB, Coit DG, Does the extent of operation influence the prognosis in patients with melanoma metastatic to inguinal nodes? *Ann Surg Oncol* 1999; 6: 263–71.
23. Hughes TM, Thomas JM, Combined inguinal and pelvic lymph node dissection for stage III melanoma. *Br J Surg* 1999; 86: 1493–8.

26

Neck dissection and parotidectomy for melanoma

Christopher J O'Brien, Jatin P Shah, Alfonsus JM Balm

INTRODUCTION

Cutaneous melanoma is a common cancer among white people, and the incidence of this disease increases with proximity to the equator and increasing levels of sun exposure. Approximately 15% of cutaneous melanomas arise on the skin of the head and neck with the face, a large and often unprotected area, most commonly involved.[1,2] Cutaneous melanomas of the head and neck, along with those around the shoulder girdle and upper trunk, may metastasize to the lymph nodes in the parotid gland and neck, and the incidence of nodal involvement is related to several factors, including tumour thickness and Clark level. Therefore the management of regional nodes in the parotid gland and neck is an integral part of the overall treatment of many patients with melanoma in this region.

The aim of this chapter is to describe the indications for and techniques of parotidectomy and neck dissection and also to detail expected therapeutic outcomes.

LYMPHATIC DRAINAGE OF THE HEAD AND NECK

Over recent years there has been increasing interest in patterns of lymphatic drainage. The advent of lymphoscintigraphy and sentinel node biopsy has led to a re-evaluation of traditional teachings, and new insights into lymphatic pathways have been gained.[3] In relation to the head and neck, there still is controversy over just how predictable lymphatic drainage pathways really are. The principal lymph node groups are shown in Figure 26.1 and the contents of each level are listed in Table 26.1. In addition to these levels, important lymph nodes are found in the parotid gland, along with the occipital region, the post-auricular region and the jugular node (see Figure 26.1).

Lymphadenectomy in the head and neck may involve parotidectomy or dissection of one or more of the named lymph node levels in the neck or both.[4,5] The importance of the external jugular node and occipital nodes has recently become apparent, but the clinical importance of the post-auricular nodes, which

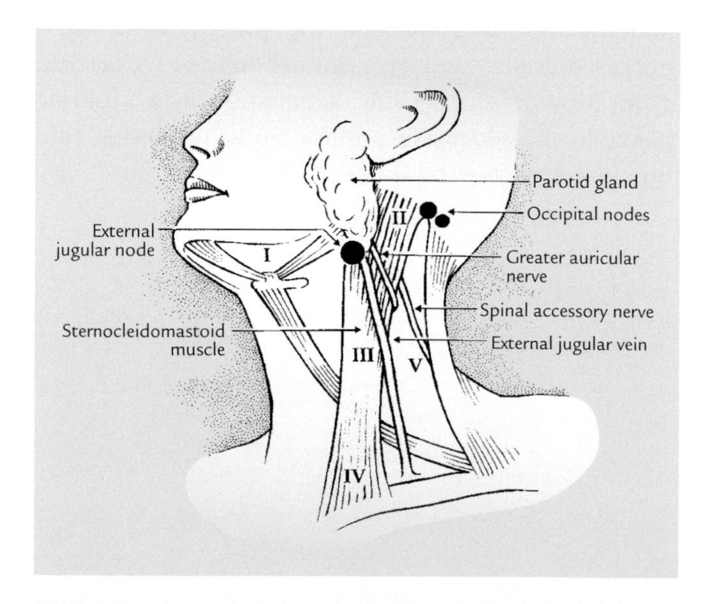

Figure 26.1 *Diagrammatic representation of the neck showing lymph node levels (Roman numerals) along with the external jugular lymph node and occipital nodes.*

are often identified as sentinel nodes on lymphoscintigraphy, is unclear.[6]

There is a body of opinion that suggests that likely patterns of metastatic spread via lymphatics in the head and neck are unpredictable, but this is contrary to the experience of the authors.[7,8]

Table 26.2 lists the at risk nodal groups that are related to particular anatomical sites in the head and neck. These traditionally understood patterns of lymphatic drainage are based on clinical experience and were used by one of the authors (COB) for 106 elective lymphadenectomies for cutaneous head and neck melanomas.[4] While elective lymphadenectomy is no longer standard practice and is not recommended by the authors, it was previously the policy at the Sydney Melanoma Unit for patients with melanomas thicker than 1.5 mm, since there was evidence from retrospective data that elective removal of clinically uninvolved lymph nodes might confer a survival benefit. The strategy used in carrying out the 106 elective dissections, with or without parotidectomy, is depicted in Figure 26.2 and is consistent with the clinically predicted patterns of lymphatic spread shown in Table 26.2. There were only three recurrences outside the dissected fields, indicating a 3% failure rate for clinical prediction. In that study no patient presented with post-auricular node involvement, no patient had post-auricular nodes dissected and, at a minimum of 2 years' follow up, no patient subsequently failed in post-auricular nodes.

The selective dissections carried out in the previously mentioned study conformed very closely with operations recommended by Shah et al., who described the distribution of pathologically involved lymph nodes among 111 patients who had radical neck dissections for cutaneous melanoma.[9] On the basis of the correlation of pathological findings with primary melanoma site, recommendations were made about which nodal groups were at risk for melanoma at different sites.

Despite the clinicopathological correlations of these two studies, a subsequent study from the Sydney Melanoma Unit suggested that likely patterns of lymphatic spread shown by lymphoscintigraphy were different from those predicted clinically.[6] In this study of 97 patients who had lymphoscintigrams for head and

Table 26.1 *Lymph node levels of the neck*

Level I	Submandibular and submental nodes
Level II	Upper jugular, upper spinal accessory, and jugulodigastric nodes
Level III	Middle jugular nodes
Level IV	Lower jugular nodes, including supraclavicular
Level V	Posterior triangle nodes (distributed along spinal accessory nerve)

Table 26.2 *Correlation of at risk nodal groups with primary melanoma site*

Site	Nodes at risk
* Face, forehead, anterior scalp	Parotid, levels I–III
* Posterior scalp, posterior upper neck	Occipital nodes, levels II–V
* Coronal scalp, ear, preauricular skin	Parotid, levels I–V
* Lower neck	Levels III–V

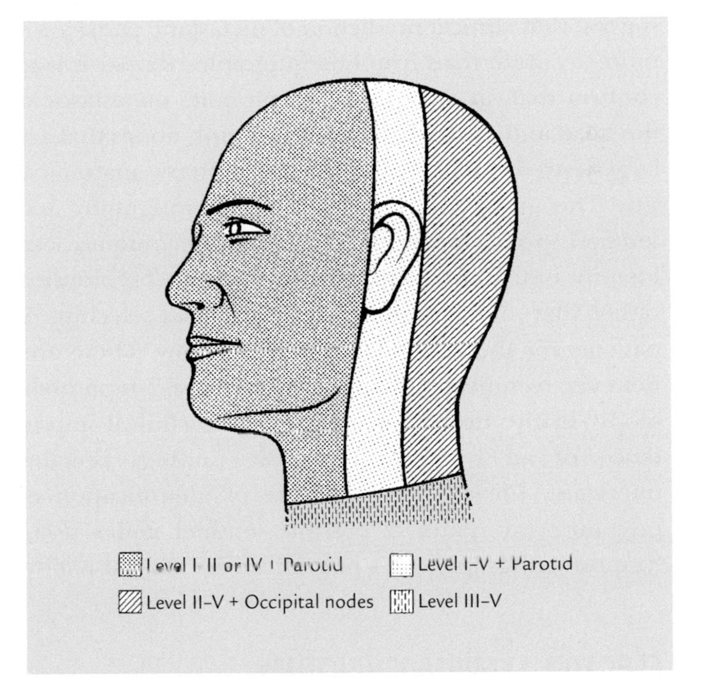

Figure 26.2 *Diagrammatic representation of the head and neck showing the lymph node groups removed by elective selective lymphadenectomy for primary melanomas in four regions: the anterior scalp, forehead, face, and anterior neck; the coronal scalp, ear and coronal upper neck; the posterior scalp and posterior upper neck; and the lower cervical region.*

neck melanomas, there was a 34% rate of disagreement between the lymphoscintigraphic findings and clinically predicted patterns. The commonest cause for discordancy was the frequent identification of post-auricular nodes as sentinel nodes on lymphoscintigraphy. There were also occurrences of contralateral spread. These and other reports concerning lymphoscintigraphy have fuelled the debate about the accuracy of clinically predicted lymphatic pathways.[7,8] However, a further recent study from the Sydney Melanoma Unit correlated clinical, operative, and pathological findings among 169 patients who had lymphadenectomy for head and neck melanomas, in which pathologically positive nodes were identified.[10] The pathological distribution of nodes conformed to the clinically predicted patterns depicted in Table 26.2 in 93% of cases. Furthermore, no patient presented with contralateral spread and the incidence of involvement of post-auricular nodes was only 1.5% (3 of 169). Interestingly also, 68% of patients had involvement of the nodal group nearest to the primary melanoma site, and 59% had only a single lymph node involved.

In reviewing these issues it is not our purpose to suggest that clinical prediction of metastatic pathways is more accurate than lymphoscintigraphy. Rather it is to confirm that, in most cases, lymph node metastases in the head and neck will develop in lymph nodes that are largely predictable, based on the primary anatomical site. The great advantage of lymphoscintigraphy and sentinel node biopsy is that these techniques can identify individual lymph nodes that can be biopsied rather than nodal regions, and this allows selection of patients for therapeutic lymphadenectomy. There are, however, technical difficulties with sentinel lymph node biopsy in the head and neck, and the clinical importance of all lymphoscintigraphic findings remains uncertain. Clearly, the high rate of identification of post-auricular nodes as possible sentinel nodes using lymphoscintigraphy does not reflect the clinical reality.

ELECTIVE LYMPHADENECTOMY

There is no evidence from a randomized clinical trial that elective removal of lymph nodes in the parotid or neck leads to a survival benefit. There has not been a specific study of patients with head and neck melanomas, but other prophylactic lymphadenectomy trials have not yielded positive results.[11–13] Certainly, elective lymphadenectomy is associated with the potential for a considerable increase in morbidity, length of hospital stay and cost.

It is recognized that patients with pathological lymph node involvement have a high likelihood of developing systemic metastatic disease and dying, and it was believed that spread to regional lymphatics was often the first step in the metastatic process. The aim of elective lymphadenectomy is to remove microscopically involved lymph nodes that are not palpable, before the metastatic disease can spread from the lymph node to distant sites. The naive optimism of this view has largely evaporated. It is clear that patients with thicker melanomas can develop haematogenous metastases without lymph node involvement, while patients with clinically palpable lymph node involvement frequently have distant metastases at the time of their presentation. It is therefore likely that any benefit from elective lymph node dissection would accrue to only a small number of patients.[1,14]

The advent of lymphoscintigraphy and sentinel node biopsy has not necessarily increased the likelihood of conferring a benefit to patients with subclinically involved lymph nodes, but it has greatly simplified the means of identifying those patients who may derive benefit from having their regional metastatic disease treated in its earliest stage.[15] Instead of carrying out prophylactic neck dissection or parotidectomy on all patients with melanomas thicker than 1 mm or 1.5 mm, sentinel node biopsy allows identification of patients with microscopically involved sentinel nodes, and these patients can then be selected for therapeutic lymphadenectomy. Other patients will have undergone a minimal procedure and, if their sentinel node is negative and the procedure has been carried out in a technically correct fashion, it is unlikely that they will subsequently fail in regional nodes.

The clinical benefit of sentinel node biopsy is still uncertain, and the results of a large multicentre trial are awaited. In the meantime, elective lymphadenectomy cannot be recommended except in limited circumstances. If a melanoma overlies a specific lymph node region, for example the parotid gland, submandibular triangle or posterior triangle, experience indicates that lymphoscintigraphy and blue dye injection at the time of sentinel node biopsy are likely to obscure possible sentinel nodes. It may be reasonable in this setting to remove the immediately adjacent or underlying nodes at the time of excision of the melanoma. Also, if resection of a primary melanoma involves excision of a large amount of skin necessitating the use of a local flap, it may be reasonable to remove the lymph nodes underlying the skin flap. Finally, in the treatment of locally recurrent melanoma it may be reasonable to carry out an elective lymphadenectomy of draining nodes since the incidence of lymph node involvement is higher in this setting. In none of these situations is there any evidence that survival will be improved, however removal of local lymph nodes may provide more effective locoregional treatment.

THERAPEUTIC LYMPHADENECTOMY

Parotidectomy

Clinical involvement of lymph nodes in the parotid gland (Figure 26.3) or neck requires surgical intervention.

It has already been said that elective lymphadenectomy cannot be supported as part of standard practice. There are occasions, however, when parotidectomy may be carried out in the absence of clinically palpable disease in the parotid gland. Such a parotidectomy would be indicated when a therapeutic neck dissection was planned for clinically palpable disease in the neck, arising from a primary site that also had potential to drain to the parotid gland, such as on the forehead, ear, or face. In this setting, although such a procedure may be regarded as being a therapeutic neck dissection combined with an elective parotidectomy, to avoid difficulties with terminology it is best to regard the entire lymphadenectomy as being a therapeutic procedure because it is carried out in the presence of clinically involved lymph nodes. Similarly, neck dissection is very often combined with therapeutic parotidectomy when there is clinically palpable disease in the parotid gland but not in the neck. Again the entire procedure would be regarded as being a therapeutic lymphadenectomy removing the clinically palpable disease in the parotid gland together with the adjacent at risk nodal groups in the neck.

Most cutaneous melanomas of the head and neck involve the forehead and face,[1,2] and, when these are combined with melanomas affecting the anterior scalp, coronal scalp and ear, it can be seen that a large proportion of these tumours have the potential to metastasize to the parotid gland. Most parotid lymph nodes

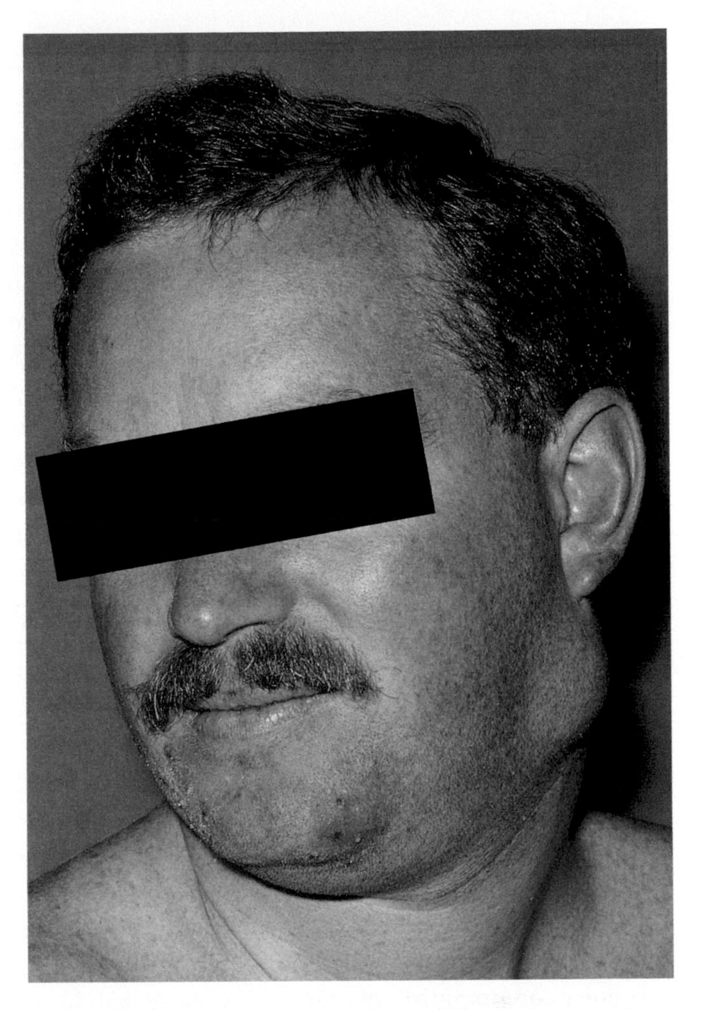

Figure 26.3 *30-year-old man with a rapidly growing mass in the tail of the left parotid gland, proved on fine needle aspiration biopsy to be metastatic malignant melanoma.*

are located in the superficial part of the parotid gland and are, in general, deep to the parotid fascia.[5,16] Lymph nodes related to the parotid gland may extend from the level of the zygomatic arch to the upper third of the sternocleidomastoid muscle. Parotid lymph nodes in the lowermost part of the gland lie in the superficial plane, similar to the external jugular lymph node, and, in some cases, they may be one and the same.

Anatomical studies of the distribution of lymph nodes in the parotid gland have demonstrated that up to 20 nodes can be found in the superficial lobe of the gland while between zero and four nodes can be shown in the deep part of the gland.[16,17] Superficial parotidectomy therefore may not encompass all lymph nodes, although, in a previous study by O'Brien et al., superficial parotidectomy was found to be an effective elective procedure in that there were no recurrences in the deep lobe after a negative superficial parotidectomy.[5]

When clinical disease is present in the parotid gland there will usually be a history of a pre-existing cutaneous melanoma. This is not always the case, but the diagnosis will, in general, be confirmed by preoperative fine needle aspiration biopsy in either setting.[18] Rarely, a patient may come to surgery for a clinically benign parotid lump, and, after removal of the lump by parotidectomy, a diagnosis of metastatic melanoma may be made. Although this situation is uncommon it does create a therapeutic dilemma for the treating surgeon, and a decision will need to be made whether or not further surgery to the parotid gland or neck should be carried out or whether radiotherapy to the parotid bed and neck should be recommended.

Imaging before therapeutic parotidectomy

Before therapeutic parotidectomy it is appropriate to carry out chest radiography to exclude pulmonary metastases. The role of imaging directed at the parotid gland and neck is unclear. Most superficially located mobile parotid lumps, benign or malignant, do not require preoperative imaging. The principal indications for computed tomography (CT) of the parotid gland are when a parotid mass is: (1) massive; (2) fixed; (3) clinically malignant, as evidenced by facial nerve paralysis, skin involvement or associated cervical lymphadenopathy; (4) recurrent. The value of CT scanning in these settings is that it provides information about relational anatomy and may predict the likely necessity for facial nerve sacrifice and reconstruction.

In addition to imaging of the parotid gland, consideration may be given to CT scanning of the clinically negative neck to identify impalpable but radiologically suspicious lymph nodes.[19] Furthermore, patients with metastatic disease in the parotid gland have a relatively high likelihood of having or developing distant metastatic disease and consideration should be given to systemic imaging. This is most accurately carried out by means of positron emission tomography (PET), which has been identified as being more accurate than total body CT scanning for subclinical metastatic disease.[20] The presence of a positive PET scan may not obviate the need for therapeutic parotidectomy, since every effort should be made to achieve locoregional control of disease. The presence of systemic metastases, however, should mitigate against very radical surgery, which is unlikely to be curative. It is currently unclear whether or not every therapeutic parotidectomy should be combined with a neck dissection. In general we recommend that at least a supraomohyoid dissection should be carried out.

Surgical technique

The technique of parotidectomy has been widely described. The standard incision is placed in the preauricular crease and carried behind the ear with a generous curve to avoid a contracture at this site. It is neither necessary nor appropriate to extend the postauricular component of the incision too high since necrosis of the skin edge at this point may occur. The incision is then carried forward into the neck in an appropriate skin crease and then anteriorly in a gentle curve to facilitate elevation of a cervical skin flap, giving access to the lymph nodes in the upper neck. A further 'lazy S' extension from the lowermost part of the neck incision can then be carried over the clavicle to allow anterior and posterior flaps to be elevated, facilitating comprehensive neck dissection (Figure 26.4).

The associated neck dissection may involve preservation of the sternomastoid muscle and spinal accessory nerve (Figure 26.5) or, depending on the clinical status of the neck, the sternomastoid muscle and internal

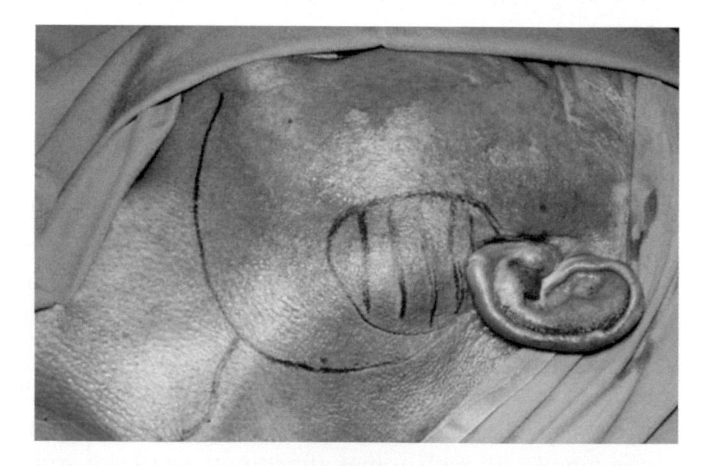

Figure 26.4 *Operative photograph of 50-year-old man with a large mass of metastatic melanoma in the left parotid gland. The incisions for combined parotidectomy and neck dissection are shown.*

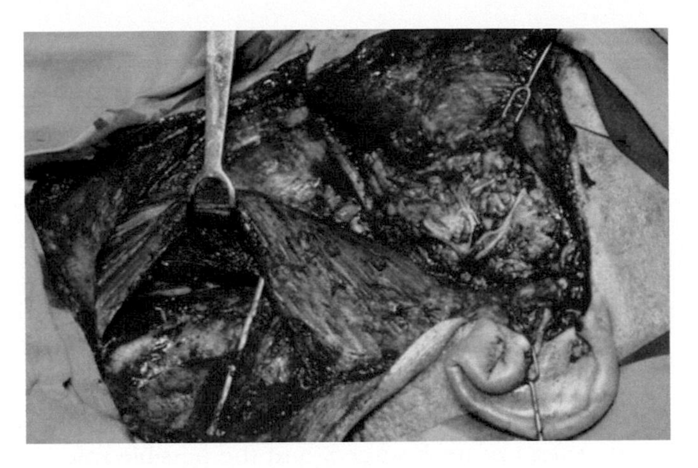

Figure 26.5 *Intraoperative photograph of parotidectomy and modified radical neck dissection showing preservation of the facial nerve, the sternomastoid muscle, and spinal accessory nerve.*

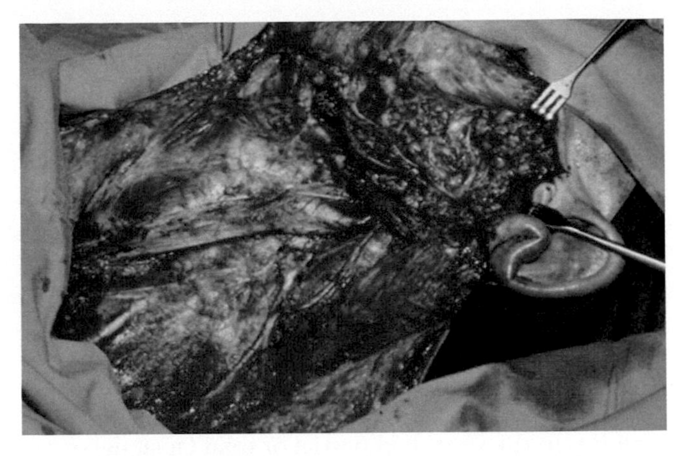

Figure 26.6 *Combined parotidectomy and modified radical neck dissection showing preservation of the facial nerve and spinal accessory nerve, however, the sternomastoid muscle and internal jugular vein have been removed.*

jugular vein may be sacrificed. However, every attempt should be made to preserve the spinal accessory nerve whenever possible (Figure 26.6).

In most situations the metastatic disease in the parotid gland will lie in the superficial lobe, allowing safe resection by means of a superficial parotidectomy. This operation is also termed 'lateral parotid lobectomy' and also occasionally 'subtotal parotidectomy' by some authors. If there is no evidence of direct involvement of the facial nerve, this should be preserved.

There is some controversy as to whether or not the deep lobe should be resected. It is the view of the authors that a total parotidectomy, with superficial and deep lobes in continuity, preserving the facial nerve, is difficult to achieve. If the deep lobe is not directly involved with metastatic disease the additional benefit of removing this tissue is doubtful.[21] It is possible, however, that microscopic subclinical disease may be present in the deep lobe, and so there is a potential source of failure at this site. Whether or not the deep lobe tissue is best treated by excision or adjuvant radiotherapy remains unclear, although the authors believe that adjuvant radiotherapy provides the potential benefit of destroying tumour cells both around the facial nerve and in the deep lobe.

It is our view that therapeutic parotidectomy for metastatic melanoma should not be carried out by the occasional parotid surgeon. Identification of the facial nerve in the course of parotidectomy is clearly an important technical step, although, in experienced hands, this should not create any difficulty. Suffice to say that the single most useful landmark that may assist in identification of the facial nerve is the tympanomastoid fissure.[22] The principal sequelae after parotidectomy for melanoma are similar to those related to any parotidectomy. Sacrifice of the greater auricular nerve is nearly always necessary, although occasionally a posterior branch of this structure may be preserved. It is important therefore to warn the patient of the likelihood of numbness over the ear and face. The risk of temporary facial nerve weakness will depend on the extent of parotidectomy, and whether or not it is necessary to sacrifice the main trunk of the facial nerve or any of its branches.[23] Even when all branches are carefully dissected and preserved, temporary weakness maybe expected in 15% or more of patients, although permanent weakness is uncommon, affecting fewer than 5% of patients.[23] The addition of neck dissection to parotidectomy greatly increases the likelihood of injury to the marginal mandibular branch of the facial nerve, and dysfunction of this structure is frequently long lasting.[4,23] Although this complication is one of the considerations that mitigates against the use of elective lymphadenectomy, in the therapeutic setting the risk is more acceptable. The patient nonetheless needs to be warned of this possible complication. Frey's syndrome, or gustatory sweating, is common after any form of parotidectomy, affecting 30% or more of patients. The problem may take one or two years to develop, is rarely debilitating, and, in the past, has been difficult to treat. More recently, intradermal injection of Botulinum toxin A (Botox) has proved effective in controlling symptoms.

Adjuvant radiotherapy

There remains some controversy over whether or not surgery alone is adequate treatment for metastatic melanoma involving the parotid gland. Caldwell and Spiro reported the Memorial Hospital experience with parotidectomy for melanoma and, among 65 patients treated there was only one recurrence among the 27 patients (3.8%) with pathological involvement with melanoma in the parotid gland.[24] These authors did not use postoperative radiotherapy, but nearly half of the patients in the study had partial or total facial nerve sacrifice indicating a relatively aggressive surgical approach. By contrast, O'Brien et al. reported five recurrences among 25 patients with histologically positive melanoma in the parotid gland.[5] Among the five patients with recurrent disease were: one of 16 patients treated with combined surgery and radiotherapy, and four of nine patients who had surgery alone. The authors of that paper concluded that radiotherapy should be combined with surgery when metastatic melanoma is present in the parotid gland. There are no data from a prospective randomized clinical trial that can definitively answer the question about whether or not adjuvant radiotherapy improves the outcome after parotidectomy for melanoma.

PAROTIDECTOMY AND NECK DISSECTION

When there is clinical disease in the parotid gland but no clinical disease in the neck from a cutaneous melanoma of the forehead or face, the minimal appropriate neck dissection that should be combined with the parotidectomy is a supraomohyoid neck dissection. This is based on the potential for the primary melanoma to metastasize to the submandibular triangle along with the upper and middle jugular node groups (levels I–III). Similarly, when the primary site involves the coronal scalp or ear and there is clinical metastatic disease in the parotid, the appropriate neck dissection is a comprehensive dissection of levels I–V. Melanomas of the posterior scalp rarely metastasize to the preauricular component of the parotid gland, however, occasionally, a metastasis to a parotid lymph node lying below or behind the ear may occur, in the absence of metastatic disease in the occipital triangle or levels II–V. In this setting, the appropriate parotid operation would involve identification of the facial nerve and superficial parotidectomy encompassing the metastatic disease in the posteroinferior part of the gland along with a neck dissection encompassing occipital and post-auricular lymph nodes and levels II–V.

Therapeutic neck dissection

When there is clinically palpable metastatic melanoma in the neck, a therapeutic neck dissection is indicated. The principal issues in this setting concern the appropriate extent of neck surgery and the possible role for adjuvant radiotherapy.

Patients with clinical metastatic melanoma require a comprehensive neck dissection. A selective dissection in this setting is likely to be associated with an increased risk of recurrence because, once metastatic lymphadenopathy is present, any lymph node level may be involved. In the previously mentioned study of Shah et al., which analyzed the distribution of pathologically involved lymph nodes in radical neck dissection specimens, levels II–IV were most commonly involved, but 23% of patients had disease in level I and 19% had involvement of level V.[9] O'Brien et al. also found that, among 175 patients undergoing various forms of neck dissection for melanoma, there was a 23% recurrence rate with therapeutic selective neck dissection whereas, among patients undergoing modified radical neck dissection, that is a comprehensive procedure preserving at least the spinal accessory nerve, the recurrence rate was 0%.[4] In the same study, there was a 14% recurrence rate in the dissected neck after radical neck dissection, but these patients had more advanced disease.

Although radical neck dissection is often regarded as being the gold standard for the surgical management of metastatic cancer of the neck, the disability related to this procedure is considerable, especially the loss of trapezius muscle innervation. This leads to a painful sagging shoulder and inability to elevate the arm above the horizontal plane (Figure 26.7). When metastatic disease does not directly involve the spinal accessory nerve every attempt should be made to preserve this structure (Figure 26.6). The dissection required during preservation of the accessory nerve may contribute to temporary dysfunction of the nerve leading to shoulder weakness in up to 50% of patients, however the vast majority will recover within about 12 months allowing return of normal shoulder function (Figure 26.8). The cause of nerve injury during modified radical neck dissection can be ischaemia along with direct local trauma due to rough handling or retraction.

The surgical techniques for comprehensive neck dissections, either radical or modified radical, are well described, and surgeons will have personal preferences in relation to incisions and whether or not the dissection technique involves the use of diathermy or scalpel. The specific technical points requiring attention in all neck dissections include gentle handling of all tissues, including the skin, meticulous haemostasis since there should be virtually no necessity for blood transfusion, and the use of suction drainage postoperatively to assure good adherence of the skin flaps to the operative bed. The use of perioperative antibiotics for clean surgery of this type is generally unnecessary, and, although there is no evidence that it makes a significant difference, wound irrigation at the end of the procedure is used by the authors.

The decision to carry out a less than comprehensive neck dissection in the presence of clinically palpable disease should be taken with caution. However, with a posteriorly located primary melanoma and occipital or posterior triangle metastatic disease, it is probably reasonable to dissect levels II–V, sparing the contents of the submandibular triangle (Figure 26.9). In every neck dissection for melanoma the external jugular node should be resected. Whether or not occipital or postauricular nodes are included should depend on the clinical findings and the site of the primary melanoma.

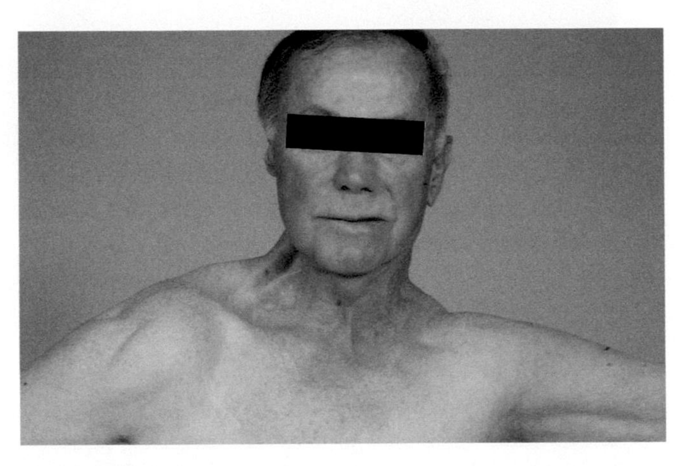

Figure 26.7 *67-year-old man with right shoulder weakness and inability to elevate the right arm above the horizontal after radical neck dissection.*

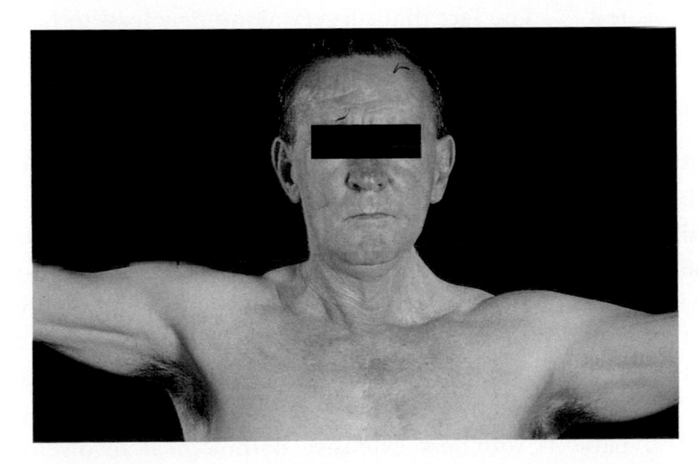

Figure 26.8 *56-year-old man after a left comprehensive neck dissection, which preserved the spinal accessory nerve. Good function of the left shoulder has been retained.*

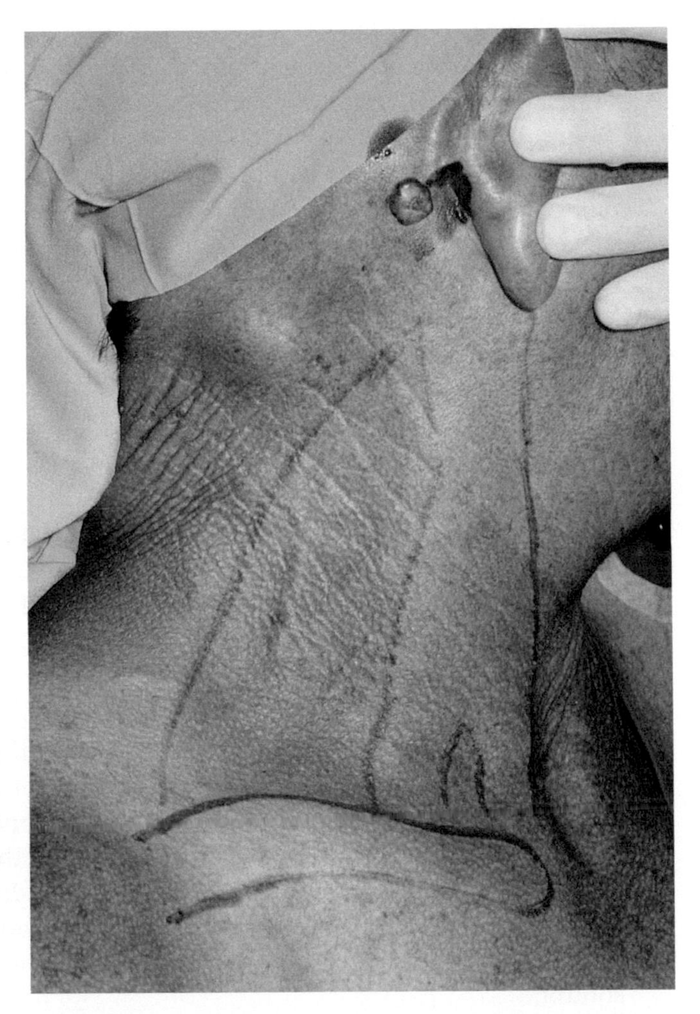

Figure 26.9 *Large malignant melanoma with superficial spreading and nodular components in the right post-auricular region of a 59-year-old man with obvious occipital nodal metastasis.*

The complications of neck dissection are not peculiar to melanoma surgery and include: postoperative haematoma requiring reoperation and evacuation, chyle leak necessitating reoperation, wound infection, skin flap necrosis, and unintentional injury to nerves, for example the vagus nerve (causing hoarseness), the phrenic nerve (causing hemi-diaphragm elevation), the hypoglossal nerve (causing ipsilateral tongue weakness and tongue wasting), the marginal mandibular nerve (causing ipsilateral lower lip weakness), and the accessory nerve.

The management of postoperative chyle leak depends on the timing of the development of the leakage and its volume. If on the first or the second postoperative day a high volume leak, 200 ml or more, is encountered, then early reoperation is indicated. If a low volume leak, say 50–100 ml per day, is encountered on the third or fourth postoperative day then a conservative approach is reasonable. This should entail commencement of a fat free diet consisting principally of fruit and vegetables. This should lead to clearing of the milky appearance of the chyle and a reduction in volume over the next three to four days. A persistent leak that prevents removal of neck drains and discharge from hospital should be treated surgically by reoperation, identification of the thoracic duct, and either ligation or oversewing. One of the authors (AJB) advocates a conservative approach from the outset, using nutritional modification with medium chain triglycerides or even total parenteral nutrition.[25]

In general the overall complication rate from neck dissection should be less than 5%, and the mortality directly attributable to surgery should be less than 1%.

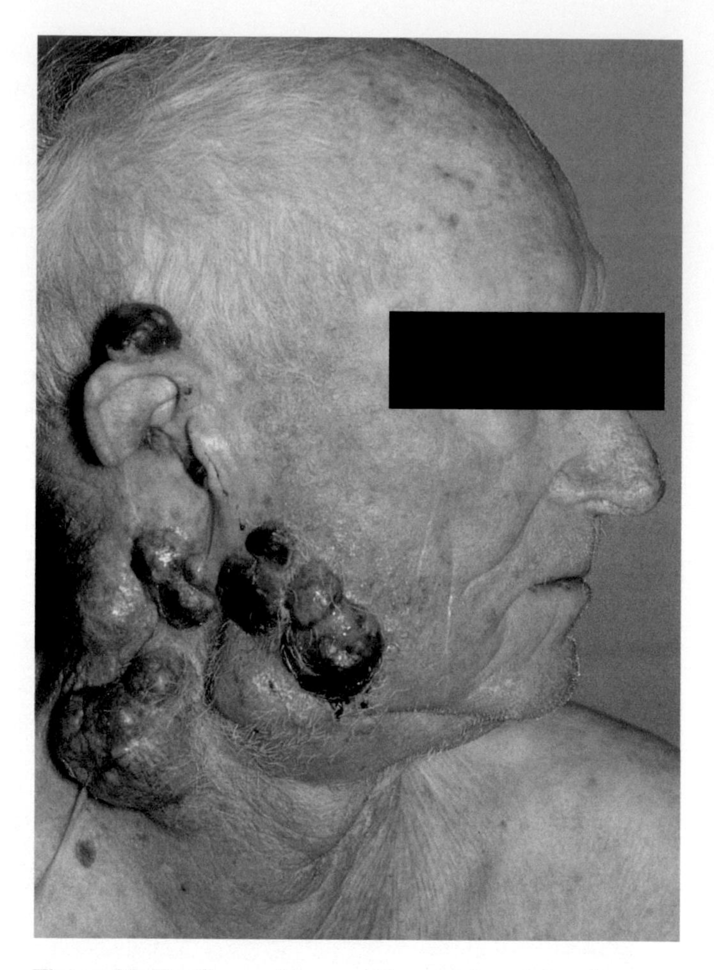

Figure 26.10 *67-year-old man with multiple nodules of recurrent malignant melanoma in the right neck, parotid, and periauricular region after previous wide excision of melanoma of the ear, parotidectomy, and neck dissection.*

Adjuvant radiotherapy

Most patients who die from metastatic malignant melanoma have disseminated disease with, in general, cancer controlled at the primary site and regional lymph nodes. Development of recurrent disease in the parotid bed or neck can cause significant morbidity (Figure 26.10) and significantly worsen prognosis, and so every attempt should be made to achieve regional control.

The recurrence rate in the dissected neck after therapeutic neck dissection may be 30% and Singletary et al. noted increasing recurrence rates as the number of positive nodes increased, with a regional recurrence rate of up to 44% when involved nodes were 'matted'.[1,26] The fact that surgery alone may lead to failure suggested a possible role for adjuvant radiotherapy, and this has already been mentioned in relation to parotidectomy.

The use of a hypofractionated schedule for radiotherapy has been shown to reduce the incidence of recurrence in the dissected neck at both the Sydney Melanoma Unit and the MD Anderson Hospital, Houston. Using six fractions of 550 cGy postoperatively O'Brien et al. reported a recurrence rate of only 6.5% among patients with melanoma in the parotid gland or neck compared with a rate of almost 19% among patients with less extensive pathological involvement who did not receive radiotherapy.[27] Figure 26.11 shows the cumulative control rates in this non-randomized study, in which 67% of irradiated patients had multiple

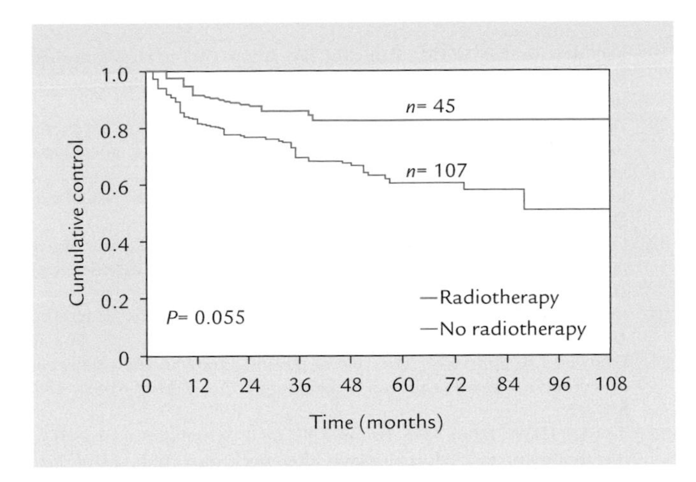

Figure 26.11 *Kaplan-Meier curves showing control rates in the parotid gland and neck among irradiated and non-irradiated patients with metastatic malignant melanoma. A trend to improved regional control among irradiated patients approached but did not reach statistical significance (reproduced with permission from O'Brien et al.,* Head Neck *1997; 19: 589–94).*[27]

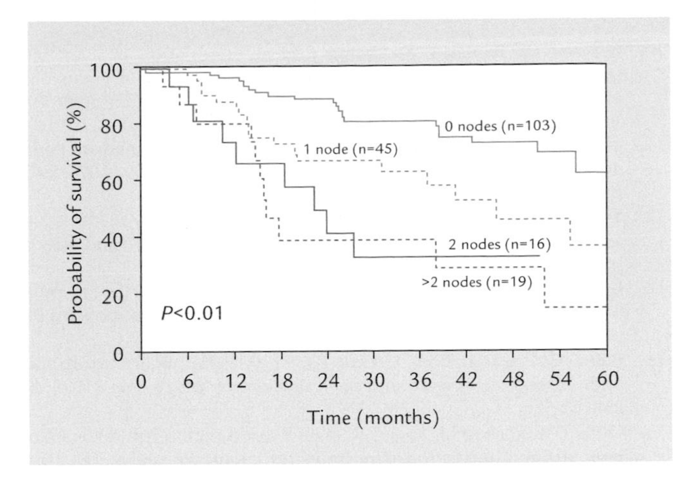

Figure 26.12 *Kaplan-Meier curves showing survival of patients based on the extent of lymph node involvement. Patients with positive nodes had a significantly worse survival, which further deteriorated significantly with involvement of multiple nodes (reproduced with permission from O'Brien et al.,* Head Neck *1995; 17: 232–41).*[4]

nodes and 48% had extracapsular spread compared with 43% and 19%, respectively, in the non-irradiated groups. Ang et al. at the MD Anderson Hospital, Houston, have also shown improved local control with the use of adjuvant hypofractionated radiotherapy and have combined this technique with 'limited' neck dissection to achieve very high rates of regional control.[28]

There are no data from a prospective randomized clinical trial which support a significant benefit from adjuvant radiotherapy, and it is recognized that there is a potential for significant long term side effects from this treatment regimen, particularly dense fibrosis and induration of normal soft tissues.

At present it is probably reasonable to recommend adjuvant radiotherapy to those patients with multiple positive nodes and extranodal spread of melanoma, to patients with metastatic melanoma in the parotid gland, and to patients who have undergone an incomplete neck dissection. It is unlikely that adjuvant radiotherapy will have a significant impact on survival, but improved locoregional control remains a worthwhile aim.

CLINICAL OUTCOME

Figure 26.12 depicts cumulative survival results for patients with pathologically confirmed melanoma in the parotid or neck.[3] Median survival rates for patients with one, two and more than two positive nodes were 46 months, 22 months, and 16 months, respectively. Survival at 5 years was less than 40% for patients with positive nodes, compared with better than 60% survival among those who had negative nodes, despite high rates of locoregional control. The presence of nodal involvement influences prognosis so significantly that prognostic factors related to the primary melanoma become irrelevant once regional spread has occurred.

REFERENCES

1. O'Brien CJ, Coates AS, Petersen-Schaefer K, et al, Experience with 998 cutaneous melanomas of the head and neck over 30 years. *Am J Surg* 1991; 162: 310–14.
2. Kane WJ, Yugueros P, Clay RP, et al, Treatment outcome for 424 primary cases of clinical stage I cutaneous malignant melanoma of the head and neck. *Head Neck* 1997; 19: 457–65.
3. Thompson JF, Uren RF, Shaw HM, et al, Location of sentinel nodes in patients with cutaneous melanomas: new insights into lymphatic anatomy. *J Am Coll Surg* 1999; 189: 195–206.
4. O'Brien CJ, Petersen-Schaefer K, Ruark D, et al, Radical, modified and selective neck dissection for cutaneous malignant melanoma. *Head Neck* 1995: 17: 232–41.
5. O'Brien CJ, Petersen-Schaefer K, Papadopoulos T, et al, Evaluation of 107 therapeutic and elective parotidectomies for cutaneous melanoma. *Am J Surg* 1994; 168: 400–3.
6. O'Brien CJ, Uren RF, Thompson JF, et al, Prediction of potential metastatic sites in cutaneous head and neck melanoma using lymphoscintigraphy. *Am J Surg* 1995; 170: 461–6.
7. Wells KE, Cruse CW, Daniels S, et al, The use of lymphoscintigraphy in melanoma of the head and neck. *Plast Reconstr Surg* 1994; 93: 757–61.
8. Norman J, Cruse CW, Espinosa C, et al, Redefinition of cutaneous lymphatic drainage with the use of lymphoscintigraphy for malignant melanoma. *Am J Surg* 1991; 162: 432–7.
9. Shah JP, Kraus DH, Dubner S, et al, Patterns of regional lymph node metastases from cutaneous melanomas of the head and neck. *Am J Surg* 1991; 162: 320–3.

10. O'Brien CJ, Pathak I, McMahon J, et al, Correlation of anatomic primary site with location of lymph node metastases in cutaneous melanoma of the head and neck (abstract). *Aust NZ J Surg* 2000; 70: A87 (supplement).
11. Veronesi U, Adams J, Bandiera D, et al, Inefficacy of immediate node dissection in stage I melanoma of the limbs. *New Engl J Med* 1977; 297: 627–30.
12. Sim F, Taylor W, Pritchard D, et al, Lymphadenectomy in the management of stage I malignant melanoma: a prospective randomised study. *Mayo Clin Proc* 1986; 61: 697–705.
13. Balch C, Soong SJ, Bartolucci A, et al, Efficacy of an elective regional lymph node dissection of 1 to 4 mm thick melanomas for patients 60 years of age or younger. *Ann Surg* 1996; 224: 255–66.
14. Balm AJM, Kroon BBR, Gregor RT, et al, Value of elective lymph node dissection in head and neck melanoma. *Diagn Oncol* 1993; 3: 263–7.
15. Ollila DW, Foshag LJ, Essner R, et al, Parotid region lymphatic mapping and sentinel lymphadenectomy for cutaneous melanoma. *Ann Surg Oncol* 1999; 6: 150–4.
16. Barr LC, Skene AI, Fish S, et al, Superficial parotidectomy in the treatment of cutaneous melanoma of the head and neck. *Br J Surg* 1994; 81: 64–5.
17. McKean ME, Lee K, McGregor IA, The distribution of lymph nodes in and around the parotid gland: an anatomical study. *Br J Plast Surg* 1985; 38: 1–5.
18. Balm AJM, Kroon BBR, Hilgers FJM, et al, Lymph node metastases in the neck and parotid gland from an unknown primary melanoma. *Clin Otolaryngol* 1994; 19: 161–5.
19. Van den Brekel MWM, Pameijer FA, Koops W, et al, Computed tomography for the detection of neck node metastases in melanoma patients. *Eur J Surg Oncol* 1998; 24: 51–4.
20. Damian DL, Fulham MJ, Thompson E, et al, Positron emission tomography in the detection and management of metastatic melanoma. *Melanoma Res* 1996; 6: 325–9.
21. Jecker P, Hartwein J, Metastasis to the parotid gland: is a radical surgical approach justified? *Am J Otolaryngol* 1996; 17: 102–5.
22. O'Brien CJ, Malka VB, Mijailovic M, Evaluation of 242 consecutive parotidectomies performed for benign and malignant disease. *Aust NZ J Surg* 1993; 63: 870–7.
23. Bron LP, O'Brien CJ, Facial nerve function after parotidectomy. *Arch Otolaryngol Head Neck Surg* 1997; 123: 1091–6.
24. Caldwell CB, Spiro RH, The role of parotidectomy in the treatment of cutaneous head and neck melanoma. *Am J Surg* 1988; 156: 318–22.
25. de Gier HHW, Balm AJM, Bruning PF, et al, Systematic approach to the treatment of chylous leakage after neck dissection. *Head Neck* 1996; 72: 947–351.
26. Singletary SE, Byers RM, Shallenberger, et al, Prognostic factors in patients with regional cervical node metastases from cutaneous malignant melanoma. *Am J Surg* 1986; 152: 371–5.
27. O'Brien CJ, Petersen-Schaefer K, Stevens GN, et al, Adjuvant radiotherapy following neck dissection and parotidectomy for metastatic malignant melanoma. *Head Neck* 1997; 19: 589–94.
28. Ang KK, Peters LJ, Weber RS, et al, Post operative radiotherapy for cutaneous melanoma of the head and neck. *Int J Radiation Biol Phys* 1994; 30: 795–8.

27

Lymphatic mapping and sentinel lymph node biopsy: the concept

Donald L Morton, John F Thompson

INTRODUCTION

Although thickness, ulceration, anatomical site, and other features of a primary melanoma are important for determining prognosis, the tumour status of the regional lymph nodes remains the most significant indicator of outcome in patients with clinically localized cutaneous malignant melanoma.[1] According to the National Cancer Database from the Commission on Cancer of the American College of Surgeons and the National Cancer Society, the 5-year survival rate is 77% for patients with localized cutaneous melanoma but only 50% for those with regional nodal disease.

Given the undisputed importance of the regional lymph nodes in patients with primary melanomas, it is startling to realize that the management of these nodes has been an unresolved source of controversy for over 100 years. In 1892, Snow recommended routine complete lymph node dissection in melanoma patients who had no clinical evidence of regional metastasis.[2] His proposal for early or elective complete lymph node dissection (ELND) assumed that metastatic melanoma progressed sequentially from primary site to regional lymph nodes and then to more distant sites. Thus early removal of regional nodes by ELND should interrupt the metastatic cascade.[1]

Despite extensive retrospective and/or nonrandomized data favouring ELND, no prospective randomized trial has conclusively shown a survival benefit, even in patients with lesions of intermediate thickness (0.76–4.0 mm).[3–6] Moreover, even if ELND is limited to patients with intermediate thickness primary melanomas, only about 20% of this group will have nodal involvement.[1] The remaining 80% of patients undergoing ELND will be unnecessarily placed at risk for acute wound problems, chronic lymphoedema, nerve injury, and anaesthetic complications. This potential morbidity is a strong argument against routine use of a surgical procedure that can benefit only 20% of its recipients.

In 1990, Morton et al. introduced sentinel lymphadenectomy as a minimally invasive alternative to routine ELND.[7] This highly specific nodal sampling technique is based on the premise that a lymphatic channel draining a primary melanoma can carry malignant cells from the tumour to the first or 'sentinel' node (SN) in the lymphatic chain. The tumour cells can lodge in the subcapsular sinus of this SN and proliferate into a nodal metastasis. Because the SN is defined as the first nodal site of tumour cells metastasizing through draining lymphatics, excision and histopathological analysis of this node should indicate the tumour status of all regional lymph nodes. More than one lymphatic channel may drain a cutaneous melanoma; thus there may be more than one SN; about 25% of patients will have two or more SNs. Each of these SNs may receive drainage from one or more lymphatic channels. However, a single channel usually drains into only one SN, and it is rare for a channel to bifurcate before reaching the regional node field. The overall process is a sequential and remarkably orderly progression of melanoma nodal metastases.[8,9]

The preferential establishment of a metastatic colony in the first draining lymph node (the SN) is supported by evidence that metastatic melanoma is relatively contained in its initial stages.[10] Investigators from the John Wayne Cancer Institute (JWCI) reported that nodes anatomically closest to a primary melanoma are immunosuppressed and are the site of early metastases.[11,12] They suggested that tumour cells or their immunomodulatory products may downregulate lymph node function, creating an environment that favours the growth and proliferation of metastatic colonies.[12] Selective immune downregulation might explain the prognostic importance of the number of tumour positive regional lymph nodes, insofar as immunosuppression (and therefore metastatic potential) increases with tumour burden.[1,13] A focused and profound immune suppression of the first draining lymph node might allow a small primary melanoma to establish metastasis in that node, i.e. the SN.

CUTANEOUS LYMPHOSCINTIGRAPHY TO IDENTIFY THE REGIONAL LYMPHATIC BASIN(S) DRAINING A PRIMARY MELANOMA

Over 200 years ago Sappey, a professor of anatomy in Paris, defined a band of 2 cm in width, which encircles the trunk at the umbilicus; lesions above this line were predicted to drain to the axillary nodes and those below to the inguinal nodes. Sappey's work was valuable, but his conclusions were oversimplified. Not all truncal lesions follow Sappey's rule; certain midline lesions, particularly those in the umbilical area or near the midline of the back, can drain to any area. Lesions in the head and neck area are even more variable and unpredictable. Lymphatic drainage from the scalp, ear, and face cannot be predicted by anatomical site; lesions anterior to the ear do not always drain through the parotid gland or directly to the anterior cervical nodes, and lesions posterior to the ear may not drain to the post-auricular nodes or to posterior cervical nodes. This tendency for ambiguous lymphatic drainage has been advanced as one argument against ELND, particularly in patients with non-extremity primary melanomas.

Morton's group suggested that cutaneous lymphoscintigraphy provides an answer to the dilemma, because this technique can identify the lymphatic basins draining a primary cutaneous melanoma. Cutaneous lymphoscintigraphy had its origins in the early 1950s, when Sherman and Ter-Pogossian used interstitial injections of radioactive colloidal gold to document the lymphatic pathways from cutaneous sites.[14] In 1977, Morton's group used gold 198 to show the drainage pathways to regional nodal basins from cutaneous melanomas arising on the trunk or proximal extremities.[15,16] Although these techniques were accurate, colloidal gold was soon abandoned as a scanning agent because of its high level of local radiation. The subsequent development of technetium labelled dextran and human serum albumin for cutaneous lymphoscintigraphy has made this procedure a safe and accurate method of detecting lymphatic pathways from a primary melanoma site to the regional lymph nodes. Although several radiopharmaceutical agents have been used for lymphoscintigraphy, the only agents currently available in the United States are ^{99m}Tc-sulfur colloid and ^{99m}Tc-human serum albumin. ^{99m}Tc-nanocolloid of albumin is widely used in Europe, and ^{99m}Tc-antimony trisulphide colloid is commonly used in Australia.

As the location of a cutaneous melanoma moves from the distal extremity to the trunk and the head and neck region, historical anatomical guidelines become increasingly inaccurate for identifying the primary lymphatic drainage basin(s).[17] Thus cutaneous lymphoscintigraphy is particularly useful for melanomas arising in an axial location on the trunk or the head and neck, because these skin sites may drain to one or more lymphatic areas.[18–20] It can also identify the 5–10% of patients who have aberrant in-transit lymph nodes that are on the lymphatic channel but outside the drainage basin.[17,21] However, although lymphoscintigraphy can show the drainage patterns from the primary to the regional lymph node field(s) and even to nodes in that field, it cannot differentiate tumour-containing nodes from normal or reactive nodes.

INTRAOPERATIVE MAPPING TO IDENTIFY THE SENTINEL NODE IN THE REGIONAL LYMPHATIC DRAINAGE BASIN

The success of lymphoscintigraphic mapping of the basin(s) draining a primary cutaneous melanoma suggested that it might be possible to visualize the pattern of drainage to nodes within the basin intraoperatively by injecting a vital dye at the site of the primary. Thus Morton's initial description of intraoperative SN mapping was the logical extension of the lymphoscintigraphy studies begun in the 1970s.[7] In 1977, his group introduced the concept of selective lymphadenectomy of the deep iliac/obturator lymph nodes directed by the pathological status of Cloquet's node and the superficial inguinal nodes.[16] At about the same time, Cabanas used the term 'sentinel node' in penile cancer to indicate a node detected by lymphangiography in an anatomical location fixed adjacent to the inferior epigastric vein.[22] His observations were not uniformly confirmed by other investigators, and the technique was not widely adopted. It is important to realize that his technique assumed an anatomically fixed site for the SN. This is not consistent with the often variable lymphatic drainage patterns from melanoma, breast cancer, and other solid neoplasms whose lymphatic drainage is determined by the anatomical site of the primary within the organ and by the normal variations in lymphatic anatomy. For these neoplasms, the SN is the first draining node, which is not in a fixed position and which is not necessarily the node closest to the primary tumour.[23] According to Morton's concept, the identity of the SN is established by its function, not its location.

A feline model was used by Morton's group to investigate the feasibility of staining the lymphatic pathways to the sentinel node.[24] When they compared various vital dyes for intraoperative lymphatic mapping (LM), patent blue-V and isosulfan blue dyes were found to be the best agents for identifying the drainage patterns in a regional lymphatic basin. When injected intradermally, these agents rapidly entered the lymphatics; their bright blue colour was readily visible and allowed easy identification of each lymphatic channel and its path to the SN.

Clinical results of intraoperative lymphatic mapping and sentinel lymphadenectomy (LM/SL) were first reported in the literature in 1992.[25] In this study, Morton's group undertook LM/SL in 237 lymphatic basins of 223 patients, all of whom subsequently underwent complete lymph node dissection. A SN was identified in 194 (82%) lymphatic basins. Forty patients (21%) had tumour positive SNs. Only two lymphatic basins had tumour negative SNs in the presence of tumour positive non-sentinel nodes, a false negative rate of 1%. Remarkably similar accuracy rates were achieved in early corroborative studies for other centres in the United States and Australia.[8,9] After extensive phase II trials to validate the consistency and accuracy of SN mapping, Morton's group, followed by investigators at other cancer centres, abandoned routine use of complete nodal dissection.[18,19,26] They now undertake complete lymphadenectomy only in patients whose SNs contain tumour cells.[27]

Almost inevitably, the use of radioisotopes was extended from preoperative localization of the SN to intraoperative identification of this node. Alex et al. in 1993 reported a preclinical/clinical study in which technetium-99m labelled colloid and a gamma probe were used to label and detect the SN in cats and then in 10 melanoma patients.[28] During the same year, JWCI investigators developed their clinical technique of intraoperative radiolymphoscintigraphy using one of three radiopharmaceuticals, and in 1994 Essner et al. reported the JWCI experience with ^{99m}Tc labelled albumin to the Society of Surgical Oncology.[29] Initially, the radiopharmaceutical was injected intraoperatively with isosulfan blue dye at the primary site. The hand-held gamma probe was then used to determine the radioactive count over a background site, over the afferent lymphatic channels, over the skin site marked during preoperative lymphoscintigraphy, and over each blue stained node before and after its excision. The count ratio derived from these measurements was used to identify blue stained nodes and distinguish sentinel from non-sentinel nodes. Currently, JWCI investigators avoid intraoperative injection of the radiocolloid by performing surgery 1–4 hours after preoperative lymphoscintigraphy.[27] A radioactive count ratio (SN:background) ≥ 2 corroborates that a blue stained node is actually the SN. At the Sydney Melanoma Unit a single dose of radioisotope is also used for both preoperative lymphoscintigraphy and intraoperative SN identification, but the surgery is routinely performed on the day after the lymphoscintigram.[30] It has been found that sufficient radioactivity usually remains in the SN to permit its intraoperative localization with a gamma probe up to 30 hours after injection of radiolabelled colloid at the primary melanoma site.

KINETICS OF THE AGENTS USED FOR LYMPHATIC MAPPING

Correct identification of the SN depends on the kinetics of the tracking agent. In the preclinical studies of Morton's group, many of the vital dyes initially tested were abandoned, largely because of their rapid diffusion into surrounding tissues.[24] Dyes that are not adequately retained by the lymphatic vessels will not reach and intensely stain the SN.

Kinetics is a particular issue with radiocolloids. Glass et al. at the JWCI evaluated the properties of three agents available in the United States, all of which feature the advantages of a ^{99m}Tc label.[31] They found that lymphatic transit was affected by particle size. Thus Tc-HSA moved faster than particulate agents such as Tc-AC and Tc-SC, and it washed out faster from the sites of injection. This meant that the interval between injection and SN localization was shorter. Particulate agents showed more nodal retention, as measured by qualitative scoring of nodal visualization and by the greater number of nodes visualized in delayed versus early images.

Largely because of these kinetic variations, lymphatic mapping with radiocolloidal agents will not realize its full potential until it is standardized. Investigators at different centres continue to use a wide variety of radiocolloidal agents: human serum albumin, albumin colloid, sulphur colloid, antimony trisulphide colloid, and stannous phytate. In addition, because the number of radioactive ('hot') nodes will vary with the radiopharmaceutical and with the interval between its injection and the surgical procedure, the definition of the SN will always be ambiguous when lymphatic mapping is performed with radiopharmaceuticals alone. The SN should be among the hot nodes if all hot nodes are removed, but not all hot nodes are SNs (Figures 27.1 and 27.2).[31,32] This is why probe directed mapping serves only as a useful adjunct to dye directed mapping, and visualization of the blue dye remains the gold standard for identifying SNs.[30,33,34]

HISTOPATHOLOGICAL VALIDATION OF THE SENTINEL NODE CONCEPT

Although the standard histological evaluation of a lymph node for regional metastasis relies on haematoxylin and eosin (H&E) staining of a single section, immunohistochemical (IHC) staining of serial sections can increase the rate of detection of nodal metastases. In the early 1980s, Morton and colleagues found that S-100 protein was present in melanomas,[35] and Cochran et al. determined that it could be used as an exquisitely sensitive marker for melanoma.[36] Immunohistochemical staining using antibodies to S-100 identified tumour cells missed by conventional H&E staining of regional lymph nodes. This very detailed examination requires more work on the pathologist's part and is therefore not practical for the large nodal specimens removed during ELND. It is, however, suitable for focused analysis of the small number of nodes removed during LM/SL.

In the landmark SN study of Morton et al., metastatic tumour cells were detected only by IHC in 45% (17/38) of tumour positive SN specimens.[25] Did this increased

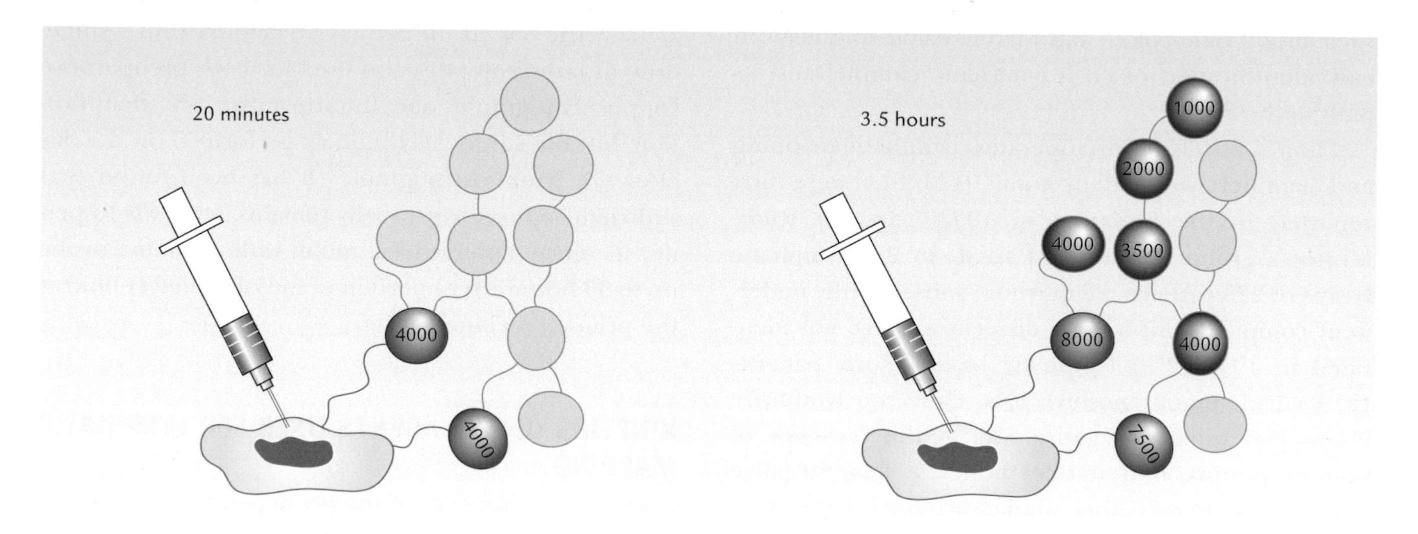

Figure 27.1 *Kinetics of lymphatic mapping using a radiopharmaceutical. Twenty to 30 minutes after injection of a radiopharmaceutical at the site of the primary melanoma, radioactivity will be localized only in the sentinel node* (blue*). Several hours after injection, radioactivity may be found in additional (non-sentinel) nodes* (red*) as the radiopharmaceutical progresses along the lymphatic chain. In contrast, blue dye rapidly dilutes out and rarely stains any node except the sentinel node blue. Numbers indicate radioactivity in counts/unit time. Reproduced with permission from Morton et al.,* J Am Coll Surg *1999; 189: 214–23.*[32]

rate of identification of metastases reflect the biologic significance of the SN or the sensitivity of the histopathological technique? To answer this question, Morton's group examined non-sentinel nodes by permanent section examination using H&E and IHC with antibodies to S-100 protein, HMB-45, and NKI/C3. Of 3079 non-sentinel nodes removed from 194 node basins during completion lymphadenectomy, only 2 (0.06%) contained metastatic tumour when every SN in the same basin was tumour free. Thus the false negative rate of the procedure was <1%.

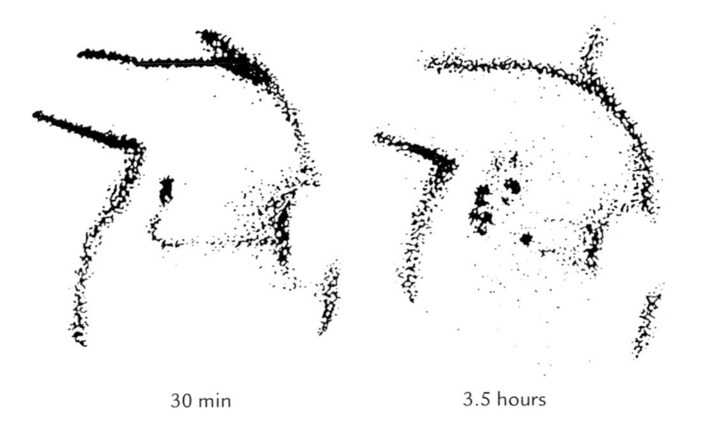

Figure 27.2 *Variation between early and delayed nodal uptake of radiocolloid (Tc-SC) in a patient with a primary melanoma behind left scapula. Early image* (left) *shows both afferent lymphatic channel and sentinel node. In delayed image* (right)*, the afferent lymphatic channel is no longer delineated, and the tracer has migrated to several axillary nodes, obscuring identification of the sentinel node. Reproduced with permission from Glass et al.,* J Nucl Med *1998; 39: 1185–90.*[31]

Sophisticated histopathological techniques including the examination of multiple sections and the use of IHC support the concept that the SN is the lymph node most likely to harbour metastatic disease in melanoma patients who have regional nodal metastasis. But is the node examined truly the SN? Tumour status cannot reliably be used to confirm the identity of an SN because of course not all SNs will contain metastases. At present, the identity of the SN is determined intraoperatively by the surgeon, based on blue staining and radioactivity. The pathologist records blue coloration as evidence of an excised node's sentinel status, but the blue dye often dissipates before the node reaches the laboratory. In addition, the whole lymph node may not be blue stained; colour can be localized to less than half of the node, making it difficult to identify the portion of the nodal microanatomy most likely to contain metastases. Further, as mentioned above, the definition of an SN by its radioactivity is subject to considerable variation. Finally, the intensity of both dye and radiocolloids is time dependent.[31] For these reasons, Morton's group has been investigating the role of carbon dye as an intraoperative adjunct to isosulfan blue dye and radiocolloid for histological confirmation of the SN.[37] The relatively large size of carbon particles makes them less time dependent, i.e. less likely to pass through the SN to non-sentinel nodes along the lymphatic chain (Figure 27.3).

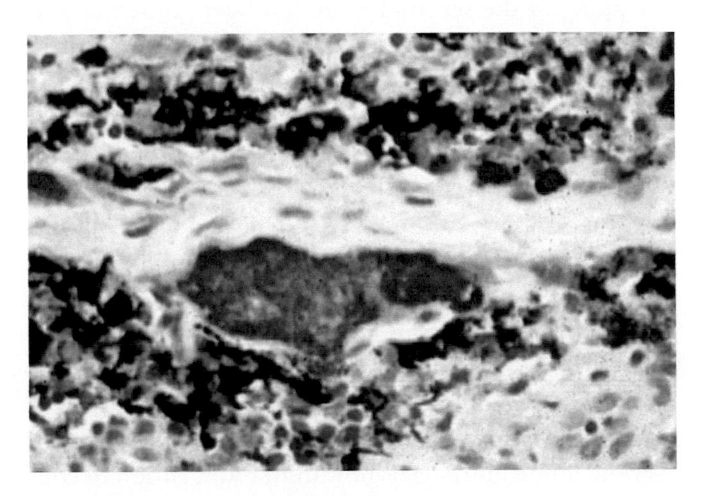

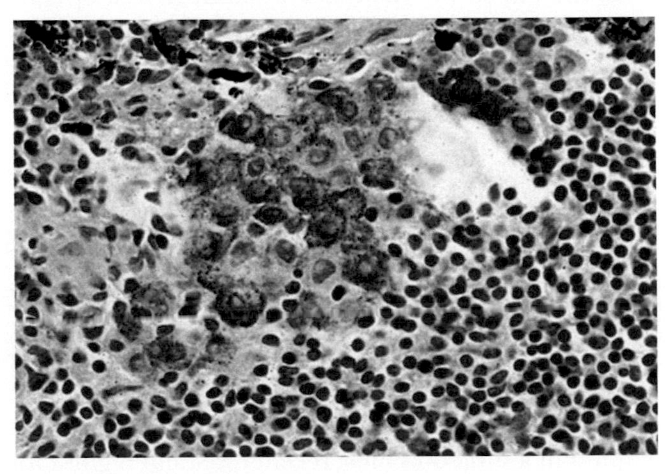

Figure 27.3 *Photomicrographs of SN sections after LM/SL using isosulfan blue dye, radiocolloid, and carbon dye.* Left: *Carbon dye* (black*), 2+, and melanoma micrometastasis* (brown*) are both located in the paratrabecular sinus (HMB-45 immunohistochemical stain, ×400).* Right: *Carbon dye* (black*), 1+, and adjacent melanoma micrometastasis* (brown*) are located in the subcapsular sinus (HMB-45 immunohistochemical stain, ×400). As expected, neither the blue dye nor the radiocolloid is visible on these sections. Reproduced with permission from* Cancer *(in press) Haigh et al.*[37]

Mapping with carbon dye alone is not practical because the high concentrations required for visualization during mapping would obscure identification of cancer cells on stained sections of excised nodes. In their animal studies, JWCI investigators found that a combination of isosulfan blue dye and carbon dye allowed intraoperative identification of blue stained SNs and light microscopic confirmation of black carbon particles within stained sections of these nodes.[38] Thompson's group in Sydney found that it is possible to measure the amounts of antimony sulphide in sentinel and non-sentinel nodes using a mass spectrometer. This technique too can thus confirm that a node is a true SN, after preoperative lymphoscintigraphy involving injection of antimony sulphide colloid labelled with technetium-99m.

CONSISTENCY, ACCURACY, AND THE TEAM APPROACH

The appealing simplicity of the SN concept tends to obscure the fact that mastery of LM/SL requires considerable practice. In the initial studies of Morton et al., three surgeons who had varying experience with dye directed mapping identified a blue-stained SN in 82% of lymphatic basins overall, but the success rate was highest (96%) for the surgeon with the most experience and lowest (72%) for the surgeon with the least experience.[25] The accuracy of LM/SL was recently examined in an international multicentre trial by comparing it with the JWCI experience.[27] The results from participating centres in Australia, the United States, and Europe were remarkably similar and consistent in regard to rate of SN identification and incidence of nodal metastases. The rate of SN identification was lower when LM was performed using blue dye alone (95.2%) versus a combination of blue dye and radiocolloid (99.1%) ($P = 0.014$), indicating that the two techniques are complementary.

LM/SL studies clearly show that successful mapping of regional lymphatic anatomy is directly related to the surgeon's experience. The rate of SN identification is highest in a surgeon's most recent cases and highest for the surgeon who has performed the most mapping procedures. Thus, although experienced investigators at the JWCI, the Sydney Melanoma Unit and other centres have proved that high rates of SN identification are possible, each surgeon must ascend a learning curve to acquire technical expertise in LM/SL. Ascent of the learning curve for LM/SL usually requires completion of approximately 30 cases.[39] During this learning phase the surgeon should routinely perform complete lymph node dissection after LM/SL to monitor the rate of false negative SNs. It should be noted that the surgeon's learning curve is applied in a multidisciplinary context; lymphatic mapping requires a committed team of nuclear medicine physicians, surgeons and pathologists who are expert in the application of their respective specialties to this technique.

SUMMARY

Intraoperative lymphatic mapping is based on the hypothesis that lymph from a primary solid neoplasm drains initially to one or more SNs, which are therefore the first nodes at risk for harbouring occult metastatic disease. These SNs can be excised and examined by using serial sectioning and immunohistochemical staining, techniques that would be impractical and costly if applied to all lymph nodes removed during conventional lymphadenectomy. According to the SN hypothesis, if metastases are present they will be found in the SN. Thus a complete lymphadenectomy is necessary only if the SN contains tumour.

Since Morton et al. introduced LM/SL for primary cutaneous melanoma in 1990, there has been tremendous interest in the sentinel node concept.[7] Lymphatic mapping of the sentinel node has been undertaken in patients with breast cancer, vulvar cancer, thyroid cancer, colon cancer, and gastrointestinal cancer.[40–44] Results confirm that the sentinel node concept may be universally applicable to all solid neoplasms which metastasize via the lymphatics.[23]

In melanoma, studies have established that LM/SL is safe, accurate, and reproducible when undertaken by an experienced multidisciplinary team of professionals from nuclear medicine, surgical oncology and pathology. As yet, however, no prospective randomized multi-institutional trial has shown that it results in a survival benefit for patients with any tumour type. Among the several multicentre trials now under way, closest to completion is a 5-year phase III study of LM/SL in patients with melanoma.[27] This trial randomizes patients with clinically localized melanoma to wide excision and nodal observation or to wide excision and LM/SL, followed by complete lymphadenectomy if the SN contains tumour (Figure 27.4). Results will indicate the prognostic significance of SN micrometastasis and whether there is a survival benefit of lymphadenectomy for melanoma patients with a tumour positive SN. Even if it transpires that LM/SL has no therapeutic benefit, the more accurate prognostic and staging information provided by this technique will probably indicate its continued use for all patients entering adjuvant therapy trials.

LM/SL is of potential diagnostic and prognostic value but it will not have direct therapeutic relevance unless it can be demonstrated that early excision of tumour involved nodes confers a survival benefit. Unless a tumour metastasizes to the regional nodes before distant sites, then a tumour positive SN is merely a marker for the metastatic phenotype. Hopefully, blood and tissue analyses using molecular and immunological markers will confirm the sequential passage of tumour cells to regional lymph nodes and then to distant sites, thereby creating a therapeutic window of opportunity for lymphadenectomy while the tumour cells are confined to SNs. As a therapeutic procedure, LM/SL is still investigational because its effect on survival has not yet been determined. However, its minimally invasive approach coupled with highly sensitive immunological and molecular techniques for pathological assessment has created a rational framework for management of the regional lymph nodes.

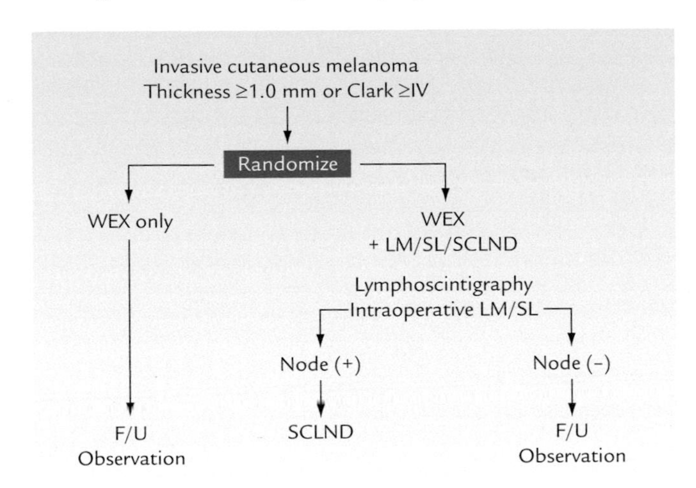

Figure 27.4 *MSLT study design. Patients are assigned in a 60:40 distribution to wide excision (WEX) plus LM/SL and selective complete lymph node dissection (SCLMD) or to WEX alone. All patients are followed for overall survival as the primary end point. F/U = follow up. Reprinted with permission from Morton et al.,* Ann Surg *1999; 230: 453–63.*[27]

REFERENCES

1. Morton DL, Wanek L, Nizze JA, et al, Improved long-term survival after lymphadenectomy of melanoma metastatic to regional nodes. Analysis of prognostic factors in 1134 patients from the John Wayne Cancer Clinic. *Ann Surg* 1991; 214: 491–9.
2. Snow H, Melanotic cancerous disease. *Lancet* 1892; 2: 872.
3. Sim FH, Taylor WF, Ivins JC, et al, A prospective randomized study of the efficacy of routine elective lymphadenectomy in management of malignant melanoma. *Cancer* 1978; 41: 948–56.
4. Veronesi U, Adamus J, Bandiera DC, et al, Inefficacy of immediate node dissection in stage I melanoma of the limbs. *N Engl J Med* 1977; 297: 627–30.
5. Veronesi U, Adamus J, Bandiera DC, et al, Delayed regional lymph node dissection in stage I melanoma of the skin of the lower extremities. *Cancer* 1982; 49: 2420–30.
6. Balch CM, Soong SJ, Bartolucci AA, et al, Efficacy of an elective regional lymph node dissection of 1 to 4 mm thick melanomas for patients 60 years of age and younger. *Ann Surg* 1996; 224: 255–63.
7. Morton D, Cagle L, Wong J, et al, Intraoperative lymphatic mapping and selective lymphadenectomy: technical details of a new procedure for clinical stage I melanoma. *Presented at the Annual Meeting of the Society of Surgical Oncology.* Washington, DC, 1990.
8. Reintgen D, Cruse CW, Wells K, et al, The orderly progression of melanoma nodal metastases. *Ann Surg* 1994; 220: 759–67.
9. Thompson JF, McCarthy WH, Bosch CM, et al, Sentinel lymph node status as an indicator of the presence of metastatic melanoma in regional lymph nodes. *Melanoma Res* 1995; 5: 255–60.
10. Cochran AJ, Wen DR, Farzad Z, et al, Immunosuppression by melanoma cells as a factor in the generation of metastatic disease. *Anticancer Res* 1989; 9: 859–64.
11. Cochran AJ, Pihl E, Wen DR, et al, Zoned immune suppression of lymph nodes draining malignant melanoma: histologic and immunohistologic studies. *J Natl Cancer Inst* 1987; 78: 399–405.
12. Hoon DS, Korn EL, Cochran AJ, Variations in functional immunocompetence of individual tumour-draining lymph nodes in humans. *Cancer Res* 1987; 47: 1740–4.
13. Callery C, Cochran AJ, Roe DJ, et al, Factors prognostic for survival in patients with malignant melanoma spread to the regional lymph nodes. *Ann Surg* 1982; 196: 69–75.
14. Sherman A, Ter-Pogossian M, Lymph node concentration of radioactive colloid gold following interstitial injection. *Cancer* 1953; 6: 1238–40.
15. Robinson DS, Sample WF, Fee HJ, et al, Regional lymphatic drainage in primary malignant melanoma of the trunk determined by colloidal gold scanning. *Surg Forum* 1977; 28: 147–8.
16. Holmes EC, Moseley HS, Morton DL, et al, A rational approach to the surgical management of melanoma. *Ann Surg* 1977; 186: 481–90.
17. Thompson JF, Uren RF, Shaw HM, et al, Location of sentinel lymph nodes in patients with cutaneous melanoma: new insights into lymphatic anatomy. *J Am Coll Surg* 1999; 189: 204–6.
18. Bostick P, Essner R, Sarantou T, et al, Intraoperative lymphatic mapping for early-stage melanoma of the head and neck. *Am J Surg* 1997; 174: 536–9.
19. Morton DL, Wen DR, Foshag LJ, et al, Intraoperative lymphatic mapping and selective cervical lymphadenectomy for early-stage melanomas of the head and neck. *J Clin Oncol* 1993; 11: 1751–6.
20. Ollila DW, Foshag LJ, Essner R, et al, Parotid region lymphatic mapping and sentinel lymphadenectomy for cutaneous melanoma. *Ann Surg Oncol* 1999; 6: 150–4.
21. Uren RF, Howman-Giles R, Thompson JF, et al, Interval nodes: the forgotten sentinel nodes in patients with melanoma. *Arch Surg* 2000; 135: 1168–72.
22. Cabanas RM, An approach for the treatment of penile carcinoma. *Cancer* 1977; 39: 456–66.
23. Bilchik AJ, Giuliano A, Essner R, et al, Universal application of intraoperative lymphatic mapping and sentinel lymphadenectomy in solid neoplasms. *Cancer J Sci Am* 1998; 4: 351–8.
24. Wong JH, Cagle LA, Morton DL, Lymphatic drainage of skin to a sentinel lymph node in a feline model. *Ann Surg* 1991; 214: 637–41.

25. Morton DL, Wen DR, Wong JH, et al, Technical details of intraoperative lymphatic mapping for early stage melanoma. *Arch Surg* 1992; 127: 392–9.
26. Morton DL, Sentinel lymphadenectomy for patients with clinical stage I melanoma. *J Surg Oncol* 1997; 66: 267–9.
27. Morton DL, Thompson JF, Essner R, et al, Validation of the accuracy of intraoperative lymphatic mapping and sentinel lymphadenectomy for early-stage melanoma: a multicenter trial. *Ann Surg* 1999; 230: 453–63.
28. Alex JC, Weaver DL, Fairbank JT, et al, Gamma-probe-guided lymph node localization in malignant melanoma. *Surg Oncol* 1993; 2: 303–8.
29. Essner R, Foshag L, Morton DL, Intraoperative radiolymphoscintigraphy: a useful adjuvant to intraoperative lymphatic mapping and selective lymphadenectomy in patients with clinical stage I melanoma. *Presented at the Annual Meeting of the Society of Surgical Oncology*, March 1994, Houston, TX.
30. Thompson JF, Niewind P, Uren RF, et al, Single-dose isotope injection for both preoperative lymphoscintigraphy and intraoperative sentinel lymph node identification in melanoma patients. *Melanoma Res* 1997; 7: 500–6.
31. Glass EC, Essner R, Morton DL, Kinetics of three lymphoscintigraphic agents in patients with cutaneous melanoma. *J Nucl Med* 1998; 39: 1185–90.
32. Morton DL, Chan AD, Current status of intraoperative lymphatic mapping and sentinel lymphadenectomy for melanoma: is it standard of care? *J Am Coll Surg* 1999; 189: 214–23.
33. Bostick P, Essner R, Glass E, et al, Comparison of blue dye and probe-assisted intraoperative lymphatic mapping in melanoma to identify sentinel nodes in 100 lymphatic basins. *Arch Surg* 1999; 134: 43–9.
34. Morton DL, Bostick PJ, Will the true sentinel node please stand? [Editorial]. *Ann Surg Oncol* 1999; 6: 12–14.
35. Gaynor R, Irie R, Morton D, Herschman HR. S100 protein is present in cultured human malignant melanomas. *Nature* 1980; 286: 400–1.
36. Cochran AJ, Wen DR, Herschman HR, Occult melanoma in lymph nodes detected by antiserum to S-100 protein. *Int J Cancer* 1984; 34: 159–63.
37. Haigh PI, Lucci A, Turner RR, et al, Carbon dye histologically confirms the identity of sentinel nodes in cutaneous melanoma. *Cancer*, (in press).
38. Lucci A, Turner RR, Morton DL, Carbon dye as an adjunct to isosulfan blue dye for sentinel lymph node dissection. *Surgery* 1999; 126: 48–53.
39. Morton DL, Intraoperative lymphatic mapping and sentinel lymphadenectomy: community standard care or clinical investigation? *Cancer J Sci Am* 1997; 3: 328–30.
40. Giuliano AE, Jones RC, Brennan M, Statman R, Sentinel lymphadenectomy in breast cancer. *J Clin Oncol* 1997; 15: 2345–50.
41. Levenback C, Burke TW, Gershenson DM, et al, Intraoperative lymphatic mapping for vulvar cancer. *Obstet Gynecol* 1994; 84: 163–7.
42. Kelemen PR, Van Herle AJ, Giuliano AE, Sentinel lymphadenectomy in thyroid malignant neoplasms. *Arch Surg* 1998; 133: 288–92.
43. Wood TF, Tsioulias GJ, Morton DL, et al, Focused examination of sentinel lymph nodes upstages early colorectal carcinoma. *Am Surg* 2000; 66: 998–1003.
44. Tsioulias GJ, Wood TF, Morton DL, Bilchik AJ, Lymphatic mapping and focused analysis of sentinel lymph nodes upstages gastrointestinal neoplasms. *Arch Surg* 2000; 135: 926–32.

28

Sentinel node biopsy: historical aspects

Roger F Uren, David N Krag

HISTORICAL ASPECTS

The lymphatic system in humans seems to have been studied for over 2000 years, and new insights into its physiology and anatomy continue to be discovered today as we enter the third millennium. The ability of the sentinel node biopsy procedure to determine accurately the lymph node status of patients with melanoma owes much to the pioneers of research into the lymphatic system. Insights gained especially over the past 150 years have contributed directly to the success of this nodal staging technique. This chapter aims to summarize the progress of our knowledge of the lymphatic drainage system from the earliest times to present day.

The earliest mention of lymphatic vessels

Over 2300 years ago Hippocrates (460 BC to 370 BC) in one of his works spoke of a white blood resembling serous fluid which entered glands.[1] This would seem to be a clear reference to a lymphatic vessel, although it was not recognized as such.

Aristotle (384 BC to 322 BC), in his work 'History of Animals', used terms that suggested he had observed lymphatic vessels, although we cannot be sure of this.

Working in the school of anatomy in Alexandria and using live animals, it was Herophilus (300 BC) who first noticed lymphatic vessels terminating in glands in the mesentery, and Herasistratus (280 BC) who first described the milky contents of such vessels.[2] Neither of these celebrated anatomists recognized these vessels as separate from the blood vessels, with the former believing that they were veins and the latter that they were arteries. The term 'lymphatic' was not used at this time by either of these individuals. Galen mentioned their work only to rebut its significance vigorously. He believed that the absorption of food occurred via the veins of the mesentery, which passed on to the liver. Galen had attempted to confirm the findings of Herophilus experimentally but made important errors in the design of his experiment. He did not realize that the lymphatics in the mesentery are visible only during the period of digestion of food and that they will be observed only in a live animal and then only at the moment that the abdomen is opened to the air.[1] He interpreted his failure to observe the lacteal vessels as definite evidence that they did not exist, and Galen's influence was such that this dogmatic assertion was accepted as fact for 14 centuries.

In 1532 Massa described channels that began in the kidney but were not always visible.[3] These were most likely lymphatics, but he did not follow them to their draining lymph nodes, which raises doubts about the significance of his observations. At about the same time Fallope observed channels on the inferior surface of the liver which passed on to terminate in glands in the region of the pancreas.[1] These were no doubt the lymphatics of the liver. The thoracic duct was first described in the horse by Eustachius in 1563.

In 1622 Gasparo Aselli, a professor of anatomy and surgery in Pavia, Italy, operated on a live dog and rediscovered the mesenteric 'lacteals'.[4] He also showed the existence of lymphatic vessels in many different animals. He was the first to study the lymphatic system in a systematic and scientific fashion, although the vessels were still not called 'lymphatics' at this time. He thought that the lymphatics he observed in the mesentery of animals were a special type of vein which he designated 'lacteal veins' because of the milky colour of the fluid contained in them. He was the first to declare that these lacteal veins were the vessels involved in the absorption of chyle. He wrote extensively on the anatomy of the lymphatic system in the dog, cat, lamb, cow, pig, and horse. Aselli, like Herophilus, noted that the lymphatic vessels in the mesentery joined mesenteric glands, but also mistakenly thought that the 'lacteal fluid' contained in the lymphatic vessels then drained to the liver.[2] Aselli died in 1626, before his work was published and before he was able to show the existence of lacteal veins in humans. This discovery was made by Gassendi et al. in 1628 when they opened the abdomen of a female patient one hour after her death.

At this time both Riolan and Harvey, who were very influential in the contemporary scientific study of the anatomy and physiology of man, denied the presence of the 'lacteal veins' of Aselli. They took a Galenic stance, which regarded lymphatic vessels as a type of vein and not part of a separate and discrete circulation. Subsequent work by Vessling (1634), Folius and Tulpius (1639), Wallee (1641) and Pecquet (1649), however, confirmed the existence of such lymphatic vessels as separate from the arteries and veins.[2] Vessling and Rudbeck showed that lymphatic vessels were present in many parts of the body, not just the mesentery. Aselli's view of the 'lacteal veins' was thus accepted as fact, and, after 14 centuries, Galen's dogma was finally consigned to the dustbin of medical history.

Further knowledge about the circulation of lymphatic fluid was contributed by Jean Pecquet, of Dieppe, France, who in 1651 opened a living dog and found a white fluid mixing with blood in the right atrium of the heart.[1] He suspected this to be chyle and found that the white fluid had entered the subclavian vein via the 'ductus thoracicus'. He later showed that the mesenteric and other abdominal lymphatic vessels did not drain to the liver but passed onwards, to converge at the start of the thoracic duct. This confluence he called the cistern or reservoir of the chyle, which later became known as the cisterna chylae. He also accurately described the anatomical arrangement of the thoracic duct and the right lymphatic duct as they enter the confluence of the internal jugular and subclavian veins on each side almost 100 years after the description of the thoracic duct by Eustachius.[5]

The first mention of the term 'lymphatic' is attributed to Thomas Bartholin in 1653. Before this time, as mentioned above, they had usually been referred to as lacteal veins.

Discovery continued and in 1665 Olof Rudbeck of Uppsala, with Thomas Bartholin of Copenhagen and others, described valves in the lumens of lymphatic vessels. Rudbeck was also the first to declare that lymphatics are present in many tissues, not just the intestine and liver. Nuck, Hale, Meckel, Haller, and Cruikshank also confirmed a wider distribution of such vessels than had previously been described.[2]

The physiology of the lymphatic system was studied by William Hunter, who at his school of anatomy in London stressed the importance of the lymphatic system in the process of absorption of fluid from the tissues. William Hewson, one of Hunter's pupils, studied the lymphatics in fish and some amphibious animals such as turtles.[1,6] He also studied the lymphatics of birds. In humans he noted that in the limbs, the superficial and deep lymphatic systems were different. He also suggested that some lymphatic vessels in mammals entered the thoracic duct without traversing a lymph node.

William Cruikshank, who was also a pupil of William Hunter, produced an important monograph in 1786 titled 'The Anatomy of the Absorbing Vessels of the Human Body', which had the most detailed illustrations of the human lymphatics seen until that time (Figure 28.1).[7]

Paolo Mascagni, who was a professor of anatomy at Siena, Italy, was the first to stress the importance of the origin of the lymphatic vessels in the interstitial fluid, and stated that such vessels did not have any direct connection with the blood system at the tissue level.[8] He also published an atlas of the lymphatic vessels in man which in detail was a significant advance on that produced by Cruikshank (Figure 28.2).

The fruitful 1800s

In 1824 Lauth established that each lymphatic vessel had its origin from a network of smaller lymphatics.[9]

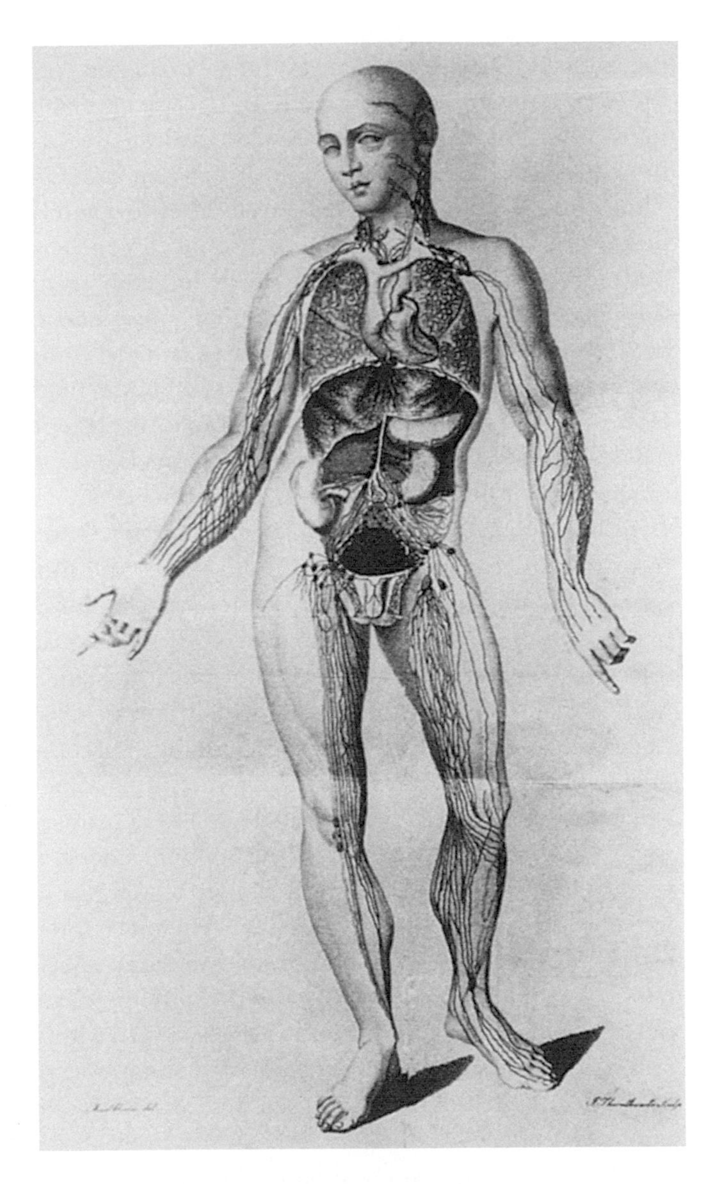

Figure 28.1 *From Cruikshank's atlas of lymphatic anatomy.*

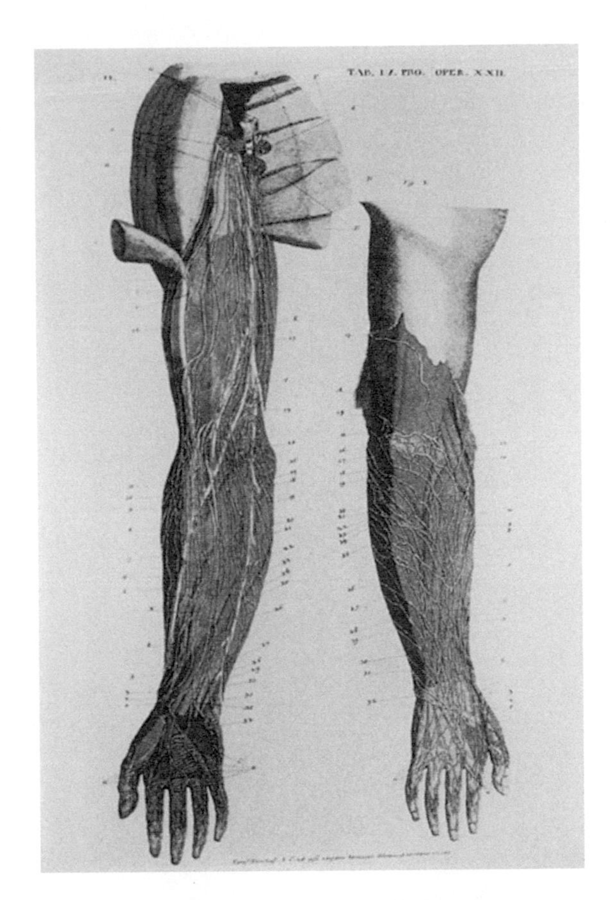

Figure 28.2 *From Mascagni's atlas of the lymphatics.*

In 1847 Sappey, a professor of anatomy in Paris, started an extensive programme of research into the lymphatics, which culminated in the publication of a large atlas in 1874.[10] Sappey injected mercury into the lymphatics of cadavers and was thus able to follow the path of lymphatic collecting vessels on their way to the draining lymph nodes. The use of mercury in the study of the lymphatics was first described by Meckel and developed by Hunter and his pupils, including Cruikshank.[2,7] Mascagni also used this technique but the method was refined by Sappey, who used it extensively.[8]

Sappey combined the information obtained in a series of cadavers into detailed drawings of the drainage pathways of lymphatic collecting vessels in every part of the body. The illustrations became classics and were the basis of the general understanding of the cutaneous lymphatics until the late 20th century (Figure 28.3). Sappey reported drainage to the axilla and groin from the skin of the trunk and showed a vertical midline zone anteriorly and posteriorly where drainage tended to overlap. A similar zone was identified passing horizontally around the waist from the umbilicus to the region of L2 vertebra posteriorly. In these zones, later called 'Sappey's lines' by others, drainage was said to be possible to either side in the case of the vertical zone or to either the groin or the axilla in the case of the horizontal zone. Outside these zones, however, Sappey stated that lymphatic drainage was always to the ipsilateral groin or axilla, depending on whether the skin site of interest was above or below the horizontal band around the waist.

Over the past 200 years further information on the physiology and microanatomy of the lymphatics has been obtained. Von Recklinghausen discovered the lymphatic endothelial cell in 1862 and showed that it

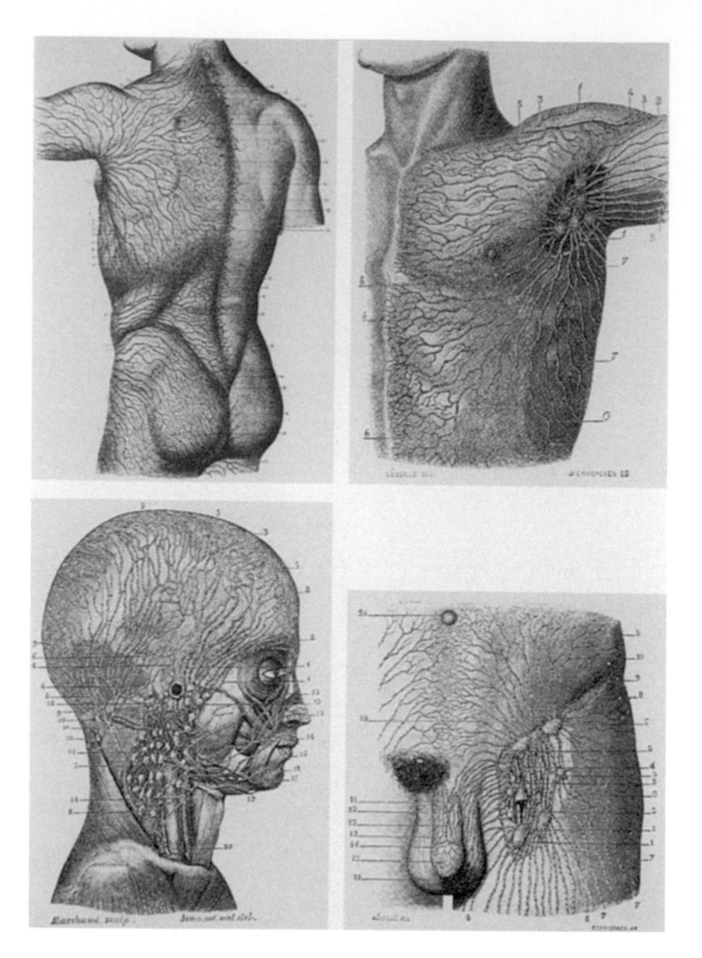

Figure 28.3 *From Sappey's atlas of the lymphatics.*

could be stained black with silver nitrate.[11] In 1894 Reaut, Regaud and Ranvier showed that every lymphatic starts as a closed ampulla within connective tissue.[12,13] Nerves in the walls of the lymphatic vessels were described by Kytmanoff in 1901.[14]

Gerota modified Sappey's approach to opacifying the lymphatic vessels by injecting coloured materials such as absolute black, cinnabar, and Prussian blue rather than mercury.[15] The advantage of this modification was that the studies could be performed on the living as well as the dead. Prussian blue was the preferred dye, made up in a solution of turpentine and sulphuric ether immediately before injection. Blue dyes continue to be important to this day in lymphatic mapping procedures, particularly during surgery.

The 20th century

In the early 1900s Bartels used modifications of Gerota's method to make important contributions to the study of lymphatic drainage in man and later, with the discovery of x rays, new methods became available to study human lymphatic vessels in the living state.[16] In the 1930s a colloidal preparation of thorium dioxide, Thorotrast, was developed. This was used in vivo and in postmortem studies. In 1939 Gray produced excellent postmortem demonstrations of the lymphatics using this method.[17] He also showed that anastomoses between lymphatic channels occurred, which could cause lymph to drain to an unexpected node field. However, it was discovered that Thorotrast caused blood dyscrasias and malignant haemangioendotheliomas of the liver and its use in patients was discontinued.[18]

In 1933 Hudack and McMaster began using vital dyes in vivo.[19] The dye was injected into the tissues and thus entered the lymphatic capillaries indirectly giving information on the lymphatic drainage of the tissues so injected. Weinberg in 1950 used the interstitial injection of vital dye to locate what he called the 'primary nodes' that drained gastric cancer, noting that the injection of dye would 'impart to them a blue colour which makes them readily identifiable'. These primary nodes were what we would now call sentinel nodes. A year later Weinberg described a similar technique in patients with bronchogenic carcinoma. He injected the root of the lung through which all the lymphatic vessels passed and then followed the stained lymphatic channels to the draining lymph nodes. This occurred within minutes, which enabled him to observe the 'mapping of the nodes by vital staining'. He used this information to minimize unnecessary surgery.

There was further application of this method in the 1950s, and several reports appeared in the surgical literature as surgeons used this approach intraoperatively as an aid to the identification of draining lymph nodes for elective lymphadenectomy.[20,21]

The technique of x ray contrast lymphangiography was developed in 1952 by Kinmonth in England and became the standard method of examining the lymphatic system in man in vivo.[22] His technique involved injecting patent blue dye subcutaneously on the dorsum of the hand or foot to highlight a lymphatic vessel. He would then dissect down to the trunk and cannulate it before injecting a radio opaque dye. This injection was directly into the lymphatic vessel. It was used in many thousands of patients, and good quality radiographs of the lymphatic collecting vessels and the draining lymph nodes were obtained. Much of the detailed knowledge that we now have of human lymphatic drainage patterns came from such studies (Figure 28.4).[23] The method used large volumes of contrast material injected directly into lymphatic capillaries with the aim of opacifying as much of the system as possible. It was most often used to assess the possibility of metastatic involvement of lymph nodes, and to do this as many nodes as possible needed to be opacified. This meant that the injections were often given some distance away from the primary tumour e.g. in the foot to visualize the groin and iliac nodes and in the hand to visualize the axillary nodes. The contrast material passed readily onward from the first node to reach other nodes. This approach is quite clearly different from the search for the sentinel node, however in some situations where the draining lymphatics had a limited path

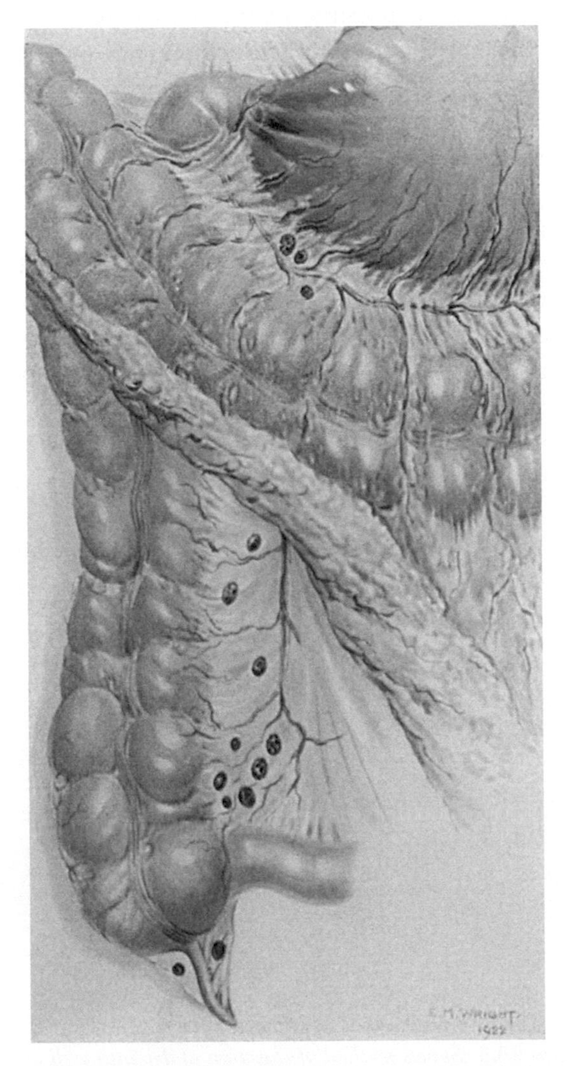

Figure 28.4 *Distribution of pigment in the lymphatic system absorbed from the appendix (so-called pigmented appendix).*

to follow direct lymphography could identify a limited number of relevant nodes in which metastatic tumour cells might lodge. Though lymphangiography could be used if there was a narrow range of lymphatic drainage from the primary site it did not have general applicability. The large injection volumes and high pressures involved were not physiological and these limitations paved the way for the development of a tracer method.

In 1950, Walker was the first to use a radiotracer to map lymphatic drainage.[24] Following this, in 1953, Sherman et al. developed the concept of lymphoscintigraphy, showing that the passage of colloidal gold could be traced from the point of intradermal injection to the draining lymph nodes.[25] This was the advent of cutaneous lymphoscintigraphy as we know it today. Initially colloidal ^{198}Au was used. This tracer had a very small particle size of about 5 nanometres, which was excellent for lymphoscintigraphy, allowing ready entry of the radiocolloid into the lumen of the initial lymphatics. The disadvantage of colloidal ^{198}Au was that it was a beta emitter, and thus tissues around the site of injection received a high radiation dose. Technetium 99m labelled colloids were developed to deal with this problem.

Sappey's concept of the lymphatic drainage of the trunk was accepted as correct for 130 years until modified somewhat by Haagensen et al., who enlarged the ambiguous zone to a 5 cm band down the midline and around the waist.[26] Sugarbaker confirmed that drainage was ambiguous from these areas, but it continued to be thought that lymph drainage from the skin of the trunk outside these ambiguous zones would predictably be to the axilla or groin.[27]

Colloidal ^{198}Au was used by Fee et al. in 1978 when they studied 32 patients with melanoma.[28] This study confirmed that lymphoscintigraphy could accurately predict the node fields that potentially contained metastatic melanoma. Nine of their patients had nodal metastases, and in every case, lymph drainage from the primary site to this node field was shown on lymphoscintigraphy. Around this time, other investigators were also using lymphoscintigraphy to map lymph drainage in patients with melanomas located on the trunk and elsewhere when drainage was considered uncertain (i.e. in Sappey's zones of uncertainty or in the head and neck region[29,30]). It was emphasized that lymphoscintigraphy could not predict whether lymph nodes contained metastases, but that it could identify which node fields were at greatest risk of harbouring occult metastases.[31] More studies began to appear that expanded the zone of uncertainty around Sappey's lines and also showed that drainage from the skin of the head and neck was quite variable.[32] The results of lymphoscintigraphy began to be used as a guide to determine which lymph node fields should be subjected to elective lymphadenectomy.[33–35] It also became increasingly apparent that drainage could sometimes be identified to node fields that would not be considered potential metastatic sites on clinical grounds.[36]

For many years, cutaneous lymphoscintigraphy was thus used to identify which node fields received lymphatic drainage from the primary melanoma site on the skin, and, therefore, which node fields were potential sites of occult metastases. With experience, it became clear that lymphoscintigraphy should be performed before wide local excision or lymphadenectomy, as it was shown that these procedures disrupted the normal lymphatic drainage pathways,[37,38] As such studies proceeded, the zones of ambiguity on the trunk and elsewhere were continually expanded as more and more exceptions to the expected patterns of lymphatic drainage were shown.[39,40] Nevertheless, lymphoscintigraphy continued to be performed only when some clinical doubt was present about the pattern of drainage. The threshold of doubt varied considerably from surgeon to surgeon, with the end result that there was considerable variation in the sites subjected to lymphadenectomy by different surgeons for lesions at the corresponding sites on the skin. Lymphoscintigraphy was not performed if the primary site was on a limb or close to an individual node field.

THE SENTINEL NODE CONCEPT

A crude map of draining lymph nodes was discovered fortuitously during surgery by Braithwaite in 1914, when he opened the abdomen of a patient who presented with acute appendicitis (Figure 28.4).[41] To his astonishment he saw jet black staining of a series of lymph nodes extending in a chain from the ileocaecal region up to the region of the duodenum and superior mesenteric artery. The nodes on the greater curvature of the stomach near the pylorus were also black. He recognized that the black pigment escaping from the appendix had found its way along the lymphatic pathways to the draining lymph nodes, which had as a result become stained a deep black colour. He deduced that if black pigment could make its way from the appendix to these draining nodes, then infection could do likewise. Over the next few years he pursued his interest in the patterns of lymphatic drainage, injecting vital dyes first in cats and then in humans so that he could follow the blue stained lymphatic vessels to the draining nodes which would also become stained. Braithwaite noted that lymph could flow via many different pathways and he referred to the draining nodes which stained with vital dye as the 'glands sentinel'. Braithwaite thus seems to have been the first person to introduce the concept of a 'sentinel node' which drains a particular part of the body (Figures 28.4–28.9).

The technique of lymphangiography described by Kinmonth, although generally used to opacify as many lymph nodes as possible in the search for metastases, could also be used to map general patterns of lymphatic drainage if the possibilities for lymph drainage were limited. This situation occurred with penile and testicular tumours. In 1963 Busch and Sayegh used this method to identify a 'primary complex' of lymph nodes which consistently received drainage from the testicle, although they did point out that there was variability in the lymphatic drainage of the testicle from one man to another.[42] They also recognized the importance of this variability for the surgical management of testicular cancer, as this raised doubts about which lymph nodes to remove at operation in an individual patient. In subsequent work they described 'primary' nodes, which first received drainage, and 'secondary' nodes, which were next in line.[43] They also noted that pedal lymphography, although identifying 'a maze of lymph nodes

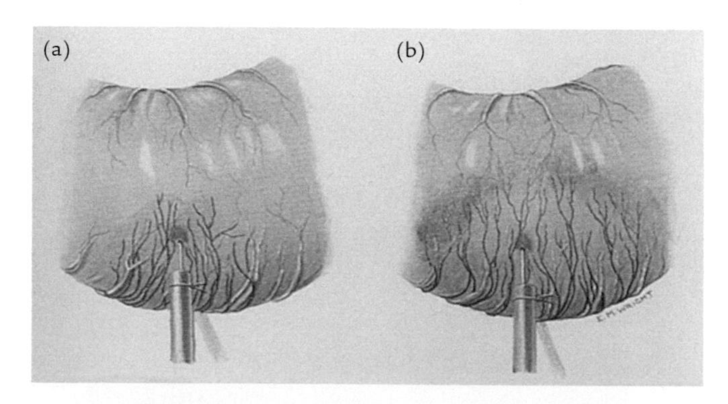

Figure 28.5 *Shows method of injection of dye into wall of stomach. Also shows that diffusion of dye injected postmortem (a) is slower and (b) less widespread than in vivo.*

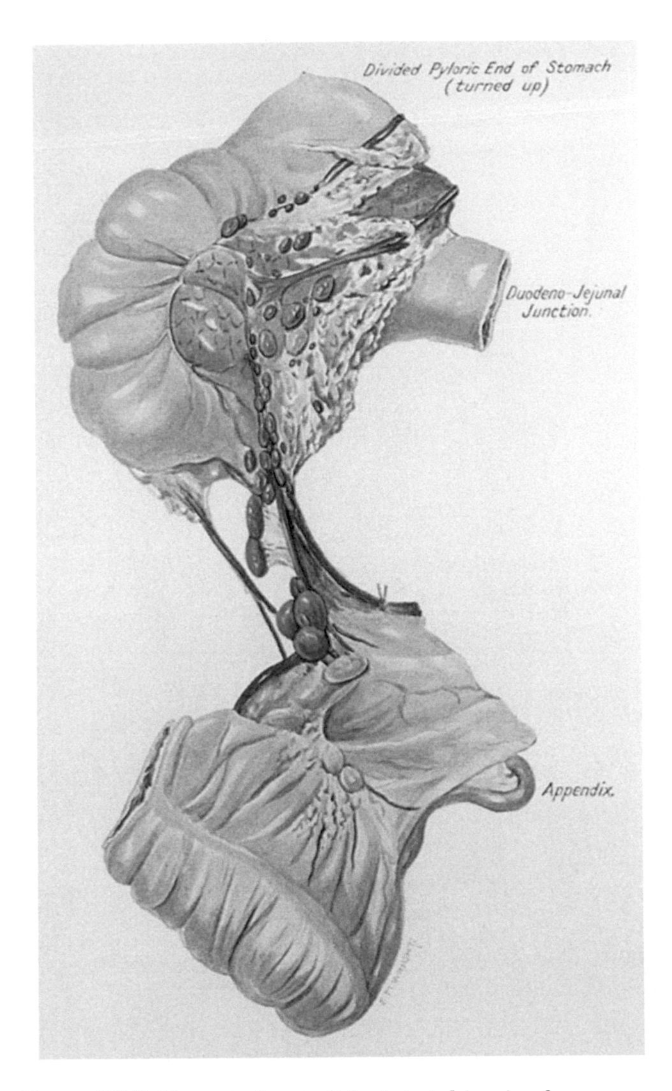

Figure 28.6 *Shows pathway of dye injected in vivo from ileocaecal junction to head of pancreas and higher.*

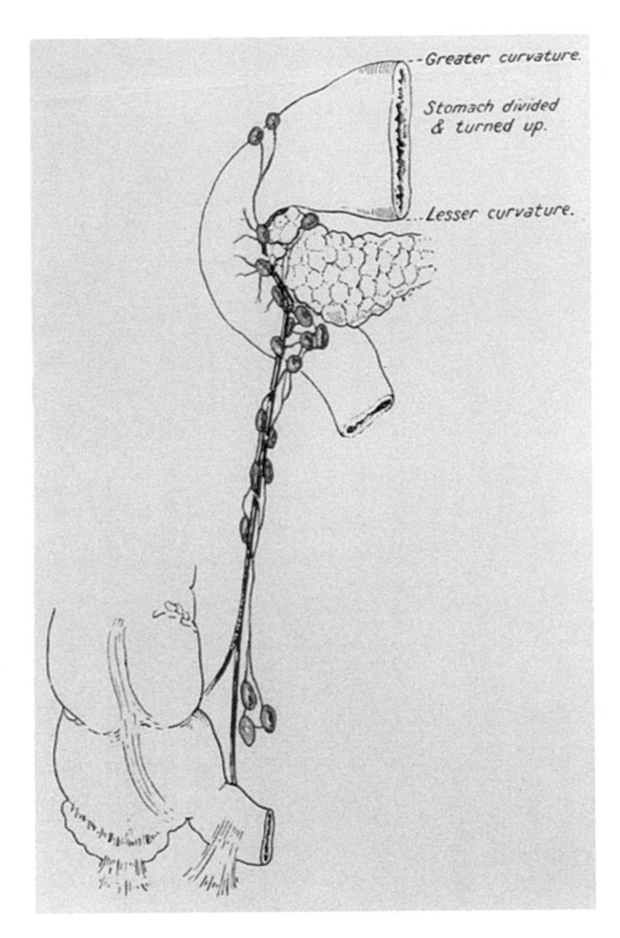

Figure 28.7 *Shows pathway of dye injected postmortem from ileocaecal junction to head of pancreas and higher.*

extending from the superficial inguinal nodes to the thoracic duct' failed to identify some of the lymph nodes opacified by direct testicular injection. They thus showed that lymph drainage from the testicle varied from patient to patient and that to identify the primary nodes selectively it was important to inject the contrast material at the site of interest. They used intraoperative x rays to guide the surgeon to the correct nodes that contained radiographic contrast. During the 1960s others performed similar studies and reached similar conclusions. Throughout these works terms are used that have echoes in our current terminology for sentinel node biopsy. It was stated in 1963 by Chiappa et al. that the lymph vessels of the testis drain the lymph to a specific lymph centre and that the metastatic emboli from a primary testicular tumour could find their first filter in this lymph centre.[44,45] In 1965 Cook et al. said that the primary lymph nodes draining the testicles were filled reliably only when the injection was made into lymph vessels directly draining the testicle.[46] Sayegh et al. using testicular lymphography, found 'a small sentinel node is immediately visualised before the main lateral nodes on each side are seen'.[47]

The term 'sentinel node' to describe the lymph nodes receiving lymphatic drainage from the penis was also used by Cabanas in 1977.[48] Cabanas had been studying the lymph drainage of a variety of tumours using lymphangiography for more than a decade. This involved a total of 250 patients with cancers of the penis, testis, breast, anus, rectum, and melanoma and lymphoma. He was interested in minimizing the extent of surgery of the groin nodes in patients with penile cancer by defining the pattern of lymphatic drainage from the penis. Cabanas observed that lymphography

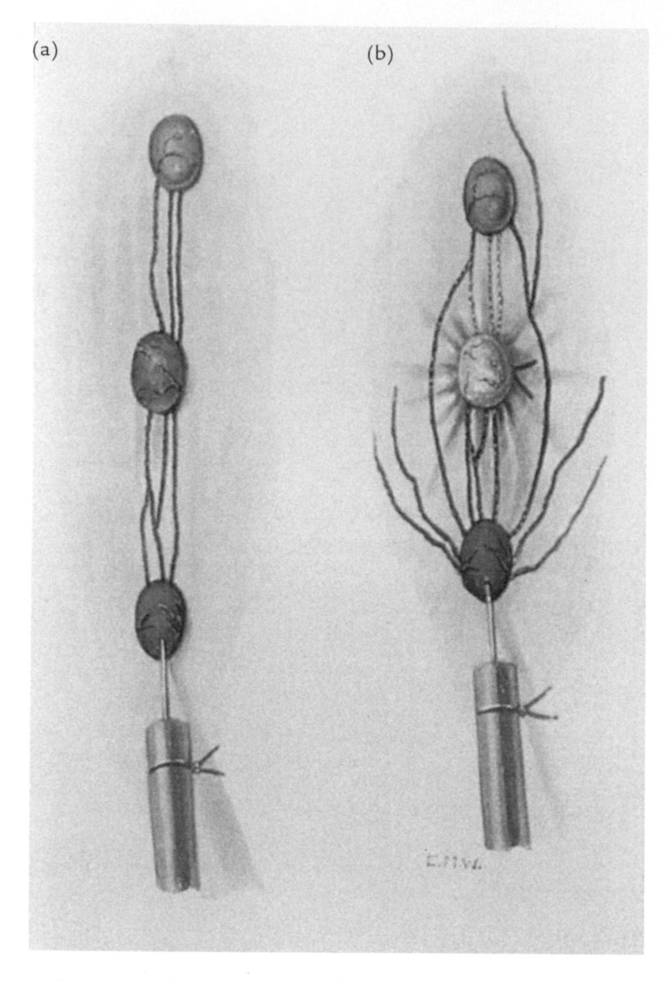

Figure 28.8 *Effect of obstruction on flow of lymph. A normal chain of lymph nodes (a), and flow around a lymph node with a ligature near its base (b). Lymph readily flows past obstructed node to next higher node.*

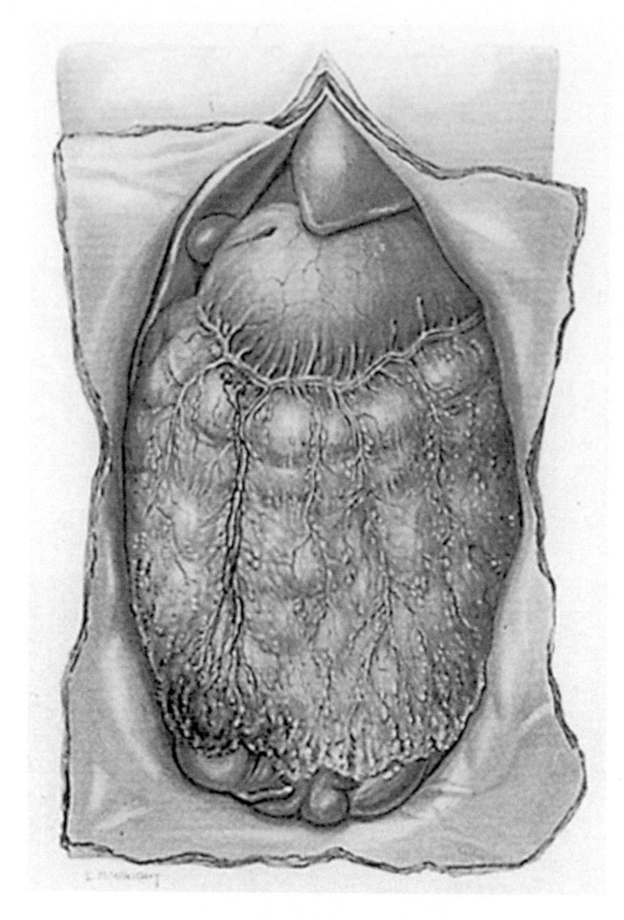

Figure 28.9 *Flow of indigo-carmine from edge of greater omentum applied with dye soaked sponge.*

performed by cannulating the dorsal lymphatic of the penis opacified a node in the superficial inguinal region lying just anterior and medial to the superficial epigastric vein. This node could also be opacified by injecting contrast into the dorsal lymphatic of the foot. This he called the sentinel node of the penis. Occasionally there was more than one node in this area but the sentinel node was the larger, more medial node in this region. He was able to identify this node in 43 patients by using the dorsal lymphatic of the penis (10 of whom also had the dorsal lymphatic of the foot injected) and in 57 patients using the dorsal lymphatic of the foot. He recommended early bilateral biopsy of this sentinel lymph node as a logical approach to the treatment of penile carcinoma. He described the technique of surgically removing this node, stating that if the sentinel node was negative a radical groin dissection could be avoided. In his hands the status of this sentinel node reliably staged the groin nodes, and he concluded that regional lymphadenectomy could be selectively performed based on the status of the sentinel lymph node. He also emphasized the unreliability of clinical palpation of the inguinal nodes as an indicator of the presence or absence of metastases. Reports began to appear, however, that biopsy of the sentinel node as described by Cabanas in patients with penile cancer sometimes missed lymph nodes that contained metastases.[49,50]

Cabanas used the term sentinel node to describe a node that regularly drained the penis and did not in his original work use any intraoperative mapping technique to locate the actual one or two nodes that drained the primary tumour site in individual patients. This was the important advance which must be attributed to Morton et al. at the John Wayne Cancer Institute in Santa Monica, California, and which is the key to the successful application of the sentinel node biopsy technique as we know it today.[51] In 1992, they described a method of mapping the lymphatic drainage from a primary melanoma site by using intradermal injections of blue dye. They had previously validated the technique in a feline model.[52] The stained lymphatic was followed surgically until the blue channel was seen entering a blue stained node in the draining node field (Figure 28.10). This node was called the 'sentinel' node. It was found that if this node was free of metastatic disease then the node field was almost invariably free of disease. The disadvantage of this approach was that the surgical technique was difficult to learn, requiring about 50 operations before a surgeon achieved reliable results. It was this study, however, which showed that the metastatic melanoma status of a whole node field could be accurately determined by selectively removing and carefully examining one or two sentinel nodes.

It is of interest that, although blue dye injection had long been used to identify lymphatics peripherally and had also been used as an aid to permit cannulation for radiological lymphangiography, the concept of tracing it to a specific lymph node or nodes had taken over 70 years to evolve from the original work of Braithwaite to be finally validated systematically by Morton et al. Their original paper, now a classic citation, was rejected by three major surgical journals in the United States before it was published in 1992. It was this publication which sparked the huge interest in sentinel node biopsy as a node staging procedure which we see today.

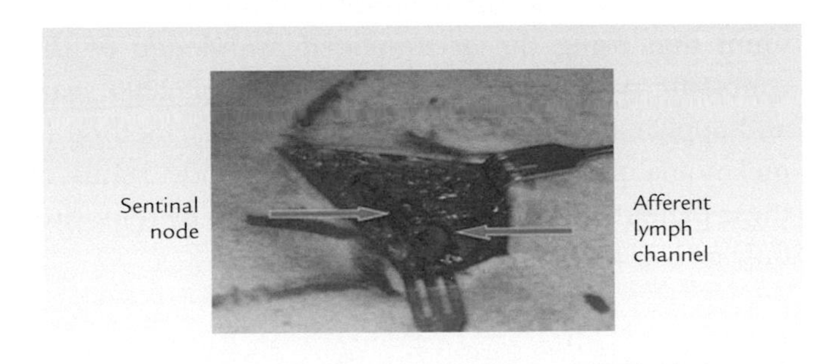

Figure 28.10 *The blue stained lymphatic vessel entering a blue stained node identifies this node as a sentinel node*

Facilitating the search for the sentinel node

The discovery by Morton et al. caused others to search for more rapid and less technically demanding methods of locating sentinel lymph nodes. After the injection of a radiolabelled colloid into the skin around a melanoma site or excision biopsy site the tracer passes via the draining lymphatics to the sentinel node or nodes where it remains for some hours. This means that the activity in the node is in high contrast to the surrounding tissues, which are essentially free of radioactivity. This is an ideal situation for the use of a handheld radiation detecting probe. Examples of such probes had been described intermittently since the late 1940s, although the original probes were based on the Geiger-Muller tube, which was very efficient for detecting beta particles (electrons) but very inefficient for detecting gamma rays.[53,54] Since most radiopharmaceuticals in nuclear medicine practice use gamma emitters because of the better radiation dosimetry, probes with better efficiency for the detection of gamma emitters were developed. Solid state detectors and scintillation detectors were both tried. In the late 1980s commercial vendors began to market probes for radio immuno guided surgery, which used cadmium telluride or sodium iodide scintillation detectors.[55] Alex et al. described the use of a ^{99m}Tc labelled colloid in combination with such a gamma detecting probe to locate the sentinel node in patients with melanoma[56] (Figure 28.11). This technique was much simpler than the original method described by Morton et al. Radiocolloid was injected intradermally around the excision biopsy site and after a brief delay of 10–20 minutes the regional node field was 'scanned' by using a gamma detecting probe to locate the one or two 'hot' sentinel nodes. This technique accurately determined the lymph node status in their patients, and there were no patients who had micrometastases in regional lymph nodes if the sentinel node was normal. This technique could be taught to surgeons over several days of training. Several studies by Krag and colleagues were published in the early 1990s that attested to the accuracy of sentinel node biopsy with the intraoperative use of a gamma detecting probe.[56–59]

Uren et al. showed that the standard lymphoscintigraphy technique, which had been in routine use to determine which node fields drained melanoma primary sites, could be modified to allow the exact location of the sentinel nodes to be marked on the skin[60,61]

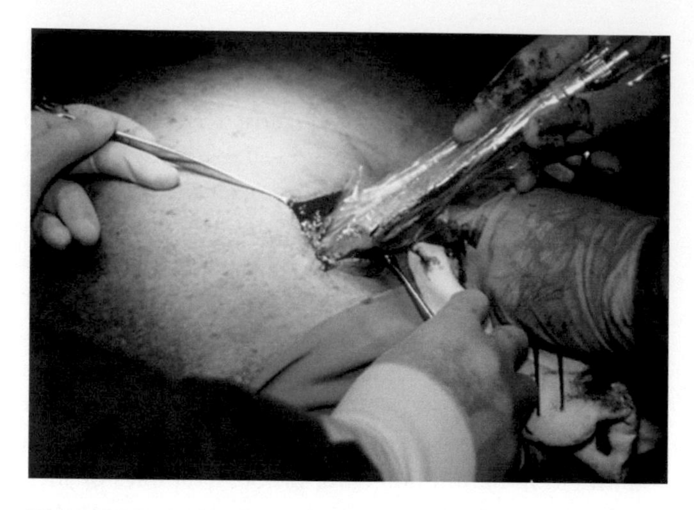

Figure 28.11 *The gamma detecting probe inside a sterile sheath aids in directing surgery towards the radiolabelled sentinel node and confirms that the node field drops to background activity after the sentinel node has been excised.*

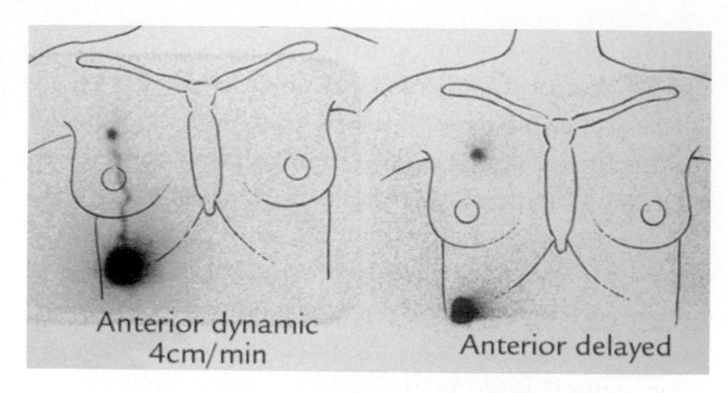

Figure 28.12 *High resolution lymphoscintigraphy identifies the lymphatic vessel reaching the sentinel node, the same vessel the surgeon sees staining blue at surgery. Unusual drainage pathways and interval nodes are also detected in this way.*

(Figure 28.12). The depth of the node deep to the skin mark could also be measured using lymphoscintigraphy. This information could then be used to aid in rapid surgical location of sentinel nodes. The surgeon would inject blue dye around the excision biopsy site and then make an incision at the site of the sentinel node as marked during lymphoscintigraphy. He would dissect down to the depth reported and find the blue lymphatic channel entering the blue stained sentinel node. A further advantage of preoperative lymphoscintigraphy was that unusual drainage pathways were defined, and the location of any interval nodes identified between the primary melanoma site and the draining node field could be marked, ensuring that all sentinel nodes were biopsied in each patient.[62] Surgeons require a shorter training period to accurately identify and excise the sentinel node using this method than when using the original method described by Morton et al.

Using lymphoscintigraphy to determine the location of sentinel nodes in this way has led to the discovery of several unusual and previously unknown pathways for lymphatic drainage of the skin.[63–68] It is now clear that when faced with an individual patient with a melanoma, there are, in fact, very few, if any, places on the skin of the human body that have completely unambiguous drainage, and in any case this concept is now redundant because the location of the sentinel node has become the main application of lymphatic mapping of the skin. Several large surgical studies have now confirmed that sentinel node status is an accurate reflection of node field status in melanoma patients.[59,69,70]

Most now accept that the best method of locating the sentinel nodes at the time of surgery is to use a combination of preoperative lymphoscintigraphy, blue dye injection just before anaesthesia, and intraoperative use of a gamma probe to assist in locating the blue and 'hot' node or nodes and show that the node field returns to background levels of activity after the presumptive sentinel nodes have been removed.[71,72] The delay between the injection of tracer and surgery will vary with different protocols; but there is enough radioactivity remaining in the sentinel nodes to allow the gamma probe to be used up to 24 hours after injection of the tracer. There are some advantages in this next day surgical approach. There is less radiation safety concern for operating theatre staff and no requirement for radiation licensing of the surgeon. Further, the node:background ratio rises with time, which facilitates the location of 'hot' nodes using the gamma detection probe intraoperatively.[71]

It is now clear at the beginning of the third millennium that using the accumulated knowledge of the lymphatic system gained over a period of 2000 years and applying it to the sentinel node biopsy method in melanoma patients allows the lymph node status of these patients to be determined accurately by removing only one or two sentinel nodes.

THE FUTURE

There are several areas where improvements could be made which would enhance the accuracy of lymphatic mapping and the sentinel node biopsy procedure. Firstly, an improved radiopharmaceutical could be produced. The perfect tracer would be one that showed almost complete migration from the injection site via the lymphatics to the sentinel node and was then trapped in the sentinel node for at least 24 hours. This would allow smaller doses to be used and would also remove the problem of radiation artefact from the injection site obscuring sentinel nodes in nearby node fields. With all of the dose in the sentinel node, detection using a gamma detecting probe during surgery would be enhanced and simplified as there would be little background radiation. Some promising tracers are currently under investigation. One theoretically attractive approach is to use receptor binding non-particulate tracers, which move rapidly from the injection site through the lymph channels to the sentinel nodes but then bind strongly to the node as a result of the receptor binding to lymphoid tissue.[73] This approach may also lead to less tracer passing on to second tier lymph nodes.

High resolution gamma camera collimators also improve the quality of lymphoscintigraphy, ensuring that there is no star artefact as a result of septal penetration. Such collimators ideally are microcast collimators and not folded metal. Septa should be of a thickness adequate to keep septal penetration below 1% at 140 KEV energies.

The intraoperative detection of the sentinel nodes would be helped by improvements in the design of gamma detecting devices. These could include smaller handheld probes for greater flexibility and also the development of a hand held gamma camera or imaging system. There are several possibilities for such a device. A small solid state detector of about 10 cm by 10 cm would allow confirmation that the nodes seen on lymphoscintigraphy are the same nodes present at the time of surgery. Such a 10 cm by 10 cm image would also allow confirmation that the sentinel nodes had been removed successfully. A system along these lines has been described for breast imaging using scintillators coupled to solid state photodiode arrays, although this device remains rather bulky for intraoperative use.[74] Such devices would also be very useful to locate the sentinel node during surgery in areas where the skin mark may not overlie the node when the patient is in the operative position. This is particularly a problem in the head and neck area.

CONCLUSIONS

Knowledge of the lymphatic system has evolved slowly over hundreds of years, and surprisingly, new insights continue to be gained today. This body of knowledge has reached the point where, by using high quality lymphatic mapping in individual patients, we are able to locate the lymph nodes that receive direct lymphatic drainage from a primary tumour site, remove them surgically, and therefore accurately determine the patient's lymph node status with minimum surgery. Cutaneous lymphatic mapping using lymphoscintigraphy and gamma detecting probes has come of age and is now finding routine application in patients with melanoma. Defining the patterns of lymphatic drainage and locating the sentinel lymph nodes is having a direct impact on the surgical management of these patients.

REFERENCES

1. Hewson W, *The works of William Hewson.* (ed, Gulliver G) F.R.S. London: The Sydenham Society, 1846.
2. Delamere G, Poirier P, Cuneo B, The lymphatics. In: *A Treatise of Human Anatomy* (ed. Charpy PPaA), Westminster Archibald Constable and Co Ltd, 1903.
3. Massa N, *Lib Introd Anat,* 1532.
4. Aselli G, *De lactibus sive lacteis venis.* Milan: J B Bidellius, 1627.
5. Pecquet J, *New anatomical experiments* (English translation). London: O Pulleyn, 1653
6. Hewson W, *Experimental inquiries on the blood, with some remarks on it and an appendix relating to the lymphatic system in birds, fishes and amphibious animals.* London, 1771.
7. Cruikshank W, *The anatomy of the absorbing vessels of the human body.* 1786.
8. Mascagni P, *Vasorum lymphaticorum corporis humani historia et ichnographia.* P Carli: Sienna, 1787.
9. Lauth, *Essai sur les vaisseaux lymphatiques.* Strasbourg, 1824.
10. Sappey MPC, *Anatomie, physiologie, pathologie des vaisseaux lymphatiques consideres chez l'homme et les vertebres.* (eds DeLahaye A, Lecrosnier E), Paris, 1874.
11. Recklinghausen FDv, *Die Lymphgefässe und ihre Beziehung zum Bindegewebe.* Berlin: A Hirschwald, 1862.
12. Regaud, Origine des vaisseaux lymphatiques de la mamelle. *C R Soc Biol* 1894; 20: 495.
13. Ranvier, Chyliferes du rat. *C R Acad Sciences* 1894; 12: 621.
14. Kytmanoff, Ueber die Nervenendigungen in den Lymphgefassen der Säugethiere. *Anat Anzeig* 15, 1901.
15. Gerota, Zur Technik der Lymphgefassinjection. Eine neue Injectionsmasse fur Lymphgefasse. *Polychrom Injection Anat Anzeiger* 1896; 12; 210.
16. Bartels P, Das Lymphgefässsystem. In: *Handbuch der Anatomie des Menschen.* (ed. Bardeleben Kv), Gustav Fischer: Jena, 4th part; vol 3; 1909.
17. Gray JH, The relation of lymphatic vessels to the spread of cancer. *Br J Surg* 1939; 26: 462.
18. Horta JD, DaMotta LC, Abbatt JD, Roriz ML, Malignancy and other late effects following administration of Thorotrast. *Lancet* 1965; 2: 201.
19. Hudack S, McMaster PD, The lymphatic participation in human cutaneous phenomena. *J Exp Med* 1933; 57: 751.
20. Strug LH, Leon W, Cohn IJ, Vital staining of lymphatics during surgery. WB Saunders: Philadelphia, *Surg Forum Am Coll Surg,* 1954.
21. Haagensen CD, Feind CR, Herter FP, et al, *The lymphatics in cancer.* Philadelphia: WB Saunders, 1972.

22. Kinmonth J, Lymphangiography in man; a method of outlining lymphatic trunks at operation. *Clin Sci* 1952; 11: 13–20.
23. Clouse ME, Wallace S, eds. *Lymphatic imaging. Lymphography, computed tomography and scintigraphy.* 2nd ed. Baltimore: Williams and Wilkins, 15–21. Harris JHJ, ed. Golden's Diagnostic Radiology, 1985.
24. Walker L, Localization of radioactive colloids in lymph nodes. *J Lab Clin Med* 1950; 36: 440–9.
25. Sherman AI, Ter-Pogossian M, Tocus EC, Lymph node concentration of radioactive colloidal gold following interstitial injection. *Cancer* 1953; 6: 1238–40.
26. Haagansen CD, Feind CR, Herter FP, et al, Lymphatics of the trunk. In: *The lymphatics in cancer.* (ed. Haagansen CD). Philadelphia: WB Saunders, 1972: 437–58.
27. Sugarbaker EV, McBride CM, Melanoma of the trunk: the results of surgical excision and anatomic guidelines for predicting nodal metastasis. *Surgery* 1976; 80: 22–30.
28. Fee HJ, Robinson DS, Sample WF, et al, The determination of lymph shed by colloidal gold scanning in patients with malignant melanoma: a preliminary study. *Surgery* 1978; 84: 626–32.
29. Meyer CM, Lecklitner ML, Logic JR, et al, Technetium-99m sulfur-colloid cutaneous lymphoscintigraphy in the management of truncal melanoma. *Radiology* 1979; 131: 205–9.
30. Sullivan DC, Croker BP, Harris CC, et al, Lymphoscintigraphy in malignant melanoma: 99m-Tc antimony sulfur colloid. *Am J Roentgenol* 1981; 137: 847–51.
31. Munz DL, Altmeyer P, Sessler MJ, Axillary lymph node groups—the center in lymphatic drainage from the truncal skin in man. Clinical significance for management of malignant melanoma. *Lymphology* 1982; 15: 143–57.
32. Wanebo HJ, Harpole D, Teates CD, Radionuclide lymphoscintigraphy with technetium 99m antimony sulfide colloid to identify lymphatic drainage of cutaneous melanoma at ambiguous sites in the head and neck and trunk. *Cancer* 1985; 55: 1403–13.
33. Reintgen DS, Sullivan D, Coleman E, et al, Lymphoscintigraphy for malignant melanoma—surgical considerations. *Am J Surg* 1893; 49: 672–8.
34. Eberbach MA, Wahl RL, Argenta LC, et al, Utility of lymphoscintigraphy in directing surgical therapy for melanomas of the head, neck, and upper thorax. Surgery 1987; 102: 433–9.
35. Kramer EL, Sanger JJ, Golomb F, et al, The impact of intradermal lymphoscintigraphy on surgical management of clinical stage I truncal melanoma. *J Dermatol Surg Oncol* 1987; 13: 508–15.
36. Logic JR, Balch CM, Defining lymphatic drainage patterns with cutaneous lymphoscintigraphy. In: *Cutaneous melanoma: clinical management and treatment results worldwide.* (eds. Balch CM, Milton GW, Shaw HM, Soong S-J). Philadelphia: JB Lippincott, 1985: 159–70.
37. Rees WV, Robinson DS, Holmes EC, Morton DL, Altered lymphatic drainage following lymphadenectomy. *Cancer* 1980; 45: 3045–9.
38. Jonk A, Kroon BBR, Mooi WJ, Hoefnagel CA, Contralateral inguinal lymph node metastasis in patients with melanoma of the lower extremities. *Br J Surg* 1989; 76: 1161–2.
39. Eberbach MA, Wahl RL, Lymphatic anatomy: functional nodal basins. *Ann Plast Surg* 1989; 22: 25–31.
40. Norman J, Cruse W, Espinosa C, et al, Redefinition of cutaneous lymphatic drainage with the use of lymphoscintigraphy for malignant melanoma. *Am J Surg* 1991; 162: 432–7.
41. Braithwaite LR, The flow of lymph from the ileocaecal angle, and its possible bearing on the cause of duodenal and gastric ulcer. *Br J Surg* 1923; XI: 7–26.
42. Busch FM, Sayegh ES, Roentgenographic visualization of human testicular lymphatics: a preliminary report. *J Urol* 1963; 89: 106–10.
43. Busch FM, Sayegh ES, Chenault OW, Some uses of lymphangiography in the management of testicular tumors. *J Urol* 1964; 490–3.
44. Chiappa S, Galli G, Barbaini S, et al, La lymphographic peroperatoire dans les tumeurs du testicule. *J Radiol Electr* 1963; 44: 613.
45. Chiappa S, Uslenghi C, Bonadonna, et al, Combined testicular and foot lymphangiography in testicular carcinoma. *Surg Gynecol Obstetr* 1966; 13: 10–14.
46. Cook FE, Lawrence DD, Smith JR, Gritti EJ, Testicular carcinoma and lymphangiography. *Radiology* 1965; 84: 420–7.
47. Sayegh E, Brooks T, Sacher E, Busch F, Lymphangiography of the retroperitoneal lymph nodes through the inguinal route. *J Urol* 1966; 95: 102–7.
48. Cabanas RM, An approach for the treatment of penile carcinoma. *Cancer* 1977; 39: 456–66.
49. Bouchot O, Bouvier S, Bochereau G, Jeddi M, Cancer of the penis: the value of systematic biopsy of the superficial inguinal lymph nodes in clinical N0 stage patients. *Prog Urol* 1993; 3: 228–33.
50. Pettaway CA, L PL, Dinney CPN, et al, Sentinel lymph node dissection for penile carcinoma: the MD Anderson Cancer Center experience. *J Urol* 1995; 154: 1999–2003.
51. Morton DL, Wen D-R, Wong JH, et al, Technical details of intraoperative lymphatic mapping for early stage melanoma. *Arch Surg* 1992; 127: 392–9.
52. Wong JH, Cagle LA, Morton DL, Lymphatic drainage of skin to a sentinel lymph node in a feline model. *Ann Surg* 1991; 214: 637–41.
53. Moore GE, Use of radioactive diiodofluorescein in the diagnosis and localization of brain tumors. *Science* 1948; 107: 569–71.
54. Selverstone B, Solomon AK, Sweet WH, Location of brain tumors by means of radioactive phosphorus. *JAMA* 1949; 140: 227–8.
55. Arnold MW, Schneebaum S, Berens A, et al, Radioimmunoguided surgery challenges traditional decision making in patients with primary colorectal cancer. *Surgery* 1992; 112: 624–30.
56. Alex JC, Weaver DL, Fairbank JT, et al, Gamma-probe-guided lymph node localization in malignant melanoma. *Surg Oncol* 1993; 2: 303–8.
57. Alex JC, Krag DN. Gamma probe guided localization of lymph nodes. *Surg Oncol* 1993; 2: 137–43.
58. Krag DN, Weaver DL, Alex JC, Fairbank JT, Surgical resection and radiolocalization of the sentinel lymph node in breast cancer using a gamma probe. *Surg Oncol* 1993; 2: 335–40.
59. Krag DN, Meijer SJ, Weaver DL, et al. Minimal-access surgery for staging of malignant melanoma. *Arch Surg* 1995; 130: 654–8.
60. Uren RF, Howman-Giles RB, Shaw HM, et al, Lymphoscintigraphy in high risk melanoma of the trunk: predicting draining node groups, defining lymphatic channels and locating the sentinel node. *J Nucl Med* 1993; 34: 1435–40.
61. Uren RF, Howman-Giles RB, Thompson JF, et al, Lymphoscintigraphy to identify sentinel nodes in patients with melanoma. *Melanoma Res* 1994; 4: 395–9.
62. Uren RF, Thompson JF, Howman-Giles RB, *Lymphatic drainage of the skin and breast: locating the sentinel nodes.* Amsterdam: Harwood Academic Publishers, 1999.
63. Uren RF, Howman-Giles RB, Thompson JF, et al, Lymphatic drainage from peri-umbilical skin to internal mammary nodes. *Clin Nucl Med* 1995; 20: 254–5.
64. Uren RF, Howman-Giles RB, Thompson JF, et al, Lymphatic drainage to triangular intermuscular space lymph nodes in melanoma on the back. *J Nucl Med* 1996; 37: 964–6.
65. Uren RF, Howman-Giles R, Thompson JF, Quinn MJ, Direct lymphatic drainage from the skin of the forearm to a supraclavicular node. *Clin Nucl Med* 1996; 21: 387–9.
66. Uren RF, Roberts J, Howman-Giles RB, Thompson JF, Direct lymphatic drainage from the skin of the elbow to an interpectoral node. *Reg Cancer Treat* 1996; 9: 100–2.
67. Uren RF, Howman-Giles RB, Thompson JF, Lymphatic drainage from the skin of the back to intra-abdominal lymph nodes in melanoma patients. *Ann Surg Oncol* 1998; 5: 384–7.
68. O'Brien CJ, Uren RF, Thompson JF, et al, Prediction of potential metastatic sites in cutaneous head and neck melanoma using lymphoscintigraphy. *Am J Surg* 1995; 170: 461–6.
69. Ross MI, Reintgen D, Balch CM, Selective lymphadenectomy: emerging role for lymphatic mapping and sentinel node biopsy in the management of early stage melanoma. *Semin Surg Oncol* 1993; 9: 219–23.
70. Thompson JF, McCarthy WH, Bosch CMJ, et al, Sentinel lymph node status as a indicator of the presence of metastatic melanoma in regional lymph nodes. *Melanoma Res* 1995; 5: 255–60.
71. Thompson JF, Niewind P, Uren RF, et al, Single-dose isotope injection for both preoperative lymphoscintigraphy and intraoperative sentinel

lymph node identification in melanoma patients. *Melanoma Res* 1997; 6: 500–6.
72. Pijpers R, Borgstein PJ, Meijer S, et al, Sentinel node biopsy in melanoma patients: dynamic lymphoscintigraphy followed by intraoperative gamma probe and vital dye guidance. *World J Surg* 1997; 21: 788–93.
73. Vera DR, Wisner ER, Stadalnik RC, Sentinel node imaging via a nonparticulate receptor-binding radiotracer. *J Nucl Med* 1997; 38: 530–5.
74. Patt BE, Iwanczyk JS, Rossington Tull C, et al, High resolution CsI(Tl)/Si-PIN detector development for breast imaging. *IEEE Trans Nucl Sci* 1998; NS-45: 2126–31.

29

The sentinel lymph node biopsy procedure: identification with blue dye and a gamma probe

Richard Essner, John F Thompson, Omgo E Nieweg

INTRODUCTION

Controversy surrounding the surgical management of the regional lymph nodes in early stage melanoma began over 100 years ago. In 1892, Herbert L Snow in his lecture on melanotic cancerous disease advocated wide excision and elective lymph node dissection (ELND) as a method of controlling metastatic lymphatic permeation.[1] His recommendation that treatment of melanoma should routinely include excision of the draining lymph nodes was based on his studies, suggesting that there was a direct connection between the primary site and the regional lymph nodes. Vigorous debate over the role of ELND for patients with early stage melanoma has continued since Snow first proposed this management approach. Although multiple retrospective studies have implied a survival benefit for patients undergoing ELND as well as wide excision of the primary tumour site, the therapeutic benefit of removing clinically normal lymph nodes has never been proved by randomized prospective studies.[2–12] Although ELND is considered a valuable staging procedure, its cost, morbidity, and overall low yield of tumour containing nodes have led most surgeons to abandon this procedure as a routine part of patient care. Yet the tumour status of the regional lymph nodes is universally recognized as being exceedingly important for determining prognosis and selecting patients for adjuvant therapy trials.[13,14]

As a result of their dissatisfaction with ELND, Morton et al. developed the technique of intraoperative lymphatic mapping and sentinel lymphadenectomy (LM/SL). This minimally invasive procedure allowed the surgeon to map the route of lymphatic drainage from the primary site to the regional lymph nodes and then selectively to excise the first (sentinel) lymph node on each lymphatic pathway. Because sentinel lymph nodes have been shown to be the most likely site for metastases, focused histological examination of the sentinel nodes leads to highly accurate staging of the node field. Patients with metastases (who are therefore most likely to benefit) can then undergo selective complete lymph node dissection (SCLND), and those without metastases are spared the expense and morbidity of this major surgical procedure.

INITIAL EXPERIENCE WITH BLUE DYE ONLY

In 1990 Morton et al. first proposed (and published two years later) the technique of LM/SL as a minimally invasive alternative to ELND for patients with clinically uninvolved regional lymph nodes.[15,16] They hypothesized that the dermal lymphatics provided a direct connection from the primary melanoma to the regional lymph field and that a sentinel node could be identified by tracing the afferent lymphatics to the point of entry into the node. The sentinel node should therefore be the first regional site of metastasis; if the sentinel nodes do not contain tumour cells from a primary melanoma, then other nodes in that lymph node field should also be free of micrometastatic disease.

LM/SL was performed in 223 patients by intradermal injection of a vital dye at the primary site. Patients with primary melanomas on the torso or head and neck underwent preoperative lymphoscintigraphy to determine the directions of lymph flow and the node fields at risk of containing metastases. A blue stained sentinel node was identified in 194 (82%) of 237 regional lymphatic drainage basins (Figure 29.1). All 223 patients underwent CLND regardless of the pathology of the sentinel node to verify the accuracy of the procedure. Of these specimens, 40 (21%) contained metastases in at least one lymph node. In only two of 194 SCLND specimens were non-sentinel nodes the exclusive site of regional metastases, a false negative rate of 1%. These results are quite remarkable, considering that in most cases preoperative lymphoscintigraphy was not used and the kinetics of the blue dye had not been well defined.[17]

Occult regional metastases were identified by both standard haematoxylin and eosin (H&E) staining and newer immunohistochemical techniques. Fifty-seven per cent of nodal metastases were found using conventional techniques; the remainder were identified by immunohistochemical staining alone.[18,19] Using immunohistochemical staining with an antiserum to S-100 protein, Cochran et al. had previously shown that 29% of lymph nodes stained negative with H&E actually contained metastatic melanoma.[19] The 3338 lymph nodes excised in the LM/SL patients were stained with the melanoma specific murine monoclonal antibody NKI/C3 to confirm the presence of melanoma cells. Few additional metastases were found by serial sectioning of the nodes compared with just examining the bivalved faces. The role of additional sectioning of the sentinel nodes is unknown.[20]

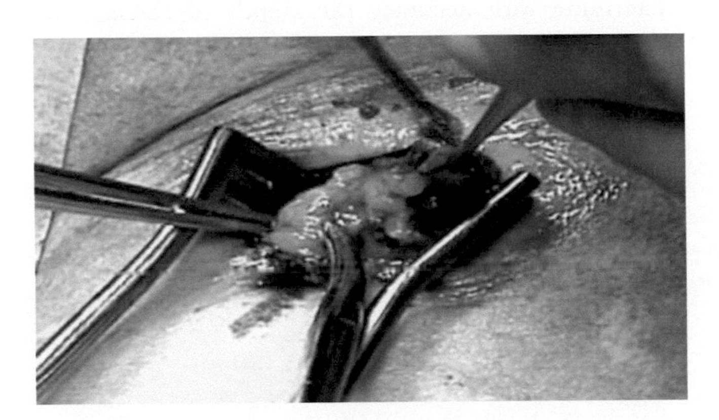

Figure 29.1 *Blue stained lymph node obtained from sentinel node biopsy of the groin. A blue stained sentinel lymph node is identified during LM/SL approximately 10–15 min after intradermal injection of 1.0 cc of isosulfan blue around the primary melanoma site.*

LM/SL is a relatively difficult technical procedure, but its learning curve is steep. In an initial 58 cases, Morton identified only 81% of blue stained sentinel nodes; but during the next 58 cases, his rate of sentinel node identification increased to 96%, and it now approaches 100%. The surgeon with the most experience with the procedure achieved an early success rate of 96%, while the surgeon with the least experience had the lowest level of success, 72% ($P<0.01$). The gradual improvement in the rate of sentinel node detection is partially based on increased experience with the technique. Blue stained afferent lymphatics and nodes can be difficult to identify, and most surgeons have little experience in dissecting lymphatic channels before performing LM/SL.

In 1993, Morton's group reported their experience of LM/SL for head and neck melanoma that drained to the cervical lymph nodes.[21] All patients had preoperative cutaneous lymphoscintigraphy. At the time of surgery blue dye alone was used to identify the sentinel nodes. The sentinel node was found in 71 (90%) of the 79 patients. Most of the missed sentinel nodes were from the occipital, post-auricular, or parotid basins where the blue dye is difficult to identify. There were no regional recurrences in those patients with tumour negative dissections during a mean follow up of 27 months. Although preoperative lymphoscintigraphy was used in all cases, this early experience with LM/SL showed the intrinsic difficulty with LM/SL for melanomas of the head and neck. The lymphatic drainage from primary melanomas in this region cannot be predicted from the anatomical location of the primary, and sentinel nodes embedded in the parotid gland, deep within the neck muscles, adjacent to the numerous facial vessels or in the thick soft tissue of the posterior neck, can be difficult to identify and remove.[22,23]

In 1993 Morton's group also reported their experience with LM/SL for melanoma of the lower torso and extremities that drained to the groin.[24] One hundred and twenty-eight patients had LM/SL performed. Preoperative lymphoscintigraphy was used only for non-extremity primaries. Sentinel nodes were identified in 96% of the 51 patients who had complete groin dissections and in 98% of the next 77 patients who had a LM/SL procedure alone. The incidence of false negative dissections was <1%. Even with this high rate of success with LM/SL in this node field, preoperative lymphoscintigraphy is now employed in all cases. In 12% of LM/SL procedures lymphatic drainage was to two lymph nodes, but in most cases a single sentinel node was identified just inferior to the inguinal ligament. However, some of the sentinel nodes were located at the apex of the femoral triangle, and not uncommonly two sentinel nodes were identified, usually on either side of the femoral vein. Although some may consider lymphoscintigraphy to be unnecessary for some primary tumours on the extremities, preoperative knowledge of the number and site of sentinel nodes is extremely valuable in all patients. The routine use of this procedure also helps to identify the occasional aberrant sentinel lymph node in the groin, the popliteal fossa or even the contralateral groin.[25]

Reintgen and associates from the Moffitt Cancer Center were the first group to confirm the original results of Morton et al.[26] Forty-two patients underwent LM/SL, all having undergone preoperative lymphoscintigraphy, with a blue stained lymph node found in each regional node field (100% accuracy). In eight of the cases metastases were found in the sentinel lymph node and in seven of the eight (88%) the sentinel lymph node was the exclusive site of disease. None of the remaining 34 patients had metastases in either sentinel or non-sentinel nodes. Their initial experience re-emphasized the importance of preoperative lymphoscintigraphy for localizing the site of the sentinel nodes. They also validated Morton's hypothesis that the sentinel node was reflective of the tumour status of the entire regional node field.

Shortly afterwards Thompson et al. at the Sydney Melanoma Unit reported their experience with LM/SL.[27] One hundred and eighteen patients underwent preoperative lymphoscintigraphy to identify the 120 node fields at risk. At the time of surgery, blue stained sentinel lymph nodes were located in 105 of the 120 fields (88%). In 18 of the 22 fields (82%) with metastatic disease the sentinel node was the exclusive site of metastasis. Their rate of false negative LM/SL (1.9%) was no different from that reported in Morton's series. Thompson et al. confirmed the steep learning curve associated with this procedure. In the first half of their experience, confident sentinel node identification was achieved in 74% of cases, but this rose to 92% during the second half.

A number of other investigators subsequently reported their experience with LM/SL using blue dye alone (Table 29.1).[26–28] Most investigators had no prior experience with LM/SL but achieved accuracy rates of at least 90%. These high success rates were undoubtedly the result of more rapid learning of the technique through the experience gained and shared by Morton and the other early pioneers of this procedure.

In Morton's initial experience the axilla and neck basins were the most difficult in which to identify sentinel lymph nodes. The anatomy of the axilla and neck often makes it difficult for the nuclear medicine physician to accurately mark the site of the sentinel node even when the patient is positioned as for surgery. It has been found that the two dimensional lymphoscintigraphy images sometimes lack sufficient information to determine with accuracy the depth of the sentinel

Table 29.1 *Initial experience with blue dye alone for sentinel lymph node biopsy. Accuracy rates of sentinel node identification were based on visual verification of blue stained lymph nodes alone. Listed are the authors, year of publication, number of subjects, basin sites and accuracy rates of sentinel node identification*

Investigators	No. of participants	Basins	Accuracy rate (%)
Morton et al. 1992[15]	223	All	82
Morton et al. 1993[21]	72	Neck	90
Essner et al. 1993[24]	128	Groin	97
Reintgen et al. 1994[26]	42	All	100
Thompson et al. 1994[27]	118	All	96
Karakousis et al. 1996[28]	55	All	93

lymph node from the skin.[29] If the blue stained afferent lymphatic is lacerated during surgery, as a result of not knowing the appropriate depth for dissection, the blue node can be extremely difficult to identify. It has also been found that patients who have undergone wide excision of the primary with margins ⩾1.5 cm or have had any procedure that disrupts the lymphatic drainage are not candidates for LM/SL.[30]

DEVELOPMENT OF GAMMA PROBE DIRECTED SENTINEL LYMPH NODE BIOPSY

While the early success with blue dye alone led to a large number of centres adopting LM/SL, it was clear that the learning phase involved too many cases for most surgeons to become proficient in using this technique alone. The routine use of cutaneous lymphoscintigraphy and gamma probe directed LM/SL not only improved the accuracy rate but also diminished the length of the learning phase.

Routine use of preoperative lymphoscintigraphy in all cases has also played a significant role in decreasing the incidence of missed sentinel nodes. In the United States the most commonly employed agents are technetium labelled (^{99m}Tc) albumin colloid (AC) (Cis-US, Inc, Bedford, MA), ^{99m}Tc filtered (20 μm) sulfur colloid (SC) (Cis-US, Inc) or ^{99m}Tc human serum albumin (HSA) (Amersham Medi-physics, Arlington Heights, IL).[31–33] Approximately 18.5–30 MBq (500–800 μCi) of radiopharmaceutical is injected intradermally at the primary melanoma site. A scintillation camera is used to document the drainage pattern from the primary site via dermal lymphatics to the regional nodes. The skin overlying the sentinel node is marked. Because there is some variation in the transit time between the various pharmaceuticals the nuclear medicine physician performing the procedure must be careful to differentiate the sentinel node from non-sentinel nodes, by observing the dynamic images. It is the experience of the John Wayne Cancer Institute (JWCI) that sentinel nodes can usually be identified by 30 minutes (depending on the agent used and the distance from the primary to the regional nodes), and often by 4 hours the sentinel node can no longer be differentiated from the adjacent non-sentinel nodes (Figure 29.2).[31] Lymphoscintigraphy is usually performed on the day of surgery to allow the radiopharmaceutical to be used for sentinel node identification. Lymphoscintigraphy is used to determine the regional lymph node field at risk for metastases and is particularly helpful in sites on the head and neck or torso, which often have unexpected lymph drainage. Norman et al. showed that up to 59% of primaries from these regions will have unexpected patterns of drainage.[32]

In a recent study Glass et al. found that in over 50% of the cases they reviewed, more than one sentinel node was identified in the draining node field.[31] Uren et al. have previously reported a similar finding.[33] Because blue dye seems to travel along the same pathways as the radiopharmaceuticals, lymphoscintigraphy is critical for the accuracy of the LM/SL technique.[33,34]

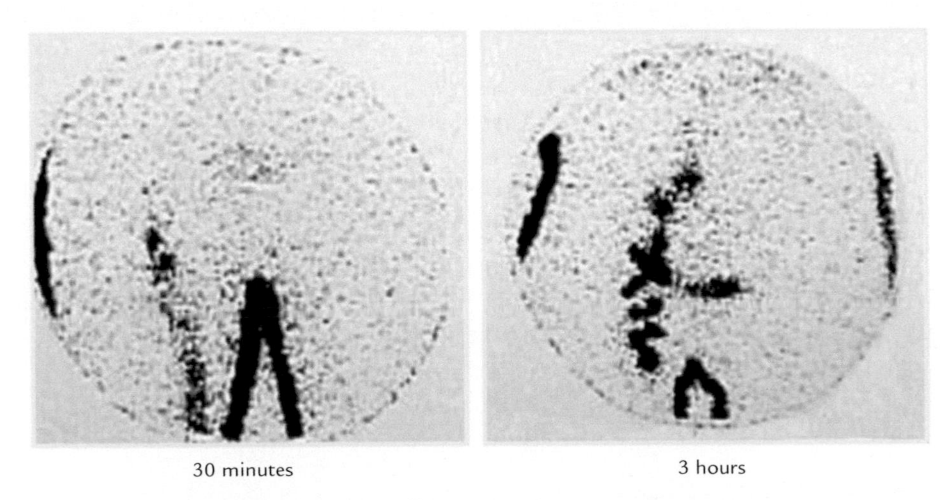

Figure 29.2 *Cutaneous lymphoscintigraphy with filtered ^{99m}Tc sulfur colloid from a lower extremity primary. Cutaneous lymphoscintigraphy with filtered ^{99m}Tc SC injected intradermally around the calf primary site was performed with images obtained at 30 min and subsequently at 3h. The 30 min image shows two inguinal lymph nodes whereas more delayed images showed multiple nodes. In the 3h image the two lymph nodes are obscured by the other hot nodes.*

Using the information obtained from lymphoscintigraphy, Krag et al. reported a high success rate for sentinel node identification with the use of a radiopharmaceutical alone for gamma probe directed LM/SL (Table 29.2).[35] One hundred and twenty-one patients underwent LM/SL, most with radiopharmaceutical alone. A sentinel node was defined as having at least 15 counts in 10 seconds and a count ratio three times background. Ninety-eight per cent of patients had a 'successful' LM/SL procedure. Yet the interval between injection of the radiopharmaceutical and surgery ranged from 15 minutes to 24 hours. The mean follow up for these patients was 220 days. With this variation in technique and no clear definition of background, we suspect that the true sentinel node may not always have been properly identified.

In 1994 the group at the JWCI devised the technique of combined blue dye and radiopharmaceutical directed LM/SL.[36] Radiolymphoscintigraphy was performed using the combination of blue dye injected intraoperatively with 18.5 MBq (approximately 500 μCi in 0.5–1.0 ml of volume) of ^{99m}Tc HSA at the primary site. A handheld gamma probe (Neoprobe Corp, Dublin, OH) was used to follow the radioactivity into the regional node field. Morton's group originally tested this combined method in 30 patients. Thirty-four lymph node fields were identified by preoperative lymphoscintigraphy. At least one sentinel lymph node was identified in each field; the blue dye identified 36 sentinel lymph nodes and the gamma probe detected all 36 nodes plus an additional six nodes. Overall, blue stained lymph nodes had roughly twofold higher radioactive counts than adjacent non-blue lymph nodes and up to eightfold higher levels of radioactivity than the lymph node field or background. Although none of the sentinel lymph nodes contained metastatic disease this study showed the utility of the handheld gamma probe to help identify blue stained sentinel lymph nodes and the close concordance between the findings from blue dye and radiopharmaceutical techniques.

The JWCI experience with LM/SL for early stage melanoma of the head and neck employing both blue dye and radiopharmaceutical has recently been updated. Bostick et al. reported 117 patients undergoing LM/SL with either blue dye alone (94 cases) or in combination with a radiopharmaceutical (23 cases) for probe directed LM/SL.[37] The accuracy rate for blue dye directed LM/SL was 92% (only slightly better than the earlier report) but improved to 96% with the combination of blue dye and radiopharmaceutical. The probe was useful for helping to identify sentinel nodes in difficult sites such as the post-auricular, occipital, and parotid areas. Ten per cent of patients had drainage to two areas. Eighty-nine per cent of the patients avoided complete neck dissection after undergoing a tumour negative LM/SL procedure. There have been no regional lymph node recurrences over a median follow up period of 46 months (range 1 to 125 months). The

Table 29.2 *Accuracy rates of probe directed sentinel lymph node biopsy. Accuracy rates for identification of sentinel lymph nodes were based upon the presence of blue dye in the nodes and/or demonstration of radioactivity with the use of a handheld gamma probe. In many of these studies the concurrent use of blue dye and radiopharmaceuticals makes it difficult to determine the true accuracy rate of either technique alone*

Investigators	No. of participants	Accuracy rate (%)
Krag et al. 1995[35]	121	98
Pijpers et al. 1995[41]	41	100
Mudun et al. 1996[42]	13	100
Albertini et al. 1996[43]	106	96
Thompson et al. 1997[38]	21	100
Bostick et al. 1997[39]	23	98
Leong et al. 1997[44]	163	98
Essner et al. 2000[40]	247	98

improved accuracy rate probably relates to increased experience with LM/SL for this part of the body but also to the use of the handheld gamma probe. While the probe helped improve the accuracy rate of LM/SL, radioactivity in adjacent second tier lymph nodes in the cervical basin can lead to the removal of an excessive number of nodes.

A major difficulty with the combined technique proved to be the logistic and regulatory problem of injecting radiopharmaceuticals in the operating room. Thompson et al. at the Sydney Melanoma Unit overcame this difficulty by introducing a single dose isotope injection technique for both preoperative lymphoscintigraphy and intraoperative sentinel node identification.[38] They found that it was possible to detect residual radioactivity in sentinel nodes after lymphoscintigraphy the previous day and soon adopted this as their standard protocol.

WHAT IS THE BEST RADIOPHARMACEUTICAL?

Glass et al. at the JWCI examined the use of the three most commonly employed radiopharmaceuticals for lymphoscintigraphy in the hope it would provide some guidance as to which agents would be best suited for intraoperative probe directed LM/SL.[31] They compared the three agents (^{99m}Tc AC, ^{99m}Tc SC, and ^{99m}Tc HSA) for their utility in identifying the afferent lymphatics and sentinel lymph nodes. Using early (up to 30 minute) images the three agents were found to be equally effective for identifying the sentinel nodes. On average two lymph nodes were identified in each basin. When they delayed their images up to 4 hours after injection of radiopharmaceutical the average number of nodes visualized did not change significantly. However, there seemed to be a wide variation in the number of lymph nodes seen by lymphoscintigraphy from patient to patient: ^{99m}Tc AC (range 1–7), ^{99m}Tc SC (range 1–14), and ^{99m}Tc HSA (range 0–9). The results from these experiences led them to examine the utility of all three radiopharmaceuticals for radiolymphoscintigraphy.

Bostick et al. reviewed the JWCI experience with LM/SL and radiolymphoscintigraphy in 100 lymph node basins from 87 patients with primaries from a variety of sites.[39] All patients underwent lymphoscintigraphy with one of the three commonly used radiopharmaceuticals. LM/SL was performed with either concurrent injection of blue dye and ^{99m}Tc HSA or ^{99m}Tc SC injected up to 4 hours before the operative procedure. One hundred and thirty-six blue stained and radioactive lymph nodes and eight additional non-blue stained but hot nodes were removed in 98 lymph node basins (success rate 98%). A handheld gamma probe was used to determine the radioactive counts over the blue nodes, adjacent non-blue nodes, and at an irrelevant background site. Ninety-two per cent of the blue stained lymph nodes had an in vivo to background count ratio of ≥ 2, and 87% had in vivo count ratios ≥ 3. Seventeen sentinel nodes from 15 basins contained metastases: 16 were located with blue dye and gamma probe, and one was found with blue dye alone. None of the tumour positive lymph nodes were identified with gamma probe alone. Using the definition of a radioactive sentinel node as having an in vivo count ratio ≥ 2 a success rate of 85% would be achieved. When the in vivo count ratio was increased to ≥ 3 to improve the specificity of the technique the success rate decreased to 78%. The concordance between the two techniques was not 100%. Not all blue stained lymph nodes will have an elevated count ratio, and, conversely, not all nodes with an elevated count ratio will be blue. In fact when they examined the in vivo count ratios for all the blue stained lymph nodes they noted a wide variation ranging from <1 to 100:1. Similar results were observed when the ex vivo count ratio of the nodes was examined, suggesting that the radiopharmaceuticals alone can be misleading for LM/SL. Both of the radiopharmaceuticals were found to give similar count ratios for radiolymphoscintigraphy and led to surgical excision of a similar number of lymph nodes. At the JWCI there has been little difficulty in performing lymphoscintigraphy and LM/SL on the same day, but logistically this approach can be difficult.

Essner et al. from the JWCI subsequently reviewed an expanded series of patients from their centre who underwent radiolymphoscintigraphy using one of three techniques: (1) intraoperative injection of blue dye and ^{99m}Tc HSA with lymphoscintigraphy performed at least 24 hr earlier, (2) same day lymphoscintigraphy and LM/SL with a single injection of ^{99m}Tc filtered SC, or (3) prior day lymphoscintigraphy with filtered ^{99m}Tc SC.[40] Preoperative lymphoscintigraphy identified 299 drainage basins from the 247 patients. Sentinel nodes were located using the combined technique of blue dye plus radiopharmaceuticals in 142 (97%) of 146 basins using HSA, 119 (98%) of 121 basins using same day SC, and 32 (100%) of 32 basins using prior day SC. A total of 463 sentinel lymph nodes were identified from the 293 lymph basins (average 1.6 sentinel nodes/basin). Although there were no differences in accuracy rates by the three techniques, same day injections of SC led to the greatest in vivo node to background ratios ($P<0.0001$) and the greatest fall off in counts from in vivo to the postexcision basin ($P<0.0001$) (Figure 29.3). JWCI surgeons have now adopted same day lymphoscintigraphy and LM/SL with SC as their method of choice, as the high level of concurrence of blue dye and radioactivity and large fall off of counts provides reassuring confirmation that all sentinel lymph nodes have been removed.

The technique now used routinely at the Sydney Melanoma Unit involves a single injection of ^{99m}Tc antimony trisulfide colloid injected about 24 hours before LM/SL.[38] In their early experience with this method Thompson et al. identified sentinel nodes in all 21 cases and 42 of the 46 (91%) lymph nodes identified by lymphoscintigraphy were found during surgery. Count ratios of hot nodes to the background node field ranged from >147:1 to 0.2:1, and three of five lymph nodes with count ratios <3:1 were blue stained. Antimony trisulfide is a small particle colloid (10–40 nm) well suited for LM/SL , but this agent is not currently available for use in the United States.

Other investigators have used an assortment of methods to perform radiolymphoscintigraphy and define a radioactive sentinel lymph node (Table 29.3).[35,39–44] Other JWCI data suggest that the in vivo count ratios for blue stained lymph nodes can vary almost 100-fold even when surgery is uniformly performed within 4 hours after injection of the radiopharmaceutical.[39] Although the use of radiopharmaceutical and probe alone for LM/SL would simplify the technique, the results from these studies suggest ^{99m}Tc SC is not perfect for this procedure. Although larger sized particles such as ^{99m}Tc SC and AC would be expected to be trapped in the afferent

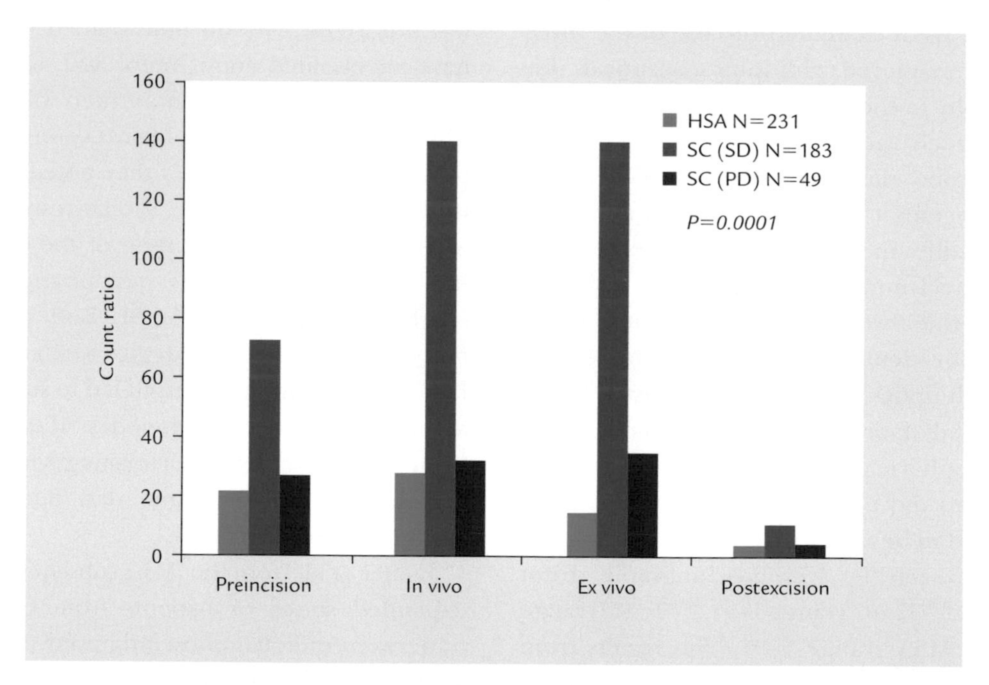

Figure 29.3 *Relative count ratios identified by three techniques of radioscintigraphy. 247 patients underwent LM/SL by one of three techniques: intraoperative injection of blue dye and ^{99m}Tc HSA (HSA), intraoperative injection of blue dye and filtered ^{99m}TcSC (SC(SD)), or intraoperative injection of blue dye and prior day lymphoscintigraphy with filtered ^{99m}Tc SC (SC(PD)). Count ratios were calculated for each site from the absolute counts divided by an irrelevant background count. The mean count ratio and standard deviation for each of the three techniques: HSA, SC(SD), SC(PD), respectively, were (1) preincision: 21 ± 68, 71 ± 123, 26 ± 26; (2) in vivo: 27 ± 65, 139 ± 216, and 31 ± 39; (3) ex vivo: 14 ± 40, 139 ± 247, and 34 ± 46; and (4) postexcision: 2 ± 3, 10 ± 17, and 3 ± 4. sentinel nodes found by SC(SD) had significantly higher in vivo (P <0.0001) and ex-vivo count (P <0.0001) ratios than sentinel nodes localized by HSA or SC(PD). The drop in count ratios after excision of the sentinel nodes (in vivo to postexcision) was greater (P <0.0001) with SC(SD) than the other two techniques. Adapted from Essner et al.[40]*

lymphatics of the nodes, some of the particles pass through to adjacent lymph nodes. Similarly, experience with ^{99m}Tc HSA has shown that this agent passes quickly from the primary to the sentinel node and there onwards to adjacent non-sentinel nodes. The ideal radiopharmaceutical for this procedure would be one that travels quickly from the primary site to the sentinel node and concentrates without leakage to adjacent lymph nodes. Until the kinetics of the radiopharmaceuticals are better defined for LM/SL, or better agents are developed, we recommend that these agents not be employed without blue dye.[45–50]

Most investigators now combine the use of blue dye and radiopharmaceuticals for LM/SL. Preoperative lymphoscintigraphy is performed using one of the colloid agents on the same day as surgery (or if not possible, then the day before). At the time of surgery the handheld gamma probe directs the surgeon to the site of the blue stained sentinel node. Occasionally the probe will lead the surgeon to an unexpected blue stained lymph node.[51,52] We have found the concordance between the two techniques to be at least 80%. There are various methods for defining a radioactive sentinel lymph node, but a blue stained lymph node remains the gold standard for this procedure.

The technique of LM/SL has now been shown by a number of investigators to be a reliable indicator of the tumour status of the regional lymph nodes. Based on these studies LM/SL has become a popular alternative to conventional ELND and is becoming a widely used procedure for staging the regional lymph nodes.[53] Yet, the successful performance of LM/SL is critically dependent on the experience and cooperation of the multidisciplinary team of surgeon, pathologist, and nuclear medicine physician. We recommend that each sentinel node team complete a learning phase of at least 15 cases (and perhaps up to 50) before LM/SL becomes the routine procedure at any centre.[54,55] Studies to date clearly indicate that successful retrieval of the sentinel nodes is directly related to the surgeon's experience. While progressing through the learning phase the surgeon must perform complete lymph node dissections to monitor his or her own false negative rate. Although the reported rates of missed sentinel nodes are extremely low, node field recurrences as late as 5 years after negative LM/SL have been reported.[53,56–58] The true accuracy rate of this technique has yet to be determined for the occasional user. Although this procedure has become increasingly popular its therapeutic value is unproved, and the results of clinical trials must be awaited.

CLINICAL TRIALS OF LYMPHATIC MAPPING AND SENTINEL NODE BIOPSY

Two major studies are examining the utility of LM/SL. In 1994 Morton et al. at the JWCI initiated an international multicentre randomized prospective trial, the Multicenter Selective Lymphadenectomy Trial (MSLT), comparing wide excision and LM/SL to wide

Table 29.3 *Proposed 'standard' definitions of radioactive sentinel lymph nodes. Radioactive sentinel nodes have been defined by various methods by a variety of investigators. The range of definitions may relate to the differences in techniques employed by each surgeon*

Investigators	Definition
Krag et al. 1995[35]	15 counts/10 sec and in vivo ratio ≥3 background
Pijpers et al. 1995[41]	LN w/ highest counts
Mudun et al. 1996[42]	300–3000 counts/10 sec and in vivo SN to background ratio ≥3
Albertini et al. 1996[43]	In vivo SN to background ratio ≥2 or ex vivo SN to NSN ratio ≥10
Thompson et al. 1997[38]	≥3:1 ratio LN to residual basin background
Bostick et al. 1997[39]	In vivo SN to background ratio ≥2
Leong et al. 1997[44]	In vivo SN to background ratio ≥3
Essner et al. 2000[40]	In vivo SN to background ratio ≥2

excision alone in patients with clinical stage I melanoma (localized disease). Patients with intermediate (1–4 mm) thickness melanoma who have not had a wide excision (with >1.5 cm margins), a skin graft, or any other procedure that would alter the lymphatic drainage are eligible. SCLND is performed only when lymphatic drainage fields contain tumour positive sentinel nodes. The purpose of this study is to determine the therapeutic benefit of LM/SL and the true accuracy of the technique at multiple international melanoma centres.[59] The experience from the MSLT to date has paralleled the experience at the JWCI and has shown that the combined blue dye and radiopharmaceutical technique seems to work best for LM/SL. Patient accrual to this trial was completed in 2002. The outcome ot the trial will determine whether LM/SL eventually becomes the standard of management for patients with clinical stage I melanoma, making conventional ELND unnecessary, and providing a better outcome than the alternative 'wait and see' approach.

A second randomized prospective trial, the Sunbelt Melanoma Trial, examines the efficacy of LM/SL as treatment for tumour positive regional lymph nodes. This study compares patients with one tumour positive lymph node determined by conventional H&E or

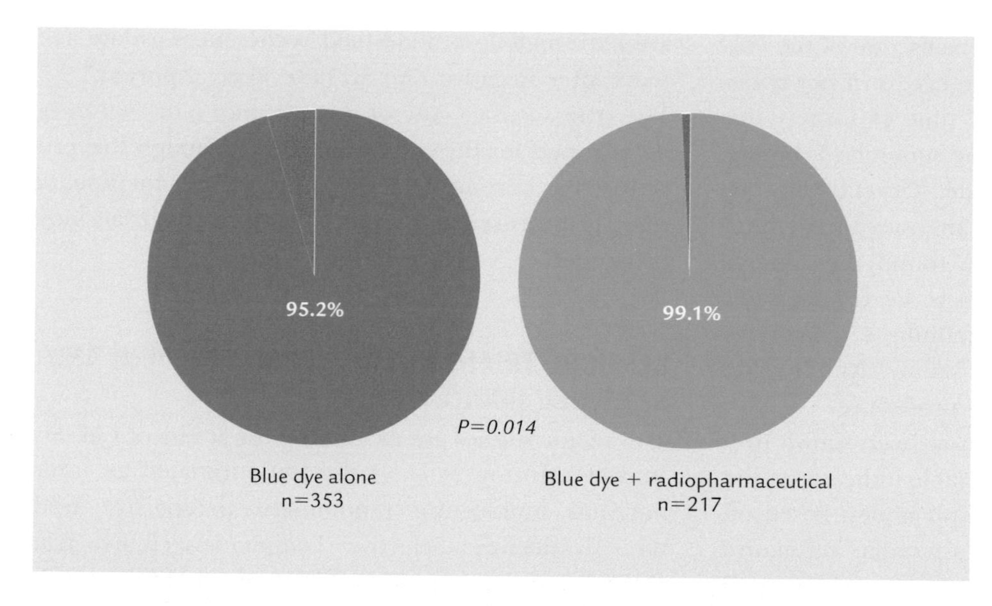

Figure 29.4. *Experience of the Multicenter Selective Lymphadenectomy Trial with LM/SL. The accuracy of sentinel node identification was significantly (P = 0.014) higher with blue dye and radiopharmaceuticals (99.1%) than with blue dye alone (95.2%). Adapted from Morton et al.*[59]

Table 29.4 *Variety of techniques used for radiolymphoscintigraphy. A variety of definitions have been employed for defining a radioactive sentinel. These definitions are based on the use of different radiopharmaceuticals, injected at different times before surgery and with or without blue dye*

Investigators	Blue dye	Radiopharmaceuticals	Time after injection
Krag et al. 1995[35]	±	Sulfur colloid, human serum albumin	15 min–24h
Pijpers et al. 1995[41]	+	Colloid albumin	2–18h
Mudun et al. 1996[42]	–	Filtered sulfur colloid	≤18h
Albertini et al. 1996[43]	+	Filtered sulfur colloid	≤4h
Thompson et al. 1997[38]	+	Antimony colloid	20–29h
Bostick et al. 1997[39]	+	Filtered sulfur colloid, human serum albumin	≤4h
Leong et al. 1997[44]	+	Filtered sulfur colloid	<7h
Essner et al. 2000[40]	+	Filtered sulfur colloid, human serum albumin Filtered sulfur colloid	≤4h >18h

immunohistochemical techniques (followed by complete lymph node dissection) to observation or treatment with adjuvant interferon-α (Schering-Plough, Kenilworth, NJ). A second group of patients who have a tumour positive sentinel lymph node by reverse transcriptase polymerase chain reaction (RT-PCR) alone are randomized to observation, complete lymph node dissection, or complete lymph node dissection and interferon-α. The organizers of this study anticipate that the results of this trial will provide further insights into the therapeutic value of LM/SL for patients with a single tumour positive lymph node identified by either routine techniques or RT-PCR.[60,61]

It is anticipated that the value of LM/SL will continue to increase as more insight is gained into the molecular biology of melanoma and the significance of micrometastatic disease. While it is tempting for the oncology community to assume that the LM/SL procedure will alter the ultimate outcome for patients, and make complete lymph node dissection unnecessary even in those patients with positive sentinel nodes, we must not be too quick to change our management approaches until the results of the ongoing clinical trials are available.[51,62,63] Certainly a standardized approach to sentinel node dissection, with preoperative lymphoscintigraphy, and use of both the blue dye and gamma probe at the time of surgery, should allow the procedure to be performed reproducibly and accurately.

ACKNOWLEDGEMENTS

Supported in part by the Saban Family Foundation, Los Angeles, and The Melanoma Foundation of the University of Sydney.

REFERENCES

1. Snow H, Melanotic cancerous disease. *Lancet* 1892; 2: 872.
2. McCarthy WH, Shaw HM, Milton GW, Efficacy of elective lymph node dissection in 2,347 patients with clinical stage I malignant melanoma. *Surg Gynecol Obstet* 1985; 161: 575–80.
3. Morton DL, Wanek L, Nizze JA, et al, Improved long-term survival after lymphadenectomy of melanoma metastatic to regional nodes: analysis of prognostic factors in 1134 patients from the John Wayne Cancer Institute. *Ann Surg* 1991; 214: 491–501.
4. Balch CM, Soong S-J, Murad TM, et al, A multifactorial analysis of melanoma. III. Prognostic factors in melanoma patients with lymph node metastases (stage III). *Ann Surg* 1981; 193: 377–88.
5. Callery C, Cochran AJ, Roe DJ, et al, Factors prognostic in patients with malignant melanoma spread to the regional lymph nodes. *Ann Surg* 1982; 196: 69–75.
6. Balch CM, Soong S-J, Milton GW, et al, A comparison of prognostic factors and surgical results in 1,786 patients with localized (stage I) melanoma treated in Alabama, USA and New South Wales, Australia. *Ann Surg* 1982; 196: 677–84.
7. Veronesi U, Adamus J, Bandiera DC, et al, Inefficacy of immediate node dissection in stage I melanoma of the limbs. *New Engl J Med* 1977; 297: 627–30.
8. Veronesi U, Adamus J, Bandiera DC, et al, Delayed regional lymph node dissection in stage I melanoma of the skin of the lower extremities. *Cancer* 1982; 49: 2420–30.
9. Sim FH, Taylor WF, Pritchard DJ, Soule EH, Lymphadenectomy in the management of stage I malignant melanoma: a prospective randomized study. *Proc Mayo Clin* 1986; 61: 697–705.
10. Balch CM, Soong S-J, Bartolucci AA, et al, Efficacy of an elective regional lymph node dissection of 1 to 4mm thick melanomas for patients 60 years of age and younger. *Ann Surg* 1996; 224: 255–66.
11. Cascinelli N, Morabito A, Santinami M, et al, Immediate or delayed dissection of regional nodes in patients with melanoma of the trunk: a randomised trial. *Lancet* 1998; 351: 793–6.
12. Rompel R, Garbe C, Buttner P, et al, Elective lymph node dissection in primary malignant melanoma: a matched-pair analysis. *Melanoma Res* 1995; 5: 189–94.
13. Kirkwood JM, Strawderman MH, Ernstoff MS, et al, Interferon alfa-2b adjuvant therapy of high-risk resected cutaneous melanoma: the eastern cooperative group trial EST 1684. *J Clin Oncol* 1996; 14: 7–17.
14. Morton DL, Barth A. Vaccine therapy for malignant melanoma. *CA Cancer J Clin* 1996; 46: 225–44.
15. Morton DL, Wen D-R, Wong JH, et al, Technical details of intraoperative lymphatic mapping for early stage melanoma. *Arch Surg* 1992; 127: 392–9.
16. Cochran AJ, Wen DR, Morton DL, Management of the regional lymph nodes in patients with cutaneous malignant melanoma. *World J Surg* 1992; 16: 214–21.
17. Wong JH, Cagle LA, Morton DL, Lymphatic drainage of skin in a sentinel lymph node in a feline model. *Ann Surg* 1991; 214: 637–41.
18. Cochran AJ, Wen DR, Herschman HR, Occult melanoma in lymph nodes detected by antiserum to S-100 protein. *Int J Canc* 1984; 34: 159–63.
19. Cochran AJ, Wen DR, Morton DL, Occult tumour cells in the lymph nodes of patients with pathological stage I malignant melanoma: an immunohistochemical study. *Am J Surg Path* 1988; 12: 612–8.
20. Heller R, Becker J, Wasselle J, et al, Detection of submicroscopic lymph node metastases in patients with melanoma. *Arch Surg* 1991; 126: 1455–60.
21. Morton DL, Wen D-R, Foshag LJ, et al, Intraoperative lymphatic mapping and selective cervical lymphadenectomy for early-stage melanomas of the head and neck. *J Clin Oncol* 1993; 11: 1751–6.
22. Shah JP, Kraus DH, Dubner S, Sarkar S, Patterns of regional lymph node metastases from cutaneous melanoma of the head and neck. *Am J Surg* 1991; 162: 320–3.
23. Wanebo HJ, Harpole D, Teates CD, Radionuclide lymphoscintigraphy with technetium 99m antimony sulfide colloid to identify lymphatic drainage of cutaneous melanoma of ambiguous sites in the head and neck and trunk. *Cancer* 1985; 55: 1403–13.
24. Essner R, Wen DR, Cochran AJ, et al, Lymphatic mapping and selective lymph node biopsy: an alternative to elective lymphadenectomy for early-stage melanomas of the trunk and lower extremities. *Proc Am Soc Clin Oncol* 1993; 12: 391.
25. Thompson JF, Saw RP, Colman MH, et al, Contralateral groin node metastasis from lower limb melanoma. *Eur J Canc* 1997; 33: 976–7.
26. Reintgen D, Cruse CW, Wells K, et al, The orderly progression of melanoma nodal metastases. *Ann Surg* 1994; 220: 759–67.
27. Thompson JF, McCarthy WH, Bosch CMJ, et al, Sentinel lymph node status as an indicator of the presence of metastatic melanoma in regional lymph nodes. *Melanoma Res* 1995; 5: 255–60.
28. Karakousis CP, Velez AF, Spellman JE Jr, Scarozza J, The technique of sentinel node biopsy. *Eur J Surg Oncol* 1996; 22: 271–5.
29. Robinson DS, Sample WF, Fee HJ, et al, Regional lymphatic drainage in primary malignant melanoma of the trunk determined by colloidal gold scanning. *Surg Forum* 1977; 28: 147.
30. Kelemen PR, Essner R, Foshag LJ, Morton DL, Lymphatic mapping and sentinel lymphadenectomy after wide local excision of primary melanoma. *J Am Coll Surg* 1999; 189: 247–52.

31. Glass EC, Essner R, Morton DL, Kinetics of three lymphoscintigraphic agents in patients with cutaneous melanoma. *J Nucl Med* 1998; 39: 1185–90.
32. Norman J, Cruse CW, Espinosa C, et al, Redefinition of cutaneous lymphatic drainage with the use of lymphoscintigraphy for malignant melanoma. *Am J Surg* 1991; 162: 432.
33. Uren RF, Howman-Giles R, Thompson JF, et al, Lymphoscintigraphy to identify sentinel lymph nodes in patients with melanoma. *Melanoma Res* 1994; 4: 395–9.
34. Essner R, The role of lymphoscintigraphy and sentinel node mapping in assessing patient risk in melanoma. *Sem Oncol* 1997; 24: S4-10.
35. Krag DN, Meijer SJ, Weaver DL, et al, Minimal-access surgery for staging of malignant melanoma. *Arch Surg* 1995; 130: 654–60.
36. Essner R, Foshag L, Morton DL, Intraoperative radiolymphoscintigraphy: a useful adjunct to intraoperative lymphatic mapping and selective lymphadenectomy in patients with clinical stage I melanoma. Presented at the Annual Meeting of the Society of Surgical Oncology, Houston, TX, March 17–20, 1994.
37. Bostick P, Essner R, Sarantou T, et al, Intraoperative lymphatic mapping for early-stage melanoma of the head and neck. *Am J Surg* 1997; 174: 536–9.
38. Thompson JF, Niewind P, Uren RF, et al, Single-dose isotope injection for both preoperative lymphoscintigraphy and intraoperative sentinel lymph node identification in melanoma patients. *Melanoma Res* 1997; 7: 500–6.
39. Bostick P, Essner R, Glass E, et al, Comparison of intraoperative lymphatic mapping in melanoma to identify sentinel nodes in 100 lymphatic basins. *Arch Surg* 1999; 134: 43–9.
40. Essner R, Bostick PJ, Glass EC, Standardized probe-directed sentinel node dissection in melanoma. *Surgery* 2000; 127: 26–31.
41. Pijpers R, Collet GJ, Meijer S, Hoekstra OS, The impact of dynamic lymphoscintigraphy and gamma probe guidance on sentinel node biopsy in melanoma. *Eur J Nucl Med* 1995; 22: 1238–41.
42. Mudun A, Murray DR, Herda SC, et al, Early stage melanoma: lymphoscintigraphy, reproducibility of sentinel node detection, and effectiveness of the intraoperative gamma probe. *Radiology* 1996; 199: 171–5.
43. Albertini JJ, Cruse CW, Rapaport D, et al, Intraoperative radiolymphoscintigraphy improves sentinel lymph node identification for patients with melanoma. *Ann Surg* 1996; 223: 217–24.
44. Leong SPL, Steinmetz I, Habib FA, et al, Optimal selective sentinel lymph node dissection in primary malignant melanoma. *Arch Surg* 1997; 132: 666–73.
45. Lingam MK, Mackie RM, McKay AJ, Intraoperative identification of SLN in patients with malignant melanoma. *Br J Canc* 1997; 75: 1505–8.
46. Van Der Veen H, Hoekstra OS, et al, Gamma probe-guided sentinel node biopsy to select patients with melanoma for lymphadenectomy. *Br J Surg* 1994; 81: 1769–70.
47. Joseph E, Messina J, Glass FL, et al, Radioguided surgery for the ultrastaging of the patient with melanoma. *CA Cancer J Clin* 1997; 3: 341–5.
48. Loggie BW, Hosseinian AA, Watson NE, Prospective evaluation of selective lymph node biopsy for cutaneous malignant melanoma. *Am Surg* 1997; 63: 1051–8.
49. Nathanson SD, Avery M, Anaya P, et al, Lymphatic diameters and radionuclide clearance in a murine melanoma model. *Arch Surg* 1997; 132: 311–15.
50. Wong JH, Terada K, Ko P, Coel MN, Lack of effect of particle size on the identification of the sentinel node in cutaneous malignancies. *Ann Surg Oncol* 1997; 5: 77–80.
51. Nieweg OE, Kapteijn BAE, Thompson JF, Kroon BBR, Lymphatic mapping and selective lymphadenectomy for melanoma: not yet standard therapy. *Eur J Surg Oncol* 1997; 23: 397–8.
52. Nieweg OE, Jansen L, Kroon BBR, Technique of lymphatic mapping and sentinel node biopsy for melanoma. *Eur J Surg Oncol* 1998; 24: 520–4.
53. Essner R, Conforti A, Kelley MC, et al, Efficacy of selective lymphadenectomy as a therapeutic procedure for early-stage melanoma. *Ann Surg Oncol* 1999; 6: 442–9.
54. Morton, DL. Intraoperative lymphatic mapping and sentinel lymphadenectomy: community standard care or clinical investigation? *Cancer J Sci Am* 1997; 3: 328–30.
55. Reintgen D, Balch CM, Kirkwood J, Ross M, Recent advances in the care of the patient with malignant melanoma. *Ann Surg* 1997; 225: 1–14.
56. Essner R, Conforti A, Kelley MC, et al, Cost-conscious management of the inguinal nodes in early-stage melanoma. *Melanoma Res* 1997; 7: S29.
57. Gershenwald JE, Colome MI, Lee JE, et al, Patterns of recurrence following a negative sentinel lymph node biopsy in 243 patients with stage I or II melanoma. *J Clin Oncol* 1998; 16: 2253–60.
58. Gershenwald JE, Thompson W, Mansfield PF, et al, Multi-institutional melanoma lymphatic mapping experience: the prognostic value of sentinel lymph node status in 612 stage I or II melanoma patients. *J Clin Oncol* 1999; 17: 976–83.
59. Morton DL, Thompson JF, Essner R, et al, Validation of the accuracy of intraoperative lymphatic mapping and sentinel lymphadenectomy for early-stage melanoma: a multicenter trial. *Ann Surg* 1999; 230: 453–65.
60. Shrivers SC, Wang X, Li W, et al, Molecular staging of malignant melanoma. Correlation with clinical outcome. *JAMA* 1998; 280: 1410–15.
61. Bostick PJ, Morton DL, Turner RR, et al, Prognostic significance of occult metastases detected by sentinel lymphadenectomy and reverse transcriptase-polymerase chain reaction in early-stage melanoma. *J Clin Oncol* 1999; 17: 3238–44.
62. Glass LF, Messina J, Glass J, et al, The results of complete lymph node dissections in 88 melanoma patients with positive sentinel nodes. *Melanoma Res* 1997; 7: S104.
63. Thompson JF, Uren RF. What is a 'sentinel' lymph node? *Eur J Surg Oncol* 2000; 26: 103–4.

30

Lymphoscintigraphy

Roger F Uren, Cornelis A Hoefnagel

INTRODUCTION

Lymphatic mapping using lymphoscintigraphy for sentinel lymph node biopsy in melanoma patients can be placed in context by considering previous discoveries that have led to the current practice of nuclear medicine in this important area of surgical oncology. This begins with the earliest attempts to study the patterns of lymphatic drainage of the skin and continues with the more recent development of radiocolloids for high quality lymphoscintigraphy and the evolution of techniques to accurately map lymphatic drainage patterns in individual patients.

LYMPHATIC MAPPING OF THE SKIN

Early studies

Using mercury injections in cadavers, Cruikshank and Mascagni and about 100 years later, Sappey and his followers Poirier, Cuneo, and Delamere extensively documented the lymphatic drainage of the skin and other parts of the body.[1–4]

In reference to lymphatic drainage of the trunk Sappey stated, 'In no part of the trunk or head have I seen any vessel spring from the side opposite to that to which it belonged.' This was a concept embraced by most practitioners until the past few years. However, 100 years before Sappey's work was published, Mascagni had reported that 'lymphatic vessels of the right side of the lumbar and dorsal regions may arise from the left side and vice versa'. Sappey simply declared that he was in error. We now know that Mascagni was correct. Poirier, Cuneo, and Delamere also realized that there were ambiguities in truncal drainage pathways in some situations.[4] In the head and neck region these authors, like Sappey, described a complex but predictable pattern of lymphatic drainage to particular node groups depending on the part of the skin injected. They also did not believe that drainage could occur across the midline or deviate significantly from these described pathways.

The work of those careful researchers who showed variations in the lymphatic drainage of the trunk was essentially ignored. Presumably the elegant illustrations in Sappey's atlas, as well as his statements, which denied the occurrence of such ambiguous drainage, persuaded most practitioners to accept his view. Thus knowledge and understanding of the lymphatic drainage of the skin was thought to be 'complete' and fairly static for about 100 years, with most practitioners exclusively following the strict teachings of Sappey until very recently. In 1953 Sherman and Ter-Pogossian described a new technique called lymphoscintigraphy, which allowed the lymphatic drainage patterns in individual patients to be accurately mapped.[5] When this technique was applied to patients with melanoma and other malignancies on the trunk, it soon became clear that Sappey's lines did not hold true in every patient.

Many subsequent workers confirmed the extreme variability of the lymphatic drainage from the skin of the trunk.[6–9] Norman et al. defined and expanded new zones of ambiguity based on this increasing store of knowledge, and Eberbach tried to combine data from several authors to illustrate further the extensive overlap of areas which drain to the various node fields.[10,11] It has only been with increasing experience with lymphoscintigraphy that it has been confirmed that there are many variations in the lymphatic drainage of the skin in humans, with clinically predictable drainage from very few sites on the body.[12]

RADIOPHARMACEUTICALS FOR LYMPHOSCINTIGRAPHY

The first radiocolloid for lymphoscintigraphy

The concept of lymphoscintigraphy was developed by Walker in 1950.[13] The original radiocolloid used for lymphoscintigraphy was gold-198 colloid, which had a very desirable uniform colloid size of 5–10 nm, but the beta emissions associated with this tracer caused very high and therefore undesirable radiation doses at the site of injection.

Technetium 99m (^{99m}Tc) labelled radiocolloids

The development of ^{99m}Tc with its high photon flux and low radiation dose spurred the development of radiocolloids labelled with this isotope. The tracer ^{99m}Tc sulphur colloid with a range of particle size of 50–2000 nm and an average size of 300 nm was used first, but the large particle size and slow clearance from the injection site encouraged the development of technetium colloids with a smaller particle size. Two radiocolloids, ^{99m}Tc stannous phytate and ^{99m}Tc antimony sulphide colloid, were investigated as agents for lymphoscintigraphy in humans.[14] In this study Kaplan concluded that ^{99m}Tc antimony sulphide colloid was the agent of choice for lymphoscintigraphy. It migrates rapidly through the lymphatic vessels to the draining node field, and yet there is excellent retention in the lymph nodes for up to 24 hours. It provides a comprehensive map of the lymphatic system of the skin and it accurately reflects the physiological lymphatic drainage in an individual patient. Antimony sulphide colloid has particles of relatively uniform size, most with diameters in the 10–15 nm range although some do range up to 40 nm. This colloid is also very stable, with the particles remaining at their initial size for at least 5 hours. Such antimony sulphide colloid particles are an ideal size to pass freely into the lymphatic capillaries via the 10–25 nm clefts between overlapping cells and the intercellular gaps, which can be considerably larger than this.

Excellent results can also be obtained using ultrafiltered ^{99m}Tc rhenium sulphur colloid, which produces a significant number of particles in the 50 nm range.[15] Similarly ^{99m}Tc nanocolloid, which is a colloid of albumin, migrates well after intradermal injection, and excellent scans are produced in most patients. This tracer has a range of particle size (3–80 nm) but 77% are less than 30 nm.[16] Other tracers that have been used include ^{99m}Tc human serum albumin colloid, ^{99m}Tc microaggregated albumin, ^{99m}Tc macroaggregated albumin, and mouse antibodies labelled with ^{99m}Tc, although none of these seem to be as satisfactory as the three tracers mentioned above. Thus it seems that the ideal radiocolloid for lymphoscintigraphy is any colloid with particles in the 5–75 nm range.

Variations in the drug approval regulations in different countries have led to some nations not having direct clinical access to any of the three ideal radiocolloids mentioned earlier. This situation is the case in the United States, for example, where clinicians have been forced to do the best they can with ^{99m}Tc sulphur colloid, which elsewhere is used almost exclusively as a liver scanning agent. Tc sulphur colloid has a wide range of particle sizes as mentioned above with a mean of 300 nm. If the particles are pushed through a 0.2 micron filter, particles over 200 nm can effectively be removed, but the colloid must be used soon after filtering as the particle size increases slowly over a 5-hour period, unlike antimony sulphide, which has a stable particle size over this period. Such filtered sulphur colloid is favoured by some as, because of its larger size, it tends to be retained well by the sentinel node.[17] This is in contrast to ^{99m}Tc human serum albumin which as a non-particulate tracer migrates more rapidly on to the second tier nodes and the systemic circulation. The size of the ^{99m}Tc sulphur colloid particles remains a concern, however, and does limit movement of this tracer into the lymphatic capillaries. Some of the smaller particles will freely enter the lymphatics via the intercellular clefts and gaps, but the larger range of particle sizes will have to rely on pinocytosis or physical factors to open up the gaps between endothelial cells before they can gain entry to the lymphatic lumen. This has led many to use larger volumes of injectate in an effort to achieve adequate labelling of the sentinel nodes. The particles in the 100–200 nm range find that the elastin fibrous matrix of the interstitium poses a barrier to their free movement before they can even reach the lymphatic capillary. This means that there is greater retention of this tracer at the injection site and less migration to the draining lymph nodes. There is some evidence, at least in vitro, that the size of the particles in ^{99m}Tc sulphur colloid is affected by the serum it comes into contact with in the patient.[18,19] The particles may increase or decrease in size. This has not been shown with ^{99m}Tc antimony sulphide colloid or ^{99m}Tc albumin nanocolloid.[15] The size distribution of ^{99m}Tc sulphur colloid is also altered by the method of preparation.[20] The number of labelled particles in the less than 400 nm range is maximized by using a reduced heating time protocol (heat for 3 minutes and cool for 2 minutes, rather than the usual heat for 10 minutes and cool for 5 minutes). This results in just over 70% of the particles being less than 400 nm in diameter compared with about 40% with the longer protocol. It is also advantageous to use technetium from a generator with a long ingrowth time (greater than 72 hours), as this also favourably increases the particle size distribution profile towards the smaller particles. Filtered ^{99m}Tc sulphur colloid and ^{99m}Tc albumin colloid, which have been passed through a 0.2 micron filter do, however, seem in clinical practice to be adequate for lymphoscintigraphy with reasonably rapid passage through the lymph channels and good retention in sentinel lymph nodes.[20] A recent study by Wong et al. suggested that particle size was not important in identifying the sentinel node and stated a preference for ^{99m}Tc sulphur colloid because there was less movement of this colloid onwards to second tier lymph nodes compared with the other tracer they studied, ^{99m}Tc human serum albumin.[21] However, whenever ^{99m}Tc sulphur colloid has been directly compared with the smaller tracers, it has been found that with sulphur colloid fewer channels are seen on dynamic images, fewer draining nodes fields per patient are identified and fewer sentinel nodes per node field are located.[22] We remain concerned therefore that, although a 'successful' sentinel node biopsy procedure may seem to be completed using microfiltered ^{99m}Tc sulphur colloid, not all true sentinel nodes will be detected in all patients.

^{99m}Tc human serum albumin is frequently used in the United States for lymphoscintigraphy. Its non-particulate nature means that it enters the lymphatic capillaries rapidly via the intercellular clefts and gaps and does show rapid movement through the lymphatic channels.[23] However, because of its non-particulate nature it may move rapidly on from the sentinel node to second tier nodes, which is a significant disadvantage when the purpose of lymphoscintigraphy is to locate the sentinel lymph nodes.[17] Sometimes it passes completely through the sentinel node so that on delayed lymphoscintigraphic scans no activity is seen in the sentinel nodes at all.[20]

The ideal radiocolloid for lymphatic mapping

On the basis of the anatomical and physiological features of lymphatic capillaries and lymph nodes it would seem that the optimal particle size for interstitial lymphoscintigraphy with inert colloids is a diameter of 5–75 nm, so that the tracer can freely enter the lymphatic system but also be well retained in the draining lymph nodes. There is extensive experience with ^{99m}Tc antimony sulphide colloid and nanocolloid of albumin labelled with ^{99m}Tc, and both give good results.[12,16] Both also have excellent retention in the draining sentinel nodes, and both of these agents have been registered specifically for lymphoscintigraphic use in humans. These are thus the best tracers to use for lymphatic mapping, if they are available. As mentioned earlier, in some countries these or equivalent tracers are not available, and, in clinical practice, particles of ^{99m}Tc sulphur colloid that have been passed through a 0.2 micron filter also seem adequate for cutaneous lymphoscintigraphy.[24] It is difficult to state dogmatically that any particular radiocolloid is 'the best' tracer to use for sentinel lymph node biopsy. Whichever tracer is used, it is important that each institution develop optimal protocols in terms of lymphoscintigraphic imaging, blue dye injection, and gamma probe use during surgery to maximize the success rate in locating the sentinel lymph node using the colloid available for patient use at that institution. We would counsel, however, that if antimony sulphide colloid or nanocolloid are available these should be used in preference to sulphur colloid, as there remains some doubt that all true sentinel nodes will be identified when using sulphur colloid.

LYMPHOSCINTIGRAPHY

High quality lymphoscintigraphy is a vital and integral part of the sentinel lymph node biopsy procedure in patients with melanoma.[12] It depends on several important factors:

(1) entry of the injected radiocolloid into the lumen of the initial lymphatic capillary;
(2) free movement of the tracer along the lymphatic vessel to the draining sentinel node;
(3) retention of the radiocolloid in the sentinel node for an adequate period of time;
(4) the ability to distinguish sentinel nodes from second tier nodes;
(5) the technique of lymphoscintigraphy and appropriate imaging protocols which ensure that all sentinel nodes are identified, regardless of their location;
(6) accurate marking of the surface location of the sentinel node; and
(7) radiation dosimetry needs to be acceptable for the clinical application of the technique.

Entry of the injected radiocolloid into the lumen of the initial lymphatic capillary

The successful use of lymphoscintigraphy as part of the sentinel lymph node biopsy procedure in patients with melanoma revolves around the ability of lymphoscintigraphy to produce an accurate map of the pattern of lymphatic drainage from a melanoma or excision biopsy site to the draining lymph nodes. For this to occur requires that the radiocolloid gains ready access to the lumen of the initial lymphatic capillaries. A consideration of the microanatomy of the initial lymphatics and their relationship with the interstitium reveals that the particle size of the radiocolloid is a critical factor determining the ease with which these tracers enter the lymphatic system.[12] Once inside the lumen of the lymphatic, any particle and even whole cells will then pass on, eventually reaching the sentinel node because of the system of valves in the lumen of lymphatic vessels, which ensures that the movement of lymph is essentially unidirectional towards the draining lymph nodes.

The effect of particle size

Particles up to 1–2 nm in diameter will tend to enter the venous blood system directly. Particles between 5 nm and 25 nm enter lymphatic capillaries via the gaps between cell junctions and the intercellular clefts formed by overlapping cells, which even when closed measure 10–25 nm across. The uptake rate of particles into lymphatic capillaries is independent of particle size within the range 6–18 nm, presumably because of these gaps and clefts.[25] Above this size the interstitial elastin matrix begins to pose a barrier to the movement of particles and their uptake into lymphatic capillaries. Particles up to 75 nm in diameter may gain entry into the lymphatic lumen by pinocytosis.[26] Such particles can enter invaginations in the outer wall of the endothelial cell called caveolae and then be transported in vesicles through the cell cytoplasm to the luminal wall before being extruded into the lumen of the lymphatic capillary. It is not clear how important a role pinocytosis has in the movement of radiocolloid particles from the interstitium to the lymphatic capillary lumen in cutaneous lymphoscintigraphy.

The matrix of reticular and elastin fibres, that makes up the connective tissue surrounding lymphatic capillaries begins to pose a physical barrier to particles in the 70–100 nm range.[12] Above this diameter particles will find this connective tissue lattice increasingly difficult to penetrate. Some particles in the 25–100 nm range will gain entry to the lymphatic capillaries via the very large gaps that can occasionally be seen between cells de novo and via the effects of movement and tension in the soft tissues. Massage of the area is an excellent method of opening up the gaps between overlapping lymphatic endothelial cells and thus enhancing entry of radiocolloids into the lumen of the initial lymphatics. Such movement causes tension on the elastin fibrils that attach the outside of the endothelial cells to the collagen fibres of the connective tissue matrix, causing the gaps between the lymphatic endothelial cells to open.[27] This method of entry into the lumen of the lymphatics can also be enhanced by using larger volumes of injectate, which increase the interstitial pressure. An increase in interstitial pressure from 10 to 40 cm H_2O significantly increases the rate of uptake of particles into the terminal lymphatics and also increases the production of lymph fluid and the volume of lymphatic flow.[25] When performing lymphoscintigraphy, the volume of injectate will therefore be an important factor in determining the rate of movement of tracer into the lymphatic capillaries. This fact can be used to partially overcome the disadvantages of using colloids with large particle sizes such as ^{99m}Tc sulphur colloid. If larger volumes of tracer are used, more of the tracer will migrate through the lymphatics.

Increased injection pressure does not, however, increase net velocity of lymph flow, and the increased volume of lymph flow in this circumstance seems to be achieved by dilatation of the lymphatic channels and the opening up of other lymphatic capillaries.[25] These other lymphatic channels, which are opened up to achieve the higher flow when large injection volumes are used, may not have drained the original injection site under physiological conditions. Such new lymphatic channels may thus drain to lymph nodes that would not normally drain the primary site. This raises a potential problem when using large injection volumes during cutaneous lymphoscintigraphy to locate sentinel lymph nodes, since the fundamentals of the tracer method demand that the system under study not be perturbed by the study itself. We therefore favour small (0.05–0.1 ml) volumes of radiocolloid at each injection site to allow the true lymphatic physiology to be studied and to minimize any disturbance of the system. If large volumes are used there is the potential for colloid to drain to nodes which do not normally drain the primary tumour site. Inaccurate identification of nodes that under physiological conditions would not receive lymph from the tumour site being studied defeats the purpose of sentinel node biopsy.

Larger particles (hundreds of nm) will remain trapped in the interstitial space for some time.[14,28–31] Such large particles rely almost exclusively on mechanical factors to gain entry into the lymphatic capillary lumen by opening up the gaps in intercellular junctions, as mentioned above. It is important to emphasize that accurate sentinel lymph node biopsy requires high quality lymphoscintigraphy to clearly delineate the draining lymphatic vessels as they pass to and reach the sentinel node/nodes (Figure 30.1).[12] These vessels will not be visualized on scans unless an adequate number of radiolabelled particles are present in their lumen. If large particle radiocolloids are used too few radiolabelled particles gain entry to the lymphatic lumen to allow it to be imaged on dynamic studies. These channels seen on lymphoscintigraphy are the same channels that the surgeon observes staining blue when he injects blue dye around the excision biopsy site just before operating. The sentinel nodes can thus be confidently identified as the lymph nodes receiving direct lymphatic drainage via one of these lymphatic vessels seen on the dynamic images.

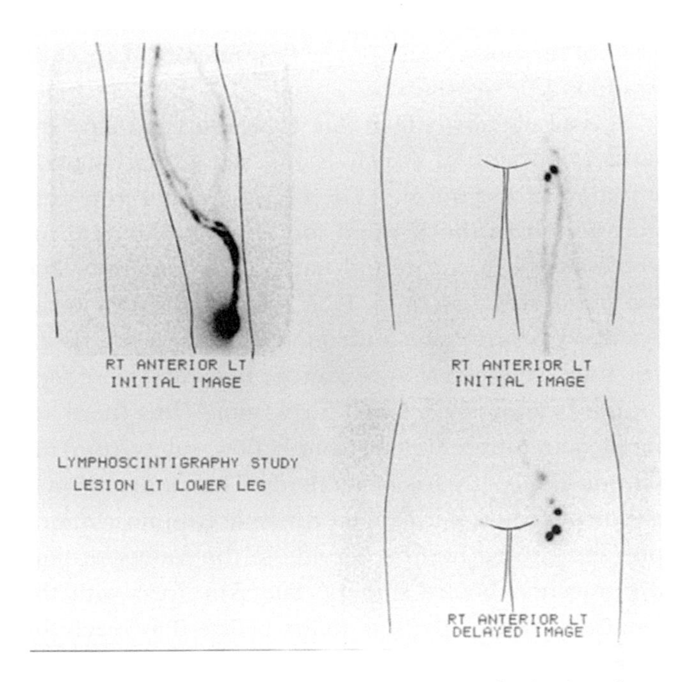

Figure 30.1 *Initial dynamic lymphoscintigraphy (top) and delayed (below) images in a patient with an excision biopsy site on the lower left shin above the ankle. On dynamic imaging three lymphatic collecting vessels are seen passing to the left groin, two medial to, and one lateral to the knee. The anterior groin dynamic phase shows the two medial vessels meeting two sentinel nodes and the lateral vessel bypassing these and proceeding on to a third higher sentinel node, which is faint on this early image. These are the same vessels the surgeon sees staining blue following blue dye injection preoperatively. The anterior delayed image shows the three bright sentinel nodes and faint activity in second tier nodes higher in the groin. There was no drainage to popliteal nodes.*

Free movement of the tracer along the lymphatic vessel to the draining sentinel node

Once particles gain entry to the lumen of a lymphatic capillary they seem to move freely in one direction towards the draining lymph nodes. There is very little if any retrograde flow of lymph. The movement of tracers along lymphatic capillaries is surprisingly fast. The rate of flow of ^{99m}Tc human serum albumin in lymphatics following intradermal injection has been measured by Nathanson et al.[23] They found the average flow rate of this non-particulate tracer in a total of 17 patients was 10.4±7.3 cm/min. The movement of ^{99m}Tc antimony sulphide colloid through the lymphatic capillaries after intradermal injection has also been measured in 198 patients with primary melanoma sites on various parts of the body.[32] An average flow rate of 4.4 cm/min was found.

Several factors affect this flow rate, perhaps the most important of which is the site of intradermal injection of the tracer.[32] The fastest average flow rates were found in the leg and foot at 10.2 cm/min, followed by the forearm and hand at 5.5 cm/min, and the thigh at 4.2 cm/min. Flow on the posterior trunk averaged 3.9 cm/min and on the anterior trunk 2.8 cm/min, while the slowest average flow rates were seen on the head and neck at 1.5 cm/min. Thus there are significant differences in lymph flow rates from the skin of different parts of the body. This information is important when performing dynamic lymphoscintigraphy and can be used as a guide to the timing of blue dye injection before surgery. The skin areas with the longest lymphatic paths to follow before they reach the draining node fields seem to have the fastest lymph flow. Flow rates from the trunk were similar front and back, at about 30–40% of the flow rate from the leg. The slowest rates of flow occurred from the skin of the head and neck and arm or shoulder. An absence of flow on the early dynamic images was most common for the shoulder or arm, the head and neck and the thigh.

Inflammation will increase both the production of lymph and the rate of lymph flow. This is commonly present in the skin when lymphoscintigraphy is performed after excision biopsy of a primary melanoma. Experience suggests that this does not cause any change in the ability of lymphoscintigraphy to detect the true sentinel node. There may be an advantage in performing lymphoscintigraphy in this situation, as the enhanced lymph flow may actually facilitate identification of the sentinel node.

Having the patient exercise the limb after injection of radiocolloid to it will increase the rate of flow of tracer through the lymphatic channels, as will massaging the injection site. However, as imaging protocols in melanoma call for immediate dynamic imaging which must be performed with the patient lying still under the gamma camera, this option is not practical for most patients undergoing cutaneous lymphoscintigraphy. Exercise and gentle massage are a useful adjunct when injecting blue dye preoperatively, and both can be used with good effect in patients having a sentinel node biopsy procedure using a gamma detection probe without lymphoscintigraphy.

Metastatic involvement

If the lymphatic channels are partly or completely blocked by metastatic tumour deposits this will certainly decrease the flow of radiocolloid through the system and may decrease the number of nodes visualized on delayed scans and induce collateral lymph flow through other vessels that do not normally drain the primary tumour site. This is usually not a practical problem when performing cutaneous lymphatic mapping to locate sentinel nodes, as this procedure is performed only in patients who do not have clinically palpable metastatic lymph nodes.

Previous surgery

Previous lymphatic or lymph node surgery has a profound effect on lymphatic drainage. There may simply be a decrease in the number of lymph channels and lymph nodes seen, progressing through to overt lymphoedema with no channels, dermal backflow, and no uptake whatsoever in lymph nodes. In patients with melanoma on the lower limbs previous surgical interference with the groin lymph nodes may induce lymphatic flow across the pubic area to nodes in the contralateral groin. These nodes then become the sentinel nodes in such patients.

It has been appreciated for some time that lymphoscintigraphy after wide local excision in patients with melanoma is unreliable, sometimes resulting in no migration of the radiocolloid in the disrupted lymphatics. Therefore in patients with melanoma it is preferable to perform lymphoscintigraphy before wide local excision of the biopsy site. There are two good reasons for this approach: (1) wide local excision will have an unpredictable effect on the pattern of lymphatic drainage, and (2) surgery within 24 hours after lymphoscintigraphy removes the skin that has received the highest dose of radiation from the radiocolloid. This can be as high as 0.45 Gy if there is no migration of the tracer.

Retention of the radiocolloid in the sentinel node for an adequate period of time

Foreign particles carried with the lymph flow are mostly phagocytosed in the lymph nodes.[15] The uptake and retention of radiocolloids in the draining lymph nodes is a complex physiological process, and it important to emphasize that lymph nodes are not simple mechanical filters. This misconception can lead to the erroneous conclusion that large particles over 100–200 nm will be trapped in sentinel nodes and that small particles 5–75 nm in diameter will not be trapped and will pass on rapidly to other lymph nodes. Colloid particles are phagocytosed in the lymph nodes after they have been recognized as foreign or have been coated with opsonins and thus recognized. The phagocytic cells are macrophages, which are concentrated especially in the subcapsular and medullary sinuses.[33] The surface charge of the particle and the agent used as a stabilizer in the production of the colloid will affect the rate of phagocytosis.[18] The rate of opsonization can also be markedly increased by the use of sterically stabilized nanocolloids.[34] The rate of phagocytosis of such colloids is greatly increased, so that up to 40% of the injected dose is trapped in the draining lymph nodes. Uptake in the draining lymph nodes can also be increased by using receptor binding radiotracers.[35]

Of the tracers that have been used clinically for lymphoscintigraphy the highest levels of uptake in the draining lymph nodes have been achieved with colloidal gold and ^{99m}Tc antimony sulphide colloid. Two hours after interstitial injection, uptake in lymph nodes averages 8% and 6% of the injected dose respectively for these two agents.[30] For other small particle size colloids such as stannous colloid and rhenium sulphide colloid uptake is 1–2%. The colloids with larger particles such as sulphur colloid show approximately one third of this uptake in the lymph nodes because very little of the injected tracer leaves the injection site.[15] This is a direct result of the difficulty such large particles have in gaining entry into the lumen of the initial lymphatic capillary. Using ^{99m}Tc nanocolloid, Kapteijn et al. found an average of 0.69% of the injected dose in sentinel lymph nodes and 0.23% in non-sentinel, second tier nodes 24 hours after intradermal injection.[16]

The retention of ^{99m}Tc antimony sulphide colloid in the sentinel node is also excellent, and at 24 hours after injection the sentinel nodes usually remain by far the most radioactive nodes.[36] This is especially true in the axilla, although even in the groin after lower limb injections, where activity in second tier nodes is more common, the sentinel node is usually the hottest node and remains so over 24 hours (Figure 30.2). It should be remembered, however, when using ^{99m}Tc nanocolloid of albumin or ^{99m}Tc antimony sulphide colloid that sometimes a second tier node may be hotter than a sentinel node in the same node field. Thus the tracer activity in the node alone cannot be used as the sole method of identifying a sentinel node. It is important to identify the lymphatic vessel entering the sentinel node on lymphoscintigraphy and this is the key reason that lymphoscintigraphy is a vital and integral part of the sentinel node biopsy procedure (Figure 30.3).

If the lymph nodes are replaced by metastatic tissue then it is theoretically possible that radiocolloid will not be accumulated in the node and that a sentinel node could be missed. In practice this does not seem to be a significant problem since the sentinel node biopsy procedure is usually not performed when there are palpable nodal metastases. It remains possible, however, that non-palpable sentinel nodes containing metastasis could be missed in this way.

The ability to distinguish sentinel nodes from second tier nodes

A second tier lymph node is any node which receives lymph flow which has previously passed through the physiological filter function of a sentinel node.

There is a variable incidence of tracer movement onward from sentinel nodes to second tier nodes. This correlates directly with the speed of lymph flow from a particular skin region.[37] High lymph flow is associated with an increased incidence of activity in second tier nodes. Thus second tier nodes are more common in the groin than elsewhere, since higher lymph flow rates are more common in lymph channels draining the leg (see Figures 30.1 and 30.2). However, high flow rates are occasionally seen in other parts of the body, thus obvious second tier activity can sometimes be seen in the axilla as well as the groin. Several features are important in helping to distinguish sentinel nodes from second tier nodes. The best way to identify a sentinel node on lymphoscintigraphy is to identify a lymph channel entering the node on dynamic imaging. If a lymph channel can be seen passing directly to a node from the injection site during the dynamic phase of lymphoscintigraphy, that is clearly a sentinel node regardless of the amount of tracer which migrates to the node. Sentinel nodes vary in the intensity of tracer uptake, and occasionally sentinel nodes will be 'colder' than second tier nodes in the same node field.

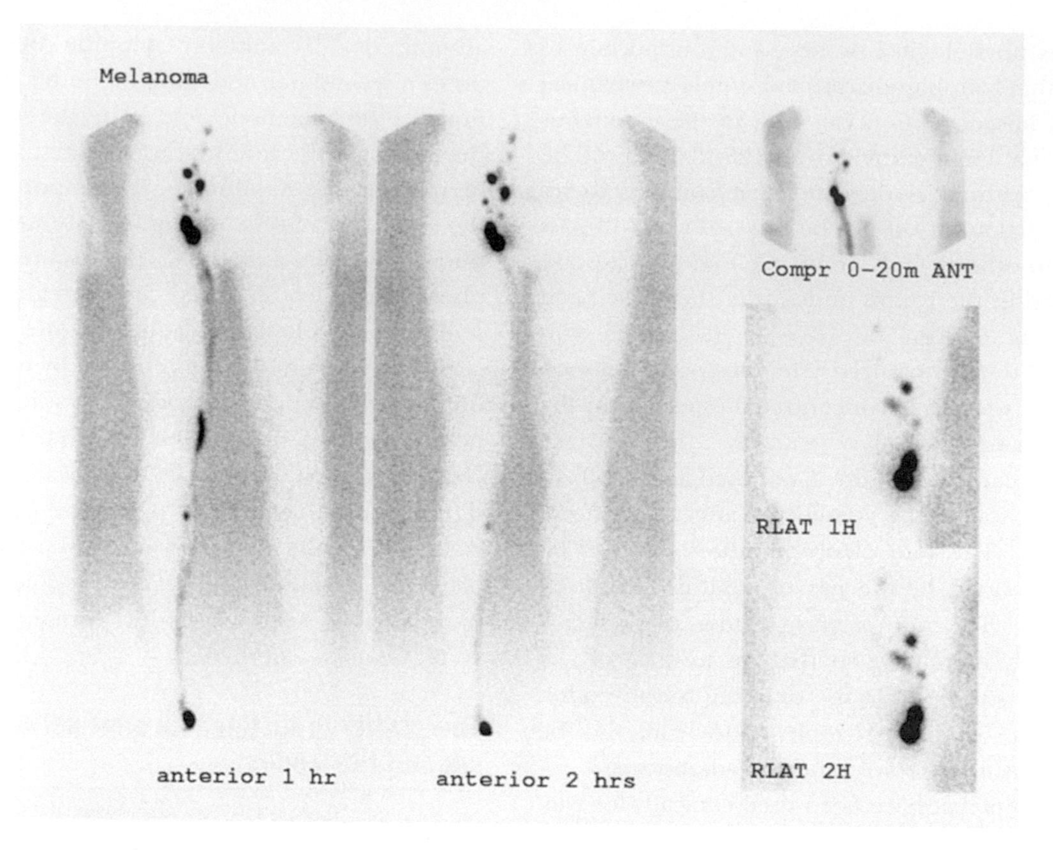

Figure 30.2 *Lymphoscintigraphy in a patient with a melanoma near the right ankle shows two lymphatic vessels passing to the right groin to meet two sentinel nodes, although second tier activity is also seen on early images (top right). On delayed scans the two sentinel nodes remain the brightest nodes in this patient. Typically the number of sentinel nodes matches the number of lymphatic vessels seen on dynamic imaging but this is not always the case, as vessels can bifurcate or join together in the thigh. A lymphatic lake is also noted lying along the path of one of the lymph vessels below the right knee. This fades in activity with time, which is the typical finding in such lymphatic lakes, and its nature was confirmed at surgery. These should not be confused with interval nodes which do not fade.*

Sometimes no movement of tracer is seen on the dynamic image, and activity in a particular node field is only evident on delayed imaging (Figure 30.4). In this situation other methods are needed to identify second tier nodes.

Second tier nodes tend to be more central in the same node field or lie in a node field which is more central on the lymphatic pathway to the thoracic duct. For example, a sentinel node in the distal inguinal area may drain to a second tier node higher in the groin area (see Figures 30.1 and 30.2), and a sentinel node in the inguinal area may have a second tier node in the iliac or obturator area.

Any node seen on delayed scans that is more peripheral to a sentinel node seen on dynamic imaging must be considered as another sentinel node and marked as such. Likewise a node that is seen only on delayed imaging but which lies lateral to or medial to a known sentinel node – for example, in the groin must be considered another sentinel node unless a channel can be seen passing onwards from the sentinel node to the other node. When in doubt, it is best to mark a second tier node as a potential sentinel node, as with the lymphatics and nodes on view and using blue dye during surgery the surgeon can determine whether this node receives the dye after it has passed through a sentinel node or directly from the primary tumour site. In this way the node will then be correctly classified as a second tier node in the first instance or as another sentinel node in the second situation.

Occasionally two lymphatic channels will seem to reach a single sentinel node in a node field, but at about the same time tracer is seen passing beyond this node to a second node higher in the same field (Figure 30.5). In the groin under these circumstances a lateral view is useful, as it may show that there are two separate

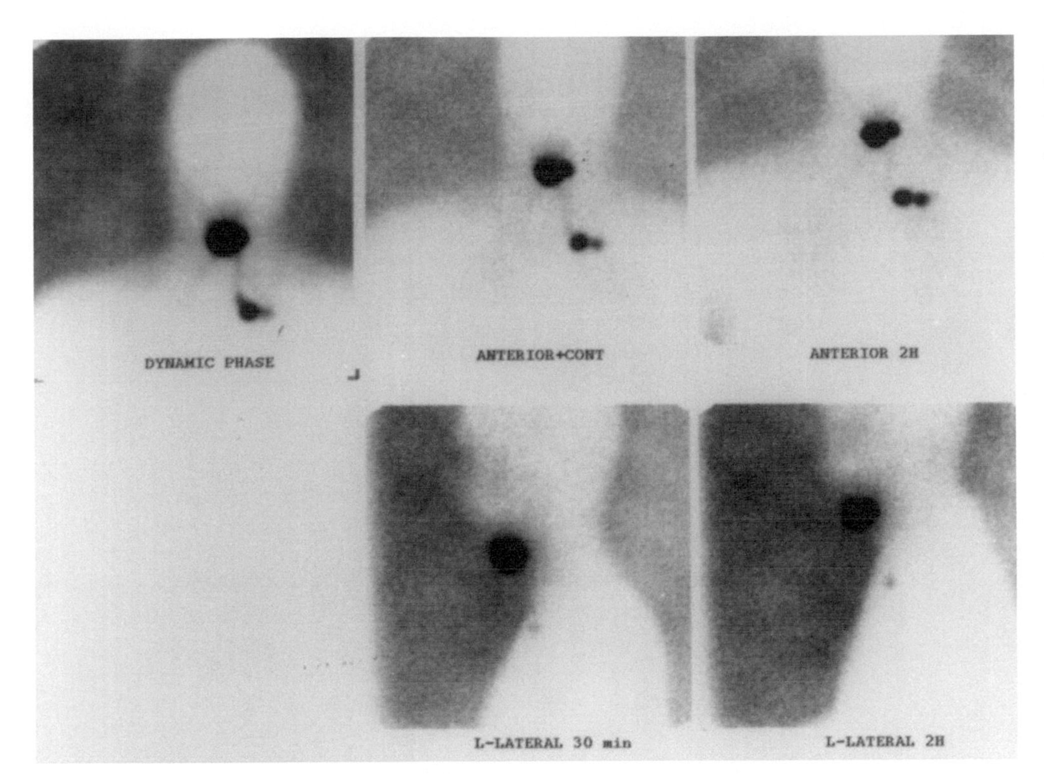

Figure 30.3
Lymphoscintigraphy in a patient with a melanoma under the chin. Dynamic imaging shows a single lymph vessel passing to a sentinel node in the left supraclavicular region. Tracer also passes rapidly on to a second tier node lateral to the sentinel node. Though this second tier node is quite 'hot' on delayed imaging there is only one sentinel node in this patient. Using counts/unit time to define a sentinel node with a gamma detecting probe in this patient would lead to unnecessary removal of the second tier node.

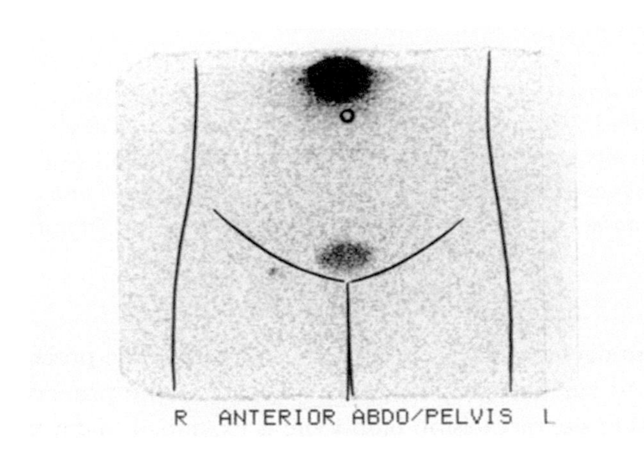

Figure 30.4 *Delayed lymphoscintigraphy image anteriorly over the groin in a patient with a melanoma on the back just above the level of the umbilicus. Faint activity is seen in a sentinel node in the right groin. Even though dynamic imaging showed no drainage to the right groin with dominant channels passing up to the axillae, the right groin node is clearly a separate sentinel node. The speed with which tracer reaches a node is irrelevant in determining whether it is a sentinel node.*

lymph channels one deep to the other passing to two separate sentinel nodes. However, occasionally doubt will still remain. In this situation both nodes must be marked and the true status of the higher node checked at the time of surgery. If a separate blue channel is seen bypassing the first node and passing directly to the higher node, then by definition this is a second sentinel node. Sometimes, the anatomical arrangement of the afferent lymphatic vessel and the lymph node means that the lymph is only partly subjected to the physiological filter function of the node and some of the lymph fluid will pass on to the next node without passing through the sentinel node.[38] This will be seen on lymphoscintigraphy as the rapid appearance of a second node more centrally in the node field after an apparently single channel has entered a sentinel node. When this is seen on lymphoscintigraphy the second node must also be marked as a potential second sentinel node. The resolution limitations of lymphoscintigraphy mean that these situations can only be confirmed at operation. As a general rule second tier nodes have less activity than sentinel nodes, but this is not universally the case.

If all of the above techniques are used it will be unusual for a second tier node to be mistaken for a sentinel node.

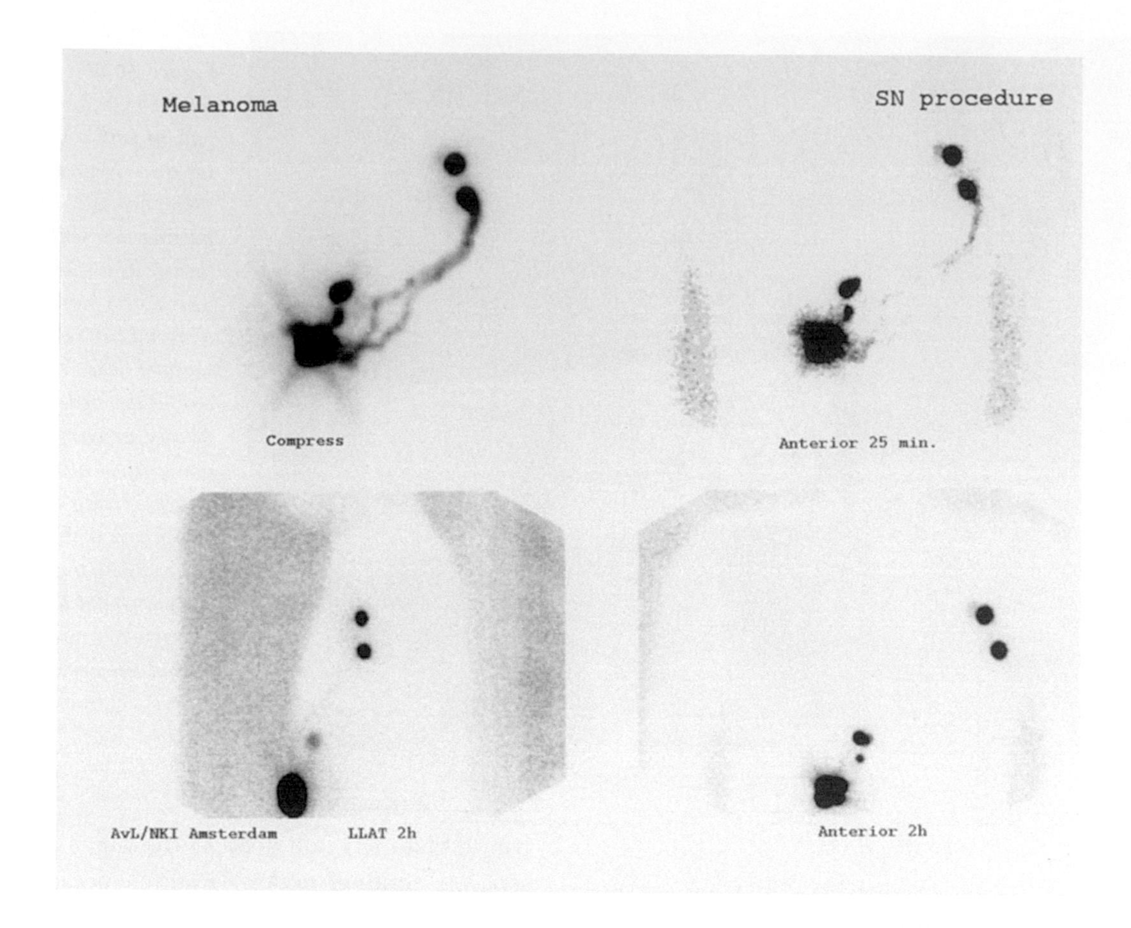

Figure 30.5 *Lymphoscintigraphy in a patient with a melanoma on the anterior trunk. Dynamic imaging shows two lymph vessels passing towards the left axilla where they seem to converge on a single sentinel node, but on the early scans a second higher axillary node appears simultaneously and as bright as the first node. This suggests that one of the lymph vessels has actually bypassed the first node and that there are in fact two sentinel nodes in the left axilla. This situation will need to be clarified at operation, but both nodes should be marked as potential sentinel nodes. There are also two interval nodes (also sentinel nodes) lying in the subcutaneous fat just above the melanoma site.*

THE TECHNIQUE OF LYMPHOSCINTIGRAPHY

Injecting the tracer

For cutaneous lymphoscintigraphy the chosen radiopharmaceutical is administered by intradermal injection. The study should be performed in an air-conditioned environment with the temperature maintained at not less than 21–22°C. If the room is cold, lymph flow will be decreased and an unsuccessful study will be more likely. The procedure should be fully explained to the patient before starting so that he or she is relaxed and comfortable about what is to happen. It is particularly important to warn the patient that each injection will sting for a few seconds, to minimize the risk of sudden movement during the injection and dislodgement of the injection needle. After the procedure has been explained to the patient the primary lesion site or excision biopsy site is examined to determine the number of injections that will be required to produce an accurate result. The injections should surround the site of the melanoma or be placed on both sides of the excision biopsy scar to surround the area that originally contained the melanoma. Most patients will require four to six intradermal injections. Once the number of injections that will be needed has been determined, the patient should be told how many injections to expect. Gloves should always be worn during the injection procedure. If possible the test should not be performed after wide local excision, as this disturbs the lymphatic drainage and renders the test less reliable. The specific activity we use is 5 MBq in 0.05 ml and this is the preferred volume for each injection. A fine 25 gauge or 27 gauge needle is used after the skin is cleaned with an alcohol wipe. There is usually pain at the site of injection. This can be quite intense, especially on the face, hands, and feet. The most intense discomfort seems to occur with injections on the sole of the foot. When the injection is started a small bleb appears or the skin blanches at the site of injection as a very high interstitial pressure is generated. Because of this it is very important that a gauze swab be placed over the needle before it is withdrawn from the skin; failure to do so will result in both the injector and the skin around the injection site being sprayed with tracer and the patient's interstitial fluid. To avoid the needle being dislodged from the skin prematurely and to avoid such contamination, it is worthwhile to have an assistant hold the hand or foot still during injection as it is a normal reflex to withdraw the limb from a source of pain. It is also advisable to place a large impervious incontinence sheet containing a cut out window over the lesion site before injection to help avoid contamination of the surrounding skin of the patient, as this could confound later interpretation. Any swab used during tracer injection will become heavily contaminated with the tracer and should be discarded with the 'hot' waste and not with normal biological waste. The time of starting the intradermal injection should be noted, so that the rate of lymph flow can be determined accurately on the early dynamic scans. The net injected dose may be calculated by subtracting the residual activity in the syringe and on the swabs from the total activity in the syringe prior to injection.

Imaging the patient

Injection of tracer should be completed as quickly as the situation allows and a dynamic acquisition commenced. Ten frames at 1 minute per frame is adequate to allow the rate of lymph flow to be measured in cm/min. This is a useful aid to the surgeon performing sentinel node surgery as it helps in timing the injection of blue dye before the induction of anaesthesia. The early dynamic study is also an essential part of lymphoscintigraphy before sentinel node surgery, as it allows the confident identification of sentinel nodes by tracing lymphatic channels as they drain directly to them. Lymph channels should thus be followed until they reach the draining node field or fields. For the head and neck and the axilla lateral views are often helpful at this stage to identify multiple sentinel nodes. Dynamic images are usually acquired for a total of 20 minutes. The lymphatic channels are best appreciated by summing the individual dynamic frames to produce a composite dynamic image or by performing a separate 5 minute static acquisition at the end of the dynamic phase.

Delayed scans are then performed at 2½ hours after injection of tracer. These delayed scans should include all node fields that can possibly receive drainage from the injection site. It is important during this phase of the study that unusual drainage pathways are detected. These include direct drainage to:

(1) the triangular intermuscular space from the skin of the back;[39]
(2) paravertebral nodes from the loin posteriorly;[40,41]
(3) a right or left costal margin interval node and then on to internal mammary nodes from periumbilical skin;[42]
(4) supraclavicular fossa nodes from the forearm and wrist;[43]
(5) interpectoral nodes from the forearm;[44]
(6) post-auricular nodes from the face and anterior scalp;[45]
(7) level IV and V cervical nodes from the scalp;[45]
(8) nodes across the midline, especially on the back and the face;[40,45]
(9) occipital, parotid and level II cervical nodes from the base of the neck;[45]
(10) axillary nodes from the base of the neck;[45] or
(11) retroperitoneal nodes from the skin of the loin.[41]

Each static acquisition should be for 5–10 minutes to ensure that even very faint sentinel nodes are detected. Most workers use a transmission source to outline the patient during delayed imaging. This gives the surgeon some anatomical guidelines when he or she views the scans in theatre the next day. However, there are potential problems when using a transmission source. If the primary melanoma site is on a part of the skin from which drainage can be ambiguous – for example, the trunk or head and neck – we strongly advise that during this delayed imaging phase a set of images be obtained without the transmission source in place. This is to ensure that all faint sentinel nodes in new node fields not suspected on dynamic imaging are found. Sometimes on the dynamic phase no lymph channel will be seen draining to a particular node field but on delayed scanning a faint but definite node will be seen (Figure 30.4). If this is in a new node field it is by definition a true sentinel node. Such faint nodes are likely to be obscured by scattered radiation through the patient if a transmission source is used.

Accurate marking of the surface location of the sentinel node

Once all the appropriate node fields have been scanned, the sentinel nodes in each node field should be marked. This is done by finding the surface location of the node with the help of a surface marker and then permanently marking this location using a pinpoint tattoo of carbon black ink and a small cross of Castellani's paint or other indelible ink (Figure 30.6). It is very important that the marking be performed with the patient in exactly the same position as that anticipated to be used during surgery. Failure to ensure this will mean that the skin mark will not overlie the node. The depth of the node beneath the skin can also be measured using an orthogonal view and by briefly imaging with a small radioactive point source placed on the skin at the site of the surface mark. The depth can then be measured electronically on the acquisition computer system or manually on the film.

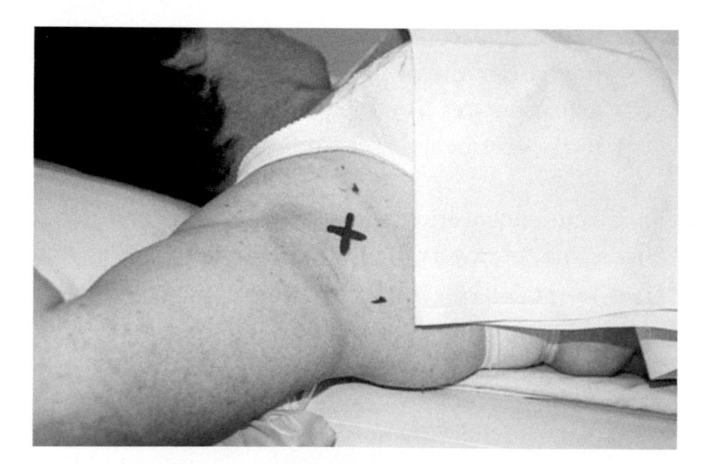

Figure 30.6 *After delayed imaging the surface location of the right axillary sentinel node in this patient is marked on the skin with an 'X' using carbon black ink for a central point tattoo and Castellani's paint. The two other small black marks are guide points made during the marking procedure. The lower mark was made with the arm above the head and notice how far away from the actual node location this is with the arm in the operative position.*

Radiation dosimetry

When ^{99m}Tc radiopharmaceuticals are injected into the interstitial space the radiation dosimetry depends upon the rate of clearance of the tracer from the point of injection. Clearance of radiocolloids from the interstitial space is quite slow, and thus there is a significant radiation dose delivered to the site of injection. A lesser dose is received by the lymph nodes which drain the point of injection and a very small dose is received by the reticuloendothelial system (RES), particularly the liver, which ultimately traps the colloid particles after they reach the blood stream.

Bronskill measured the width of the injection site and the normalized count rate following intramuscular injection of ^{99m}Tc antimony sulphide colloid in the subcostal area.[46] This allowed an estimate of the clearance of the tracer from the injection site over time. He found a biological half clearance time from this injection site of 20.6 hours. This meant that 5 hours after injection, 84.5% of the activity remained at the injection site, 2% was in the draining internal mammary lymph nodes and the remaining 13.5% was in the RES, mainly the liver. From these data Bronskill calculated an absorbed dose at the centre of the injection site of 0.456 Gy for an injected activity of 20 MBq (45.6 rads for 0.5 mCi). He also estimated the absorbed dose for a typical lymph node to be less than 0.2 Gy. Biological half clearance times from other sites were also measured. These were found to be 5.2 hours for the web space between the first and second toes, 9.4 hours for the web space between the second and third fingers, and greater than 36 hours for perianal injections. Maximum dose estimates for these areas were 75 mGy/MBq for the toe web space, 84 mGy/MBq for the finger web space, and 43 mGy/MBq for the perianal area. Bronskill did not specifically measure the absorbed dose for the intradermal injection of this tracer.

Glass et al. did measure the washout half times after intradermal injection for ^{99m}Tc albumin colloid, ^{99m}Tc human serum albumin and ^{99m}Tc sulphur colloid (both of the colloids had been filtered through a 0.2 micron filter).[24] They found half times from the injection site averaged 7.5±6.4 hours, 4.3±1.4 hours and 13.9±12.7 hours respectively for the three agents. These clearance half times imply lower doses at the injection site than those calculated by Bronskill. If one assumes a worst case scenario of no migration of tracer from the injection site after intradermal injection, maximum absorbed doses using 5 MBq of ^{99m}Tc antimony sulphide colloid at each injection site would be in the order of 0.45 Gy assuming a volume of distribution of 1 cc. This is below the threshold dose for deterministic radiation effects and thus no erythema or other effect should be observed. When lymphoscintigraphy is performed to locate the sentinel nodes preoperatively, with our protocol the injections are given intradermally around the excision biopsy site the day before wide local excision of the biopsy site. The radiation dose at the injection site, which accounts for most of the absorbed dose, thus becomes irrelevant as this tissue is excised within 24 hours of tracer injection.

There is also no risk to the surgical team or histopathologists handling the surgical specimens as these activities usually take place the day after lymphoscintigraphy, by which time several physical half lives for ^{99m}Tc have expired.

PATTERNS OF LYMPHATIC DRAINAGE OF THE SKIN

The sentinel nodes that receive direct lymphatic drainage from the skin may lie in any of the following node fields.

The patterns of flow are not predictable in any individual, but some useful information can be obtained by looking at the frequency with which lymph flows from particular parts of the skin to the various node fields. This may serve as a guide to which areas should be examined initially during dynamic imaging.

Box 30.1 ***Lymph node fields draining the skin***

Axillary	Pelvic (obturator and external iliac)
Epitrochlear	Popliteal
Interpectoral	Cervical (levels I–V) and supraclavicular (part of level V)
Paravertebral	Preauricular
Retroperitoneal	Post-auricular
Triangular intermuscular space	Occipital
Costal margin	
Internal mammary	
Groin	

Trunk

As mentioned earlier, it is now clear that 'Sappey's lines' cannot be relied on to predict the pattern of lymphatic drainage in an individual patient.

Lymphoscintigraphy was first performed in patients with cutaneous melanoma to define the draining node field or fields for radical lymph node dissection in patients who had lesions in areas considered likely to have ambiguous drainage. These were mainly lesions on the trunk or the head and neck. We, like others, quickly observed the enormous variability in lymphatic drainage patterns from patient to patient from similar areas of the trunk, and our potentially ambiguous zones on the trunk rapidly got larger and larger until we came to regard almost any lesion on the trunk as having potentially ambiguous drainage. In 1992, when Morton et al. described a method of locating the sentinel lymph node in patients with melanoma using injections of blue dye, lymphoscintigraphy began to be used to locate the sentinel nodes in each draining node field as well as to define the drainage pattern in each patient.[47] This meant that the technique was relevant for all patients and was performed in patients who had what was thought previously to be unambiguous drainage such as from the upper and lower limbs. As a result, data on the lymphatic drainage of the skin for over 2000 patients with lesion sites all over the body have been accumulated.[12]

The data show that drainage in the directions indicated by Sappey's lines is more likely to be correct for lesions on the anterior trunk than for those on the posterior trunk. Drainage across the midline is not common from the anterior trunk but is frequent from the posterior trunk and often from a site well away from the midline. Drainage across Sappey's horizontal line around the waist from sites on the low back to the axilla is also not uncommon, and drainage from above Sappey's line to the groin nodes can also occur. Drainage from the skin of the trunk usually includes the axilla, but exceptions occur.

Unusual patterns of lymphatic drainage occur from the trunk of some patients. In 20% of cases, lymphatics drain from the periumbilical area to a right or left costal margin interval node before passing towards the midline and then through the chest wall to internal mammary nodes.[42]

In some patients, lymphatics drain from the skin of the back to nodes in the triangular intermuscular space node field.[39] This drainage can be unilateral or bilateral. Drainage to this node field is perhaps the most important unusual pathway to look for when performing lymphoscintigraphy to locate sentinel nodes. If drainage to this node field is overlooked, then sentinel nodes will be missed in up to one in ten patients with melanomas on the back.

Some patients have lymphatic channels that pass from the skin of the posterior loin superiorly towards the midline and then through the body wall to paravertebral lymph nodes and finally upwards towards the thoracic duct. A lymph channel may also be seen to pass directly through the body wall in the posterior loin to nodes in the retroperitoneal space, with onward drainage from there to paravertebral nodes.[41] Most of these patients also have some drainage to the usual node fields in the axilla and groin, but occasionally there is exclusive drainage to paravertebral nodes, with no drainage at all to the axilla or groin (Figure 30.7).[48]

Interval nodes in the subcutaneous tissue of the trunk are most common low in the mid-axillary line, along channels passing towards the axilla (Figure 30.8). They are also found along the back, as channels passing up and towards the midline before traversing the body wall to paravertebral nodes. Interval nodes are also often seen along the path of channels passing up towards posterior triangle (level V cervical) nodes from sites on the upper back (Figure 30.9), and on the posterior buttocks in the line of channels heading towards groin nodes from sites on the low back. In a series of 731 patients with primary sites on the trunk, 610 of them on the posterior trunk, and 121 on the anterior trunk, the patterns of lymphatic drainage were as shown in Table 30.1.

Posterior trunk

Of those who showed drainage to the axilla in this group of patients with posterior trunk primary sites, there were 186 patients (33.5%) who showed bilateral axillary drainage (Figure 30.10). Of those who showed drainage to groin nodes there were 16 (26.2%) who

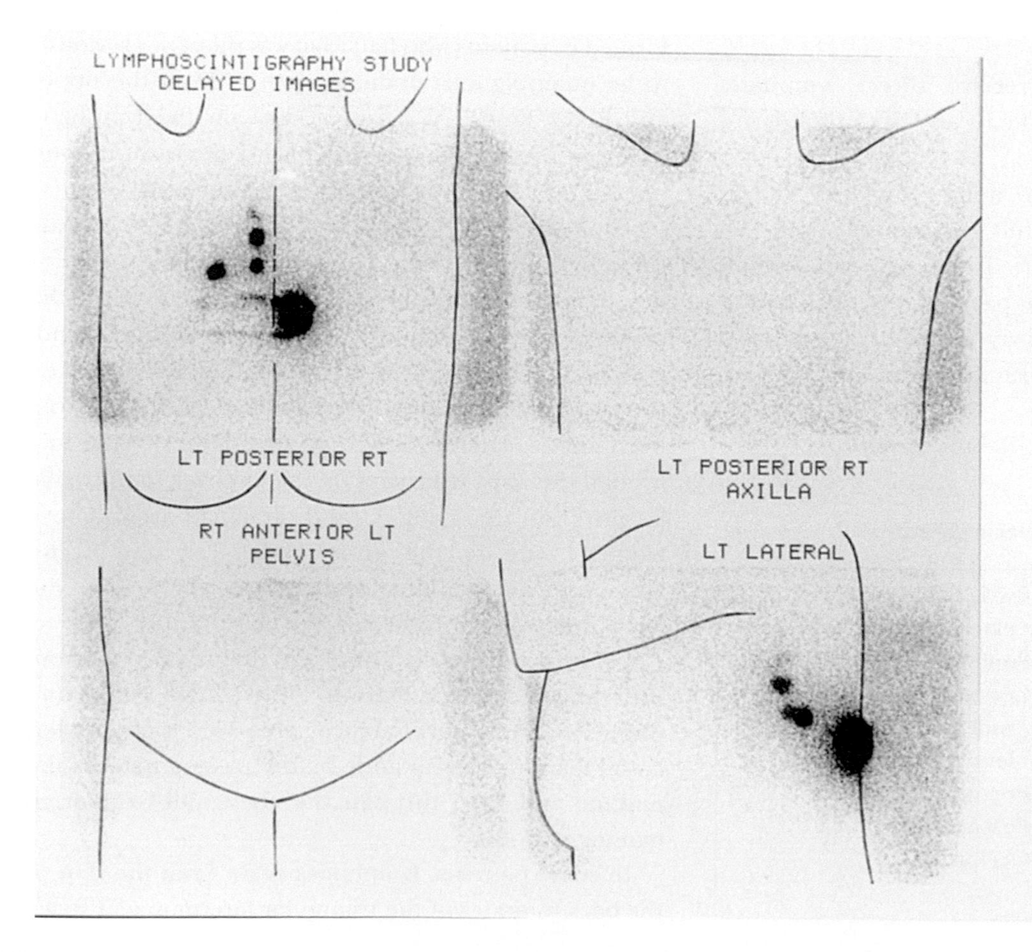

Figure 30.7 *Delayed lymphoscintigraphy images in a patient with a melanoma on the lower back just to the right of midline. There is no drainage whatsoever to the axilla or groin. Drainage is through the posterior body wall exclusively to nodes in the left retroperitoneal and paravertebral regions. A node biopsy in the groin or axilla in this patient would be futile.*

Table 30.1 *Melanoma of the trunk. Drainage on lymphoscintigraphy*

Draining node field	Anterior trunk (N=121) (%)	Posterior trunk (N=610) (%)
Axilla	81	91
Groin	18	10
Triangular intermuscular space	0	9
Paravertebral	0	2.5
Cervical level II	<1	0
Cervical level III	2.5	<1
Cervical level IV	<1	1
Cervical level V	6	21
Supraclavicular (part of level V)	6	14
Occipital	0	<1
Costal margin	4	0
Interval nodes	5	9

(Adapted from reference 12)

had bilateral groin node drainage. The incidence of drainage from the posterior trunk to triangular intermuscular space sentinel nodes was about 9%, but this may underestimate the true incidence of drainage to this node field, as the earlier studies were performed using an imaging protocol that did not specifically look for sentinel nodes in this node field. Drainage to nodes in this field is now consistently seen in approximately 11% of patients with melanomas on the back. In the 15 patients who showed drainage through the posterior abdominal wall directly to paravertebral nodes there were three who also showed drainage to retroperitoneal nodes. Eight of the patients with drainage to the triangular intermuscular space showed drainage to these nodes bilaterally, and 10 patients showed drainage to supraclavicular nodes bilaterally. Five of the 40 patients with drainage to posterior triangle nodes (cervical level V) had bilateral drainage to these nodes.

Anterior trunk

In patients with anterior trunk primary sites who showed drainage to the axilla, 21 (21.4%) had bilateral drainage while only one had bilateral drainage to the supraclavicular fossa. A noticeable difference between anterior and posterior trunk drainage is the significantly smaller percentage of patients with anterior trunk primary sites who show drainage to the supraclavicular fossa, 6% for the anterior trunk versus 14% for the posterior trunk. Drainage from the anterior trunk to the triangular intermuscular space was not expected and was not found. No drainage was seen to level V cervical nodes or occipital nodes, and it seems that direct drainage to paravertebral nodes does not occur from the anterior trunk. Drainage from the skin of the anterior trunk directly to internal mammary nodes seems to be very rare and was not observed in this particular series. However, drainage to internal mammary nodes did occur from periumbilical skin via a costal margin interval node in some patients. Interval nodes were seen less often on the anterior trunk compared with the posterior trunk.

Base of the neck

The skin around the base of the neck is an area that has particularly unpredictable drainage patterns. Drainage can occur to supraclavicular nodes, occipital nodes, cervical nodes (level II–V) (Figure 30.11), triangular intermuscular space nodes, and axillary nodes. It is not uncommon for lymph channels to pass over the shoulder from the back to supraclavicular nodes. The drainage pattern from the base of the neck area usually involves multiple draining node fields (Figure 30.12). In a series of 154 patients with primary melanoma sites in this area the findings were as shown in Table 30.2.

In 24 patients (15.6%) drainage was to both axillae, 11 had bilateral drainage to the supraclavicular fossae, three had bilateral drainage to level V cervical nodes, one had bilateral drainage to level IV cervical nodes, and one had bilateral drainage to triangular intermuscular space sentinel nodes. Thus a total of 26% of patients with primary sites in this region showed bilateral drainage to particular node fields. Drainage from the posterior base of neck to both supraclavicular fossae was possible from only a very small area of the skin of the upper back around the midline. In 124 patients the

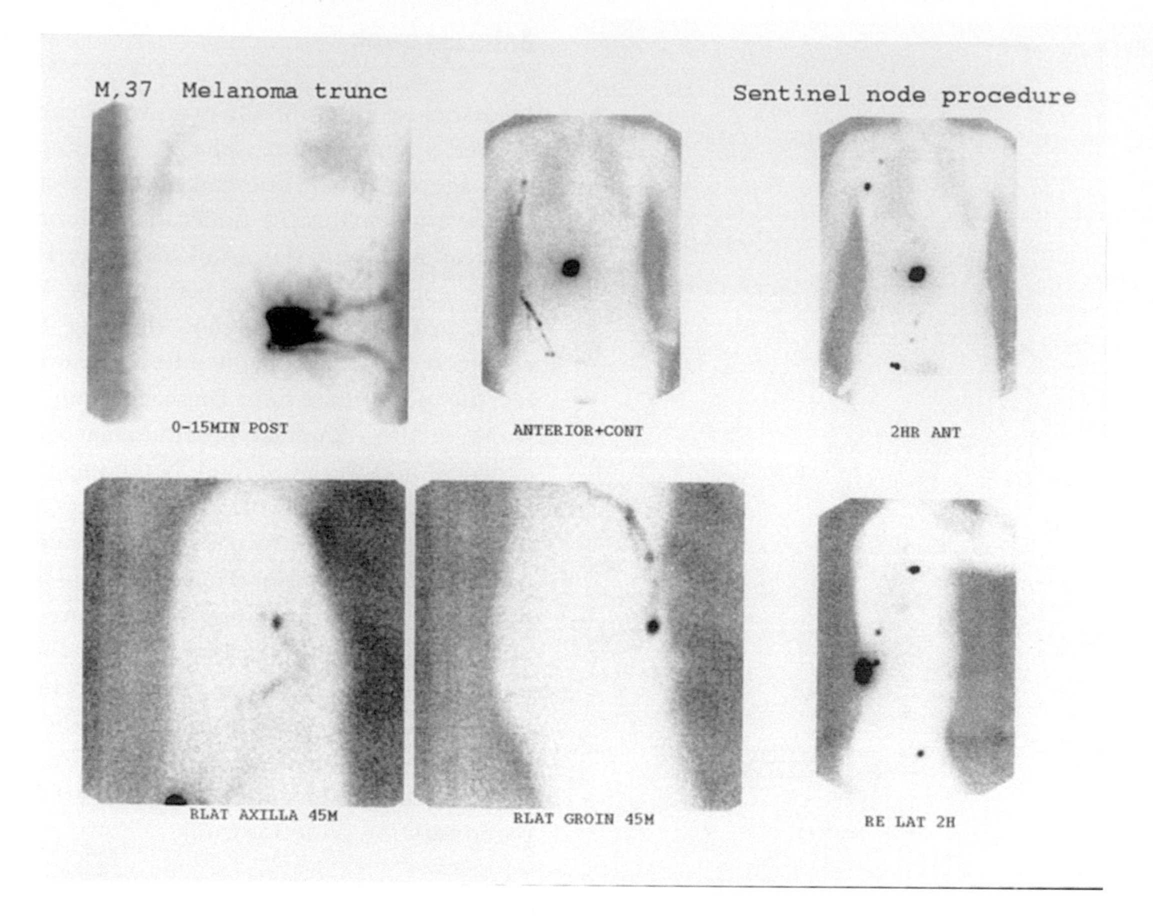

Figure 30.8 *Lymphoscintigraphy in a patient with a melanoma on the right posterior trunk. One lymph vessel passes to the right axilla to a single sentinel node and two lymph vessels pass to the right groin to two sentinel nodes side by side. Interval nodes are also present on the posterior right trunk and the lateral right trunk. This is a common site for interval nodes along the path of lymphatic vessels draining the posterior trunk and passing up towards the axilla.*

primary site was on the posterior aspect of the base of the neck and 53 of these (43%) showed drainage over the shoulders to sentinel nodes in the supraclavicular fossa. Seven of these patients (6%) had drainage over the shoulders to anterior cervical nodes at level III or IV. There was drainage across the midline in 40 patients (32%) to sentinel nodes in a total of 53 node fields.

In the 30 patients who had primary sites on the base of the neck anteriorly there were 6 (20%) who showed drainage across the midline. Five (17%) showed drainage up the neck to cervical level II or III nodes (Figure 30.11), and 25 (83%) showed drainage down to the axilla. Axillary drainage was bilateral in three patients, one patient had bilateral drainage to supraclavicular nodes, and one patient had bilateral drainage to cervical level III nodes.

Head and neck

In the past, guidelines have been proposed for clinical prediction of lymphatic drainage patterns from the skin of the head and neck.[49,50] These have suggested that drainage from the face is to ipsilateral parotid and level I–III cervical nodes, from the anterior scalp to parotid and level I–III nodes, from the posterior scalp to occipital and level II–V nodes, and from the coronal midline scalp to parotid and level I–V nodes. Drainage from the skin of the anterior upper neck would be expected to be to parotid and level I–IV nodes, while the anterior lower neck would be expected to drain to level III–V nodes. Drainage from the skin of the posterior upper neck would be expected to be to occipital and level II–V nodes, while drainage from the posterior lower neck is

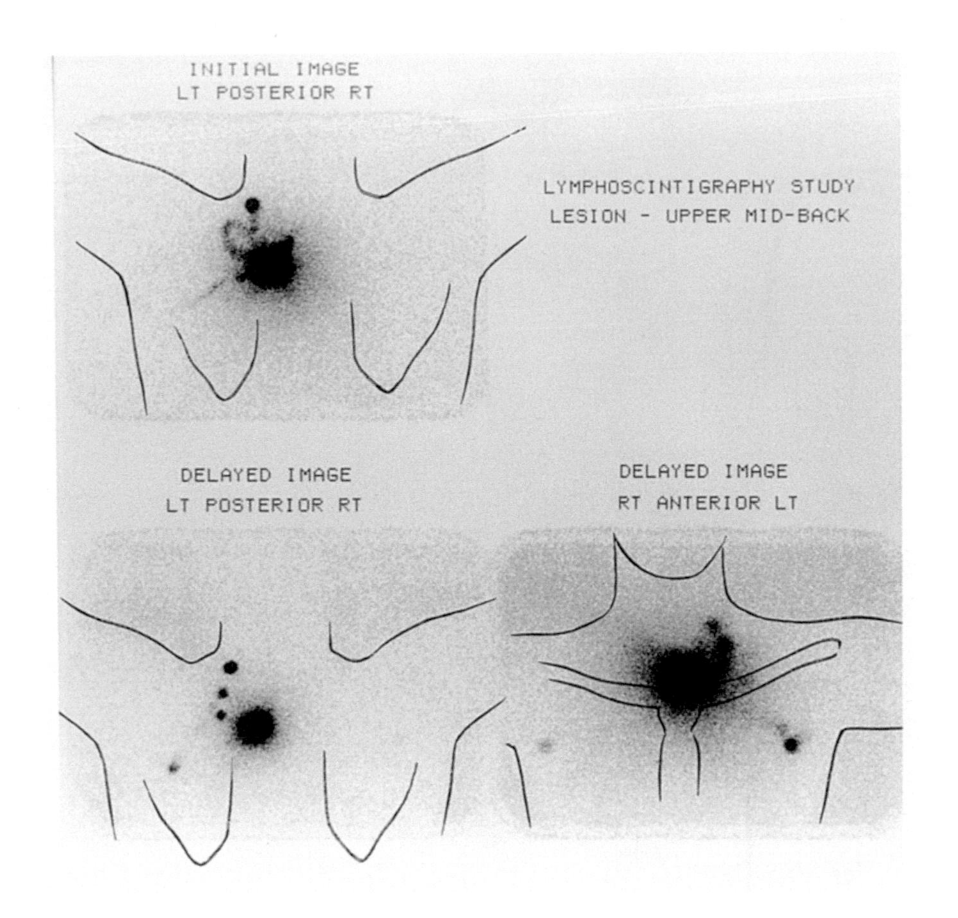

Figure 30.9 *Lymphoscintigraphy in a patient with a melanoma on the upper back just to the left of midline. Dynamic imaging (top) shows lymphatics passing up towards the left neck base posteriorly as well as a vessel passing to the left axilla. Delayed images show a series of interval nodes on the left upper back as well as a single sentinel node in the left axilla (and faint second tier activity). There is also a faint single sentinel node in the right axilla even though no vessel was detected passing to this node field on early imaging. Delayed scans must include all potential draining node fields, not just those which were shown to receive a lymph vessel on dynamic scans.*

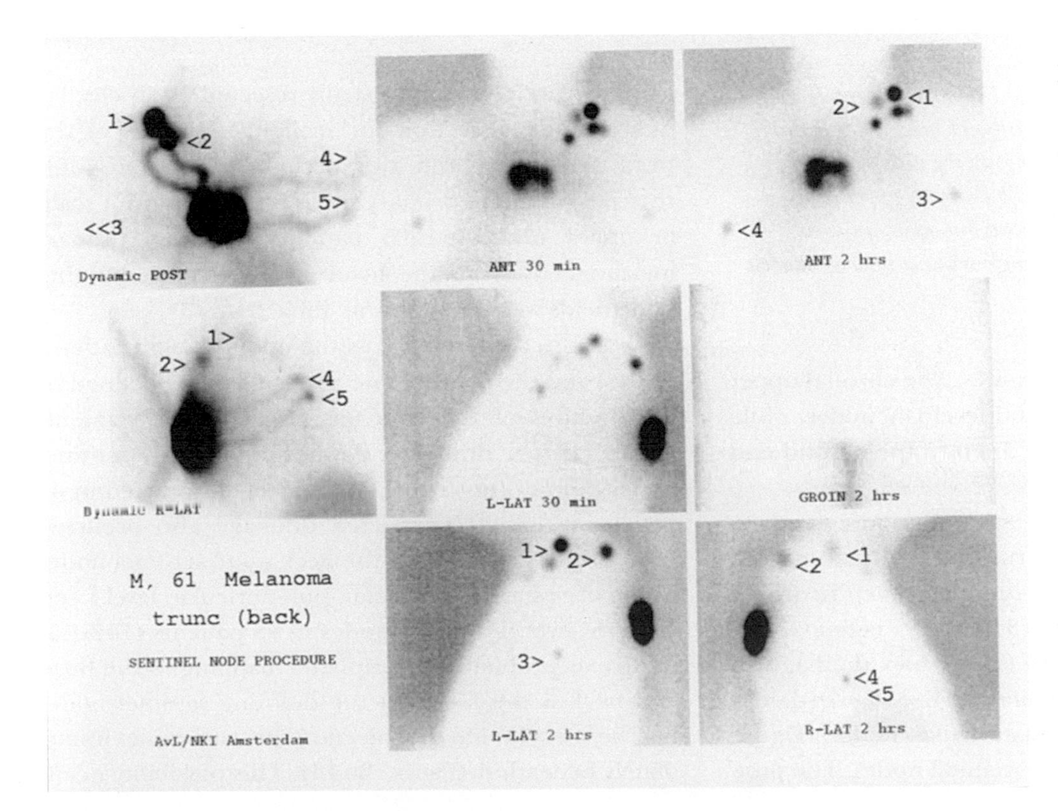

Figure 30.10 *Lymphoscintigraphy in a patient with a melanoma lying between the scapulae. Lymphatic drainage in this area can be very complex as in this patient. Five separate lymph vessels are seen passing to five sentinel nodes, two in the right axilla, one in the left axilla, and two in the left supraclavicular region. High quality lymphoscintigraphy is essential to sort out such complex patterns of lymphatic drainage.*

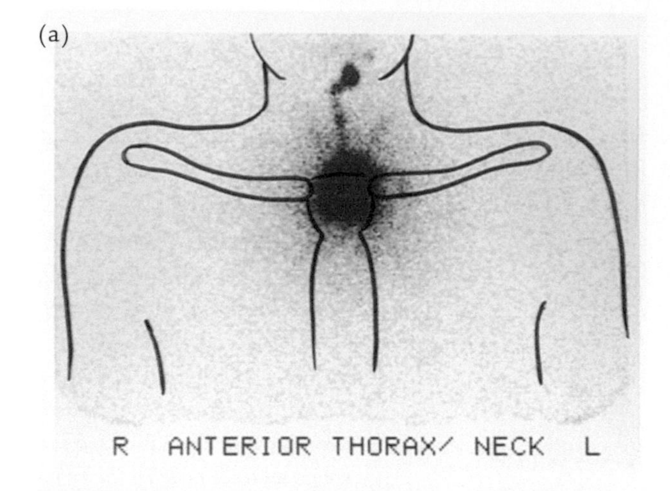

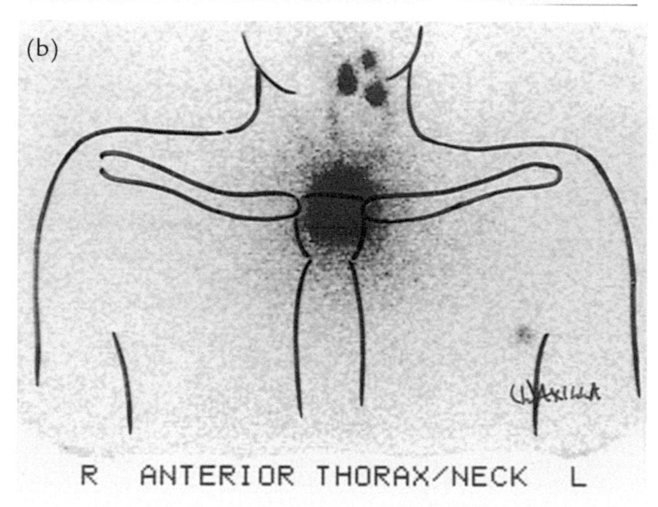

Figure 30.11 *Dynamic and delayed lymphoscintigraphy in a patient with melanoma at the suprasternal notch. The dynamic scan shows two lymph vessels passing up the neck to sentinel nodes which lay in the left submandibular and upper cervical regions. Flow up the neck is unexpected but occurs in some patients. This patient also had a single sentinel node in the left axilla.*

predicted to be to level III–V nodes. The coronal upper neck would include parotid and level I–V nodes, while the ear would be expected to drain to the parotid and level I–V nodes.

However, when lymphoscintigraphy was used to examine lymphatic flow patterns in the head and neck it was found that lymphatic drainage was discordant with clinical prediction in 33 (34%) of 97 patients studied.[45] A total of 21 patients (22%) had drainage to nodes other than the parotid and the five standard neck levels. In 13 this was to post-auricular nodes (Figure 30.13), and in five this was to occipital nodes. The post-auricular nodes are not usually resected in an elective radical node dissection for malignant disease of the head and neck, and the occipital nodes are only resected when the primary site is on the posterior scalp or upper neck. In 205 patients who had primary melanoma sites on the head and neck, the draining node fields were as shown in Table 30.2.

Table 30.2 *Melanoma of the head and neck. Drainage on lymphoscintigraphy*

Draining node field	Head and neck (N=205) (%)	Base of neck (N=154) (%)
Preauricular (parotid)	39	0
Post-auricular	13	0
Occipital	11	1
Cervial level I	18	0
Submental (part of level I)	2	0
Cervical level II	62	1
Cervical level III	14	3
Cervical level IV	17	5
Cervical level V	32	62
Supraclavicular (part of level V)	14	44
Axilla	3	87
Triangular intermuscular space	0.5	7
Interval nodes	3.5	6

Drainage occurred across the midline in 30 patients (15%), and the coronal line across the head defined by the position of the ears was crossed in 27 patients (13%). Direct drainage down the neck to sentinel nodes beyond those normally expected occurred in 42 patients (21%). Unexpected drainage also occurred from primary sites low in the neck up to sentinel nodes in the occipital, preauricular, post-auricular, level I cervical, or level II cervical nodes in 28 patients (14%). A particular problem for lymphatic mapping in the head and neck is the fact that the draining sentinel nodes may lie very close to the injection site, sometimes immediately beneath it (Figure 30.14). This possibility needs to be excluded during surgery and will not always be detected during imaging.

It is thus clear that any attempt to make clinical predictions about lymphatic drainage pathways in patients with head and neck melanomas is unrealistic. If these predictions are used to determine the site and extent of lymph node surgery the surgeon will fail to remove nodes potentially containing metastatic disease in one

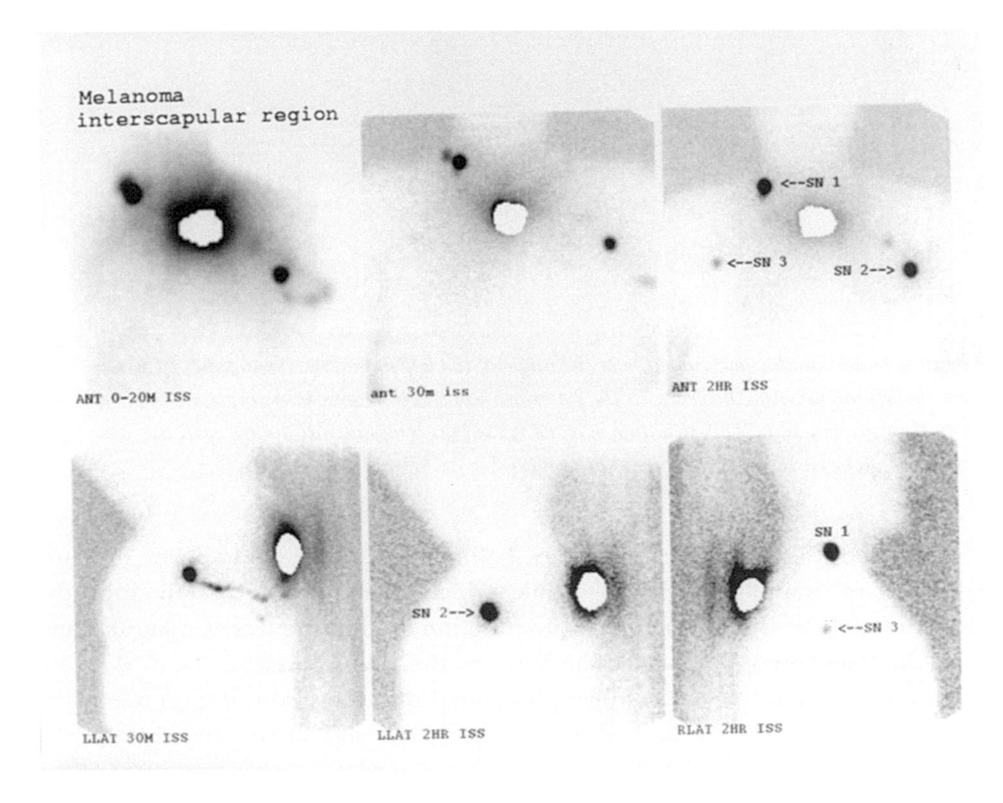

Figure 30.12
Lymphoscintigraphy in a patient with a melanoma on the upper back close to the midline. Drainage from such sites usually involves multiple node fields as in this case. Drainage over the shoulder to neck nodes from this area is very common and this patient also has bilateral axillary drainage.

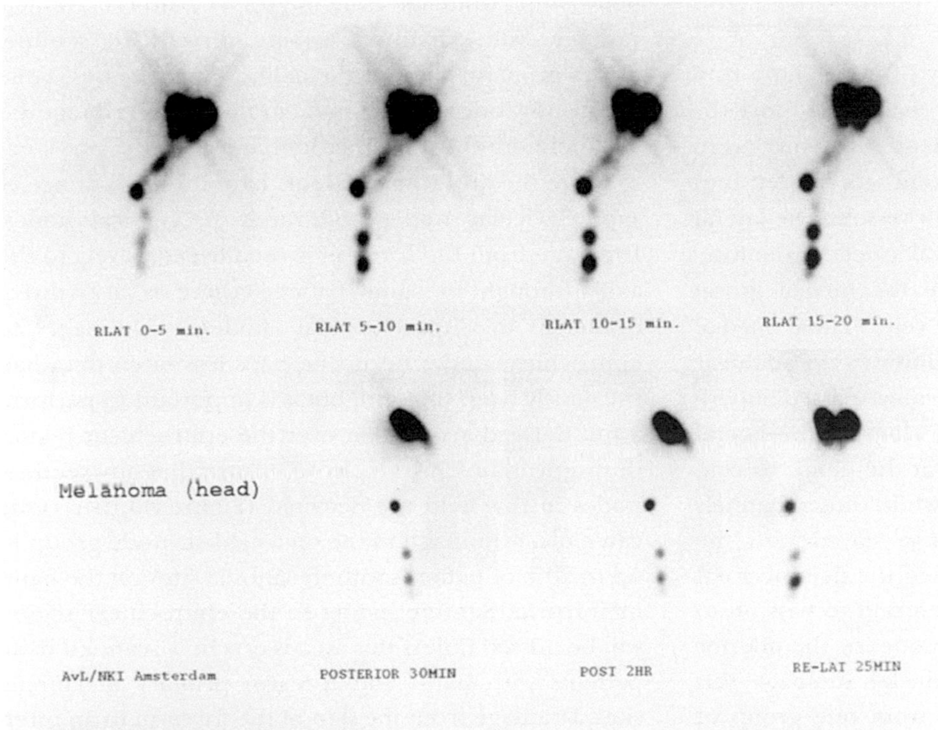

Figure 30.13
Lymphoscintigraphy in a patient with a melanoma on the right lateral parietal scalp. Two lymphatic vessels are seen, one passing behind the right ear to a post-auricular node and one passing anterior to the ear to an upper cervical node. Both are thus sentinel nodes. A third node lower in the right cervical chain also seems bright early, and in this situation it is wise to mark such a node as a potential sentinel node as sometimes the contents of a lymphatic vessel are not subject to the full filter function of a node with some lymph passing on unfiltered. This would need to be checked at surgery.

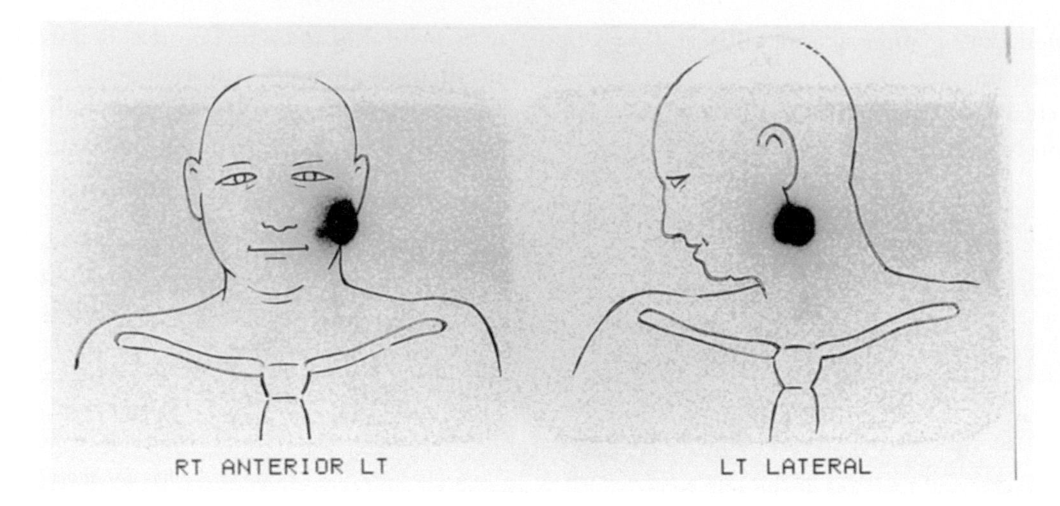

Figure 30.14 *Delayed lymphoscintigraphy in a patient with a melanoma over the angle of the left mandible. No activity in nodes separate from the injection site is evident on the left lateral view, however, in the anterior view tracer is seen in a single sentinel node in the upper cervical chain immediately deep to the injection sites. This situation may be missed on lymphoscintigraphy, and the area beneath an injection site in the neck always needs to be checked for blue nodes at surgery.*

in three patients. As with many other body sites, it seems that rational surgical management of draining lymph nodes in patients with malignant disease that spreads via the lymphatics is not possible unless preoperative lymphatic mapping using lymphoscintigraphy is performed.

Upper limb

Standard accounts of the anatomy of upper limb lymphatic vessels have been largely based on work by Rouviere.[51] Superficial and deep systems were described, and the superficial system was divided into lateral and medial groups of lymph vessels. The lateral group was said to pass up the lateral aspect of the forearm with the cephalic vein while the medial group passed medially with the basilic vein. These medial channels were said to pass sometimes to epitrochlear nodes above the elbow, although most passed superiorly to the lateral axillary nodes. Many of the lateral group were said to pass medially at the elbow to continue on with the medial group, while those channels which persisted in a lateral course stayed with the cephalic vein and eventually reached the deltopectoral nodes. Efferent channels were then said to pass on to the subclavicular (apical) axillary nodes or the inferior cervical nodes. A complex system of drainage was described, with channels passing from one group of axillary nodes to the next. Most passed finally to the apical nodes before continuing on to form the subclavian trunk, which itself drains directly into the jugular trunk, the junction of the internal jugular and subclavian vein, or the thoracic duct.[52]

On lymphoscintigraphy most skin sites on the upper limb drain to the axilla and direct drainage to the deltopectoral nodes is not seen. As in other parts of the body lymph drainage from the upper limb is extremely variable, with channels passing directly to sentinel nodes in many parts of the axilla. There is most commonly only one sentinel node in the axilla (average 1.3 sentinel nodes) with upper limb injections.[53]

From the arm some patients have direct drainage to supraclavicular nodes and rarely to cervical nodes. Drainage from the forearm is usually exclusively to the axilla though in some patients there is also direct drainage to supraclavicular nodes.[43] Drainage to epitrochlear nodes occurs perhaps less often than had previously been thought, but it is important to perform a full delayed acquisition over the epitrochlear region during lymphoscintigraphy to ensure that any sentinel nodes in this field are detected (Figure 30.15).[54] One can expect drainage to the epitrochlear node group in up to 20% of patients with melanoma sites on the hand or forearm. Sentinel nodes in the epitrochlear region will be missed unless this area is carefully scanned in all patients with hand and forearm primary melanoma sites. Drainage from the skin of the forearm to an interpectoral or intraclavicular node is rare.[44]

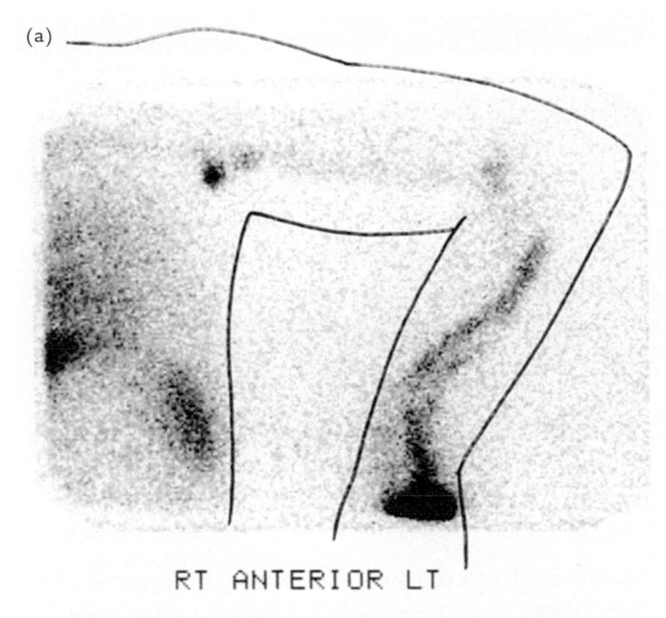

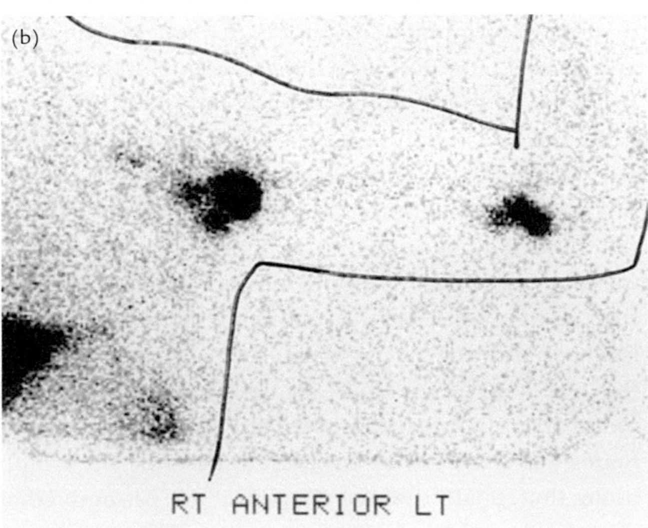

Figure 30.15 *Lymphoscintigraphy in a patient with a melanoma on the left wrist. The early dynamic image (a) shows two lymph vessels passing up the arm, one to the left epitrochlear region, and one to the left axilla. The delayed image (b) shows a sentinel node in the left epitrochlear region and another in the left axilla, with some second tier activity in the axilla.*

In a series of 298 patients with primary melanoma sites on the upper limbs and shoulders (using a vertical line in a sagittal plane through the axilla to define the limits of the upper limb and shoulder versus the trunk) there were 206 patients with lesion sites on the anterior upper limb or shoulder and 92 with posterior lesion sites. The draining node fields seen in these patients are summarized in Table 30.3.

Table 30.3 *Melanoma of the upper limb. Drainage on lymphoscintigraphy*

Draining node field	Upper limb (N=205) (%)
Axilla	97
Supraclavicular	7
Epitrochlear	4
Interpectoral	<1
Triangular intermuscular space	<1
Cervical level V	<1
Interval nodes	5

(Adapted from reference 12)

Of the 21 patients who had drainage to a sentinel node in the supraclavicular fossa there were four whose primary site was on the forearm.

Lower limb

Conventional descriptions of the patterns of lymphatic drainage from the lower limb have been based largely on radiographic lymphography.[55,56] These reports have described the lymphatic vessels of the lower limb as consisting of superficial (subcutaneous) prefascial and deep subfascial systems. The superficial system has anterior and posterior vessels. Injection on the dorsum of the foot, which is the usual site for lymphography, displays the anterior system and usually does not cause opacification of the deep subfascial system. It is said that the medial side of the dorsum of the foot drains via anterior lymphatic vessels along the path of the long saphenous vein, while the lateral aspect of the dorsum of the foot drains via vessels that pass anteriorly and laterally below the knee. Lateral vessels tend towards the medial side of the leg just proximal to the knee, again following the long saphenous vein to the inguinal nodes.[52] The lymphatics branch frequently and above the knee towards the groin there are often bifurcations. The posterior superficial system is displayed on lymphography by injecting a lymph vessel below the lateral malleolus. Clouse has stated that there are fewer lymph channels here and that they accompany the short saphenous vein to the popliteal fossa, where they enter the popliteal nodes.[52] From here efferent vessels turn anteromedially to become deep subfascial vessels and then pass with deep blood vessels on the medial aspect of the thigh to inguinal nodes. The deep subfascial system is not usually relevant in a consideration of cutaneous lymphatic flow, as valves direct flow from the deep to the superficial system and flow in the opposite direction is rare. As expected, lymphatic drainage from the lower limb is exclusively to the ipsilateral groin except when the patient has had prior surgery on the groin nodes, and in this situation lymphatic channels may be seen passing across the pubis to contralateral groin nodes.[57,58]

The above information about the lymphatic vessels of the leg has been derived almost exclusively from subcutaneous injections made into the dorsum of the foot. In lymphoscintigraphy, however, the site of injection of the tracer is determined by the site of the melanoma, thus lymphatic drainage from all parts of the skin of the lower limb has been studied. There is a general tendency for the lymph channels to pass medially, but there is a great variation in the path taken by these channels in different patients. Lymphatic channels from the leg commonly pass both medially and laterally up the lower limb. Drainage to the popliteal nodes has been observed from the skin of the dorsum of the foot, the sole of the heel, the medial heel, and the lower calf on the medial side. This is a considerably more extensive distribution of sites than that suggested by Clouse, who found popliteal drainage only from the skin of the posterolateral heel.

As is the case with drainage to the epitrochlear region, drainage to the popliteal fossa will be missed unless a full 10 minute acquisition is performed over this node field on delayed imaging. Relying on the presence of tracer in this area on the persistence scope is inadequate. Drainage to the popliteal fossa can be expected in approximately 15% of patients with melanoma sites on the leg and foot.

Channels from the leg branch often in the anterior thigh and multiple sentinel nodes in the groin after lower limb injections are the rule rather than the exception.[53] The average number of sentinel nodes seen in the groin after lower limb injections is 3.3. It is quite common for channels to bypass nodes near the apex of the femoral triangle to drain directly into higher inguinal nodes.

Another consistent feature of lymphatic mapping in the lower limb is that second tier lymph nodes are frequently seen, often on the early dynamic phase component of the study.[37] This is in contrast to the axilla where sentinel nodes are often the only nodes seen to contain tracer and even at 24 hours can remain the only significantly radioactive nodes.[36] The high incidence of second tier lymph nodes in the groin is associated with high lymph flow velocities, as mentioned earlier, and it has already been mentioned that lymph flow rates from the lower limb are the highest seen in the skin.[32]

THE 'SENTINEL' LYMPH NODE IN MELANOMA

Definition of a sentinel node

The term 'glands sentinel' was used by Braithwaite in the early 1900s and many others used similar terms to describe the lymph node or nodes that received blue dye and stained blue after interstitial injection of blue dye at surgery. The term 'sentinel' lymph nodes was also used in the medical literature to refer to the nodes in the deep inferior cervical group into which the subclavian lymphatic trunks sometimes drained just before they joined the thoracic duct or right lymphatic duct. These nodes were the last possible lymph node filter before the lymph fluid contents entered the venous circulation at the confluence of the internal jugular and subclavian veins. Thus the nodes were the final 'sentinel' for the entry of metastatic cells into the circulation.[59] The term 'sentinel' nodes was also used by Cabanas to describe the lymph nodes that usually drained the penis.[60] He proposed that these nodes, which lay in the superficial inguinal area associated with the superficial epigastric vein, would be the ones to harbour metastases if any were present in lymph nodes. He described good survival if these nodes were excised and were negative for metastases on histology. Others found a significant false negative rate, with recurrence occurring in other, 'non-sentinel' nodes during follow up.[61,62] All of these studies involved a standard dissection of the medial group of superficial inguinal nodes, and no dye or radiotracer was used. In these studies, there was also no intraoperative method employed to locate draining nodes. This is not the concept of the sentinel node as we know it today.

A sentinel node was defined by Morton et al. as the first lymph node to receive drainage from a lesion site.[47] This definition is open to misinterpretation, especially if there is more than one sentinel node. We prefer the definition 'any lymph node receiving direct lymphatic drainage from a lesion site', as this essentially describes the physiology of the sentinel node concept itself as seen on dynamic lymphoscintigraphy and includes all possible scenarios, including multiple sentinel nodes and interval nodes.[53] It also removes the concept of time from the definition, as this can become confusing if one sentinel node receives tracer rapidly and another sentinel node receives tracer slowly. They both remain sentinel nodes if they receive the tracer directly from the lesion site.

There is usually only one sentinel node in node fields which drain the skin of the trunk, though there may be multiple node fields draining certain parts of it. The axilla and groin both average 1.3 sentinel nodes when drainage occurs from the skin of the trunk.

Multiple sentinel nodes are more likely to occur in the groin with lower limb lesion sites and in the cervical, occipital, preauricular and post-auricular node fields with lesion sites on the head and neck. With lesion sites on the lower limb there are on average 3.3 sentinel nodes in the groin. For the head and neck there are on average 2.7 sentinel nodes per patient and 85% of patients have multiple sentinel nodes.[12]

These multiple sentinel nodes in individual node fields reflect the varying physiology of the lymphatic system in different parts of the body and are not an artefact caused by the use of a particular colloid. If multiple sentinel nodes are not being found in the groin with leg injections in a significant number of patients, this indicates poor mapping of the lymphatic system by the radiocolloid being used. Some researchers seem to be concentrating on removing one or two 'hot' nodes rather than seeking accurately to map the pattern of lymphatic drainage from the primary site and then locating and excising the sentinel nodes, which will almost always be the 'hottest' nodes in the node field. It needs to be remembered, however, that less 'hot' second tier nodes will sometimes remain behind in the node field after a successful sentinel node biopsy. Alternatively on occasions a sentinel node will have only a small amount of tracer compared with other sentinel nodes in the field, and such complex situations need high quality lymphoscintigraphy for clarification. They cannot be accurately resolved using a gamma probe alone.

During surgery whenever possible the sentinel node lying deep to the 'X' marked on the skin during lymphoscintigraphy is confirmed as the node receiving a blue lymphatic channel and itself staining blue. A gamma detection probe can also be used during surgery to confirm that the sentinel node thus found is 'hot' and that the residual node field count is low after it has been removed.

Interval nodes

Interval nodes are lymph nodes draining a tumour site which lie between that site and a recognized node field. They receive lymphatic drainage directly from the lesion site and are therefore, by definition, sentinel nodes. Such interval nodes when they are sentinel nodes have the same likelihood of harbouring micrometastases as sentinel nodes located in standard node fields and a sentinel node biopsy procedure that ignores interval nodes will be incomplete.[63]

DRAINAGE TO MULTIPLE NODE FIELDS

Multiple node fields draining a single skin site are common on the trunk and also for lesion sites around the base of the neck and around the midline of the body, both anteriorly and posteriorly. The skin sites that drain to two or more node fields tend to be congregated around the midline of the trunk, in a band around the waist, across the shoulders posteriorly, and in the head and neck region. Drainage to three node fields is seen in a similar distribution over the posterior trunk and in the periumbilical area anteriorly as well as the head and neck, but drainage to four or more node fields is seen only occasionally in the head and neck and from very restricted areas of the trunk.[12] These truncal areas lie between the scapulae and at around L2 level near the midline (where Sappey's lines cross) on the back and in the periumbilical area on the anterior trunk.

THE OPTIMAL METHOD OF SENTINEL NODE BIOPSY IN MELANOMA

Preoperative lymphoscintigraphy allows any unusual drainage patterns to be identified and anticipated at the time of surgery. The speed of lymphatic transport of the colloid is recorded. The draining node fields are identified and all interval nodes and sentinel nodes are located and marked on the skin. This is true even if drainage to a particular sentinel node is very slow or if it has only a small amount of radioactivity. Before the induction of anaesthesia blue dye is injected intradermally around the lesion or excision biopsy site. The timing of this injection is determined by the speed of lymph flow observed during lymphoscintigraphy. If flow is slow, the dye is injected earlier and the patient is encouraged to exercise the body part to enhance lymphatic drainage. During surgery the sentinel node is identified, beneath the mark made on the skin at lymphoscintigraphy, as a node receiving at least one blue channel and staining blue. The search for the sentinel node during surgery is facilitated by intraoperative use of a gamma probe. The gamma probe helps to ensure that the search for the sentinel node remains on track, especially when the patient is obese (in an axilla the sentinel node may be 10 cm or more deep to the skin mark). The gamma probe is also useful to document a fall in residual node field counts to background levels after the sentinel node has been removed. We are convinced that the use of all three techniques together is the most accurate method of ensuring that all sentinel nodes are identified preoperatively and removed at the time of surgery.

THE FUTURE

New ^{99m}Tc labelled tracers for lymphatic mapping

The ideal radiocolloid for lymphoscintigraphy would migrate completely from the intradermal injection site and be retained completely by the sentinel lymph nodes. Such an agent is not yet available.

In an effort to further improve visualization of lymphatic channels and sentinel lymph nodes, however, some novel approaches have recently been described. New radiotracers using receptor binding agents or surface engineered nanospheres to increase phagocytosis in the regional lymph nodes have been developed.[34,35] Vera et al. have developed a non-particulate receptor binding radiotracer that has excellent retention in the sentinel nodes, thus potentially offering the advantages of both rapid flow through lymph channels of the non-particulate agents such as human serum albumin and the good node retention of the particulate agents such as antimony sulphide colloid.[35] Moghimi et al. have used copolymers sterically to stabilize nanospheres.[34] This dramatically increases the opsonization of these agents in the lymph nodes so that up to 40% of the injected dose is trapped in sentinel node macrophages. Such a high percentage of the injected dose reaching draining lymph nodes also suggests that clearance from the injection site has been enhanced, perhaps by an increase in lymphatic capillary uptake of these agents through their opsonization and active transport into the capillary by pinocytosis. Developments such as these may lead to better tracers becoming available for lymphoscintigraphy in the future.

Collimators

High resolution collimators are best for lymphoscintigraphy and microcast collimators are preferable to folded metal collimators as they have less star artefact caused by septal penetration of high activity from the injection site. Ideally septal penetration should be less than 1% at 140 Kev energy. This will prevent the occurrence of star artefact.

CONCLUSIONS

Lymphatic mapping using high resolution lymphoscintigraphy is now the essential first step for accurate identification and removal of the sentinel lymph nodes in patients with melanoma. It allows any unusual lymph drainage pathways to be identified and ensures that sentinel nodes will not be overlooked, even when they are in unusual node fields or are interval nodes lying along the path of a lymphatic vessel. Experience has shown that micrometastases are present in such sentinel nodes with an incidence similar to that seen in sentinel nodes located in standard node fields. This in essence is the key to the importance of lymphoscintigraphy in sentinel node biopsy. It ensures that all true sentinel nodes are identified in each patient and that sentinel nodes are not overlooked because they might lie in an unusual location. Knowledge of the accurate surface location of the sentinel nodes before surgery simplifies the surgical procedure and shortens the time required under anaesthesia. If preoperative lymphoscintigraphy is not performed, it is inevitable that sentinel nodes will be missed in some patients, negating the fundamental objective of sentinel node biopsy as a staging procedure.

REFERENCES

1. Cruikshank W, *The anatomy of the absorbing vessels of the human body.* 1786.
2. Mascagni P, Vasorum lymphaticorum corporis humani historia et ichnographia. P Carli, Sienna. 1787.
3. Sappey MPC, Anatomie, physiologie, pathologie des vaisseaux lymphatiques consideres chez l'homme at les vertebres. DeLahaye A, Lecrosnier E, (eds). Paris. 1874.
4. Delamere G, Poirier P, Cuneo B, The lymphatics. In: *A treatise of human anatomy.* (ed Charpy PPaA) Westminster: Archibald Constable and Co Ltd, 1903: 301.
5. Sherman AI, Ter-Pogossian M, Tocus EC, Lymph node concentration of radioactive colloidal gold following interstitial injection. *Cancer* 1953; 6: 1238–40.
6. Fee HJ, Robinson DS, Sample WF, et al, The determination of lymph shed by colloidal gold scanning in patients with malignant melanoma: a preliminary study. *Surgery* 1978; 84: 626–32.
7. Meyer CM, Lecklitner ML, Logic JR, et al, Technetium 99m sulfur-colloid cutaneous lymphoscintigraphy in the management of truncal melanoma. *Radiology* 1979; 131: 205–9.
8. Sullivan DC, Croker BP, Harris CC, et al, Lymphoscintigraphy in malignant melanoma: ^{99m}Tc antimony sulfur colloid. *Am J Roentgenol* 1981; 137: 847–51.
9. Bergqvist L, Strand S, Hafstrom L, et al, Lymphoscintigraphy in patients with malignant melanoma: a quantitative and qualitative evaluation of its usefulness. *Eur J Nucl Med* 1984; 9: 129–35.
10. Norman J, Cruse W, Espinosa C, et al, Redefinition of cutaneous lymphatic drainage with the use of lymphoscintigraphy for malignant melanoma. *Am J Surg* 1991; 162: 432–7.
11. Eberbach MA, Wahl RL, Lymphatic anatomy: functional nodal basins. *Ann Plast Surg* 1989; 22: 25–31.
12. Uren RF, Thompson JF, Howman-Giles RB, *Lymphatic drainage of the skin and breast: locating the sentinel nodes.* Amsterdam, Harwood Academic Publishers, 1999.
13. Walker L, Localization of radioactive colloids in lymph nodes. *J Lab Clin Med* 1950; 36: 440–9.
14. Kaplan WD, Davis MA, Rose CM, A comparison of two technetium-99m-labeled radiopharmaceuticals for lymphoscintigraphy. *J Nucl Med* 1979; 20: 933–7.
15. Bergqvist L, Strand S-E, Persson BRR, Particle sizing and biokinetics of interstitial lymphoscintigraphic agents. *Semin Nucl Med* 1983; 8: 9–19.
16. Kapteijn BAE, Nieweg OE, Muller SH, et al, Validation of gamma probe detection of the sentinel node in melanoma. *J Nucl Med* 1997; 38: 362–6.
17. Nathanson SD, Anaya P, Karvelis KC, et al, Sentinel lymph node uptake of two different technetium-labeled radiocolloids. *Ann Surg Oncol* 1997; 4: 104–10.
18. Frier M, Phagocytosis. In: *Progress in radiopharmacology.* (ed Cox PM) Amsterdam: Elsevier/North Holland Biomedical Press, 1981: 249–60.
19. Dornfest BS, Lenehan PF, Reilly TM, Effects of sera of normal, anemic and leukemic rats on particle size distribution of ^{99m}Technetium-sulfur colloid in vitro. *J Reticuloendothel Soc* 1977; 21: 317–29.
20. Alazraki NP, Eshima D, Eshima LA, et al, Lymphoscintigraphy, the sentinel node concept, and the intraoperative gamma probe in melanoma, breast cancer, and other potential cancers. *Semin Nucl Med* 1997; 27: 55–67.
21. Wong JH, Terada K, Ko P, Coel MN, Lack of effect of particle size on the identification of the sentinel node in cutaneous malignancies *Ann Surg Oncol* 1998; 5: 77–80.
22. Tonakie A, Yahanda A, Sondak V, Wahl RL, Reproducibility of lymphoscintigraphic drainage patterns in sequential TC-99M HSA and TC-99M sulfur colloid studies: implications for sentinel node identification in melanoma. *J Nucl Med* 1998; 39: 25P.
23. Nathanson SD, Nelson L, Karvelis KC, Rates of flow of technetium 99m-labeled human serum albumin from peripheral injection sites to sentinel lymph nodes. *Ann Surg Oncol* 1996; 3: 329–35.
24. Glass EC, Essner R, Morton DL, Kinetics of three lymphoscintigraphic agents in patients with cutaneous melanoma. *J Nucl Med* 1998; 39: 1185–90.
25. Swartz MA, Berk DA, Jain RK, Transport in lymphatic capillaries. I. Macroscopic measurements using residence time distribution theory. *Am J Physiol* 1996; 270: H324–9.
26. Yoffey JM, Courtice FC, *Lymphatics, lymph and the lymphomyeloid complex.* London: Academic Press, 1970.
27. Casley-Smith JR, *Lymph and lymphatics in microcirculation.* Kaley G, Altura BM, ed. University Park Press, 1977: 423–502.
28. Aspegren K, Strand SE, Persson BRR, Quantitative lymphoscintigraphy for detection of metastases to the internal mammary lymph nodes. Biokinetics of ^{99m}Tc-sulphur colloid uptake and correlation with microscopy. *Acta Radiol Oncol* 1978; 17: 17–26.
29. Ege GN, Warbick A, Lymphoscintigraphy: a comparison of 99Tc(m) antimony sulphide colloid and 99Tc(m) stannous phytate. *Br J Radiol* 1979; 52: 124–9.
30. Strand SE, Persson BRR, Quantitative lymphoscintigraphy I: basic concepts for optimal uptake of radiocolloids in the parasternal lymph nodes of rabbits. *J Nucl Med* 1979; 20: 1038–46.
31. Nagai K, Ito Y, Otsuka N, et al, Experimental studies on uptake of ^{99m}Tc-antimony sulfide colloid in RES. A comparison with various ^{99m}Tc-colloids. *Int J Nucl Med Biol* 1981; 8: 85–9.
32. Uren RF, Howman-Giles RB, Thompson JF, et al, Variability of cutaneous lymphatic flow rates. *Melanoma Res* 1998; 8: 279–82.
33. Nopajaroonsri C, Simon GT, Phagocytosis of colloidal carbon in a lymph node. *Am J Pathol* 1971; 65: 25–42.
34. Moghimi SM, Hawley AE, Christy NM, et al, Surface engineered nanospheres with enhanced drainage into lymphatics and uptake by macrophages of the regional lymph nodes. *FEBS Lett* 1994; 344: 25–30.
35. Vera DR, Wisner ER, Stadalnik RC, Sentinel node imaging via a nonparticulate receptor-binding radiotracer. *J Nucl Med* 1997; 38: 530–5.
36. Thompson JF, Niewind P, Uren RF, et al, Single-dose isotope injection for both preoperative lymphoscintigraphy and intraoperative sentinel lymph node identification in melanoma patients. *Melanoma Res* 1997; 6: 500–6.
37. Uren RF, Howman-Giles RB, Thompson JF, Demonstration of second tier lymph nodes during preoperative lymphoscintigraphy for melanoma: Incidence varies with primary tumour site. *Ann Surg Oncol* 1998; 5: 517–21.
38. Ludwig J, Ueber kurschlusswege der lymphbahnen und ihre beziehungen zur lymphogen krebsmetastasierung. *Path Microbiol* 1962; 25: 329.
39. Uren RF, Howman-Giles RB, Thompson JF, et al, Lymphatic drainage to triangular intermuscular space lymph nodes in melanoma on the back. *J Nucl Med* 1996; 37: 964–6.
40. Uren RF, Howman-Giles RB, Shaw HM, et al, Lymphoscintigraphy in high risk melanoma of the trunk: predicting draining node groups, defining lymphatic channels and locating the sentinel node. *J Nucl Med* 1993; 34: 1435–40.
41. Uren RF, Howman-Giles RB, Thompson JF, Lymphatic drainage from the skin of the back to intra-abdominal lymph nodes in melanoma patients. *Ann Surg Oncol* 1998; 5: 384–7.
42. Uren RF, Howman-Giles RB, Thompson JF, et al, Lymphatic drainage from peri-umbilical skin to internal mammary nodes. *Clin Nucl Med* 1995; 20: 254–5.
43. Uren RF, Howman-Giles R, Thompson JF, Quinn MJ, Direct lymphatic drainage from the skin of the forearm to a supraclavicular node. *Clin Nucl Med* 1996; 21: 387–9.
44. Uren RF, Roberts J, Howman-Giles RB, Thompson JF, Direct lymphatic drainage from the skin of the elbow to an interpectoral node. *Reg Cancer Treat* 1996; 9: 100–2.
45. O'Brien CJ, Uren RF, Thompson JF, et al, Prediction of potential metastatic sites in cutaneous head and neck melanoma using lymphoscintigraphy. *Am J Surg* 1995; 170: 461–6.
46. Bronskill MJ, Radiation dose estimates for interstitial radiocolloid lymphoscintigraphy. *Semin Nucl Med* 1983; 13: 20–5.
47. Morton DL, Wen D-R, Wong JH, et al, Technical details of intraoperative lymphatic mapping for early stage melanoma. *Arch Surg* 1992; 127: 392–9.
48. Uren RF, Howman-Giles RB, Thompson JF, McCarthy WH, Exclusive lymphatic drainage from a melanoma on the back to intraabdominal lymph nodes. *Clin Nucl Med* 1998; 23: 71–3.
49. Robbins KT, Medina JE, Wolfe GT, et al, Standardizing neck dissection terminology. Official report of the Academy's committee for head and neck surgery and oncology. *Arch Otolaryngol Head Surg* 1991; 117: 601–5.

50. O'Brien CJ, Petersen-Schaefer K, Ruark D, et al, Radical, modified, and selective neck dissection for cutaneous malignant melanoma. *Head Neck* 1995; 17: 232–41.
51. Rouviere H, *Anatomy of the human lymphatic system.* Ann Arbor, MI: Edwards Brothers, 1938.
52. Clouse ME, Wallace S, eds, *Lymphatic imaging. Lymphography, computed tomography and scintigraphy.* 2nd ed. Baltimore: Williams and Wilkins: 1985: 15–21.
53. Uren RF, Howman-Giles RB, Thompson JF, et al, Lymphoscintigraphy to identify sentinel nodes in patients with melanoma. *Melanoma Res* 1994; 4: 395–9.
54. Hunt JA, Thompson JF, Uren RF, et al, Epitrochlear lymph nodes as a site of melanoma metastasis. *Ann Surg Oncol* 1998; 5: 248–52.
55. Kinmonth JB, Taylor GW, Harper RK, Lymphography: a technique for its clinical use in the lower limb. *BMJ* 1955; 1: 940.
56. Browse NL, Normal lymphographic appearances of the lower limb and axilla. In: *The lymphatics: diseases, lymphography and surgery.* (ed Kinmouth JB) Baltimore: Williams and Wilkins, 1972: 70.
57. Jonk A, Kroon BBR, Mooi WJ, Hoefnagel CA, Contralateral inguinal lymph node metastasis in patients with melanoma of the lower extremities. *Br J Surg* 1989; 76: 1161–2.
58. Thompson JF, Saw RP, Colman MH, et al, Contralateral groin node metastasis from lower limb melanoma. *Eur J Cancer* 1997; 33: 976–7.
59. Haagensen CD, Feind CR, Herter FP, et al, *The lymphatics in cancer.* Philadelphia: W B Saunders: 583.
60. Cabanas RM, An approach for the treatment of penile carcinoma. *Cancer* 1977; 39: 456–66.
61. Bouchot O, Bouvier S, Bochereau G, Jeddi M, Cancer of the penis: the value of systematic biopsy of the superficial inguinal lymph nodes in clinical N0 stage patients. *Prog Urol* 1993; 3: 228–33.
62. Pettaway CA, L PL, Dinney CPN, et al, Sentinel lymph node dissection for penile carcinoma: the MD Anderson Cancer Center experience. *J Urol* 1995; 154: 1999–2003.
63. Uren RF, Howman-Giles R, Thompson JF, et al, Interval nodes: the forgotten sentinel nodes in melanoma patients. *Arch Surg* 2000; 135: 1168–72.

31

Sentinel lymph node biopsy: results to date

Douglas Reintgen, Merrick I Ross, Richard Essner

INTRODUCTION

There is an epidemic of melanoma in the United States and in 2000, 47,700 people were diagnosed with the disease.[1] Melanoma is a tumour that affects people who are young and in the most productive years of their lives, constituting a major public health problem for the United States and other countries. The care of patients with melanoma has changed in the past 10 years. With the development of new lymphatic mapping techniques to reduce the cost and morbidity of nodal staging, the emergence of more sensitive assays for occult melanoma metastases, and the identification of interferon-α-2b as an effective adjuvant treatment for the treatment of patients with melanoma at high risk for recurrence, nodal staging for this disease becomes more important.[2]

Lymphatic mapping and sentinel lymph node (SLN) biopsy for melanoma involve a more conservative operation that causes less morbidity but also provides a mechanism for more accurate staging to occur. This chapter will detail the results to date with this new technology.

MELANOMA MAPPING

Prognostic factors for cutaneous melanoma

Prognostic factor determination is important in order to stratify and analyze results of treatment accurately and determine which patients may benefit from more intensive therapy. Many factors are known to predict the risk for metastatic disease in melanoma. When evaluating treatments it becomes important to account for prognostic factors that can accurately categorize patients into different risk groups for metastatic disease. Otherwise differences (or lack of differences) between treatment regimens may not be due to the treatments themselves but may merely reflect imbalances of prognostic factors.

The most powerful predictor of survival for patients with melanoma is the presence or absence of lymph node metastases. Once patients develop metastatic melanoma to their regional nodes, prognostic factors based on the primary melanoma contribute very little to the prognostic model. The presence of lymph node metastases decreases the 5-year survival of patients by approximately 40% compared with those who have no evidence of nodal metastases. Much time, effort and expense has been involved in the identification of prognostic factors based on characteristics of the primary tumour. Yet, in multiple regression analysis performed on many collected populations in the literature, the lymph node status of the patient with melanoma is by far the most powerful factor predicting recurrence and survival. Primary tumour variables such as Breslow thickness, ulceration, primary site, and sex may add to the prognostic model, but only after nodal status is considered. Recently, a new staging system has been proposed for melanoma. Primary site variables such as tumour thickness and ulceration of the primary continue to influence regional nodal metastasis and survival.[3] A patient with a deep ulcerated melanoma who is node negative has a survival very similar to a patient with documented stage III melanoma.

Sentinel node technology enables the surgeon to map the cutaneous lymphatic flow from the primary tumour and identify the SLN in the regional basin that allows better nodal staging of the melanoma patient. Use of this procedure, as initially proposed by Morton et al., has shown that the SLN is the first site of metastatic disease; if the SLN is histologically negative, then the remainder of the lymph nodes in the basin are also likely to be histologically negative.[4–7] Intraoperative mapping and sentinel lymphadenectomy also allow for a detailed pathological examination of the SLN, since the examination is limited to one or two nodes. This advance allows the pathologist to examine the node by serial section and use immunohistochemistry to look for micrometastatic disease. A more intensive pathological examination of one or two SLNs, rather than routine examination of all the regional lymph nodes, may more accurately identify patients with micrometastatic lymph node metastases, since metastatic melanoma in the SLN may be very low volume disease (Figure 31.1).

Elective node dissection for staging and treatment

Elective lymph node dissection (ELND) has in the past been the mainstay of the surgeon's armamentarium for nodal staging of the patient with melanoma. This approach refers to the removal of clinically negative nodes, as opposed to therapeutic dissection, which is performed to remove nodes when they are grossly involved with tumour. There is a lack of consensus as to whether ELND actually extends the survival of the melanoma patient or whether it serves solely as a staging procedure. A number of prospective randomized trials have failed to show an improvement in survival for patients with melanoma randomized to receive ELND as treatment versus the control population who were treated by wide local excision (WLE) only as their primary surgical treatment.[8,9] However, retrospective studies based on large databases suggested that there were subpopulations of patients with melanoma who benefited.[10,11] Perhaps this controversy has been laid to rest with the reporting of results of the Intergroup Melanoma Trial, in which only patients with intermediate thickness melanomas (tumour thickness between 1.0 mm and 4.0 mm) were eligible. In addition, this was the first prospective trial that required preoperative lymphoscintigraphy in all patients to identify and remove all basins at risk for metastatic disease. Without this preoperative test to provide a map for the surgeon, ELND may be misdirected in greater than 50% of the head and neck and trunk dissections. In addition, in 5% of the melanoma population, in-transit nodal areas (defined as nodes outside the classic anatomical basin between the primary site and the regional nodes) may be missed.[12] These in-transit nodes are equally at risk for metastatic disease.[13]

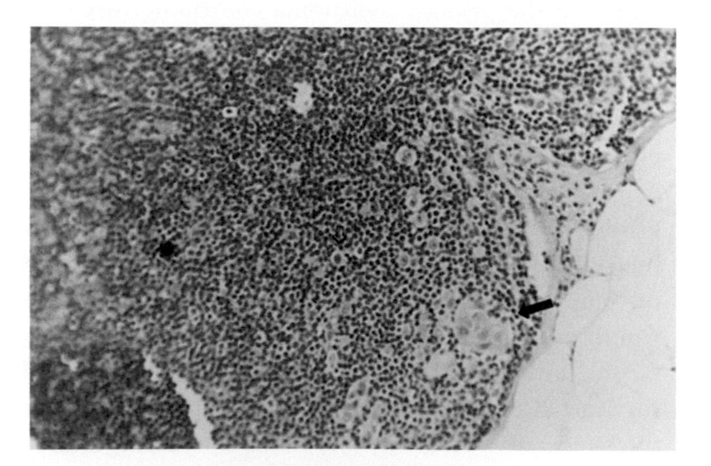

Figure 31.1 *Photomicrograph of a bivalved sentinel lymph node with an H&E stain. Metastatic melanoma can invade into the regional basin as low volume disease. There are small clusters of metastatic cells (closed arrow) as well as single cells (open arrow) invading into the substance of the sentinel node.*

In the Intergroup Melanoma Trial, overall survival was not significantly different for those patients who received WLE of their primary site and observation of the regional basins versus those patients who received a WLE and ELND as their surgical treatment. However, two defined subsets of patients had a significant increase in overall survival with ELND. Patients with melanomas between 1.1 mm and 2.0 mm or patients younger than 60 years of age experienced a survival benefit with the addition of ELND as part of their primary surgical treatment.[14] The tumour thickness stratification was part of the original design of the trial, but the benefit by age was only apparent with subgroup analysis in a retrospective fashion. In a more recent update from the Intergroup Melanoma Trial, now with follow up out to 10 years, there continues to be widening of the curves between those who received ELND as part of their primary treatment versus those in whom the regional basin was simply observed. The *P* value for the difference between the curves has fallen to 0.09 with the longer follow up. The point remains that the only patients ELND can possibly benefit are those with nodal disease. Now there is a relatively low morbidity procedure to perform, an SLN biopsy, to ascertain which patients are node positive or negative.

Because of the results from the Balch study and the interferon-α-2b study that was the impetus for FDA approval of this drug as the first effective adjuvant treatment, one can argue that patients with a defined risk of nodal metastases should have a nodal staging procedure. For national trials the level for consideration of nodal staging is those patients with melanomas ≥1.0 mm in thickness. Patients with melanomas that are thinner than this (0.76–1.0 mm) have a 6–10% incidence of nodal metastases when lymphatic mapping is performed and a more detailed examination of the SLN is undertaken.[15]

Sentinel lymph node biopsy as a staging procedure

A new procedure has been developed to assess the status of the regional lymph nodes more accurately and decrease the morbidity and expense to the healthcare system of ELND. The technique, termed intraoperative lymphatic mapping and sentinel lymphadenectomy, relies on the concept that regions of the skin have specific patterns of lymphatic drainage not only to the regional lymphatic basin, but also to a specific sentinel lymph node (SLN) in the basin. Morton et al. initially proposed the technique using a vital blue dye injected at the primary site and showed that in animal studies and human trials, the SLN was the first node in the lymphatic basin to which the primary melanoma consistently drains.[4,5] With the blue dye, the surgeon gets a visual clue as to where these first nodes in the chain of lymphatics are located. Morton showed that defined patterns of lymphatic drainage allowed determination of the first node in the basin (the SLN) that received lymphatic flow from the primary site. He went on to hypothesize that the presence or absence of metastatic melanoma in the SLN will accurately reflect the disease status in the remaining regional lymph nodes. Complete nodal staging could thus be obtained with an SLN biopsy.

Choice of vital dye

Morton et al. investigated a number of vital dyes for their potential applicability in cutaneous lymphatic mapping. These included methylene blue (American Regent Lab, Shirley, NY), isosulfan blue (1% in aqueous solution; United States Surgical Corporation, Norwalk, CT), patent blue-V (Laboratoire Guerbert, France), Cyalume (American Cyanamid Co, Bound Brook, NJ) and fluorescein dye. All substances tested were known to be non-toxic in vivo and were injected intradermally as provided by the supplier. The patent blue-V and isosulfan blue dyes produced the best results among the substances tested for their accuracy in identifying the regional lymphatic drainage pattern in the cat.[16] These dyes rapidly entered the lymphatics with minimal diffusion into the surrounding tissue. The bright blue colour of the dyes was readily visible and allowed easy identification of the exposed lymphatics. Isosulfan blue has worked extremely well for SLN mapping. In some patients with thin skin, the afferent lymphatics can be seen through the skin after the injection of isosulfan blue (Figure 31.2). Additionally, when entering the lymph node the vital blue dye stains part of the node blue, which is easily discernible from the surrounding non-SLNs. In contrast, the other dyes were proved to be unsatisfactory and abandoned because of their rapid diffusion into surrounding tissue and insufficient retention by the lymphatic channels to stain the SLN. The fluorescent dyes fluorescein and Cyalume were readily visualized but required a dark room for optimal

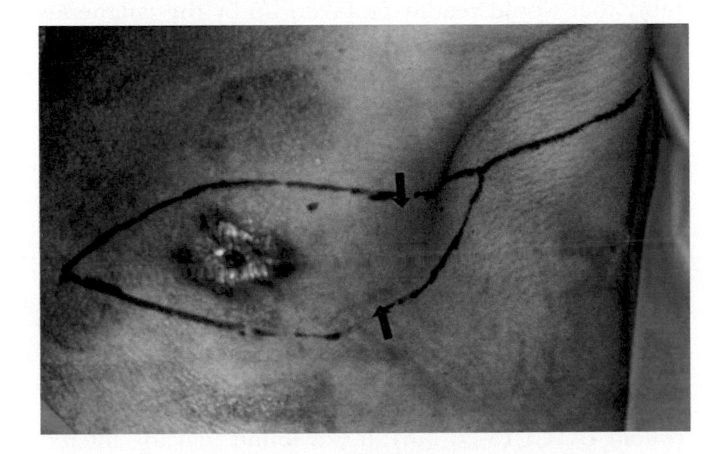

Figure 31.2 *Intraoperative photograph. The vital blue dye has been injected into the skin around the melanoma biopsy scar. This patient has thin skin, and the afferent lymphatics leading to the sentinel node in the axilla can be visualized (arrows).*

visualization. Additionally, because of their diffusion into the surrounding tissue, background fluorescence made these agents unacceptable. Methylene blue proved to have relatively poor retention by the lymphatics and thus the SLN stained only faintly.

The use of the vital blue dyes has rarely been associated with any significant complications. Allergic reactions have not occurred in large experiences, although they have been reported in the literature.[6,7] There can be retention of the blue dye at the primary site for over a year, with gradual fading of the dye with time. However, patients can be left with a permanent tattoo if the injected dye is not removed with the wide local excision (WLE) of the primary site or with the lumpectomy in the breast cancer patient. Fortunately, in the head and neck area where a permanent tattoo would be unacceptable, the richness of the cutaneous lymphatics allows for a rapid clearance of the blue dye from the skin and subcutaneous tissues. A small amount of residual dye left behind after the WLE has not been a problem and has rapidly disappeared. All patients report the presence of dye in the urine during the first 24 hours and the dye can interfere with transcutaneous oxygen monitoring during anaesthesia.

Choice of radiocolloid

Little work has been performed to determine which radiocolloid is most optimally suited for either preoperative or intraoperative mapping. The ideal radiocolloid for intraoperative SLN mapping should have the characteristics of an appropriate particle size and stability that would readily be taken up by the cutaneous lymphatics and deposited and perhaps trapped or concentrated in the SLN. A uniform dispersion of small particles (<100 nm) is necessary for the colloid to translocate from the intradermal injection site to the lymphatic channels and the SLN. The ideal radiocolloid should also have a short half life that will not complicate the handling of the excised specimen. Technetium (^{99m}Tc) labelled compounds, because they are gamma emitters, satisfy most of these requirements. In a direct comparison between filtered and unfiltered ^{99m}Tc sulfur colloid (SC) and ^{99m}Tc antimony trisulfide colloid (ATC) (3–30 nm), it was found that the filtered ^{99m}Tc SC showed a faster transport rate to the nodal basin and a lower radiation dosimetry for liver, spleen, and whole body compared with ^{99m}Tc ATC. Unfiltered ^{99m}Tc sulfur colloid has a relatively large particle size (100–1000 nm), and particle migration from the injection site in some series is slower. However, other investigators have found that this radiocolloid is slow to flow through the first SLN to higher secondary nodes, which is advantageous.[17]

In comparisons of the quality of the lymphoscintigrams between ^{99m}Tc human serum albumin (HSA), ^{99m}Tc stannous phylate, and ^{99m}Tc ATC, the latter colloid gave superior images for preoperative lymphoscintigraphy.[18] In a direct comparison between ^{99m}Tc HSA and filtered ^{99m}Tc SC, it was found in an animal model that ^{99m}Tc SC was actually concentrated in the SLN over a period of 1–2 hours, whereas the ^{99m}Tc HSA rapidly passed through the SLN.[19] The ability of the SLN to concentrate the ^{99m}Tc SC provided better localization ratios at the time of intraoperative mapping, increased the success rate of localization, made the technique easier and thus was a superior reagent.[19]

The Sydney Melanoma Unit (SMU) prefers to use ^{99m}Tc antimony trisulfide colloid (ATC), since it seems to have a smaller more uniform particle size that allows rapid migration into the lymphatic channels, but appropriate trapping and retention by the SLN.[20] The use of this compound in Sydney has allowed the injection of the radiocolloid and the imaging to be performed the day before the operation. These investigators find that 'hot' spots in the regional basin are maintained even if 24 hours have elapsed from the time of the injection. The counts of radioactivity in the basin over the hot spot (i.e. over the SLN) are decreased due to the expenditure of four half lives of the technetium, and some pass through of the radiocolloid, but the ratios of activity in the SLN versus neighbouring non-SLNs are similar. ^{99m}Tc ATC has been removed from the market in the United States and is not currently available there for clinical use.

Clinicians at Moffitt Cancer Center (MCC) have recommended filtered technetium sulfur colloid using a 0.2 micron filter. This particle size gives good images on lymphoscintigraphy and is trapped and concentrated in the SLN over a period of time so that the hot spot of activity in the SLN actually increases compared with surrounding tissue for 2–6 hours after injection, making the SLN easier to find. It also has an advantage as the primary sites get closer to the regional basin, which is the case most often with breast cancer mapping. Only 1–5% of the injected activity from the primary site is delivered to the SLNs. Even if a WLE is done first, there may be so much 'shine through' activity from the primary site that it makes finding the SLN in the basin almost impossible with radiocolloid mapping alone. In this instance, the blue dye becomes more important. Using unfiltered technetium sulfur colloid only contributes to a larger shine through problem.

Results to date for lymphatic mapping for melanoma

In the initial report by Morton et al., they were able to identify the SLN in 194 of 237 lymphatic basins and found that 40 specimens (21%) contained metastatic melanoma detectable by routine histological examination with haematoxylin and eosin (H&E) stains (12%) or only by immunohistochemical staining (9%). 'Skip metastases', defined as a negative SLN but with a higher node or nodes in the basin being positive, can only be measured in those patients with metastatic disease in their regional basin. One must examine closely the patients with metastatic disease. Metastases were present in 47 of 259 (18%) SLNs, while non-SLNs were the exclusive site of metastases in only two of 3079 nodes from 194 dissections, a false negative rate of 1% (false negative rate based on nodes and not patients as the unit of analysis). An analysis by patients shows that of 40 patients with histologically positive nodes, SLN mapping identified 38 of them (a 5% false negative rate). Only one SLN drained a particular primary site in 72% of basins. Two SLNs were found in 20% of the basins and 8% of the basins contained three or more SLNs. The success rate in SLN identification ranged from 72% to 96% depending on where the surgeon was on the learning curve. Groin mappings accounted for the highest success rate, with successful SLN identification in 89% of attempts. Seventy-eight per cent of the time an SLN could be identified in the axilla in this study, in which only the vital blue dye was used for mapping. A learning curve of 60 cases was thought to be necessary from this initial report, thereby confining the procedure's applicability to major medical centres treating large numbers of melanoma patients. Nevertheless, this new technique accurately identified patients with occult lymph node metastases who might benefit from radical lymphadenectomy.[4,5]

These data have been confirmed by numerous other institutions, including the MCC, MD Anderson Cancer Center, the Sydney Melanoma Unit (SMU), and the University of Vermont.[6,7,21–23] These studies have confirmed an orderly progression of melanoma nodal metastases. The data from these surgical studies for patients with melanoma showed that the pattern of nodal metastases from cutaneous primary sites is not random. The SLNs in the lymphatic basins can be individually identified and they reflect the presence or absence of melanoma metastases in the remainder of the nodal basin.

The second report to confirm these results came from a collaboration between the MD Anderson Cancer Center and MCC. In the initial study of 42 patients with intermediate thickness melanomas, an SLN biopsy was followed by a complete node dissection to confirm the low incidence of 'skip' metastases in this population. Thirty-four patients had histologically negative SLNs, with the rest of the nodes in the basin also being negative. Thus, no patients in this study had skip metastases. Eight patients had a positive SLN, with seven of the eight having the SLN as the only site of disease. Nodal involvement was compared between the SLN and the non-SLN based on the binomial distribution and the null hypothesis of equality in distribution of nodal metastases. The probability of this distribution of lymph node metastases occurring by chance was 0.008, proving that the SLN was the first and favoured site of metastatic disease.[5] All patients underwent preoperative lymphoscintigraphy to define all basins at risk for metastatic disease and intraoperative mapping was performed using isosulfan blue. The technical failure rate in this series was 10%.

Krag et al., from the University of Vermont, used radiocolloid for intraoperative mapping after they found that using the vital blue dye could be difficult if not impossible.[24] In 1995, a group headed by these investigators reported on a series of 100 patients with melanomas arising in a wide variety of primary sites. All patients had lymphoscintigraphy from 1 to 24 hours before intraoperative mapping and SLN excision. A handheld gamma probe (C Trak, Care Wise Medical Products, Morgan Hill, CA) aided in the accurate identification and excision of the SLN. Incisions were made directly over the hot spot, minimizing dissection which was further guided by the gamma probe. The presence of high levels of radioactivity in the excised lymph node easily identified it as a SLN. The presence of additional radioactivity in the basin detected by the gamma probe was a sensitive indicator of additional SLN(s) that were then also excised. The absence of radioactivity in the basin after lymph node excision confirmed that all the SLN(s) had been removed. A successful localization of the SLNs was accomplished in 98% of the patients, a marked increase compared with previously reported localization rates.

Krag and associates have recently updated their experience with their melanoma consortium to confirm Morton's original finding.[23] Between February 1993 and October 1994, 121 patients with invasive melanomas and clinically negative nodes were enrolled in an intraoperative mapping study using only a handheld gamma probe and injection of unfiltered ^{99m}Tc sulfur colloid, ^{99m}Tc human serum albumin or Microlite (Dupont, Billerica, MA) around the primary site. Surgeons were successful in the identification of the SLN in 97.6% of the patients. In 36% of the patients in whom a combination of vital blue dye and radiocolloid was used, all the blue stained SLNs were also hot with the radiocolloid. In four patients the blue dye was not identified in any of the lymph nodes and thus the mapping would have been unsuccessful if this was the only mapping technique used. Preoperative lymphoscintigraphy was used in 93% of the patients with a technical failure rate of 10%. These patients did not have successful imaging of the radiolabelled SLN, but with the use of the handheld gamma probe, 9 of 12 patients had an SLN identified at the time of the operation. This would suggest that the handheld gamma probe is more sensitive at identifying the SLN compared with a scintillation camera that accumulates data for imaging over a period of 2–6 minutes. With the handheld gamma probe, activities and resultant localization ratios are accumulated in seconds. This is probably also the explanation of why on preoperative lymphoscintigraphy, after a period of time between the injection of radiocolloid and the imaging (1–2 hours), multiple nodes may be imaged. But with intraoperative mapping, the SLN can be readily identified and multiple nodes are not found to be hot. This observation holds true even if the intraoperative mapping occurs 2–4 hours after the lymphoscintigram. Multiple hot nodes are not identified as long as ^{99m}Tc SC is used as the mapping agent.[20] In Krag's series, 15 patients (12.4%) had micrometastatic disease, with 10 patients having the SLN as the only site of metastases. With a minimum follow up of 220 days, there has been one regional nodal recurrence in a SLN negative patient.[22]

With the addition of intraoperative radiolymphoscintigraphy to vital blue dye lymphatic mapping,[23,25,26] the SLN localization becomes easier and more widely applicable. In the initial study from MCC combining the vital blue dye and radiocolloid mapping techniques, 450 μCi of technetium labelled sulfur colloid was used with the standard isosulfan blue and injected at the site of the primary cutaneous melanoma. A gamma probe (Neoprobe, Dublin, OH, Navigator, USSC, Norwalk, CT) was used to trace lymphatic channels from the primary site to lymph nodes in the regional lymphatic basin.

This study consisted of 106 consecutive patients with cutaneous melanomas greater than 0.76 mm thickness at all primary site locations. A total of 200 SLNs and 142 neighbouring non-sentinel nodes (non-SLNs) were harvested from 129 basins in 106 patients. When correlated with the vital blue dye mapping, 70% of the SLNs demonstrated blue dye staining while 84% of SLNs were defined as being hot by radioisotope localization. With the use of both intraoperative mapping techniques, identification of the SLN was possible in 96% of the nodal basins sampled. Micrometastases were identified in SLNs in 15% of the patients by routine histology while two patients had micrometastatic disease in a hot but not blue stained node. These data suggest that the radiocolloid localization identifies more SLNs, some of which are clinically important since they contain micrometastatic disease.[27] Morton's group supported these findings when they used a combination of the vital blue dye and radiocolloid mapping technique (^{99m}Tc HSA) to increase the surgeon's accuracy in identification of the SLN.[26] In a series of 30 patients with melanoma from all primary sites, the SLN stained blue and was the site of highest radioactivity in 27 (90%). In 5 of 13 patients undergoing a groin dissection, radiolymphoscintigraphy identified two SLNs in the drainage basin. In each case, the presence of the second inguinal SLN was suggested by the high radioactivity in the basin after removal of the first node and not by the blue dye. After excision of the second node, basin radioactivity decreased to background levels. These investigators concluded that radiolymphoscintigraphy can be a useful adjunct to vital dyes for intraoperative mapping and can be used not only to confirm blue dye identification of the first node, but also signal the presence of additional SLNs not easily identified with the dye technique alone.

The use of the radiocolloid and a handheld gamma probe for intraoperative mapping allows identification of the location of the SLN through the skin, before making a skin incision.[28] This permits many of the procedures to be performed under local anaesthesia without the need for extensive skin flaps. According to Morton et al. an acceptable level of skill using blue dye alone requires approximately 60 cases, a number of cases that is more than many surgeons see in their entire career.[4,5] In contrast, the gamma probe guided resection of radiolabelled lymph nodes is readily mastered and can be incorporated into a variety of clinical settings with successful localization rates even after minimal experience.

In a subsequent trial from MCC using isosulfan blue and ^{99m}Tc SC as mapping agents, only those patients who had a positive SLN were subjected to a complete node dissection.[25] With follow up of 3 years, there have been two recurrences in regional basins in patients who had a previous negative SLN biopsy. No abnormal cells could be identified with serial sectioning and immunohistochemical staining of the SLN block, however, both patients' SLNs demonstrated gene expression for the melanoma associated proteins tyrosinase detected by reverse transcriptase-polymerase chain reaction (RT-PCR), suggesting that micrometastatic disease was missed with the more conventional methods of examination.[29]

In another report, the Sydney Melanoma Unit (SMU) described a success rate of 87% in identifying the SLN. There was a learning curve in that the success rate in their last 100 patients was 97%. In total, cutaneous lymphoscintigraphy (Figure 31.3) was performed in 800 patients with melanoma from the SMU and had been used as a guide for subsequent SLN harvesting. Twenty-three per cent of the patients were found to have micrometastatic disease. Initially, frozen sections for occult metastases were performed on the SLN, but a false negative rate of 9% caused this group of clinicians to abandon the frozen sections in favour of permanent sections. With this approach the pathologist is allowed 2–5 days to perform a detailed examination of the SLN, an examination that may include serial sectioning, immunohistochemical staining, and possibly RT-PCR assays for occult metastases. In the SMU, patients who are found to have a positive SLN are subsequently returned to the operating room (OR) for a complete node dissection. Using the technique of preoperative lymphoscintigraphy followed by intraoperative mapping using a combination of a vital blue dye and a radiocolloid (^{99m}Tc ATS) with a handheld gamma probe, a 1.9% false negative SLN rate was reported.[30]

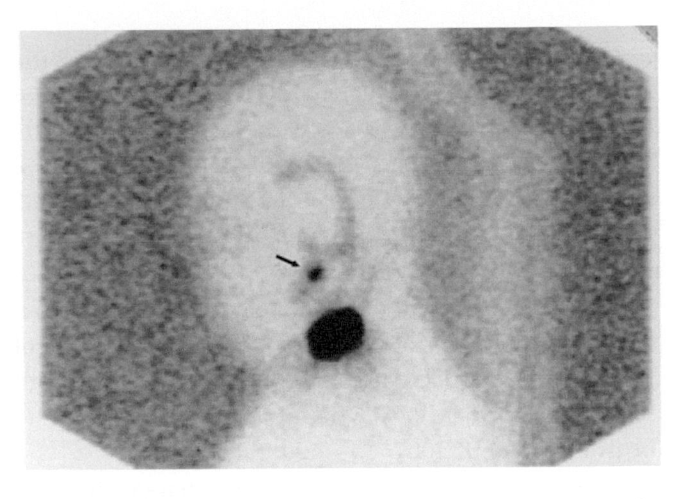

Figure 31.3 *Preoperative lymphoscintigraphy in a patient with an intermediate thickness melanoma of the left neck. Approximately 450 μCi are injected into the skin around the primary melanoma, and the patient is scanned. The outline of the body is produced with a cobalt flood source for anatomical orientation. The study shows flow to a sentinel lymph node in the upper left neck, around the parotid gland (arrow).*

To date, over 6000 melanoma patients have undergone lymphatic mapping and SLN biopsy at MCC, MD Anderson Cancer Center, and the John Wayne Cancer Institute. The success rate of identifying an SLN among the three institutions approaches 99%. Combination mapping techniques, using both vital blue dye and radiocolloid, are being used at all three centres. The groin continues to have the highest SLN identification rate, followed by the axilla and the head and neck (cervical) region. Approximately 20% of patients are found to have micrometastatic disease with haematoxylin and eosin staining. With the addition of immunohistochemical staining with S-100, an additional 8–10% of the patients are identified to have evidence of nodal spread. The recurrence rate in the mapped basin after a negative SLN biopsy ranges from 1–4.5%, with most of the recurrences due to a failed pathological examination rather than a failed surgical technique. More follow up is needed to determine the long term failure rate of the procedure.

A National Cancer Institute (USA) sponsored prospective trial is currently being performed that randomizes patients to receive either WLE of the primary melanoma site versus WLE and SLN biopsy of the regional lymphatic basins at risk for metastases.[31] The end point of the study is whether this surgical strategy can extend the survival of the melanoma patient. The study differs from the previous randomized trials addressing the efficacy of ELND since only a percentage of the patients with melanomas greater than 1.0 mm will receive a complete node dissection. As of May 2002, over 2000 patients have been accrued to this study. Survival data from this trial are not expected to be available until 2007.

This information is being used to change the standards for melanoma surgical care so that only those patients with evidence of nodal metastatic disease are subjected to the morbidity and expense of a complete node dissection.[8–11] These studies show accurate pathological staging, no decrease in standards of care, and a reduction of morbidity (no lymphoedema, early return to work or normal activity) with a less aggressive, rational, surgical approach and lower costs for the healthcare system.[32] The status of the SLN can then be used as a prognostic factor to identify which patients need the more radical complete regional node dissection.

REFERENCES

1. Parker SL, Tong T, Bolden S, Wingo PA, Cancer Statistics 1996. *CA Cancer J Clin* 1996; 46: 5–27.
2. Kirkwood JM, Strawderman MH, Ernstoff MS, et al, Adjuvant therapy of high-risk resected cutaneous melanoma: the Eastern Cooperative Oncology Group Trial EST 1684. *J Clin Oncol* 1996; 14: 7–17.
3. Teng S, Powers A, Cruse CW, et al, Validation of the proposed new AJCC staging system for malignant melanoma. 53rd Annual Meeting of the Society of Surgical Oncology, New Orleans, LA, March, 2000 (abstract).
4. Morton DL, Wen DR, Wong JH, et al, Technical details of intraoperative lymphatic mapping for early stage melanoma. *Arch Surg* 1992; 127: 392–9.
5. Morton DL, Wen DR, Cochran AJ, Management of early-stage melanoma by intraoperative lymphatic mapping and selective lymphadenectomy or 'watch and wait.' *Surg Oncol Clin North Am* 1992; 1: 247–59.
6. Reintgen DS, Cruse CW, Berman C, et al, The orderly progression of melanoma nodal metastases. *Ann Surg* 1994; 220: 759–67.
7. Ross M, Reintgen DS, Balch C, Selective lymphadenectomy: emerging role of lymphatic mapping and sentinel node biopsy in the management of early stage melanoma. *Semin Surg Oncol* 1993; 9: 219–23.
8. Veronesi U, Adamus J, Bandiera DC, et al, Inefficacy of immediate node dissection in stage I melanoma of the limbs. *N Engl J Med* 1977; 297: 627.
9. Sim FH, Taylor WF, Pritchard DJ, et al, Lymphadenectomy in the management of stage I malignant melanoma: a prospective randomized study. *Mayo Clin Proc* 1986; 61: 697.
10. Balch CM, Soong S-J, Milton GW, et al, A comparison of prognostic factors and surgical results in 1,786 patients with localized (stage I) melanoma treated in Alabama, USA, and New South Wales, Australia. *Ann Surg* 1982; 196: 677.
11. Reintgen DS, Cox EB, McCarthy KS, et al, Efficacy of elective lymph node dissection in patients with intermediate thickness primary melanoma. *Ann Surg* 1983; 198: 379–85.
12. Roozendaal GK, de Vries JDH, van Poll D, et al, Sentinel nodes outside lymph node basins in melanoma. 53rd Annual Meeting of the Society of Surgical Oncology, New Orleans, LA, March, 2000, (abstract).
13. Reintgen DS, Albertini J, Berman C, et al, Accurate nodal staging of malignant melanoma. *Cancer Control: J Moffitt Cancer Center* 1995; 2: 405–14.
14. Balch CM, Soong S-J, Bartolucci AA, et al, Efficacy of an elective regional lymph node dissection of 1 to 4 mm thick melanomas for patients 60 years of age and younger. *Ann Surg* 1996; 224: 255–66.
15. Gershenwald J, Sumner W, Porter G, et al, Role of sentinel lymph node biopsy in patients with thin (<= 1.0 mm) cutaneous melanoma. 53rd Annual Meeting of the Society of Surgical Oncology, New Orleans, LA, March, 2000, (abstract).
16. Wong JH, Cagle LA, Morton D, Lymphatic drainage of skin to a sentinel lymph node in a feline model. *Ann Surg* 1991; 214: 637–41.
17. Tanabe KK, Lymphatic mapping and epitrochlear node dissection for melanoma. *Surgery* 1997; 121: 101–4.
18. Hung JC, Wiseman GA, Wahner HW, et al, Filtered technetium-99m-sulfur colloid evaluated for lymphoscintigraphy. *J Nucl Med* 1995; 36: 1895–1900.
19. Nathanson SD, Anaya P, Eck L, Sentinel lymph node uptake of two different radio nuclides. 49th Cancer Symposium, The Society of Surgical Oncology, 1996, (abstract).
20. Uren RF, Howman-Giles RB, Thompson JF, et al, Lymphoscintigraphy in melanoma patients. The Sixth World Congress on Cancers of the Skin. Argentina, 1995 (abstract).
21. Thompson JF, McCarthy WH, Bosch C, et al, Sentinel lymph node status as an indicator of the presence of metastatic melanoma in regional lymph nodes. *Melanoma Res* 1995; 5: 255–60.
22. Krag DN, Meijer SJ, Weaver DL, et al, Minimal-access surgery for staging of melanoma. *Arch Surg* 1995; 130: 654–60.
23. Krag D, Meijer S, Weaver D, et al, Minimal access surgery for staging regional nodes in malignant melanoma. 48th Cancer Symposium, Society of Surgical Oncology, Boston, 1995, (abstract).
24. Alex JC, Weaver DL, Fairbank JT, et al, Gamma-probe-guided lymph node localisation in malignant melanoma. *Surg Oncol* 1993; 2: 303–8.
25. Albertini J, Cruse CW, Rapaport D, et al, Intraoperative radiolymphoscintigraphy improves sentinel lymph node identification in melanoma patients. *Ann Surg* 1996; 223: 217–24.
26. Essner R, Foshag L, Morton D, Intraoperative radiolymphoscintigraphy: a useful adjunct to intraoperative lymphatic mapping and selective lymphadenectomy in patients with clinical stage 1 melanoma. 48th Cancer Symposium, Society of Surgical Oncology, Houston, TX, 1994, (abstract).
27. Costello D, Teng S, Puleo C, et al, The natural history of patients with malignant melanoma who have a negative sentinel lymph node biopsy. 48th Cancer Symposium, Society of Surgical Oncology, Houston, TX, 1994, (abstract).
28. Norman J, Wells K, Kearney R, et al, Identification of lymphatic basins in patients with cutaneous melanoma. *Semin Surg Oncol* 1993; 9: 224–7.
29. Wang X, Heller R, VanVoorhis N, et al, Detection of submicroscopic metastases with polymerase chain reaction in patients with malignant melanoma. *Ann Surg* 220: 768–74.
30. Thompson JF, McCarthy WH, Robinson E, et al, Sentinel lymph node biopsy in 102 patients with clinical stage 1 melanoma undergoing elective lymph node dissection. 47th Cancer Symposium, Society of Surgical Oncology, March 1994, Houston, TX (abstract).
31. Multicenter Selective Lymphadenectomy Trial. National Cancer Institute Grant No. PO1 CA29605–12
32. Reintgen DS, Einstein A. The role of research in cost containment. *Cancer Control: J Moffitt Cancer Center* 1995; 2: 429–31.

32

Sentinel lymph node biopsy: unresolved questions

Omgo E Nieweg, Roger F Uren, John F Thompson

INTRODUCTION

It is amazing to look back and observe the amount of work that was accomplished on lymphatic mapping and sentinel node biopsy in the 10-year period 1991–2000. A literature search found 140 papers in peer reviewed journals on lymphatic mapping in melanoma. More than half of these publications came from seven institutions: the John Wayne Cancer Institute, the H Lee Moffitt Cancer Center, the Netherlands Cancer Institute, the Free University Hospital in Amsterdam, the Sydney Melanoma Unit, the University of Vermont, and the MD Anderson Cancer Center.

The hypothesis of stepwise spread of melanoma through the lymphatic system has matured, and its correctness has been established.[1,2] How to do the procedure in the nuclear medicine department has been described, and the pathology techniques that should be applied are well established. It is also clear that surgeons should have the technique with both the blue dye and the gamma ray detection probe in their repertoire to find all sentinel nodes on the one hand and to avoid removing non-sentinel nodes unnecessarily on the other.[3]

This chapter focuses on the unresolved questions (Box 32.1). Issues that will be addressed include the definition of a sentinel node, lymphoscintigraphy, the learning phase, pathology, sensitivity, regional control, and the potential survival benefit.

Box 32.1 ***Unresolved issues***

Definition of a sentinel node
Lymphoscintigraphy
Learning phase
Pathology
Sensitivity
Regional control
Survival

DEFINITION

Morton and Cochran said that a sentinel node is the lymph node nearest the site of the primary melanoma, on the direct drainage pathway (Figure 32.1).[1] This definition accurately reflects the concept of stepwise spread of cancer through the lymphatic system. However, this definition is based on a concept, and is not always of help in clinical practice. For example, how to act in the familiar situation where early lymphoscintigraphic images show overlapping lymphatic channels? How does the definition help the surgeon who is confronted with a cluster of radioactive nodes? It is not surprising that various investigators have modified Morton's original definition of a sentinel node and changed it to be more helpful in the interpretation of lymphoscintigraphic images or in the operating room (Box 32.2). Attempts to improve the practical applicability of the definition are to be encouraged but should not have led to the current confusing situation with different investigators recommending widely diverging definitions.[4–6]

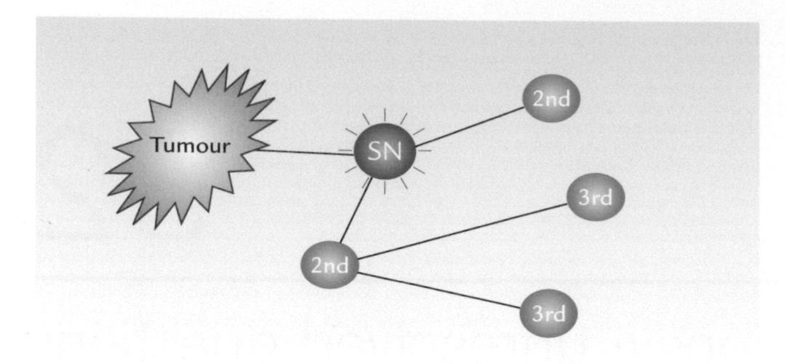

Figure 32.1 *The sentinel node (SN) is a lymph node on a direct drainage pathway from the primary tumour. Subsequent lymph nodes are second and third tier nodes.*

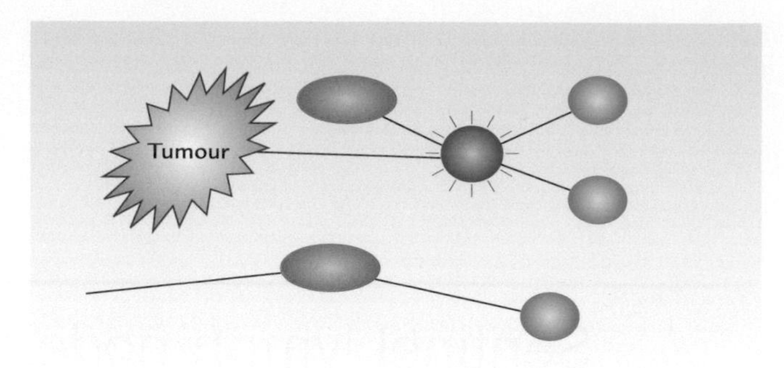

Figure 32.2 *Lymph from the primary tumour region does not necessarily travel to the nearest node.*

Box 32.2 ***Definitions of a sentinel lymph node***

A sentinel lymph node is:
- the lymph node nearest the primary tumour
- the first lymph node depicted on the lymphoscintigraphic images
- the 'hottest' lymph node
- a radioactive lymph node
- a lymph node that is more radioactive than the background
- a lymph node that is more radioactive than other lymph nodes
- a blue lymph node

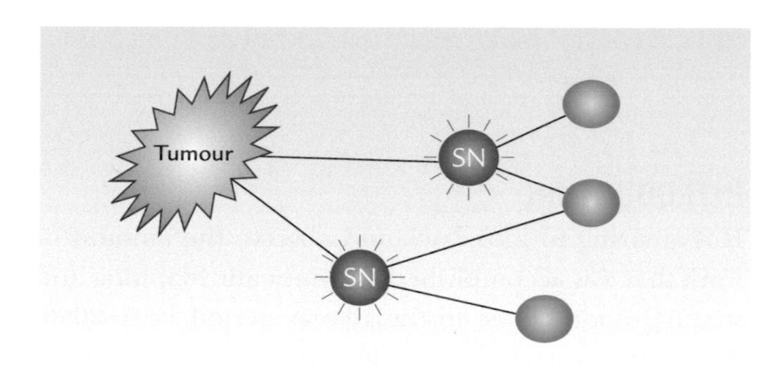

Figure 32.3 *Two lymphatic channels originating in the primary tumour running to two different sentinel lymph nodes (SN).*

Definitions have been based on anatomy, on lymphoscintigraphic features, and on radioactivity or vital dye content of lymph nodes. Some investigators have defined the sentinel node as the lymph node closest to the primary lesion. This anatomically oriented definition does not take into consideration the physiology of lymph drainage. The node closest to the primary tumour is the first one to be involved only when it receives direct drainage from the injection site (Figure 32.2).

In the situation where more nodes than one take up the radioactive tracer, some investigators consider only the first node that is visualized on the lymphoscintigraphic images to be the sentinel node. However, a lymphatic channel may divide or there may be multiple lymphatic channels originating in the region of the primary tumour passing to different lymph nodes (Figure 32.3). One of these nodes may be depicted on the scintigraphy images before another because of preferential drainage even though all these nodes are directly at risk of receiving tumour cells.

Not all of the radiolabelled tracer that reaches the sentinel lymph node is retained in that node. Some of the tracer may pass through and move on to second tier nodes. This occurs especially when lymph flow is rapid. Faced with a multitude of 'hot' nodes on the images, some surgeons tend to regard only the hottest node as the sentinel node. That definition has several drawbacks. Again, there can be more nodes than one to receive direct drainage from a tumour site. Furthermore, the amount of tracer that is accumulated by a node depends not only on its position in the drainage order but also on parameters such as lymph flow rate. One of the reasons for a node to receive a sparse lymph supply is that the flow to that particular node is hampered by metastatic disease obstructing its ingress. Nodal size is another parameter that determines the amount of radioactivity that is accumulated: a large second tier node may accumulate more of the tracer than a small first tier node.

Another relevant point is that the brightness of a node on the images not only depends on the amount of radionuclide in that node but also on its distance from the gamma camera. Deeper nodes seem less 'bright' because the gamma rays are attenuated as they pass through more soft tissue. Although the inverse square law of physics is not fully applicable when a gamma camera with a collimator is used, the situation is such that of two nodes with an equal amount of a radionuclide, the node closest to the gamma camera is depicted as the hottest one (Figure 32.4). Thus, there are several reasons not to use its brightness on the scintigram to decide whether a lymph node is a sentinel node.

Some surgeons define a sentinel node as any radioactive node. They tend to remove every radioactive node that can be identified with the gamma ray detection probe. This point of view does not acknowledge the fact that some of the tracer may pass through the sentinel (first tier) node and lodge in second tier nodes that are not directly at risk of harbouring metastatic disease. The result is the unnecessary removal of too many nodes.

A seemingly more refined approach is to use the probe and define a sentinel node as a node that contains proportionally more radioactivity than the background: the sentinel node to background ratio. However, this definition is also flawed. The amount of radioactivity that is accumulated in a lymph node depends on numerous factors, some of which are associated with the type of colloid particles that are used, such as their size, their surface characteristics, and stability. The size of the lymph node, macrophage avidity for the tracer, and the lymph flow rate clearly play a part as well. Lymph flow depends on factors like physical exercise, ambient temperature, medication, massaging of the injection site, and hydration of the patient. Lymph flow rate also varies systematically with the location of the primary melanoma, the most rapid flow being seen from the legs and arms.[7] Because so many parameters are involved, it is not surprising that tracer uptake in a sentinel node is highly variable. In a study of 60 melanoma patients, uptake in the sentinel node ranged from 0.0013% to 6.8% of the injected tracer dosage.[8]

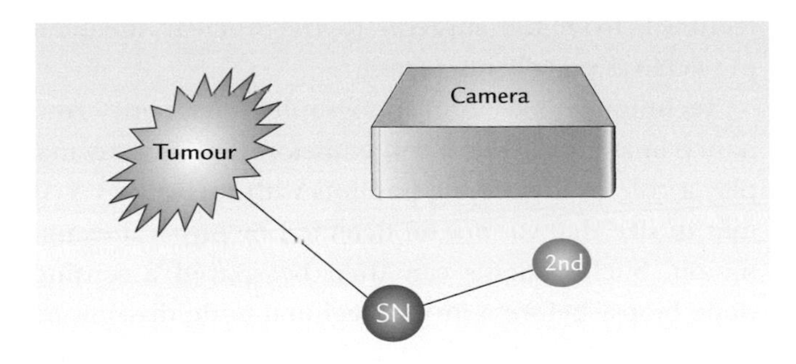

Figure 32.4 *If a sentinel node and a second tier node contain an equal amount of radioactivity, the latter will be brighter on the lymphoscintigraphy image when it is situated closer to the gamma camera.*

The background count rate is also not the solid denominator that it seems to be. Where is the probe placed to determine the background? Many surgeons obtain a background reading in the lymphatic field. Such a reading is notoriously variable and depends on the distance to the radioactive node, the distance from the injection site, and the angle at which the device is held. A background reading with a shield attached to the probe is considerably higher than a reading obtained with a collimator. A reading without shield or collimator is even higher.

Defining the sentinel node based on the sentinel node to non-sentinel node ratio also has its drawbacks. This approach implies that one has to find a non-sentinel node first and then evaluate the other nodes with the probe to determine whether they exceed the designated count rate. Additional exploration is performed. This approach also requires a definition of the characteristics of a non-sentinel node. How many counts are acceptable for a node to be considered non-sentinel node? Based on these considerations, one cannot but conclude that the definition of a sentinel node should not be based solely on factors measurable with the gamma ray detection probe.

The definition of a sentinel node being a blue node does not acknowledge the fact that the vital dye is not always retained in the first tier lymph node. At a certain point in time, there will be a string of subsequent blue nodes, of which only the first is directly at risk of having accumulated tumour cells.

There is obviously no consensus on the definition of a sentinel lymph node at this time. Morton's original definition accurately reflects the concept of stepwise spread of cancer through the lymphatic system but is not always helpful in the practical clinical situation. A definition that encompasses all possible scenarios is 'any lymph node that receives direct lymphatic drainage from a primary tumour site'.[6] The best approach may be to adhere to this definition and to use all the available detection techniques in the repertoire to find the sentinel node(s). The scintigraphy images indicate the area to explore, the location and the number of expected sentinel nodes. The gamma ray detection probe can pinpoint the location of the radioactive sentinel nodes. Careful dissection of the blue lymphatic channels lays out the drainage pattern and identifies the node(s) that receive drainage directly from the primary lesion. When the blue dye approach fails, it is best to err on the safe side and remove the radioactive nodes that potentially receive direct drainage from the primary lesion site. If it is unclear whether a particular node is on a direct drainage pathway and thus whether it is by definition a sentinel node, that uncertainty should be admitted. But that node must be excised and should be submitted for pathologic examination as a potential sentinel lymph node.

LYMPHOSCINTIGRAPHY

The need for preoperative dynamic and static lymphoscintigraphy has been uniformly agreed upon. Most nuclear medicine physicians use ^{99m}Tc labelled colloids.

The optimum size of the colloid particles is a topic of debate. Larger particles may be more avidly accumulated in the first tier node and less likely to pass through and move on to subsequent nodes. Smaller particles better delineate the lymphatic vessels because they are quicker to clear the injection site. Other tracer characteristics are less often discussed but also deserve attention: the volume to be injected, specific activity, protein composition, particle shape and surface characteristics (Box 32.3). Within a few years, there may be non-particulate tracers that are accumulated in a lymph node through other mechanisms. Characteristics that investigators are looking for in new tracers are quick and complete accumulation in the lymphatic vessels and complete absorption in the lymph node on the direct drainage pathway (see Chapter 30).

Box 32.3 ***Tracer characteristics that have a role***

- Particle size
- Volume
- Specific activity
- Protein composition
- Particle shape
- Surface characteristics

The reproducibility of lymphoscintigraphy has been the subject of two studies. The results were similar, with a reproducibility of 88% and 85%.[9,10] Thus, lymph flow may be variable and this may result in different drainage patterns when scintigraphy is performed on different occasions. This phenomenon is of some concern and may explain some of the false negative results that have been reported. Future studies need to address this important issue.

Despite paying attention to every detail of the lymphoscintigraphy, there is sometimes a discrepancy between the number of sentinel nodes that is indicated by the images and the definitive number of sentinel nodes found during the operation when the blue lymph vessels are dissected and the drainage pattern is laid out. A study correlating the nuclear medicine reports and operative notes revealed a different number of sentinel nodes in 46 of 200 patients (23%).[11] Scintigraphy may suggest either too few nodes or too many nodes. Most discrepancies in the number of sentinel nodes is apparently caused by the limited resolution of the gamma camera, and for this reason it is important to use the highest resolution collimator available in the department. Super high resolution collimators are preferred. Nevertheless, there will be occasions when the situation is unclear on lymphoscintigraphy and will become clear only at surgery when the field is exposed to visual inspection. Because resolution is not likely to improve substantially in the near future, scintigraphic images should be interpreted with caution. It is important for the surgeon to review the images together with the nuclear medicine physician. However, feedback from the surgeon to the nuclear medicine physician is equally important.

Techniques like ultrasonography, magnetic resonance imaging and positron emission tomography may play a role in identifying patients with metastases 3–10 mm in size that cannot be detected by physical examination. Such patients can then be spared a sentinel node biopsy before a formal regional node dissection.

LEARNING PHASE

The surgical procedure has been fairly well established: both the blue dye technique and the gamma ray detection probe technique should be in the repertoire. A matter that has not been resolved is the learning phase. Surgeons who want to embark on lymphatic mapping should ideally attend a course and do a number of procedures under the guidance of an experienced surgeon. It is difficult to determine how many cases they should do before an adequate level of skill has been attained. To determine whether the sentinel node is found is not the problem but to determine the negative predictive value of that node is difficult. Axillary node dissection is the standard of care in breast cancer but prophylactic regional node dissections have been all but abandoned in patients with melanoma. The melanoma surgeon lacks the convenience of the completion regional node dissection that provides feedback on one's performance. False negative results may not declare themselves for several years, at which time a palpable metastasis may be found in the very nodal basin from which a tumour free sentinel node has been previously removed.

The conclusion from a study by the Multicenter Selective Lymphadenectomy Trial Group was that doing 30 cases is enough to acquire the desired expertise.[12] However, this study was done by a group of specialized surgeons who are part of dedicated multidisciplinary groups. All these surgeons had considerable experience before they embarked on their 30 case learning phase for the trial.

PATHOLOGY

It would be ideal to determine the tumour status of the sentinel node intraoperatively, so that subsequent regional node dissection can be carried out immediately. Unfortunately, frozen section examination of the sentinel node cytology has been shown to be unreliable.[13,14] A further disadvantage of frozen section is the wasted operating theatre time while the result is awaited. The time reserved for a complete lymph field dissection remains unused in some 80% of the patients. There is consensus on the need for serial sectioning and immunohistochemistry.[15] These techniques each raise the sensitivity some 10–20%.

The reverse transcriptase-polymerase chain reaction (RT-PCR) is an extremely sensitive and specific technique to establish the presence of messenger RNA from melanoma cells.[16] In theory, RT-PCR can detect a single melanoma cell among millions of normal cells. In practice, the technique is hampered by technical problems that limit its sensitivity. It seems reasonable to expect that these problems will be solved in the next few years and that RT-PCR will find its way into clinical practice.

SENSITIVITY, REGIONAL CONTROL, SURVIVAL

When reporting the sensitivity of sentinel node biopsy, investigators should follow the accepted practice in statistics and diagnostic sciences in order to facilitate the comparison of results. The sensitivity of a diagnostic procedure is:

$$\frac{\text{number of true positive findings}}{\text{number of true positive findings} + \text{number of false negative findings.}}$$

Many surgeons calculate the percentage of false negative results not only for those who have involved lymph nodes but for the entire group of patients. This approach inevitably presents a rosy picture of the sensitivity.

Following on from the previous discussion of the learning phase, the sensitivity of lymphatic mapping is currently unknown. The false negative rate will become evident within the next few years when large studies with conscientious follow up mature sufficiently. The results at the Netherlands Cancer Institute are not encouraging in this respect. A series of 200 patients was followed for an average of 32 months. The sensitivity was 89%, with a false negative rate of 11%.[17] A World Health Organization study looking at 829 patients with a median follow up of 29 months revealed an even more disappointing false negative rate of 22.1% (sensitivity 77.9%).[14] These numbers are worrying. Most of the false negative cases occurred early in the two series, so one may blame the poor results on lack of experience. However, more false negative results may emerge in the more recent series of patients with longer follow up.

Is a complete node dissection always necessary when the sentinel node contains a micrometastasis? Probably not. Criteria need to be developed to determine when a completion regional node dissection should or should not be performed. Breslow thickness of the primary lesion and size of the metastasis may play a part in the decision process.[11,18,19]

It makes sense to perform a superficial inguinal node dissection when a superficial inguinal sentinel node is involved with metastatic disease. But what about a deep node dissection? Is it beneficial to remove the iliac and obturator nodes as well? For the time being, it seems reasonable to do so when a lateral scintigraphy image indicates that the second tier node is situated above the level of the inguinal ligament or when additional superficial nodes are affected and/or Cloquet's node is involved.

Regional control with lymphatic mapping and the potential survival benefit are subjects of two ongoing randomized trials. The Multicenter Selective Lymphadenectomy Trial will complete accrual in 2002. It will take several years for the results to mature. The Sunbelt Melanoma Trial is the second randomized trial. This trial is also looking at the effect of adjuvant therapy with interferon. It may be difficult to justify lymphatic mapping in clinical practice if these trials show that the outcome is not improved. However, that does not necessarily mean that the procedure will fall into oblivion. There is no doubt that lymphatic mapping improves staging and provides important prognostic information. Therefore, lymphatic mapping should be an essential element in the selection of patients for trials of adjuvant treatment, presuming that the above mentioned trials do not show a worsened outcome. Sentinel node positive patients seem a likely target for adjuvant treatment. As soon as effective adjuvant treatment becomes available, its value needs to be assessed in sentinel node positive patients.

CONCLUDING REMARKS

The work that has been done over the past 10 years has answered a number of important questions but has also generated new issues that need to be addressed– for example, the fundamental matter of how to define a sentinel node. A number of crucial questions about selective lymphadenectomy in relation to regional control and survival are unresolved at this time, but answers should be available in the next few years. Better tracers and more accurate pathological evaluation can be foreseen in the more distant future.

REFERENCES

1. Morton DL, Wen D, Wong JH, et al, Technical details of intraoperative lymphatic mapping for early stage melanoma. *Arch Surg* 1992; 127: 392–9.
2. Reintgen D, Cruse CW, Wells K, et al, The orderly progression of melanoma nodal metastases. *Ann Surg* 1994; 220: 759–67.
3. Nieweg OE, Jansen L, Kroon BBR, Technique of lymphatic mapping and sentinel node biopsy for melanoma. *Eur J Surg Oncol* 1998; 24: 520–4.
4. Morton DL, Bostick PJ, Will the true sentinel node please stand? *Ann Surg Oncol* 1999; 6: 12–4.
5. Balch CM, Ross MI, Sentinel lymphadenectomy for melanoma—is it a substitute for elective lymphadenectomy? *Ann Surg Oncol* 1999; 6: 416–7.
6. Thompson JF, Uren RF, What is a 'sentinel' lymph node? *Eur J Surg Oncol* 2000; 26: 103–4.
7. Uren RF, Thompson JF, Howman-Giles RB, *Lymphatic drainage of the skin and breast: locating the sentinel lymph nodes.* Amsterdam: Harwood Academic Publishers, 1999.
8. Kapteijn BAE, Nieweg OE, Muller SH, et al, Validation of gamma probe detection of the sentinel node in melanoma. *J Nucl Med* 1997; 38: 362–6.
9. Kapteijn BAE, Nieweg OE, Valdés Olmos RA, et al, Reproducibility of lymphoscintigraphy for lymphatic mapping in patients with cutaneous melanoma. *J Nucl Med* 1996; 37: 972–5.
10. Mudun A, Murray DR, Herda SC, et al, Early stage melanoma: lymphoscintigraphy, reproducibility of sentinel node detection, and effectiveness of the intraoperative gamma probe. *Radiology* 1996; 199: 171–5.
11. Jansen L, Sentinel node biopsy: evolving from melanoma to breast cancer. Thesis, University of Amsterdam, 2000.
12. Morton DL, Thompson JF, Essner R, et al, Validation of the accuracy of intraoperative lymphatic mapping and sentinel lymphadenectomy for early-stage melanoma: a multicenter trial. Multicenter Selective Lymphadenectomy Trial Group. *Ann Surg* 1999; 230: 453–63.
13. Tanis PJ, Boom RPA, Schraffordt Koops, et al, Intraoperative examination of the sentinel node in malignant melanoma and breast cancer. *Ann Surg Oncol* 2001; 8: 221–6.
14. Cascinelli N, Belli F, Santinami M, et al, Sentinel lymph node biopsy in cutaneous melanoma: the WHO melanoma program experience. *Ann Surg Oncol* 2000; 7: 469–74.
15. Cochran AJ, The pathologist's role in sentinel lymph node evaluation. *Semin Nucl Med* 2000; 30: 11–17.
16. Wang X, Heller R, VanVoorhis N, et al, Detection of submicroscopic lymph node metastases with polymerase chain reaction in patients with malignant melanoma. *Ann Surg* 1994; 220: 768–74.
17. Jansen L, Nieweg OE, Peterse JL, et al, Reliability of sentinel lymph node biopsy for staging melanoma. *Br J Surg* 2000; 87: 484–9.
18. Joseph E, Brobeil A, Glass F, et al, Results of complete lymph node dissection in 83 melanoma patients with positive sentinel nodes. *Ann Surg Oncol* 1998; 5: 119–25.
19. Borgstein PJ, Pijpers HJ, Van Diest P, et al, Staging early lymphatic metastases in melanoma: the case for super-selective lymph node dissection. Society of Surgical Oncology, 51st Annual Meeting, San Diego 1998; PO57 (abstract).

33

Cutaneous melanoma in childhood: incidence and prognosis

Helen M Shaw, John F Thompson

INTRODUCTION

Whether or not melanomas arising in childhood are fundamentally different in their aetiology and behaviour from melanomas occurring in the adult population has been a matter of considerable uncertainty for several decades. The question, of course, has important implications for the diagnosis and treatment of melanomas in children. Do the clinical features of a childhood melanoma differ from those in an adult and should a different treatment strategy be followed?

Various risk factors for the development of melanomas in childhood are described in the literature, including giant congenital naevi, Xeroderma pigmentosum, immune deficiency and a family history of melanoma (although the latter is true for many adult melanoma patients too). However, only a small proportion of the pre-pubertal children who do present with a histologically definite melanoma have one of these risk factors, and in most series no predisposing condition can be identified for the great majority of childhood melanoma cases.

Even the incidence of cutaneous melanoma in children and the prognosis of the disease in younger age groups are, and have always been, difficult to assess. There are several reasons for these difficulties, which have been discussed in recent articles.[1,2] The first and most fundamental difficulty is that there is no general agreement on the definition of a child. Some series have included patients up to 18 years of age, whereas other studies have considered a child to be younger than 12 years of age (i.e. pre-pubertal). The latter seems a much more logical definition, particularly when the exponential increase in the incidence of melanoma known to commence at the age of 12 is considered (see Figure 33.1). In previous studies of childhood melanoma, only a small proportion of children have been in this pre-pubertal age bracket. Yet any series which includes many teenagers is unlikely to produce results of relevance to the truly paediatric population of patients with melanoma.

This highlights the second difficulty, which is that melanoma is a very rare entity in pre-pubertal children, with an age-standardized incidence rate of <1/100,000/year, even in countries such as Australia, which has the highest overall incidence rate of melanoma in the world. Most published series have not been population based but are rather experiences from large institutions, which has inevitably created a significant referral bias.

The third problem is that many early series included children in whom the diagnosis of melanoma was not assessed according to more stringent recent guidelines. The main cause of early diagnostic difficulty was the continued confusion between true melanoma and the benign Spitz naevus. This resulted in an overdiagnosis of melanoma and skewed prognosis favourably. Because of this diagnostic confusion, some reviews only included those melanomas associated with melanoma metastases, thereby skewing prognosis in the opposite direction. Histological features, particularly tumour thickness and ulceration, which are now recognized as the two major prognostic indicators, were not reported in most early series of childhood melanoma.

Lastly, in more recent reviews, follow up was not sufficiently long to allow accurate estimation of prognosis. It is generally agreed that 5-year survival is not synonymous with cure, particularly in children who now tend to be diagnosed with melanoma at a very early biological stage.

To demonstrate some of the difficulties associated with the assessment of incidence and prognosis in children, 22 cases of invasive cutaneous melanoma in children younger than 12 years of age were drawn from the records of two large referral centres for melanoma in New South Wales, Australia – the Sydney Melanoma Unit (SMU) and the Newcastle Melanoma Unit (NMU).

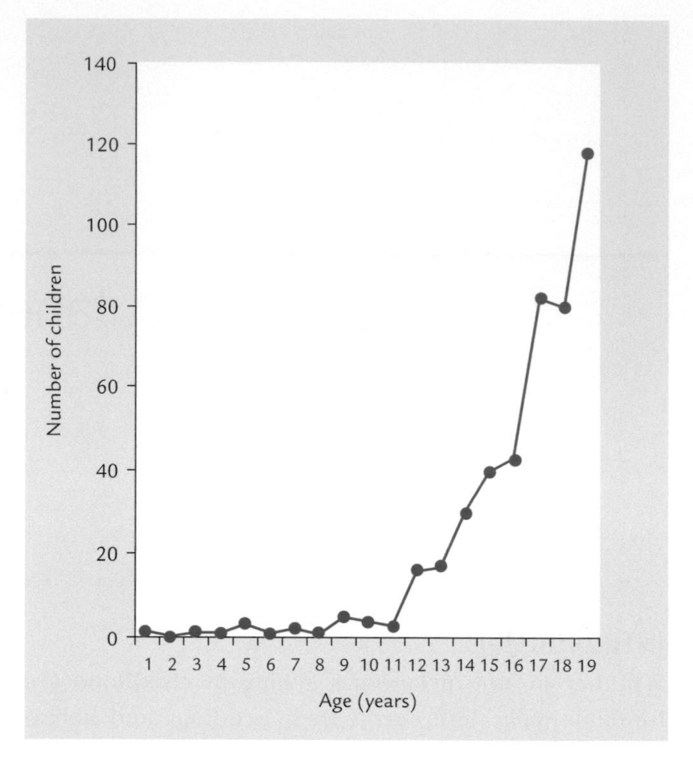

Figure 33.1 *The incidence of childhood and adolescent melanoma according to age (Sydney and Newcastle Melanoma Units, 1950–1999).*

DATA COLLECTION

Twenty-two cases of cutaneous melanoma in patients younger than 12 years of age at the time of first definitive treatment were drawn from the databanks of the two aforementioned major referral centres, 20 cases from the SMU and two cases from the NMU. Although the actual pubertal status in these children was unknown, this age group was arbitrarily chosen to be representative of 'pre-pubertal' children. Also taken into consideration was the previously mentioned fact that at around the age of 12 the start of an exponential increase in the incidence of melanoma manifests (Figure 33.1).

Not included in the present review was one case of non-cutaneous melanoma in a child (an iris melanoma in a 10-year-old girl[3] and an in situ melanoma of the fingernail in a 6-year-old boy). The SMU databank documents 16,280 patients treated at the Royal Prince Alfred, the St Vincent and the Sydney Hospitals, Sydney, between January 1950 and December 1999; the NMU databank documents 4369 patients treated at the Royal Newcastle, the Wallsend and the Mater Hospitals, Newcastle, between January 1981 and December 1999. More than half of these patients were treated since January 1989. In order to minimize the chance of a misdiagnosis, the only cases included in the present review were those in which histological slides of primary lesions or melanoma metastases were available for review by SMU and NMU pathologists, who are highly experienced in the diagnosis of melanoma. In order to compare the data from this present series with data from a population based registry, all cases of cutaneous melanoma in patients younger than 12 years of age recorded between January 1989 and December 1998 in New South Wales were obtained from the population based New South Wales Central Cancer Registry (NSWCCR) (Coates M, personal communication). This time period was chosen arbitrarily, being the most recent available from the NSWCCR and abiding by the Cancer Council Ethics Committee regulations.

None of the 22 cases of childhood cutaneous melanoma in the present series were associated with giant congenital naevi, Xeroderma pigmentosum or documented immune deficiency. A family history of melanoma was present only in Case 13. The clinical and histological details of the 22 cases are summarized in Table 33.1.

CLINICAL CHARACTERISTICS

There were similar numbers of girls and boys (12 and 10, respectively). The most common anatomical site of the primary melanoma was on the trunk in boys and on

Table 33.1 *Sydney and Newcastle Melanoma Units childhood melanoma data (1950–1999)*

Case no.	Age	Sex*	Year of diagnosis	Site	Stage	Thickness	Status
Sydney Melanoma Unit							
1	7	M	1954	Calf	1	NA	Dead
2	9	F	1956	Face	2	5.00	Dead
3	6	F	1970	Flank	1	2.40	Dead
4	9	F	1971	Neck	1	NA	Dead
5‡	5	F	1972	Thigh	1	1.40	Dead
6	9	M	1973	Abdomen	1	0.60	Alive
7	5	M	1973	Thorax	1	0.70	Alive
8	10	F	1979	Thorax	1	0.30	Alive
9§	8	F	1980	Arm	1	NA	Alive
10	7	F	1981	Arm	1	2.00	Alive
11	11	M	1984	Thorax	1	0.70	Alive
12	10	F	1986	Thorax	1	0.75	Alive
13	4	M	1989	Thorax	1	0.55	Alive
14	10	M	1989	Thorax	1	0.54	Alive
15	5	M	1991	Ear	1	3.00	Alive
16	9	M	1995	Neck	1	4.50	Alive
17	1	F	1996	Arm	1	7.00	Alive
18	10	F	1996	Forehead	1	1.84	Dead
19	3	M	1997	Scalp	1	8.00	Alive
20	9	F	1998	Ear	1	2.50	Alive
Newcastle Melanoma Unit							
21	11	M	1981	Scalp	1	0.60	Alive
22	11	F	1982	Shoulder	1	1.00	Alive

* M, Male; F, female.
NA, Not available.
‡ Metastasizing Spitz naevus-like malignant melanoma.
§ Curetted initially, then developed lymph node metastases after 12 months.

an extremity in girls. The second most common site in both sexes was on the head or neck. Mean ages of the girls and boys were similar (7.9 and 7.4 years of age, respectively).

INCIDENCE

The ratios of childhood melanoma to adult melanoma diagnosed between 1989 and 1998 from the present series and the patients recorded by the NSWCCR series

(Table 33.2) were compared. The ratio for the SMU/NMU series (8/10,471; 0.08%) was a little lower than for the NSWCCR (22/23,804; 0.10%), suggesting a minor referral bias.

DIFFICULTIES IN HISTOLOGICAL DIAGNOSIS

Ten of the 23 children recorded as having melanoma by the NSWCCR were treated at the SMU (Table 33.2) and in three of these 10 cases (Cases 3, 9 and 21), the evidence for a diagnosis of melanoma was considered insufficient on review by highly experienced SMU pathologists (Table 33.2).

These pathologists concluded that the first case of the NSWCCR series (Case 3) was, '... either a proliferating benign melanocytic lesion or malignant melanoma. Ploidy studies are not conclusive but tend to favour a borderline or benign lesion.' The second case of the NSWCCR series (Case 9) provided even more diagnostic difficulties, the conclusion being that, '... suggestive of malignancy are mitoses (up to 6/mm^2, occasionally deep), poor maturation, an area of necrosis, and projection into a lymphatic vessel. On the other hand, the mitoses and the inflammatory infiltrate could be reactive to the ulceration, mitoses appear abnormal and there is no convincing epidermal invasion. A malignant melanoma with a maximum thickness of about 2.0 mm, Clark level IV, cannot be excluded. Nor is there sufficient evidence to confirm a diagnosis of malignancy, the alternative being an irritated atypical compound naevus. Also, any ploidy study results cannot be considered absolute.' Subsequent ploidy studies on this case revealed no significant aneuploidy. However, there were increased numbers of S phase cells and rare cells with DNA ploidy above the tetraploid region were noted. The conclusion of SMU pathologists in the third case of the NSWCCR series (Case 21) was that there was not enough evidence to go beyond the diagnosis of an atypical cellular blue naevus. Because of the uncertain diagnosis in these three cases they were not included in the SMU series. Case 18 of the SMU series again presented considerable diagnostic difficulty. Initially diagnosed as a benign atypical compound melanocytic naevus by two pathologists in New Zealand, this child subsequently developed recurrences within 5 months and regional lymph node metastases within 12 months. An SMU pathologist's unbiased opinion without knowledge of these metastases was again, 'An unusual asymmetrical compound melanocytic lesion'. This opinion was later altered to, 'A minimal deviation melanoma with one or two satellites in lymphatics', in light of her subsequent clinical history. The girl died 2 years after initial diagnosis from widespread metastases.

Table 33.2 *New South Wales Central Cancer Registry childhood melanoma data (1989–1998)*

Case no.	Age	Sex	Year of diagnosis
1$^+$	4	M	1989
2$^+$	10	M	1989
3^{++}	11	M	1989
4	8	F	1990
5$^+$	5	M	1991
6	10	F	1991
7	0	M	1991
8	4	M	1992
9^{++}	9	M	1992
10	10	F	1992
11	11	M	1992
12	11	F	1993
13	11	M	1994
14$^+$	9	M	1995
15$^+$	1	F	1996
16	7	F	1996
17$^+$	3	M	1997
18	8	M	1997
19	9	M	1997
20	11	M	1997
21^{++}	4	F	1998
22	5	M	1998
23$^+$	9	F	1998

$^+$ Treated at SMU.
$^{++}$ Treated at SMU but not unequivocally diagnosed as melanoma.

The consensus of opinion in Case 19 of the SMU series involving four of its pathologists was that this

3-year-old boy had an '8 mm thick Spitz naevus-like, or minimal deviation melanoma', and that this lesion had 'uncertain malignant potential'. This boy remained free of disease 30 months after diagnosis. A similar consensus of opinion was made in Case 20 of the SMU series and this girl remained free of disease 24 months after diagnosis.

TREATMENT

Treatment of all 22 children from the SMU and NMU series, except one (Case 9), included at least a wide local excision of their primary lesion. One child (Case 2) who first presented for treatment of melanoma with palpable nodes (stage III, AJCC/UICC) underwent, in addition, a therapeutic regional lymph node dissection. In SMU Cases 5, 10 and 17, an elective lymph node dissection was performed for their intermediate to thick primary melanomas. No lymph node biopsies were undertaken in Cases 15, 16, 18 and 19, despite the fact that these children had intermediate to thick primary lesions. This was mainly because of inability to accurately predict the lymphatic drainage pathways from these lesions and the equivocal nature of the diagnosis of melanoma. A lymph node biopsy in Case 20 proved to be negative.

PROGNOSIS

The histological slides of the primary tumours for three of the first nine children in the SMU series (Cases 1, 4 and 9), all diagnosed prior to 1981, were unavailable for review of tumour thickness (Table 33.1). However, the diagnosis of melanoma in each of these children was unequivocal since they all subsequently developed metastatic melanoma. Five of these 9 children subsequently died of their disease (Table 33.1). The disease-free interval was short (<39 months) in all but one 5-year-old girl (Case 5), whose history is of particular interest. The primary lesion in this child was originally diagnosed as melanoma despite her age. This diagnosis was subsequently substantiated by her death from metastatic melanoma after a disease-free interval of 12 years. However, on unbiased review of the primary lesion for the purpose of a previous review,[4] the diagnosis was considered equivocal. The experienced pathologists thought it more likely that the lesion was an atypical Spitz naevus rather than a Spitz naevus-like malignant melanoma. All histological slides of primary lesions in the 11 children diagnosed since 1981 at the SMU were available for review and median tumour thickness was found to be 2.0 mm (Table 33.1). Ten of these children were alive with no sign of recurrence as at June 2000 and the remaining 10-year-old girl (Case 18) developed local recurrences within 4 months of diagnosis, regional lymph node recurrences within 12 months and died from widespread metastases 23 months after diagnosis. Both childhood cases from the NMU had tumours <1.01 mm in thickness and both are currently alive with no sign of recurrence (Table 33.1).

GENERAL CONSIDERATIONS WHEN REVIEWING THE LITERATURE

Clinical characteristics

The slight female preponderance recorded in the present series has also been noted by others.[5–8] In the present series, as in others,[5,8–10] the most common anatomical sites were similar to those in adults: the trunk in boys and the extremities in girls. However, in both sexes there was a high proportion of head and neck lesions – the pathology reports on most of these cases comment on their 'Spitz naevus-like' nature. It is interesting to speculate whether this distribution was due to the fact that Spitz naevi preferentially involve the head and neck region.[11]

Incidence and prognosis

Several factors must be considered, the first being the definition of 'childhood' melanoma. The incidence of melanoma in patients younger than 12 years of age is extremely low but the rate rises sharply after this age, as our data illustrate in Figure 33.1. These increases are apparent from the most recent data from Queensland, which has the highest overall age-standardized incidence of melanoma in the world: 0.1/100,000/year in the 0–4 years age group to 3.0/100,000/year in the 10–14 years age group.[12] Similar sharp increases around this age have also been reported recently in Scandinavia.[8,10] Again, increases in the 10–14 years age group are evident in the NSWCCR data, but the actual sharp increase appears to occur at 14 years rather than 12 years as in

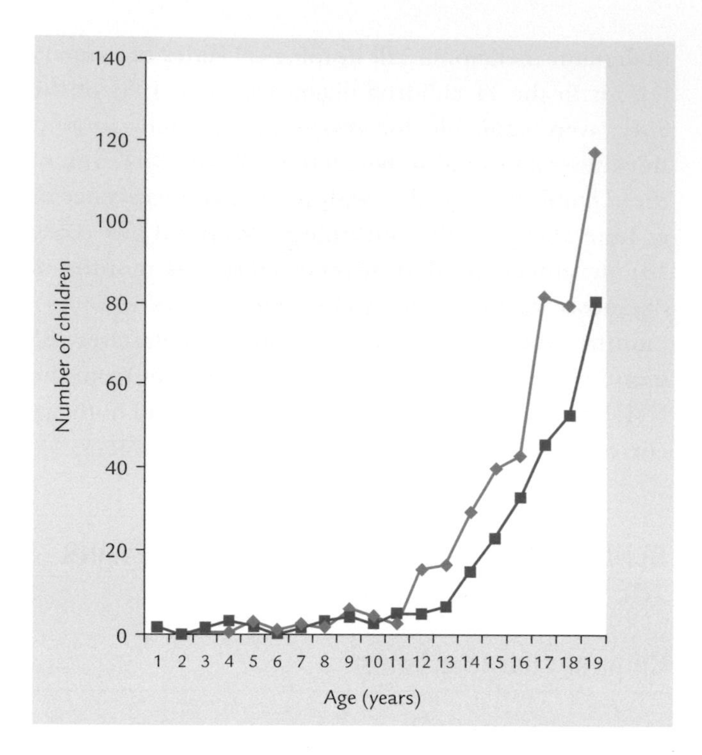

Figure 33.2 *The incidence of childhood and adolescent melanoma according to age [Sydney and Newcastle Melanoma Units, 1950–1999 (◆) versus New South Wales Central Cancer Registry, 1989–1998 (■)].*

the SMU/NMU series (Figure 33.2). This may be the result of either referral bias or the reticence among non-expert pathologists to attribute the diagnosis of melanoma to very young children. Most 'childhood' melanomas reported in the literature are in patients older than 12 years of age, with some larger series defining melanoma patients younger than 21 years of age as being children or 'juveniles'.[7,11,13–18]

Changing time frames and histological diagnoses

Because of the rarity of melanoma in children, most series span several decades in order to accumulate sufficient cases to report.[1,13,15,19–21] Inherent in the use of such extended time frames are errors in estimates of incidence and prognosis created by changing diagnostic and treatment policies during these periods. The main cause of diagnostic difficulties has been the frequent occurrence of the benign but malignant-appearing Spitz naevus. Before Spitz's classic description of juvenile melanoma,[22] and more specific delineation of its features,[23] it was believed that melanoma had a uniformly benign course in children.[24] Because of the inclusion of Spitz naevi in many series, there was overdiagnosis of melanoma, prognosis was skewed favourably, and associated mortality was underestimated. Soon after, there were reports indicating that this benign entity was clinically and histopathologically distinguishable from melanoma.[25–27] Due to continued reluctance to consider a diagnosis of melanoma in children, there was a tendency to include only metastasizing melanomas in early reports. Thus, metastasis and/or death was regarded as the ultimate 'gold standard' and the only objective criterion for diagnosing true childhood melanoma.[28] There resulted a skewing in the opposite direction, towards a very unfavourable prognosis for childhood melanoma, as was reported in a Scandinavian review in 1966.[29] Only including those cases that demonstrated malignancy by metastasis, the calculated 3-year survival rate in children with regional lymph node disease equated to the 5-year survival rate in adults at a similar stage of disease (*c.* 26%).

Another example of the difficulty in establishing the histological differential diagnosis of melanoma in children over the years has been highlighted in another Scandinavian review.[30] This illustrates the problem of using cancer registry figures, in Scandinavia at least, where the extraordinarily high figure of almost 95% of cases registered as melanoma were reclassified as Spitz naevi or other benign tumours on review of the histological slides.[31–33]

In more recent times, there has evolved an even more precise appreciation of the distinction between Spitz naevi (both typical and atypical) and melanoma.[1,4] This has allowed better estimates of both incidence and prognosis to be made. However, it is now accepted that, in rare cases, Spitz naevi metastasize. Barnhill et al.[1] have stressed the rarity of the Spitz naevus associated with death or widespread metastases by reviewing the nine cases reported in the literature, which includes Case 5 of the present series. It is interesting to note that none of the high risk factors recently proposed to objectively grade Spitz naevi[34] were evident in the lethal tumours of Cases 5 and 18: age greater than 10 years, diameter of the primary lesion >10 mm, presence of ulceration, Clark level V invasion and mitotic rate >6 mm^2. Nonetheless, almost all Spitz naevi follow a benign course. It is thus essential to distinguish between the two entities in any study which seeks to estimate prognosis.

DIFFICULTIES ENCOUNTERED IN THIS REVIEW

Various aspects of six difficulties associated with determining melanoma incidence and prognosis in children as itemized by Barnhill et al.[1] were evident in the present series of 22 children.

Rarity

The rarity of this disease in patients younger than 12 years of age in any one particular review is reflected by the fact that in recent years (1989–1998) only 0.08% of the total number of melanoma patients recorded in the two major treatment centres in NSW occurred in patients in this age group.

Referral bias

That a referral bias was probably experienced by these two institutions is evident from the fact that 0.08% is marginally lower than the proportion recorded by the population based NSWCCR (0.10%) over the same time period.

Histological differential diagnosis

That difficulty in establishing a histological differential diagnosis is still a problem is evident from the fact that three of the 10 'melanomas' recorded by the NSWCCR over this recent time period were diagnosed, on review by SMU pathologists, as being benign.

Metastasizing melanoma

It is significant that the first five cases of melanoma in children from the SMU databank all died from their disease. Most of these cases were added to the melanoma databank after they had developed their metastases, underscoring the early problems associated with attributing a diagnosis of melanoma to a young child.

Prognostic indicators

The problems experienced by others in obtaining histological slides for review of tumour thickness and other prognostic indicators in early cases of melanoma in children were also encountered in the present review, with three of the nine cases being unavailable.

Follow up and estimation of survival rates

The follow up in the present series was longer than in most other reviews, with 11 of the 16 survivors having been followed up for >10 years. Despite this, the wide range of primary tumour thicknesses in these children did not permit valid estimates of survival to be made in subgroups of the patients.

CONCLUSIONS

The overall impression gleaned from this series conforms with the most recent reports on patients of this age group that the clinical diagnostic features and prognosis in children with melanoma are similar to those in adults with equivalent disease.[1,9,18,30,35,36] Pre-existing conditions reported as increasing the risk of melanoma in children, such as a family history of melanoma, a giant congenital naevus, Xeroderma pigmentosum or immune deficiency, were not evident in the present series.[17,19,37–39] Nor was there evidence to support the contention that there tend to be longer disease-free intervals before relapse in children than in adults.[40] Just as diagnostic features and prognosis are similar in children and adults, available evidence suggests that the treatment of melanomas in children should also be the same as in adults.

ACKNOWLEDGEMENTS

The authors thank the following for their contributions to this review:

Drs SW McCarthy, KA Crotty, AA Palmer and ABP Ng from the Department of Anatomical Pathology, Royal Prince Alfred Hospital; Dr G Roberts from Hampson Pathology, Newcastle. The financial assistance of the Melanoma Foundation of the University of Sydney is gratefully acknowledged.

REFERENCES

1. Barnhill RL, Flotte TJ, Fleischli M, Perez-Atayde A, Cutaneous melanoma and atypical Spitz tumors in childhood. *Cancer* 1995; 76: 1833–45.
2. Milton GW, Shaw HM, Thompson JF, McCarthy WH, Cutaneous melanoma in childhood: incidence and prognosis. *Australas J Dermatol* 1997; 38 (suppl): S44–S48.
3. Stanford DG, Hart R, Thompson JF, Ocular melanoma in childhood: a case report and review of the literature. *Aust NZ J Surg* 1993; 63: 727–31.
4. Crotty KA, McCarthy SW, Palmer AA et al, Malignant melanoma in

childhood: a clinicopathologic study of 13 cases and comparison with Spitz nevi. *World J Surg* 1992; 16: 179–85.

5. McWhirter WR, Dobson C, Childhood melanoma in Australia. *World J Surg* 1995; 19: 334–6.
6. Spatz A, Ruiter D, Hardmeier T et al, Melanoma in childhood: an EORTC–MCG multicenter study on the clinico-pathological aspects. *Int J Cancer* 1996; 68: 317–24.
7. Zhu N, Warr R, Cai R et al, Cutaneous malignant melanoma in the young. *Br J Plast Surg* 1997; 50: 10–14.
8. Berg P, Lindelof B, Differences in malignant melanoma between children and adolescents. *Arch Dermatol* 1997; 133: 295–7.
9. Riuz-Maldonado R, Orozco-Covarrubias ML, Malignant melanoma in children. *Arch Dermatol* 1997; 133: 363–71.
10. Karlsson P, Boeryd B, Sander B et al, Increasing incidence of cutaneous malignant melanoma in children and adolescents 12–19 years of age in Sweden 1973–92. *Acta Derm-Venereol Suppl (Stockh)* 1998; 78: 289–92.
11. Saenz NC, Saenz-Badillos J, Busam K et al, Childhood melanoma survival. *Cancer* 1999; 85: 750–4.
12. Whiteman D, Valery P, McWhirter W, Green A, Incidence of cutaneous childhood melanoma in Queensland, Australia. *Int J Cancer* 1995; 63: 765–8.
13. Pratt CB, Palmer MK, Thatcher N, Crowther D, Malignant melanoma in children and adolescents. *Cancer* 1981; 47: 392–7.
14. Peters MS, Goellner JR, Spitz naevi and malignant melanomas of childhood and adolescence. *Histopathology* 1986; 10: 1289–302.
15. Reintgen DS, Seigler HF, Juvenile malignant melanoma. *Surg Gynecol Obstet* 1989; 168: 249–53.
16. Rao BN, Hayes FA, Pratt CB et al, Malignant melanoma in children: its management and prognosis. *J Pediatr Surg* 1990; 25: 198–203.
17. Novakovic B, Clark WH, Fears TR et al, Melanocytic nevi, dysplastic nevi, and malignant melanoma in children from melanoma-prone families. *J Am Acad Dermatol* 1995; 33: 631–6.
18. Nassan A, Al-Nafussi A, Quaba A, Cutaneous malignant melanoma in children and adolescents in Scotland, 1979–1991. *Plast Reconstr Surg* 1996; 98: 442–6.
19. Boddie AW, Smith JF, McBride CM, Malignant melanoma in children and young adults: effect of diagnostic criteria on staging and end results. *South Med J* 1978; 71: 1074–8.
20. Vennin P, Baranzelli MC, Demaille MC, Desmons F, Les melanomes malins de l'enfant et de l'adolescent. Huit observations. *Presse Med* 1985; 14: 529–32.
21. Mehregan AH, Mehregan DA, Malignant melanoma in childhood. *Cancer* 1993; 71: 4096–103.
22. Spitz S, Melanomas of childhood. *Am J Pathol* 1948; 24: 591–609.
23. McWhorter HE, Woolner LB, Pigmented nevi, juvenile melanomas, and malignant melanomas in children. *Cancer* 1954; 7: 564–85.
24. Pack GT, Anglem TJ, Tumors of the soft somatic tissues in infancy and childhood. *J Pediatr* 1939; 15: 372–400.
25. Trozak DJ, Rowland WD, Hu F, Metastatic malignant melanoma in prepubertal children. *Pediatrics* 1975; 55: 191–204.
26. Stromberg BV, Malignant melanoma in children. *J Pediatr Surg* 1979; 14: 465–7.
27. Boddie AW, McBride CM, Melanoma in childhood and adolescence. In: *Cutaneous Melanoma.* (eds Balch CM, Milton GW, Shaw HM, Soong S-J). Philadelphia: Lippincott, 1985: 63–70.
28. Lerman RI, Murray D, O'Hara JM et al, Malignant melanoma of childhood. A clinicopathologic study and a report of 12 cases. *Cancer* 1970; 25: 436–49.
29. Skov-Jensen T, Hastrup J, Lambrethsen E, Malignant melanoma in children. *Cancer* 1966; 19: 620–6.
30. Handfield-Jones SE, Smith NP, Malignant melanoma in children, *Br J Dermatol* 1996; 134: 607–16.
31. Saksela E, Rintala A, Misdiagnosis of prepubertal malignant melanoma. *Cancer* 1968; 22: 1308–14.
32. Malec E, Lagerlof B, Malignant melanoma of the skin in children registered in the Swedish Cancer Registry during 1959–1971. *Scand J Plast Reconstr Surg* 1977; 11: 125–9.
33. Partoft S, Osterlind A, Hou-Jensen K, Drzewiecki KT, Malignant melanoma of the skin in children (0 to 14 years of age) in Denmark, 1943–1982. *Scand J Plast Reconstr Surg* 1989; 23: 55–8.
34. Spatz A, Calonje E, Handfield-Jones S, Barnhill RL, Spitz tumors in children. A grading system for risk stratification. *Arch Dermatol* 1999; 135: 282–5.
35. Tate PS, Ronan SG, Feucht A et al, Melanoma in childhood and adolescence: clinical and pathologic features of 48 cases. *J Pediatr Surg* 1993; 28: 217–23.
36. Bartoli C, Bono A, Zurrida S et al, Childhood cutaneous melanoma. *J Dermatol* 1994; 21: 289–93.
37. Scalzo DA, Hida CA, Toth G et al, Childhood melanoma: a clinicopathological study of 22 cases. *Melanoma Res* 1997; 7: 63–8.
38. Greene MH, Clark WH, Tucker MA et al, High risk of malignant melanoma in melanoma-prone families with dysplastic nevi. *Ann Intern Med* 1985; 102: 458–65.
39. Ceballos PI, Ruiz-Maldonado R, Mihm MC. Melanoma in children. *N Engl J Med* 1995; 332: 656–62.
40. Davidoff AM, Cirricione C, Seigler HF, Malignant melanoma in children. *Ann Surg Oncol* 1994; 1: 278–82.

34

Desmoplastic and neurotropic melanoma

Michael Quinn, Kerry Crotty

INTRODUCTION

In 1971, Conley et al.[1] described a group of seven patients in whom, following the appearance of a generally inconspicuous pigmented skin lesion, there developed an invasive spindle cell tumour with extreme desmoplasia. This malignant tumour was interpreted as an unusual variant of spindle cell melanoma that produced or elicited the production of abundant collagen and was named desmoplastic malignant melanoma (DM) (Figure 34.1). DM are rare melanomas that present diagnostic challenges for both clinicians and pathologists because they often lack the typical features of melanoma.

In 1979, Reed and Leonard[2] reported 19 cases of DM with neuroma-like qualities, which they termed desmoplastic neurotropic melanoma (DNM) (Figure 34.2). Since these initial reports, many more cases of DM and DNM have been described, including a series of 128 cases from the American Armed Forces Institute of Pathology published in 1995.[3] In the same year a review summarized the features of all 327 cases previously reported and added a further 28 cases.[4] Then, in 1998, the Sydney Melanoma Unit (SMU) published a series of 280 cases accrued in a single institution over a 10-year period.[5]

INCIDENCE

The SMU cases represented 4.1% of the 6791 patients entered on the SMU database during that period, but this figure is likely to be higher than the population

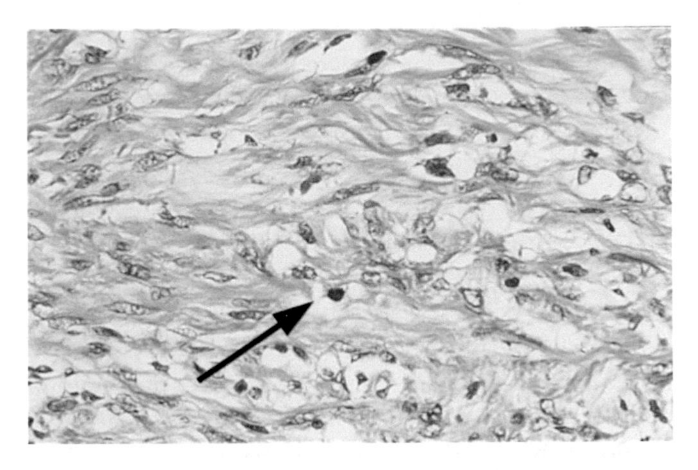

Figure 34.1 *Desmoplastic melanoma showing scant spindled melanocytes embedded in a collagenous stroma. The arrow points to a mitosis. (Photograph courtesy of Dr Stanley McCarthy.)*

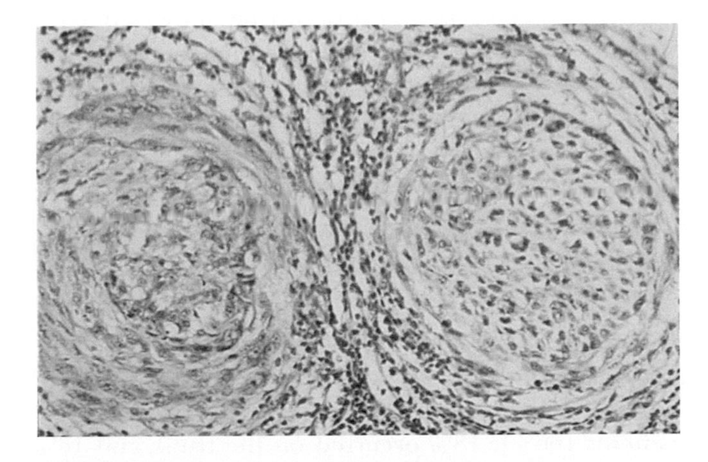

Figure 34.2 *Neurotropic melanoma showing infiltration around a nerve. (Photograph courtesy of Dr Stanley McCarthy.)*

based incidence of DM, as the SMU is a tertiary referral centre for all stages of melanoma and, as such, its database is biased towards more advanced forms of melanoma. Carlson et al.[4] suggested that DM represent *c*.1% of all melanomas. The true incidence is probably somewhere between the two figures.

PRESENTATION

There is no doubt that DM is difficult to diagnose. Smithers et al.[6] noted that 67% of tumours were non-pigmented. Not surprisingly, the diagnosis of melanoma was suspected in only 15 of 45 patients: five presented as subcutaneous nodules and of the others 21 were nodular and 15 palpably irregular. Even on initial histopathology the diagnosis was suspected in only 35 of the 45 cases.

Patients with DM are older than those with other cutaneous melanomas, with the SMU series having a median age at diagnosis of 61.5 years (range 24–91 years). This is similar to previous series,[2,6–13] excluding individual case reports, in which the median age of the 263 patients was 64 years (range 17–91 years).

DM occurs more often in males than in females; the SMU series contained 178 males and 102 females, a ratio of 1.75:1. This compares to previously published series containing 278 males and 181 females, a ratio of 1.55:1.[3,7–16] This male predominance is similar to that found with other cutaneous melanomas. The New South Wales Central Cancer Registry showed a similar male predominance. In 1995, 61.1% of melanomas diagnosed in the state of NSW were in male patients, a ratio of 1.55:1.

DM has been reported as occurring more frequently on the head and neck, i.e. in areas of increased sun exposure: this was confirmed by the SMU series. The head and neck was the most common site for DM in both sexes (106 patients; 37%): other sites included the upper limb (69 patients; 24.6%), the trunk (67 patients; 23.9%) and the lower limb (32 patients; 11.4%). The lower leg was the only site more common in women than in men; this is a site of increased sun exposure in women compared with men.

In previously published series[2–4, 6–9, 11–13,16,17] the head and neck was the most common site for DM, with 217 patients (66%): 18% occurred on the trunk and 16% on the limbs. Interestingly, in the SMU series, when specific subsites on the head and neck were considered, the lesions occurred on the cheeks in 45 patients (13.6%), with a similar incidence on the lips and nose, with 16 and 14 patients, respectively. When DNM was specifically addressed in the SMU series, of the 106 patients who had the head and neck recorded as the anatomical site, 44 (41.5%) had DNM, which is an increased proportion compared to other sites. This may be related to the increased density of nerves in this region.

HISTOLOGICAL CHARACTERISTICS

The median thickness of the tumours in the SMU series was 2.5 mm (range 0.2–18 mm). This is much thicker than the median thickness of 1.0 mm for other cutaneous melanomas presenting to the SMU after 1986. From amalgamated series where thickness was tabulated, the median was 3.85 mm (range 0.32–18 mm) in 73 patients.[11,12,17] The Queensland series showed an even thicker median of 4.3 mm (range 0.45–16 mm) in 58 patients.[15]

Clark's level of invasion was assessed in 260 of the SMU patients and compared to a total of 205 patients in other published series.[4,6] It was level V in 88 SMU and 100 comparison patients, level IV in 144 SMU and 98 other patients, level III in 15 SMU and four other patients and level II in 13 SMU and three other patients.

This overall increased thickness and greater depth of invasion implies either a delay in diagnosis for this type of melanoma or more rapid progression of the disease. In 53 (20.8%) of the 262 patients where histology slides were available, the melanoma was ulcerated. In two other series where ulceration was recorded, ulceration was present in one (8.3%) of 12[9] and five (18.5%) of 27[4] cases.

Although DM has an increased thickness compared to other cutaneous melanoma, and ulceration is normally associated with thicker melanomas, the level of ulceration was only slightly increased in DM and DNM. Ulceration was present in 17% of all SMU patients treated after 1986. This relatively low level of ulceration in desmoplastic melanomas is suggestive of a poor ability of the intraepidermal component to invade towards the surface of the epidermis and cause ulceration.

Where pigmentation was assessed clinically in a review of previously published series,[4] it was found to be present in 68 (27.7%) of 245 patients. The SMU series looked at overall microscopic pigmentation, which was recorded as present even if the amount was focal or slight. Melanin pigment was noted to be present in 130 (54.6%) of 238 patients. However, no differentiation was made between pigmentation present in the epidermal component compared to the dermal spindle cell component, which is often said to be amelanotic.

Four publications have addressed microscopic pigmentation in the dermal component. Ainstey et al.[17] found melanin pigment in four of 25 patients, two with only a few positive cells, one had pigment within an infiltrated nerve and one only within the superficial component of the dermal tumour. Reiman et al.[8] found no melanin pigment in the spindle cell component and a Fontana stain was negative for pigment in the eight cases tested. Kossard et al.[7] found pigmentation present in the dermal component of one of eight patients. Finally, Skelton et al.[3] found no melanin pigment in 28 cases.

The mitotic count was assessable on the slides of 256 patients in the SMU series: 71 (27.7%) of these patients had a low mitotic rate ($<1/mm^2$), 119 had an intermediate mitotic rate ($1–4/mm^2$) and 66 had a high mitotic rate ($>4/mm^2$). Mitoses were said to be infrequent in three other papers.[3,7,8] In Carlson's series,[4] where the actual count was given for each of 28 patients, 10 had a low mitotic rate, 12 had an intermediate rate and four had a high mitotic rate. In another series,[9] the mitotic count of the dermal spindled component was found to be low in seven patients, intermediate in six patients and high in only one patient. This is in keeping with the original reports of the spindled component being bland, leading to difficulties in diagnosing a malignant process and in differentiating the lesion from an evolving scar.

Regression was tabulated in Carlson's series[4] and noted to be complete in four (15%) and partial in one of 28 patients. The presence of lymphocytic aggregates amongst the tumour cells is a useful clue to the diagnosis of DM.[7,9]

HISTOLOGICAL TYPES

Some DM occur without an atypical epidermal component. Reed and Leonard[2] were the first to note this, describing three types: one associated with lentigo maligna, the second associated with a minimal deviation melanoma variant and a third arising de novo. Jain and Allen[16] also noted a de novo type, a category associated with an atypical intraepidermal melanocytic component and a nerve-centred desmoplastic melanoma.

The SMU currently classifies DM into three types:

(a) Type 1 – DM associated with a classical histogenetic melanoma subtype such as superficial spreading melanoma (Figure 34.3);
(b) Type 2 – DM associated with a scant atypical junctional melanocytic proliferation (Figure 34.4);

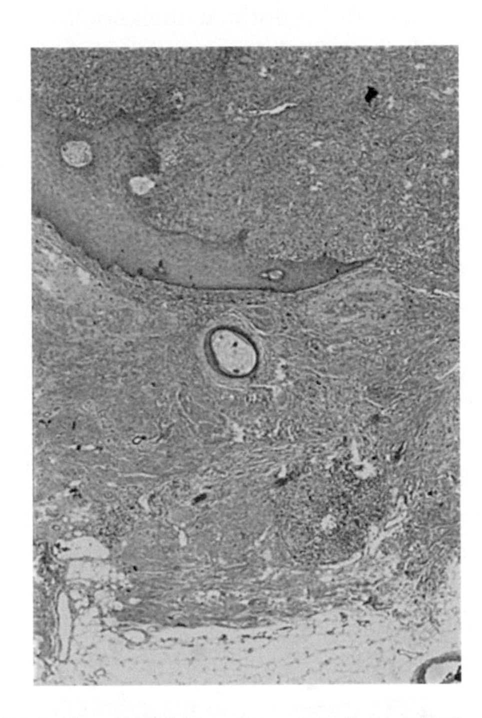

Figure 34.3 *Type 1 DM beneath a more classical melanoma. The clue to the presence of the subtle DM is the lymphoid follicle. The more classical melanoma is composed of large pleomorphic epithelioid cells. A downgrowth of epidermis appears to separate the two types of melanoma.*

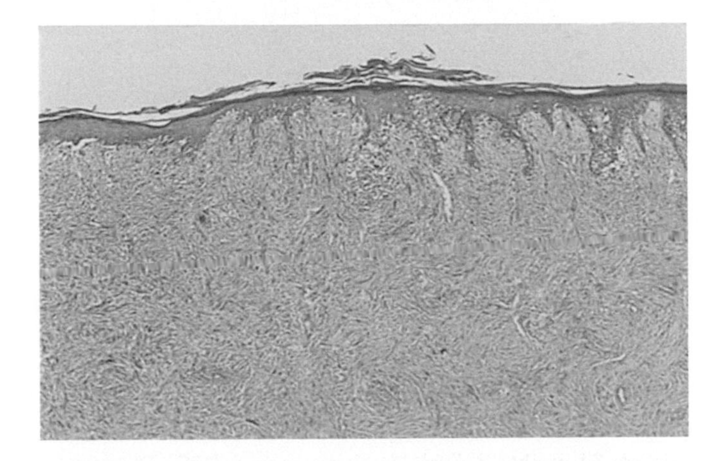

Figure 34.4 *Type 2 DM. There is only a scant junctional component. In the dermis there is a subtle proliferation of spindled melanocytes.*

(c) Type 3 – de novo DM apparently arising in the dermis or subcutaneous tissue, with no overlying epidermal component (Figure 34.5).

Carlson et al.[4] in their review and series had 139 type 1 cases out of a total of 257. These included 82 lentigo maligna melanomas, 54 superficial spreading melanomas and three nodular melanomas. The SMU series, which specifically attempted to identify the classical subtype, found 47 (16.8%) superficial spreading melanomas, 46 (16.4%) lentigo maligna melanomas, 14 (5%) nodular melanomas and three (1.1%) acral lentiginous melanomas. This is a markedly increased incidence of lentigo maligna melanoma compared to an overall incidence of 4% in all cutaneous melanomas. Carlson et al's[4] review also noted 59 cases (23%) as having an atypical lentiginous intraepidermal melanocytic component, which would be type 2 in the SMU classification. Finally, Carlson et al. noted 54 cases (21%) where there was no intraepidermal component, i.e. type 3, the de novo type.

Carlson et al.[4] in their own series examined whether the dermal component was continuous or discontinuous (i.e. with a Grenz zone) with the epidermal component. This contiguity, with transgression of the epidermal basement membrane, was identified in 10 cases (36%). These tumours were noted to be thinner and usually had an identifiable classical epidermal component, mostly lentigo maligna. In the group with a Grenz zone separating the dermal and epidermal components, the mean thickness was 4.6 mm and was associated with lentiginous melanocytic proliferation in most cases. The final group of four cases had no epidermal component, being the thickest group, with a mean thickness of 6.9 mm. It is interesting to contemplate a possible progression of increasing depth with gradual disappearance in content and definition of the epidermal component.

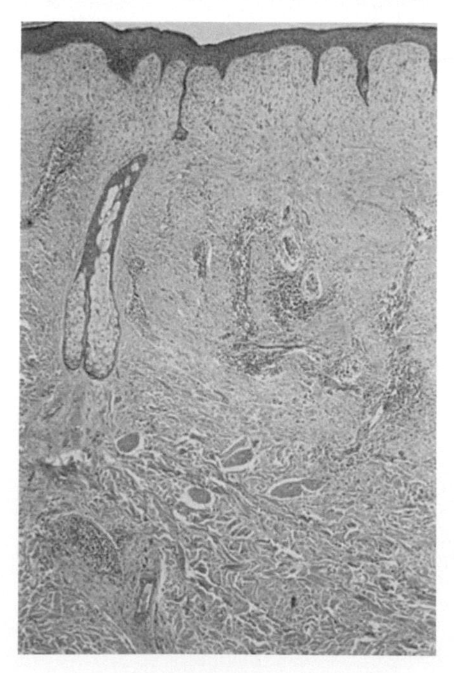

Figure 34.5 *Type 3 desmoplastic melanoma (DM). There is no junctional component – the DM is in the dermis only. The clue to the presence of the DM is the collections of lymphocytes. (Photograph courtesy of Dr Stanley McCarthy.)*

IMMUNOHISTOCHEMISTRY

With difficulty in both a diagnosis especially in the absence of melanocytic pigmentation, and in distinguishing tumour margins, immunohistochemistry plays an important role in diagnosis.

S-100 staining is usually positive. In the SMU series, where 114 cases had S-100 stained slides available for review, all were positive for S-100. In the series and review by Carlson et al.,[4] 198 of 206 cases stained positive for S-100. Vimentin was positive in 48 of 49 cases. Non-specific enolase was positive in 25 of 47 cases and HMB-45 was positive in only 11 of 47 cases. Staining by HMB-45 was of the epidermal component or in epithelioid cells in the superficial dermis. When electron microscopy was used to examine the ultrastructural features of DM, premelanosomes and melanosomes were found in only six of 42 cases.

Desmoplasia and neurotropism

Many authors consider neurotropism a variant of desmoplasia. The SMU series specifically separated DM from DNM and found that 190 of 280 patients exhibited desmoplasia alone whereas 90 of 280 patients had desmoplasia with neurotropism. Smithers et al.[6] and Reed and Leonard[2] also divided the tumours with nerve involvement into neurotropic and neural transforming (where the tumour takes on a neuroid appearance or neurosarcomatous change). Smithers et al.[15] later applied stricter criteria to desmoplasia and only noted this as being present if >50% of the tumour was fibrosed; they found that eight cases were neurotropic without desmoplasia. In Baer's series of 27 patients there were 11 patients with desmoplasia and neurotropism, and five patients with neurotropism only.[14] Jain and Allen[16] had neurotropism in 24 of 45 patients, with one of the nerve-centred tumours being neurotropic only. Neurotropism can thus exist without desmoplasia.

DIFFERENTIAL DIAGNOSIS

The main histopathological differential diagnoses include scars and fibrosing reparative reactions, fibrohistiocytic tumours and sclerosing blue naevi, which are often positive for HMB-45. Differentiating between a scar and a DM is the most common problem in diagnosis. Scarring is common in melanocytic lesions because of trauma and previous biopsies. Scarring is differentiated from DM by the more ordered pattern of spindle cell proliferation in scar tissue, with fibroblasts parallel to the skin surface and blood vessels perpendicular to the surface. S-100 is often useful in distinguishing scar tissue from DM, but scars may contain regenerating nerve twigs and other cells that may be S-100 positive. Mitoses may also be present in scar tissue.

CLINICAL BEHAVIOUR AND OUTCOME

It was originally suggested that desmoplastic melanoma had a high local recurrence rate and poor survival. More recent series began to suggest that this was not so, especially when there was no neurotropism present. Smithers et al.[6] showed a 5-year survival rate of 63% for DM >4 mm thick. This compares to a 5-year survival rate of 37% for all cutaneous melanomas >4 mm thick from the SMU database.

The SMU series attempted to determine prognostic variables and survival outcomes. All patients were staged on presentation according to the UICC/AJCC staging system: 79 patients (28.2%) were stage I, 185 patients (66.1%) were stage II, 12 patients (4.3%) were stage III and one patient was stage IV. Three patients were unable to be staged and 14 patients were lost to follow up. An overall survival curve was constructed, based on the Kaplan Meier product limit method (Figure 34.6). The overall survival rate at 5 years was 72.2% with 28.6% of patients still at risk. The overall survival at 10 years was 52% with 2.5% of patients still at risk. Median survival had not been reached (survival range 0.2–133 months).

The effects of clinical and histological variables on survival were compared by univariate analysis by

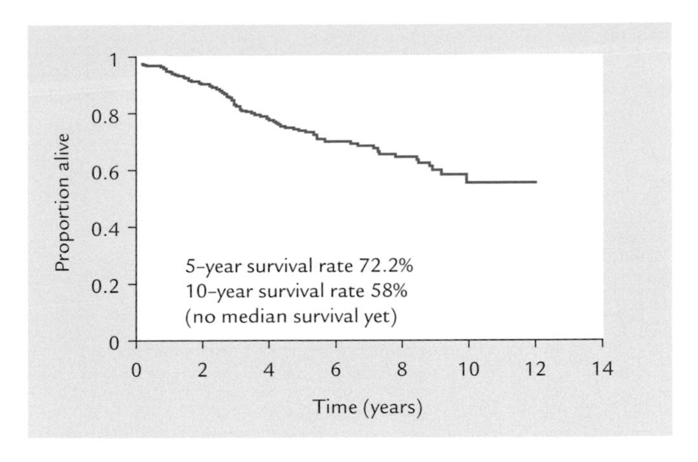

Figure 34.6 *Overall survival of patients with desmoplastic and neurotropic melanoma.*

determining the statistical difference between survival curves from log rank tests. There were significant associations with high mitotic rate ($P < 0.001$), male gender ($P = 0.016$), older age group ($P = 0.001$), thickness categorized by T classification ($P = 0.012$) and ulceration ($P = 0.023$). Site was significant as a heterogeneous group, of which the head and neck site was the worst performer. A multivariate Cox proportional hazards model of possible characteristics affecting survival was then constructed. High mitotic rate was found to be significant ($P = 0.011$). Notably, there was no difference in survival between DM and DNM – the overall survival rate at 5 years was 72.2% for both. This was slightly higher than the 68% overall survival in Skelton et al's study.[3] However, when compared stage for stage, the 5-year survival rate for stages I and II (90%) was higher for DM and DNM when compared with all cutaneous melanomas at the SMU, for which the survival rate was 79% at 5 years.

Disease recurrence occurred in 28.6% of SMU patients. Local recurrence occurred in 31 patients, of which 13 were DM and 18 were DNM. Regional recurrence occurred in 26 patients (21 DM and five DNM). Systemic recurrence occurred in 38 patients (24 DM and 14 DNM). A disease-free survival curve (Figure 34.7) was constructed for patients with local, regional and systemic recurrence. At 5 years, 62% of patients were disease free: within 2 years of presentation, recurrence had occurred in 78.2% of the patients who ultimately experienced recurrence.

Time-to-treatment failure was subjected to univariate analysis and found to be significantly shorter in association with high mitotic rate ($P < 0.001$), a narrow excision margin ($P < 0.001$), head and neck site

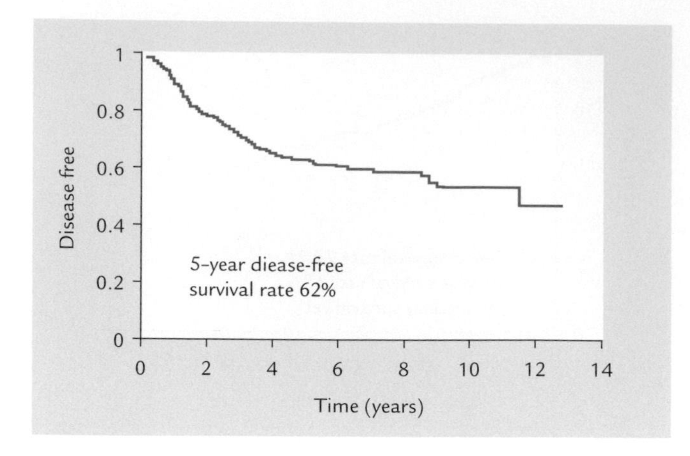

Figure 34.7 *Disease-free suvival for 280 patients with desmoplastic and desmoplastic neurotropic melanoma.*

($P = 0.001$), neurotropism ($P = 0.043$) and thickness categorized by T classification ($P = 0.003$). Multivariate analysis of possible characteristics affecting time-to-treatment failure found thickness ($P = 0.012$), mitotic rate ($P < 0.001$), and an excision margin of <1 cm compared with an excision margin of >2 cm to be significant ($P = 0.001$).

The reported high rate of local recurrence[11,16] was addressed in the SMU series by logistic regression analysis. When the margins were histologically positive, there was recurrence of all lesions that were not re-excised. When patients with excision margins of <1 cm and >2 cm were compared, the local recurrence rate was significantly greater ($P = 0.001$) for those with a <1 cm margin. When those with excision margins of 1–2 cm and >2 cm were compared, there was no significant benefit for the greater margin, however, the odds ratio for recurrence in the 1–2 cm margin group compared with the >2 cm group was 2:1. Skelton et al.[3] also found an excision margin of <1 cm a significant predictor of local recurrence.[3] Neurotropism was also found to be significant in predicting local recurrence, as had been found previously.[18]

The 11% local recurrence rate is higher than the 3.2% previously reported for a collected series of all forms of melanoma treated at multiple centres.[19] However, it was not as high as the mean recurrence rate of 49% recorded in a previously published review of local recurrence for DM and DNM patients.[4] In the SMU series, when the local recurrence rates for DM and DNM patients were separated, 6.8% of DM patients had local recurrence, compared with 20% of DNM patients.

The local recurrence rate of 6.8% for DM patients is marginally higher than the 6% upper range limit of the collected series of all cutaneous melanomas mentioned above. However, the median tumour thickness in this series was 2.5 mm and when comparison was made with the local recurrence rate of 6.6% for tumours classified as T3 (i.e. those 1.5–4 mm in thickness) treated at the SMU, DM did not appear to have an increased recurrence rate.

An interesting finding is that regional lymph node involvement at the time of diagnosis, and as the site of first recurrence, is relatively infrequent in DM and DNM: this had been noted previously.[4,6,8,9,16] Although DM and DNM present as thicker tumours, and the presence of lymph node metastases is usually directly related to melanoma thickness, only 4% of cases in the SMU series presented with stage III disease. Of all cutaneous melanoma patients who presented to the SMU, *c.* 20% had stage III disease. A decreased incidence of subsequent regional lymph node recurrence in DM and DNM (8.2%) when compared with other cutaneous melanoma (11.9%) was unexpected.

The SMU study also confirmed the previous finding[6,10,12,16] that recurrence in DM and DNM occurs sooner than after other melanomas, with 78.2% of observed recurrences occurring within 24 months.

PATHOGENESIS

The origin of DM is controversial. Those associated with classical melanoma or atypical melanocytic hyperplasia may be considered as variants of classical melanoma. However, the existence of a subtype arising de novo in the dermis is not well explained by regression of a pre-existing epidermal component, given the absence of regression in the majority of these subtypes.

It is postulated that the presence of collagen in DM may arise from fibroblasts or from the spindled melanoma cells. Valensi,[20] in electron microscopy studies, showed the presence of macular desmosomes in DNM. Similar structures are also seen in the fibroblasts from specialized fibrous structures, including fetal tendon. From[21] described collagen within spindled melanoma cells, which may represent differentiation into a fibrogenic type cell. Basic fibroblast growth factor has been implicated in the aetiology of DM.[23,24] Desmoplasia found in association with other tumours is often thought of as a host response to the presence of the tumour.[25] While this may be true for desmoplastic melanoma, alternative theories suggest a tumour origin for the desmoplasia. Melanoma cells acting as adaptive fibroblasts may be considered responsible for collagen synthesis in DM because of the ultrastructural findings of fibroblastic and myofibroblastic differentiation, and the presence of collagen within rough endoplasmic reticulum of tumour spindle cells.[21]

Conversely, Fearns and Dowdle[26] suggested that melanoma cells induce collagen synthesis in host fibroblasts, showing a twofold increase in collagen synthesis when the human melanoma cell line UCT-Mel7 was added to a culture of human fibroblasts. This was further shown to require direct contact between the two cell types. The human melanoma cell line UCT-Mel7 may represent a consistent in vivo model of DM. When injected into nude mice it consistently results in a desmoplastic tumour resembling desmoplastic melanoma. This tumour has an unusual phasic growth pattern in nude mice, whereas typical melanoma cell lines when injected into nude mice grow progressively, without development of a host response. This phasic growth pattern of UCT-Mel7 is characterized by initial limited growth, then a period of prolonged dormancy and finally progression, with a rapidly growing lethal tumour. This is interesting given the finding in the SMU study that the most significant prognostic indicator was a high mitotic rate, perhaps indicative of the final phase of growth.

Reed and Leonard[2] have suggested that the spindle cells of DM do not have the full malignant potential of the large epithelioid cells often seen in more classical melanomas. This is further supported by the finding that regional and systemic metastases of DM often resemble classical melanoma.[2,3,9,10,21] This suggests that the spindle cells of DM have the ability to invade locally but may require further stimuli to attain metastatic potential. Because the tumour cell in DM appears to have the capability of melanocytic, nerve sheath and fibroblastic differentiation,[1] carcinogenic stimulation at various stages of migration and differentiation could account for the wide range of phenotypic and behavioural expression manifested by this tumour, with varying amounts of desmoplasia and neurotropism in combination or separately. Not only would this order of events explain the histogenesis of DM, but the arrest of a primitive precursor cell in the dermis may also account for the category of DM that does not have an overlying epidermal component.

ORIGIN OF NEUROTROPISM

The neurotropin receptor (p75NTR) and one of its ligands, nerve growth factor, reportedly regulate the migration of Schwann cells along embryonic nerves. There is a strong correlation between expression of p75NTR and the desmoplastic phenotype, suggesting that the propensity of these melanomas for neurotropism involves p75 and its ligands.[27]

In the SMU study, neurotropism was only found at a thickness >1.5 mm and in Clark level IV and V tumours. It may be that this nerve growth factor only becomes significant at the level of the reticular dermis when the density or type of nerve fibres is sufficient to activate it. Two patients are recorded on the SMU database as initially having thin melanomas (<1.5 mm in thickness) and with no evidence of desmoplasia or neurotropism. Both tumours recurred locally as thicker tumours, with marked neurotropism present. This phenomenon was previously noted by Ainstey et al.[17] and would suggest that these tumours became neurotropic once the required depth had been attained.

CRANIAL NEUROPATHIES

Gentile and Donovan[21] reported the first cranial neuropathy associated with DNM. Following this there were a number of other reports:[2,7,8,11,12,17,18] Jain and Allen[16] reported nine cases and Smithers et al.[6] reported four. These neuropathies usually involve branches of the trigeminal nerve. The mortality of this event is high, although recently there have been anecdotal reports that the involved nerve may be surgically removed to the gasserian ganglion leading to possible increased survival. An alternative method is to biopsy the affected nerve till it is clear on pathological examination, then follow this with irradiation of the distal cutaneous nerve distribution. In this manner, the present authors have treated one patient who had involvement of the supraorbital nerve at the foramen from a melanoma excised from the anterior scalp.

RADIOTHERAPY AND NEUROTROPIC MELANOMA

There are some reports of these melanomas being treated by radiotherapy. Kossard et al.[7] had one patient who had no recurrence following excision and radiotherapy but another patient who required re-excision after radiotherapy following incomplete excision. Jain and Allen[16] had three cases that arose in areas of previous irradiation. Smithers et al.[15] reported two patients with inoperable recurrences who appeared to have a complete local response to radiotherapy but died of disease elsewhere.

Radiotherapy is currently recommended at the SMU for patients with primary neurotropic melanoma of the head and neck where the melanoma has been completely excised. Although there are no studies showing a benefit, in the SMU experience with melanoma of the lip, of five patients who had local recurrence, four patients had neurotropism and none had had adjuvant radiotherapy. Of five patients with neurotropic melanoma who have had adjuvant radiotherapy, none has had local recurrence.

REFERENCES

1. Conley J, Lattes R, Orr W, Desmoplastic malignant melanoma (a rare variant of spindle cell melanoma). *Cancer* 1971; 28: 914–36.
2. Reed RJ, Leonard DD, Neurotropic melanoma. A variant of desmoplastic melanoma. *Am J Surg Path* 1979; 3: 301–11.
3. Skelton HG, Smith KJ, Laskin WB et al, Desmoplastic malignant melanoma. *J Am Acad Dermatol* 1995; 32: 717–25 (see Comments).
4. Carlson JA, Dickersin GR, Sober AJ, Barnhill RL, Desmoplastic neurotropic melanoma. A clinicopathologic analysis of 28 cases. *Cancer* 1995; 75: 478–94.
5. Quinn MJ, Crotty K, Thompson JF et al, Desmoplastic and desmoplastic neurotropic melanoma, experience with 280 patients. *Cancer* 1998; 83: 1128–35.
6. Smithers BM, McLeod GR, Little JH, Desmoplastic, neural transforming and neurotropic melanoma: a review of 45 cases. *Aust NZ J Surg* 1990; 60: 967–72.
7. Kossard S, Doherty E, Murray E, Neurotropic melanoma. A variant of desmoplastic melanoma. *Arch Dermatol* 1987; 123: 907–12.
8. Reiman HM, Goellner JR, Woods JE, Mixter RC, Desmoplastic melanoma of the head and neck. *Cancer* 1987; 60: 2269–74.
9. Walsh NM, Roberts JT, Orr W, Simon GT, Desmoplastic malignant melanoma. A clinicopathologic study of 14 cases. *Arch Pathol Lab Med* 1988; 112: 922–7.
10. Egbert B, Kempson R, Sagebiel R, Desmoplastic malignant melanoma. A clinicohistopathologic study of 25 cases. *Cancer* 1988; 62: 2033–41.
11. Beenken S, Byers R, Smith JL et al, Desmoplastic melanoma. Histologic correlation with behavior and treatment. *Arch Otolaryngol – Head Neck Surg* 1989; 115: 374–9.
12. Devaraj VS, Moss AL, Briggs JC, Desmoplastic melanoma: a clinicopathological review. Br J Plast Surg 1992; 45: 595–8.
13. Weinzweig N, Tuthill RJ, Yetman RJ, Desmoplastic malignant melanoma: a clinicohistopathologic review. *Plast Reconstr Surg* 1994; 95: 548–55.
14. Baer SC, Schultz D, Synnestvedt M, Elder DE, Desmoplasia and neurotropism. Prognostic variables in patients with stage I melanoma. *Cancer* 1995; 76: 2242–7.
15. Smithers BM, McLeod GR, Little JH, Desmoplastic melanoma: patterns of recurrence. *World J Surg* 1992; 16: 186–90.
16. Jain S, Allen PW, Desmoplastic malignant melanoma and its variants. A study of 45 cases. *Am J Surg Pathol* 1989; 13: 358–73.
17. Ainstey A, McKee P, Jones EW, Desmoplastic malignant melanoma: a clinicopathological study of 25 cases. *Br J Dermatol* 1993; 129: 359–71.
18. Bruijn JA, Mihm Jr MC, Barnhill RL, Desmoplastic melanoma. *Histopathology* 1992; 20: 197–205.
19. Ames FC, Balch CM, Reintgen DS, Local recurrences and their management. In: *Cutaneous melanoma.* 2nd edn. (eds Balch CM, Houghton AN, Milton GW et al). Philadelphia: JB Lippincott, 1992: 287–94.
20. Valensi QJ, Desmoplastic malignant melanoma: a light and electron microscopy study of two cases. *Cancer* 1979; 43: 1148–55.
21. From L, Hanna W, Kahn HJ et al, Origin of desmoplasia in desmoplastic malignant melanoma. *Hum Pathol* 1983; 4: 1072–80.
22. Gentile RD, Donovan DT, Neurotropic melanoma of the head and neck. *Laryngoscope* 1985; 95: 1161–6.
23. Al-Alousi S, Carlson JA, Blessing K et al, Expression of basic fibroblast growth factor in desmoplastic melanoma. *J Cutan Pathol* 1996; 23: 118–25.
24. Sherman L, Stocker KM, Morrison R et al, Basic fibroblast growth factor acts intracellularly to cause the transdifferentiation of avian neural crest-derived Schwann cell precursors into melanocytes. *Development* 1993; 118: 1313–26.
25. Liotta LA, Tumour extracellular matrix. *Lab Invest* 1982; 47: 112–13.
26. Fearns C, Dowdle EB, The desmoplastic response: induction of collagen synthesis by melanoma cells in vitro. *Int J Cancer* 1992; 50: 621–7.
27. Kanik AB, Yaar M, Bhawan J, p75 nerve growth factor receptor staining helps identify desmoplastic and neurotropic melanoma. *J Cutan Pathol* 1996; 23: 205–10.

35

Radiation therapy in locally advanced melanoma

Graham Stevens

INTRODUCTION

There is growing interest in the use of radiation in the management of locally advanced melanoma. In particular, the role of radiation therapy as an adjunct to surgery is being actively investigated. This interest stems from a combination of factors, including:

- reports of high local relapse rates following surgery alone;
- an appreciation of surgical and pathological features that predict increased risk of local failure;
- the extreme morbidity of uncontrolled local failure;
- reports that adjunctive radiation therapy improves local control;
- recognition of prolonged survival in a proportion of patients with locally advanced melanoma.

On the other hand, it is well recognized that the combination of aggressive surgery and radiation therapy increases the risk of treatment-related complications and that recurrence of melanoma in these patients manifests frequently as a systemic disease.

As a result of these complex and overlapping factors, the management of patients with locally advanced melanoma is frequently difficult. There are no modern randomized clinical trials of the use of radiation therapy to guide management. At the Sydney Melanoma Unit (SMU), a multidisciplinary approach to optimize treatment has been adopted for many years. The aim of this chapter is to address the issue of locoregional relapse and to present a scheme for the appropriate introduction of radiation therapy into the management of locally advanced melanoma.

For melanoma, in common with many other malignancies, the term 'locally advanced' is ill-defined. It is used predominantly as an operational utility rather than as a formal definition and has been applied to AJCC/UICC stages I–III melanoma.

LOCAL RECURRENCE RATES FOLLOWING SURGERY ALONE

Most patients with localized melanoma are managed appropriately with surgery alone. Retrospective surgical series have, however, allowed identification of patients at increased risk of locoregional relapse following excision of primary melanomas and/or dissection of regional nodes.

In relation to the primary melanoma, the incidence of local recurrence is generally very low (1% in one series).[1] However, the risk rises considerably for thick melanomas and for those displaying desmoplasia, neurotropism or lymphatic invasion. For melanomas >4 mm, the recurrence rate was 12% for a recent series[2] but was 24% for an older series of head and neck primaries.[3] Recurrence rates of 20–50% have been reported for desmoplastic neurotropic melanomas.[4,5] Lymphatic invasion was followed by in-transit metastases or satellitosis in >90% of cases, compared with 2% without lymphatic invasion.[6]

For regional nodal disease, a number of factors predict for increased failure in the nodal basin. Higher recurrence rates have been reported in the neck (35–45%) than either the axilla (25–30%) or the groin (10–20%).[7,8] Recurrence within the parotid was 18.7% when parotid nodes were positive and superficial parotidectomy was performed.[9] The indication for surgery is predictive for local recurrence rates, with recurrence rates of 34–50% following therapeutic dissections and 3–16% following elective dissections.[2,7,10,11] Increasing number and/or size of involved nodes have been found to correlate with increased risk of failure, with 60–80% recurrence rates for multiple nodes involved or nodes >6 cm in diameter.[7] Extracapsular extension (ECE) (up to *c.* 60% local failure for ECE versus *c.* 15% without ECE)[7,11,12] and connective tissue invasion (28% local failure)[12] are of particular importance in this respect. Data from a selection of reports relating to these factors are listed in Table 35.1.

Using multivariate analysis, two series have shown that ECE was the only independent predictor of recurrence in the neck.[7,11] That the number of nodes was a significant variable on univariate analysis but was not significant on multivariate analysis may relate to a higher incidence of ECE with increasing nodal involvement (31% ECE with more than three positive nodes versus 19% with less than three positive nodes).[11]

The experience of the surgeon has also been proposed as a factor in recurrence in the neck following neck dissection.[11] For neck dissections performed initially at tertiary referral melanoma centres, neck recurrences were *c.* 4%, compared with *c.* 25% in patients referred to these centres following neck dissection elsewhere. However, selection bias may contribute to this large difference.

RADIATION BIOLOGY OF MELANOMA

A brief review of the radiation biology of melanoma may be useful at this point, to provide an explanation for the unusual radiation fractionation schedules that have been used by some workers. This has been an area of intense interest and investigation for the past 30 years and many excellent reviews have been published.[13–16] A more detailed discussion of this topic is presented in Chapter 51.

There is substantial evidence from laboratory[17] and clinical[18,19] data that the radiation response of

Table 35.1 *Factors influencing relapse in lymph node bed following dissection*

Variable	Relapse %						Reference
Site of nodal bed	Neck	Axilla		Groin			
	43	28		23			7
	33	24		10			8
Indication for surgery	Elective			Therapeutic			
	3			16			11
	9			34			9
	16			50			10
Extracapsular extension	Absent			Present			
	23			63			7
	15			28			12
	9			24			11
Number of involved nodes	≤3	≤4	>3	>4	3–6	>6	
	15		8				11
	24				42	80	7
		10		20			50
Size of largest node (cm)	<3	>3					
	24	>40					7
Institution	Tertiary melanoma			Other			
	4.0			22			11
	4.5			27			51

melanomas is, on average, more sensitive to changes in the size of the daily radiation dose than most other tumour types. This is represented graphically (Figure 51.1) as a 'curvier' dose–response curve than is found for most tumours, and quantitatively as a lower α/β ratio in the linear–quadratic mathematical model. This means that melanomas are more likely to respond to radiation when the radiation is delivered as a small number of large doses, in so-called hypofractionated schedules. It needs to be stressed that this is an average situation and there is wide variation between different melanoma cell lines and tumours, with a spectrum that overlaps with other tumour types[20] and ranges from the most sensitive to the most resistant tumours.

Many clinical trials of melanoma have utilized a hypofractionated radiation schedule. The optimal dose per fraction, to maximize the therapeutic ratio, has been determined as 4–6 gray (Gy),[21] but there remains controversy,[22] as a randomized clinical trial showed equivalence of conventional and hypofractionated schedules.[23] Also, hypofractionation has the potential to cause severe late complications[24] due to the similarity between the responses of melanomas and late-reacting normal tissues.

That melanoma is, on average, a radioresponsive tumour has now been evident for 30 years or more. It is clear that some of the previous uncertainty related to the wide range of sensitivities of melanoma compared with many common epithelial tumours. This has presented difficulties in the choice of a uniform treatment schedule and has been hampered by the lack of effective predictive tests of radiation sensitivity for individual tumours. Despite the steady accumulation of data attesting to the efficacy of radiation in the treatment of melanoma, the concept that melanoma is unresponsive to radiation and that radiation has only a limited role in its management has become ingrained in surgical training. Comments such as 'Radiation therapy has no role as an adjuvant to surgery for localized disease that is treatable by wide excision . . .',[25] 'Radiotherapy is strictly palliative and has been used for brain and bone metastases',[26] 'Melanoma is considered to be weakly radiosensitive'[27] and 'High dose per fraction radiation produces a better response rate than low-dose, large-fraction therapy'[28] can be found in current surgical textbooks. These ideas arose from early reports of poor responses to radiation.[29] In many cases patients had locally advanced or metastatic lesions that would be considered incurable and difficult to control by any modality. Despite reports of curative treatment of melanoma with radiation,[30,31] melanoma became a 'surgical' disease and the supposed futility of radiation was reinforced by the continued referral of patients with large, unresectable tumours. Radiation has been an effective treatment for primary melanoma and response rates of 70% for gross tumours treated by radiation are reported routinely.

ADJUVANT RADIATION THERAPY

As there are no modern randomized clinical trials comparing the local control rates of surgery alone versus surgery and adjuvant radiation therapy, evidence for a benefit of adjuvant radiation therapy is limited to prospective and retrospective single institution data. Attempts to initiate and accrue patients to randomized trials have had limited success, partly because patients with locally advanced melanoma are also candidates for trials of systemic agents. In particular, radiation has the theoretical risk of impairing the patient's immune response in trials of immunotherapy.

Most experience with adjuvant radiation relates to reported control of lymph node regions, with experience in elective nodal irradiation, postoperative irradiation and preoperative irradiation. There are few reports relating to the adjuvant use of radiation in treatment of the primary melanoma.

Irradiation of nodal regions

Elective nodal irradiation

As a component of a larger study of 174 patients, 79 patients with primary melanomas >1.5 mm thick of the head and neck with a clinically negative neck were treated with 30 Gy in five fractions.[32] The local control rate was excellent.

Postoperative irradiation

The only randomized clinical trial included 56 patients who were randomized between therapeutic lymph node dissections alone and surgery followed by adjuvant irradiation.[33] The radiation was delivered as a split course schedule of two cycles of 25 Gy in 14 fractions, separated by 3–4 weeks. (This is an unusual treatment schedule which would not be used currently.) There was a trend towards improved survival in the radiation arm, (which the authors attributed to an imbalance in patient characteristics), but no comparison of local control.

Most reports have based the use of postoperative irradiation on the operative and pathological findings following full nodal dissection. Johansen et al.[34] reported their experience, in which primary or nodal regions were treated using 24 Gy in three fractions (on days 0, 7 and 21) for gross residual tumour (nine patients) and histopathological findings of positive margins, extracapsular lymph node extension and large or multiple involved nodes (22 patients). Infield recurrence was 22% for microscopic disease and 44% for gross disease.

Burmeister et al.[35] irradiated 26 patients postoperatively for multiple involved nodes, ECE or tumour spillage, and 31 patients for unresectable nodal disease, using a variety of radiation schedules. Infield recurrences were 12 and 26% for microscopic and unresectable disease, respectively. Local control was improved for fraction sizes >4 Gy and total doses >30 Gy. However these data are difficult to interpret as no fractionation schedules were provided. Complications were reported to be minimal and were unrelated to radiation treatment parameters. Similarly, Fenig et al.[36] gave adjuvant postoperative irradiation to 25 patients with extensive nodal involvement of the neck, axilla or groin. A variety of treatment schedules were used. The local control rate at 3 years was 84%, with no difference according to fraction size. As with the previous authors, this finding is difficult to evaluate, as the actual treatment schedules were not given.

Strom and Ross[37] irradiated the axillae of 28 patients postoperatively for gross residual disease, multiple involved nodes, large nodes or ECE. The hypofractionated schedule of 30 Gy in five fractions was used for 13 of 28 patients. Local control was 95% for microscopic disease and 43% for gross disease. Arm oedema occurred in three patients without recurrent tumour. Storper et al.[38] reported on a group of 44 patients with residual or recurrent melanoma treated with various combinations of surgery and/or radiation. The addition of postoperative radiation did not alter survival, which was the main end point. Little can be taken from this publication, however, as the treatment groups were not comparable and radiation was administered to patients with larger tumours.

Corry et al.[39] irradiated nodal regions (neck, axilla or groin) of 113 patients, 42 with microscopic disease and 71 with gross disease. The indications for adjuvant treatment were multiple involved nodes, extracapsular spread and recurrent disease. Following adjuvant treatment, 74% had relapsed by 5 years. Of the 20% of these patients who had initial relapse in the nodal basin, approximately one half failed outside the radiation field. By contrast, most initial failures were at the treated site when there was gross disease and the 5-year relapse-free survival was 4%. The radiation schedule for adjuvant treatment was 50 Gy in 25 fractions, with a variety of schedules used to treat gross disease. Lymphoedema (nine patients) and 'severe' fibrosis (five patients) were found but the treatment arms of these patients were not specified.

Other authors have concluded that there is either no role for postoperative irradiation following nodal dissection, or that its role is limited. Shen et al.[11] analyzed recurrence in the neck of 196 patients with positive nodes from melanoma of the head and neck. On multivariate analysis, only ECE predicted for increased cervical recurrence ($P = 0.03$); neither the number of involved nodes (three or fewer versus more than three) nor the size of the nodes (palpable versus impalpable) was significant. The authors concluded that the presence of ECE may justify adjuvant irradiation. Fuhrmann et al.[40] performed a retrospective matched-pair analysis of 58 patients who had received adjuvant irradiation against 58 who were treated with nodal dissection alone. The indications for irradiation were: more than two involved nodes, any node >1 cm in diameter, or ECE. Radiation doses were 50–65 Gy in fraction sizes of 2–3.8 Gy for most patients. Recurrence rates were 15% in the irradiated group and 21% in the matched, non-irradiated group. There was no breakdown of the recurrence rate in the presence of ECE. Severe limb oedema occurred in 45% of the irradiated group, compared with 12% in the surgery-only group. These authors concluded that there was no basis to support a recommendation for adjuvant irradiation. Conversley, Lee et al.[7] suggested that adjuvant irradiation should be considered for patients with a wide range of clinical and pathological features, including neck node involvement, ECE, more than three positive, palpable nodes, and nodes >3 cm diameter.

The SMU experience

The SMU experience was updated in early 2000, with a series of 172 patients who received postoperative adjuvant irradiation to nodal regions. The nodal basins treated were neck in 50%, axilla in 34%, inguinal in 13% and multiple regions in 3%. The indications for treatment of nodal regions were adverse surgical and/or pathological findings following initial dissection in 127 patients and recurrent disease in 45 patients: these indications are listed in Table 35.2. As expected, many patients had more than one indication for treatment. A small number received postoperative radiation for other indications, including involved parotid nodes (see below).

Most patients received a hypofractionated schedule of 30–33 Gy in six fractions over 2.5 weeks. Treatment techniques varied according to the region treated. The neck was usually treated with 7–9 MV electrons, dosed to the 90% isodose. A photon wedge-pair technique was used when the treatment volume included the submental and submandibular regions. The axilla and drain sites were treated with parallel opposed fields. The supraclavicular region was included if more than three positive nodes were found in the axilla. Extensive use was made of shielding to protect lung and soft tissues around the shoulder. The groin was treated using photons or electrons. If the surgical scar extended up the abdominal wall, a further electron or orthovoltage field was added.

Table 35.2 *Indications for treatment of nodal regions*

	No. of patients	%
Initial resection		
Multiple nodes involved	16	9
Extracapsular extension	24	14
Node >3 cm	9	5
Connective tissue deposits	10	6
Close or positive margins	3	2
Parotid node(s) involved	11	6
Perineural/vascular/ lymphatic spread	2	1
Initial operation elsewhere*	2	1
Clinical trial+	3	2
Multiple indications	43	25
Other	4	3
Recurrent nodal disease	45	26

*Incomplete dissection, with decision not to reoperate.
+Patients entered onto clinical trial comparing surgery ± RT.

In keeping with an earlier report,[41] the infield recurrence rate was 11%. Infield recurrence was increased in patients who developed metastatic disease ($P=0.04$), had an interval of more than 6 weeks from surgery to the start of radiation ($P=0.02$) and had radiation treatment extending over >18 days ($P=0.05$). There was no influence of dose per fraction, although most had a standard treatment schedule. Infield failure was not increased specifically by the histopathological findings of more than three positive nodes, largest node >3 cm, extracapsular spread, matted nodes, connective tissue deposits or positive surgical margins.

The acute radiation effects were limited to skin and mucosa, except for two patients who developed transient jaw pain following parotid and neck irradiation. There was moist desquamation in skin folds. There were two main types of late complication. Firstly, arm oedema requiring a compressive stocking occurred in *c.* 60% of patients who had axillary dissection and postoperative irradiation. Secondly, most patients had progressive fibrosis of soft tissues within the radiation field. This was most evident in the axilla and consisted of soft tissue induration and restriction of shoulder movement. The relative contributions of surgery and radiation have not been determined. Two patients had late complications following neck irradiation; one suffered severe fibrosis, the other developed mastoiditis and hearing loss.

The median survival was 22 months and the 5-year survival rate was 37%. The 5-year survival rate was influenced strongly by infield recurrence (0 and 44% for patients with and without local relapse respectively, $P=0.004$) and also by the number of positive nodes (19 and 51% for three or fewer and more than three positive nodes respectively).

Patients found to have involved parotid nodes receive postoperative irradiation routinely, as O'Brien et al.[9] found reduced local relapse (6.5%) relative to a contemporary cohort with fewer risk factors for recurrence (18.7%).

The neck has been irradiated following limited dissection of palpable adenopathy alone, without a full dissection. A group of 76 patients received postoperative radiation therapy using a schedule of 30 Gy in six fractions following a limited dissection.[32] A high proportion had either more than three positive nodes or a node >3 cm in diameter. The 5-year local control rate in the neck was *c.* 90% and was not reduced by the adverse findings of multiple or large nodes, or ECE.

At the SMU, a number of patients, predominantly elderly with considerable co-morbidity, have been treated similarly: to date, there have been no locoregional failures. This concept has been extended by Byers,[42] with the suggestion that the finding of a positive 'sentinel' lymph node in a clinically negative neck may provide the indication for neck irradiation. This approach is worthy of further study in the neck, as it may provide a less morbid alternative to neck dissection. There is no experience reported for the axilla and groin.

At the time of writing, there are two randomized clinical trials proposed to test the benefit of postoperative adjuvant radiation following lymph node dissection at which positive nodes are identified histologically. An ECOG/RTOG trial will compare interferon-α, either alone or with postoperative irradiation, following neck dissection for head and neck melanoma. A Trans-Tasman Radiation Oncology Group (TROG) trial, (an Australasian multicentre organization) will compare postoperative irradiation (48 Gy in 20 daily fractions) to no further treatment in melanoma patients with cervical, axillary or groin nodal involvement.

Preoperative irradiation

Preoperative irradiation of the neck was reported for a small number of patients with palpable lymphadenopathy.[32] The radiation schedule was 24 Gy in four fractions over 2 weeks. The results of the preoperative group were not reported separately from the main cohort of patients treated with postoperative radiation.

Preoperative irradiation has been utilized infrequently at the SMU in the treatment of locally advanced melanoma. Although its use has been highly individualized, there have been two broad indications. More commonly, it has been delivered to primary and/or nodal disease considered to be marginally operable. The 'adjuvant' radiation schedule (33 Gy in six fractions) was used, as there was no intention to sterilize the gross disease. Surgery was delayed 4–6 weeks after completion of radiation. In all cases there was impressive shrinkage of tumour, permitting excision with clear margins, and no wound complications. The second indication has been rapidly growing recurrent primary tumours, often with satellite nodules. Due to the high risk of extensive subclinical tumour infiltration, preoperative radiation was delivered to sterilize the margins of the surgical field. Surgery was performed when the acute skin reaction subsided.

Irradiation of primary melanoma

There is little information relating to the use of adjuvant irradiation of the primary melanoma site, although data suggesting an impact of adjuvant irradiation were available in 1958, when Dickson[43] substituted post-excision radiation for radical surgery. At the SMU, 46 patients have received adjuvant postoperative irradiation to the primary site: the sites of these primary melanomas are listed in Table 35.3. Of these, the indication for radiation was neurotropism in 27 patients, following either initial resection or recurrence. Other indications were close or positive surgical margins where re-excision would be mutilating, and tumours with rapid or multiple recurrences. As with irradiation of nodal regions, many patients had more than a single indication for treatment.

Most were treated with the same adjuvant schedule of 33 Gy in six fractions over 2.5 weeks, using electrons or orthovoltage photons. The local recurrence rate was

Table 35.3 *Anatomical sites of primary melanomas receiving adjuvant irradiation*

	No. of patients	%
Head and neck		
Nasal skin	7	15
Scalp	8	17
Cheek	5	11
Lip	4	9
Periauricular skin	7	15
Periorbital skin	3	7
Forehead	1	2
Skin of neck	1	2
Limbs	6	13
Trunk	4	9

14% and was not affected by neurotropism. The acute and late toxicities were unremarkable. The median survival time and 5-year survival rate of this group were 54 months and 49%, respectively.

The value of adjuvant irradiation in neurotropic melanomas has not been assessed formally. Gallardo and Juillard[44] reported a series of 32 patients with neurotropic melanoma. The local recurrence rate after initial surgery was 41%: recurrent tumours were re-excised – 10 had adjuvant radiation, including three with positive margins. Local control was maintained in all patients, compared with further local failure in all patients who were not irradiated. Investigation of the use of adjuvant irradiation following initial excision should be considered.

The use of radiation therapy as an alternative to excision of primary or recurrent melanoma was reported in early years[45] and also more recently.[46,47] Local control rates have been excellent in circumstances where elderly patients with, predominantly, facial lesions would have required extensive surgery.

Gross disease

At the SMU, there were 28 patients who were irradiated postoperatively for gross residual disease. Of these, 18 had disease in nodal regions and 10 in relation to the primary site. Most received a hypofractionated schedule of 36 Gy in six fractions over 2.5 weeks, a higher dose than the usual schedule for adjuvant treatment. The local control rate was 50%, within the range of 43–74% reported by others.[34,35,37] The median survival was 11 months, with a 5-year survival rate of only 15%.

It is clear that different strategies are required for the management of unresectable gross disease. Hyperthermia has been reported as effective in this setting. Using a schedule of three fractions of 8–9 Gy delivered in 8 days, the complete response rate was 35% for radiation alone compared with 65% for the addition of heat, despite the minimum temperature being achieved in only 14% of lesions.[48] Although an entire nodal basin could not be treated in this manner, a boost to gross disease using the combination could be envisaged. Unfortunately, few centres have the expertise and equipment for hyperthermia. The use of concurrent chemoradiation has been reported as effective in melanoma[49] but no comparative studies have been performed.

SUMMARY

Subsets of patients at high risk of locoregional failure have been identified from retrospective review of surgical series, mainly relating to melanoma of the head and neck. Most have used the adverse pathological findings that have been identified in the treatment of squamous carcinoma as the basis for postoperative irradiation of melanoma. In nodal regions, these include multiple involved nodes, large nodes, extracapsular spread and connective tissue invasion. In primary sites, neurotropic behaviour has been identified in particular.

Studies incorporating adjuvant irradiation have shown improved local control compared with historical surgical series. Infield relapse rates of 10–15% are reported for adjuvant treatment, but rise to *c.* 50% when gross disease remains. No particular histopathological features were associated with higher local recurrence rates in the SMU series, but a significant effect of ECE has been reported by others. Hypofractionated schedules have been favoured but one report found no benefit in using higher doses per fraction. There is no evidence that hypofractionation results in higher complication rates than conventional schedules but meaningful comparison between studies is difficult. A reduced time from surgery to adjuvant irradiation may decrease local failure.

It should be emphasized that there are no randomized data to either confirm the benefit of adjuvant treatment for particular pathological features or determine the optimal fractionation. These issues are being addressed by proposed multicentre studies. Until these randomized clinical trials are performed, it seems reasonable to recommend adjuvant postoperative radiation therapy to patients with these adverse pathological features.

In most cases, the indication for postoperative irradiation has been based on surgical and pathological findings. This inevitably means that the patient receives both a dissection and a course of radiation, increasing the possibility of treatment-related complications. The parameters influencing late toxicity have not been determined, and the incidence and severity of late toxicity vary greatly across different reports. These differences are certainly multifactorial and, by analogy with other tumour types (e.g. breast cancer), relate not only to the surgical and irradiation techniques but also to the surveillance programmes used to detect and manage complications.

Table 35.4 *Recommendations for adjuvant postoperative radiation therapy*

Following lymph node dissection
Multiple positive nodes
Large nodes
Extracapsular spread
Matted nodes
Melanoma deposits in connective tissue
Recurrence following previous dissection
Following excision of primary
Rapid or multiple recurrences
Close or positive margins not amenable to re-excision
Recurrence of neurotropic melanoma
? Following initial resection of melanoma with neurotropism or lymphatic invasion

To avoid the potential complications of aggressive treatment using two modalities, the combination of limited dissection and irradiation for palpable adenopathy should be explored. In the case of clinically negative nodes, biopsy of a positive sentinel node could be followed by radiation rather than node dissection.

There has been no suggestion to date that adjuvant radiation improves survival. This would be difficult to compare across different reports, as staging procedures vary widely. At the SMU, identification of subclinical metastases by PET scanning has, on an individual patient basis, influenced a decision regarding the use of adjuvant radiation.

REFERENCES

1. Cohn-Cedermark G, Mansson-Brahme E, Rutquist LE et al, Outcomes of patients with local recurrence of cutaneous malignant melanoma: a population-based study. *Cancer* 1997; 80: 1418–25.
2. Heaton KM, Sussman JJ, Gershenwald JE et al, Surgical margins and prognostic factors in patients with thick (>4mm) primary melanoma. *Ann Surg Oncol* 1998; 5: 322–8.
3. O'Brien CJ, Coates AC, Petersen-Schaefer K et al, Experience with 998 melanomas of the head and neck over 30 years. *Am J Surg* 1991; 162: 310–14.
4. Quinn MJ, Crotty KA, Thompson JF et al, Desmoplastic and desmoplastic neurotropic melanoma. *Cancer* 1998; 83: 1128–35.
5. Beenken S, Byers R, Smith JL et al, Desmoplastic melanoma. *Arch Otolaryngol Head Neck Surg* 1989; 115: 374–9.
6. Borgstein PJ, Meijer S, van Diest PJ, Are locoregional cutaneous metastases in melanoma predictable? *Ann Surg Oncol* 1999; 6: 315–21.
7. Lee RJ, Gibbs JF, Proulx GM et al, Nodal basin recurrence following lymph node dissection for melanoma: implications for adjuvant radiotherapy. *Int J Radiat Oncol Biol Phys* 2000; 46: 467–74.
8. Bowsher WG, Taylor BA, Hughes LE, Morbidity, mortality and local recurrence following regional node dissection for melanoma. *Br J Surg* 1986; 73: 906–8.
9. O'Brien CJ, Petersen-Schaefer K, Stevens G et al, Adjuvant radiotherapy following neck dissection and parotidectomy for metastatic malignant melanoma. *Head Neck* 1997; 19: 589–94.
10. Byers RM, The role of modified neck dissection in the treatment of cutaneous melanoma of the head and neck. *Arch Surg* 1986; 121: 1338–41.
11. Shen P, Wanek LA, Morton DL, Is adjuvant radiotherapy necessary after positive lymph node dissection in head and neck melanomas? *Ann Surg Oncol* 2000; 7: 554–9.
12. Calabro A, Singletary SE, Balch CM, Patterns of relapse in 1001 consecutive patients with melanoma nodal metastases. *Arch Surg* 1989; 124: 1051–5.
13. Habermalz HJ, Irradiation of malignant melanoma: experience in the past and present. *Int J Radiat Oncol Biol Phys* 1981; 7: 131–3.
14. Geara FB, Ang KK, Radiation therapy for malignant melanoma. *Surg Clin N Am* 1996; 76: 1383–97.
15. Cooper JS, The evolution of the role of radiation therapy in the management of mucocutaneous malignant melanoma. *Hematol/Oncol Clin N Am* 1998; 12: 849–62.
16. Schmidt-Ullrich RK, Johnson CR, Role of radiotherapy and hyperthermia in the management of malignant melanoma. *Sem Surg Oncol* 1996; 12: 407–15.
17. Barranco SC, Romsdahl MM, Humphrey RM, The radiation response of human malignant melanoma cells grown in vitro. *Cancer Res* 1971; 31: 830–3.
18. Hornsey S, The relationship between total dose, number of fractions and fraction size in the response of malignant melanoma in patients. *Br J Radiol* 1978; 51: 905–9.
19. Overgaard J, Overgaard M, Vegby Hansen P, von der Maase H, Some factors of importance in the radiation treatment of malignant melanoma. *Radiother Oncol* 1986; 5: 183–92.
20. Rofstad EK, Radiation biology of malignant melanoma (review). *Acta Radiol* 1986; 25: 1–10.
21. Bentzen SM, Overgaard J, Thames HD et al, Clinical radiobiology of malignant melanoma. *Radiother Oncol* 1989; 16: 169–82.
22. Trott K, The optimal dose per fraction for the treatment of malignant melanomas. *Int J Radiat Oncol Biol Phys* 1991; 20: 905–7.
23. Sause WT, Cooper JS, Rush S et al, Fraction size in external beam radiation therapy in the treatment of melanoma. *Int J Radiat Oncol Biol Phys* 1991; 20: 429–32.
24. Fletcher GH, Hypofractionation: lessons from complications. *Radiother Oncol* 1991; 20: 10–15.
25. Clunie GJA, Tjandra JJ, Francis DMA (eds) *Textbook of Surgery.* Blackwell: 1997: 421.
26. Jarrell BE, Carabasi RA, *Surgery (National Medical Series for Independent Study)*, 3rd edn. Wilkins and Williams: 1996: 490.
27. Blackbourne LH, Fleischer KJ (eds) *Advanced Surgical Recall.* Wilkins and Williams: 1997: 645.
28. Schwartz E, *Principles of Surgery*, 7th edn. McGraw-Hill: 1999: 527.
29. Adair FE, Treatment of melanoma: report of four hundred cases. *Surg Gynecol Obstet* 1936; 62: 406–9.
30. Harwood AR, Cummings BJ, Radiotherapy for malignant melanoma: a re-appraisal. *Cancer Treat Rev* 1981; 8: 271–82.
31. Harwood AR, Dancuart F, Fitzpatrick PJ, Brown T, Radiotherapy in nonlentiginous melanoma of the head and neck. *Cancer* 1981; 48: 2599–605.
32. Ang KK, Byers RM, Peters LJ et al, Regional radiotherapy as adjuvant treatment for head and neck malignant melanoma. *Arch Otolaryngol Head Neck Surg* 1990; 116: 169–72.
33. Creagan ET, Cupps RE, Ivins JC et al, Adjuvant radiation therapy for regional nodal metastases from malignant melanoma. *Cancer* 1978; 42: 2206–10.
34. Johanson CR, Harwood AR, Cummings BJ, Quirt I, 0–7–21 Radiotherapy in nodular melanoma. *Cancer* 1983; 51: 226–32.
35. Burmeister BH, Smithers BM, Poulsen M et al, Radiation therapy for nodal disease in malignant melanoma. *World J Surg* 1995; 19: 369–71.
36. Fenig E, Eidelevich E, Njuguna E et al, Role of radiation therapy in the management of cutaneous malignant melanoma. *Am J Clin Oncol* 1999; 22: 184–6.
37. Strom EA, Ross M, Adjuvant radiation therapy after axillary lymphadenectomy for metastatic melanoma: toxicity and local control. *Ann Surg Oncol* 1995; 2: 445–9.

38. Storper IS, Lee SP, Abemayor E, Juillard G, The role of radiation therapy in the treatment of head and neck cutaneous melanoma. *Am J Otolaryngol* 1993; 14: 426–31.
39. Corry J, Smith J, Bishop M, Ainslie J, Nodal radiation therapy for metastatic melanoma. *Int J Radiat Oncol Biol Phys* 1999; 44: 1065–9.
40. Fuhrmann D, Lippold A, Borrosch F et al, Should adjuvant radiotherapy be recommended following resection of regional lymph node metastases of malignant melanomas? *Br J Dermatol* 2001; 144: 66–70.
41. Stevens G, Thompson JF, Firth I et al, Locally advanced melanoma: results of postoperative hypofractionated radiation therapy. *Cancer* 2000; 88: 87–93.
42. Byers RM, Treatment of the neck in melanoma. *Otolaryngol Clin N Am* 1998; 31: 833–9.
43. Dickson RJ, Malignant melanoma: a combined surgical and radiotherapeutic approach. *Am J Roentgenol* 1958; 79: 1063–70.
44. Gallardo D, Juillard G, Efficacy of radiation therapy in the local control of desmoplastic melanoma. Proceedings of the 36th Annual ASTRO Meeting, 1999.
45. Hellriegel W, Radiation therapy of primary and metastatic melanoma. *Ann NY Acad Sci* 1963; 100: 131–41.
46. Newman C, Wagner RF, Gordon W, Sanchez RL, Radiation therapy as an alternate therapy for locally recurrent acral lentiginous malignant melanoma. *Arch Dermatol* 1992; 128: 19–21.
47. Christie DRH, Tiver KW, Radiotherapy for melanotic freckles. *Australas Radiol* 1996; 40: 331–3.
48. Overgaard J, Gonzalez Gonzalez D, Hulshof MC et al, Randomised trial of hyperthermia as adjuvant to radiotherapy for recurrent or metastatic malignant melanoma. European Society for Hyperthermic Oncology. *Lancet* 1995; 345: 540–43.
49. Rosenthal MA, Bull CA, Coates AS et al, Synchronous cisplatin infusion during radiotherapy in the treatment of metastatic melanoma. *Eur J Cancer* 1991; 27: 1564–6.
50. Singletary SE, Byers RM, Shallenberger R et al, Prognostic factors in patients with regional cervical nodal metastases from cutaneous malignant melanoma. *Am J Surg* 1986; 152: 371–5.
51. Santini H, Byers RM, Wolf PF, Melanoma metastatic to cervical and parotid nodes from an unknown primary site. *Am J Surg* 1985; 150: 510–12.

36

Isolated limb perfusion for melanoma: technical aspects

H Schraffordt Koops, FJ Lejeune, BBR Kroon, JM Klaase, HJ Hoekstra

INTRODUCTION

The principle of regional perfusion using cytostatic drugs stems from an observation reported by Klopp et al.[1] in 1950. These investigators found that pain was alleviated and tumour volume decreased after small doses of nitrogen mustard (chlormethine) were injected directly into the regional arterial blood flow. The best results were obtained when venous return from the treated area was blocked. In 1959, Creech et al.[2] combined this vascular isolation procedure with extracorporeal circulation using a pump oxygenator. The isolated limb perfusion (ILP) technique was designed to obtain maximal tumour kill and minimal systemic toxicity. In 1956, Luck[3] reported that melphalan (L-phenylalanine mustard) was an effective agent in the treatment of melanomas in mice. Since then, melphalan has been the most widely used cytostatic agent for the treatment of extremity melanoma by ILP. In 1967, Cavaliere et al.[4] laid the foundations for ILP with hyperthermia when they described the selective susceptibility of cancer cells to high temperatures. Two years later, in 1969, Stehlin[5] described ILP under mild hyperthermic (39–40°C) conditions; this continues to be the most commonly used ILP technique. In 1992, Liénard et al.[6] reported promising results in melanoma patients treated by ILP using tumour necrosis factor (TNF).

PERFUSION TECHNIQUE

General endotracheal anaesthesia is used. Mild hyperthermic perfusion requires the extremity to be kept warm during the operation. For this reason, the limb is covered after skin preparation with a sterile warm-water-circulation blanket (paediatric size blanket roll), set at 40°C. The patient is positioned on the operation table so that an isolating bandage or tourniquet can be placed around the base of the limb.

The entire limb is prepped with a chlorhexidine scrub (this includes the abdomen, perineum and hip for lower limb perfusions, and the axilla, anterior chest, shoulder and neck for upper limb perfusions). The limb should be kept in the operating field to monitor temperature and blood flow. Lower limb perfusions are normally performed via the external iliac artery and vein. These are approached through a paramedian incision (Figure 36.1). The vessels are then approached through the retroperitoneal space, and an iliac and obturator lymph node dissection is performed. For external iliac perfusion, the inferior epigastric, circumflex and obturator vessels are ligated or clipped, and the internal iliac artery is temporarily occluded to improve isolation. The external iliac artery and vein are secured by placing rubber tapes around them.

The patient is then given heparin at a dosage of 200 IU/kg (3.3 mg/kg body weight). After 2 minutes have elapsed, the vessels are occluded with vascular clamps, a small incision is made in the anterior surface of the vein, and a flexible vinyl catheter is introduced. The same procedure is followed for the artery. A 14–16 FG catheter is generally used for an artery and a 18–22 FG catheter for a vein. However, the patient anatomy will indicate the proper diameter. Catheters are secured with rubber tapes and rubber tubing to prevent dislodgement during perfusion (Figure 36.2).

Collateral vessels of the skin and subcutaneous tissue are occluded with the aid of an Esmarch rubber bandage. A Steinmann pin is inserted into the iliac crest, and the rubber bandage is twisted around this pin and the upper thigh. The tips of the catheters should be located just caudal to this bandage.

The sterile tubing of an extracorporeal circuit, containing a pump oxygenator and heat exchanger, is primed with lactated Ringer's solution and whole blood in a ratio of 2:1, to which heparin has been added (Figures 36.3 and 36.4). Increasing the haematocrit of the perfusate to physiological levels by using whole blood can achieve a physiological tissue oxygenation at relatively low flow rates.[7]

The flow rate within the extracorporeal circuit and isolated limb is adjusted to 35–40 ml/l limb volume/minute. There is only one modular rotating pump for the arterial line, venous blood being recovered by gravity. Depending on systemic leakage, which is correlated with the flow rate,[8] the pump flow may vary considerably and can range from 150 to 750 ml/minute. It is important that the fluid level in the reservoir of the oxygenator is kept stable; therefore, the fluid level in the reservoir should be observed continuously during the perfusion period. The flow rate may go down to as little as 150 ml/minute in iliac perfusion in some cases, without jeopardizing results and without additional toxicity, provided the oxygen saturation levels do not drop <60%. In the past few years, it has been learnt from experiments with dogs that tissue perfusion during extracorporeal circulation differs from that in the non-perfused limb. Adequate tissue oxygenation could be

Figure 36.1 *Technique of lower extremity perfusion. a, iliac perfusion via the external iliac artery and vein; b, lymph node dissection and femoral perfusion; c, popliteal perfusion.*

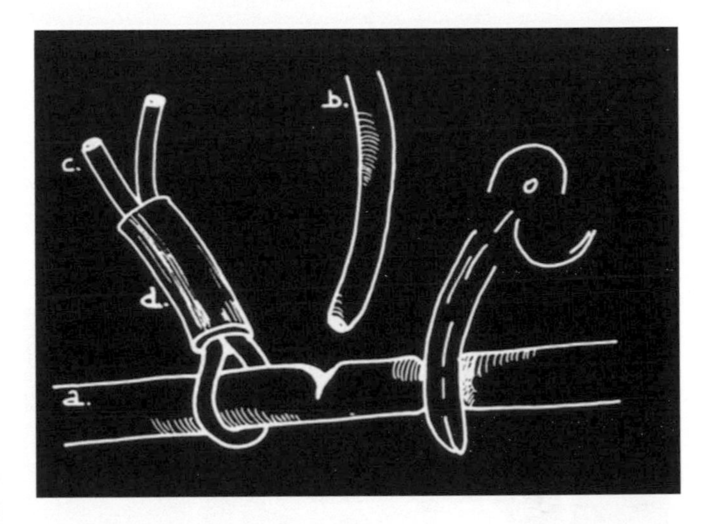

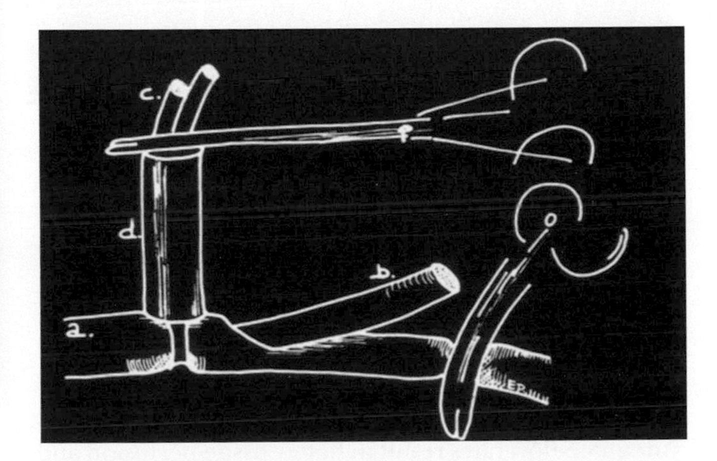

Figure 36.2 *Technique of catheter cannulation into the vessel. a, vessel; b, catheter; c, rubber tape; d, rubber tubings.*

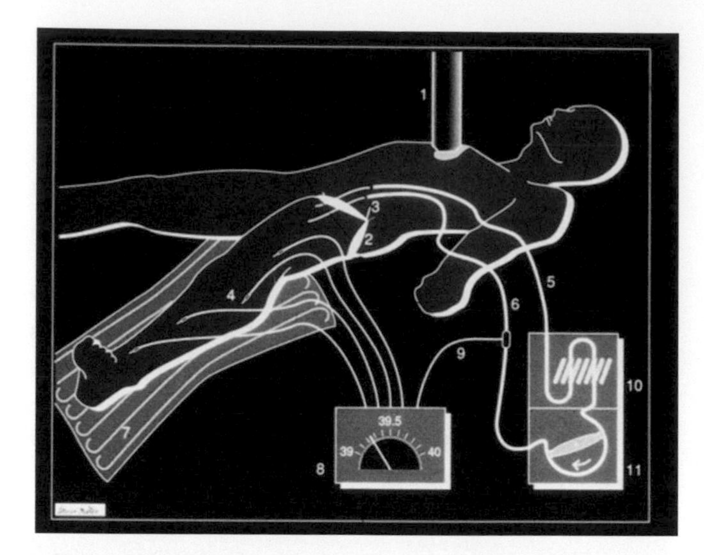

Figure 36.3 *Scheme of an iliac perfusion. 1, scintillation detector; 2, rubber tourniquet; 3, pin in the iliac crest; 4, muscle/subcutaneous thermometer; 5, venous line; 6, arterial line; 7, warm-water blanket; 8, temperature measurement; 9, temperature arterial blood; 10, bubble oxygenator and heat exchanger; 11, single/roller pump.*

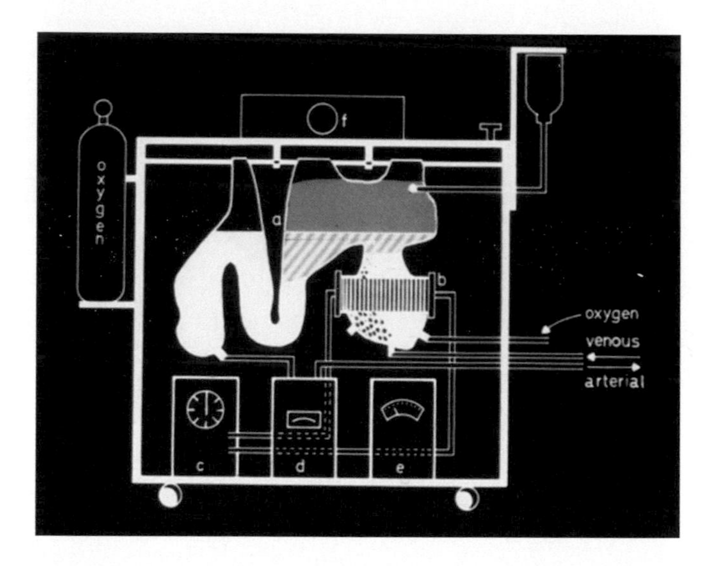

Figure 36.4 *The basic elements of the circuit are a roller pump, an oxygenator with an integrated reservoir, a heat exchanger, the interconnecting tubing and the perfusate. a, bubble oxygenator; b, heat exchanger; c, water bath for heating blood; d, roller pump; e, thermometer; f, balance.*

maintained only when the perfusion pressure was not <15 mmHg below systemic mean arterial pressure. Adequate flow rates result in better tissue perfusion and less drug toxicity.[9] An additional advantage of sufficient flow is that high tissue temperatures are attained more quickly. Low and inadequate flow rates are usually the result of improper placement of the catheters (e.g. when the catheter tip is just at the level of a venous valve) or incorrect positioning of the tourniquet. Adjustment of the catheter tip positions and/or adjustment of the tourniquet position may improve the flow rate, although minimization of systemic leakage should always be the top priority.

Limb temperatures are monitored by four thermistor probes inserted through the skin into the subcutaneous tissue and the muscles of the upper and lower parts of the limb. Administration of drug is started when the subcutaneous tissue temperature of the lower part of the limb reaches 38°C. With the help of the water-circulation blanket and heating of the perfusate, the limb temperature is then adjusted to the required temperature. The authors prefer a tissue temperature of 39–40°C (so-called 'mild' hyperthermia).

Any leakage to the systemic circulation can be monitored using a radioactive tracer. A small calibration dose of ^{131}I-albumin and a dose of ^{99}mTc-albumin are injected into the systemic circulation, while a larger dose of ^{131}I-albumin is injected into the extracorporeal circuit (10 times the calibration dose). Leakage from the perfusion region to the remainder of the body is indicated by the increased radioactivity in the systemic circulation, measured by means of a scintillation detector placed over the heart.[10] Leakage can be detected quantitatively and corrective measures undertaken.

The cytostatic is injected into the oxygenator or slowly into the arterial line (e.g. during one circulation time of the circuit), so that mixing can occur quickly. At the completion of the perfusion, after 60–90 minutes, a thorough washout is performed to remove drug and toxic end products from the isolated area. The rinse is performed using an indifferent fluid (e.g. isotonic saline). The tourniquet is released, the catheters withdrawn and the vessels repaired. The heparinization is reversed with 1.65 mg protamine chloride/kg body weight, or according to clotting time. Protamine sulfate is avoided because of hypotension that can occur during reversion.

The wound is closed and vacuum suction drains are left in the wound. At completion of the operation, a prophylactic fasciotomy of the lateral compartment of the lower leg is performed in some centres, to prevent compression of nerves as a result of oedema.[11] This is done via a 2 cm incision halfway between knee and ankle, and lateral to the fibula.

For femoral perfusions, the cannulas are introduced immediately below Poupart's ligament; this technique may require an inguinal lymph node dissection. For a femoral perfusion, the vena saphena can be used as an entry point for cannulating the femoral vein. For popliteal perfusion, the cannulas are introduced at the level of the adductor canal (Figure 36.1). The technique for femoral and popliteal perfusion is the same in principle as for an iliac perfusion. In the case of a popliteal perfusion, a blood pressure cuff can be used for occlusion of skin vessels instead of an Esmarch bandage.

For upper limb perfusion (Figure 36.5), an arm board is used for abduction of the extremity. The proximal portions of the axillary artery and vein are exposed. The pectoralis major muscle can be freed from the humerus to expose the vessels better. The pectoralis minor muscle can also be divided at its insertion. An axillary lymph node dissection may be performed because follow up examination of the axilla can be difficult and unreliable due to the presence of scar tissue caused by the perfusion operation. For distally located tumours a brachial perfusion can be performed, introducing the cannulas at the level of the brachial vessels.

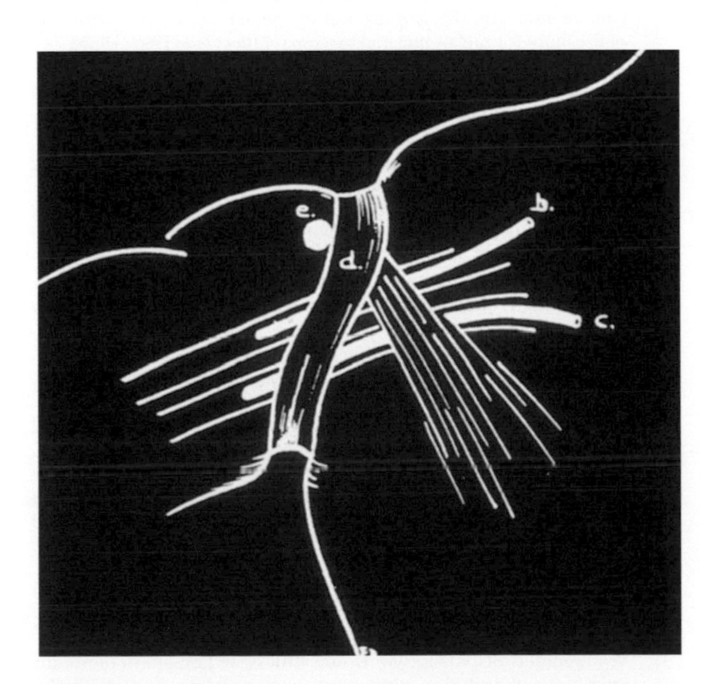

Figure 36.5 *Technique of upper extremity perfusion. b, arterial catheter; c, venous catheter; d, Esmarch bandage; e, Steinmann pin in the head of the humerus.*

In upper limb perfusions, smaller catheters are used than for the leg, usually a 12 or 14 FG catheter for the artery and a 16–18 FG catheter for the vein. Collateral vessels of the skin are occluded with an Esmarch bandage. A Steinmann pin is inserted into the head of the humerus, and the rubber bandage is twisted around this pin and the upper arm. The nerve plexus is protected by gauze sponges between the skin and the rubber bandage. For a brachial perfusion a tourniquet is applied around the upper arm. It is the authors' practice to perfuse for 60–90 minutes after the cytostatic drug has been injected.

To protect sensitive parts of the perfused limb (such as the hand or foot) from excessive toxic cytostatic reaction, Esmarch bandages can be wrapped tightly around the hand or the foot, in cases where there is no foot or hand involvement by the tumour.[12] This will reduce capillary flow in these areas and will result in less damage to the tissues by the cytostatic agent.

CHEMOTHERAPEUTIC AGENTS

Melphalan (L-phenylalanine mustard) is the drug most widely used for regional perfusion, either alone or in combination with other drugs, for patients with melanoma.

In the authors' institutions, the melphalan dosage has been calculated on the basis of the limb volume, as suggested by Wieberdink et al.[13] Prior to surgery, the arm or leg is immersed in water to determine the exact volume. For upper limb perfusions the standard dose of melphalan is 13 mg/l perfused tissue and for lower limb perfusions 10 mg/l perfused tissue. TNF, which seems to increase the number of complete responses in combination with melphalan, but is without proven impact on the limb recurrence-free interval, has a recommended dose regimen of 3 mg for an upper limb and 4 mg for a lower limb. The perfusion time varies for both drugs, being 90 minutes for TNF and 60 minutes for melphalan. The administration of TNF, the cytokine that is always used in combination with melphalan, is started when the subcutaneous tissue temperature of the lower part of the limb reaches 38°C.

Thrombosis prophylaxis is started the day after perfusion and continued until the patient is fully mobilized. Antibiotics are not routinely given in either the pre- or postoperative periods.

COMPLICATIONS

Tissue reactions in the extremity are seen *c.* 2 days after a hyperthermic perfusion. In most cases, the perfused extremity becomes red, warm, and slightly oedematous. The red discoloration fades to brown and over 3 months gradually turns to light brown. After 6 months, there is normally no visible evidence of the changes caused by perfusion. In a few cases, other local manifestations are seen (e.g. temporary loss of nails, drying or blistering of the skin of palms or soles, and inhibition of hair growth on the extremity). However, more severe tissue reactions, in the form of blistering of the skin, muscle damage and, rarely, a compartment syndrome may occur. This may lead to chronic limb function impairment, especially of the ankle.[14,15] Risk factors for more severe acute regional toxicity have recently been identified, with tissue temperatures >40°C and a high melphalan peak concentration being the most important.[16] With increased experience and improvement of isolation techniques, severe bone marrow depression (i.e. leucopenia and thrombocytopenia) should no longer occur.

The most common vascular complications described in the literature are thrombophlebitis, venous thrombosis and pulmonary embolism. It seems plausible that high heparin doses, used during the authors' perfusions, and postoperative thromboprophylaxis limit these complications, because they are very uncommon in the authors' centres.

Most patients undergoing ILP using TNF will experience a short-lived 'sepsis-like' systemic reaction over the first few hours following termination of the perfusion, due to the fact that, notwithstanding an optimal washout, a small amount of this very toxic cytokine will enter the systemic circulation. These reactions may be characterized by fever, a slight increase in cardiac output, a slightly diminished peripheral resistance, a minor activated clotting system abnormality and a slightly increased alveolar–arterial oxygen tension gradient. Normally, these events do not need to be monitored during the intensive care unit period. However, more severe 'sepsis-like' reactions may occur in some patients. Maintenance of adequate fluid hydration should be the main goal in this situation. In the case of a mild 'sepsis-like' reaction (systolic arterial pressure decreasing to 90 mmHg) treatment with vasoactive drugs, e.g. a dopamine infusion, should be considered. Moderate to severe 'sepsis-like' reactions should be treated with the appropriate therapeutic measures applicable for this clinical situation.[18]

CONCLUSIONS

ILP is a highly specialized surgical technique that requires special equipment not only for the perfusion but also for monitoring perfusate leak to the systemic circulation.[17] With an appropriate perfusion strategy, most perfusions can be performed with essentially no leakage, so that >80% of perfusions are performed with <2% of perfusate exposure to the systemic circulation.[18]

REFERENCES

1. Klopp C, Alford T, Bateman J et al, Fractionated intra-arterial cancer chemotherapy with methyl bisamine hydrochloride. A preliminary report. *Ann Surg* 1950; 132: 811–32.
2. Creech O, Ryan R, Krementz E, Treatment of malignant melanoma by isolation perfusion technique. *JAMA* 1959; 169: 339.
3. Luck J, Action of P-di(2–chloroethyl)-amino-L-phenylalanine on Harding Passey mouse melanoma. *Science* 1956; 123: 984.
4. Cavaliere R, Ciocatoo E, Giovanella B et al, Selective heat sensitivity of cancer cells. Biochemical and clinical studies. *Cancer* 1967; 20: 1351–81.
5. Stehlin JS, Hyperthermic perfusion with chemotherapy for cancers of the extremity. *Surg Gynecol Obstet* 1969; 129: 305–8.
6. Liénard D, Lejeune F, Delmotte J et al, High dose of TNF α in combination with IFN-gamma and melphalan in isolation perfusion of the limbs for melanoma and sarcoma. *J Clin Oncol* 1992; 10: 52–60.
7. Klaase JM, Kroon BBR, Slooten GW van et al, Comparison between the use of whole blood versus a diluted perfusate in regional isolated perfusion by continuous monitoring of transcutaneous oxygen tension: a pilot study. *J Invest Surg* 1994; 7: 249–58.
8. Klaase JM, Kroon BBR, Geel AN van et al, Systemic leakage during isolated limb perfusion for melanoma. *Br J Surg* 1993; 80: 1124–6.
9. Fontijne WPJ, Mook PH, Schraffordt Koops H et al, Improved tissue perfusion during pressure regulated hyperthermic regional isolated perfusion. A clinical study. *Cancer* 1985; 55–7: 1455–61.
10. Daryanani D, Komdeur R, Ter Veen J, et al, Continuous leakage measurement during hyperthermic isolated limb perfusion. *Ann Surg Oncol* 2001; 8: 566–72.
11. Schraffordt Koops H, Prevention of neural and muscular lesions during hyperthermic regional perfusion. *Surg Gynecol Obstet* 1972; 135: 402–3.
12. Thompson JF, Lai DTM, Ingvar C, Kam PCA. Maximising efficacy and minimising toxicity in isolated limb perfusion for melanoma. *Melanoma Res* 1994; 4 (Suppl 1): 45–50.
13. Wieberdink J, Benckhuizen C, Braat RP et al, Dosimetry in isolation perfusion of the limb by assessment of perfused tissue volume and grading of toxic tissue reactions. *Eur J Cancer Clin Oncol* 1982; 18: 905–10.
14. Olieman AFT, Schraffordt Koops H, Geertzen JHB et al, Functional morbidity of hyperthermic isolated regional perfusion of the extremities. *Ann Surg Oncol* 1994; 1: 382–8.
15. Vrouwenraets BC, Klaase JM, Kroon BBR et al, Long-term morbidity after regional perfusion with melphalan for melanoma of the limbs: the influence of acute regional toxic reactions. *Arch Surg* 1995; 130: 43–7.

16. Vrouwenraets BC, Klaase JM, Nieweg OE, Kroon BBR, Toxicity and morbidity of isolated limb perfusion. *Semin Surg Oncol* 1998; 14: 224–31.
17. Fraker DL, Hyperthermic regional perfusion for melanoma of the limbs. In: *Cutaneous Melanoma* (eds Balch ChM, Houghton AN, Sober AJ, Soong S-J) St Louis, MO: Quality Medical Publishing, Inc, 1998; 281–300.
18. Van Ginkel RJ, Limburg PC, Piers DA, Koops HS, Hoekstra HJ, Value of continuous leakage monitoring with radioactive Iodine-131-labeled human serum albumin during hyperthermic isolated limb perfusion with tumor necrosis factor-alpha and melphalan. *Ann Surg Oncol* 2002; 9: 355–63.

37

Isolated limb perfusion for melanoma: results and complications

Bart C Vrouenraets, Bin BR Kroon, Omgo E Nieweg, John F Thompson

INTRODUCTION

In 1957, Creech et al.[1] introduced the technique of isolated limb perfusion (ILP) in the treatment of melanoma. The main advantage of ILP is that by isolating a limb from the rest of the body, a high dose of anticancer drug (usually melphalan) can be delivered to a tumor-bearing region, thereby minimizing systemic exposure to the drug and subsequent generalized toxicity. The concept of ILP offers therapeutic advantages especially in the treatment of tumors with a relatively high tendency for locoregional recurrence, such as melanoma.

The value of ILP remains controversial because of the shortcomings of most studies of its use. Published results of ILP are typically limited to survival data, lack control groups, frequently contain small numbers of perfused patients, and often report results after only a short follow up period.[2] In many studies, the stage of disease and extent of associated surgery are not clearly defined. Also, little attention has been paid to the side effects of ILP, although the complication rate can be substantial. Authors usually confine themselves to remarking that increased experience, standardization of the ILP technique and technological improvements have permitted reduction of the most serious complications to a mimimum.[3–5]

RESULTS

Prophylactic isolated limb perfusion (ILP) as an adjuvant to local excision of primary melanoma

In a number of patients, melanoma recurs locoregionally because of the microscopic involvement of local tissues, regional lymphatics and soft tissues between the primary tumor and the regional lymph node basin.[6–8] Theoretically, the concept of treating an entire limb in an effort to eliminate these clinically undetectable tumor deposits makes sense, but can ILP really eliminate microscopic metastatic cells not removed by primary surgery, thereby preventing regional recurrence and, most importantly, improving survival? Numerous retrospective studies addressing this issue have been reported, using both historical and matched controls, with contradictory results: benefits could either not be demonstrated,[9–11] or could be shown only in rather small subgroups of patients with more deeply invasive melanomas.[12–15] The pitfalls of using retrospective studies to assess the impact of ILP on outcome were amply illustrated by two reports from The Netherlands.[16,17] A group of patients from Groningen treated with wide excision and ILP with melphalan was retrospectively compared to a similar group of patients from Sydney treated with wide excision only.[16] The study was confined to women with a melanoma on the lower limb with a Breslow thickness of ≥1.5 mm and a Clark level of IV or V; none underwent lymph node dissection. The two groups were similar in age, Breslow thickness, Clark level, ulceration and location of the primary lesion. Women with a melanoma of the leg (excluding the foot) who had been treated by adjuvant ILP had a significantly better 10-year disease-free survival rate (77 versus 45%), a significantly higher 10-year overall survival rate (81 versus 60%) and fewer locoregional recurrences (22 versus 54%) than women treated by excision only. Subsequently, the same patients from Groningen were compared with another matched group of patients who had not been perfused, from a nearby region in The Netherlands and Germany.[17] The selection criteria to match these two groups were: tumor location not in proximal third of upper arm or leg, a Clark level of III–IV, and a Breslow thickness of ≥1.5 mm. In contrast to the previous comparison, no effect attributable to ILP was demonstrated in time to limb recurrence, time to regional lymph node metastases, time to distant metastasis, disease-free interval or survival. This latter study by Franklin et al.[17] is theoretically superior to the former, as variations in factors such as skin complexion and sun exposure were reduced to a minimum, patient groups were considerably larger and the authors performed a multivariate analysis to correct for all the relevant prognostic factors.

The problem of performing adequate prospective randomized trials is well illustrated by two small prematurely closed trials, containing 37 and 30 patients each, that both appeared to support the use of adjuvant ILP for high-risk primary melanoma.[18–20] Both studies can be criticized severely for the small numbers of patients, the high recurrence rates in the control arms and the lack of a multivariate analysis of the data.

It was not until more than 25 years after the introduction of ILP that the first well-designed prospective study was commenced. This multi-institutional trial was conducted by the European Organisation for Research and Treatment of Cancer (EORTC) Melanoma Cooperative Group, the World Health Organization (WHO) Melanoma Program, and the North American Perfusion Group (NAPG) between 1984 and 1994, with 16 participating centers.[21] Patients with a melanoma of at least 1.5 mm in thickness were randomized to wide local excision with ILP or wide local excision alone. The decision to perform elective lymph node dissection was left to local policy. ILP was performed with melphalan, 10 mg/l of tissue for the lower limbs and 13 mg/l of tissue for the upper limbs. Perfusion was performed under 'mild' hyperthermic conditions (38–40°C) for a duration of 1 hour. Of 832 evaluable patients, 412 were randomized to wide excision only and 420 to wide excision plus 'mild' hyperthermic ILP with melphalan. Median patient age was 50 years, 68% of patients were female, 79% of melanomas were located on a lower limb and 47% had a thickness ≥3 mm. After a median follow up of 6.4 years there was a trend for a longer disease-free interval after ILP. The difference was significant only for the patients who had not undergone elective lymph node dissection. The impact of ILP was clearly on the occurrence – as first site of progression – of in-transit metastases, which were reduced from 6.6 to 3.3%, and of regional lymph node metastases, with a reduction of 16.7 to 12.6%. However, there was no benefit of ILP in terms of time to distant metastasis or survival. Side effects were higher after ILP and, although transient in most patients, there were two amputations for toxicity. Treatment costs were increased considerably by ILP and hospital stay was prolonged by 70%; also increased operating theatre time and additional staff and equipment were required to perform ILP.[21]

Because of the outcome of this well-conducted prospective trial, prophylactic ILP with melphalan cannot be recommended as an adjunct to wide excision in high-risk primary limb melanoma. It does not make sense to use a laborious and expensive procedure that carries a risk of morbidity to prevent or delay locoregional recurrences in only a small percentage of patients without improving survival. Such recurrences can generally be managed with local excision(s) or therapeutic lymph node dissection.

Prophylactic isolated limb perfusion (ILP) as an adjuvant to excision of recurrent melanoma

According to some authors, adjuvant ILP has a role in the treatment of patients with recurrent melanoma of the limbs.[22–25] In comparison to the reported 8–50% 5-year survival rate following surgical excision alone for locoregional limb recurrences,[26] large series suggest that ILP improves survival (28–73%) (Table 37.1).[3,26–32] These observations, however, are subject to the criticisms inherent in all retrospective analyses without

Table 37.1 *Five- and 10-year survival rates after local surgery with or without prophylactic isolated limb perfusion (ILP) in patients with locoregionally recurrent melanoma of the limbs*

Reference (year)	No. of patients*	5-year survival (%)			10-year survival (%)			LRR†
		II	IIIA	IIIAB	II	IIIA	IIIAB	(%)
Local surgery								
26 (1963)	75	–	50‡	8	–	–	–	–
Local surgery + ILP§								
27 (1980)	116	–	–	–	–	–	–	50
28 (1988)	117	75	70	36	–	50	23	–
29 (1988)	110	74	67	40	63	45	34	38
30 (1994)	216	57	45	25	–	–	–	45
3 (1994)	324	80	36	23	61	30	17	–
31 (1994)								
Rome	112	80‖	54	21	–	54	21	49
Milan	215	–	46	33	–	26	19	36
Mean	–	*73*	*48*	*28*	*62*	*37*	*21*	*43*

* MD Anderson staging system for melanoma: II, local recurrence/satellitosis; IIIA, in-transit metastases (≥3 cm from primary lesion, scar or skin graft); IIIAB, in-transit and regional lymph node metastases.
† Limb recurrence rate.
‡ II+IIIA.
§ Only series of >100 patients are listed.
‖ Di Filippo et al.,[32] (1989).

controls, i.e. the apparently improved survival may be purely a result of patient selection.

Moreover, a significant number of these patients will fail and again succumb to locoregionally recurrent disease, despite prophylactic ILP. After ILP and resection of all macroscopic tumor tissue, limb recurrence rates are reported to be of the order of 36–50% in large series.[27,29–31] The majority of these recurrences occur within 2–3 years of ILP,[27,29–31] the median duration of the limb recurrence-free interval is between 5 (MD Anderson stage IIIAB) and 9 (stage II) months.[30] On the other hand, meticulous removal of in-transit metastases cures the disease often enough to make it difficult to compare the effectiveness of any adjuvant treatment.[33]

In six retrospective comparative studies of patients with recurrent melanoma, a significant advantage of ILP over excision alone could not be convincingly demonstrated.[9,34–39] In only three of these studies did ILP decrease the locoregional failure rate significantly;[37–39] survival was affected in only one study.[39] Definite conclusions cannot be drawn because the treatment groups were too small, follow up periods were too short, and the treatment groups were neither homogeneous nor matched for important prognostic factors, such as site of the primary tumor, stage of disease, number of lesions, number of previous limb recurrences, tumor thickness and Clark level of the primary melanoma.[30,32,40]

In 1991, the Swedish Melanoma Study Group published the results of a prospective randomized trial involving 69 patients with recurrent melanoma (either local recurrences, satellitosis or in-transit metastases).[41] These patients were randomly allocated to radical surgery (36 patients) or radical surgery plus ILP with melphalan, using limb temperatures of 40–41.5°C (33 patients). Stratification was employed for localization to an upper or lower limb. With a mean observation time of 39 months, the tumor-free survival time was enhanced in the ILP group from 10 to 17 months ($P = 0.04$). The type of recurrence was similar in both groups but further recurrences within the limb were fewer in the ILP group: six versus 10 local recurrences, six versus nine in-transit metastases and three versus five regional lymph node metastases. Again, an overall survival advantage could not be demonstrated ($P = 0.28$). The authors concluded that ILP cannot be recommended as an adjuvant to excision of recurrent melanoma except in prospective randomized studies with a non-perfused control arm.[41] Because these future studies must achieve prolonged survival, large international trials will be needed. Until that time, prophylactic ILP as an adjunct to excision of recurrent melanoma cannot be recommended.

Therapeutic isolated limb perfusion (ILP) in locally advanced melanoma

With the advent of ILP, the need for amputation to control extensive limb melanoma has been reduced substantially.[42] Nowadays, such ablation is required only rarely for extensive or deeply infiltrative lesions associated with severe pain, bleeding and odor not responding to ILP.[43,44] Although the main indication for ILP has traditionally been these in-transit metastases not amenable to local surgery,[45,46] data on objective response rates in large series are rather scarce. All series in the literature that contained at least 10 patients with measurable disease are summarized in Tables 37.2–37.4: most data apply to recurrent disease and some include neglected primaries.

With ILP using melphalan, an average complete remission rate of *c.* 54% can now be obtained (Table 37.2) (Figures 37.1 and 37.2).[2] Complete remission rates have tended to improve over the years. ILP at the beginning of the perfusion era was associated with lower remission rates and complete remission rates have increased by *c.* 10% since 1988.[2,46] This may be attributed not only to the fact that most of the early ILPs were probably performed under less effective hypothermic conditions,[46] but also because ILP schedules have become more sophisticated. After ILP with melphalan, irrespective of tissue temperature, the median duration of complete remission ranges between 9 and 19 months, depending on the follow up period.[40,47] When complete remission is achieved, further limb recurrence develops in *c.* 44% of patients (range 24–54%) (Table 37.2)[2] after a relatively short median interval of 5–10 months.[32,40,48,49]

Strategies have been developed to improve the complete remission rate, such as multiple ILP schedules, application of hyperthermia, use of cytostatic agents other than melphalan and the introduction of biological response modifiers. It is interesting to note that the complete response rates of 'controlled' normothermic ILP (tissue temperature between 37 and 38°C) and of ILP performed under 'mild' hyperthermic conditions (39–40°C) are within the same wide range (39–76%).[40,48,50–52] Only by using borderline 'true' hyperthermia (41–42°C),[32,53,54] or by performing multiple ILPs,[55] do these complete response rates seem to improve significantly. No other drug is as effective as melphalan in the ILP setting, either as a single agent or in a multiple-agent regimen (Table 37.3).[2,56]

A recent development has been the introduction of recombinant tumor necrosis factor-alpha (TNF-α) to ILP (Table 37.4). The combination of this agent with interferon-gamma (IFN-γ) and melphalan was first used by Lejeune's group in Brussels.[57,58] Complete remission was achieved in 17 of 19 patients with melanoma treated for stage IIIA or IIIAB disease, with the majority having five or more melanoma nodules after failure of a previous ILP with either melphalan or cisplatin.[57,58] However, in a multicenter randomized phase II study,[59] response rates after ILP with the combination TNF-α, melphalan and, in half of the patients, IFN-γ, the complete remission rate was 73%. Limb recurrence or progression was observed in 59% of these patients, with a median time to recurrence/progression of 405 days. The addition of IFN-γ somewhat increased the complete remission rate from 69% with TNF-α and melphalan to 78% with the three-drug regimen. The corresponding times to local recurrence/progression were 327 and >498 days, respectively. The data from this study were compared with those of 103 patients with similar stage III regionally recurrent melanoma who were treated with standard melphalan ILP between 1980 and 1988 by the same teams. Melphalan ILP alone produced a lower complete response rate (52%), with a somewhat shorter median time to local recurrence/progression of 338 days. These data suggest that TNF-α associated with melphalan may be superior to melphalan alone in the ILP setting, especially in bulky disease, and that IFN-γ demonstrates a marginal additional benefit in terms of response rates.

Data from similar studies in Italy showed lower complete response rates with TNF-α, with or without IFN-γ, in the range of 50–70% (Table 37.4),[60–64] and most patients did not present with disease as bulky as that treated by Liénard et al.[57,58] Regional relapse rates ranged from 15 to 50%,[61–64] with relapses occurring after only a short median period of 6 months (range 3–14 months) following ILP.[61–64] These figures and the Italian results after 'borderline' hyperthermic (41–42°C) ILP with melphalan alone were considered to be essentially the same,[25,31,35,60,64] although the short follow up of the TNF-α series does not allow any definite conclusions to be drawn.

Table 37.2 *Complete response rates in patients with melanoma after isolated limb perfusion (ILP) with melphalan*

Reference (year)*	No. of patients	Complete response rate (%)	Tissue temperature (°C)	Limb recurrence rate (%)[†]
137 (1966)	10	40		50
36 (1975)	19	53	40[‡]	40
138 (1977)	14	21	40–42[‡]	
27 (1980)	80	26	39–40	
139 (1983)	15	7	>38	
47 (1983)	23	65	39–41	
140 (1985)	22	81	40	
53 (1985)	26	81	40.5–42	24
141 (1990)	41	49		
50 (1990)	35	60	39–40	
48 (1991)	17	76	39	47
54 (1992)	11	64	41–42	
142 (1992)	10	90	42–43[§]	
143 (1992)	70	36	40	
31 (1994)				
Rome	112	44	41–41.8	49
Milan	138	59	41–41.8	36
40 (1994)				
Single	73	44	37–38	46
Multiple	47	70	37–38	
51 (1995)	103	52	37–40	
144 (1995)	85	40	41.5	
52 (1996)	103	76	38–40	27
145 (1996)	16	56	40.5–42	
49 (1997)	105	74	40.5–41.5	54

*Only series of ≥10 patients are included.
[†] In patients with complete remission.
[‡] Temperature of heat exchanger.
[§] Hyperthermia and melphalan sequentially.

Although the complete remission rate of ILP in melanoma has increased considerably in the last decade, most studies have a relatively short follow up, without mention of the long-term durable complete response rate. In the few studies that do supply this information, the limb relapse rate after a complete remission is a disappointing 40–50%, and the corresponding limb disease-free interval is of only a short

Table 37.3 *Complete response rates in patients with melanoma after isolated limb perfusion with drugs other than melphalan*[36,66–73]

Reference (year)*	No. of patients	Complete response rate (%)	Drugs
36 (1975)	28	36	Thiotepa, melphalan
146 (1976)	54	13	Thiotepa, actinomycin D, melphalan
147 (1983)	12	17	Cisplatin
148 (1984)	14	0	Vindesine, dacarbazine, cisplatin
149 (1986)	19	32	Nitrogen mustard
150 (1987)	24	13	Dacarbazine
151 (1988)	12	0	Mouse monoclonal antibody R24
152 (1993)	24	33	Cisplatin
153 (1995)	10	10	Interleukin-2 and LAK† cells

*Only series of ≥10 patients are included.
† Lymphokine-activated killer.

Table 37.4 *Complete response rates in patients with melanoma after isolated limb perfusion with melphalan, tumor necrosis factor-alpha (TNF-α) and interferon-gamma (INF-γ)*

Reference (year)*	No. of patients	Complete response rate (%)	IFN-γ	Limb recurrence rate (%)†
57 (1992)	29	90	Yes	
154 (1994)	53	91	Yes	33
60 (1995)	47	57	In 12	
61 (1995)	10	50	–‡	
155 (1996)				
TNF-α 4 mg	25	76	Yes	53
TNF-α 6 mg	11	36	Yes	25
59 (1999)	64	73	In 32	–

*Only series of ≥10 patients are included.
† In patients with complete remission.
‡ Temperature ≥41°C.

duration. It also remains difficult to assess what proportion of patients with irresectable melanoma can obtain good palliation with ILP, as most reports do not indicate whether responses were obtained in locally inoperable melanoma or, as probably was the case in many series, in recurrent disease deliberately left in situ to monitor the effect of ILP. Because the macroscopic tumor burden (as expressed by the number of lesions, the total tumor surface area and the nodal status) is an important prognostic factor for tumor response and limb recurrence-free interval,[32,40] the local control rates in several reports are probably too optimistic for patients with locally inoperable melanoma.

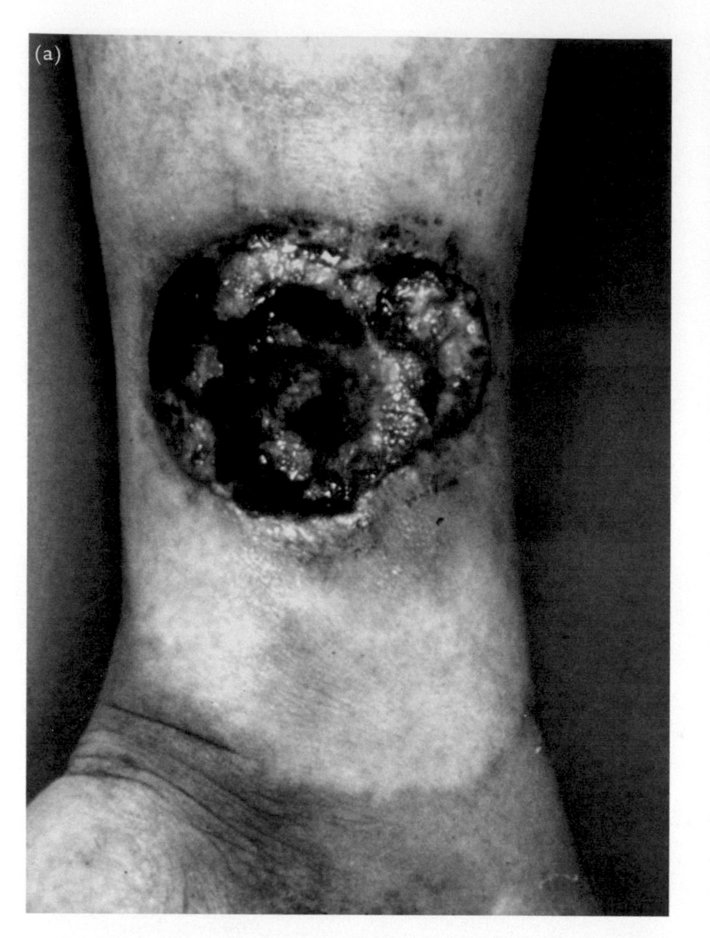

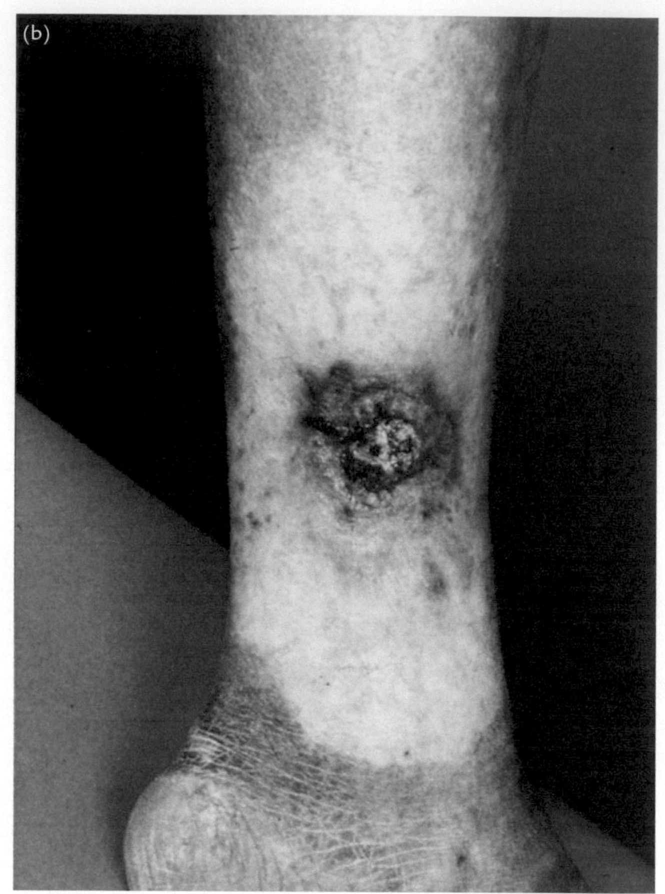

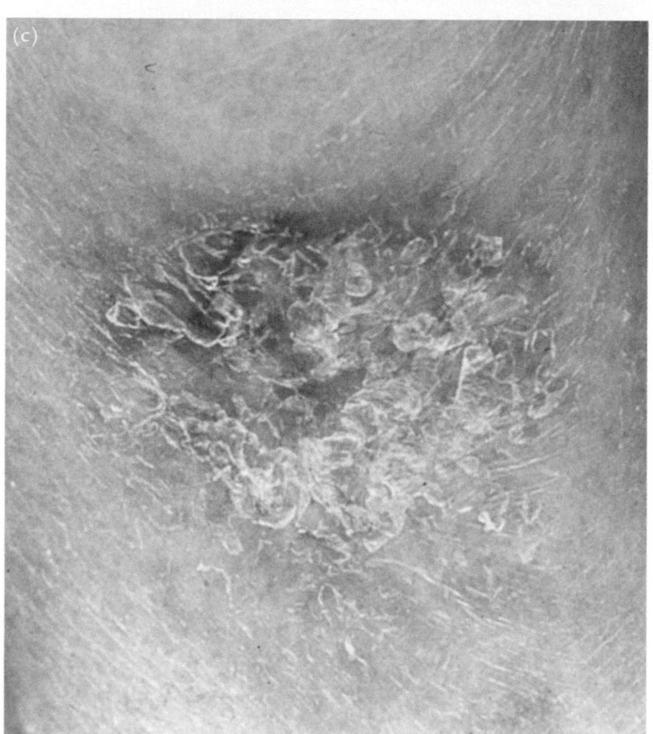

Figure 37.1 *(a) Neglected primary melanoma with bone involvement. (b) Partially regressed melanoma 3 months after ILP. (c) Complete remission 6 months after ILP.*

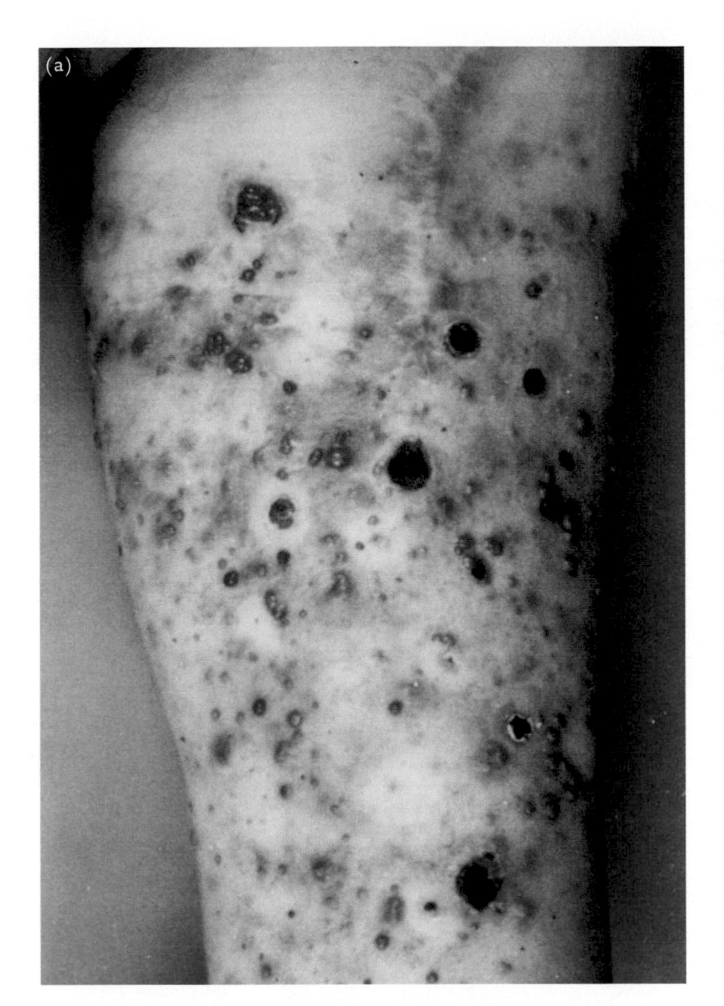

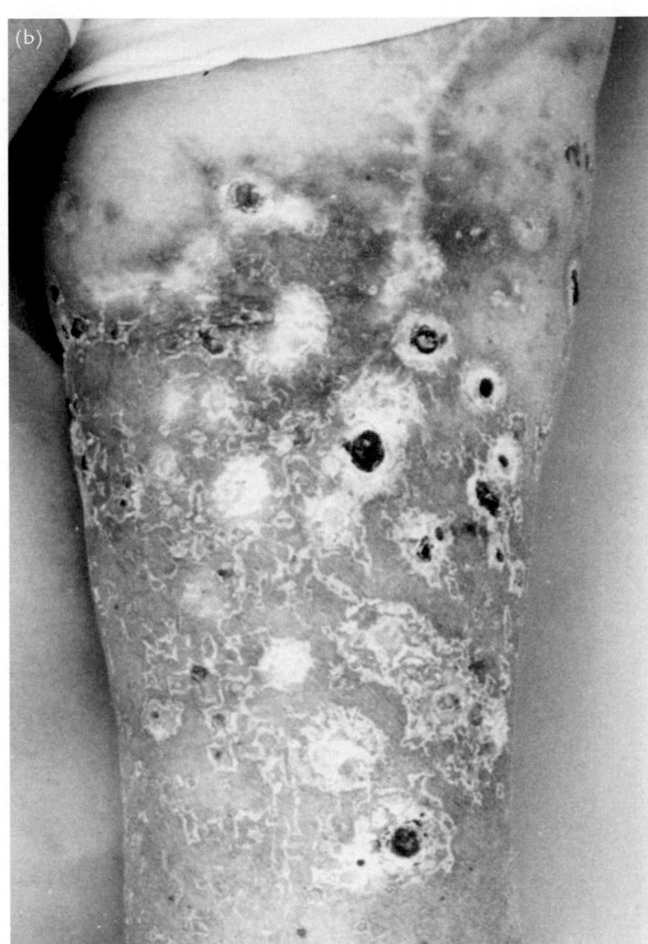

Figure 37.2 *(a) Extensive in-transit metastases of the left upper leg. (b) Six weeks after ILP with melphalan the metastases have almost disappeared, resulting in a complete remission some weeks later.*

Repeat isolated limb perfusion for recurrent melanoma of the limbs

Melanoma recurring locoregionally after ILP constitutes a therapeutic dilemma. Isolated limb recurrences can be successfully managed by excision[65] or, when they are multiple and small, by laser ablation.[66–68] When lesions are too numerous, too large or recurring too rapidly, repeat ILP can still result in high complete remission rates of 44–74%.[49,69–71] However, the subsequent limb recurrence rate after repeat ILP is high (71%) and the limb recurrence-free interval relatively short (11 months).[70] Since for repeat ILP more intensive schedules are usually used, toxicity is somewhat more pronounced.[70,71]

COMPLICATIONS

The side effects of ILP can be separated into acute toxic reactions in the perfused tissues, neurological and vascular complications, systemic toxicity and long-term morbidity. These complications can be caused by the cytostatic agent, usually melphalan, the application of hyperthermia, or ILP technique-related factors.

Acute regional toxicity

Slight edema, erythema and pain in a warm limb commonly develop within 48 hours after ILP with melphalan, and usually resolve within 14 days. The redness fades to brown, which gradually becomes lighter over a period of 3–6 months. Usually, there is no visible

Table 37.5 *Acute regional toxicity grading system according to Wieberdink et al.*[72]

Grade I	No reaction
Grade II	Slight erythema and/or edema
Grade III	Considerable erythema and/or edema with some blistering; slightly disturbed motility permissible
Grade IV	Extensive epidermolysis and/or obvious damage to the deep tissues, causing definite functional disturbances; threatening or manifest compartmental syndrome
Grade V	Reaction which may necessitate amputation

evidence of any change after *c.* 6 months. Other local manifestations are sometimes seen (e.g. temporary loss of nails, drying or blistering of skin of the palm of the hand or sole of the foot, inhibition of hair growth on the extremity, or transient neuralgia) but all recover over time.

A grading system for these toxic reactions in the normal tissues after ILP with melphalan was introduced by Wieberdink et al.[72] in 1982 (Table 37.5) (Figures 37.3 and 37.4). From published data of large series, one can conclude that moderate to severe acute skin/soft tissue reactions (grades III–V according to Wieberdink et al.)[72] occur in 7–37% of patients.[73,74]

Problems with the Wieberdink grading system are that it is more or less subjective and mixes reactions

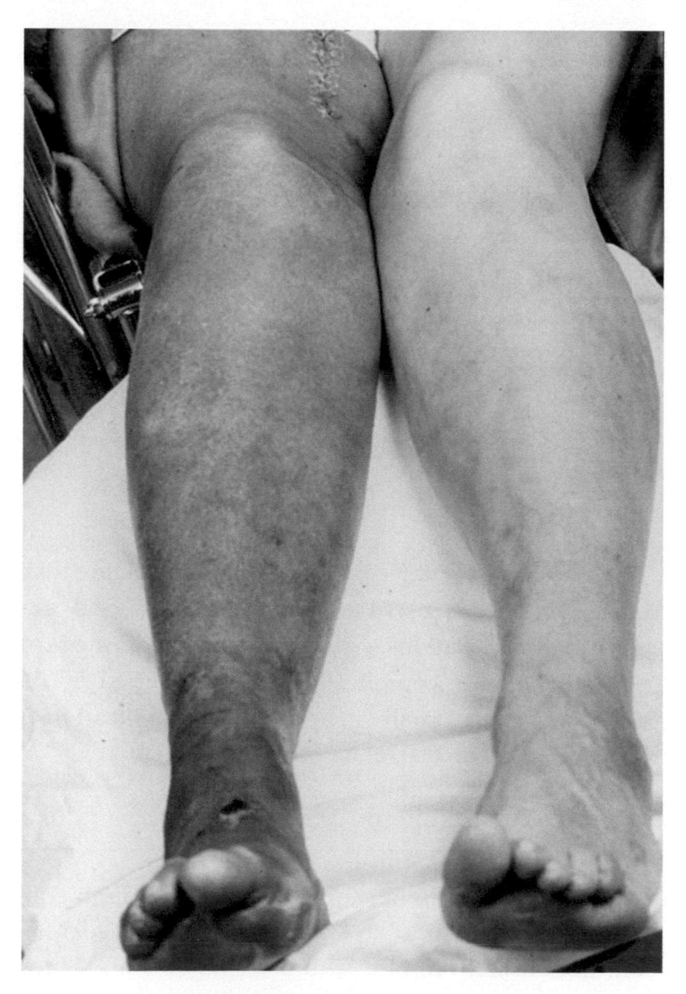

Figure 37.3 *Grade II acute regional toxicity reaction with erythema and edema.*

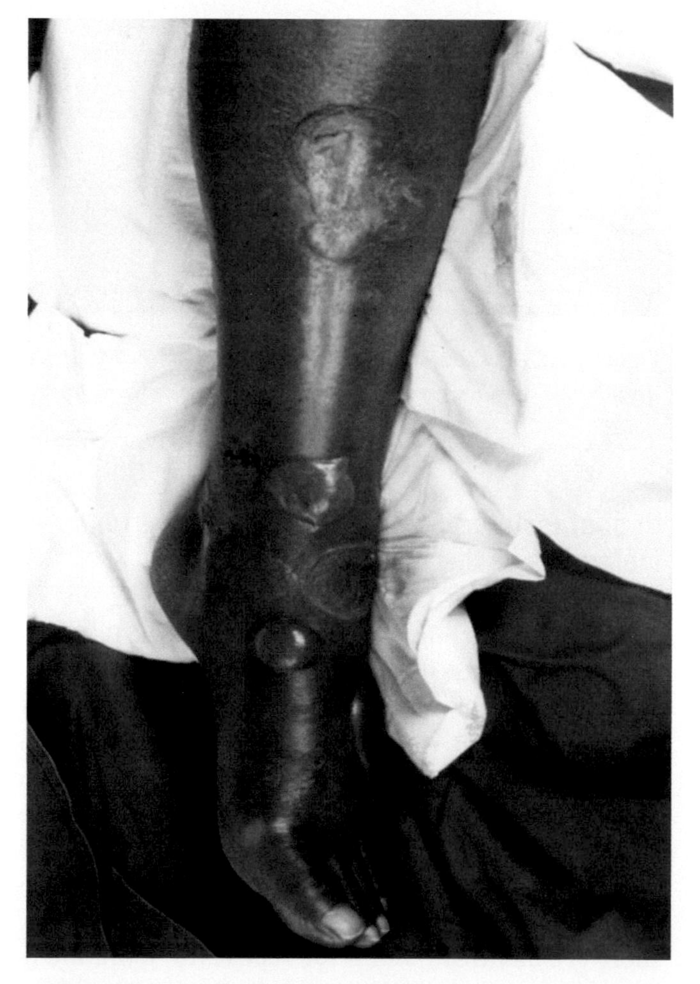

Figure 37.4 *Grade III reaction with considerable erythema, edema and blistering.*

of skin, soft tissues and nerves, which can all have a different etiology (e.g. due to the cytostatic drug and/or ILP-related factors). To establish a more objective and refined acute regional toxicity grading system, one could add creatine kinase (CK) levels, intracompartmental pressure, limb circumference measurements, and neurological examination.[75] The duration of a reaction could also be taken into account.[72,75] Pain could be described according to a standard pain score. Long-term morbidity should be recorded separately.

Although a dose–response relationship is likely, there is no evidence that more severe toxicity (grades III–V) is associated with a higher response rate or improved outcome.[76] Grade IV and V toxicity lead to permanent tissue damage and should be avoided at all cost. Wieberdink grade II toxicity usually resolves completely,[75,77] and probably indicates that the highest acceptable dose has been given.[72]

Factors influencing acute regional toxicity

A correlation has been demonstrated between acute regional toxicity and pharmacokinetic parameters (such as total melphalan dose, melphalan peak concentration, concentration at equilibrium, and area under the curve), tissue temperatures, sex, venous blood gas values of the perfusate, level of isolation, and perfusate flow rate.[72,78–80]

1. *Pharmacokinetic parameters*

Wieberdink et al.[72] reported a uniform degree of toxicity in limbs perfused with a fixed dose of melphalan per liter of tissue volume and normothermia (37–38°C). For upper limb ILP, this dose is 13 mg/l of perfused tissue and for lower limbs 10 mg/l of perfused tissue.[72,81] This dosage system eliminates variable factors, e.g. body weight, age, type of skin complexion, hair color, and decreases the risk of severe toxicity. Still, severe toxicity or absence of toxicity is occasionally seen.[4,9,78,82]

Recently, it has been demonstrated that toxicity is closely related to the melphalan peak concentration in the perfusate,[78–80] which, in turn, is determined by perfusion circuit volume and drug dosage. This finding highlights the importance of standardizing and optimizing not only the drug dosage but also the priming volume. Results obtained using a dye-dilution technique, which permits immediate calculation of the perfusion circuit volume, have revealed considerable interpatient variation in circuit volume measurements, corresponding with a wide range of melphalan peak concentrations, and may explain unexpected severe reactions.[82]

2. *Tissue temperatures*

Especially above 41°C, the thermal enhancement ratio of melphalan describes a steep upward curve,[83] with a significant increase in the risk of severe toxicity above 40°C.[73,80,83] The first clinical results obtained with 'true' hyperthermic (42.5–43.0°C) ILP were satisfactory in terms of tumor control.[84,85] However, a high incidence of major complications was observed (postoperative deaths, non-functional limbs, and arterial thrombosis requiring amputation). Therefore, at present, it is generally accepted that tissue temperatures should not exceed 42°C during ILP.[86,87]

With borderline 'true' hyperthermia (41–42°C), major complications have been seen in some institutions,[83] but not in others.[86,87] Explanations for this discrepancy have been sought in factors such as melphalan peak concentrations, the perfusate pH, and the maximum temperature of the perfusate.[86,87] Also, leakage of melphalan to the systemic circulation, leading to an unintentional dose reduction, may have played a role in limiting regional toxicity.[75] Some investigators using borderline 'true' hyperthermia inject the melphalan when tissue temperatures reach 38–40°C, and raise temperatures subsequently.[82] Since the melphalan concentration decreases rapidly,[81,88] a high melphalan concentration with concurrent high temperature, and potentiation of melphalan by heat, is avoided.

Mild hyperthermic conditions (38–40°C) do not seem to increase toxicity significantly.[75,89]

3. *Sex*

Women are at increased risk for developing toxicity.[73,77] This female risk factor may be attributed to the fact that women have a lower muscle/fat ratio than men. Since there is a higher melphalan uptake in muscle as opposed to fat,[90] the muscle tissue of female patients is exposed to a relatively higher dose of melphalan. Also, young patients with good limb musculature and minimal fat tolerate higher doses better than those with flabby muscles and increased fatty tissue.[3]

4. *Physiological conditions in the perfused limb*

Adequate oxygenation during ILP appears to be essential to provide a sufficient cellular energy supply to maintain cellular integrity. Hypoxic or anoxic conditions increase the permeability of blood vessels by damaging endothelial cells and impairing the tolerance of normal cells to melphalan. This leads to edema and necrosis of muscle and skin.[91] In vitro studies have shown that both a low level of oxygenation and a low pH increase cytotoxicity by melphalan, the magnitude of the enhanced toxic effect being greatest when hypoxia and acidic pH are combined.[92] This is probably due to an increased drug uptake and, consequently, greater exposure to it. Secondly, a small decrease in extracellular pH could increase the stability of melphalan by reducing the rate of hydrolysis.[93] Therefore, reduced oxygenation and a low pH during ILP might contribute to melphalan toxicity.[73,92]

5. *Isolation level*
An explanation for proximal isolation level as a risk factor for more severe toxicity is the fact that, at these levels, the absolute melphalan dose is higher, while usually no increased perfusate volume is used compared to more distal brachial and femoropopliteal isolation levels.[73,75] This results in higher melphalan peak concentrations, a condition demonstrated to be associated with more severe toxicity, as previously stated.

Prevention of severe acute regional toxicity

1. *Drug scheduling*
By using larger priming volumes and by prolonged injection or fractionated administration of melphalan, its peak concentration can be lowered without decreasing the absolute dose. The melphalan peak concentration can also be lowered by injecting the cytostatic into the venous reservoir of the oxygenator, instead of directly into the arterial line, so that mixing can occur first.[82]

One can also consider tailoring the dose of melphalan to meet the needs of individual patients, e.g. reducing drug doses by 10% for an obese extremity and increasing them by 10% for a muscular extremity.[79]

2. *Physiological conditions in the perfused limb*
Periods of oxygen depletion are inevitable during cannulation of the vessels and during re-establishment of the normal circulation at the end of the procedure. As these hypoxic periods may impair the tolerance of the normal tissues to melphalan by lowering tissue oxygenation and pH, they should be kept as short as possible.[72]

In ILP, a lowered hematocrit and elevated tissue temperatures generally account for a four to six times higher perfusion flow than normal to meet the oxygen demands of the normal tissues.[94] As high flow rates cause systemic leakage, and high venous pressures result in an increased incidence of edema and localized toxicity,[72,82] many ILP centers make use of high arterial oxygen tensions to meet oxygen needs.[92] In theory, a physiological drawback of high arterial oxygen tensions during ILP may be the production of oxygen-derived free radicals and gaseous microemboli, increased blood cell damage, and constriction of arterioles, all of which result in increased tissue toxicity. Physiological conditions seem to be guaranteed when a perfusate with a physiological hematocrit is used,[95,96] and this can have a protective effect against limb toxicity.[95]

3. *Distal tourniquet*
An important aspect of morbidity following ILP is the toxic effect on the foot or hand, with early pain and edema, and later epidermolysis and desquamation of the sole or palm (Figure 37.5). These sequelae sometimes cause considerable discomfort for several weeks, and prevent the patient from walking without difficulty or from using the hand for normal activities. Loss of nails may cause further discomfort. All these effects can be prevented by the simple maneuver of wrapping the foot or hand tightly with an Esmarch rubber bandage immediately before injection of the cytostatic drug into the perfusion circuit (Figure 37.6).[74] This technique is applicable, of course, only when the distal part of the limb is not affected by the disease.

4. *Monitoring creatinine kinase (CK) patterns*
Muscle damage as a result of ILP is a common phenomenon,[97,98] and acute renal failure due to severe rhabdomyolysis can occur.[99] Three CK patterns following ILP have been identified:[97] a normal CK pattern was defined by values that remained within normal limits; an early peak CK pattern was defined by values that peaked between the first and fourth post-ILP day; a late peak CK pattern was defined by values that peaked after the fifth post-ILP day. A clear association between a late peak CK pattern and severe limb toxicity has been demonstrated. In one series,[97] severe limb toxicity did

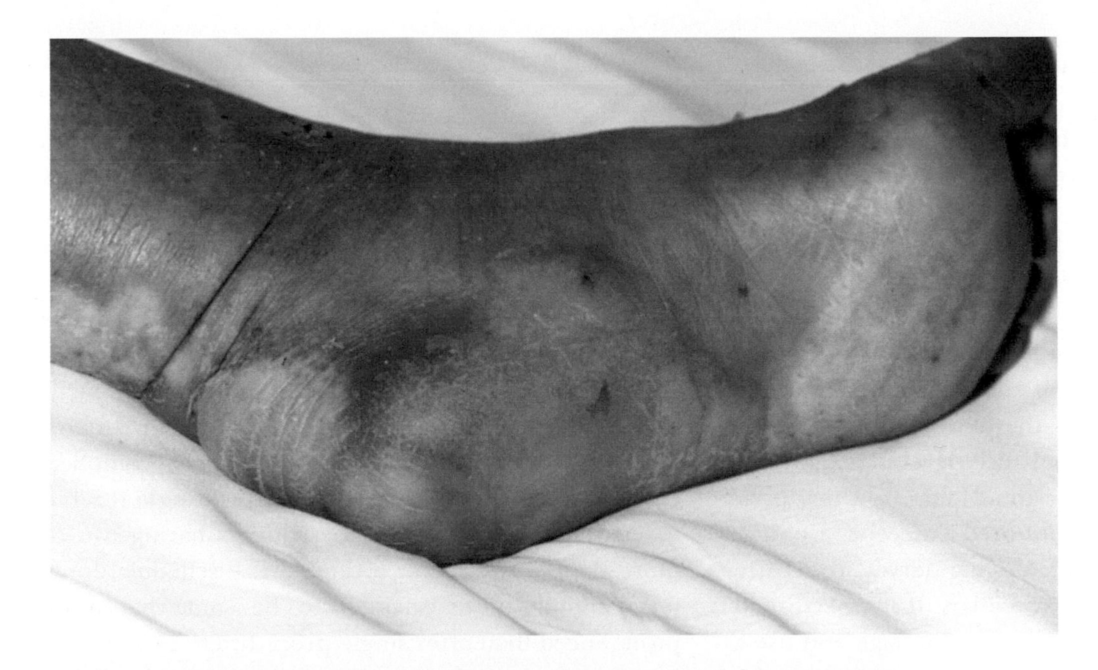

Figure 37.5 *Painful blistering of the sole 2 weeks after ILP.*

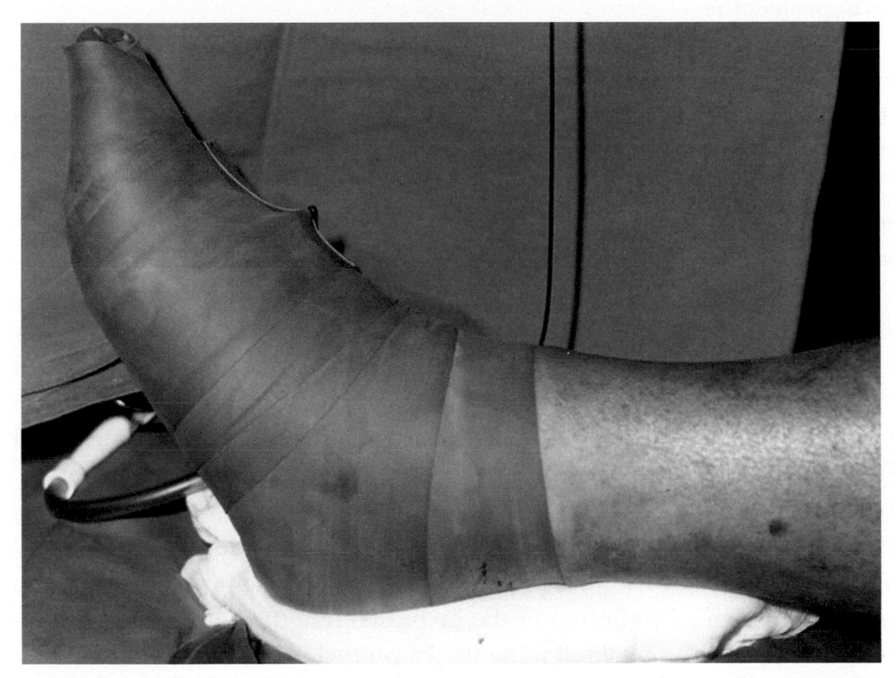

Figure 37.6 *The Esmarch rubber bandage around the foot of the perfused lower limb.*

not occur if CK values remained <1000 IU/l from the second post-ILP day onwards; however, in seven out of 15 limbs, severe toxicity developed when CK values exceeded 1000 IU/l on the second to fifth post-ILP days. Therefore, routine CK measurements following ILP are clinically useful, and close observation of a limb is required when the CK value exceeds 1000 IU/l after the first post-ILP day.[97,98] Also a rise in white blood cell count after the second post-ILP day can be an indicator of impending toxicity.[98]

5. *Prophylactic fasciotomy*

There is no agreement on the value of a routine prophylactic fasciotomy after ILP for prevention of a clinical or subclinical compartment compression syndrome, which may lead to late fibrosis and neuropathy.[100,101]

Neuropathy

One of the most troublesome side effects after ILP is neuropathy, which has been reported in a wide range

(1–48%) of perfused patients.[102] It can be caused by the drug, by a compartment compression syndrome or, in most cases, by pressure-induced damage resulting from a too tightly applied isolating bandage, especially at the axillary level.[102]

In axillary ILP, there is little control on the exerted pressure, because use is made of an elastic rubber Esmarch bandage which is wrapped around the root of the limb with rather uncontrolled force. The brachial plexus lacks the protection of enveloping muscular and subcutaneous tissues and is therefore especially prone to damage. At more distal ILP levels, isolation is achieved using an inflatable tourniquet in which pressure can be carefully monitored, thereby avoiding excessive pressure on the underlying nerves. To reduce the risk of nerve damage in axillary ILP, one should carefully apply the isolating rubber bandage and use a thick gauze pad underneath the bandage to protect the underlying brachial plexus.[102]

A causative role of the isolating tourniquet in the occurrence of neuropathy after ILP has been questioned.[34] Some authors noticed the development of edema in the regional muscles after ILP, leading to an acute compartment compression syndrome usually 2–3 days after ILP, and this was presumed to be the causative factor of the neuropathy.[100] Based on this observation, routine prophylactic fasciotomy was advocated after ILP.

Vascular complications

ILP has no effect upon macrovasculature of the perfused limb.[103] However, patients selected for ILP should be evaluated as to their potential for development of vascular complications: patients with severe arteriosclerotic disease are not suitable for this procedure.[103,104] In a large series,[105] the incidence of thrombosis at the arteriotomy site was 2.5% in 356 patients but re-exploration prevented serious morbidity in all cases.

Deep vein thrombosis can occur and is extremely difficult to diagnose clinically, since the effects of ILP itself mask the classical symptoms. Some authors routinely carry out Doppler flow studies in the post-ILP period.[106] However, the risk of venous thrombosis is probably limited by systemic anticoagulation postoperatively and early mobilization with the wearing of a graduated compression stocking.

Repeat ILP

Repeat ILP can be technically more difficult owing to the scar tissue produced by the previous procedure. Nevertheless, complications from the additional ILP generally relate to the drugs and hyperthermia, and not the surgical technique.[55,107] Authors usually advise performing repeat ILP in the same limb through more proximal arterial and venous sites, to avoid vascular complications.[3] An increase in acute regional toxicity and complication rates has been observed in patients undergoing repeat ILP.[3,108] One or more complications occurred in 28% of patients with a single ILP but the risk increased to 51% for patients having two or more ILPs.[108] Also, after a double ILP schedule, long-term complications seemed to be somewhat more pronounced than after single procedures.[55]

Regional lymph node dissection

Some postoperative complications of ILP can be at least partly attributed to a regional lymph node dissection that has been performed concomitantly. In these situations, lymphedema occurs frequently, although it can usually be controlled with properly graduated elastic stocking support.[77] The high percentage of lymphedema after concomitant regional lymph node dissection in lower limb ILP led some authors to treat their patients in two stages, with the lymph node dissection performed 4–6 weeks after ILP. This resulted in fewer complications.[109]

Healing of the lymphadenectomy wound is adversely affected by ILP, with wound infection and prolonged lymph discharge occurring frequently.[9,110] This is also reflected in the increased length of time spent in hospital following the combined procedure.[110] However, in one series,[111] ILP did not increase the morbidity of a regional lymph node dissection.

Long-term morbidity

In one large series, 44% of 367 patients showed some degree of objective or subjective morbidity 1 year after ILP.[77] Most had lymphedema (28%), but this was often related to a regional lymph node dissection performed at the same time. Acute regional toxic reactions had a causative effect on the incidence of long-term morbidity. Moderate to severe acute regional toxic reactions (grades III–V according to Wieberdink et al.)[72] were strongly linked to the occurrence of muscle atrophy or fibrosis and limb malfunction (Figure 37.7).

Only three other studies focused on the issue of functional morbidity.[112–114] The study by Van Geel et al.,[113] described 57 patients with a median follow up period of 5 years after ILP. There was only one case of severe subjective problems in the perfused limb. However, objective investigation showed lymphedema or atrophy in 20% of the 15 upper limbs and in 36% of the 42 lower limbs. In the upper limb, a disturbed mobility of the joints was found in four cases. In the lower limb, the ankle showed severe functional restriction in >25% of the cases. These results were confirmed by others,[114] reporting that functional impairments mainly concerned ankle mobility after ILP. Atrophy of the musculature of the lower leg was also common after iliac ILP. When perfused patients were compared to patients treated by wide excision only, however, no extra morbidity was seen after ILP in one series.[112]

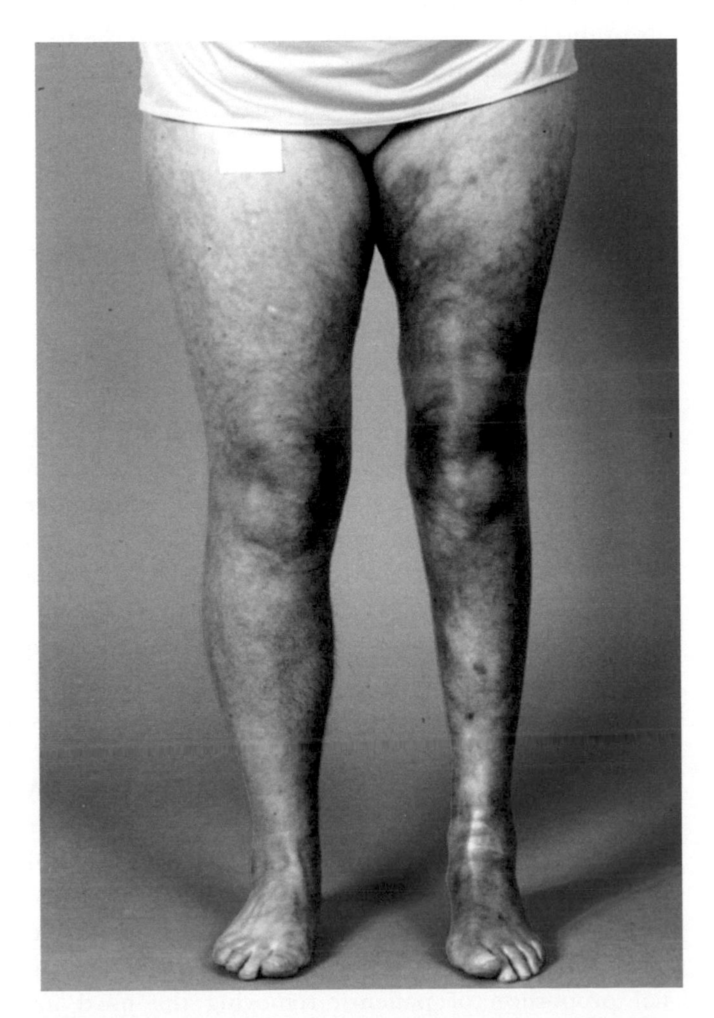

Figure 37.7 *Atrophy of the left lower limb 6 months after ILP.*

Systemic toxicity

Toxicity after systemic administration of melphalan includes bone marrow depression, hair loss, maculopapular rashes, pruritus, and gastrointestinal toxicity such as nausea and vomiting, diarrhea and stomatitis.[93] The concentration of melphalan in the perfusion circuit is *c.* 10 times higher than the concentration in blood after the maximum-tolerated dose for systemic administration.[115] During ILP, the melphalan peak concentration is *c.* 150 times higher in the perfusate than in the systemic circulation.[116] Therefore, optimal isolation of the limb is of utmost importance to avoid leakage of the drug into the systemic circulation. Total leakage values during ILP of up to 15% do not necessarily cause severe systemic toxicity.[117] After melphalan is given as a single dose at the start of ILP, the concentration of melphalan in the perfusate declines rapidly during the early phase of drug circulation; there is a 40–50% decrease after 10 minutes and after 30 minutes almost all melphalan has accumulated in the tissues.[81,88,115] Therefore, it is not surprising that melphalan toxicity to the bone marrow is related to leakage during the first 5–10 minutes of ILP.[118] Hence, melphalan should not be administered until hemodynamics have stabilized and no leakage of the perfusate into the systemic circulation is observed. In general, it is advisable to stop the ILP if the systemic leakage exceeds 10–20%. Risk factors associated with systemic leakage are a proximal level of isolation, a small diameter of the venous cannula, not ligating the internal iliac vein in iliac ILP,[119] and high limb venous pressures.[82] To reduce systemic leakage, these factors should be taken into account.

Mortality rates after ILP with melphalan range from 0 to 9%,[120,121] with reported deaths mainly occurring in the early years of ILP experience. Mortality usually results from pulmonary emboli, cardiac failure, renal failure or bone marrow depression.

Bone marrow depression is reported in up to 59% of perfused patients.[120] The maximum depression is usually reached during the second postoperative week, and peripheral blood counts begin to improve *c.* day 14, thereafter rising steadily. Apart from drug leakage, the total dose of melphalan has also been reported to influence bone marrow depression.[120] Despite very careful washout procedures at the end of ILP, systemic peak concentrations of melphalan have been observed after reconnection of the perfused limb to the systemic circulation.[119] This fraction of melphalan may derive from poorly flushed intravascular components of the limb or via release of tissue-bound drug.

Nausea and vomiting during the first 24 postoperative hours are common and these symptoms can be particularly distressing after ILP at the iliac level (which requires a sizeable incision through the musculature of the iliac fossa) because they cause a great deal of additional pain. It appears that the combination of melphalan, anesthetic agents, major surgery and postoperative narcotic analgesics given to control pain, is a powerful emetogenic stimulus. Also, pain itself and the release of toxic products from the perfused limb may be involved. Ondansetron, given intravenously at the time of anesthetic induction, has recently been reported to be effective in controlling nausea and vomiting in the great majority of patients after ILP.[122]

Diffuse toxic hair loss has been reported but is rare if adequate leakage control is achieved.[120]

ILP with drugs other than melphalan

Melphalan combined with TNF-α

Initially, high-dose TNF-α in ILP did not appear to add any regional toxicity compared to ILP with melphalan alone. Grade II skin toxicity (erythema) occurred in 24 of 31 patients and grade III skin toxicity (blistering) in the other seven patients.[57] In later reports, however, the rapidity of onset, the overall duration and the degree of most regional side effects appeared to be more prominent with TNF-α added to melphalan.[123] In one series,[124] a higher incidence of grade III reactions after ILP with TNF-α (36%) compared to normothermic or 'mild' hyperthermic ILP with melphalan alone (16%) was found. This was probably due to the higher temperature level (39–40 versus 37–38°C) at which the melphalan was administered in the TNF-α ILP, resulting in thermal enhancement of melphalan. Escalation of the TNF-α dose to 6 mg resulted in significant edema and cutaneous toxicity in some patients, and it appeared that the dose-limiting toxicity for this combination of agents had been reached.[125] Furthermore, ILP with TNF-α induces a mild, mainly sensory, neuropathy in perfused limbs, not disturbing either the functionality or the recovery time.[126]

In contrast with the negligible incidence of severe systemic side effects after modern ILP with melphalan, the complications associated with TNF-α in ILP can be impressive. Application of high doses of TNF-α, which in contrast to melphalan, maintains high stable drug levels in the perfusate throughout the ILP,[127] can lead to high systemic levels and induce a systemic inflammatory response syndrome similar to septic shock, comprising fever, chills, hypotension, and acute respiratory distress.[57,128] This toxicity is directly correlated to leakage during ILP.[128,129] When leakage is prevented and thorough washout is performed, only a short-lived (<1 hour) systemically measurable TNF-α peak is observed, and systemic toxicity is restricted to fever and limited to the day of the ILP.[130,131]

Cisplatin

Regional toxicity after ILP with cisplatin is high, with severe sensory and motor neurotoxicity.[132–134] The severity of the local toxicity seems to be related to the total amount of cisplatin administered.[132,134,135] When the temperature limit of 40°C is exceeded, regional toxicity increases dramatically.[132,134] Surprisingly, some authors use cisplatin with remarkable absence of local complications.[133,136] The reason for this discrepancy is not entirely clear but is probably due to the use of a lower dose of the drug.

CONCLUSIONS

Prophylactic ILP with melphalan cannot be recommended as an adjunct to standard excisional surgery in high-risk primary melanoma. In a large multicenter prospective randomized trial, no survival benefit was seen for the ILP-treated group, although ILP reduced the number of locoregional recurrences. In the only available small prospective randomized trial involving patients with recurrent melanoma, prophylactic ILP decreased the incidence of further locoregional metastases, compared with excision of recurrences alone. Again, no survival advantage was demonstrated. A large multicenter trial will be needed to assess whether ILP provides a survival advantage. For patients with locally inoperable limb melanoma, ILP appears to be the treatment of choice, since it results in complete disappearance of all macroscopic disease in a substantial proportion of patients, removing the need for amputation and providing palliation of symptoms.

However, high limb recurrence rates and short durations of response need improvement. Results of alternative treatments should be compared prospectively with those of ILP in this clinical situation.

A relationship between toxicity and treatment outcome has not been demonstrated for ILP with melphalan, therefore, it is important to keep the side effects of the procedure to a minimum. Risk factors for more severe acute regional toxicity have been recently identified, with tissue temperatures above 40°C and high melphalan peak concentrations being the most important. Acute regional toxicity should be mild when these risk factors are taken into account and when the normal physiological conditions in the limb are maintained during ILP. This should also decrease the incidence of long-term morbidity, especially ankle stiffness and muscle atrophy, since a relation between the severity of the acute regional tissue reactions and the occurrence of long-term morbidity has been demonstrated. A concomitant regional lymph node dissection increases the incidence of lymphedema significantly and it may therefore be useful for this operation to be delayed until the acute regional tissue reactions have subsided. It is not yet clear whether the addition of TNF-α to melphalan increases regional toxicity. In the absence of leakage to the systemic circulation during ILP, systemic toxicity is minimal, even when TNF-α is used. Compared to ILP with melphalan ± TNF-α, ILP with other drugs is less effective and is, in some cases, associated with increased regional toxicity.

REFERENCES

1. Creech Jr O, Krementz ET, Ryan RF, Winblad JW, Chemotherapy of cancer: regional perfusion utilizing an extracorporeal circuit. *Ann Surg* 1958; 148: 616–32.
2. Vrouenraets BC, Nieweg OE, Kroon BBR, Thirty-five years of isolated limb perfusion for melanoma: indications and results. *Br J Surg* 1996; 83: 1319–28.
3. Krementz ET, Carter RD, Sutherland CM et al, Regional chemotherapy for melanoma: a 35-year experience. *Ann Surg* 1994; 220: 520–35.
4. Vrouenraets BC, Klaase JM, Nieweg OE, Kroon BBR, Toxicity and morbidity of isolated limb perfusion. *Semin Surg Oncol* 1998; 14: 224–31.
5. Taber SW, Polk Jr HC, Mortality, major amputations, and leukopenia after isolated limb perfusion with phenylalanine mustard for the treatment of melanoma. *Ann Surg Oncol* 1997; 4: 440–5.
6. Cascinelli N, Bufalino R, Marolda R et al, Regional non-nodal metastases of cutaneous melanoma. *Eur J Surg Oncol* 1986; 12: 175–80.
7. Lee Y-TM, Local-regional primary and recurrent melanoma: III. Update of natural history and non-systemic treatment (1980–1987). *Cancer Treat Rev* 1988; 15: 135–62.
8. Wong JH, Cagle LA, Kopald KH et al, Natural history and selective management of in transit melanoma. *J Surg Oncol* 1990; 44: 146–50.
9. Stehlin JS, Clark RL, Melanoma of the extremities: experience with conventional treatment and perfusion in 339 cases. *Am J Surg* 1965; 110: 366–83.
10. Golomb FM, Bromberg J, Dubin N, A controlled study of the survival experience of patients with primary malignant melanoma of the distal extremities treated with adjuvant isolated perfusion. In: *Adjuvant Therapy of Cancer*, 2nd edn, (eds Jones SE, Salmon SE). New York: Grune and Stratton, 1979: 519–26.
11. McKay AJ, Lingam MK, Scott RN et al, A single center prospective study of adjuvant isolated limb perfusion. In: *Advances in the Biology and Clinical Management of Melanoma* (eds Balch CM, Fidler IJ, Kripke ML). MD Anderson Cancer Center Department of Scientific Publications: Houston, TX, 1995: 117–18 (abstract).
12. McBride CM, Smith JL, Brown BW, Primary malignant melanoma of the limbs: a re-evaluation using microstaging techniques. *Cancer* 1981; 48: 1463–8.
13. Rege VB, Leone LA, Soderberg CH et al, Hyperthermic adjuvant perfusion chemotherapy for stage I malignant melanoma of the extremity with litreature review. *Cancer* 1983; 52: 2033–9.
14. Tonak J, Hohenberger W, Weidner F, Göhl H, Hyperthermic perfusion in malignant melanoma: 5-year results. *Rec Results Cancer Res* 1983; 86: 229–38.
15. Edwards MJ, Soong S-J, Boddie AW et al, Isolated limb perfusion for localized melanoma of the extremity. *Arch Surg* 1990; 125: 317–21.
16. Martijn H, Schraffordt Koops H, Milton GW et al, Comparison of two methods of treating primary malignant melanomas Clark IV and V, thickness 1.5 mm and greater, localized on the extremities. *Cancer* 1986; 57: 1923–30.
17. Franklin HR, Schraffordt Koops H, Oldhoff J et al, To perfuse or not to perfuse? A retrospective comparative study to evaluate the effect of adjuvant regional perfusion in patients with stage I extremity melanoma with a thickness of 1.5 mm or greater. *J Clin Oncol* 1988; 6: 701–8.
18. Ghussen F, Nagel K, Groth W et al, A prospective randomized study of regional extremity perfusion in patients with malignant melanoma. *Ann Surg* 1984; 200: 764–8.
19. Ghussen F, Kruger I, Smalley RV, Groth W, Hyperthermic perfusion with chemotherapy for melanoma of the extremities. *World J Surg* 1989; 13: 598–602.
20. Fenn NJ, Horgan K, Johnson RC et al, A randomized controlled trial of prophylactic isolated cytostatic perfusion for poor-prognosis primary melanoma of the lower limb. *Eur J Surg Oncol* 1997, 23: 6–9.
21. Schraffordt Koops H, Vaglini M, Suciu S et al, Prophylactic isolated limb perfusion for localized, high-risk limb melanoma: results of a multicenter randomized phase III trial. *J Clin Oncol* 1998; 16: 2906–12.
22. Yeung RSW, Recurrent cutaneous melanoma: a surgical perspective. *Semin Oncol* 1993; 20: 400–18.
23. Bowers GJ, Copeland EM, Surgical limb perfusion for extremity melanoma. *Surg Oncol* 1994; 3: 91–102.
24. Singletary SE, Balch CM. Recurrent regional metastases and their management. In: *Cutaneous Melanoma* (eds Balch CM, Houghton AN, Milton GW et al). London: JB Lippincott, 1992: 427–35.
25. Cavaliere R, Di Filippo F, Giannarelli D et al, Hyperthermic antiblastic perfusion in the treatment of local recurrence or 'in-transit' metastases of limb melanoma. *Semin Surg Oncol* 1992; 8: 374–80.
26. Treidman L, McNeer G, Prognosis with local metastasis and recurrence in malignant melanoma. *Ann NY Acad Sci* 1963; 100: 123–30.
27. Rosin RD, Westbury G, Isolated limb perfusion for malignant melanoma. *Practitioner* 1980; 244: 1031–6.
28. Stehlin JS, Greeff PJ, De Ipolyi PD et al, Heat as an adjuvant in the treatment of advanced melanoma: an immune stimulant? *Houston Med J* 1988; 4: 61–82.
29. Baas PC, Schraffordt Koops H, Hoekstra HJ et al, Isolated regional perfusion in the treatment of local recurrence, satellitosis and in-transit metatstases of extremity melanoma. *Reg Cancer Treat* 1988; 1: 33–6.

30. Klaase JM, Kroon BBR, Van Geel AN et al, Limb recurrence-free interval and survival in patients with recurrent melanoma of the extremites treated with normothermic isolated perfuson. *J Am Coll Surg* 1994; 178: 564–72.
31. Cavaliere R, Cavaliere F, Deraco M et al, Hyperthermic antiblastic perfusion in the treatment of stage IIIA–IIIAB melanoma patients: comparison of two methods. *Melanoma Res* 1994; 4 (Suppl 1): 5–11.
32. Di Filippo F, Calabro A, Giannarelli D et al, Prognostic variables in recurrent limb melanoma treated with hyperthermic antiblastic perfusion. *Cancer* 1989; 63: 2551–61.
33. Lee Y-TM, Loco-regional recurrent melanoma: II. Non-systemic treatments (1964–1979). *Cancer Treat Rev* 1988; 15: 105–33.
34. McBride CM, Clark RL, Experience with L-phenylalanine mustard dihydrochloride in isolation-perfusion of extremities for malignant melanoma. *Cancer* 1971; 28: 1293–6.
35. Santinami M, Belli F, Cascinelli N et al, Seven years experience with hyperthermic perfusions in extracorporeal circulation for melanoma of the extremities. *J Surg Oncol* 1989; 42: 201–8.
36. Cox KR, Survival after regional perfusion for limb melanoma. *Aust NZ J Surg* 1975; 45: 32–6.
37. Singletary SE, Tucker SL, Boddie AW, Multivariate analysis of prognostic factors in regional cutaneous metastases of extremity melanomas. *Cancer* 1988; 61: 1437–40.
38. Reintgen DS, Cruse CW, Wells KE et al, Isolated limb perfusion for recurrent melanoma of the extremity. *Ann Plast Surg* 1992; 28: 50–54.
39. Brobeil A, Berman C, Cruse CW et al, Efficacy of hyperthermic isolated limb perfusion for extremity-confined recurrent melanoma. *Ann Surg Oncol* 1998; 5: 376–83.
40. Klaase JM, Kroon BBR, Van Geel AN et al, Prognostic factors for tumor response and limb recurrence-free interval in patients with advanced melanoma of the limbs treated with regional isolated perfuson with melphalan. *Surgery* 1994; 115: 39–45.
41. Hafström L, Rudenstam C-M, Blomquist E et al, Regional hyperthermic perfusion with melphalan after surgery for recurrent malignant melanoma of the extremities. *J Clin Oncol* 1991; 9: 2091–4.
42. Kapteijn BA, Klaase JM, Van Geel AN et al, Results of regional isolated perfusion in locally inoperable melanoma of the limbs. *Melanoma Res* 1994; 4: 135–8.
43. Kourtesis GJ, McCarthy WH, Milton GW, Major amputations for melanoma. *Aust NZ J Surg* 1983; 53: 241–4.
44. Jacques DP, Coit DG, Brennan MF, Major amputation for advanced malignant melanoma. *Surg Gynecol Obstet* 1989; 169: 1–7.
45. Rampen FHJ, Towards a rational perfusion strategy for malignant melanoma. *Eur J Surg Oncol* 1985; 11: 117–78.
46. Kroon BBR, Regional isolation perfusion in melanoma of the limbs: accomplishments, unsolved problems, future. *Eur J Surg Oncol* 1988; 14: 101–10.
47. Lejeune FJ, Deloof T, Ewalenko P et al, Objective regression of unexcised melanoma in-transit metastases after hyperthermic isolation perfusion of the limbs with melphalan. *Rec Results Cancer Res* 1983; 86: 268–76.
48. Neades GT, Evans WD, Mansel RE, Choice of agent and predicton of systemic toxicity in isolated hyperthermic limb perfusion. *Reg Cancer Treat* 1991; 3: 252–5.
49. Thompson JF, Hunt JA, Shannon KF, Kam PC, Frequency and duration of remission after isolated limb perfusion for melanoma. *Arch Surg* 1997; 132: 903–7.
50. Kettelhack C, Kraus T, Hupp T et al, Hyperthermic limb perfusion for malignant melanoma and soft tissue sarcoma. *Eur J Surg Oncol* 1990; 16: 370–5.
51. Lejeune FJ, High dose recombinant tumor necrosis factor (rTNFα) administered by isolation perfusion for advanced tumors of the limbs: a model for biochemotherapy of cancer. *Eur J Cancer* 1995; 31A: 1009–16.
52. Lingam MK, Byrne DS, Aitchison T et al, A single centre's 10 year experience with isolated limb perfusion in the treatment of recurrent malignant melanoma of the limb. *Eur J Cancer* 1996; 32A: 1668–73.
53. Storm FK, Morton DL, Value of hyperthermic limb perfusion in advanced recurrent melanoma of the lower extremity. *Am J Surg* 1985; 150: 32–5.
54. Kroon BBR, Klaase JM, Van Geel BN, Eggermont AMM, Application of hyperthermia in regional isolated perfusion for melanoma of the limbs. *Reg Cancer Treat* 1992; 4: 223–36.
55. Klaase JM, Kroon BBR, Van Geel AN et al, A retrospective comparative study evaluating the results of a single-perfusion versus double-perfusion schedule with melphalan in patients with recurrent melanoma of the lower limb. *Cancer* 1993; 71: 2990–4.
56. Thompson JF, Gianoutsos MP, Isolated limb perfusion for melanoma: effectiveness and toxicity of cisplatin compared with that of melphalan and other drugs. *World J Surg* 1992; 16: 227–33.
57. Liénard D, Lejeune FJ, Ewalenko P, In transit metastases of malignant melanoma treated by high dose rTNFα in combination with interferon-γ and melphalan in isolation perfusion. *World J Surg* 1992; 16: 234–40.
58. Liénard D, Ewalenko P, Delmotte J-J et al, High-dose recombinant tumor necrosis factor alpha in combination with interferon gamma and melphalan in isolation perfusion of the limbs for melanoma and sarcoma. *J Clin Oncol* 1992; 10: 52–60.
59. Liénard D, Eggermont AM, Schraffordt Koop H et al, Isolated limb perfusion with tumor necrosis factor-alpha and melphalan with or without interferon-gamma for the treatment of in-transit metastases: a multicentre randomized phase II study. *Melanoma Res* 1999; 9: 491–502.
60. Santinami M, Chiti A, Deraco M et al, Does αTNF improve complete responses in perfusion of IIIA–IIIAB limb's melanoma? VII. International Congress on Regional Cancer Treatment, Wiesbaden, 1995: 94 (abstract).
61. Di Filippo F, Rossi RC, Anza M et al, Hyperthermic antiblastic perfusion with TNF-alpha and melphalan in the treatment of stage II–III limb melanoma. VII. International Congress on Regional Cancer Treatment, Wiesbaden, 1995: 89 (abstract).
62. Vaglini M, Belli F, Ammatuna M et al, Treatment of primary or relapsing limb cancer with high-dose alpha-tumor necrosis factor, gamma-interferon, and melphalan. *Cancer* 1994; 73: 483–92.
63. Vaglini M, Santinami M, Manzi R et al, Treatment of in-transit metastases from cutaneous melanoma by isolation perfusion with tumor necrosis factor-alpha (TNF-α), melphalan and interferon-gamma (IFN-γ): dose-finding experience at the National Cancer Institute of Milan. *Melanoma Res* 1994; 4 (Suppl 1): 35–8.
64. Vaglini M, Carraro O, Belli F et al, αTNF + L-PAM for stage IIIA–IIIAB extremities' melanoma. *Eur J Surg Oncol* 1994; 20: 322–3 (abstract).
65. Feldman AL, Alexander Jr HR, Bartlett DL et al, Management of extremity recurrences after complete responses to isolated limb perfusion in patients with melanoma. *Ann Surg Oncol* 1999; 6: 562–7.
66. Hill S, Thomas JM, Use of carbon dioxide laser to manage cutaneous metastases from malignant melanoma. *Br J Surg* 1996; 83: 509–12.
67. Lingam MK, McKay AJ, Carbon dioxide laser ablation as an alternative for cutaneous metastases from malignant melanoma. *Br J Surg* 1995; 82: 1346–8.
68. Strobbe LJ, Nieweg OE, Kroon BBR, Carbon dioxide laser for cutaneous melanoma metastases: indications and limitations. *Eur J Surg Oncol* 1997; 23: 435–8.
69. Vaglini M, Ammatuna M, Belli F et al, Evaluation of a second isolated perfusion for melanoma of the limbs. *Melanoma Res* 1993; 3: 100 (abstract).
70. Klop WMC, Vrouenraets BC, Van Geel BN et al, Repeat isolated limb perfusion with melphalan for recurrent melanoma of the limbs. *J Am Coll Surg* 1996; 182: 467–72.
71. Bartlett DL, Ma G, Alexander HR et al, Isolated limb reperfusion with tumor necrosis factor and melphalan in patients with extremity melanoma after failure of isolated limb perfusion with chemotherapeutics. *Cancer* 1997; 80: 2084–90.
72. Wieberdink J, Benckhuijsen C, Braat RP et al, Dosimetry in isolation perfusion of the limbs by assessment of perfused tissue volume and grading of toxic tissue reactions. *Eur J Cancer Clin Oncol* 1982; 18: 905–10.
73. Klaase JM, Kroon BBR, van Geel AN et al, Patient and treatment related factors associated with acute regional toxicity after isolated perfusion for melanoma of the extremities. *Am J Surg* 1994; 167: 618–20.
74. Thompson JF, Lai DTM, Ingvar C et al, Maximizing efficacy and minimizing toxicity in isolated limb perfusion for melanoma. *Melanoma Res* 1994; 4 (Suppl 1): 45–50.

75. Vrouenraets BC, Kroon BBR, Klaase JM et al, Severe acute regional toxicity after normothermic or 'mild' hyperthermic isolated limb perfusion with melphalan for melanoma. *Melanoma Res* 1995; 5: 425–31.
76. Vrouenraets BC, Hart GA, Eggermont AMM et al, Relation between limb toxicity and treatment outcomes after isolated limb perfusion for recurrent melanoma. *J Am Coll Surg* 1999; 188: 522–30.
77. Vrouenraets BC, Klaase JM, Kroon BBR et al, Long-term morbidity after regional isolated perfusion with melphalan for melanoma of the limbs: the influence of acute regional toxic reactions. *Arch Surg* 1995; 130: 43–7.
78. Liénard D, Lejeune F, Autier Ph et al, Physiological and pharmacokinetics parameters in isolaton perfusion of the limbs. In: *Malignant Melanoma: Medical and Surgical Management* (eds Lejeune FJ, Chaudhuri PK, Das Gupta T). New York: McGraw-Hill, 1994: 241–8.
79. Klaase JM, Kroon BBR, van Slooten GW, Benckhuijsen C, Relation between calculated melphalan peak concentrations and toxicity in regional isolated perfusion for melanoma. *Reg Cancer Treat* 1992; 4: 309–12.
80. Thompson JF, Eksborg S, Kam PCA et al, Determinants of acute regional toxicity following isolated limb perfusion for melanoma. *Melanoma Res* 1996; 6: 267–71.
81. Benckhuijsen C, Kroon BBR, van Geel AN, Wieberdink J, Regional perfusion treatment with melphalan for melanoma in a limb: an evaluation of drug kinetics. *Eur J Surg Oncol* 1988; 14: 157–63.
82. Thompson JF, Good PD, Kam PCA, Hyperthermic isolated limb perfusion in the treatment of melanoma: technical aspects. *Reg Cancer Treat* 1994; 1: 147–54.
83. Kroon BBR, Klaase JM, van Geel BN, Eggermont AMM, Application of hyperthermia in regional isolated perfusion for melanoma of the limbs. *Reg Cancer Treat* 1992; 4: 223–36.
84. Cavaliere R, Ciocatto EC, Giovanella BC et al, Selective heat sensitivity of cancer cells: biochemical and clinical studies. *Cancer* 1967; 20: 1351–81.
85. Stehlin Jr JS, Hyperthermic perfusion with chemotherapy for cancers of the extremities. *Surg Gynecol Obstet* 1969; 129: 305–8.
86. Pace M, Galli A, Bellacci A, Local and systemic toxicity in 'borderline true' hyperthermic isolated perfusion for lower limb melanoma. *Melanoma Res* 1995; 5: 371–6.
87. Cavaliere R, Cavaliere F, Deraco M et al, Hyperthermic antiblastic perfusion in the treatment of stage IIIA–IIIAB melanoma patients: comparison of two methods. *Melanoma Res* 1994; 4 (Suppl 1): 5–11.
88. Thompson JF, Kam PCA, Razan, Yau DF, Clinical pharmacokinetics of melphalan in isolated limb perfusion: compartmental modelling and moment analysis. *Reg Cancer Treat* 1994; 8: 83–7.
89. Klaase JM, Kroon BBR, Eggermont AMM et al, A retrospective comparative study evaluating the results of mild hyperthermic versus controlled normothermic perfusion for recurrent melanoma of the extremities. *Eur J Cancer* 1995; 31A: 58–63.
90. Scott RN, Blackie R, Kerr DJ et al, Melphalan in isolated limb perfusion for malignant melanoma, bolus or divided dose, tissue levels, the pH effect. In: *Progress in Regional Cancer Therapy* (eds Jakesz R, Rainer H). Berlin: Springer, 1990: 195–200.
91. Wieberdink J, *Physiological Considerations Regarding Isolation Perfusion of the Extremities.* Meppel: Krips Repro, 1978.
92. Vrouenraets BC, Kroon BBR, van de Merwe SA et al, Physiological implications of hyperbaric oxygen tensions in isolated limb perfusion using melphalan: a pilot study. *Eur Surg Res* 1996; 28: 235–44.
93. Furner RL, Brown RK, L-Phenylalanine mustard (L-PAM): the first 25 years. *Cancer Treat Rep* 1980; 64: 559–74.
94. Fontijne WPJ, Mook Ph, Elstrodt JM et al, Isolated hindlimb perfusion in dogs: the effect of perfusion pressures on the oxygen supply (p_tO_2 histogram) to the skeletal muscle. *Surgery* 1985; 97: 278–84.
95. Krementz ET, Saha S, Limb perfusion with melphalan for melanoma by increased dose and dilution compared to standard technique: a pilot study. *Reg Cancer Treat* 1989; 2: 233–7.
96. Klaase JM, Kroon BBR, van Slooten GW et al, Comparison between the use of whole blood versus a diluted perfusate in regional isolated perfusion by continuous monitoring of transcutaneous oxygen tension: a pilot study. *J Invest Surg* 1994; 7: 249–58.
97. Lai DTM, Ingvar C, Thompson JF, The value of monitoring serum creatine phosphokinase following hyperthermic isolated limb perfusion for melanoma. *Reg Cancer Treat* 1993; 1: 36–9.
98. Vrouenraets BC, Kroon BBR, Klaase JM et al, Value of laboratory tests in monitoring acute regional toxicity after isolated limb perfusion. *Ann Surg Oncol* 1997; 4: 88–94.
99. Rauschecker HF, Osterloh B, Acute renal failure following hyperthermic isolation perfusion of the left leg. *Anticancer Res* 1987; 7: 451–4.
100. Schraffordt Koops H, Prevention of neural and muscular lesions during hyperthermic regional perfusion. *Surg Gynecol Obstet* 1972; 135: 401–3.
101. Hohenberger P, Finke LH, Schlag PM, Intracompartmental pressure during hyperthermic isolated limb perfusion for melanoma and sarcoma. *Eur J Surg Oncol* 1996; 22: 147–51.
102. Vrouenraets BC, Eggermont AMM, Klaase JM et al, Long-term neuropathy after regional isolated perfusion with melphalan for melanoma of the limbs. *Eur J Surg Oncol* 1994; 20: 681–5.
103. Klein ES, Walden R, Ben-Ari GY, Peripheral blood flow studies following isolated limb perfusion with cisplatin. *Reg Cancer Treat* 1993; 3: 137–9.
104. Muchmore JH, Krementz ET, Kerstein MD, Noninvasive evaluation of peripheral vasculature following regional hyperthermic chemotherapeutic perfusion. *Am Surg* 1987; 53: 94–6.
105. Klicks RJ, Vrouenraets BC, Nieweg OE, Kroon BBR, Vascular complications of isolated limb perfusion. *Eur J Surg Oncol* 1998; 29: 288–91.
106. Rosin DR, Isolated limb perfusion: past experience and present studies using a minimal-access approach. *Melanoma Res* 1994; 4 (Suppl 1): 51–7.
107. Klop WMC, Vrouenraets BC, van Geel AN et al, Repeat isolated limb perfusion with melphalan for recurrent melanoma. *J Am Coll Surg* 1996; 182: 467–72.
108. Krementz, ET, Ryan RF, Carter RD et al, Hyperthermic regional perfusion of the limbs. In: *Cutaneous Melanoma: Clinical Management and Treatment Worldwide* (eds Balch CH, Milton GW). Philadelphia: Lippincott, 1985: 171–90.
109. Lejeune FJ, Deloof T, Ewalenko P et al, Objective regression of unexcised melanoma in-transit metastases after hyperthermic isolation perfusion of the limbs with melphalan. *Rec Results Cancer Res* 1983; 86: 268–76.
110. Bulman AS, Jamieson CW, Isolated limb perfusion with melphalan in the treatment of malignant melanoma. *Br J Surg* 1980; 67: 660–2.
111. Baas PC, Schraffordt Koops H, Hoekstra HJ et al, Groin dissection in the treatment of lower-extremity melanoma: short-term and long-term morbidity. *Arch Surg* 1992; 127: 281–6.
112. Olieman AFT, Schraffordt Koops H, Geertzen JHB et al, Functional morbidity of hyperthermic isolated regional perfusion of the extremities. *Ann Surg Oncol* 1994; 1: 382–8.
113. van Geel AN, van Wijk J, Wieberdink J, Functional morbidity after regional isolated perfusion of the limbs for melanoma. *Cancer* 1989; 63: 1092–6.
114. Vrouenraets BC, In't Veld GJ, Nieweg OE, Van Slooten GW, Van Dongen JA, Kroon BBR, Long-term functional morbidity after mild hyperthermic isolated limb perfusion with melphalan. *Eur J Surg Oncol* 1999; 25: 503–8.
115. Briele HA, Djuric M, Jung DT et al, Pharmacokinetics of melphalan in clinical isolation perfusion of the extremities. *Cancer Res* 1985; 45: 1885–9.
116. Scott RN, Kerr DJ, Blackie R et al, The pharmacokinetic advantages of isolated limb perfusion with melphalan for malignant melanoma. *Br J Cancer* 1992; 66: 159–66.
117. Hoekstra HJ, Naujocks T, Schraffordt Koops H et al, Continuous leakage monitoring during hyperthermic isolated regional perfusion of the lower limb: techniques and results. *Reg Cancer Treat* 1992; 4: 301–4.
118. Neades GT, Evans WD, Mansel RE, Choice of agent and prediction of systemic toxicity in isolated hyperthermic limb perfusion. *Reg Cancer Treat* 1991; 3: 252–1.
119. Klaase JM, Kroon BBR, van Geel AN et al, Systemic leakage during isolated limb perfusion for melanoma. *Br J Surg* 1993; 80: 1124–6.

120. Sonneveld EJA, Vrouenraets BC, van Geel BN et al, Systemic toxicity after isolated limb perfusion with melphalan for melanoma. *Eur J Surg Oncol* 1996; 22: 521–7.
121. Taber SW, Polk Jr HC, Mortality, major amputations, and leukopenia after isolated limb perfusion with phenylalanine mustard for the treatment of melanoma. *Ann Surg Oncol* 1997; 4: 440–5.
122. Thompson JF, Malouf DJ, Merzliakov S, Kam PCA, Efficacy of single-dose ondansetron in the prevention of post-operative nausea and vomiting following isolated limb perfusion with cytostatic agents. *Reg Cancer Treat* 1993; 4: 177–82.
123. Fraker DL, Alexander HR, Isolated limb perfusion with high-dose tumor necrosis factor for extremity melanoma and sarcoma. In: *Important Advances in Oncology 1994* (eds DeVita VT, Hellman S, Rosenberg SA). Philadelphia: JB Lippincott, 1994: 179–92.
124. Vrouenraets BC, Eggermont AMM, Hart AAM et al, Regional toxicity after isolated limb perfusion with melphalan and tumor necrosis factor α versus toxicity after melphalan alone. *Eur J Surg Oncol* 2001; 27: 390–5.
125. Yang JC, Fraker DL, Thom AK et al, Isolation perfusion with tumor necrosis factor-α, interferon-γ, and hyperthermia in the treatment of localized and metastatic cancer. *Rec Results Cancer Res* 1995; 138: 161–5.
126. Drory VE, Lev D, Groozman GB et al, Neurotoxicity of isolated limb perfusion with tumor necrosis factor. *J Neurol Sci* 1998; 158: 1–4.
127. Gérain J, Liénard D, Ewalenko P, Lejeune FJ, High serum levels of TNFα after its administration for isolation perfusion of the limbs. *Cytokine* 1992; 4: 585–91.
128. Zwaveling JH, Maring JK, Clarke FL et al, High plasma tumor necrosis factor (TNF)-α concentrations and a sepsis-like syndrome in patients undergoing hyperthermic isolated limb perfusion with recombinant TNF-α, interferon-γ, and melphalan. *Crit Care Med* 1996; 24: 765–70.
129. Thom AK, Alexander HR, Andrich MP et al, Cytokine levels and systemic toxicity in patients undergoing isolated limb perfusion with high-dose tumor necrosis factor, interferon gamma, and melphalan. *J Clin Oncol* 1995; 13: 264–73.
130. Swaak AJG, Liénard D, Schraffordt Koops H et al, Effects of recombinant tumor necrosis factor alpha (rTNFα) in cancer: observations of the acute phase protein reaction and immunoglobin synthesis after high dose rTNFα administration in isolated limb perfusions in cancer patients. *Eur J Clin Invest* 1993; 23: 812–18.
131. Vrouenraets BC, Kroon BBR, Ogilvie AC et al, Absence of severe systemic toxicity after leakage-controlled isolated limb perfusion with TNFα and melphalan. *Ann Surg Oncol* 1999; 6: 405–12.
132. Thompson JF, Gianoutsos MP, Isolated limb perfusion for melanoma: effectiveness and toxicity of cisplatin compared with that of melphalan and other drugs. *World J Surg* 1992; 227–33.
133. Coit DG, Isolation limb perfusion for melanoma: current trends and future direction. *Melanoma Res* 1994; 4 (Suppl 1): 57–60.
134. Busse O, Aigner K, Wilimzig H, Peripheral nerve damage following isolated extremity perfusion with cis-Platinum. *Rec Results Cancer Res* 1983; 86: 264–7.
135. Guchelaar H-J, Hoekstra HJ, de Vries EGE et al, Cisplatin and platinum pharmacokinetics during hyperthermic isolated limb perfusion for human tumors of the extremities. *Br J Cancer* 1992; 65: 898–902.
136. Papa MZ, Klein E, Karni T et al, Regional hyperthermic perfusion with cisplatin following surgery for malignant melanoma of the extremities. *Am J Surg* 1996; 171: 416–20.
137. Irvine WT, Luck RJ, Review of regional limb perfusion with melphalan for malignant melanoma. *BMJ* 1966; 1: 770–4.
138. Hansson JA, Simert G, Vang J, The effect of regional perfusion treatment on recurrent melanoma of the extremities. *Acta Chirurgica Scandinavica* 1977; 143: 33–9.
139. Jönsson P-E, Hafström L, Hugander A, Results of regional hyperthermic perfusion for primary and recurrent melanomas of the extremities. *Rec Results Cancer Res* 1983; 86: 277–82.
140. Minor DR, Allen RE, Alberts D et al, A clinical and pharmacokinetic study of isolated limb perfusion with heat and melphalan for melanoma. *Cancer* 1985; 55: 2638–44.
141. Hohenberger W, Isolation perfusion for malignant melanomas: established facts and parameters to be clarified. In: *Progress in Regional Cancer Therapy* (eds Jakesz R, Rainer H) Berlin: Springer, 1990: 182–7.
142. Kroon BBR, Klaase JM, Van de Merwe SA et al, Results of a double perfusion schedule using high-dose hyperthermia and melphalan sequentially for recurrent melanoma of the limbs: a pilot study. *Reg Cancer Treat* 1992; 4: 305–8.
143. Mattson J, Hafström L, Rudenstam C-M, Tumor response: influence of time, temperature and flow in regional hyperthermic perfusion. *Eur J Surg Oncol* 1992; 18 (Suppl 1): 62–3 (abstract).
144. Bryant PJ, Balderson GA, Mead P, Egerton WS, Hyperthermic isolated limb perfusion for malignant melanoma: response and survival. *World J Surg* 1995; 19: 363–8.
145. Decian F, Mondini G, Demarchi R et al, Conventional isolated hyperthermic antiblastic perfusion in the treatment of recurrent melanoma. *Anticancer Res* 1996; 16: 2017–24.
146. Golomb FM, Perfusion of melanoma: 133 isolated perfusions in 114 patients. *Panminerva Med* 1976; 18: 8–10.
147. Aigner K, Hild P, Henneking K, Paul E, Hundeiker M, Regional perfusion with cis-Platinum and Dacarbazine. *Rec Results Cancer Res* 1983; 86: 239–45.
148. Aigner K, Jungbluth A, Link KH et al, Die isolierte hypertherme Extremitäten Perfusion mit Vindesin, Dacarbazin und Cis-Platin bei der Behandlung maligner Melanoma. *Onkologie* 1984; 7: 348–53.
149. Shiu MH, Knapper WH, Fortner JG et al, Regional isolated limb perfusion of melanoma in-transit metatstases using mechlorethamine (nitrogen mustard). *J Clin Oncol* 1986; 4: 1819–26.
150. Vaglini M, Belli F, Marolda R et al, Hyperthermic antiblastic perfusion with DTIC in stage IIIA-IIIAB melanoma of the extremities. *Eur J Surg Oncol* 1987; 13: 127–9.
151. Coit D, Houghton A, Cordon-Cardo C et al, Isolation limb perfusion with monoclonal antibody R24 in patients with malignant melanoma. *Ann Meeting Am Soc Clin Oncol* 1988; 7: 962 (abstract).
152. Coit DG. Hyperthermic isolation limb perfusion (HILP) with cisplatin (CDDP) for metastatic intransit melanoma: a phase I–II trial. *Melanoma Res* 1993; 3 (Suppl 1): 98 (Abstract).
153. Vaglini M, Belli F, Santinami M et al, Isolation perfusion in extracorporeal circulation with interleukin-2 and lymphokine-activated killer cells in the treatment of in-transit metastases from limb cutaneous melanoma. *Ann Surg Oncol* 1995; 2: 61–70.
154. Liénard D, Eggermont AMM, Schraffordt Koops H et al, Isolated perfusion of the limb with high-dose tumor necrosis factor-alpha (TNF-α), interferon-gamma (IFN-γ) and melphalan for melanoma stage III: results of a multi-centre pilot study. *Melanoma Res* 1994; 4 (Suppl 1): 1–26.
155. Fraker DL, Alexander HR, Andrich M, Rosenberg SA, Treatment of patients with melanoma of the extremity using hyperthermic isolated limb perfusion with melphalan, tumor necrosis factor, and interferon gamma: results of a tumor necrosis factor dose-escalating study. *J Clin Oncol* 1996; 14: 479–89.

38

Isolated limb infusion for melanoma

John F Thompson, Peter CA Kam, Johannes HW de Wilt, Per Lindnér

INTRODUCTION

Metastatic melanoma confined to a limb has been treated by isolated limb perfusion (ILP) with melphalan for more than four decades. The advantages of treating patients with recurrent limb melanoma in this way, by administering high-dose regional chemotherapy whilst avoiding serious systemic side effects, are clearly established.[1,2] Complete remission (CR) can be obtained in approximately 50% of patients and partial remission (PR) in another 35–40% of patients with ILP using high-dose melphalan.[1–3] Unfortunately, the ILP technique involves a complex and invasive operative procedure. Several attempts were made to achieve similar results more simply, such as by direct intraarterial infusion[4] or by 'tourniquet infusion' with partial venous outflow occlusion,[5,6] but these all failed to achieve remission rates comparable to those obtained with ILP.

In 1994, Thompson et al.[7] reported a simple yet effective alternative to the ILP procedure, which they called isolated limb infusion (ILI). ILI is essentially a very low flow ILP, performed via percutaneously placed catheters without oxygenation of the perfusate. Like ILP, it achieves high-dose regional therapy with cytotoxic agents but avoids troublesome systemic side effects. Results obtained by ILI using melphalan and actinomycin D have been similar to those obtained by conventional ILP.[8]

ISOLATED LIMB INFUSION PROTOCOL

Preoperative management

From the time of admission to hospital, patients receive antithrombotic prophylaxis (aspirin 300 mg daily and subcutaneous heparin 5000 IU every 8 hours). Preoperative limb volume measurements are made using a simple water-displacement method, as described by Wieberdink et al.[9] Markings that indicate tissue volumes are made on the limb at multiple levels.

Image-guided placement of vascular catheters

Percutaneous arterial and venous access via the common femoral artery and vein in the contralateral groin is achieved using a standard Seldinger technique. Under radiological imaging, guide wires are placed into the artery and vein of the affected limb. A straight 8 FR catheter with 10 side holes near its tip (William A Cook Pty Ltd, Brisbane, Australia) is inserted over the guide wire in the vein. A straight 6 FR catheter is inserted through a standard radiological sheath and then advanced over the guide wire into the artery of the affected limb. When angulation of the arterial catheter occurs at the bifurcation of the aorta a long sheath, which also crosses the aortic bifurcation, is used to increase rigidity and prevent kinking at that point.

For lower limb ILI, the catheter tips are positioned in the popliteal artery and vein distal to the adductor hiatus, just proximal to the knee (Figure 38.1). For the

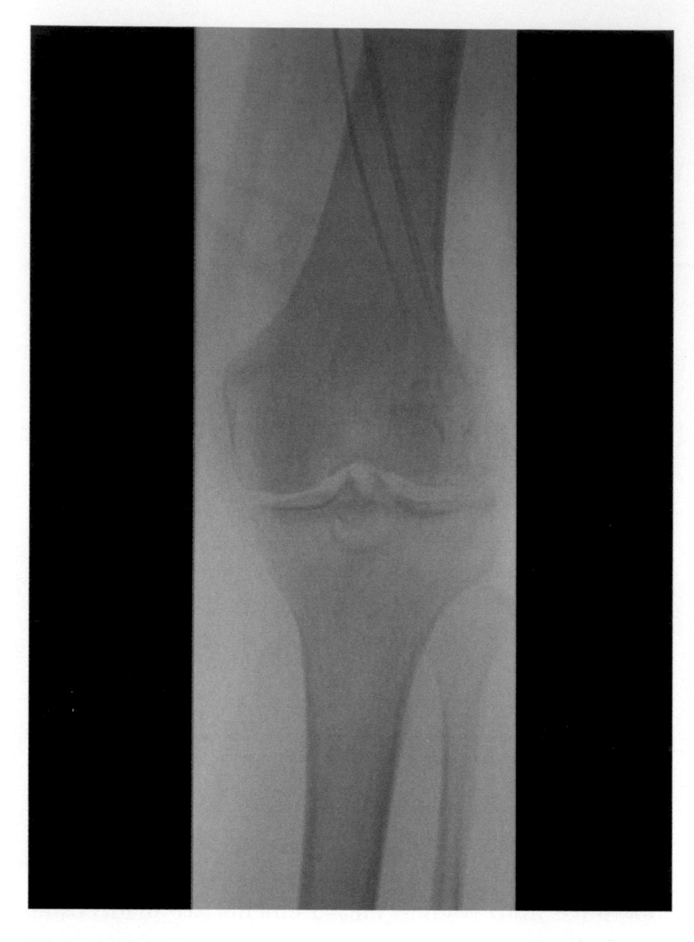

Figure 38.1 *Angiogram of a lower limb showing the tips of the infusion catheters positioned in the popliteal artery and vein distal to the adductor hiatus, just proximal to the knee.*

upper limb, the catheter tips are positioned in the brachial artery and basilic vein just above the elbow. Low-dose heparin via the catheters is started immediately after placement and continued until commencement of the ILI procedure. The patient is kept warm using a metallic space blanket, with additional warm blankets on top.

Intraoperative management

The operating theatre temperature is maintained at 28–30°C. As soon as the patient arrives in the anaesthetic room, a hot-air blanket (Bair Hugger™, Augustine Medical, Eden Prairie, Minnesota, USA), with the air temperature set at 41°C, is placed over the patient, ensuring that the affected limb is completely covered by the device. These manoeuvres are designed to keep the patient's body core temperature >36°C.

Once in the operating theatre, the patient is anaesthetized and fully heparinized (3 mg/kg IV). A single 5 mg IV dose of tropisetron, a $5HT_3$ antagonist, is administered as prophylaxis against postoperative nausea and vomiting. A second hot-air blanket (air temperature again 41°C) is wrapped around the diseased limb and kept in place around it for the duration of the ILI.

At the commencement of the procedure in the operating theatre, intraarterial papaverine (30–60 mg) is injected directly into the popliteal or brachial artery via the arterial catheter. A pneumatic tourniquet is then positioned at an appropriate level around the thigh or arm, and subcutaneous and intramuscular temperature monitoring probes are inserted into the calf or forearm.

If it is not affected by the disease process, an Esmarch bandage is applied to the foot or hand to exclude it from effects of the cytotoxic agents. When there is no tumour distal to the knee or elbow, a second pneumatic tourniquet is applied around the calf or forearm to exclude limb tissue that does not require drug exposure. The volume of limb tissue distal to the thigh or arm tourniquet and proximal to the distal tourniquet or Esmarch bandage (if used) is then estimated with the aid of the preoperative limb volume measurements marked on the limb.

The cytotoxic drugs melphalan (7.5 mg/l of tissue to be infused; range 5–10 mg/l) and actinomycin D (75 μg/l of tissue; range 50–100 μg/l) are added to 400 ml heparinized normal saline that has been warmed to 40°C. The pneumatic tourniquet around the thigh or arm is inflated, and the prepared cytotoxic drug solution is rapidly infused into the isolated limb via the arterial catheter using a pressurized infusion bag and a standard intravenous fluid pump set. The infusate is then continuously recirculated using a syringe and a low-resistance (wide bore), high-flow three-way stopcock (Level 1 Technologies Inc, Rockland, MA, USA), by repeatedly withdrawing blood from the venous catheter and reinjecting it into the arterial catheter (Figure 38.2). A blood warmer modified to enable it to be set at 41°C is incorporated into the extracorporal circuit (Figure 38.3) to assist with progressive limb warming.

After 30 minutes (range 20–40 minutes), the limb vasculature is flushed with 500–1000 ml of Hartmann's solution (at room temperature) via the arterial catheter. Effluent (venous blood) from the limb is extracted from the venous catheter using a syringe and three-way stopcock, and discarded. The heating blanket around the affected limb is removed. When the effluent is clear, the arterial and venous catheters are removed and protamine is administered intravenously to reverse the effects of residual heparin. Firm pressure is applied to the groin at the exit sites of the catheters using an inflatable occluder device (Femo Stop II™, RADI Medical Systems, Uppsala, Sweden) and maintained until complete haemostasis is achieved.

Postoperative management

The patients are kept in bed with the treated limb elevated for at least 48 hours postoperatively, then mobilized if limb discomfort and swelling are not excessive. Serum creatine phosphokinase levels are measured daily and limb toxicity is assessed clinically using the Wieberdink scale (Table 38.1). Subcutaneous heparin (5000 IU every 8 hours) is continued during the stay in hospital. This is normally 6–7 days, because peak limb toxicity occurs very predictably on the fourth or fifth postoperative day. On discharge, the patients are instructed to continue taking aspirin (100–150 mg daily) for 3 months.

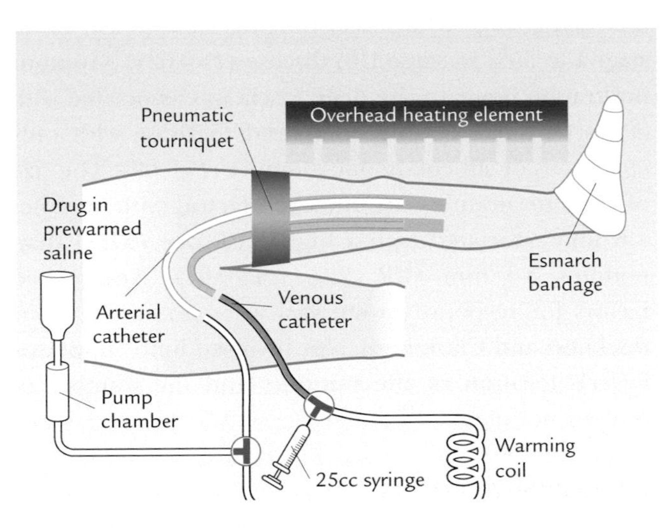

Figure 38.2 *Schematic representation of an isolated limb infusion procedure.*

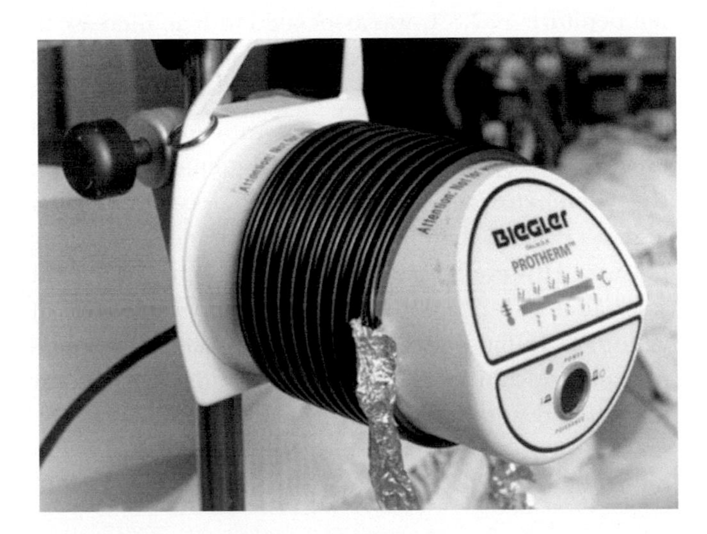

Figure 38.3 *Blood-warming coil to prevent cooling of the perfusate.*

PRECLINICAL STUDIES OF ISOLATED LIMB INFUSION

Several regional perfusion models have been developed in animals to elucidate mechanisms of action and explore ways to improve efficacy (see Chapter 39). Most models in dogs, as well as in rats, have mimicked the ILP technique[10–13] and used a surgical approach in the groin to cannulate the femoral artery and vein. The rat model developed by Wu et al.[14] has more similarities with the ILI technique because the renal vessels are used to cannulate the femoral vessels, without the need for exploration of the groin. A tourniquet applied in the groin prevents leakage of administered agents to the systemic circulation, which is also comparable to the ILI technique in humans. Several studies were performed in nude rats carrying a human melanoma xenograft on the perfused limb to assess optimal perfusion conditions. It was demonstrated that intratumoral uptake of melphalan is higher when the perfusion rate is high and the perfusate has low melphalan binding capacity (i.e. no albumin).[15] When these prerequisites in perfusate conditions were implemented, tumour growth

Table 38.1 *Limb toxicity according to Wieberdink et al.*[9]

Grade	Toxic limb reactions
I	No visible effect
II	Slight erythema and/or oedema
II	Considerable erythema and/or oedema
IV	Extensive epidermolysis and/or obvious damage to deep tissues with a threatened or actual compartment syndrome
V	Severe tissue damage requiring limb amputation

was decreased and survival increased.[16] In another study it was found that tissue melphalan concentrations increased when the cytotoxic drugs were slowly infused during the ILI procedure, compared to administration as a bolus injection at the beginning.[17] Results of these and other animal studies provide information which cannot easily be obtained in clinical situations and are therefore important for planning future improvements of regional perfusion techniques such as ILI.

CLINICAL EFFICACY OF ISOLATED LIMB INFUSION

Patients treated by isolated limb infusion

From November 1992 to August 1998, 207 ILI procedures were performed on 135 patients with recurrent or advanced melanoma at the Sydney Melanoma Unit (SMU) in Sydney, Australia. This group comprised 55 males and 80 females with a mean age of 66 years (range 36–91 years). A single ILI was performed in 72 patients and 56 patients were treated according to an elective double ILI protocol, with the second ILI performed 3–4 weeks after the first.

Only cutaneous disease was present in the affected limb in 51% of the patients, only subcutaneous disease in 18% and cutaneous plus subcutaneous disease in 31%. The mean number of tumour nodules in the limb was 10 (range 1–200) and their mean diameter was 5.5 mm (range 1–50 mm).

Limb toxicity after ILI was Wieberdink grade I in 1% of patients, grade II in 41%, grade III in 53%, grade IV in 5% and grade V in 0%. There was no mortality related to the procedure.

Responses after isolated limb infusion

In a prospective study of 128 patients, the overall response (OR) rate was 85%. A CR occurred in 53 patients (41%), a PR in 55 (44%), stable disease (SD) in 15 patients (12%) and five (4%) had progressive disease.[18] The median duration of CR was 42 months (range 12–68 months), whereas the duration of PR was 9 months (range 4–20 months). When relapses occurred, most (96%) occurred within 22 months. After a median follow-up of 18 months, median overall survival was 34 months (range 13–>72 months). Of the 135 patients who were treated, 69 died and of these 33 did not have any progression of limb disease. Patients in whom a CR was achieved had a significantly longer median survival time of 42 months (range 13–>72 months) compared to those who achieved a PR, and had a median survival time of 32 months (range 12–53 months) (*P*=0.04).

Prognostic factors

Patient-related factors

Patients over 70 years of age had a better OR rate than younger patients (*P*=0.05). Disease stage was also a significant predictor for response rate, duration of response and survival. The CR rate declined with increasing stage of disease, ranging from 100% CR in stage I to 35% in stage IIIb disease (*P*=0.03).[19] Tumour infiltration beneath the deep fascia was associated with a shorter survival time compared to those with only cutaneous or subcutaneous tumours (*P*=0.03). The size of tumour nodules are another factor, with nodules <6 mm associated with a higher CR rate (57%) than nodules >6 mm (CR 32%) (*P*=0.01). Non-related factors for response or survival were primary tumour thickness and Clark level, sex, involved limb (upper or lower), location of the tumours and the number of tumour nodules.

Intraoperative factors

Tourniquet time and the final subcutaneous temperature of the treated limb were found to be important prognostic factors for patient survival. A subcutaneous temperature >37.8°C was associated with an increase in survival rate (*P*=0.006), and a trend towards prolongation of the duration of CR and PR. A tourniquet time >40 minutes was also associated with longer survival time (*P*=0.05). The CR rate in patients with grade III–IV limb toxicity was 49%, which was significantly higher (*P*=0.04) than in patients with grade I–II toxicity (31%). However, greater limb toxicity was not associated with prolongation of survival or duration of CR or PR. Initial limb temperature, infusion time, melphalan concentration and severity of acidosis or hypoxia did not influence response or survival.

Limb temperatures during isolated limb infusion

There is good evidence of a synergistic effect between hyperthermia and melphalan in enhancing the therapeutic effects of ILP.[1] An independent cytotoxic effect of hyperthermia during ILP was demonstrated many years ago by Cavaliere et al.[20] True hyperthermia of the treated limb, with tissue temperatures >41°C, is rarely achieved during ILI because of the relatively low flow rate through the infusion circuit caused by the high resistance of the narrow calibre arterial and venous catheters. Normothermia with final subcutaneous temperatures >37.5°C can be consistently achieved in the limbs undergoing ILI, but only by taking meticulous care to avoid body and limb cooling in the immediate preoperative period (Figure 38.4). A blood-warming coil incorporated in the external circuit to heat the circulating limb infusate is also essential to achieve and maintain satisfactory tissue temperature of limbs undergoing ILI. Routine intraarterial administration of papaverine into the arterial catheter maximizes cutaneous blood flow during the initial phase of infusion to enhance drug delivery to tumours in and on the skin. However, it is likely that maximal cutaneous vasodilation occurs within a few minutes of limb isolation as a result of progressive hypoxia, acidosis and hypercarbia in the isolated limb.

Pharmacokinetics of melphalan during isolated limb infusion

During ILI, the plasma concentration of melphalan decays in a mono-exponential manner, suggesting a rapid uptake of melphalan by the tissues (Figure 38.5).[19] This is consistent with the findings of in vitro studies using human melanoma cells in which it was demonstrated that uptake of melphalan by the tumour cells is a rapid, active, sodium- and temperature-dependent process that reaches a plateau after *c.* 10 minutes due to saturation of the uptake mechanism.[21] During ILI, the mean residence time and $T_{1/2}\beta$ of melphalan were 21–35 minutes and 15–25 minutes, respectively.[19]

Studies with ILP in humans and animal models have demonstrated similar pharmacokinetics, with rapid melphalan uptake in the first minutes of perfusion.[22,23]

Tourniquet times

Tourniquet times of up to 40 minutes for ILI procedures did not cause any adverse effects and tourniquet times >40 minutes were associated with longer survival.[18] This phenomenon could be explained by the potential synergism of hypoxia with melphalan. Ischaemia of variable duration produced by inflation of the tourniquet prior to the infusion would be expected to enhance the cytotoxic effects of melphalan, with further enhancement by the acidosis. Hypoxia increases the cytotoxic effects of melphalan by 1.5 times, and the combination of hypoxia and acidosis would further increase the cytotoxic effects of melphalan by *c.* three times.

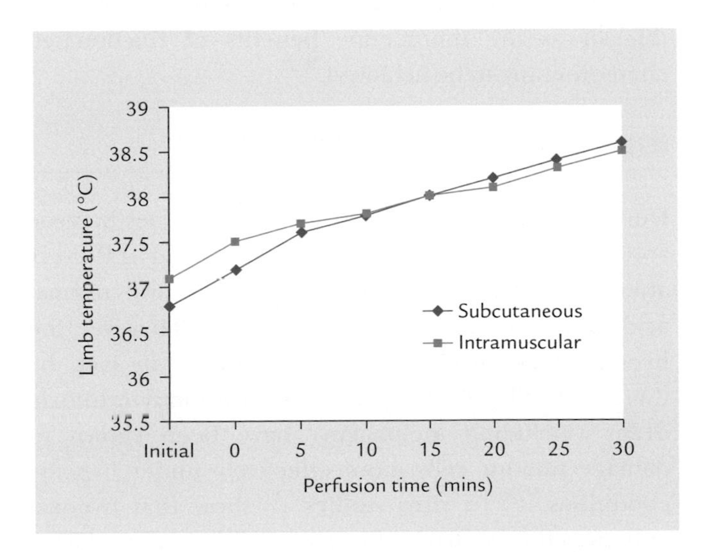

Figure 38.4 *Typical temperature graph during isolated limb infusion. The 'initial' temperatures were those recorded before drug infusion. Those at time '0' were at the completion of drug infusion.*

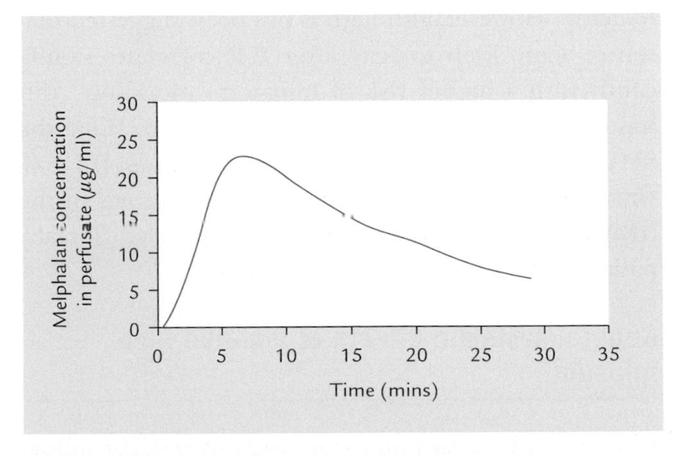

Figure 38.5 *Typical melphalan concentration graph during isolated limb infusion.*

MORBIDITY AFTER ISOLATED LIMB INFUSION

Local effects of isolated limb infusion

Erythema of the skin and mild oedema of the limb tissues develop within 24 hours, reach a peak after 4–5 days and then begin to subside. A ring of intense inflammation in the skin surrounding or overlying tumour deposits often becomes apparent within 48 hours. Some tumour involution is usually discernible within 7–10 days. However, complete disappearance of tumour nodules may take many weeks or even months.

Careful clinical monitoring for signs of compartment syndrome is important, as well as daily monitoring of serum creatine phosphokinase (CK) levels. When clinical signs of compartment syndrome are apparent, or CK levels rise to >1000 IU/l, a fasciotomy is indicated. However, the last 150 consecutive ILI using melphalan and actinomycin D were performed without the need for a fasciotomy.

Hair growth in the area of the treated limb exposed to the cytotoxic agent ceases for up to 3 months. If the foot or hand had not been excluded by an Esmarch bandage or pneumatic tourniquet from exposure to the cytotoxic infusate, loss of original toe- or fingernails occurs 3–4 months after the ILI. These effects are identical to the effects observed after conventional ILP.[24,25]

Limb toxicity grade III or IV was experienced in 52% of the patients treated with an ILI, which is considerably higher than in a recent large ILP series in which only 24% experienced grade III or greater toxicity.[26] In this group's experience at the SMU, using conventional ILP, 35% of 135 patients developed grade III or greater limb toxicity.[27] However, although it has been suggested that severe acute limb toxicity after ILP correlates significantly with a higher risk of long-term morbidity,[2] this has not been observed in patients treated by ILI at the SMU. In the 74 patients who experienced post-ILI toxicity of grade III or grade IV severity, symptoms in the treated limb were not recorded as a problem for any patient at follow-up after 1 year.

General/systemic effects of isolated limb infusion

Postoperative nausea and vomiting rarely occur following ILI when routine antiemetic prophylaxis with tropisetron, a $5HT_3$ antagonist, is used. Serious systemic adverse effects such as bone marrow depression are not observed following ILI because inflation of the pneumatic tourniquet reliably prevents systemic drug leakage and meticulous flushing of the limb prior to the release of the tourniquet removes most of the cytotoxic drug remaining in the vascular compartment (blood) of the treated limb.

ADVANTAGES OF ISOLATED LIMB INFUSION

Technical aspects

The ILI technique is technically much simpler and yet has an efficacy that is similar to that of ILP in the treatment of limb melanoma.[3,7,8] Complex and expensive equipment (e.g. roller pump, oxygenator) is not required, and the number of medical, nursing and technical support personnel is low, thereby reducing the costs considerably. The total operating theatre time rarely exceeds 60 minutes (compared to 3–5 hours for an ILP), making it possible to treat up to three patients by ILI in a single morning or afternoon operating-theatre session.

ILI is a less invasive procedure than ILP, since the vascular catheters are placed percutaneously, thus avoiding the need for surgical exposure and open cannulation of major blood vessels: this results in reduced morbidity. Repeat ILI can readily be performed and this allows the therapeutic benefits of fractionated chemotherapy to be achieved.[28,29]

Hypoxia and acidosis of infusate

During ILI the infusate progressively becomes hypoxic and acidotic (Figure 38.6), whereas during ILP every attempt is made to maintain hyperoxic and normal acid–base conditions of the perfusate.[8,30] However, the hypoxic state produced during ILI may, in fact, be therapeutically advantageous, because many cytotoxic drugs (including melphalan) have been shown to damage tumour cells more effectively under hypoxic conditions.[31,32] In vitro studies[31,33] show that hypoxia enhances the cytotoxic effects of melphalan by a factor of 1.5. The cytotoxic effects of melphalan are further increased by a factor of 2.3–3.5 when hypoxia and acidosis are combined,[31,34] due to enhanced cellular uptake of melphalan, and, in addition, the rate of

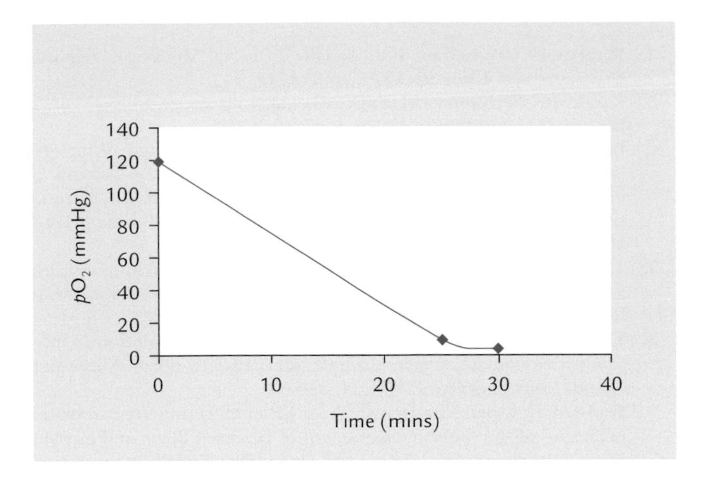

Figure 38.6 *Typical graph of* pO_2 *in perfusate during isolated limb infusion.*

hydrolysis of melphalan is reduced by acidosis. Antitumour effects of melphalan increased in a hypoxic animal ILP model when it was compared to oxygenated melphalan perfusions.[22] Aigner and Kaevel[35] have suggested that low-flow perfusion and induced hypoxia also provide more uniform distribution of cytotoxic agents throughout tissues in which vascular isolation has been achieved.

Blood transfusion requirements

Homologous blood transfusion is not required with the ILI procedure, thus avoiding the infection risks, immunological suppression and costs associated with transfusion. In contrast, homologous blood is routinely used for ILP to prime the perfusion circuit, and additional blood must often be added to the isolated circuit to maintain the reservoir volume.

Vascular disease

ILI can safely be used to treat melanoma on the limb in patients with major occlusive peripheral disease, whereas this is a contraindication to ILP. When there is complete arteriosclerotic occlusion of the superficial femoral artery it is still possible to perform an ILI with the arterial catheter tip positioned in the distal profunda femoris artery. Likewise, if the superficial femoral vein is thrombosed, the venous catheter tip can be positioned in the profunda vein. The collateral arterial and venous circulation connections between profunda femoral territory and superficial femoral/popliteal territory enables adequate low-flow perfusion of the entire limb with fairly uniform drug distribution. In routine ILI of the lower limb, the catheters are placed in the superficial femoral artery and vein, with retrograde flow in collateral blood vessels to perfuse the tissues in the mid and distal thigh that are normally supplied by the profunda femoral vessels.

ISOLATED LIMB INFUSION MODIFICATIONS

Fractionated chemotherapy

The simplicity and low morbidity of ILI make it readily possible to perform repeated ILI to achieve fractionated chemotherapy. Repeat exposure to the chemotherapeutic agent within a short period may eliminate most or all residual tumour. Tumour cells partially damaged by the first exposure to cytotoxic drugs are likely to be more vulnerable to the cytotoxic drugs on the second or subsequent exposures. Consequently, tumour cell damage should be maximized whereas toxic side effects on normal tissue are minimized.[36]

In a study to determine the value of fractionated chemotherapy in ILI, 47 patients underwent a planned double ILI.[29] In this elective double ILI protocol the aim was to perform the second ILI 3–4 weeks after the first procedure. However, in the 47 patients the actual interval between the ILIs ranged from 2 to 8 weeks (mean 4.2 weeks) for logistic reasons. A CR was achieved in 18 of the 44 assessable patients (41%), PR in 21 (47%) and SD in five patients (21%). The median duration of response after double ILI (taken from the time of the first ILI) was 18 months (range 6–60 months). Thus, no significant difference in response rate or duration of response from a single ILI protocol was demonstrated. When a CR was achieved with a double ILI protocol, the median duration of CR of 60 months (range 15–∞ months) was significantly longer than the median PR duration of 7 months (range 4–18 months).

Kroon et al.[37] used a double ILP schedule to assess the value of fractionated chemotherapy but, because of the complex nature of ILP, the complication rate was high and the logistic difficulties encountered were daunting.

There was no significant difference in the duration of survival in patients treated according to the double

ILI protocol compared to that following the single ILI control group. Patients who achieved a CR after the double ILI protocol survived for longer than those who achieved a PR [mean 43 months (range 18–∞ months) versus 12 months (range 9–24 months)]. Most recurrences occurred within 22 months.

Repeat isolated limb infusion due to disease progression after the first ILI

Fourteen patients initially treated with an ILI received a second ILI due to progression of disease,[29] with a median interval between the two treatments of 14 months (range 4–19 months). The OR rate in these 14 patients was 79%, not significantly different from the OR rate obtained after the first ILI, but the CR rate was lower (one of 14 patients versus six of 14 patients). The median duration of response was 5 months (range 4–11 months) after the second ILI compared to 6 months (range 3–9 months) after the first treatment, which was not significantly different. These results are similar to those reported by Klop et al.[38] and Feldman et al.[39] following repeat ILP for limb disease recurrence.

FUTURE PROSPECTS

The simplicity and non-invasive nature of ILI, resulting in low morbidity rates, makes it possible to perform more than two sequential ILIs or repeated ILIs. The risk of significant systemic drug leakage is extremely low, and this makes it a valuable model for testing new and existing drugs without the risk of systemic side effects. In a pilot study of patients treated with the alkylating agent fotemustine, an OR rate in the treated limb of 92% was achieved, but the procedure was associated with severe local toxicity.[40] It is possible that other chemotherapeutic agents or cytokines with serious systemic toxic effects, such as tumour necrosis factor, may be safely administered using the ILI technique.

REFERENCES

1. Thompson JF, Lai DT, Ingvar C, Kam PC, Maximizing efficacy and minimizing toxicity in isolated limb perfusion for melanoma. *Melanoma Res* 1994; 4S: 45–50.
2. Vrouenraets BC, Nieweg OE, Kroon BBR, Thirty-five years of isolated limb perfusion: indications and results. *Br J Surg* 1996; 83: 1319–28.
3. Thompson JF, Hunt JA, Shannon KF, Kam PC, Frequency and duration of remission after isolated limb perfusion for melanoma. *Arch Surg* 1997; 132: 903–7.
4. Karakousis CP, Kanter PM, Lopez R et al, Modes of regional chemotherapy. *J Surg Res* 1979; 26: 134–41.
5. Karakousis CP, Kanter PM, Park HC et al, Tourniquet infusion versus hyperthermic perfusion. *Cancer* 1982; 49: 850–8.
6. Bland KI, Kimura AK, Brenner DE et al, A phase II study of the efficacy of diamminedichloroplatinum [cisplatin] for the control of locally recurrent and intransit malignant melanoma of the extremities using tourniquet outflow-occlusion techniques. *Ann Surg* 1989; 209: 73–80.
7. Thompson JF, Waugh RC, Saw RPM, Kam PCA, Isolated limb infusion with melphalan for recurrent limb melanoma: a simple alternative to isolated limb perfusion. *Reg Cancer Treat* 1994; 7: 188–92.
8. Thompson JF, Kam PC, Waugh RC, Harman CR, Isolated limb infusion with cytotoxic agents: a simple alternative to isolated limb perfusion. *Semin Surg Oncol* 1998; 14: 238–47.
9. Wieberdink J, Benckhuijsen C, Braat RP et al, Dosimetry in isolated perfusion of the limbs by assessment of perfused tissue and grading of toxic reactions. *Eur J Cancer Clin Oncol* 1982; 18: 905–10.
10. Fontijne WP, de Vries J, Mook PH et al, Improved tissue perfusion during pressure-regulated hyperthermic regional isolated perfusion in dogs. *J Surg Oncol* 1984; 26: 69–76.
11. Pfeiffer T, Krause U, Thome U et al, Tissue toxicity of doxorubicin in first and second hyperthermic isolated limb perfusion – an experimental study in dogs. *Eur J Surg Oncol* 1997; 23: 439–44.
12. Manusama ER, Nooijen PTGA, Stavast J et al, Synergistic antitumour effect of recombinant human tumour necrosis factor alpha with melphalan in isolated limb perfusion in the rat. *Br J Surg* 1996; 83: 551–5.
13. Manusama ER, Stavast J, Durante NMC et al, Isolated limb perfusion with TNF alpha and melphalan in a rat osteosarcoma model: a new anti-tumour approach. *Eur J Surg Oncol* 1996; 22: 152–7.
14. Wu ZY, Smithers BM, Roberts MS, Tissue and perfusate pharmacokinetics of melphalan in isolated perfused rat hindlimb. *J Pharmacol Exp Ther* 1997; 282: 1131–8.
15. Wu ZY, Smithers BM, Parsons PG, Roberts MS, The effects of perfusion conditions on melphalan distribution in the isolated perfused rat hindlimb bearing a human melanoma xenograft. *Br J Cancer* 1997; 75: 1160–6.
16. Wu ZY, Roberts MS, Parsons PG, Smithers BM, Isolated limb perfusion with melphalan for human melanoma xenografts in the hindlimb of nude rats: a surviving animal model. *Melanoma Res* 1997; 7: 19–26.
17. Wu ZY, Smithers BM, Roberts MS, Melphalan dosing regimens for management of recurrent melanoma by isolated limb perfusion: application of a physiological pharmacokinetic model based on melphalan distribution in the isolated perfused rat hindlimb. *Melanoma Res* 1997; 7: 252–64.
18. Lindner P, Doubrovsky A, Kam PCA, Thompson JF, Prognostic factors after isolated limb infusion with cytotoxic agents for melanoma. *Ann Surg Oncol* (in press).
19. Thompson JF, Ramzan I, Kam PCA, Yau DF, Pharmacokinetics of melphalan during isolated limb infusion for melanoma. *Reg Cancer Treat* 1996; 9: 13–16.
20. Cavaliere R, Ciocatto EC, Giovanella BC et al, Selective heat sensitivity of cancer cells. Biochemical and clinical studies. *Cancer* 1967; 20: 1351–81.
21. Parsons PG, Carter FB, Morrison L, Regius Mary Sister, Mechanism of melphalan resistance developed in vitro in human melanoma cells. *Cancer Res* 1981; 41: 1525–34.
22. de Wilt JHW, Manusama ER, van Tiel ST et al, Prerequisites for effective isolated limb perfusion using tumour necrosis factor alpha and melphalan in rats. *Br J Cancer* 1999; 80: 161–6.
23. Benckhuijsen C, Kroon BB, van Geel AN, Wieberdink J, Regional perfusion treatment with melphalan for melanoma in a limb: an evaluation of drug kinetics. *Eur J Surg Oncol* 1988; 14: 157–63.
24. Vrouenraets BC, Kroon BB, Klaase JM et al, Severe acute regional toxicity after normothermic or 'mild' hyperthermic isolated limb perfusion with melphalan for melanoma. *Melanoma Res* 1995; 5: 425–31.
25. Vrouenraets BC, Klaase JM, Nieweg OE, Kroon BB, Toxicity and morbidity of isolated limb perfusion. *Semin Surg Oncol* 1998; 14: 224–31.

26. Vrouenraets BC, Hart GA, Eggermont AM et al, Relation between limb toxicity and treatment outcomes after isolated limb perfusion for recurrent melanoma. *J Am Coll Surg* 1999; 188: 522–30.
27. Thompson JF, Eksborg S, Kam PC et al, Determinants of acute regional toxicity following isolated limb perfusion for melanoma. *Melanoma Res* 1996; 6: 267–71.
28. Thompson JF, Kam PCA, Saw RPM et al, Isolated limb infusion for melanoma: results of an elective double infusion protocol. *Reg Cancer Treat* 1995; 8: 122–7.
29. Lindner P, Colman M, Kam PCA, Thompson JF, Double isolated limb infusion with cytotoxic agents for recurrent and metastatic limb melanoma. Submitted for publication.
30. Thompson JF, Good PD, Kam PCA, Hyperthermic isolated limb perfusion in the treatment of melanoma: technical aspects. *Reg Cancer Treat* 1994; 7: 147–54.
31. Siemann DW, Chapman M, Beikirch A, Effects of oxygenation and pH on tumor cell response to alkylating chemotherapy. *Int J Radiat Oncol Biol Phys* 1991; 20: 287–9.
32. van de Merwe SA, van den Berg AP, Kroon BB et al, Modification of human tumour and normal tissue pH during hyperthermic and normothermic antiblastic regional isolation perfusion for malignant melanoma: a pilot study. *Int J Hyperthermia* 1993; 9: 205–17.
33. Chaplin DJ, Acker B, Olive PL, Potentiation of the tumor cytotoxicity of melphalan by vasodilating drugs. *Int J Radiat Oncol Biol Phys* 1989; 16: 1131–5.
34. Skarsgard LD, Skwarchuk MW, Vinczan A et al, The cytotoxicity of melphalan and its relationship to pH, hypoxia and drug uptake. *Anticancer Res* 1995; 15: 219–23.
35. Aigner KR, Kaevel K, Pelvic stopflow infusion [PSI] and hypoxic pelvic perfusion [HPP] with mitomycin and melphalan for recurrent rectal cancer. *Reg Cancer Treat* 1994; 7: 6–11.
36. DeVita VT, Principles of cancer management: chemotherapy. In: *Cancer Principles and Practice of Oncology*, 5th edn, (eds De Vita VT, Hellman S, Rosenberg SA). Philadelphia: Lippincott, 1997: 333–48.
37. Kroon BB, Klaase JM, van Geel BN et al, Results of a double perfusion schedule with melphalan in patients with melanoma of the lower limb. *Eur J Cancer* 1993; 29A: 325–8.
38. Klop WM, Vrouenraets BC, van Geel BN et al, Repeat isolated limb perfusion with melphalan for recurrent melanoma of the limbs. *J Am Coll Surg* 1996; 182: 467–72.
39. Feldman AL, Alexander Jr HR, Bartlett DL et al, Management of extremity recurrences after complete responses to isolated limb perfusion in patients with melanoma. *Ann Surg Oncol* 1999; 6: 562–7.
40. Bonenkamp JJ, de Wilt JHW, Watson L, Thompson JF, Fotemustine and dacarbazine in isolated limb infusion for locoregional advanced melanoma. *Melanoma Res* 2001; 11: S211.

39

Isolated limb perfusion and infusion: preclinical studies and future directions

B Mark Smithers, Johannes HW de Wilt

INTRODUCTION

Since the introduction of isolated limb perfusion (ILP) in 1958,[1] most of the changes and refinements of the technique have been made and assessed in the clinical laboratory rather than in formal preclinical studies. The evaluation of outcomes such as morbidity and tumour responses in patients and their limbs have been markers of the value of any changes that have occurred in the technique. The pharmacokinetics of cytotoxic drugs within normal limb tissues, along with cytotoxic drug concentrations in tumour deposits, have been studied during ILP.[2–4] Major attempts to validate changes in the conditions of ILP, with the aim of improving results, or to develop and refine new techniques such as isolated limb infusion (ILI),[5] would be difficult outside large multicentre studies. The distribution of cytotoxic drug(s) or solute into tissues during ILP is determined by a combination of the inherent physicochemical properties of the solute along with the tissue physiology.[6] In animal studies, the conditions of an ILP or ILI can be changed more dramatically and the pharmacokinetics and pharmacodynamics of the drugs can be more adequately assessed, as well as the physiology within the isolated limb during and after therapy.

ANIMAL MODELS

In the early days of the development of ILP, the dog was widely used as a model because it afforded easy access to large vessels, and provided the ability to assess subtle problems that occurred within the limb[7–9] and the effects of changes in perfusion techniques.[10] More recently, the dog has been used to further explore optimal perfusion flow rates and perfusion pressures,[11] as well as to assess the effects of the cytotoxic drugs dacarbazine (DTIC)[12] and cisplatin[13] used in an isolated perfusion system. The disadvantages of large animal work are its cost, the lack of a transplantable tumour to assess response and the growing pressure to decrease large animal experimentation.

In the small animal setting, rodents provide the advantages of ready animal availability, the existence of rodent-specific tumours which can be implanted onto a limb, the availability of an immunodeficient species which will allow the use of cultured human melanoma tumour xenografts, and vessels still large enough to allow cannulation and therapy. Initially, in the rodent model, low flow rates were considered necessary,[14–16] however, a reproducible model with a high flow, as would be used in the human, was subsequently developed.[17] For drug pharmacokinetic studies, animals may be sacrificed at certain times during the therapy, allowing access to information about tissue drug levels under particular conditions. Alternatively, animals may be allowed to survive following the isolated limb therapy so that an assessment of local (limb) and other morbidity can be made. The utility of the rodent model has been expanded with the development of tumour implantation on a limb to assess tumour response to therapy and drug pharmacodynamics in the tumour and normal tissues.[14,18–21] Typically, the tumours have been species-specific sarcomatous tumours.[14,19–21] However, xenografts of human cultured melanoma cells have recently been implanted successfully onto the hind limbs of nude rats, allowing an assessment of tumour response to ILP with melphalan.[18]

In the rodent models of ILP, with species-specific tumour grafts, the femoral vessels have been ligated following the perfusion. The limb survives due to the extensive collateral circulation in this region.[14,19,20] In the previously mentioned nude rat model, the femoral artery and vein are cannulated via the left renal artery and vein. Once the limb therapy has been completed the cannulae are removed and a left nephrectomy is performed. In this model, vascular networks within the implanted tumour were demonstrated using casts, blood flow in the tumour was demonstrated with ^{15}C-labelled microspheres, and tissue concentrations of melphalan in the implanted tumour and the surrounding tissues were measured. A reduction in the size of the implanted tumour was noted with higher doses of melphalan.[18]

A disadvantage of animal models using implanted tumours is the different mechanism of tumour establishment and growth compared to a true metastasis. In the study by Wu et al.,[18] the tumour blood flow was 30% of the flow in normal tissues and the melphalan concentration 40% of that in normal tissues. Despite these differences, tumour response, drug pharmacokinetics and drug pharmocodynamics can be assessed using conditions similar to those used in human ILP or ILI procedures. Another potential problem occurs if the implanted tumour is allowed to grow too large, because the deposits become necrotic in the centre and this may influence the results of studies.

PHARMACOKINETIC STUDIES

Quantitative data on drug uptake and washout during and after isolated limb therapy using different perfusate and washout conditions have been undefined in humans. These aspects have been carefully studied in the rodent model, with the aim of establishing optimal treatment conditions. When examining the pharmacokinetics of melphalan in tissues following ILP of the rat hind limb, Norda et al.[22] found increased tissue penetration of melphalan when: the pH was between 7.3 and 7.7; the perfusion temperature was 40–41.5°C; melphalan was given as a single dose into the reservoir of the extracorporeal circuit; and there was a low perfusate flow rate. Others have found the concentration of melphalan in perfusate and normal tissues to be linearly related to input concentrations, and the rate of uptake of melphalan to be higher at a temperature of 41.5°C when compared with a temperature of 37°C.[23] The melphalan uptake into perfused tissue was impaired by the use of a perfusate with high albumin content because the melphalan became protein bound. Washout of the melphalan from normal tissue, notably muscle, on the other hand, was facilitated by using solutions that had a high protein content because of the protein binding of melphalan.[23]

To assess dosing regimens, a physiological and pharmacokinetic model has been developed, based on melphalan distribution in the isolated perfused hind limb of the rat.[24] The amount of melphalan in the tissues was highest after a single bolus of the drug at the beginning of the perfusion. The tissue concentration was less after melphalan was given in divided doses over 60 minutes and further reduced if it was given as an infusion over 60 minutes. The conclusions were that a single bolus of melphalan provided longer exposure times at higher tissue concentrations and should increase the efficacy of melphalan in ILP.[24] In humans, a single bolus at the beginning of an ILP has been shown to offer improved pharmacokinetic conditions over divided doses.[25] Whether changing the method of drug delivery will influence tumour response is unknown and large numbers of patients in a randomized trial would be required to assess the value of such a change. The animal model offers the opportunity to assess the effects of tumour response to such a change in perfusion conditions in a much more direct and controlled way.

It has also been shown in human studies that toxicity following ILP with melphalan was independently related to maximum tissue temperature, peak concentration of melphalan and the area under the curve of melphalan concentration in the perfusate over 60 minutes.[26] Using the dosing regimen model,[24] an infusion over 20 minutes will offer the same area under the curve for melphalan concentration in the perfusate but will reduce the peak concentration. In an ILI, the initial infusion of melphalan occurs over *c.* 5 minutes. Using the pharmacokinetic studies of drug delivery in ILP, it would appear that this time of delivery is suitable for melphalan uptake into a melanoma metastasis during this procedure.

In animal models with implanted tumours it is possible to examine drug pharmacodynamics related to the tumour. In the model with an implanted human melanoma, the effect of a perfusate based on protein (albumin) confirmed the problem of protein binding of melphalan because there was a reduction, by a factor of three, in the concentration of melphalan in the implanted tumour when compared to a perfusate based on dextran.[27] Examining the appropriate crystalloids to use in a perfusion revealed lower melphalan hydrolysis with Hartmann's solution.[27] A study in a non-tumour-bearing animal showed that a low flow rate would increase the time of exposure of the tissues to the drug and thus suggested that this would be an optimal perfusion parameter.[22] However, it has also been shown that higher flow rates increase tumour blood flow, although this does not occur in a linear fashion.[27] Given that the flow rates in the implanted tumour were one-third of those in the skin and the subcutaneous tissues, it would appear, in the animal model, that higher flow rates of 4–8 ml/min are optimal.

As previously stated, after ILP the concentrations of melphalan in the tumours of the rat model with implanted human melanoma were less than the concentrations in the subcutaneous tissues and the skin.[18,22] Klaase et al.[4] showed a linear relationship between the tumour melphalan concentration and the area under the curve for melphalan concentrations in the perfusate over 60 minutes. Their biopsy studies post-ILP with melphalan in humans showed the tumour concentrations to be equivalent to those in muscle and over twice the concentrations seen in skin. This possibly highlights the different growth kinetics and mechanisms of drug uptake into implanted tumours compared with what has been reported in human melanoma metastases.

In an attempt to reduce the number of animals that are required to perform pharmacokinetic studies, the technique of microdialysis has recently been employed in the rat model of ILP.[28] Microdialysis is based on analytes from the interstitial compartment of the tissue being studied passing through a semipermeable membrane within a microprobe that has been inserted into the tissue. These probes can be inserted into subcutaneous tissue, muscle or an implanted tumour. The potential to use these techniques in sampling analytes from tumour and muscle have been reported,[29] as has their use in assessing cytotoxic kinetics in melanoma metastases.[30] Using the rat hind limb model of ILP, melphalan concentrations in tissues have been examined, showing a linear relationship between the tissue dialysate and tissue concentrations of melphalan, although the melphalan concentration in the dialysate was only 20% of the tissue melphalan concentration.[28]

The potential benefit of using microdialysis, in both animal and human studies, is the ability to monitor drug uptake and tissue toxicity in a dynamic fashion. This should assist in optimizing dosing and administration schedules, and in the selection of cytotoxic compounds with favourable tissue penetration characteristics. The optimal conditions for microdialysis to be used in ILP and ILI are presently being defined.[28]

DRUG THERAPY

Melphalan remains the gold standard in the management of patients with localized melanoma metastases in a limb in whom ILP or ILI is indicated. There have been many drugs used in human ILP but there are few published animal studies assessing the efficacy or pharmacokinetics of drugs other than melphalan. The effects of DTIC and cisplatin have, however, been assessed in the dog.[12,13] The studies with DTIC were performed to assess the effects of the drug on the vasculature[12] and the studies of cisplatin to assess the pharmacokinetics of the drug in a dog hind limb bearing a canine osteogenic sarcoma.[13]

More recently, tumour necrosis factor-alpha (TNF-α) has become available and, with its known major systemic toxicity in humans, it has been ideal to examine the effects of the drug in animals. A number of studies have examined the response of implanted tumours following ILP with TNF-α alone or in combination with melphalan. A clear synergism has been identified between TNF-α and melphalan[20,21,31] compared with a very poor response when TNF-α is used alone. It has been shown that the mechanism of action of TNF-α is to alter the permeability and integrity of the microvasculature. Animal studies have also shown that neutrophils play an important role in the antitumour effects induced by TNF-α.[32] In a study of a rodent-specific implanted sarcoma (metastasizing BN-175) in inbred BN rats, the optimal conditions for ILP with melphalan and TNF-α were examined.[33] Hypoxia enhanced the effects of TNF-α and melphalan alone but not as a combination. A minimum exposure time of 30 minutes was required and the lowest dose of TNF-α to produce a response was 40 μg/kg.[33] The presence of TNF-α has been shown to increase the tumour concentration of melphalan sixfold, with a corresponding improvement in response. This effect on intratumoral drug concentrations might be induced by the effects of TNF-α on the tumour vasculature and could play a significant role in the synergism between the two drugs.[34] A similar increase in tumour drug concentration was found with doxorubicin and TNF-α.[35] It has been the experience of this group that attempts to assess the effects of TNF-α in the nude rat model have been universally unsuccessful because the smallest dose of TNF-α leads to the rat's demise.

New drugs may be studied in the animal model, before human trials, with the aim of determining optimal dosing schedules, predicting tumour response rates and assessing morbidity. Studies with less toxic TNF mutants (e.g. TNF-SAM2) in combination with melphalan and doxorubicin demonstrated antitumour effects that were similar to those of the toxic recombinant human TNF-α.[36] The use of this agent might improve the safety of future clinical perfusions and could allow expansion of the use of TNF-α to other perfusion settings which are less leakage-free or involve organs more sensitive to its toxic effects. Recently, fotemustine has shown promise in cell culture studies[37] and would be an ideal cytotoxic drug to study in ILP/ILI rodent models. The animal studies also allow the assessment of drugs that do not themselves have a direct cytotoxic effect but may enhance the action of the cytotoxics that are to be used in ILP or ILI. Animal studies performed with L-NAME, a nitric oxide inhibitor affecting tumour blood flow and tumour angiogenesis, demonstrated improved tumour responses in combination with both melphalan and TNF-α.[38] The advantage of the animal studies is that the potential for a response to occur can be assessed in a short time and an optimal dosing regimen can be determined. More recently, studies have used the rodent model of ILP for implanted sarcoma as a gene therapy delivery system.[39–41] There was evidence of a clinical response in the tumour[39,41] that was superior to intravenous or intratumoral injection of the therapeutic agents in the latest study.[41]

CONCLUSIONS

The response after ILP or ILI may range from a complete response, a partial response, no response or to recurrence of disease after a complete response. Therefore, it is important and justifiable to examine ways of optimizing these procedures. It is worthwhile as well, to continue studies exploring the utility of new drugs and adjuvant treatments which may improve disease response and control. It seems sensible to continue to use the small animal model to explore proposed changes before transferring these new therapies to the clinical situation. The advantages of using animal studies appear to be: validation of a change in the conditions of established ILP or ILI techniques; validation of the use of new drugs by assessment of the drug tissue and tumour pharmacokinetics and pharmacodynamics; and assessment of an implanted tumour's response to changed conditions, or use of different drugs, by comparison with the gold standard, which is currently ILP with melphalan.

REFERENCES

1. Creech Jr O, Krementz ET, Ryan RF et al, Chemotherapy of cancer regional perfusion utilizing an extracorporeal circuit. *Ann Surg* 1958; 148: 616–32.
2. Benckhuijsen C, Kroon BB, van Geel AN et al, Regional perfusion treatment with melphalan for melanoma in a limb; an evaluation of drug kinetics. *Eur J Surg Oncol* 1988; 14: 157–63.
3. Scott RN, Blackie R, Kerr DJ et al, Melphalan concentration and distribution in tissues of tumour-bearing limbs treated by isolated limb perfusion. *Eur J Cancer* 1992; 28A: 1811–13.
4. Klaase JM, Kroon BB, Beijnen et al, Melphalan tissue concentration in patients treated with regional isolated perfusion for melanoma of the lower limb. *Br J Cancer* 1994; 70: 151–3.
5. Thompson JF, Kam PC, Waugh RC et al, Isolated limb infusion with cytotoxic agents: a simple alternative to isolated limb perfusion. *Semin Surg Oncol* 1998; 14: 238–47.
6. Wu ZY, Cross SE, Roberts MS, Influence of physicochemical parameters and perfusate flow rate on the distribution of solutes in the isolated perfused rat hindlimb determined by impulse–response technique. *J Pharmac Sci* 1995; 84: 1020–7.
7. Parkins WM, Ravdin RG, Cogins PF, Exploratory study of vascular occlusion and perfusion tehcniques for localization of action of cytotoxic drugs. *Am Coll Surg, Surg Forum* 1959; 9: 591–6.
8. Ryan RF, Krementz ET, Creech Jr O et al, Selected perfusion of isolated viscera with chemotherapeutic agents using an extracorporeal circuit. *Am Coll Surg, Surg Forum* 1958; 8: 158–161.
9. Ryan RF, Winblad JN, Hottinger GC et al, Effects of various perfusates in isolated vascular beds using extracorporeal circuit. *Am Coll Surg, Surg Forum* 1959; 9: 194–8.
10. Hottinger GC, Ryan RF, Delgado JP et al, Physiology of extracorporeal circulation. Studies on blood flow, oxygen consumption and metabolism in the isolated perfused extremity. *Am Coll Surg, Surg Forum* 1959; 10: 80–3.
11. Fontijne WPJ, de Vries J, Mook PH et al, Improved tissue perfusion during pressure-regulated hyperthermic regional isolated perfusion in dogs. *J Surg Oncol* 1984; 26: 69–76.
12. Aigner K, Hild P, Breithauipt H et al, Isolated extremity perfusion with DTIC. An experimental and clinical study. *Anticancer Res* 1983; 3: 87–93.
13. van Ginkel RJ, Hoekstra HJ, Meutstege FJ et al, Hyperthermic isolated regional perfusion with cisplatin in the local treatment of spontaneous canine osteosarcoma: assessment of short-term effects. *J Surg Oncol* 1995; 59: 169–76.

14. Turner FW, Tod M, Francis GJ et al, The technic for isolation–perfusion of the rat hind limb. *Cancer Res* 1962; 22: 49–52.
15. Yates A, Fisher B, Experimental studies in regional perfusion. *Arch Surg* 1962; 85: 827–36.
16. Buckner DM, Busch J, Economou SG, An experimental study of influences on the escape of perfusate during perfusion for cancer. *Cancer Chemother Rep* 1960; 10: 41–3.
17. Benckhuysen C, van Dijk WJ, van't Hoff SC, High-flow isolation perfusion of the rat hind limb in vivo. *J Surg Oncol* 1982; 21: 249–57.
18. Wu ZY, Roberts MS, Parsons PG et al, Isolated limb perfusion with melphalan for human melanoma xenografts in the hindlimb of nude rats: a surviving animal model. *Melanoma Res* 1997; 7: 19–26.
19. Manusama ER, Durante NMC, Marquet RL et al, Ischaemia promotes the antitumour effect of tumour necrosis factor in isolated limb perfusion in the rat. *Reg Cancer Treat* 1994; 7: 155–9.
20. Gutman M, Sofer D, Lev-Chelouche D et al, Synergism of tumor necrosis factor-alpha and melphalan in systemic and regional administration: animal study. *Invasion Metastasis* 1997; 17: 169–75.
21. Nooijen PT, Manusama ER, Eggermont AM et al, Synergistic effects of TNF-alpha and melphalan in an isolated perfusion model of rat sarcomas: a histological, immunohistochemical and electron microscopic study. *Br J Cancer* 1996; 74: 1908–15.
22. Norda A, Loos U, Sastry M et al, Pharmacokinetics of melphalan in isolated limb perfusion. *Cancer Chemother Pharmacol* 1999; 43: 35–42.
23. Wu ZY, Smithers BM, Roberts MS, Tissue and perfusate pharmacokinetics of melphalan in isolated perfused rat hindlimb. *J Pharmacol Exp Ther* 1997; 282: 1131–8.
24. Wu ZY, Smithers BM, Roberts MS, Melphalan dosing regimens for management of recurrent melanoma by isolated limb perfusion: application of a physiological pharmacokinetic model based on melphalan distribution in the isolated perfused rat hindlimb. *Melanoma Res* 1997; 7: 252–64.
25. Scott RN, Kerr DJ, Blackie R et al, The pharmacokinetic advantages of isolated limb perfusion with melphalan for malignant melanoma. *Br J Cancer* 1992; 66: 159–66.
26. Thompson JF, Kam PCA, Ramzan I et al, Clinical pharmacokinetics of melphalan in isolated limb perfusion: compartmental modelling and moment analysis. *Reg Cancer Treat* 1995; 8: 83–7.
27. Wu ZY, Smithers BM, Parsons PG et al, The effects of perfusion conditions on melphalan distribution in the isolated perfused rat hindlimb bearing a human melanoma xenograft. *Br J Cancer* 1997; 75: 1160–6.
28. Wu ZY, Smithers BM, Anderson C et al, Can tissue drug concentration be monitored by microdialysis during or after isolated limb perfusion for melanoma treatment? *Melanoma Res* 2000; 10: 47–54.
29. Palmeier RK, Lunte CE, Microdialysis sampling in tumour and muscle: study of the disposition of 3-amino-1,2,4-benzotriazine-1,4-Di-N-oxide (SR4233). *Life Sci* 1994; 55: 815–25.
30. Blochl-Daum B, Muller M, Meisinger V et al, Measurement of extracellular fluid carboplatin kinetics in melanoma metastases with microdialysis. *Br J Cancer* 1996; 73: 920–4.
31. Manusama ER, Nooijen PTGA, Stavast J et al, Synergistic antitumour effect of recombinant human tumour necrosis factor α with melphalan in isolated limb perfusion in the rat. *Br J Surg* 1996; 83: 551–5.
32. Manusama ER, Nooijen PTGA, Stavast J et al, Assessment of role of neutrophils on the antitumour effect of TNF-α in an in vivo isolated limb perfusion model in sarcoma bearing Brown Norway rats. *J Surg Res* 1998; 78: 169–75.
33. de Wilt JHW, Manusama ER, van Tiel ST et al, Prerequisites for effective isolated limb perfusion using tumour necrosis factor alpha and melphalan in rats. *Br J Cancer* 1999; 80: 161–6.
34. de Wilt JHW, ten Hagen TLM, de Boeck G et al, Tumour necrosis factor alpha increases melphalan concentration in tumour tissue after isolated limb perfusion. *Br J Cancer* 2000; 82: 1000–3.
35. van der Veen AH, de Wilt JHW, Eggermont AMM et al, TNF-α augments intratumoural concentrations of doxorubicin in TNF-α-based isolated limb perfusion in rat sarcoma models and enhances antitumour effects. *Br J Cancer* 2000; 82: 973–80.
36. de Wilt JHW, Soma G-I, ten Hagen TLM et al, Synergistic anti-tumor effect of TNF-SAM2 with melphalan doxorubicin in isolated limb perfusion in rats. *Anticancer Res* 2000; 20: 3491–6.
37. Hayes MT, Bartley J, Parsons PG, In vitro evaluation of fotemustine as a potential agent for limb perfusion in melanoma. *Melanoma Res* 1998; 8: 67–75.
38. de Wilt JHW, Manusama ER, van Etten B et al, Nitric oxide synthase inhibition results in synergistic anti-tumour activity with melphalan and tumour necrosis factor alpha-based isolated limb perfusions. *Br J Cancer* 2000; 83: 1176–82.
39. Milas M, Ferg B, Yu D et al, Isolated limb perfusion in the sarcoma-bearing rat: a novel preclinical gene delivery system. *Clin Cancer Res* 1997; 3: 2197–203.
40. de Roos WK, de Wilt JHW, van der Kaaden ME et al, Isolated limb perfusion for local gene delivery: efficient and targeted adenovirus-mediated gene transfer into soft tissue sarcomas. *Ann Surg* 2000; 232: 814–21.
41. de Wilt JHW, Bout A, Eggermont AMM et al, Adenovirus-mediated IL-3β gene transfer using isolated limb perfusion inhibits growth of limb sarcoma in rats. *Hum Gene Ther* 2001; 12: 489–502.

40

Recurrent limb melanoma: treatments other than isolated limb perfusion and infusion

Alan J McKay, Dominique S Byrne

INTRODUCTION

There are fundamental questions that need to be addressed in relation to a patient with local or loco-regional recurrence of melanoma. Some of these questions are considered in other chapters dealing with the use of isolated limb perfusion (ILP) and isolated limb infusion (ILI), but they are worthy of further reflection.

- What is the extent of the disease recurrence (i.e. number of nodules/tumour burden)?
- Is there associated regional nodal disease?
- Is there metastatic disease elsewhere?
- What other treatments have been used?

It is essential that the entire patient status is reviewed and that decisions are not based simply on the fact that there are black nodules on a limb. Clearly, the prognosis for any patient is determined by the conflict between the aggressiveness of the tumour and the effectiveness of the immune response which it elicits. Many patients with melanoma can develop local limb recurrence at intervals stretching over many years and yet not develop life-threatening disseminated disease. Such a history needs to be carefully noted, since it can influence the choice of subsequent treatment for these patients. Conversely, patients with asymptomatic local recurrence in whom there is evidence of widespread dissemination of their disease should be treated quite differently. As with every patient, it is thus important to start the management planning with a careful and detailed history. The present episode of recurrence must be placed in the context of the history of the disease from the time of first diagnosis and viewed within the context of the patient's overall prognosis.

Once the history is established, a careful physical examination is important, since further metastases may have been missed by the referring clinician or, indeed, may have become apparent only since the time of the referral. A simple example may be the discovery of lymphadenopathy in a basin other than the draining lymph nodes. Such a finding might drastically alter the treatment plan. Thereafter, it is necessary to stage the disease as accurately as possible. This usually requires computed tomography (CT) scans of the chest, abdomen and pelvis. A CT scan of the brain might also be indicated, although most clinicians would now regard this as unnecessary in the absence of symptoms suggestive of intracranial disease.

In recent years, the status of the regional nodal basin has come under increasingly close scrutiny. In a patient who has significant cutaneous recurrence, and no evidence of metastatic disease outside the limb, aggressive local treatment might be justified. However, the presence of microscopic nodal disease might influence such a decision. While the status of the sentinel lymph node is now routinely established in many major centres dealing with primary melanoma, its value in patients with cutaneous recurrence is more controversial. If it is important to know the nodal status in primary disease, there is some logic in the argument that it is even more important to know the nodal status in the presence of recurrent disease. For example, in a patient with multiple nodules which are symptomatic, ILP or ILI would be treatment options. However, if it is established that the regional nodes are involved, then the prognosis is so adversely altered that a less aggressive form of treatment, possibly with a purely palliative goal, might be more appropriate.

For the remainder of this section, it will be assumed that ILP or ILI have been considered and excluded as appropriate therapeutic options. Thus, other treatment options for cutaneous recurrence of melanoma on a limb will now be considered. These include the following:

- Local surgical excision.
- Laser ablation of tumour deposits.
- Immunotherapy.
- Cryotherapy.
- Hormonal therapy.
- Radiotherapy.
- Systemic chemotherapy.

In the present authors' practice, locoregional recurrence is treated by local excision, laser ablation or ILP in almost all cases. There will be patients in whom symptomatic local disease is part of more widespread recurrence, possibly involving many different organs. Caring for the whole patient is of paramount importance in this situation. It will occasionally be appropriate to offer aggressive local treatment, such as ILP or ILI, even in the presence of widely disseminated disease, but such an approach would be the exception rather than the rule. It is important to remember that cutaneous or soft tissue recurrences are likely to be associated with systemic disease, but it is equally important to spot the patient who has locally aggressive disease which may recur over many years without entering a truly disseminated phase.

LOCAL SURGICAL EXCISION

In considering the surgical excision of melanoma deposits, it is helpful to make the distinction between truly local recurrence and regional recurrence. In this regard, the mode of spread of melanoma is important. The typical appearance of metastatic deposits within a region of the body as satellite lesions or in-transit metastases is believed to be the result of intralymphatic spread of tumour cells, with arrest of their migration at sites situated between the primary lesion and the regional lymph nodes.[1] It is clear, therefore, that these features of the disease probably preclude successful eradication by surgical means unless the tumour deposits are confined to a small area of skin near the primary site. This is generally taken to be within a radius of 3 cm, the truly local recurrence of melanoma.

Just as with a primary melanoma, local recurrence can be treated by wide local excision, and this implies excision of all the skin and subcutaneous tissue between the scar of the primary surgery and the metastatic deposit(s), as well as a margin of tissue around the metastases. The present authors recommend a minimum clearance of 1 cm from any melanoma deposit but would also advocate that a balance be achieved between radical surgical clearance and the risk of cosmetically unacceptable or disfiguring procedures. One should bear in mind that recurrence of melanoma is an indicator of deteriorating prognosis, even when only local recurrence is evident.[2,3]

With satellite metastases and in-transit metastases, it would be naive to believe that surgical excision can achieve any significant degree of prognostic improvement. Even the most radical surgery for locally or regionally recurrent melanoma – limb amputation – is known not to improve the prognosis for these patients.[4–6] The implication is that the metastases represent only the visible part of a more widely spreading tumour. Accordingly, any excisional surgery should be limited to achieving a cosmetically acceptable and/or palliative result. Clearly, where only two or three deposits are visible/palpable, this might be achievable by excision of each of the lesions or of the group of lesions if they are in close proximity to each other. However, when the recurrence manifests itself as multiple deposits of tumour, perhaps spread over a wide area of skin, alternative means of treatment may be more appropriate (vide infra).

The management of metastases within the regional lymph nodes, often confirmed clinically by fine-needle aspiration cytology, can be awkward. When clinically evident, the usual practice is for the surgeon to remove them by dissection of the involved nodal basin.[1,7,8] However, one must bear in mind the possibility (or likelihood) that the disease has already spread beyond the nodal basin. The present authors would therefore advise that a thorough search is made, with a detailed clinical examination and imaging of the central organs, usually by CT scan, to ascertain whether there is any evidence of systemic spread of the melanoma. If so, the patient's treatment should be based principally on therapy of systemic metastases. This does not imply that no specific treatment should be undertaken for the involved lymph nodes. There are situations where, for symptomatic relief or to avoid complications such as erosion into adjacent vessels or through the skin, one might consider local radiotherapy or surgical resection of the affected nodes.[9] However, the aim of that treatment would be palliative.

When regional lymph node metastases coexist with cutaneous deposits in a limb, the surgical option is even more limited. In this situation, the present authors believe that ILP, often followed by a regional node clearance, offers the best prospect of disease control, always assuming that systemic spread of the melanoma has, as far as possible, been excluded.

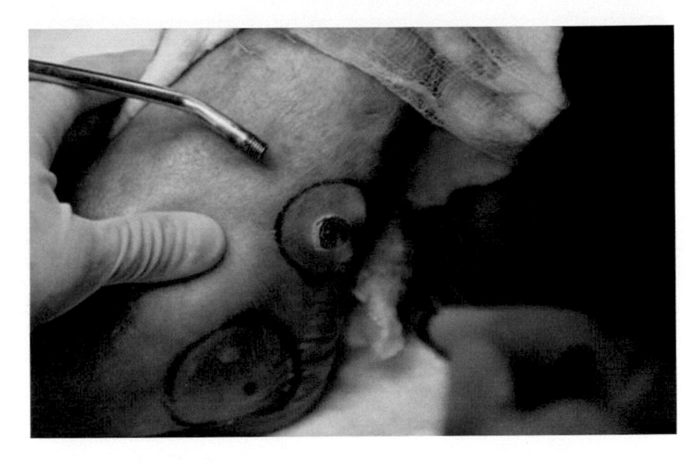

Figure 40.1 *Ablation of subcutaneous deposits of melanoma using the carbon dioxide laser. Note the need to use suction to avoid inhalation of the plume of smoke produced by the vaporization of tumour.*

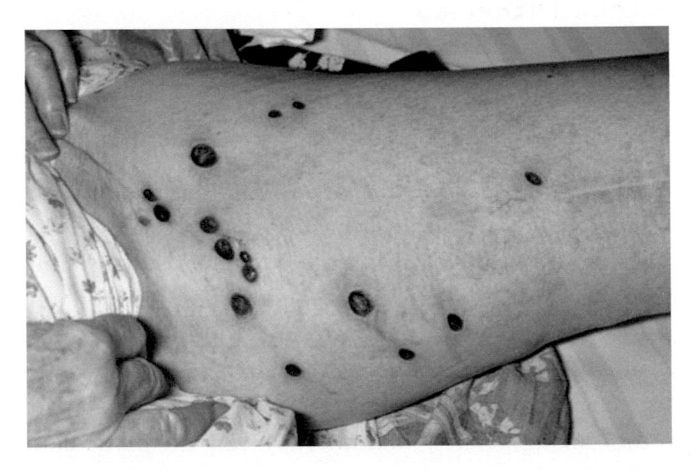

Figure 40.2 *The very localized defects created by laser ablation of melanoma deposits can be left to heal by secondary intention.*

LASER ABLATION OF MELANOMA DEPOSITS

The principal limitation of local excision of metastatic melanoma deposits is the difficulty of achieving skin closure or cover when the deposits are numerous and/or spread over a wide area of the limb. The primary closure of skin defects requires, in most cases, the formation of an elliptical defect and, since several ellipses in close proximity create considerable technical difficulties, a larger ellipse incorporating several deposits may be more desirable. However, this process is ultimately limited by the width of ellipse that would need to be excised to clear the tumour deposits. The application of a skin graft can reduce this problem, but the area which can be grafted with clinically and cosmetically acceptable results is also limited. The prospect of confining the surgical excision to the area of the tumour with a minimal rim of surrounding tissue is therefore an attractive one.

The carbon dioxide (CO_2) laser delivers very short wavelength energy and, at power settings of 10–30 W, allows a focused beam of light with a spot size of 0.5–1.0 mm to destroy tumour nodules (Figure 40.1). The energy produces vaporization of the tumour and can be used simply to ablate the smaller deposits or to excise the larger deposits very accurately without causing significant injury to the surrounding tissue (Figure 40.2). The technique also minimizes blood loss due to the cauterizing effect of the laser. The resultant defect does not require closure but can be treated simply with dressings until healing by secondary intention is complete, typically leaving circular white scars (Figure 40.3). Laser vaporization is therefore a technique which can be used to destroy a large number of tumour deposits at the same time.[10–12] While the need for general anaesthesia in many cases might be regarded as a drawback of this technique, one should bear in mind that the number of lesions which could be surgically excised at one time is very limited compared with laser ablation. In the present authors' practice, laser ablation of melanoma offers a useful therapeutic option in locoregionally recurrent melanoma, particularly when treating recurrent or residual metastases after ILP.

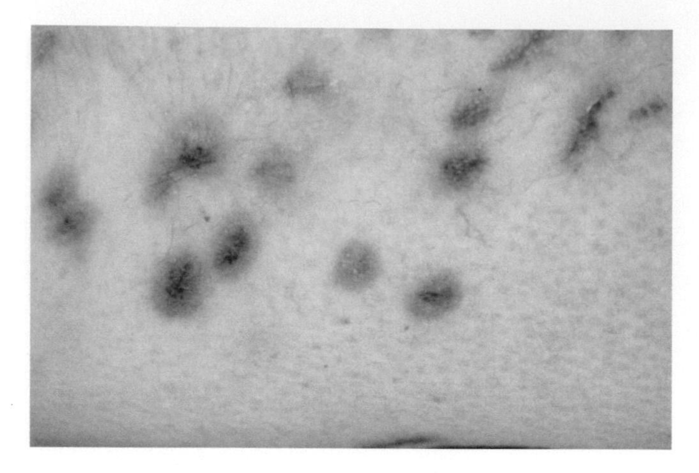

Figure 40.3 *Healed skin after laser ablation of melanoma deposits: the scars will eventually become pale.*

OTHER THERAPIES

If ILP, laser ablation and repeated local excisions have failed to control recurrent disease, what else is available? The use of systemic chemotherapy, local radiotherapy and immunotherapy have been dealt with elsewhere in this book and no amplification is really required. The present authors wish to emphasize that they make regular use of locoregional radiotherapy and have found it to be a useful modality for bulky recurrences, especially in the limbs and the iliac fossa. It is sometimes possible to revert to debulking surgery once the course of radiotherapy has been completed. As with other malignancies, radiotherapy can be particularly helpful when pain is a major problem, though melanoma, even in its advanced form, is not commonly associated with major pain-control problems, the obvious exception being when bone metastases occur.

REGIONAL IMMUNOTHERAPY

It has been known for many years that there are tumour-specific antigens on melanoma cells. Unfortunately, these antigens do not generally produce a vigorous immune response. Agents such as bacille Calmette-Guérin (BCG) or *Corynebacterium parvum* can produce a measurable increase in antibody response to melanoma antigens and, in theory, this might translate into survival benefit.[13] In practice, no such benefit has ever been determined. More specific immunization using irradiated melanoma cells, or with melanoma antigens alone or in combination with chemotherapy or radiotherapy, has been tried, once again with no survival benefit and very low local response rates in comparison with other treatment modalities.[14]

Intralesional BCG can undoubtedly produce regression of dermal nodules but it has little effect on subcutaneous nodules, involved lymph nodes or visceral metastases.[15] Bauer et al.[16] reported a complete response rate of 67% and a partial response rate of 29% using this method.[16] This method is no longer used in the present authors' practice, as it is believed that alternative methods give superior results.

Within the last decade, immunotherapy using either single or clustered monoclonal antibodies has attracted considerable attention. Isotopic labelling of antibodies demonstrated their relative tumour specificity, but adding a therapeutic dimension proved to be unrewarding. In the present authors' unit, use of labelled monoclonal antibodies within the ILP setting allowed identification of otherwise undetectable metastases within the perfused limb. However, the uptake ratios achieved between tumour and normal tissue (2.5:1–3.5:1) were lower than desired and redistribution of the antibody to the liver was observed after 24 hours. As a result, targeted therapy could not be safely undertaken.

CRYOTHERAPY

Approximately 20 years ago, cryotherapy was being proposed as the treatment of choice in many surgical conditions, from liver metastases to haemorrhoids, including recurrent melanoma. In many ways, the treatment is analogous to laser ablation in that it can be used under local or regional anaesthesia, does not require hospital admission and the extent of tissue necrosis can be controlled to an acceptable degree. There are very few reports of its use in prospective studies, but such experience as has been reported suggests that it is most effective for intradermal metastases.[17]

In units where clinicians have gained experience of the technique it remains in use, but laser ablation has largely replaced it in most major centres.

HORMONAL THERAPY

The apparent hormonal influence on the human melanocyte system, both in health (chloasma of pregnancy) and in disease (female survival advantage in melanoma), would suggest that hormone manipulation might have something to offer in the treatment of locoregional recurrence. Almost inevitably, tamoxifen has been tried in such patients, but studies have shown poor objective response rates with this drug, as well as with medroxyprogesterone acetate.[18–20] It is of interest that tamoxifen appears to produce an advantage when added to the chemotherapeutic combination of dacarbazine, carmustine (BCNU) and cisplatin, but, while the mechanism is unclear, this is believed to be due to a synergy between tamoxifen and cisplatin.[21,22] The use of corticosteroids, particularly dexamethasone, can be justified for brain secondaries of melanocytic origin, as with other types of malignancy.[23]

CONCLUSIONS

Local and locoregional recurrences can range from a single subcutaneous deposit to very extensive involvement of a region of the body without necessarily being accompanied by rapidly progressive systemic disease (Figure 40.4). It is this characteristic which creates the need for a variety of therapeutic modalities in the armamentarium of the melanoma specialist. At times, the choice of therapy may be difficult, but the present authors recommend the use of an algorithm, such as that shown in Figure 40.5, as a guide to treatment in individual cases.

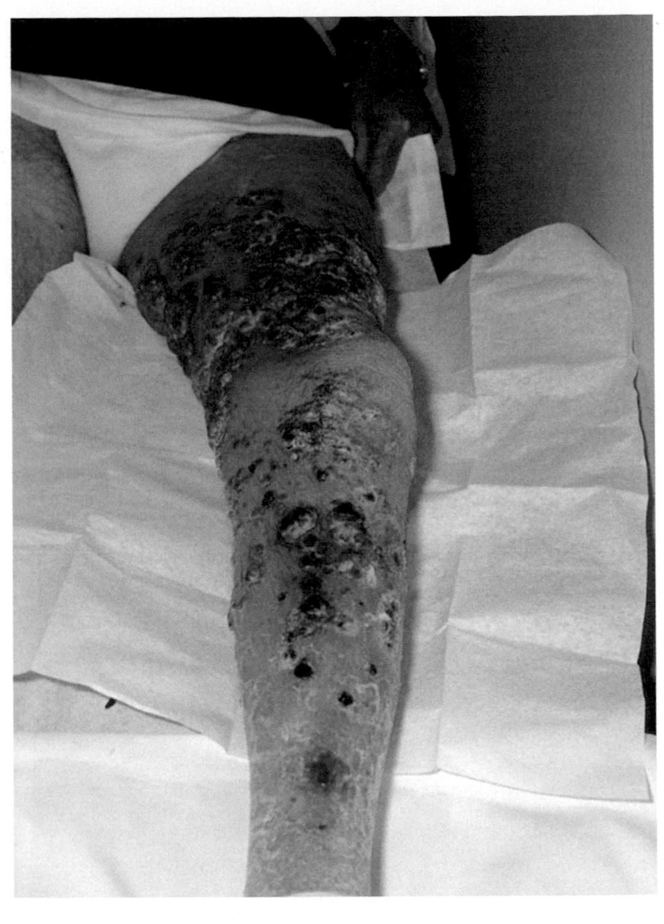

Figure 40.4 *Extensive locoregional recurrence of melanoma, in this case not accompanied by detectable systemic disease. Isolated limb perfusion is the only realistic therapeutic option in such a case.*

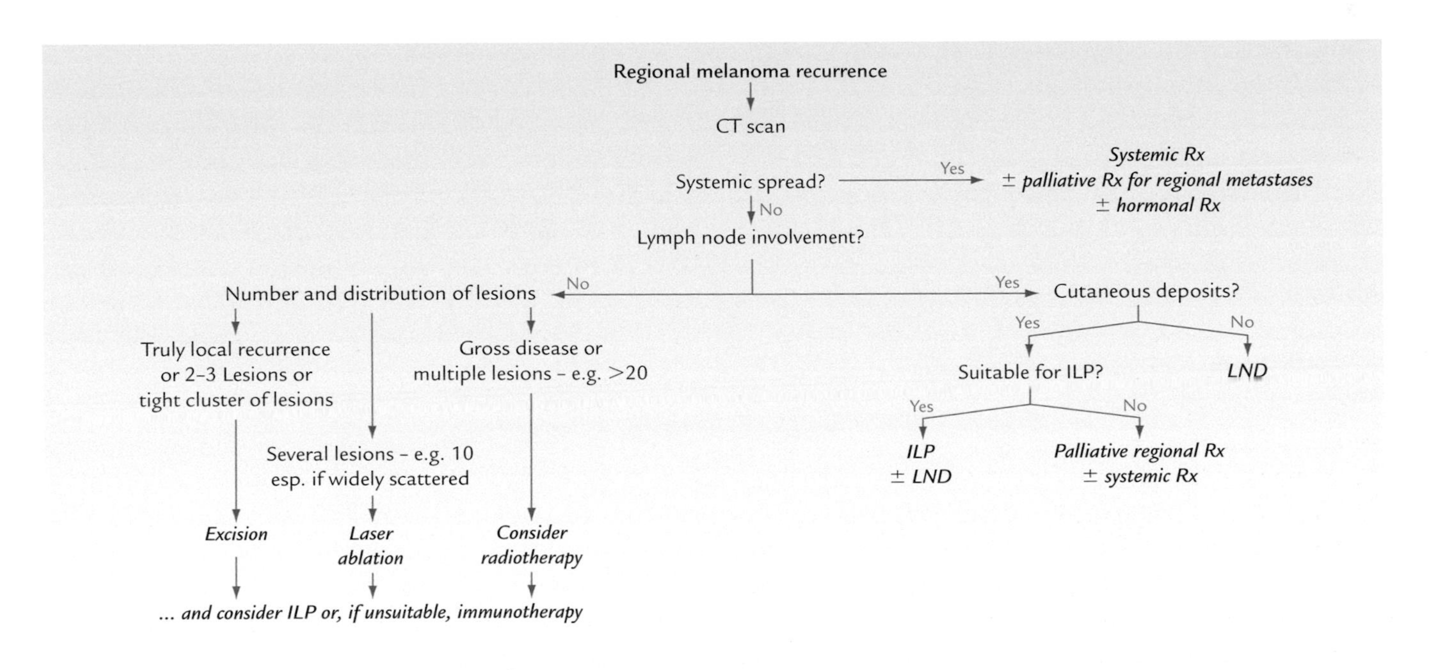

Figure 40.5 *Suggested algorithm for the management of patients with recurrent malignant melanoma.*

REFERENCES

1. Balch CM, Urist MM, Maddox WA et al, Management of regional metastatic melanoma. In: *Cutaneous melanoma. Clinical management and treatment results worldwide* (eds Balch CM, Milton GW). Philadelphia: JP Lippincott, 1985: 93–130.
2. Fortner JG, Strong EW, Mulcare RJ et al, The surgical treatment of recurrent melanoma. *Surg Clin North Am* 1974; 54: 865–70.
3. Reintgen DS, Vollmer R, Tso CY, Seigler HF, Prognosis for recurrent stage I malignant melanoma. *Arch Surg* 1987; 122: 1338–42.
4. McPeak CJ, McNeer GP, Whiteley HW, Booher RJ, Amputation for melanoma of the extremity. *Surgery* 1963; 54: 426–31.
5. Turnbull A, Shah J, Fortner J, Recurrent melanoma of an extremity treated by major amputation. *Arch Surg* 1973; 106: 496–8.
6. Cox KR, Survival after amputation for recurrent melanoma. *Surg Gynecol Obstet* 1974; 134: 720–2.
7. Veronesi U, Adamus J, Bandiera DC et al, Delayed regional lymph node dissection in Stage I melanoma of the skin of the lower extremities. *Cancer* 1978; 41: 948–56.
8. Bowsher WG, Taylor BA, Hughes LE, Morbidity, mortality and local recurrence following regional node dissection for melanoma. *Br J Surg* 1986; 73: 906–8.
9. Wanebo HJ, Binns R, Surgical treatment of recurrent and metastatic malignant melanoma. In: *Contemporary issues in clinical oncology, Volume 6: Management of advanced melanoma* (ed Nathanson L). New York: Churchill Livingstone, 1986; 185–94.
10. Lingam MK, McKay AJ, Carbon dioxide laser ablation as an alternative treatment for cutaneous metastases from malignant melanoma. *Br J Surg* 1995; 82: 1346–8.
11. Hill S, Thomas JM, Use of carbon dioxide laser to manage cutaneous metastases from malignant melanoma. *Br J Surg* 1996; 83: 509–12.
12. Strobbe LJ, Nieweg OE, Kroon BB, Carbon dioxide laser for cutaneous melanoma metastases: indications and limitations. *Eur J Surg Oncol* 1997; 23: 435–8.
13. Balch CM, Hersey P, Current status of adjuvant therapy. In: *Cutaneous melanoma. Clinical management and treatment results worldwide* (eds Balch CM, Milton GW). Philadelphia: JP Lippincott, 1985: 197–218.
14. Mastrangelo MJ, Schultz S, Kane M, Berd D, Newer immunologic approaches to the treatment of patients with melanoma. *Semin Oncol* 1988; 15: 589–94.
15. Mastrangelo MJ, Bellet RE, Berd D, Immunology and immunotherapy of human cutaneous malignant melanoma. In: *Human malignant melanoma* (eds Goldman WH, Mastrangelo MJ). New York: Grune and Stratton, 1979: 355–416.
16. Bauer R, Kopald K, Lee J et al, Long term results of intralesional BCG for locally advanced recurrent malignant melanoma. *Proc Am Soc Clin Oncol* 1990; 9: 276 (abstract).
17. Burge SM, Dawber RP, Cryotherapy for lentigo maligna [letter]. *J Dermatol Surg Oncol* 1984; 10: 910.
18. Coates AS, Durant JR, Chemotherapy for metastatic melanoma. In: (eds Balch CM, Milton GW) *Cutaneous melanoma. Clinical management and treatment results worldwide.* Philadelphia: JP Lippincott, 1985: 275–82.
19. Wagstaff J, Thatcher N, Rankin E, Crowther D, Tamoxifen in the treatment of metastatic malignant melanoma. *Cancer Treat Rep* 1982; 66: 1771.
20. Beecher R, Kloke O, Hoffken K et al, Phase II study of high dose medroxyprogesterone acetate in advanced malignant melanoma. *Br J Cancer* 1989; 59: 948.
21 McClay EF, Mastrangelo MJ, Sprandio JD, Bellet RE, Berd D, The importance of tamoxifen to a cisplatin-containing regimen in the treatment of metastatic melanoma. *Cancer* 1989; 63: 1292–5.
22. McClay EF, Albright KD, Jones JA, Christen RD, Howell SB, Tamoxifen modulation of cisplatin sensitivity in human malignant melanoma cells. *Cancer Res* 1993; 53: 1571–6.
23. Fletcher JW, George EA, Henry RE, Donati RM, Brain scans, dexamethasone therapy and brain tumours. *JAMA*; 1975; 232: 1261–3.

41

Metastatic melanoma at distant sites: follow-up

John A Olson Jr, Daniel G Coit

INTRODUCTION

The incidence of cutaneous melanoma is rising faster than any other human malignancy. In the United States of America (USA) alone, 47,700 new cases of melanoma were diagnosed during 2000. Estimates suggest that one in 72 persons born in the year 2000 in the USA will develop melanoma in their lifetime.[1] Malignant melanoma will become a major public health concern in several countries, not only with regard to diagnosis and treatment, but, as most patients are rendered disease-free after initial treatment, also with regard to patient follow-up.

As a result of increasing public awareness, most patients with melanoma now present with early stage disease curable by surgery alone.[2] Statistics from the US Surveillance, Epidemiology, and End Results (SEER) Program have shown a steady increase in 5-year survival for patients with melanoma, now >88% overall.[1] However, the biology of melanoma is complex and the course of the disease is often unpredictable. Melanoma may remain dormant for years and patients may develop distant metastases decades after the initial diagnosis. In addition, survivors of melanoma have an estimated 3–6% lifetime risk of developing a second primary melanoma.[3–5]

Melanoma is mostly a disease of young people; the median age at diagnosis is 45 years and most patients are otherwise healthy. Median survival for patients with early stage melanoma is >20 years.[1] Hence, patients with melanoma have many productive years of life at stake, and frequently face a lifetime of uncertainty.

The combination of rising incidence, young age at diagnosis, and a high but unpredictable cure rate will create a relatively large population of melanoma patients who are at risk for disease recurrence. Evidence-based strategies are required to effectively monitor these patients following primary treatment. This chapter will address post-treatment surveillance of patients with melanoma and will outline suggestions for follow-up based on the available data.

WHY FOLLOW UP PATIENTS WITH MELANOMA?

Based upon the reasonable assumption that follow-up of treated patients will identify tumor recurrences amenable to treatment, surveillance of patients after potentially curative treatment for melanoma is routine practice. Careful follow-up is also the only mechanism to define the natural history of melanoma and to document end results of new therapies. Patient education, aimed at minimizing risk and enhancing early detection of second melanomas, is another important aspect of melanoma surveillance. A final and compelling argument for surveillance is the psychosocial support and reassurance that patients derive from being followed-up.

Melanoma can be an indolent disease with an unpredictable clinical course. Locoregional and distant recurrences occurring beyond 10 years after treatment of a primary melanoma are not uncommon.[6] The potential for delayed recurrence is often cited as a reason for prolonged surveillance of melanoma patients. Survivors of melanoma are also at increased risk of a second primary melanoma. Estimates of lifetime risk vary from 3 to 6%, and are higher for patients with dysplastic nevi and/or a family history of melanoma.[7,8] The yield of dermatologic surveillance in these patients should be high relative to the general non-melanoma population, since structured, prospective surveillance for melanoma in these high-risk groups has been reported to enhance detection of subsequent thinner melanoma.[9] Melanoma survivors are also at risk for the development of other non-melanoma skin cancers and may be at slightly increased risk for other non-cutaneous malignancies.[10]

The intuitive assumption that a structured follow-up program results in improved detection of treatable recurrences has been challenged by a number of retrospective studies. These address not only who detects recurrent melanoma, but also what is the outcome after patient-detected versus physician-detected recurrences.[11–15] In general, these studies suggest that patients detect roughly half of all recurrences. Furthermore, the preponderance of data suggest that outcome after physician-detected recurrence is quite similar to that of patient-detected recurrence (see Table 41.1).

WHO RECURS?

Overall, *c.* one in four patients with localized melanoma will recur.[6] Depth of invasion directly correlates with the risk of recurrence in these patients.[16] For patients with in situ and thin (<1.0 mm) primary lesions, recurrence is infrequent. At the other end of the spectrum, patients with thick melanoma (≥4.0 mm) have an estimated 50% chance of recurrence at 5 years.[17] Additional factors that increase the risk of recurrence for early stage melanoma include tumor ulceration, axial location, older age, and male sex. Patients treated for melanoma metastatic to regional lymph nodes are at higher (40–70%) risk of recurrence.[18,19] In this group, the risk of both locoregional and distant relapse increases with increasing number of positive lymph nodes and the presence of extranodal tumor extension.[20]

WHEN DO PATIENTS WITH MELANOMA RECUR?

Time to melanoma recurrence varies inversely with tumor stage at presentation. The greatest annual risk of recurrence occurs in the first year following treatment, declining steadily over time.[21,22] Among patients with localized melanoma who recur, 55–67% become evident within 2 years, while 65–85% become apparent by 3 years after initial treatment (Figure 41.1).[16,18,23]

Time to recurrence for patients with node-negative (stage I–II) melanoma varies inversely with tumor thickness.[16] Of patients with localized melanoma followed by McCarthy et al.,[21] 95% of recurrences in patients with primary tumors <0.7 mm thick developed within 11 years; in contrast, 95% of recurrences in patients with primary tumors >3.0 mm thick occurred within 5 years. Age at diagnosis may also influence time to recurrence; patients older than the age of 50 have been found to relapse sooner than patients younger than the age of 50.[16] A small subset of patients (<7%) with thin (<1 mm) node-negative melanoma will recur 10 or more years after primary diagnosis.[6,24]

Patients who present with nodal metastases from melanoma recur earlier than those with negative lymph

Table 41.1 *Melanoma follow-up series*

Author(s) (ref. no.)	No. of patients	No. evaluable recurrences	Recurrences detected by patient (%)	Recurrences detected by physician	Survival difference
Baughan et al. (12)	331	65	41 (63)	20 (37)	*P* = NS*
Jillella et al. (13)	279	49	46 (16)	3 (3)	Not stated
Ruark et al. (14)	2268	257	185 (72)	72 (28)	*P* = 0.03
Shumate et al. (15)	1475	195	128 (66)	67 (34)	*P* = NS*
Weiss et al. (11)	261	145	99 (45)	46 (32)	Not stated
Reeves (53)	614	138	– (59)	– (41)	*P* = 0.02

*NS, Not significant.

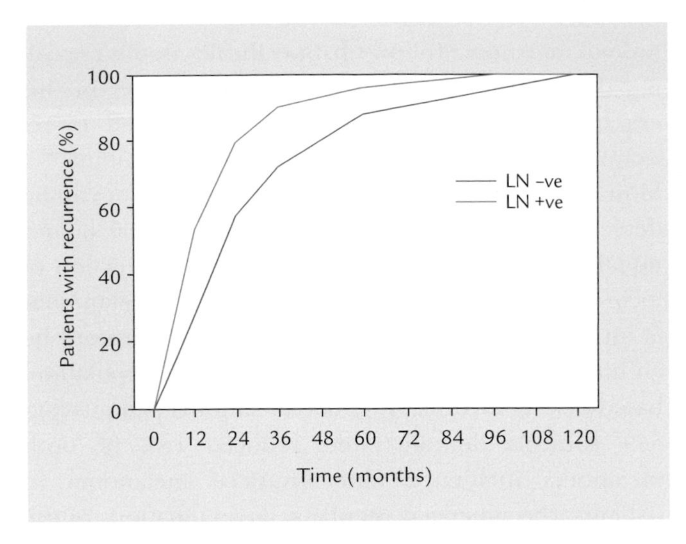

Figure 41.1 *Time course to initial melanoma recurrence after lymph node (LN) dissection, stratified by nodal status. Modified with permission from Gadd et al.,* Arch Surg *1992; 127: 1412–16.*

nodes. Eighty percent of recurrences in node-positive patients are detected within 2 years of initial treatment (Figure 41.1).[19,25]

WHERE DOES MELANOMA RECUR?

Autopsy and clinical data have shown that melanoma can spread to virtually any organ or tissue.[26] Site of melanoma recurrence depends upon both tumor biology and initial treatment. Clinical patterns of melanoma recurrence have been well described elsewhere.[21,22] Nodal recurrence is the initial site of relapse in 50–60% of patients in whom an elective lymph node dissection was not a component of primary treatment (Figure 41.2a). For patients who have had elective lymph node dissection, there is no increased rate of melanoma metastases overall, but systemic visceral

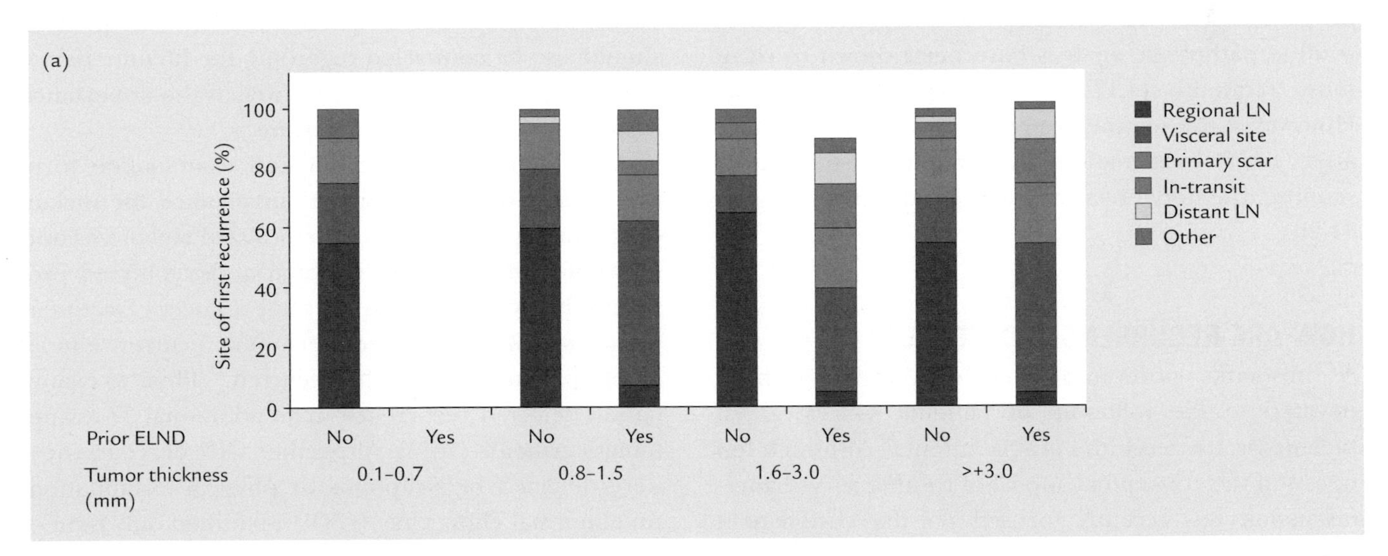

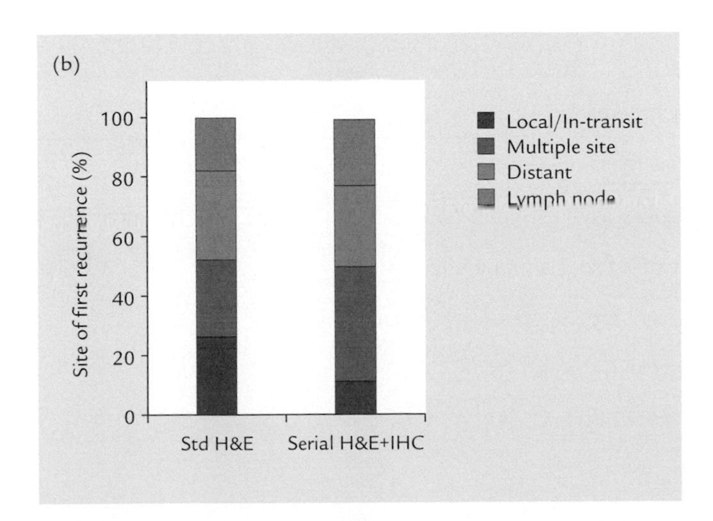

Figure 41.2 *(a) Site of first recurrence following treatment of primary melanoma in 3171 patients at the Sydney Melanoma Unit. Data are expressed as a percentage of total recurrences and are grouped according to primary tumor thickness and initial surgical treatment. Total recurrences: 662 (27%) in 2417 patients without elective lymph node dissection (ELND) and 214 (28%) in 754 patients with ELND. LN, Lymph node. (Modified from McCarthy et al,[21] with permission.) (b) Site of first recurrence following negative sentinel lymph node (SLN) biopsy in primary melanoma. Data are expressed as a percentage of total recurrences and are grouped according to the method of SLN analysis. Left-hand column: routine hematoxylin–eosin (H&E) evaluation; right-hand column: re-evaluation of routine H&E-negative SLN with serial section H&E and immunohistochemistry (IHC). Data taken with permission from Gershenwald et al.,* J Clin Oncol *1998; 16: 2253–60.*[29]

metastases predominate and regional nodal recurrences occur relatively less frequently. However, even after lymph node dissection, regional nodal disease is still observed in 2–33% of patients who recur.[19] Local and in-transit recurrence can be expected in 2–10% and 2–38% of melanoma patients, respectively. Local and in-transit recurrences occur most often in thick melanomas and those with lymphovascular invasion or satellites. The incidence of local recurrence does not appear to depend on the initial treatment of the draining nodal basin.

Visceral metastases are the initial site of relapse in *c.* 25% of all melanoma patients who recur.[6,16,21,27,28] The most common clinical sites of visceral metastases are the lung, brain, liver and gastrointestinal tract. Bone metastases are infrequently the first site of melanoma relapse.

Patterns of recurrence after sentinel lymph node biopsy (SLNB) for melanoma have recently been described.[29] Patients who have had a negative SLNB by routine pathologic analysis have been shown to recur most frequently (4.1%) in the mapped nodal basin. However, if the sentinel lymph nodes are truly negative after serial examination and immunohistochemical staining, the nodal recurrence rate is quite low (Figure 41.2b).

HOW ARE RECURRENCES DETECTED?

A substantial portion of melanoma care has been devoted to the follow-up of patients with localized melanoma treated with curative intent.[30] Although few question the conceptual appeal of routine surveillance, discussion has recently focused on the cost–benefit ratio of melanoma follow-up. Specifically, doubt regarding the yield of expensive imaging modalities in this era of cost-effective medical practice has led to re-examination of follow-up strategies for melanoma.[30,31] Most melanoma recurrences are symptomatic or can be detected by physical examination. Regular skin and nodal basin self-examination can facilitate detection of locoregional recurrences and new primary melanomas at an early stage. Patient education must therefore be an integral part of melanoma follow-up. A population-based case–control study of 650 melanoma patients and 549 controls demonstrated reduced risk of both melanoma incidence and advanced melanoma in patients who practiced regular self-examinations of the skin.[32] Visceral recurrences are more often clinically silent or produce non-specific symptoms (Table 41.2). Metastatic disease should be suspected and investigated appropriately with any new symptom that progresses in either intensity or frequency. Melanoma patients should also be counseled regarding the lifetime risk of a second primary melanoma, as well as the importance of avoiding excessive sun exposure.

A periodic history and physical examination form the cornerstone of physician surveillance for melanoma. Among 261 patients with localized melanoma and melanoma metastatic to regional nodes followed prospectively by the North Central Cancer Treatment Group, symptoms signaled melanoma recurrence in 99 of 145 patients (68%) who recurred.[11] Physical examination detected recurrence in an additional 37 asymptomatic patients (26%). Altogether, 94% of recurrences were detected by symptoms or physical examination. An abnormal chest x ray (CXR) identified only nine of

Table 41.2 *Symptoms of recurrent melanoma**

Metastatic site	Symptoms
Skin, lymph node, subcutaneous site	New mass
Lung	Usually asymptomatic (rarely, cough, dyspnea, or hemoptysis)
Gastrointestinal tract	Obstruction, pain, anemia
Liver	Weight loss, anorexia, abdominal pain
Brain	Headache, weakness
Bone	Pain, fracture

*Modified from Meyers and Balch,[52] with permission.

145 recurrences (6%) and in no patient was an abnormal laboratory test the sole indicator of recurrent disease.

Similarly, Mooney et al.[31] assessed the impact of a surveillance program using physical examination, blood tests, and CXR on 1004 patients with American Joint Committee on Cancer (AJCC) stage I or II cutaneous melanoma. Physical examination detected 72% of recurrences, constitutional symptoms indicated 17% of recurrences, and chest radiographs revealed 11% of recurrences. Blood tests did not identify any recurrence. Thus, the preponderance of data suggests that most recurrences can be identified by a directed history and physical examination during the follow-up visit. CXR detected 6–11% of recurrences in these studies.

Routine laboratory studies have limited application in surveillance of patients with melanoma. An exception may be serum lactate dehydrogenase (LDH); an isolated elevation of this serum enzyme in patients at risk is considered by many to be suggestive of metastatic disease. Khansur et al.[33] found an LDH level >300 U/l in all patients with imageable chest, lung, bone, and visceral metastases, and they concluded that LDH is a useful screening tool for metastatic disease. In contrast, Buzaid et al.[34] found the sensitivity of LDH as an indicator of distant metastases to be low, suggesting that the low tumor burden at initial recurrence in closely followed patients makes LDH a less effective screening tool. Other laboratory tests, including lipid-bound sialic acid, neuron-specific enolase, serum S-100 and 5-*S*-cysteinyldopa, have shown promise in early studies, but have not been sufficiently evaluated to be recommended.[35]

Kelley et al.[36] have reported on the predictive value of the tumor-associated antigen TA-90 in serum of patients with melanoma. In their study, the presence of the antigen in patients clinically free of disease, as measured by enzyme-linked immunosorbent assay (ELISA), was highly predictive of subsequent clinical relapse. The sensitivity and specificity of the TA-90 ELISA test were estimated at 77% and 76%, respectively. In another study, authors from the same institution postulated that the combination of TA-90 ELISA testing and a positron emission tomography (PET) scan might have a role in the routine surveillance of patients at risk for melanoma recurrence.[37] To date, however, this strategy has not been widely adopted.

Extensive radiologic testing in follow-up of asymptomatic patients is frequently unrewarding and generally not indicated. A standard posteroanterior CXR for screening asymptomatic patients is sufficiently sensitive and cost-effective to warrant routine use. In the absence of symptoms or an abnormal finding on physical examination, CXR or laboratory tests (e.g. elevated LDH), the yield of routine CT scanning is too low to be recommended for use as a screening tool. The false-positive rate of CT in the asymptomatic patient is high and often leads to additional unrewarding tests.[34] The recent successful application of FDG-PET to melanoma staging has stimulated interest in this modality as a surveillance tool.[38] Currently, the high cost and limited availability of FDG-PET preclude its use in routine screening of asymptomatic patients for recurrence.

DOES EARLY DETECTION AND TREATMENT OF RECURRENCE IMPROVE SURVIVAL?

Melanoma patients who recur are more likely to die from their disease but, in at least some patients, early detection of recurrences could lead to potentially curative therapy and prevent death from disease. Therapy for recurrent melanoma may be either curative or palliative, determined most often by site of recurrence. Isolated locoregional and solitary pulmonary metastases are the lesions most amenable to resection with curative intent, and surveillance to detect these recurrences may prove worthwhile. On the other hand, visceral, brain and bone recurrences are more often components of multiple-site, incurable recurrences. Survival for patients destined for this type of recurrence is not likely to be influenced by surveillance, and treatment for these patients is more often directed at palliation of identifiable symptoms.

Treatment options for patients with unresectable melanoma metastases are limited. Systemic therapy with dacarbazine (DTIC), either as a single agent or in combination with carmustine (BCNU), cisplatin and tamoxifen (the Dartmouth regimen), produces an overall response rate of *c.* 20–34%.[39] Complete responses to chemotherapy are infrequent (5–10%) and median survival is usually <9 months. The recent combination of chemotherapy and biologic agents, including interferon-alpha (IFN-α) and interleukin-2 (IL-2), which alone have modest activity against melanoma, has renewed interest in systemic treatment of melanoma. Early reports of biochemotherapy suggest a complete response rate of up to 21%, a partial response rate of 43%, and a median survival of almost 12 months.[40] Despite these encouraging results, there is no convincing evidence that systemic treatment of distant metastases results in prolonged survival for most patients. A detailed discussion of systemic therapy for melanoma metastases can be found elsewhere in this book.

Most series of patients treated for metastatic melanoma have shown that surgical, as opposed to nonsurgical, treatment is associated with improved survival.[41] This likely reflects the better performance status and lower tumor burden of patients with localized disease who are amenable to surgery. Subsets of patients with isolated recurrences clearly benefit from surgical treatment and presumably, therefore, surveillance.

Patients who have not undergone elective lymph node dissection or SLNB as a component of initial treatment recur most often within undissected nodal basins. These recurrences are usually amenable to resection with curative intent. Consequently, surveillance of melanoma patients who have not had lymph node dissection may be especially necessary.

Locoregional and distant non-visceral metastases represent 52–69% of melanoma recurrences, almost half of which are solitary.[42] Screening for these treatable recurrences is accomplished inexpensively with directed physical examination and the potential exists to direct curative therapy. Complete resection of locoregional and distant soft tissue metastases results in median survival of as high as 50 months, with 5-year survival rates of up to 61%.[42]

The lung is the most common visceral site of metastasis.[25] Isolated pulmonary recurrences represent 7–21% of melanoma recurrences and are potentially curable with resection. Of patients with pulmonary metastases from melanoma, 12–25% are operable and 65–96% of these are completely resected.[23,43,44] After complete resection median survival of 8–20 months is reported, with 5-year survival rates of 10–25%.[41,43,44] It is likely that resection of pulmonary metastases alters the natural course of melanoma in certain patients. Since the usual presentation of pulmonary metastases is an asymptomatic nodule on screening CXR, routine surveillance may benefit the small subgroup of patients who recur only in the lung.

Melanoma metastases to other visceral sites, including the brain, liver and gastrointestinal (GI) tract, often produce symptoms and are often components of multiple site recurrences. Brain metastases produce neurologic symptoms of mass effect. Surgical intervention in these cases is most often palliative and few long-term survivors exist, even after complete resection. Hepatic metastases as a sole site of cutaneous melanoma recurrence are uncommon. Hepatic resection for isolated ocular melanoma recurrences in highly selected patients has been reported.[45] Melanoma metastases to the GI tract most often cause either obstruction or occult bleeding. Surgical palliation is effective and, if resection is complete, can result in 5-year survival rates of up to 20% in selected patients.[46] In general, the impact of surgery on the natural history of symptomatic melanoma metastases to the brain, liver and GI tract is likely to be small, with no evidence that treating asymptomatic patients improves outcome. Therefore, routine surveillance for these recurrences is probably not worthwhile.

Based on the observation that melanoma deposits >2 cm are resistant to chemotherapy, surgical debulking of melanoma metastases followed by either biochemotherapy or immunotherapy with melanoma vaccines has been proposed. The potential benefit for this multimodality approach is presently unclear and awaits the results of ongoing clinical trials.

WHAT IS CURRENTLY PRACTICED?

There are no widely accepted uniform surveillance paradigms for patients with localized melanoma. It is often a combination of individual patient preferences and physician experience with other malignancies that influences the pattern of follow-up and follow-up schedule.

In 1991, the National Cancer Institute published a consensus statement for the follow-up of patients treated for early (<1.0 mm thick) melanoma.[47] Patients with melanoma in situ can be followed with yearly skin examinations. Those with thin melanoma and without dysplastic nevi or a family history of melanoma can be followed at 6-monthly intervals for 2 years, and then yearly. Patients with thin melanoma and dysplastic nevi and/or a family history of melanoma can be followed with history and physical examination only at 3–6-monthly intervals for at least 2 years, depending on stability of atypical moles. For all patients, education regarding skin examination and sun avoidance is appropriate. The consensus statement suggested that examination should focus on dermatologic surveillance and a locoregional physical examination; searching for clinically occult distant metastases with CXR or bloodwork is generally not recommended.

A number of studies have been published that describe follow-up of patients treated for melanoma. Kelly et al.[48] proposed a follow-up schedule based on their analysis of recurrence in 1324 clinical stage I melanoma patients who were followed for a mean of 3.5 years: patients with melanoma <0.76 mm thick be seen at 6-monthly intervals for the first year, and yearly thereafter; 0.76–1.49 mm thick, every 6 months; 1.5–4.0 mm every 3 months for the first year, every 4 months during years 2–4, and every 6 months thereafter; 4.0 mm thick, every 2–3 months for the first year, every 3 months during years 2–4, and every 6 months thereafter.

Review of 3171 patients followed at the Sydney Melanoma Unit from 2.5 to 36.2 years demonstrated an overall recurrence rate of 28%.[21] Interval to first recurrence correlated with tumor thickness and the authors proposed the following surveillance scheme based on the assumption that the physician detects at least 50% of recurrences during a routine follow-up visit: patients with tumors <0.7 mm thick, once yearly; 0.8–1.5 mm thick, every 6 months for 3 years, and yearly thereafter; 1.6–3.0 mm thick, every 2 months for the first year, every 4 months during year 2, every 6 months during year 3, every 9 months during years 4 and 5, and once yearly thereafter; >3.0 mm thick, every 1.5 months during the first year, every 2 months for the second year, every 4 months during years 3–5, and once yearly thereafter.

Romero et al.[49] proposed schedules for follow-up intervals based on a survey of eight melanoma experts. The authors suggested that regular follow-up intervals vary as follows according to thickness of the melanomas: for melanomas up to 0.75 mm thick, every 6 months for years 1 and 2, and then annually for years 3–5; for melanomas 0.76–1.50 mm thick, every 3 months for years 1 and 2, and semi-annually for years 3–5; and for melanomas >1.50 mm thick, every 3 months for years 1–3, and semi-annually for years 4 and 5. After the fifth year, all patients are examined annually for life because of the continued risk of recurrences and new primary melanomas. More frequent examinations may be appropriate for those individuals at especially high risk for developing multiple primary melanomas, such as those patients with dysplastic nevi or a strong family history of melanoma.

Recently, Poo-Hwu et al.[50] reported results of a prospective melanoma surveillance protocol involving 373 patients at the Yale Melanoma Unit. This program consisted of a patient education program and a follow-up schedule based upon the stage of disease. Of 78 recurrences, 56% were detected by physicians (asymptomatic recurrence) and 44% were discovered by patients themselves (symptomatic recurrences). Most recurrences were found within 1 (47%) or 2 (78%) years of follow-up. In this study, asymptomatic patients with a recurrence had a survival advantage over those patients with symptomatic recurrences. Based on the hazard ratio of recurrence, a follow-up schedule was proposed: stage I (melanoma thickness <1.5 mm) – annually; stage II (melanoma thickness >1.5 mm) – every 6 months for years 1 and 2, then annually; stage III (melanoma of any thickness with nodal and/or in-transit metastases) – every 3 months for year 1, every 4 months for year 2, every 6 months for years 3–5, then annually.

Uniform staging, treatment, and surveillance schemes for all stages of melanoma have recently been proposed by the National Comprehensive Cancer Network (NCCN) (Figure 41.3).[51] In the absence of clear data, opinions on the appropriate follow-up for patients with melanoma varied widely. The authors concluded that for patients with melanoma <1.0 mm thick, history and physical examination alone should be performed every 6 months for years 1 and 2, and then annually; laboratory and CXR screening were not recommended. For patients with stage I–II melanomas ≥1.0 mm thick, history and physical examination should be performed every 3–6 months for years 1–3, every 6–12 months for years 4 and 5, and then annually. Routine use of liver function tests (LFT) and CXR were acknowledged as extremely low yield, but were nevertheless included in the guidelines, to be performed at 6–12-monthly intervals at the discretion of the physician. Patients with stage III melanoma were recommended to have a history and physical examination every 3–6 months for years 1–3, every 4–12 months for years 4 and 5, and then annually. LFT, complete blood count (CBC) and CXR were included every 3–12 months at the discretion of the physician. Routine CT scans were considered inappropriate in the absence of abnormalities detected through history, physical examination, blood tests or CXR. A similar schedule was recommended for patients with stage IV melanoma. At the present authors' center the follow-up schedule proposed by the NCCN, shown in Figure 41.3 is used.

The optimal duration of follow-up for all patients with melanoma remains controversial. It is clear that most recurrences occur within 5 years of initial treatment and that the most cost-effective strategy is to follow patients during this period. Nevertheless, the potential for late recurrence (>10 years), as well as the risk of second melanoma (4%), are recognized reasons for a lifetime of at least dermatologic surveillance.

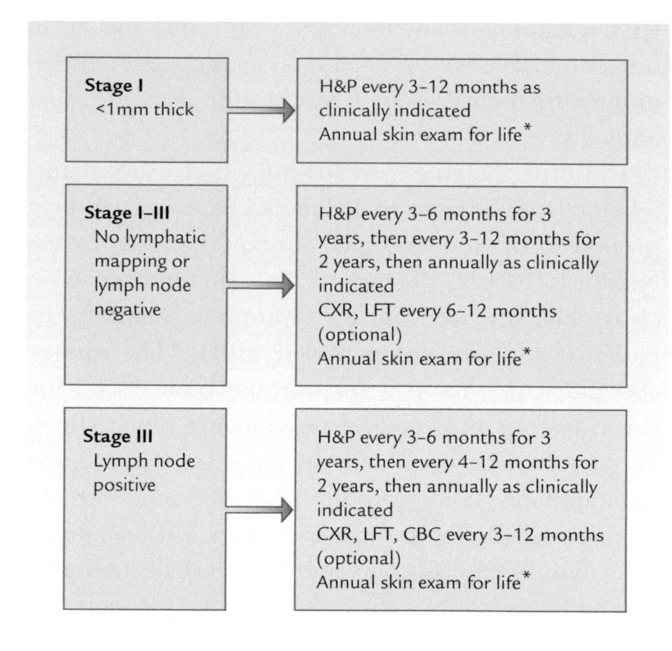

Figure 41.3 *Recommended follow-up scheme for patients with localized melanoma. H&P, Physician history and physical examination (exam), with emphasis on skin and lymph nodes; CXR, PA/lateral chest x ray; LFT, liver function tests; CBC, complete blood count. *Follow-up schedule influenced by risk of recurrence from primary, and includes other factors such as dysplastic nevus syndrome and patient anxiety. (Modified from Houghton et al,[51] with permission.)*

SUMMARY OF SURVEILLANCE FOR MELANOMA

An optimal program of staging and follow-up for melanoma will only be defined in the context of a prospective clinical trial. Until such a trial is undertaken, appropriate staging and surveillance strategies will rely upon examination of currently available retrospective data to reach a consensus. The data suggest that:

- Melanoma recurs in *c.* one-quarter of patients with localized disease; the likelihood increases with increased tumor thickness.
- The majority of recurrences develop within 3 years of initial treatment; patients with thicker primary tumors relapse earlier than those with thinner tumors.
- Most recurrences produce either symptoms or signs recognizable by patients educated in melanoma surveillance.
- Careful physician history and physical examination will identify the majority of recurrences not identified by patients.
- Periodic screening CXR may identify a small subset of patients with asymptomatic pulmonary metastases; a subset of these pulmonary recurrences will be resectable.
- Laboratory studies and CT scans detect few recurrences and often lead to unnecessary confirmatory studies.
- Treatment of melanoma recurrence may alter the natural history of melanoma in some patients.

Patient education combined with physician history and physical examination form the cornerstone of melanoma surveillance. Laboratory and radiologic investigations of asymptomatic patients are generally low in yield. The intensity of follow-up is generally higher in patients with more advanced disease, and greatest within the first 3 years following diagnosis. The optimal duration of follow-up is unclear but a lifetime of dermatologic surveillance is appropriate.

Surveillance of patients with melanoma will become an increasingly important issue as cost-effective health care is applied to the management of a growing number of those patients. In addition to detecting early recurrences amenable to curative treatment, surveillance of patients with melanoma provides data on the natural history of melanoma and documents end results of new treatments. Importantly, surveillance also adds to the melanoma patient's sense of well-being, a fact that is often underappreciated.

CONCLUSIONS

Evidence-based strategies are required to effectively follow up patients after treatment for melanoma. Patient surveillance is performed to detect recurrences amenable to further treatment and to assess treatment results. Melanoma surveillance requires careful use of resources to be cost-effective.

REFERENCES

1. Ries LAG, Kosary CL, Hankey BF et al, *SEER Cancer Statistics Review, 1973–1996.* Bethesda, MD: NIH Publications/National Cancer Institute, 1999.
2. Provost N, Marghoob AA, Kopf AW et al, Laboratory tests and imaging studies in patients with cutaneous malignant melanomas: a survey of experienced physicians. *J Am Acad Dermatol* 1997; 36: 711–20.
3. Ariyan S, Poo WJ, Bolognia J et al, Multiple primary melanomas: data and significance. *Plast Reconstr Surg* 1995; 96: 1384–9 (see comments).
4. Frank W, Rogers GS, Melanoma update. Second primary melanoma. *J Dermatol Surg Oncol* 1993; 19: 427–30.
5. Slingluff Jr CL, Vollmer RT, Seigler HF, Multiple primary melanoma: incidence and risk factors in 283 patients. *Surgery* 1993; 113: 330–9.
6. Slingluff Jr CL, Dodge RK, Stanley WE, Seigler HF, The annual risk of melanoma progression. Implications for the concept of cure. *Cancer* 1992; 70: 1917–27.
7. Kopf AW, Hellman LJ, Rogers GS et al, Familial malignant melanoma. *JAMA* 1986; 256: 1915–19.
8. Rigel DS, Rivers JK, Kopf AW et al, Dysplastic nevi. Markers for increased risk for melanoma. *Cancer* 1989; 63: 386–9.
9. MacKie RM, McHenry P, Hole D, Accelerated detection with prospective surveillance for cutaneous malignant melanoma in high-risk groups. *Lancet* 1993; 341: 1618–20.
10. Gutman M, Cnaan A, Inbar M et al, Are malignant melanoma patients at higher risk for a second cancer? *Cancer* 1991; 68: 660–5.
11. Weiss M, Loprinzi CL, Creagan ET et al, Utility of follow-up tests for detecting recurrent disease in patients with malignant melanomas. *JAMA* 1995; 274: 1703–5.
12. Baughan CA, Hall VL, Leppard BJ, Perkins PJ, Follow-up in stage I cutaneous malignant melanoma: an audit. *Clin Oncol (R Coll Radiol)* 1993; 5: 174–80.
13. Jillela A, Mani S, Nair B et al, The role of close follow-up of melanoma patients with AJCC stages I–III: A preliminary analysis. *Proc ASCO* 1995; 14: 413.
14. Ruark DS, Shaw HM, Ingvar C et al, Who detects the first recurrence in stage I cutaneous melanoma: patient or doctor? *Melanoma Res* 1993; Suppl 1: 44.
15. Shumate CR, Urist MM, Maddox WA, Melanoma recurrence surveillance. Patient or physician based? *Ann Surg* 1995; 221: 566–9 (see comments).
16. Schultz S, Kane M, Roush R et al, Time to recurrence varies inversely with thickness in clinical stage 1 cutaneous melanoma. *Surg Gynecol Obstet* 1990; 171: 393–7.
17. Kim SH, Garcia C, Rodriguez J, Coit DG, Prognosis of thickness cutaneous melanoma. *J Am Coll Surg* 1999; 188: 241–7.
18. Coit DG, Rogatko A, Brennan MF, Prognostic factors in patients with melanoma metastatic to axillary or inguinal lymph nodes. A multivariate analysis. *Ann Surg* 1991; 214: 627–36.
19. Gadd MA, Coit DG, Recurrence patterns and outcome in 1019 patients undergoing axillary or inguinal lymphadenectomy for melanoma. *Arch Surg* 1992; 127: 1412–16.
20. Calabro A, Singletary SE, Balch CM, Patterns of relapse in 1001 consecutive patients with melanoma nodal metastases. *Arch Surg* 1989; 124: 1051–5.
21. McCarthy WH, Shaw HM, Thompson JF, Milton GW, Time and frequency of recurrence of cutaneous stage I malignant melanoma with guidelines for follow-up study. *Surg Gynecol Obstet* 1988; 166: 497–502.
22. Milton GW, Shaw HM, Farago GA, McCarthy WH, Tumour thickness and the site and time of first recurrence in cutaneous malignant melanoma (stage I). *Br J Surg* 1980; 67: 543–6.
23. Gorenstein LA, Putnam JB, Natarajan G et al, Improved survival after resection of pulmonary metastases from malignant melanoma. *Ann Thorac Surg* 1991; 52: 204–10 (see comments).
24. Crowley NJ, Seigler HF, Late recurrence of malignant melanoma. Analysis of 168 patients. *Ann Surg* 1990; 212: 173–7 (see comments).
25. Balch CM, Soong SJ, Murad TM et al, A multifactorial analysis of melanoma. IV. Prognostic factors in 200 melanoma patients with distant metastases (stage III). *J Clin Oncol* 1983; 1: 126–34.
26. Patel J, Nemoto T, Rosner D et al, Axillary lymph node metastasis from an occult breast cancer. *Cancer* 1981; 47: 2923–7.
27. Gadd MA, Cosimi AB, Yu J et al, Outcome of patients with melanoma and histologically negative lymph nodes. *Arch Surg* 1999; 134: 381–7.
28. Reintgen DS, Cox C, Slingluff Jr CL, Seigler HF, Recurrent malignant melanoma: the identification of prognostic factors to predict survival. *Ann Plast Surg* 1992; 28: 45–9.
29. Gershenwald JE, Colome MI, Lee JE et al, Patterns of recurrence following a negative sentinel lymph node biopsy in 243 patients with stage I or II melanoma. *J Clin Oncol* 1998; 16: 2253–60.
30. Mooney MM, Mettlin C, Michalek AM et al, Life-long screening of patients with intermediate-thickness cutaneous melanoma for asymptomatic pulmonary recurrences: a cost-effectiveness analysis. *Cancer* 1997; 80: 1052–64.
31. Mooney MM, Kulas M, McKinley B et al, Impact on survival by method of recurrence detection in stage I and II cutaneous melanoma. *Ann Surg Oncol* 1998; 5: 54–63.
32. Berwick M, Begg CB, Fine JA et al, Screening for cutaneous melanoma by skin self-examination. *J Natl Cancer Inst* 1996; 88: 17–23 (see comments).
33. Khansur T, Sanders J, Das SK, Evaluation of staging workup in malignant melanoma. *Arch Surg* 1989; 124: 847–49.
34. Busaid AC, Tinoco L, Ross MI et al, Role of computed tomography in the staging of patients with local-regional metastases of melanoma. *J Clin Oncol* 1995; 13: 2104–8.
35. Coit D, Patient surveillance and follow-up. In: *Cutaneous melanoma,* 3rd edn (eds Balch CM, Houghton AN, Sober AJ, Soong S-J). St Louis: Quality Medical Publishing, Inc, 1998: 313–21.
36. Kelley MC, Jones RC, Gupta RK et al, Tumor-associated antigen TA-90 immune complex assay predicts subclinical metastasis and survival for patients with early stage melanoma. *Cancer* 1998; 83: 1355–61.
37. Hsueh EC, Gupta RK, Glass EC et al, Positron emission tomography plus serum TA90 immune complex assay for detection of occult metastatic melanoma. *J Am Coll Surg* 1998; 187: 191–7.
38. Rinne D, Baum RP, Hor G, Kaufmann R, Primary staging and follow-up of high risk melanoma patients with whole-body 18F-fluorodeoxyglucose positron emission tomography: results of a prospective study of 100 patients (see comments). *Cancer* 1998; 82: 1664–71.
39. Nathan FE, Mastrangelo MJ, Systemic therapy in melanoma. *Semin Surg Oncol* 1998; 14: 319–27.
40. Legha SS, Ring S, Eton O et al, Development of a biochemotherapy regimen with concurrent administration of cisplatin, vinblastine, dacarbazine, interferon alfa, and interleukin-2 for patients with metastatic melanoma. *J Clin Oncol* 1998; 16: 1752–9.
41. Coit DG, Role of surgery for metastatic malignant melanoma. *Semin Surg Oncol* 1993; 9: 239–45.
42. Sharpless SM, Das Gupta TK, Surgery for metastatic melanoma. *Semin Surg Oncol* 1998; 14: 311–18.

43. Harpole DH, Jr., Johnson CM, Wolfe WG, George SL, Seigler HF, Analysis of 945 cases of pulmonary metastatic melanoma. *J Thorac Cardiovasc Surg* 1992; 103; 743–8
44. Wong JH, Euhus DM, Morton DL, Surgical resection for metastatic melanoma to the lung. *Arch Surg* 1988; 123: 1091–5.
45. Papachristou DN, Fortner JJ, Surgical treatment of metastatic melanoma confined to the liver. *Int Surg* 1983; 68: 145–8.
46. Ollila DW, Essner R, Wanek LA, Morton DL, Surgical resection for melanoma metastatic to the gastrointestinal tract. *Arch Surg* 1996; 131: 975–9.
47. NIH, Diagnosis and treatment of early melanoma. NIH Consensus Development Conference, January 27–29 1992. *Consensus Statement* 1992; 10: 1–25.
48. Kelly JW, Blois MS, Sagebiel RW, Frequency and duration of patient follow-up after treatment of a primary malignant melanoma. *J Am Acad Dermatol* 1985; 13: 756–60.
49. Romero JB, Stefanato CM, Kopf AW, Bart RS, Follow-up recommendations for patients with stage I malignant melanoma. *J Dermatol Surg Oncol* 1994; 20: 175–8.
50. Poo-Hwu WJ, Ariyan S, Lamb L et al, Follow-up recommendations for patients with American Joint Committee on Cancer Stages I–III malignant melanoma. *Cancer* 1999; 86: 2252–8.
51. Houghton A, Coit D, Bloomer W et al, NCCN melanoma practice guidelines. National Comprehensive Cancer Network, revised 3/9/00. *Oncology (Huntington)* 1998; 12: 153–77.
52. Meyers M, Balch C, Diagnosis and treatment of metastatic melanoma. In: *Cutaneous melanoma*, 3rd edn (eds Balch CM, Houghton AN, Sober AJ, Soong S-J). St Louis: Quality Medical Publishing Inc, 1998: 325.
53. Reeves XX, Detection of melanoma recurrence by a physician is associated with prolonged patient survival. Proceedings of the 53rd Annual Cancer Symposium of the Society of Surgical Oncology, 03/16/200, New Orleans, LA, 49.

42

Diagnosis of systemic melanoma metastases: general principles

Harald J Hoekstra, Heimen Schraffordt Koops

INTRODUCTION

The incidence of cutaneous melanoma is increasing throughout the world by 5% per year. Fortunately, due to increased public awareness, cutaneous melanomas are being diagnosed at an earlier stage and, as a consequence, the melanoma mortality rate has begun to plateau.[1] Nevertheless, about 20% of all newly diagnosed melanoma patients will ultimately die of systemic metastatic disease.[2]

The greater the thickness and depth of local invasion of the melanoma, the higher the chance of lymph node and/or distant metastases. Thicker melanomas have a much higher metastatic potential and the metastases develop much earlier.[3] Melanoma can have a more variable and unpredictable outcome than almost any other malignancy. For example, thicker melanomas tend to recur locally first, whereas thinner melanomas have a greater tendency to first metastasize at distant sites.[4] Distant recurrences are usually diagnosed later than locoregional recurrences,[5] but the clinical course of systemic metastatic disease can vary widely among patients.[6]

The staging of a melanoma patient is still based on clinical examination, the tumour thickness and depth of invasion, the presence or absence of clinical or subclinical nodal involvement (sentinel lymph node biopsy), whether there are in-transit metastases, and clinical signs of systemic metastatic disease. Blood counts, liver function tests, serum lactate dehydrogenase (LDH) levels, as well as chest x rays, are routinely performed and sufficiently sensitive for screening American Joint Committee on Cancer (AJCC) stage I and II disease. Regional metastases (i.e. stage III disease) are the most common indication of metastatic melanoma. As well as a thorough medical history and physical examination, the same work-up is required as for AJCC stage I and II disease, since cost–benefit considerations and the rate of false-positive tests makes more extensive evaluations inappropriate.

The idea behind the use of computerized tomography (CT), magnetic resonance imaging (MRI) or positron emission tomography (PET), as well as serum tumour markers and the technique of reverse transcriptase polymerase chain reaction (RT-PCR), in the clinical staging, treatment and follow-up of melanoma patients is to monitor the disease (i.e. to achieve early prediction and/or detection of recurrences) and to evaluate the effects of therapy.

Eighty-five per cent of newly diagnosed cutaneous melanoma patients present with localized disease (AJCC stage I or II), 9–13% with regional disease (AJCC stage III) and only 2–6% with distant metastatic disease (AJCC stage IV). A small proportion of the patients with metastatic disease (4–12%) have metastatic melanoma from an unknown primary site.[7,8] Approximately two-thirds of patients with metastases from an unknown primary present with lymph node metastases, whereas one-third present with distant metastases. Metastases diagnosed when there is no past history of melanoma are generally considered likely to be metastatic disease from a spontaneously regressed primary tumour, or alternatively a melanoma arising de novo in a lymph node or at a visceral site.

The 10-year survival rate for stage I patients (≤1.5 mm) is *c.* 90% and that for stage IIB (>4.0 mm) *c.* 50%.[9] Microscopic disease is already present in the regional lymph nodes in 5% of the patients with melanomas 0.75–1.5 mm in thickness (AJCC stage IB) and this percentage rapidly increases to >50% in patients with primaries >4.0 mm thick (stage IIB). The presence of lymph node metastases correlates strongly with the presence of systemic disease.[10] Cutaneous melanoma patients with a tumour thickness of 4.0 mm and/or clinically involved regional lymph nodes are especially at risk for developing distant metastases, and a thorough clinical work-up is indicated to rule out distant metastases at the time of initial diagnosis. Patients with metastases in skin, subcutaneous tissue or lymph node(s) beyond the regional lymph nodes already have stage IV disease. Once melanoma has metastasized to the regional lymph nodes (AJCC stage III) or distant sites (AJCC stage IV), the cure rate drops substantially, with a 5-year survival rate of 20–40% for AJCC stage III and <5% for AJCC stage IV.[8,11] Between 14 and 18% of AJCC stage I–III patients will ultimately develop distant metastatic disease (AJCC stage IV).[7,8]

New insights were gained into lymphatic drainage pathways with the introduction of lymphoscintigraphy in the early 1990s. A new minimally invasive staging procedure, sentinel node biopsy, became available to detect nodal disease in clinically node-negative patients.[12] Preliminary data suggest that patients with a tumour-positive sentinel lymph node have a 3-year survival rate of 67%, whereas those with a negative sentinel lymph node have a 3-year survival rate of 93%.[13] The introduction of lymphoscintigraphy in the staging and treatment of AJCC stage I and II melanoma patients, as well as the use of systemic adjuvant treatment for AJCC stage III and IV patients who have been rendered disease free by surgical resection of metastases, may, in the near future, alter the risk for and outcome of systemic metastatic disease.

Melanoma can metastasize to almost every major organ and tissue. Metastases in skin or subcutaneous tissue or lymph nodes beyond the regional lymph nodes are considered to be distant metastases. In roughly half the patients who develop distant metastases, the first site of metastasis is located in the skin, subcutaneous tissues or distant lymph nodes, in one-third of patients the site of diagnosis is in the lungs, and in the remaining patients the metastases are diagnosed in the brain, liver, bone, gastrointestinal tract, heart, adrenal glands, pancreas or kidneys.[14] Visceral metastases are being identified more frequently with CT scans, MRI scans, PET scans and ultrasound examinations.

There are limited data with respect to the prognosis of patients with systemic metastatic disease. Only the number of metastatic sites and the location of those sites (visceral versus non-visceral) have been found to correlate with survival rates. No histological criteria of the primary melanoma, the previously performed treatment, nor any other clinical variables can predict the clinical course once distant metastases are encountered. Patients with recurrences in the skin, soft tissues and distant lymph nodes can sometimes be rendered disease free by surgical resection, in contrast to most other sites. The prognosis for disseminated melanoma, with a median survival ranging from 7 to 11 months and an estimated 5-year survival rate of 6%, has not changed over the last two decades.[15] There are significant differences in the expected median survival and estimated 5-year survival rates for the different metastatic sites. For cutaneous, nodal or gastrointestinal metastases, the median survival is 12.5 months and the 5-year survival rate is 14%; for pulmonary metastases the median survival is 8.3 months and the 5-year survival rate is 3% (Table 42.1).[15] The number of organs or tissues containing metastases is the most significant factor in predicting survival in patients with systemic metastatic disease.[14] Another important prognostic factor is the rate of tumour growth. Melanoma is the single most common tumour reported to regress spontaneously, but the incidence of spontaneous regression is <1%.[15,16] The majority of patients with disseminated disease ultimately die from cerebral or respiratory complications, as shown in Table 42.2.[17,18]

In patients diagnosed with systemic metastatic disease there should be a high level of suspicion for associated brain, spinal cord or meningeal metastases. There is a large discrepancy between the metastatic sites diagnosed clinically and at autopsy, and several autopsy series have demonstrated how the extent of systemic metastatic disease is frequently underestimated in melanoma patients (Table 42.3). It is clear that the site of the first manifestation of metastatic disease is an important prognostic variable.[19,20] This is not surprising, since the majority of these metastases are asymptomatic and can only be clinically diagnosed with extensive diagnostic procedures, which have no impact on the

Table 42.1 *Prognosis of disseminated melanoma according to site**

Site of metastatic disease	Median survival (months)	Five-year survival rate (%)
Overall	7–11	6
Cutaneous/nodal/gastrointestinal	12.5	14
Pulmonary	8.3	4
Liver/brain	4.4	3

*Modified with permission from Barth et al., *J Am Coll Surg* 1995; 181: 193–201.[15]

Table 42.2 *Cause of death in 355 autopsied patients with metastatic melanoma.**[17,18]

Cause of death	Incidence (range) (%)
Respiratory failure	29 (39–16)
Brain/cord complication	25 (20–32)
Cardiac failure	10 (9–10)
Liver failure	7 (7)
Infection	8 (7–10)
Miscellaneous	20 (17–26)

*Modified from Meyers ML, Balch CM, Diagnosis and treatment of metastatic melanoma. In: *Cutaneous Melanoma*, 3rd edn (eds Balch CM, Houghton AN, Sober AJ, Soong S-J. St Louis: Quality Medical Publishing, Inc, 1998: 329), with permission.

disease outcome. Routine laboratory tests such as blood analysis and chest x rays have limited value.[21] The detection of asymptomatic systemic metastatic disease during clinical staging and follow-up is increasing with the availability of ultrasound, CT, MRI, PET, serum tumour markers, and RT-PCR techniques in blood and bone marrow. Whether this will ultimately alter the disease outcome is questionable. In asymptomatic patients with clinically diagnosed nodal involvement (AJCC stage III disease), CT and/or MRI of the chest, abdomen, brain and/or other anatomical sites are only indicated if there is clinical suspicion of metastatic disease, and are therefore not performed routinely.[22] More recently, serum tumour markers for melanoma have been under investigation, including lipid-bound sialic acid (LASA-P), S-100, serum antigen-specific immune complex (ASIC), as well as RT-PCR to detect melanoma cells in blood and bone marrow.[23–30] The role of PET tracers as part of the staging procedure is currently under investigation but appears to be promising (see Chapter 44).

For physicians treating melanoma patients it is essential that they understand the biological behaviour of the disease based on the different histopathological factors, the value of conventional imaging techniques, including conventional x rays, CT, ultrasound, MRI and new imaging techniques such as PET, serum tumour markers and RT-PCR. It is also important that they understand the role of lymphoscintigraphy for the staging of melanoma patients and for determining the patterns of potential metastatic spread, the value of follow-up to detect metastatic disease, and the role of surgery and radiotherapy in the treatment of metastatic disease.

Melanoma is a disease that often affects young adults. The main reason to perform follow-up in melanoma patients is to detect, and potentially to treat local, locoregional and/or distant recurrences at an early stage, with the ultimate goal of improving the overall and/or disease-free survival. This may require additional surgery, radiotherapy, chemotherapy, immunotherapy and/or a combination of these treatments. When follow-up schedules for melanoma patients are designed to detect metastatic disease, psychosocial aspects as well as cost-effectiveness must also be taken into account.[21]

Currently, most patients are well informed about their disease by their physicians. In addition, specific information materials for melanoma patients are generally available through cancer institutes or cancer organizations. Through the internet, melanoma patients can retrieve all kinds of information about their disease through the Cancer Information Service (CIS) of the National Cancer Institute (NCI).[31] As a

Table 42.3 *Common distant sites of metastatic melanoma**

Site	Clinical series (%)	Autopsy series (%)
Skin, subcutaneous, lymph nodes	42–59	50–75
Lungs	18–36	70–87
Liver	14–20	54–77
Brain	12–20	36–54
Bone	11–17	23–49
Gastrointestinal	1–7	26–58
Heart	<1	40–45
Pancreas	<1	38–53
Adrenals	<1	36–54
Kidneys	<1	35–48
Thyroid	<1	25–39

*Modified from Meyers ML, Balch CM (Diagnosis and treatment of metastatic melanoma. In: *Cutaneous Melanoma*, 3rd edn (eds Balch CM, Houghton AN, Sober AJ, Soong S-J). St Louis: Quality Medical Publishing, Inc, 1998: 329), with permission.

result of this education and self-examination for locoregional recurrences, it is not surprising that almost all locoregional recurrences (>90%) are patient detected. Studies have shown no difference in survival between patient- or physician-detected recurrences.[32–35]

The importance of lifetime follow-up for patients with melanoma, especially for locoregional recurrences, is well recognized. There is a difference between the follow-up schedule of patients with AJCC stage I, II or III disease, based on the initial hazard rate, at a ratio of *c.* 1:2:6 (Table 42.4).[36] Each scheduled visit should include a history, physical examination, full blood count and liver function tests, with an annual chest x ray. These simple and relatively inexpensive measures will detect the common sites of metastatic disease. The serum LDH level is currently the most widely available and sensitive marker of tumour burden. Abnormalities in the blood count and liver function tests are an indication for further diagnostic evaluation. It has to be taken into account, with respect to the suggested follow-up schedule for melanoma, that the majority of the recurrences are detected by the patient themselves between follow-up visits. Local or regional recurrences are preferably treated by surgical resection. When systemic metastatic disease is diagnosed, there is

Table 42.4 *Follow-up schedule for melanoma stage I–III**

Month	Stage I⁺	Stage II⁺	Stage III⁺
3	–	–	x
6	–	x	x
9	–	–	x
12	x	x	x
16	–	–	x
18	–	x	x
20	–	–	x
24	x	x	x
30	–	–	x
36	x	x	x
42	–	–	x
48	x	x	x
54	–	–	x
60	x	x	x

x refers to patient visit; –, no visit.
*Modified from Poo-Hwu W-J et al,[36] with permission.

still a role for surgery, when possible, to render the patient disease free with the possible future treatment option of an adjuvant therapy (such as immunotherapy, chemotherapy or vaccination treatment). Sometimes, palliative surgical resection may be indicated. Although the majority of recurrences are patient detected, these follow-up recommendations may also provide a patient survival benefit. The effectiveness of such recommendations can only be evaluated in large prospective trials.

REFERENCES

1. Oliveria SA, Christos PJ, Halpern AC et al, Patient knowledge, awareness and delay in seeking medical attention for malignant melanoma. *J Clin Epidemiol* 1999; 52: 1111–16.
2. Jemal A, Thomas A, Murray T, Thun M, Cancer statistics, 2002. *CA Cancer J Clin* 2002; 52: 23–47.
3. Balch CM, Murad TM, Soong S-J et al, A multifactorial analysis of melanoma. Prognostic histopathological features comparing Clark's and Breslow's staging methods. *Ann Surg* 1978; 188: 732–42.
4. McCarthy WH, Shaw HM, Thompson JF, Milton GW, Time and frequency of recurrence of cutaneous stage I malignant melanoma with guidelines for follow-up study. *Surg Gynecol Obstet* 1988; 166: 497–502.
5. Fusi S, Ariyan S, Sternlicht A, Data on first recurrence after treatment for malignant melanoma in a large population. *Plast Reconstr Surg* 1993; 91: 94–8.
6. Amer MH, Al-Sarraf M, Vaitkevicius VK, Clinical presentation, natural history and prognostic factors in advancing malignant melanoma. *Surg Gynecol Obstet* 1979; 149: 687–92.
7. Rigel DS, Malignant melanoma: perspectives on incidence and its effects on awareness, diagnosis, and treatment. *CA Cancer J Clin* 1996; 46: 195–8.
8. Chang AE, Karnell LH, Menck HR, The National Cancer Database report on cutaneous and noncutaneous melanoma: a summary of 84,836 cases from the last decade. The American College of Surgeons Commission on Cancer and the American Cancer Society. *Cancer* 1998; 83: 1664–78.
9. Coit D, Sauven P, Brennan M, Prognosis of thick cutaneous melanoma of the trunk and the extremity. *Arch Surg* 1990; 125: 322–6.
10. Slingluff CL, Stidham KR, Ricci WR et al, Surgical management of regional lymph nodes in melanoma patients. *Ann Surg* 1994; 219: 120–30.
11. Morton DL, Wanek L, Nizze JA et al, Improved long-term survival after lymphadenectomy of melanoma to regional nodes: analysis of prognostic factors in 1134 patients from the John Wayne Cancer Clinic. *Ann Surg* 1991; 214: 491–499; discussion 499–501.
12. Morton DL, Wen DR, Cochran AJ, Management of early stage melanoma by intraoperative lymphatic mapping and selective lymphadenectomy: an alternative to routine elective lymphadenectomy or 'watch and wait'. *Surg Oncol Clin North Am* 1992; 1: 247–59.
13. Jansen L, Nieweg OE, Peterse JL et al, Reliability of sentinel lymph node biopsy for staging of melanoma. *Br J Surg* 2000; 87: 484–9.
14. Balch CM, Soong S-J, Murad TM et al, A multifactorial analysis of melanoma: IV. Prognostic factors in 200 melanoma patients with distant metastases (Stage III). *J Clin Oncol* 1983; 1: 126–34.
15. Barth A, Wanek LA, Morton DL, Prognostic factors in 1,521 melanoma patients with distant metastases. *J Am Coll Surg* 1995; 181: 193–201.
16. Houghton AN, Meyers ML, Chapman PB et al, Medical treatment of metastatic melanoma. *Surg Clin North Am* 1996; 76: 1343–54.
17. Budman DR, Camacho E, Wittes RE, The current death in patients with malignant melanoma. *Eur J Cancer* 1978; 14: 327–30.
18. Patel JK, Didolkar MS, Pickren JW, Moore RH, Metastatic patterns of malignant melanoma. A study of 216 autopsy cases. *Am J Surg* 1978; 135: 807–10.
19. Lee YT, Malignant melanoma: pattern of metastasis. *CA Cancer J Clin* 1980; 30: 137–42.
20. Lee ML, Tomsu K, Von Eschen KB, Duration of survival for disseminated malignant melanoma: report meta-analysis. *Melanoma Res* 2000; 10: 81–92.
21. Weiss M, Loprinzi CL, Creagan ET et al, Utility of follow-up tests for detecting recurrent disease in patients with malignant melanoma. *JAMA* 1995; 274: 1703–5.
22. Buzaid A, Tinoco, Ross M et al, Role of computed tomography in the staging of patients with local-regional metastases of melanoma. *J Clin Oncol* 1995; 13: 2104–8.
23. Bonfrer JM, Korse CM, Nieweg OE, Rankin EM, The luminescence immunoassay S-100: sensitive test to measure circulating S-100B: its prognostic value in malignant melanoma. *Br J Cancer* 1998; 77: 2210–14.
24. Kelley MC, Jones RC, Gupta RK et al, Tumor-associated antigen TA-90 immune complex assay predicts subclinical metastasis and survival for patients with early stage melanoma. *Cancer* 1998; 83: 1355–61.
25. Schutter EM, Visser JJ, van Kamp GJ et al, The utility of lipid-associated sialic acid (LASA or LSA) as a serum marker for malignancy. A review of the literature. *Tumour Biol* 1992; 12: 121–32.
26. McMasters KM, Sondak VK, Lotze MT, Ross MI, Recent advances in melanoma staging and therapy. *Ann Surg Oncol* 1999; 6: 467–75.
27. Shivers SC, Stall A, Goscin C et al, Molecular staging for melanoma and breast cancer. *Surg Oncol Clin North Am* 1999; 8: 515–26.
28. Mellado B, Gutierrez L, Castel L et al, Prognostic significance of the detection of circulating malignant cells by reverse transcriptase-polymerase chain reaction in long-term clinically disease-free melanoma patients. *Clin Cancer Res* 1995; 1843–8.
29. Curry BJ, Myers K, Hersey P, Polymerase chain reaction detection of melanoma cells in the circulation: relation to clinical stage, surgical treatment, and recurrence from melanoma. *J Clin Oncol* 1998; 16: 1760–9.
30. Curry BJ, Myers K, Hersey P, MART-1 is expressed less frequently on circulating melanoma cells in patients who develop distant compared with locoregional metastases. *J Clin Oncol* 1999; 17: 2562–71.
31. Http://cancernet.nci.nih.gov.
32. Shumate CR, Urist MM, Maddox WA, Melanoma recurrence surveillance. Patient or physician based. *Am Surg* 1995; 221: 566–9; discussion 569–71.
33. Baughan CA, Hall VL, Leppard BJ, Perkins PJ, Follow-up in stage I cutaneous malignant melanoma: an audit. *Clin Oncol (R Coll Radiol)* 1993; 5: 174–80.
34. Jillela A, Mani S, Nair B et al, The role of close follow-up of melanoma patients with AJCC stages I–III: a preliminary analysis. *J Clin Oncol (ASCO Proc)* 1995; 14: 413.
35. Ruark DS, Shaw HM, Ingvar C et al, Who detects the first recurrence in stage I cutaneous malignant melanoma: patient or doctor? *Melanoma Res* 1993; 3 (Suppl 1): 11.
36. Poo-Hwu W-J, Ariyan S, Lamb L et al, Follow-up recommendations for patients with American Joint Committee on Cancer Stages I–III malignant melanoma. *Cancer* 1999; 86: 2252–8.

43

Diagnosis of systemic metastatic melanoma: conventional imaging techniques

Richard Perry

INTRODUCTION

Modern imaging technology has four potential roles to play in primary melanoma management: staging clinical disease, investigation of the symptomatic patient, surveillance and clinical trial evaluation. There is, however, no consensus about the extent to which imaging should be undertaken in these settings. With the exception of the symptomatic patient, where investigation would follow conventional diagnostic algorithms, there is considerable variation in the use of imaging in melanoma. This lack of consensus is in part due to the lack of a satisfactory systemic therapy[1] and to the unpredictable distribution of metastatic melanoma.

Conventional imaging techniques encompass plain radiography and computerized axial tomography (CT), both of which generate images using x rays, ultrasound that utilizes sound energy, and magnetic resonance imaging (MRI) where images are based on the distribution of protons detected with large magnetic fields. In the following discussion, the role of these imaging techniques in staging and surveillance of melanoma will be reviewed. The second section will review the imaging characteristics of metastatic melanoma.

ROLE OF IMAGING IN STAGING AND SURVEILLANCE

The likelihood of metastases from thin melanoma is very small and staging other than clinical evaluation is probably unnecessary.[1,2] However, there have been recommendations for the use of chest x ray and/or liver function tests in stage I or II disease, but reviews of the use of plain chest radiography do not support this practice. In one study of 876 asymptomatic patients with localized melanoma, the detection rate of unsuspected pulmonary metastases was 0.1% (one patient).[3] However, 15% had suspicious findings requiring additional work-up, which were subsequently found to be benign. Other studies have shown similar results, with very low detection rates for metastases in stage I or stage II disease but a high incidence of false-positive results requiring further investigation.[2,4,5] The high false-positive rate increases morbidity and has a significant effect on patient anxiety levels, and also adversely affects the cost-effectiveness of treatment protocols.

The alternative view favours performing a chest x ray in stage I and II disease.[6–9] It is believed that *c.* 20% of all patients with melanoma have a metastasis at the time of diagnosis,[10] and that the lung is one of the earlier sites of spread. Chest x rays are easy to obtain and interpret, widely available with low cost and low risk.[8,9] The initial chest x ray can help to establish a diagnosis of metastatic disease and also provides a baseline.[8,9] When thoracic symptoms do occur, metastases is generally quite advanced and the possibility of resection, the treatment option in early disease, is not available.

More aggressive imaging investigation for staging in early disease has also been shown to be unsatisfactory. A chest x ray may be ineffective because lesion detection is limited to lesions of *c.* ≥1 cm and it has been demonstrated that CT scanning is superior to chest radiography in the detection of pulmonary metastatic disease generally.[11–13] However, studies have shown the same levels of low true-positive and high false-positive rates for CT-based staging protocols as for chest x-ray-based studies.[14] Similar results are seen in CT staging of the abdomen.[15] Consequently, imaging in stage I and II disease is likely to have a low true-positive yield and a high false-positive rate, and even a chest x ray is probably unnecessary.

In clinical stage III disease, a chest x ray and CT scan of the chest, abdomen and pelvis, and sometimes the brain, has been recommended, although again the evidence is confusing. Buzaid et al.,[14] in 89 asymptomatic patients with stage III locoregional melanoma with normal chest x rays and normal lactate dehydrogenase (LDH) levels, and having CT scans of the brain, chest and abdomen, demonstrated a true-positive rate of 7% and a false-positive rate of 22%. Kuvshinoff et al.[16] found a true-positive rate of 4.2% and a false-positive rate of 8.4%. Both studies demonstrated a zero incidence of cerebral metastases in their asymptomatic population. Alternatively, Johnson et al.[15] demonstrated a true-positive rate of 16% and a false-positive rate of 12% in 127 patients, with a 5% incidence of brain metastases. It has been suggested that, in clinical stage III disease, a CT scan of the head in the asymptomatic patient, a chest CT scan in patients with groin adenopathy, and a pelvic CT scan in the presence of axillary and cervical adenopathy are not indicated.[16] However, selective use of chest CT scans in patients with cervical adenopathy or pelvic CT scans, in the presence of groin disease,[16] and CT neck and chest scans in head and neck melanoma[6] may be of value.

The use of abdomen CT scans, despite their low yield, has been advocated for baseline information in the asymptomatic patient in this high-risk group.[6] Once again, the high level of false-positive results reinforces the observation that confirmation of metastases is required and this can generally be achieved through fine needle aspiration biopsy.[1,15]

For stage IV disease, the presence of further metastases is highly likely and further investigation may be warranted, depending on the clinical circumstances.

The issues related to surveillance are similarly clouded. Several studies have suggested that history and/or clinical examination will detect the majority of recurrences.[17–19] Routine blood analysis, chest x ray and other imaging investigations appear to be of little value.

Recommendations developed by National Institute of Health consensus panel on early melanoma for follow-up do not include imaging studies.[20] Similar recommendations have also been made in small cell carcinoma[21] and other tumours. Recommendations for imaging in staging melanoma, based on currently available studies, are summarized in Table 43.1. No imaging studies are recommended for surveillance.

IMAGING FEATURES OF METASTATIC MELANOMA

Melanoma, perhaps above all other cancers, has the capacity to metastasize in the most unpredictable way to an extraordinary number of sites with a wide variety of appearances.

Brain and spine

Melanoma is the third most common neoplasm to metastasize the brain.[22] In metastatic melanoma, the brain may be the only site of metastasis and symptoms may predate the discovery of the primary lesion. On the other hand, >10% of cerebral melanoma metastases are clinically silent.[23] Although intracerebral metastases are generally multiple, regardless of their origin, there is a relatively high incidence of solitary metastasis in melanoma,[24] offering the potential of curative resection.

CT scanning has been regarded as the first-line investigation for detection of cerebral melanoma metastases. The appearance of cerebral metastases on non-contrast CT scans varies. Metastases can be variable in size and are often hyperdense, most likely related to haemorrhage (Figure 43.1); they may also be isodense or hypodense. Cystic change or necrosis may be seen, although purely cystic metastasis appear to be uncommon. There is generally considerable cerebral oedema. The amount

Table 43.1 *Recommended imaging for melanoma staging*

Melanoma stage	Modality
1	Nil
2	Nil
3	Chest x ray, CT abdomen +/- CT chest, neck or pelvis, depending on primary
4	Appropriate modality for symptoms, chest x ray, CT thorax, CT abdomen, MRI brain

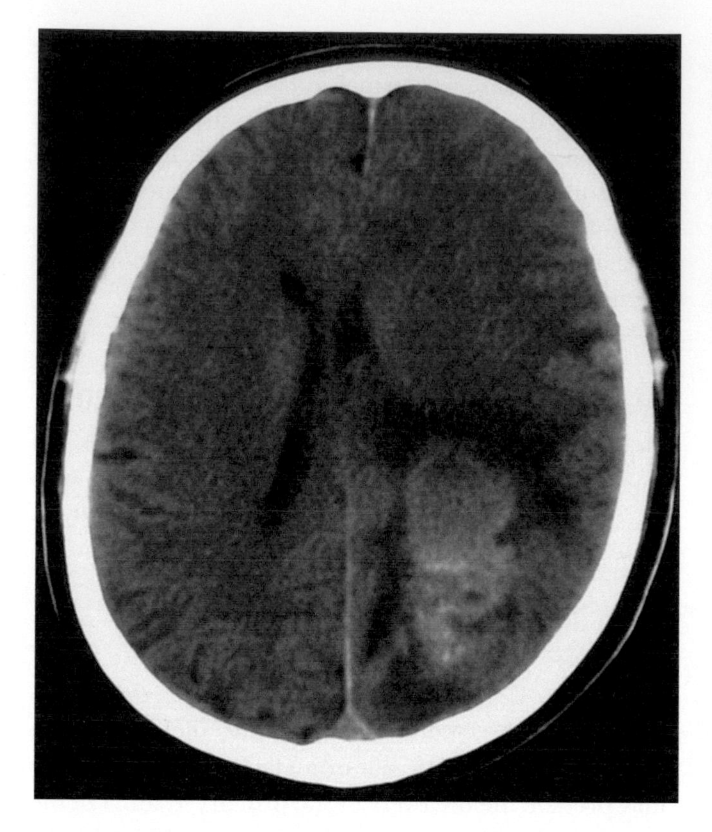

Figure 43.1 *CT scan demonstrating hyperdense metastases in the left parietal and occipital lobes.*

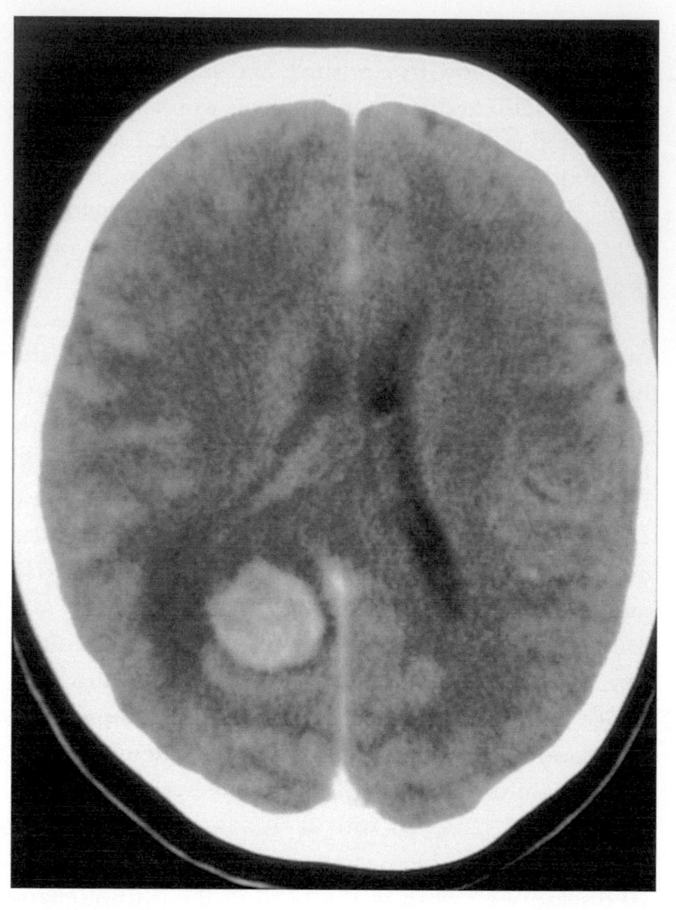

Figure 43.2 *Contrast-enhanced CT scan demonstrating an enhancing metastasis in the right occipital lobe.*

of oedema bears no relation to the size of the metastases nor to clinical symptoms. Although oedema is usually marked, it may be absent, particularly in cortical metastases.[24] Metastases may not be evident without an IV contrast agent, especially if they are small or cortical. Melanoma metastases demonstrate marked enhancement with IV contrast agents in a solid or ring-like pattern (Figure 43.2). IV contrast agents increase the sensitivity for documentation of intracerebral metastases. Metastases demonstrate enhancement because a deficient blood–brain barrier in the vascular endothelium of the involved capillary allows circulating contrast agent access to the lesion. The blood–brain barrier prevents contrast, enhancing normal brain.

However, it is now recognized that MRI, especially with an IV contrast agent, is more sensitive than CT scanning for demonstration of cerebral metastases.[25,26] Metastases are generally well demonstrated on T2-weighted images, where the lesion can be seen as a focus of variable signal intensity in a sea of high signal intensity oedema (Figure 43.3). As with CT scanning, metastases generally show marked enhancement with an MRI contrast agent (Figure 43.4). Although this is seen in both CT scanning and MRI, contrast-enhanced MRI is more sensitive than CT scanning because of an inherently higher contrast resolution.[23,25,26]

It has also been shown that higher doses of contrast agent increase the number of metastatic lesions detected. Increasing the IV MRI contrast agent dose from the standard dose (0.1 mml/kg) to double or triple dose (0.3 mml/kg) is associated with an increase of 15–43% in the detection rate. An increase in specificity, as well as in sensitivity, has also been shown.[27] It has been estimated that *c.* 10% of such cases alter patient management.[28] Certainly, with the tendency for surgery for single metastases, the presence of a small, otherwise undetected, metastases is very significant for patient management. However, cost–benefit studies have yet to be performed.

One algorithm suitable for this situation is to perform a single-dose MRI scan. Where a single metastasis is demonstrated, the study can be repeated immediately with a further double dose. If multiple metastases are

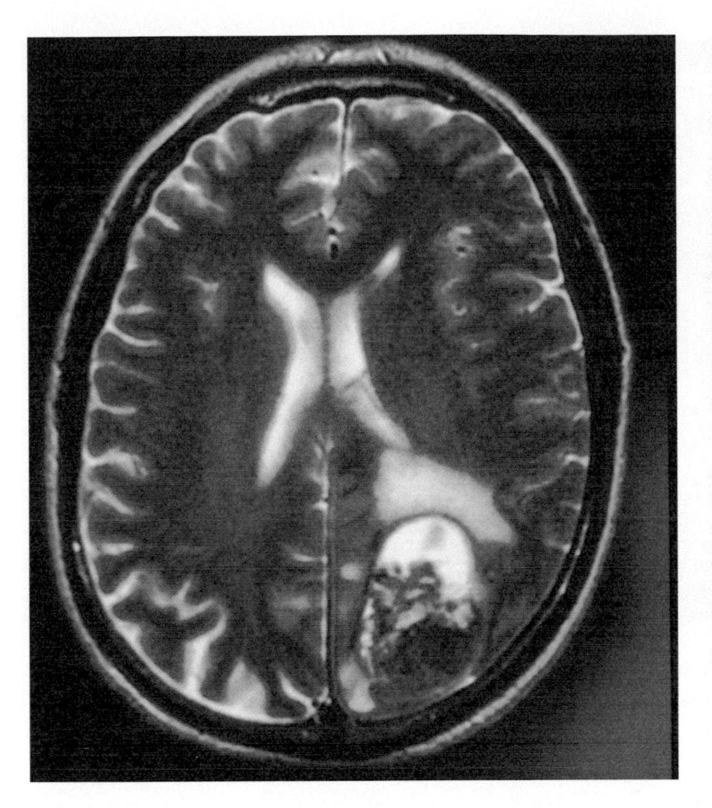

Figure 43.3 *MRI scan of the patient shown in Figure 43.1. Long TR/TE image (T2-weighted image) show metastasis in the occipital lobe with oedema in the deep white matter.*

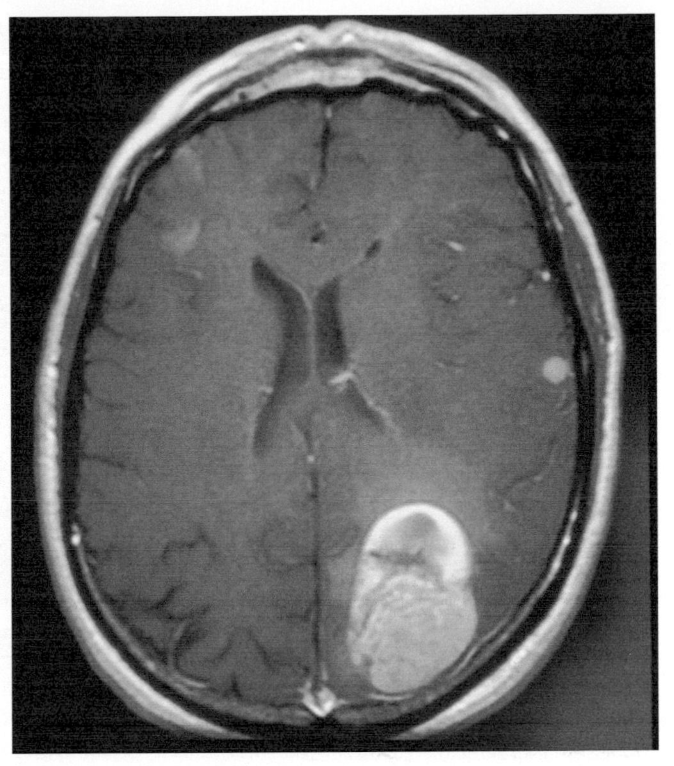

Figure 43.4 *MRI scan of the patient in Figures 43.1 and 43.3. TI image with gadolinium enhancement demonstrates two lesions. Note that the small lesion is not visible on the T2 sequence shown in Figure 43.3.*

seen on the initial single-dose study, further investigation would not normally be required.

The presence of melanin within melanoma metastases may produce characteristic appearances on MRI. MRI measures the behaviour of protons, generally the proton of hydrogen in water, in a large magnetic field to create images: i.e. an MRI image is essentially a water map. T1 and T2 relaxation times refer to properties of protons in an altering magnetic field, and their measurement forms the basis of the image. Some naturally occurring compounds have intrinsic properties that alter, at the molecular level, the magnetic field operating on the local protons and thus alter the appearance of the images obtained. These compounds are said to be paramagnetic. Stable free radicals within melanin pigment are paramagnetic and cause shortening of T1 and T2 relaxation times relative to other tissues.[24,29] Other materials demonstrating paramagnetic relaxation effects include gadolinium contrast agent and haemoglobin blood products.

Metastases, as well as primary brain tumours, tend to be hypointense to brain on T1-weighted images and hyperintense to brain on T2-weighted images, reflecting their increased water content. The effect of the paramagnetic property of melanin is that the expected signal pattern for melanoma metastases is relatively hyperintense in relation to the cortex on T1-weighted images, reflecting shortening of the T1 relaxation time (Figure 43.5a), and relatively hypointense in relation to the cortex on T2-weighted images, reflecting shortening of the T2 relaxation time (Figure 43.5b). Amelanotic metastases have a signal pattern similar to that of other brain tumours.

Melanoma metastases are also liable to haemorrhage and the presence of blood products, which are also paramagnetic, will significatly alter the signal intensity pattern. This alteration will depend on the age of the haematoma. Commonly, subacute haemorrhage is present and this will demonstrate hyperintensity on T1-weighted sequences relative to grey matter, due to methaemoglobin. In early subacute haemorrhage, with intracellular methaemoglobin, the lesion will be hypointense on T2-weighted sequences, similar to those for melanin but these lesions will become hyperintense in late subacute haemorrhage where there is cell lysis and

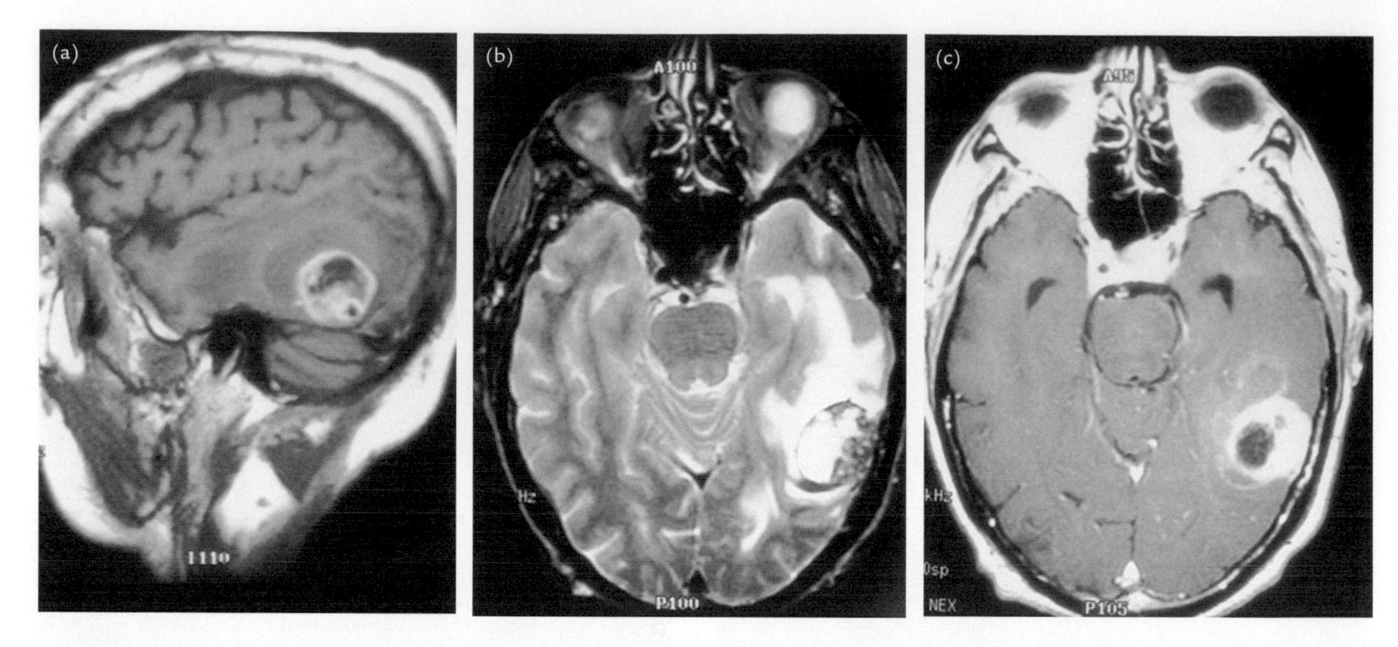

Figure 43.5 *(a) Sagittal T1-weighted image demonstrates a melanoma metastasis with a marked high signal intensity, reflecting the paramagnetic effect of melanin. (b) Axial T2-weighted image demonstrates metastasis with a hypodense periphery, consistent with melanin content. There is a medial cystic component, consistent with a haemorrhagic tumour cyst. There is considerable oedema. (c) Axial T1 image after gadolinium enhancement demonstrates faint enhancement about the cystic component with high signal due to melanin in the solid tumour.*

release of extracellular methaemoglobin.[24] Metastases rarely show the orderly progression of signal changes seen in simple cerebral haematoma.[23]

It has been shown that only a minority of melanoma metastases (25%) show the predicted specific MRI patterns.[29] However, this pattern is relatively specific for melanoma metastases and the presence of this pattern correlates to the percentage of melanotic cells present. Most melanoma metastases do not show this pattern and these metastases have been shown, histologically, to be amelanotic or to contain <10% melanotic cells.

MRI should be the imaging investigation of choice in investigation of patients with known metastatic melanoma who develop cerebral symptoms. It is also more sensitive in detecting metastases, which may be relevant in staging in asymptomatic patients where significant surgery is considered. However, use of MRI or, indeed, CT scanning in routine staging of melanoma in asymptomatic patients is not justified.

Melanoma is one of the more common causes of metastases to the spinal cord, the leptomeninges, and the spine and epidural space.[24] Metastases to the spinal cord are relatively rare but vertebral metastases with spinal cord compression are common. Although bone scans will demonstrate spinal metastases, MRI has been shown to be the investigation of choice, since it demonstrates the multilevel vertebral and epidural metastases, and those lesions causing cord compression (Figure 43.6a and b).[30,31] Myelography is invasive and will not demonstrate all levels in multilevel cord compression. Melanoma may arise primarily in the brain in the meninges and in the ventricles.[32]

Thorax

Metastases are seen in the lungs in 70% of patients in autopsy series.[33] The thorax is a common site of relapse and recurrence is often occult.[34]

CT scanning is the most accurate method in detecting metastases (Figure 43.7a and b).[11,12] As previously noted, CT scanning will be superior to chest x rays because of its improved spacial resolution. Melanoma metastases are usually multiple and, at least initially, small.[13] Feeding vessels may be seen reflecting haematogenous spread. Most lesions are in the 1–2 cm range (Figure 43.8). Metastases to the hilar and mediastinal nodes are common.

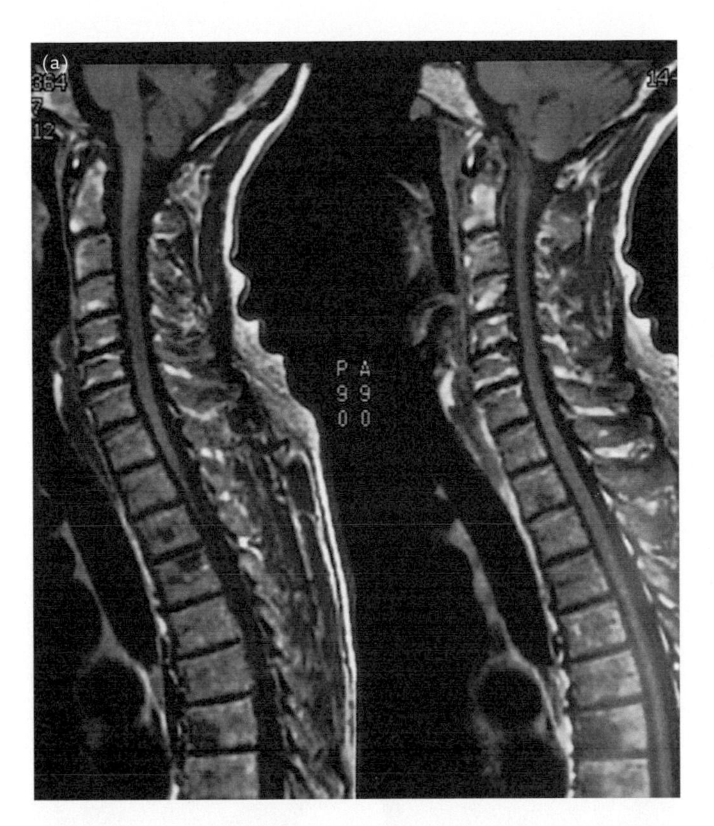

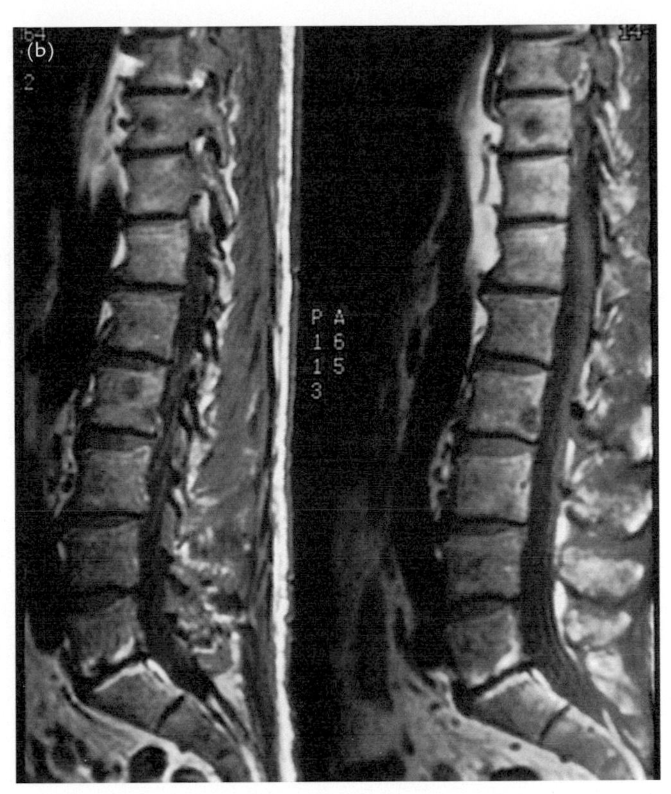

Figure 43.6 *(a) and (b) Sagittal T1-weighted images demonstrate multiple metastases, which are hypodense in the vertebrae compared to the normal vertebral body fat signal.*

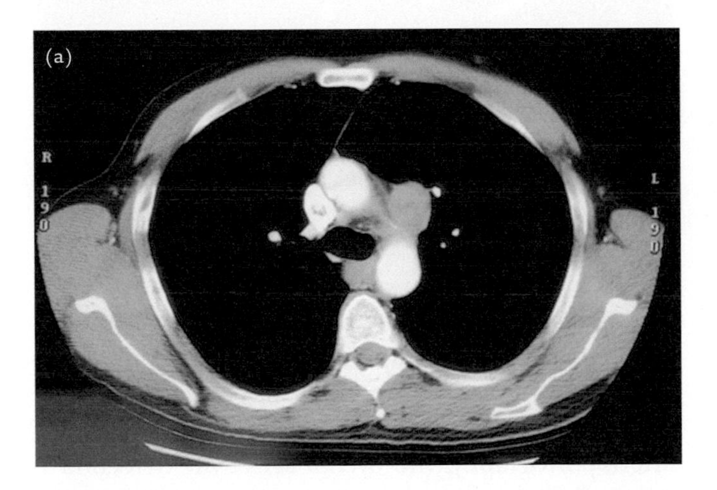

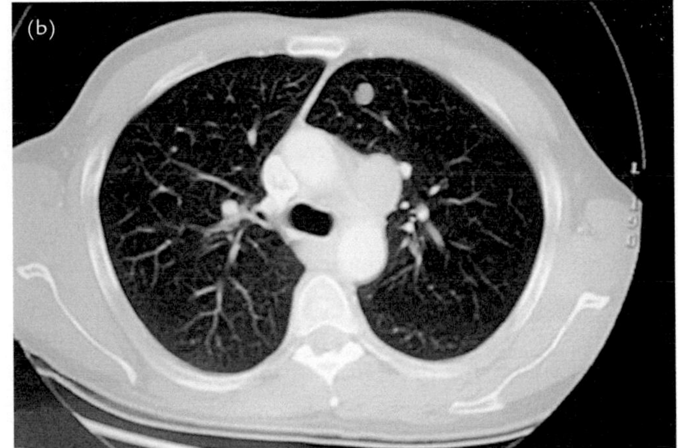

Figure 43.7 *(a) Axial CT scan of the thorax demonstrates a mass in the aortopulmonary window. Note the small subcutaneous metastases in the left anterior chest wall. (b) The same images as in (a) windowed for lung parenchyma demonstrates a pulmonary metastasis in the anterior left lung.*

Abdomen

Metastatic melanoma can involve multiple organ systems and CT scanning is an ideal imaging modality for examining these patients. Hepatic metastases have been demonstrated in clinical series in 17–22% of patients.[35,36] In autopsy series, up to 60% of patients have liver metastases:[33] their appearance on CT scans is variable, though they are generally hypodense on post-contrast images compared to surrounding liver.

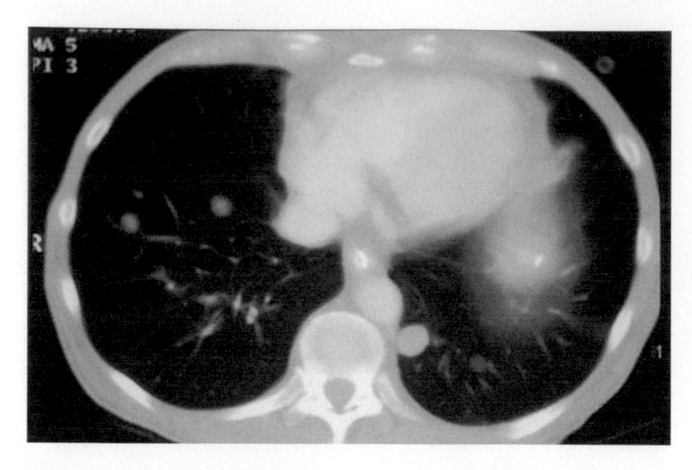

Figure 43.8 *Multiple pulmonary metastases demonstrated in the lung bases on an axial CT scan.*

Variable size, single or multiple, lesions may be seen (Figure 43.9a and b). Necrosis is not uncommon and calcification may be seen.

Conventional CT scanning protocols for liver metastasis staging involve administration of an IV iodinated contrast agent and scanning the liver during the period of portal venous enhancement. Recently developed multiphase spiral CT scanning enables scanning of the liver during variable phases of hepatic enhancement, including the arterial enhanced phase, the portal venous enhanced phase and the delayed phase. Multiphase spiral CT scanning involves delivering a relatively high volume of contrast agent at a high injection rate and scanning rapidly through the liver (20 8–10 mm sections in 15–20 seconds) at the time of hepatic artery enhancement (generally 20–25 seconds after injection) and portal venous enhancement (generally 60–80 seconds after injection.[37,38]

Although a portal venous phase is generally the most sensitive phase for detection of metastatic disease, this has been shown not to be the case where the metastases, such as melanoma, are hypervascular.[37,39] Because of this hypervascularity, melanoma metastases may be isodense, so may not be visible in the portal venous phase but may be visible during the arterial phase. A combination of the non-enhanced and portal venous phases, or the arterial and portal venous phases, are equally effective in detecting metastases.[38]

The sensitivity for the detection of metastases is *c.* 80% for helical CT scanning and 65% for conventional contrast-enhanced non-helical CT scanning. These fall to *c.* 50% for detecting metastases of *c.* 1 cm. The sensitivity

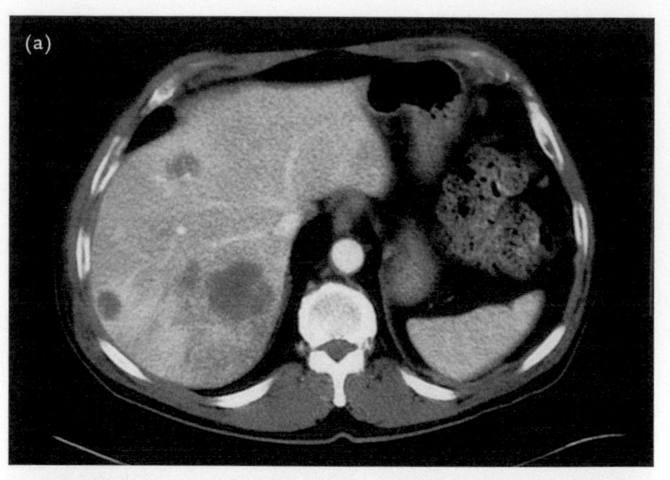

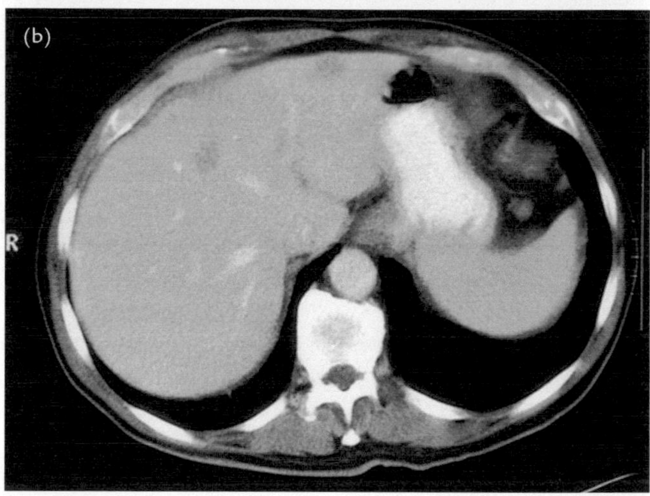

Figure 43.9 *(a) Multiple metastases in the liver on an axial contrast-enhanced CT scan. (b) The same patient as shown in (a) but a higher level demonstrates liver metastases and lesions in the omental fat anterior to the spleen in the left upper quadrant.*

thresholds can be elevated by the use of CT arteriography and arterioportography, where CT scanning is performed with contrast injected via catheters in the hepatic or superior mesenteric artery. With helical CT arterioportography, the overall sensitivity detection is >90%.[39] This technique is invasive, requiring catheterization of the hepatic and superior mesenteric arteries, and so is generally reserved for operative candidates.

Ultrasound examination is convenient, quick and inexpensive, and therefore continues to play a valuable role in detecting hepatic metastases (Figure 43.10). However, it has been shown that the false-negative rate is >50% and that there is relatively low specificity.[40] Various techniques have been proposed to increase this sensitivity, including measurement of the Doppler

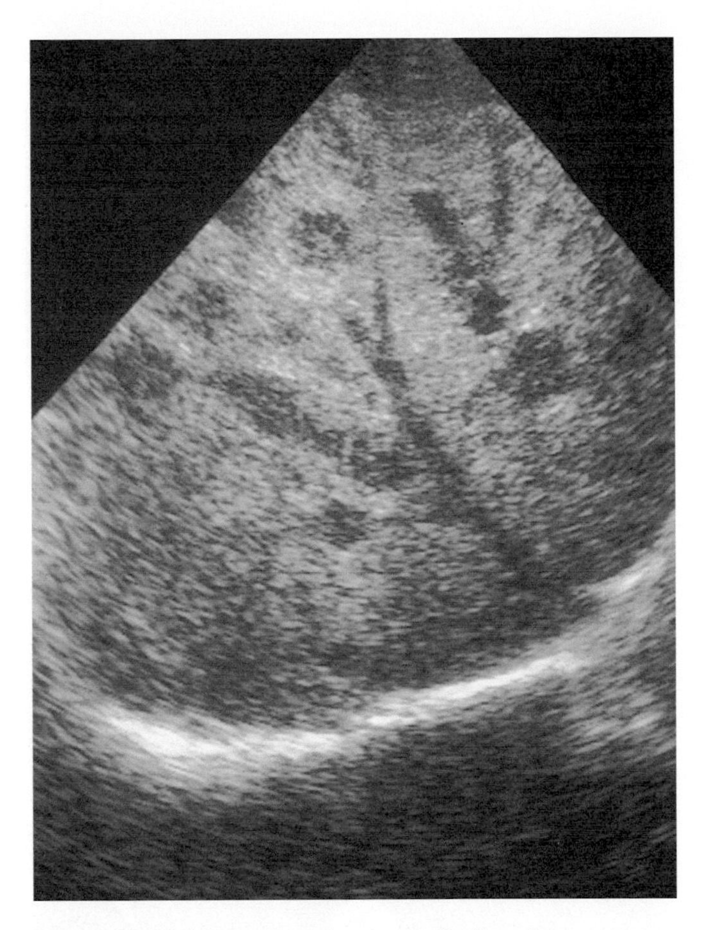

Figure 43.10 *Metastatic melanoma in the liver shown on an ultrasound scan.*

perfusion index and development of sonographic contrast agents. However, ultrasound remains highly operator and, to some extent, patient dependent. Metastases often occur outside the solid organs of the abdomen and these areas are difficult to image during routine abdominal screening ultrasound, an area where CT scanning shows significant advantage.

MRI of the liver is becoming available for use in the detection and characterization of metastases. (Figure 43.11).[38,41] There are a large number of different imaging techniques and there is no consensus on the optimal technical protocol. Commonly applied techniques include T2-weighted sequences, T1-weighted sequences with and without fat suppression, and T1-weighted breath-hold gradient echo sequences with serial acquisition after gadolinium enhancement. The T2 and immediate post-gadolinium-enhanced T1 sequences provide good lesion detection, and the T2-weighted and serial post-gadolinium T1 sequences provide lesion and tissue characterization.[41]

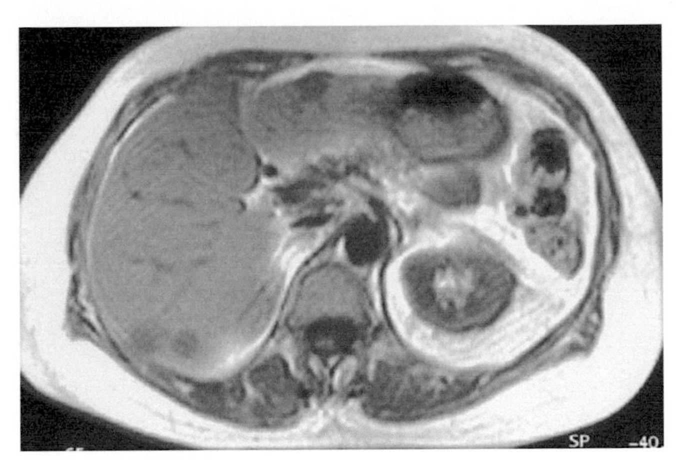

Figure 43.11 *Melanoma metastases in the right lobe of the liver on an axial T1-weighted MRI scan.*

As with CT scanning, metastases vary significantly in appearance. In general, they demonstrate low signal intensities on T1-weighted sequences and moderately high signal intensities on T2-weighted sequences. The most common feature on gadolinium enhancement is a peripheral ring enhancement on immediate post-enhanced sequences, although other patterns are also seen. Melanoma metastases may have a mixture of high and low signals on both T1- and T2-weighted sequences due to the paramagnetic property of melanin. Like lesions in the brain, this depends on the amount of melanin within the metastases.

MR imaging is as sensitive as CT scanning in detecting focal liver disease[41] and may now be, with appropriate breath-hold sequences, as sensitive as CT arterioportography.[42] However, the ability of CT scanning to cover the chest, abdomen and pelvis in a rapid (20–60 second) study means that it is currently the imaging modality of choice for staging. MRI, however, may be used to further investigate uncertain hepatic lesions. The role of MRI may be further extended by the development of liver-specific MR contrast agents. These new agents may further improve the sensitivity and specificity of MRI for metastases.

Melanoma metastases may involve the gastrointestinal tract from the oesophagus through to the rectum:[43–45] occasionally, it may be a primary site.[44] Most symptomatic metastases through the gastrointestinal tract involve the small bowel or mesentery and this is commonly found at autopsy.[45] Metastases may be seen in the submucosa, causing a submucosal endoluminal mass, in the serosa or mesentery (Figure 43.12).

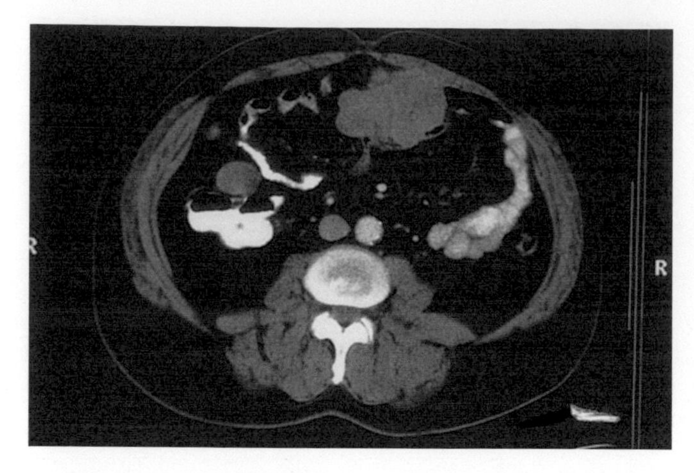

Figure 43.12 *Melanoma metastases in the mesentery in the anterior abdomen and a second lesion adjacent to the caecum.*

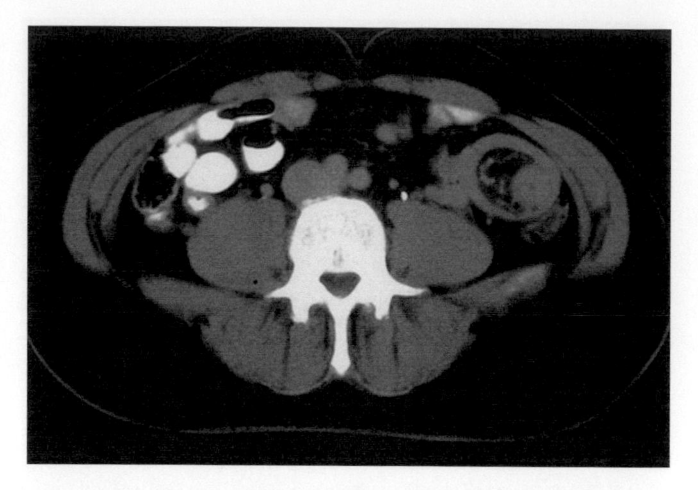

Figure 43.13 *Intussuscepting metastases without obstruction.*

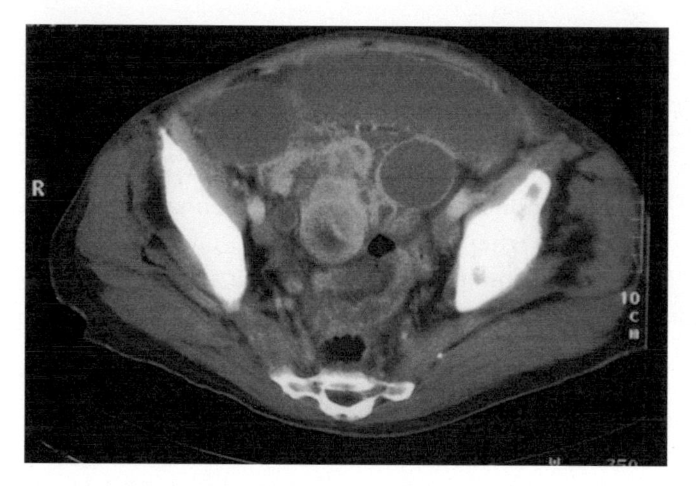

Figure 43.14 *Intussusception of small bowel metastases with small bowel obstruction.*

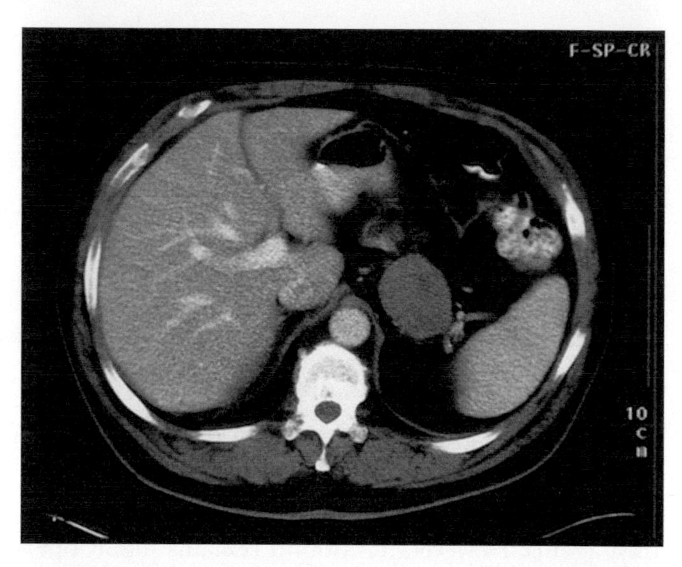

Figure 43.15 *Metastatic melanoma in the left adrenal gland.*

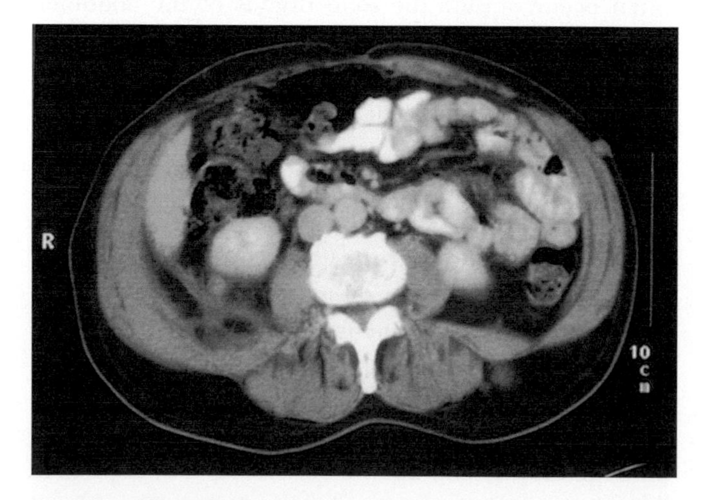

Figure 43.16 *Metastatic melanoma in right posterior pararenal space. Note the metastases in the left posterior subcutaneous fat and the left anterior subcutaneous fat.*

Intussusception is common and this may or not cause obstruction (Figures 43.13 and 43.14). Although luminal studies using barium may demonstrate these lesions well, in practice CT scanning is the technique most commonly used to identify gastrointestinal and mesenteric involvement. These may be identified as masses within the mesentery or as small masses involving the gut wall. Frequently, a mass will be demonstrated causing obstruction. The speed of image acquisition and the high sensitivity of CT scanning provides significant advantage over barium-based fluoroscopic studies. Colonic metastases are less common but can be seen.

Metastases may be seen in other solid organs, including the spleen and kidney. Adrenal metastases are commonly seen at autopsy[33] and may be bilateral (Figure 43.15). Metastases of the pararenal space have also been identified (Figure 43.16). Metastases of the pararenal space, though generally uncommon, are more commonly seen in melanoma than in other metastatic diseases.[46]

Autopsy studies show a bone metastatic rate of 23–49%. The radiological detection of metastasis is infrequent.[47,48] Two large reviews of 1677 and 1870 melanoma patients found metastases by radiological or scintigraphic means in 7 and 8%, respectively.[49,50] This discrepancy is, in part, due to the insentivity of plain x ray and scintigraphy to intramedullary metastases. A higher incidence has been reported with CT imaging, with up to 17% of patients with metastatic melanoma having axial skeletal bone metastases in one study.[51]

Metastatic melanoma bone lesions are frequently osteolytic, slightly expansile (Figure 43.17) and often involve the axial skeleton (Figure 43.18a and b). Associated soft tissue is common, but associated periosteal reaction and an identifiable tumour matrix are generally not seen. Sclerotic or blastic metastases are uncommon.

MRI is the imaging modality of choice in characterizing bone lesions, and particularly in determining the degree of marrow and soft tissue involvement. These are

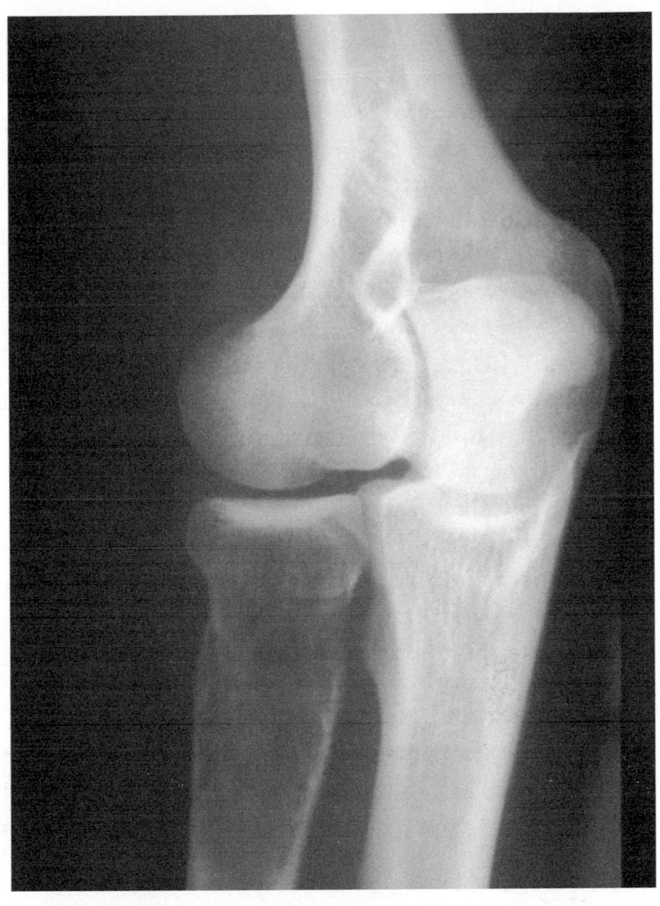

Figure 43.17 *Metastatic melanoma in the proximal radius.*

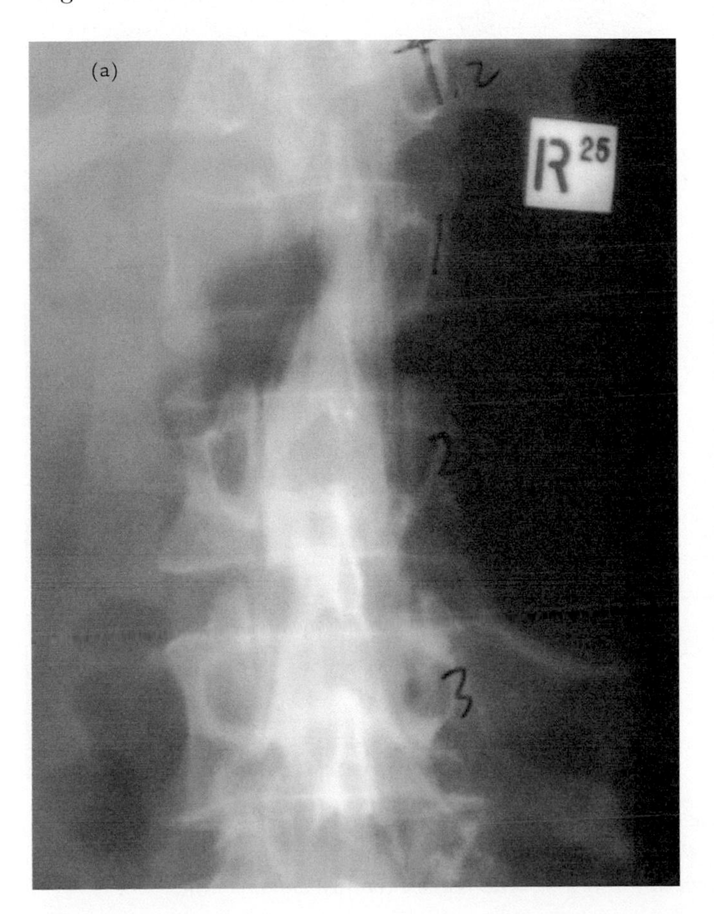

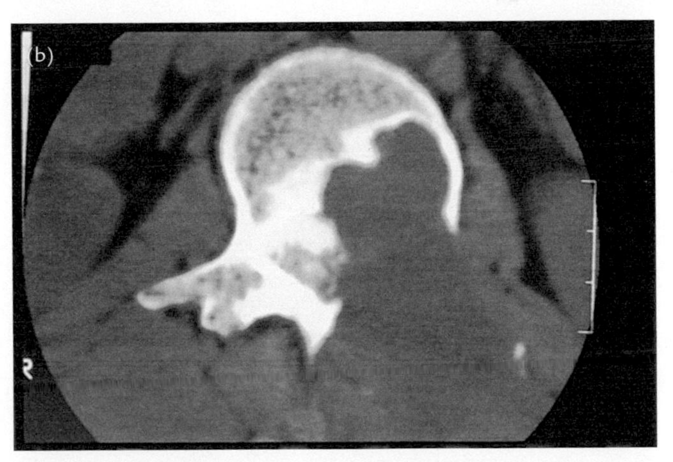

Figure 43.18 *(a) Myelogram of the lumber spine demonstrating a destructive metastasis in the right side of L1, displacing the cord to the left. (b) CT axial image of L1 after myelography, demonstrating the metastasis with a large soft tissue mass extending posterolaterally and displacing the thecal sac medially with compression. This lesion would be better imaged with MRI.*

important issues if treatment is considered as they are poorly demonstrated on plain film and CT scans. MRI is the imaging modality of choice in the spine, as previously noted. However, radionuclide bone scans cover the entire skeleton with relatively high sensitivity for metastasis and remain important where staging is required. Whole-body MRI techniques for screening bone and soft tissues are being developed and show much promise.

Metastatic melanoma may also occur in muscle (Figure 43.19).[34] These may be difficult to identify by CT scanning, even with an IV contrast agent. MRI will identify these lesions because of their altered water content and the inherently higher signal:noise ratio of MRI, especially with post-contrast enhanced T1-weighted images. MRI also provides excellent anatomical information on the location of vital structures, such as the neurovascular bundles, which will determine resectability (Figure 43.20).

Subcutaneous nodules can be seen with CT scanning, most commonly in the 5–10 mm range (Figure 43.7 and 43.16). These may represent the primary lesion or a metastasis, usually from haematogenous spread.[52]

CONCLUSIONS

Melanoma can, and does with depressing regularity, metastasize almost anywhere. A mass discovered in an unusual location may be a metastasis and, in a susceptible population, melanoma should be considered early in the diagnostic process.

MRI is the imaging modality of choice in the neuroaxis, in soft tissue lesions and in further characterizing lesions where surgical resection or other radical treatment is considered. CT remains the imaging method of choice in staging in the neck, chest and abdomen, and in investigating patients with symptoms in those areas.

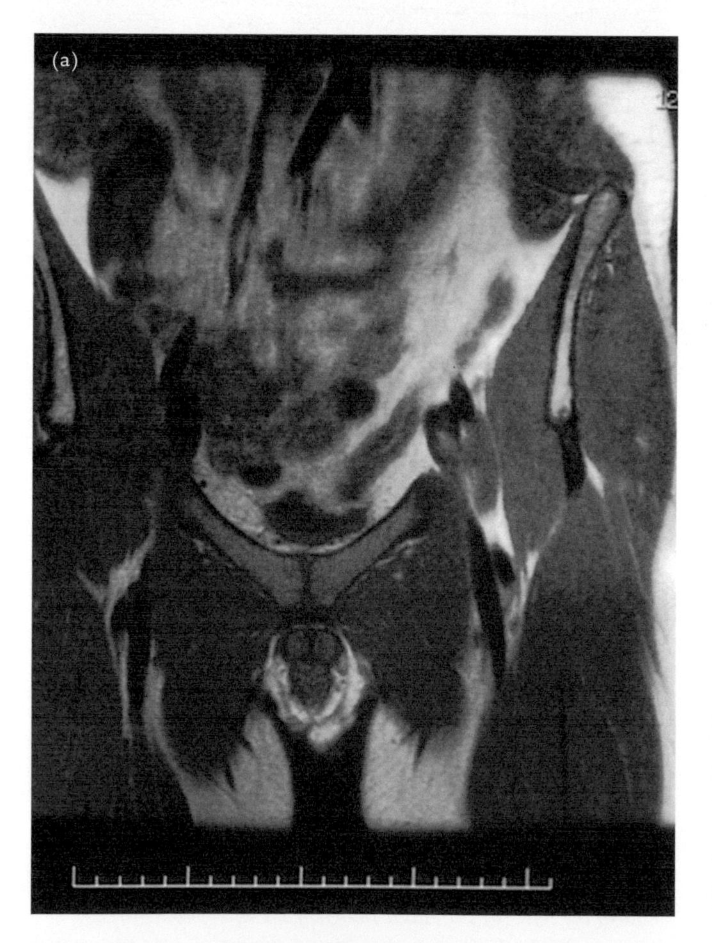

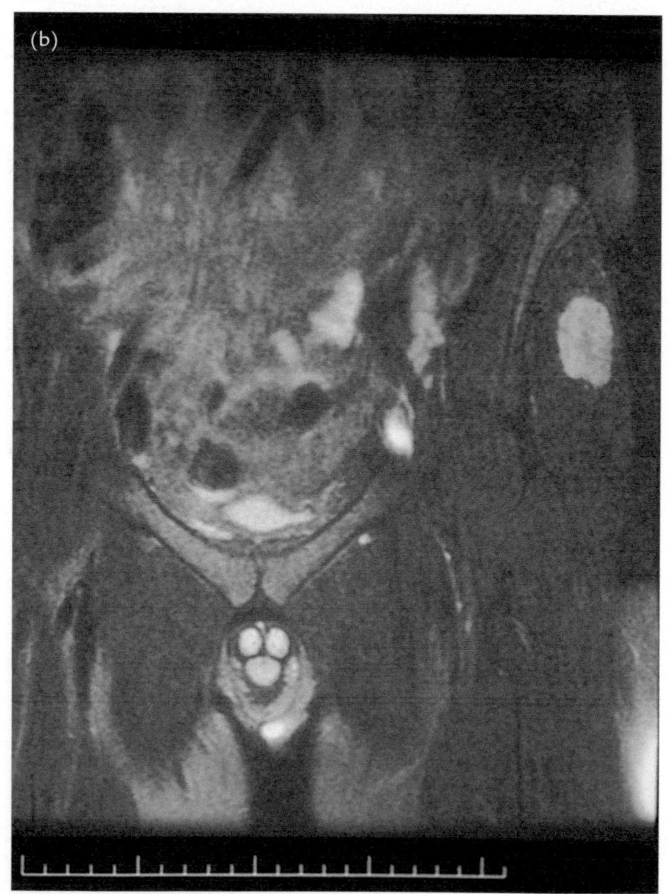

Figure 43.19 *(a) Coronal T1-weighted image demonstrates a subtle mass in the left gluteal muscle. (b) Coronal T2-weighted image demonstrates the mass well, reflecting the increased water content of the metastasis relative to muscle. (c) (see opposite page) Coronal T1-weighted image after gadolinium enhancement demonstrates the metastatisis well, with marked contrast enhancement.*

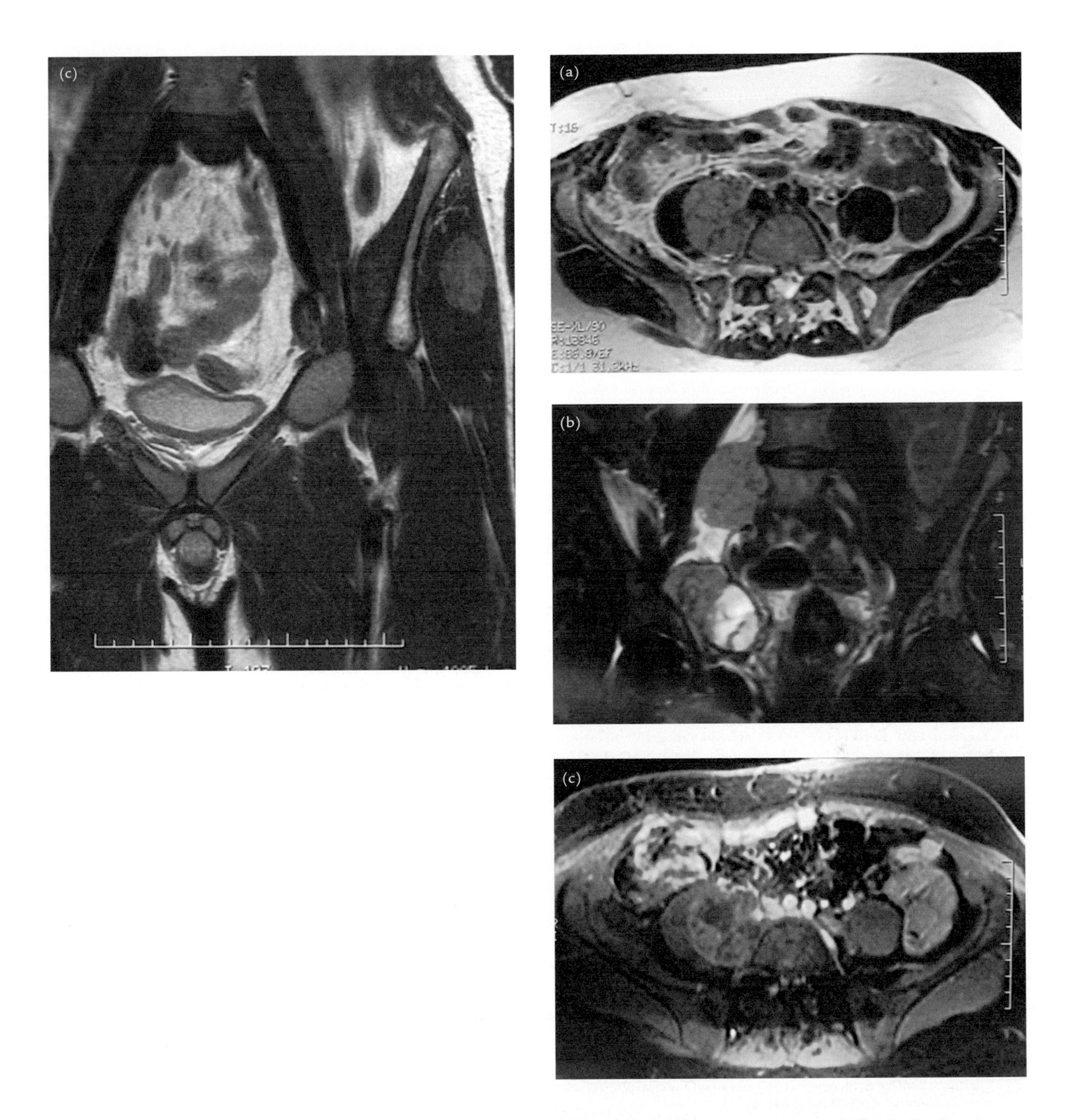

Figure 43.20 *(a) Axial T1-weighted image demonstrates a metastasis in the right psoas muscle. (b) Coronal T2-weighted image demonstrates the intrinsically higher signal of the two metastases relative to the psoas muscle, reflecting a higher water content and a cystic component in the pelvic metastasis. (c) Axial T1-weighted enhanced image demonstrates the intimate relationship of the superior lesion to the iliac veins.*

REFERENCES

1. Horgen K, Hughes LE, Review staging of melanoma. *Clin Radiol* 1993; 48: 297–300.
2. Khansor T, Saunders J, Das SK, Evaluation of staging workup in malignant melanoma. *Arch Surg* 1989; 124: 847–9.
3. Terhune MH, Swanson N, Johnson TM, Use of chest radiography in the initial evaluation of patients with localised melanoma. *Arch Dermatol* 1998; 134: 569–72.
4. Ardizzoni A, Gimaldi A, Repetto et al, Stage I–II melanoma: the value of metastatic workup. *Oncology* 1987; 44: 87–9.
5. Zartman GM, Thomas MR, Robinson WA, Metastatic disease in patients with newly diagnosed malignant melanoma. *J Surg Oncol* 1987; 35: 163–4.
6. Gershenwald JE, Buzaid AC, Ross MI, Classification and staging of melanoma. *Haematol–Oncol Clin North Am* 1998; 12: 737–65.
7. Huang CL, Provost N, Marghoob AA et al, Laboratory tests and imaging studies in patients with cutaneous malignant melanoma. *J Am Dermatol* 1998; 39: 451–63.
8. Gross A, Initial evaluation of malanoma. *Arch Dermatol* (editorial). 1998; 134: 623–4.
9. Parish LC, Witkowski JA, Melanoma and the radiograph: the sanctity of human life. *Lancet* 1998; 352: 922–3.
10. Balch CM, Cascinelli N, Drewiecki ICT et al, A comparison of pragmatic factors worldwide In. *Cutaneous melanoma* (eds Balch CM, Houghton AW, Milton AW, et al). Philadelphia: Lippincott JB, 1992: 188–99.
11. Libshitz HI, North LB, Pulmonary metastases. *Radiol Clin Am* 1982; 20: 437–51.
12. Heaston DK, Putnam CE, Rodan PA et al, Solitary pulmonary metastases in high risk melanoma patients: a prospective comparison of conventional and computed tomography. *AJR* 1983; 141: 169–74.
13. Webb WR, Gamsu G, Thoracic metastases in malignant melanoma. *Chest* 1977; 71: 176–81.
14. Buzaid AC, Sandler AB, Mani S et al, Role of computed tomography in the staging of primary melanoma. *J Clin Oncol* 1993; 11: 638–43.
15. Johnson TM, Fader PJ, Chang AE et al. Computed tomography in the staging of patients with melanoma metastatic to regional lymph nodes. *Ann Surg Oncol* 1997; 4: 396–402.
16. Kuvshinoff BW, Kurtz C, Cort DG, Computed tomography in the evaluation of patients with Stage III melanoma. *Ann Surg Oncol* 1997; 4: 252–8.
17. Weiss M, Loprinzi C, Creagan ET et al, Utility of follow-up tests for detecting recurrent disease in patients with malignant melanoma. *JAMA* 1995; 274: 1703–5.
18. Kersey PA, Iscoe NA, Gapski JA et al, The value of staging and serial follow-up investigation in patients with completely resected, primary cutaneous malignant melanoma. *Br J Surg* 1985; 72: 614–17.
19. Basseres N, Grob JJ, Richard MA, Cost effectiveness of surveillance of stage I melanoma. A retrospective appraisal on a 10 year experience in a dermatology department in France. *Dermatology* 1995; 191: 199–203.
20. Jubelwer SJ, Surveillance testing in patients with primary malignant melanoma. *W-V-Med-J* 1999; 95: 80–1.
21. Perez EA, Loprinzi CL, Sloan JA et al, Utility of screening procedures for detecting recurrence of disease after complete response in patients with small cell lung cancer. *Cancer* 1997; 80: 676–80.
22. Beresford HR, Melanoma of nervous system – treatment with corticosteroids and radiation. *Neurology* 1969; 19: 59–65.
23. Giraldi S, Wallace S, Shalen P et al, Computed tomography in malignant melanoma. *AJNR* 1980; 1: 531–5.
24. Atlas SW, Lavi E, *Intra-axial brain tumours in magnetic resonance imaging of the brain and spine*, 2nd edn. Philadelphia: Lippincott-Raven, 1996.
25. Healy ME, Hesschlink JR, Press GA, Middleton MS, Increased detection of intracranial metastases with intravenous Gd-DTPA. *Radiology* 1987; 165: 619–24.
26. Russell EJ, Geremia GK, Johnson CE et al, Multiple cerebral metastases: delectability with Gd-DTPA-enhanced MR imaging. *Radiology* 1987; 165: 609–17.
27. Abdullah ND, Mathews VP, Contrast issues in brain imaging in brain tumour. *Neuroim Clin North Am* 1999; 9: 733–49.
28. Yuh WT, Fisher DJ, Runge VM et al, Phase III multicentre trial of gadoteridol MR imaging in the evaluation of brain metastases. *AJNR* 1994; 15: 1037–51.
29. Isiklar I, Leeds NE, Fuller GN, Kumar AJ, Intracranial metastatic melanoma: correlation between MR imaging characteristics and melanin content. *AJR* 1995; 165: 1503–12.
30. Smoker WRR, Godersley JC, Nutzon RK et al, Role of MR imaging in evaluation of spinal metastatic disease. *AJNR* 1987; 8: 901–8.
31. Carmody RF, Yang DJ, Seeley GW et al, Spinal cord compression due to metastatic disease: diagnosis with MR imaging versus myelography. *Radiology* 1989; 173: 225–29.
32. Arbelaez A, Castillo M, Armao DM, Imaging features of intraventricular melanoma. *AJNR* 1999; 20: 691–3.
33. Patel JK, Didolkar MS, Pickren JW, Moore RM, Metastatic pattern of malignant melanoma. *Am J Surg* 1978; 135: 807–10.
34. Fishman EK, Kuhlman JE, Schucher LM et al, CT of malignant melanoma in the chest, abdomen, and musculoskeletal system. *Radiographics* 1990; 10: 603–20.
35. Shirkoda A, Albin J, Malignant melanoma: correlating abdominal and pelvic CT with clinical staging. *Radiology* 1987; 165: 75–8.
36. Silverman PM, Heaston DC, Koroblein M, Siegler HF, Computed tomography in the detection of abdominal metastases from malignant melanoma. *Invest Radiol* 1984; 19: 309–12.
37. Oliver III JH, Baron RL, Hepatic biphasic contrast enhanced CT of the liver: technique indications, interpretations and pitfalls. *Radiology* 1996; 201: 1–14.
38. Blake SP, Weisinger K, Atkin M, Raptopoulos V, Liver metastases from melanoma detection with multiphase contrast enhanced CT. *Radiology* 1999; 213: 92–6.
39. Paley MR, Ros PR, Hepatic metastases. *Radiol Clin North Am* 1998; 36: 349–63.
40. Abbitt PL, Ultrasonography update on liver technique. *Radiol Clin North Am* 1998; 36: 299–307.
41. Semelka RC, Mitchell GD, Reinhold C, The liver and biliary system. In: *MRI of the body* (eds Higgins CB, Hricat H, Helms CA): Lippincott Raven, 1997: 591–637.
42. Semelka RC, Cance WG, Marcos HI, Mauro MA, Liver metastases: comparison of current MR techniques and spiral CT during arterial portography for detection of 20 surgical staged cases. *Radiology* 1999; 213: 86–91.
43. McDermott VG, Low VHS, Keogen MT et al, Malignant melanoma metastases to the gastrointestinal tract. *AJR* 1996; 809–15.
44. Gollib MJ, Prowde JC, Primary melanoma of the oesophagus: radiological and clinical findings in six patients. *Radiology* 1999; 213: 97–100.
45. Das Gupta TH, Brasfield RD, Metastatic melanoma of the gastrointestinal tract. *Arch Surg* 1964; 88: 969.
46. Shirkhoda A, Computed tomography of perirenal metastases. *J Comput Assist Tomogr* 1987; 10: 435–8.
47. Resnick D, Niwayama G, Skeletal metastasis. In: *Diagnosis of bone and joint disease*, 2nd edn (eds Resnick D, Niwayama G) Philadelphia: Saunders, 1988: 3977–8.
48. Murray RO, Jacobson HG, Less common manifestations of skeletal disorders. In: *Radiology of skeletal disorders*, 2nd edn (eds Murray RO, Jacobson HG). Edinburgh: Churchill Livingstone, 1977: 1458.
49. Stewart WR, Gelberman RH, Harrelson JM, Siegler HF, Skeletal metastases in melanoma. *J Bone Joint Surg (Am)* 1978; 60A: 645–9.
50. Fon GT, Wong WS, Gold RH, Kaiser LR, Skeletal metastases in melanoma: radiologic, scintigraphic and clinical review. *AJR* 1981; 137: 103–8.
51. Patten RM, Shuman WP, Teefey S, Metastases from malignant melanoma to the axial skeleton: a CT study of frequency and appearance. *AJR* 155: 109–12.
52. Patten RM, Shuman WP, Teefey S, Subcutaneous metastases from malignant melanoma: prevalence and findings on CT. *AJR* 1989; 152: 1009–12.

44

Positron emission tomography

Jakob DH De Vries, Omgo E Nieweg, Roger F Uren

INTRODUCTION

Positron emission tomography (PET) is a relatively new diagnostic technique in nuclear medicine. PET requires advanced and expensive technology, which is not likely to be available in the average nuclear medicine department in the foreseeable future. The value of PET was initially established in neurology and cardiology. PET is now increasingly being used in oncology to diagnose metastatic disease, to monitor treatment and to provide additional functional information when conventional imaging techniques are not diagnostic. The number of PET scans in cancer patients now exceeds the number performed in other fields of medicine. Increasing demand has meant that an increasing number of hospitals have acquired this new technology, which, in turn, has led to more widespread use of PET in melanoma. This chapter describes the basic principles of PET, outlines its value in the management of melanoma patients and provides information about likely future applications.

BASIC PRINCIPLES

The basic principles of both PET scanning and conventional nuclear medicine techniques are the same. A radiopharmaceutical is administered to a patient and accumulates in its intended target tissue. This can be visualized with the aid of an imaging device. In contrast to conventional nuclear medicine, which uses single photon-emitting radionuclides, PET makes use of positron-emitting radionuclides.

A positron is a particle with a mass and a charge that are equivalent to the mass and the charge of an electron. The difference between a positron and an electron is that the charge of the former is positive, whereas the charge of the latter is negative. Certain chemical elements have unstable isotopes that emit a positron from the nucleus. The atom thereby loses its excess energy and falls back into a stable state. After ejection from the atom's nucleus, the positron travels a short distance, losing kinetic energy, before recombining with an electron to form a positronium. The positronium annihilates immediately, releasing its mass as energy in the form of two 511 keV photons emitted in opposite directions. The energy of these rays is too high for adequate detection with the type of gamma camera that is routinely used in conventional nuclear medicine. A positron camera makes use of opposing detectors that can register these two high-energy photons in a process called coincidence detection. A coincidence event will be recorded if both of the opposing detectors produce a signal within a few nanoseconds of each other. These signals are transmitted to a computer that determines where the annihilation took place, which will be along a line joining the two detectors that simultaneously recorded the signal. The computer can then generate images that can be presented as tomographic planes or whole-body images.

Among the radionuclides that emit positrons are carbon-11 (^{11}C), nitrogen-13 (^{13}N), oxygen-15 (^{15}N) and fluorine-18 (^{18}F). PET utilizes the fact that most molecules in the human body, and most medicines, contain one or more of these elements. Metabolism can be studied in vivo by substituting positron-emitting atoms for the body's own atoms of the same elements. An example will illustrate the point: ^{18}F-fluoro-2-deoxy-D-glucose (FDG) is an often-used radiopharmaceutical in PET scanning and is basically a glucose molecule in which a fluorine atom has been incorporated. After administration to the patient, the biological properties of FDG are initially the same as those of normal glucose. FDG will be absorbed by cells with high glucose consumption. Uptake of glucose and FDG into malignant cells is facilitated by an increased number of glucose transporter molecules at the cell membrane. Several genes encoding such glucose transporters are currently known. Inside the cell, FDG cannot be metabolized and remains trapped; the radiation emitted from the cell by ^{18}F allows a tumour deposit to be visualized.

In addition to visualization, modern technology also allows metabolic processes to be calculated and quantified. In theory, every body substance or drug that contains carbon, oxygen, nitrogen or fluorine can be labelled with a positron-emitting isotope without altering its molecular structure. These features place PET in a unique position for the study of metabolism in vivo.

Positron-emitting radionuclides are produced in a cyclotron. The isotopes are short-lived: the half-life ranges from a few minutes to 2 hours. An advantage of a short half-life is the limited time that a patient is exposed to radioactivity. The radiation doses in PET and conventional nuclear medicine are similar.[1,2] Another advantage of a short half-life is that a PET study can be repeated after a short interval, e.g. to assess how a treatment regimen affects tumour metabolism. The disadvantage is that there must be a cyclotron for the production of radionuclides in the near vicinity of the positron camera. Transportation over more than a limited distance is complicated because the isotopes lose their radioactivity quickly. A radiochemistry laboratory equipped with robots and thick lead shielding is needed for the synthesis of radiopharmaceuticals from the radionuclides as soon as they are produced in the cyclotron.

A fully equipped PET centre consists of a cyclotron, a radiochemistry laboratory and a positron camera. Physicists, chemists, pharmacists and physicians work closely together. It is understandable that the availability of PET is limited due to the associated high cost and complexity of the technique.

In contrast to conventional radiology techniques, PET scanning does not demonstrate anatomical structures but provides information about tissue metabolism. This means that the tumour can be depicted even when the anatomy is changed by earlier operations. PET cannot be used to visualize anatomy; other imaging techniques, like computerized tomography (CT), x rays and magnetic resonance imaging (MRI), are much more suitable for that purpose. But merging PET images and CT or MRI images can combine physiological and anatomical information. A camera has been developed that can simultaneously make CT and PET images, and fuse the separate images into one. Three-dimensional imaging is also possible.

DIAGNOSIS OF METASTATIC DISEASE

FDG is the most commonly used radiopharmaceutical in PET oncology. Melanoma cells have a great affinity for this tracer. The value of FDG-PET has been the subject of a number of studies. A meta-analysis of six studies showed a pooled sensitivity of 79% and a pooled specificity of 86% for the detection of melanoma metastases.[3] Sensitivity ranged from 66 to 93% and specificity from 78 to 95%. Comments on these PET data are that the patient populations in some studies were small and that they were heterogeneous in others.

The sensitivity is limited by the avidity of tumours for FDG, the size of tumour deposits and the characteristics of the PET camera. The uptake of FDG in melanoma cells is generally high but metastases <5 mm are often not identified.[4,5] A study by Crippa et al.[6] demonstrated that FDG-PET detected 100% of lymph node metastases >10 mm in size, 83% of metastases 6–10 mm in size and 23% of metastases ≤ 5 mm in size. False-positive scans can be caused by inflammation, surgical wounds and a variety of other clinical problems.[5,7] Using the clinical history of a patient when evaluating the scans may improve the predictive value of a positive PET scan to figures of up to 91%.[8,9]

The benefit of PET for patients with clinically localized melanoma is limited, both because 80% of these patients do not have metastatic disease and because the remainder usually have only micrometastases,[8] which PET is not capable of visualizing. In these patients, metastases usually involve lymph nodes. Holle-Robatsch et al.[10] compared PET and sentinel node biopsy in 39 patients with surgically resected melanoma >0.75 mm in

Breslow thickness. Five of the patients had metastases proved by sentinel node biopsy (13%), but PET revealed only one of these tumour deposits. A similar study of 50 patients was reported by Ackland et al.:[11] in none of the 14 patients with a tumour-positive sentinel node did PET scanning identify metastatic disease in the same location. Sentinel lymph node biopsy appears to be the most reliable technique to establish the presence of lymphatic (micro-)metastases.[12,13] Micrometastases as small as 0.0005 mm^2 can be detected with sentinel node biopsy; even a single cell is sometimes recognized.[14]

PET is more sensitive in patients with enlarged lymph nodes or established regional metastases. A retrospective study involving 20 patients with clinically suspicious lymph nodes was conducted to compare the diagnostic validity of FDG-PET and real-time ultrasonography.[15] A total of 83 lymph nodes were assessed with ultrasonography and PET; imaging results were confirmed by histologic studies or follow-up ultrasonographic examinations. The sensitivity of PET was 74% and the specificity 93%; ultrasound showed a comparable sensitivity and specificity. In a series of 95 patients with clinically evident lymph node and/or in-transit metastases, Tyler et al.[8] found that PET identified 144 of 165 tumour deposits (87%). The 21 areas of melanoma that were missed included 10 microscopic foci and nine foci <1 cm in diameter. In 39 areas, the PET scan showed increased activity that could not be associated with malignancy (79% predictive value of a positive test). The false-positive rate was 57% and inflammatory processes were the most frequent cause of these. Fifteen per cent of the PET scans led to a change in the treatment of the patient.

PET scanning is clearly superior to conventional imaging techniques for the detection of widespread disease in patients with regional metastases.[16] Distant metastases may occur anywhere in the body due to the highly variable spreading pattern of the disease; MRI, CT, chest x ray, bone scintigraphy and ultrasound are methods used to identify these locations. All these conventional techniques are employed to investigate a specific part of the body but are not useful to give a complete picture. One of the important features of whole-body PET is that it can identify all these locations and thus stage the patients more accurately. A thorough review of the literature indicated that the diagnostic accuracy of FDG-PET was better in stage IV disease than in less advanced stages.[3]

When the presence of recurrent disease has been established and important treatment decisions have to be made, it is of crucial importance to be optimally informed about the extent of the disease. PET can be used for this purpose. In a patient with distant metastasis limited to one location, surgery is usually a therapeutic option.[17] An intended surgical intervention may be postponed or abandoned when PET shows disease to be more widespread than was assumed. Tumour deposits at more than one location will mostly prompt systemic treatment, or a wait-and-see policy (Figure 44.1). Intuitively, patients in whom surgery is being contemplated for distant disease appear to be an appropriate group for PET. To the present authors' knowledge, this indication has not yet been studied in detail.

Several investigators have examined the role of PET scanning in stage IV patients. However, many of these studies are retrospective, usually concern fairly small groups of patients, the study groups contain patients with various other stages of the disease and tissue confirmation has not always been pursued. One study showed

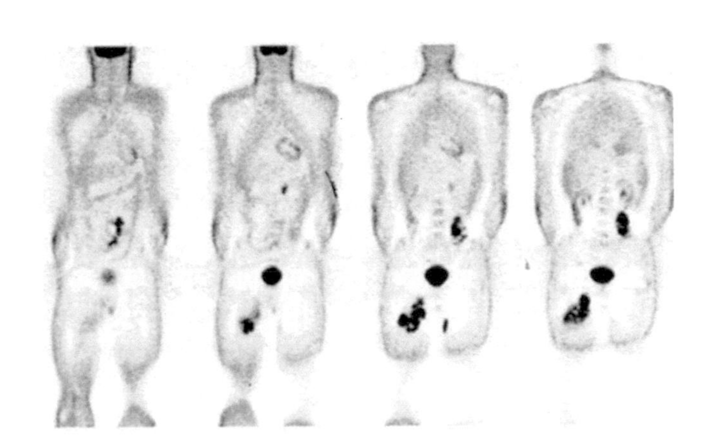

Figure 44.1 *A 29-year-old man was diagnosed with a subcutaneous in-transit metastasis from a primary melanoma on the left shoulder 9 years previously. The lesion was excised. An elevated serum S-100 level was detected during follow up. Physical examination, ultrasound of the liver, chest radiography, magnetic resonance imaging of the brain and bone scintigraphy revealed no abnormalities. A positron emission tomography (PET) scan was ordered to investigate the possibility of a surgically treatable lesion. However, the PET scan demonstrated large lesions in the left retroperitoneum and right thigh, and smaller lesions in the left upper abdominal region and left thigh. Systemic treatment was given. (PET Centre of the Free University, Amsterdam, the Netherlands).*

that FDG-PET was inferior to CT for diagnosing lung and liver metastases.[18] However, PET detected more lymph node and bone metastases than conventional imaging.[19] Another study found PET to be as sensitive as CT in the detection of lung metastases and more sensitive than CT for the detection of liver metastases.[5] A study comparing PET and CT/MRI/ultrasound did not show either up- or downstaging by PET.[18] Other investigators found that PET led to changes in the treatment plan in 8–15% of patients.[8,20] PET is not appropriate for the detection of brain metastases due to the high FDG uptake in normal brain tissue;[7,21] MRI is currently the standard imaging technique for this purpose.

FOLLOW-UP AND TREATMENT MONITORING

Melanoma patients are routinely followed using regular, careful physical examination; laboratory tests and radiographic studies are generally not recommended.[22,23] In theory, PET may reveal treatable metastases in parts of the body that are presumed to be free of disease. In practice, however, the yield is insufficient to recommend PET for routine follow-up. However, PET may be able to indicate the outcome of systemic therapy at an early phase of the treatment. This approach may be more accurate than measuring tumour size, since tumour size and tumour viability are not well correlated. Tumour metabolism investigated with PET may reveal remaining tumour deposits after completion of radiotherapy, surgery or systemic therapy. Studies exploring this potential application in melanoma patients have not been published but promising results have been demonstrated in other tumour types.[24–29]

FUTURE PROSPECTS

PET scanning is a still evolving imaging technique. In the future, equipment will improve, computers will operate faster and software will become more refined. In addition to these improvements, new radiopharmaceuticals will become available which are more specifically accumulated in tumour cells than the agents currently used: *N*[3-(4-morpholino)-propyl]-*N*-methyl-5-iodobenzylamine labelled with the single photon-emitting iodine-123 may be such an agent.[30] Uptake of melanoma-seeking tracers by normal tissue should be kept to a minimum. When successful systemic therapies are developed, there will be an increasing demand for PET scans to monitor these patients. Not only can PET be used to monitor tumour growth rate, but various other aspects of tumour physiology can potentially be investigated with it in vivo, e.g. blood perfusion, oxygen consumption, pH, and the presence of receptors for various cytokines and hormones. For instance, the study of oxygen consumption of tumours can give information about the sensitivity of tumour tissue to radiotherapy, and tumours with a low pH may also be more sensitive to chemotherapy.[31] Now that the human genome project is virtually completed, attention in research will shift towards linking genetic abnormalities to biological expressions of disease. Determining a gene expression profile may be useful to characterize tumour behaviour and help select appropriate treatment.[32] A role for PET can be foreseen in many of these areas of research.

CONCLUSIONS

PET is a new nuclear medicine technique that allows the study of metabolism in vivo. In the immediate future, PET will remain restricted to a limited number of institutions because of inherent technical and financial factors. However, PET appears to be of great value in detecting metastatic disease in patients for whom important treatment decisions have to be made,[33] but there is a need for larger prospective studies in well-defined patient populations to substantiate this. PET currently has no role in routine follow-up. Patients likely to benefit from PET have to be carefully selected because of its high cost. PET scans have to be interpreted in conjunction with the clinical history of the patient to minimize the number of false-positive findings and thereby save patients from unnecessary work-up.

New radiopharmaceuticals and more advanced equipment will probably increase the demand for PET. The ability of PET to visualize tumour biology and physiology offers vast opportunities for clinical research. PET also has the potential to obtain better knowledge of tumour behaviour in individual patients. With the advent of molecular biology based medicine, a transition is being made to incorporate information based on biochemical changes that take place in disease, frequently in the absence of changes in anatomy, into diagnostic imaging. PET can take advantage of this transition to a more functional approach and should play an increasing role in the biological profiling of individual tumours to allow more specific treatments to be instigated.

REFERENCES

1. Jones SC, Alavi A, Christman D et al, The radiation dosimetry of 2-[F-18]fluoro-2-deoxy-D-glucose in man. *J Nucl Med* 1982; 23: 613–17.
2. ICRP. *Radiation dose to patients from radiopharmaceuticals*. Pergamon Press: Oxford, 1987: 67.
3. Mijnhout GS, Hoekstra OS, van Tulder MW et al, Systemic review on the diagnostic accuracy of ^{18}F-fluorodeoxyglucose positron emission tomography in melanoma patients. *Cancer* 2001; 91: 1530–42.
4. Macfarlane DJ, Sondak V, Johnson T et al, Prospective evaluation of 2-[18F]-2-deoxy-D-glucose positron emission tomography in staging of regional lymph nodes in patients with cutaneous malignant melanoma. *J Clin Oncol* 1998; 16: 1770–6.
5. Holder WD, White RL, Zuger JH et al, Effectiveness of positron emission tomography for the detection of melanoma metastases. *Ann Surg* 1998; 227: 764–9.
6. Crippa F, Leutner M, Belli F et al, Which kind of lymph node metastases can FDG PET detect? A clinical study in melanoma. *J Nucl Med* 2000; 41: 1491–4.
7. Steinert HC, Huch Boni RA, Buck A et al, Malignant melanoma: staging with whole-body positron emission tomography and 2-[F-18]-fluoro-2-deoxy-D-glucose. *Radiology* 1995; 195: 705–9.
8. Tyler DS, Onaitis M, Kherani A et al, Positron emission tomography scanning in malignant melanoma: clinical utility in patients with Stage III disease. *Cancer* 2000; 89: 1019–25.
9. Paquet P, Henry F, Belhocine T et al, An appraisal of 18-fluorodeoxyglucose positron emission tomography for melanoma staging. *Dermatology* 2001; 67–9.
10. Holle-Robatsch S, Mirzaei S, Knoll P et al, Positron emission tomography for detecting occult lymph node metastases in patients with primary malignant melanoma stage I and II. *Melanoma Res* 2001 (Suppl 1): S183.
11. Ackland K, Healy C, O'Doherty et al, Staging of patients with primary malignant melanoma: a comparison of PET scanning and sentinel node biopsy. *Melanoma Res* 2001; 11 (Suppl 1): S105.
12. Wagner JD, Schauwecker D, Davidson D et al, Prospective study of fluorodeoxyglucose-positron emission tomography of lymph node basins in melanoma patients undergoing sentinel lymph node biopsy. *J Clin Oncol* 1999; 17: 1508–15.
13. Mijnhout GS, Pijpers R, Hoekstra OS et al, The FDG-PET scan cannot replace the sentinel node biopsy. *Cancer* 1999; 85: 1199–201.
14. Borgstein PJ, Pijpers R, van Diest P et al, Staging early lymphatic metastases in melanoma: the case for super-selective lymph node dissection. *Proceedings of the Society of Surgical Oncology 51st Cancer Symposium*, San Diego, California, March 26–7, 1998.
15. Blessing C, Feine U, Geiger L et al, Positron emission tomography and ultrasonography. A comparative retrospective study assessing the diagnostic validity in lymph node metastases of malignant melanoma. *Arch Dermatol* 1995; 131: 1394–8.
16. Eightved A, Andersson AP, Dahlstrom K et al, Use of fluorine-18 fluorodeoxyglucose positron emission tomography in the detection of silent metastases from malignant melanoma. *Eur J Nucl Med* 2000; 27: 70–5.
17. Balch CM, Palliative surgery for stage IV melanoma: is it a primary treatment? *Ann Surg Oncol* 1999; 6: 623–4.
18. Krug B, Dietlein M, Groth W et al, Fluor-18-fluorodeoxyglucose positron emission tomography (FDG-PET) in malignant melanoma. Diagnostic comparison with conventional imaging methods. *Acta Radiol* 2000; 41: 446–52.
19. Dietlein M, Krug B, Groth W et al, Positron emission tomography using 18F-fluorodeoxyglucose in advanced stages of malignant melanoma: comparison of ultrasonographic and radiological methods of diagnosis. *Nucl Med Commun* 1999; 20: 255–61.
20. Jadvar H, Johnson DL, Segall GM, The effect of fluorine-18 positron emission tomography on the management of cutaneous malignant melanoma. *Clin Nucl Med* 2000; 25: 48–51.
21. Rinne D, Baum RP, Hor G et al, Primary staging and follow-up of high risk melanoma patients with whole-body 18F-fluorodeoxyglucose positron emission tomography: results of a prospective study of 100 patients. *Cancer* 1998; 82: 1664–71.
22. Kroon BBR, Nieweg OE, Hoekstra HJ et al, Principles and guidelines for surgeons: management of cutaneous malignant melanoma. European Society of Surgical Oncology, Brussels. *Eur J Surg Oncol* 1997; 23: 550–8.
23. Shumate CR, Urist MM, Maddox WA, Melanoma recurrence surveillance. *Ann Surg* 1995; 221: 566–71.
24. Nieweg OE, Wong WH, Singletary SE et al, Positron emission tomography of glucose metabolism in breast cancer. Potential for tumor detection, staging and evaluation of chemotherapy. *Ann NY Acad Sci* 1993; 698: 423–8.
25. Minn H, Paul R, Ahonen A, Evaluation of treatment response to radiotherapy in head and neck cancer with fluorine-18 fluorodeoxyglucose. *J Nucl Med* 1998; 29: 1521–5.
26. Hawkins RA, Hoh C, Dahlbom M et al, PET cancer evaluations with FDG. *J Nucl Med* 1991; 32: 1555–8.
27. Ginkel RJ van, Hoekstra HJ, Pruim J et al, FDG-PET to evaluate response to hyperthermic isolated limb perfusion for locally advanced soft-tissue sarcoma. *J Nucl Med* 1996; 37: 984–90.
28. Kole AC, *In vivo tumor analysis, detection, staging & monitoring therapy with positron emission tomography*. PhD Thesis, University of Groningen, the Netherlands, 1998.
29. Ginkel RJ van, Kole AC, Nieweg OE et al, L-[1-11C]-tyrosine PET to evaluate response to hyperthermic isolated limb perfusion for locally advanced soft-tissue sarcoma and skin cancer. *J Nucl Med* 1999; 40: 262–7.
30. Salopek TG, Scott JR, Joshua AV et al, Radioiodinated ^{123}I-ERC-9, *N*[3-(4-morpholino)-propyl]-*N*-methyl-5-iodobenzylamine: a new potential melanoma imaging agent. *Melanoma Res* 2001; 11 (Suppl 1): S184 (abstract).
31. Chaplin DJ, Acker B, Olive PL, Potentiation of the tumour toxicity of melphalan by vasodilatating drugs. *Int J Rad Biol Phys* 1989; 16: 1131–5.
32. Tjuvajev JG, Stockhammer G, Desai R et al, Imaging the expression of transfected genes in vivo. *Cancer Res* 1995; 55: 6126–32.
33. Damian DL, Fulham MJ, Thompson E, Thompson JF, Positron emission tomography in the detection and management of metastatic melanoma. *Melanoma Res* 1996; 6: 325–9.

45

Diagnosis of systemic metastatic melanoma: blood tests and markers

Eddy C Hsueh

INTRODUCTION

Between 1973 and 1995, the incidence of melanoma in the United States increased at a faster rate than any other malignant neoplasm.[1] Nationwide, approximately 47,700 individuals developed melanoma and 7700 died from this cancer in the year 2000.[2] Distressingly, melanoma tends to develop when a patient is in his or her prime (35.4% are between the ages of 35 and 54); the median age at diagnosis is 56 years of age. Each death from melanoma corresponds to an average of 19.3 years of life lost, one of the highest for any cancer. Because of its resistance to chemotherapy and radiation therapy, melanoma has been treated primarily by surgery. Although melanoma is surgically curable in its early (localized) stages, the 5-year survival rate of patients with regional and distant metastases [American Joint Committee on Cancer (AJCC) stage III and IV melanoma] is poor (40% and <6%, respectively).[3]

A major factor contributing to the poor prognosis of patients with metastatic melanoma is the lack of an effective surveillance strategy. Close observation with careful history and physical examination has been the best, and most cost-effective, surveillance tool,[4] but physical examination can neither predict nor trace the pattern of distant spread.[5] This is evident in the dichotomy between clinical and autopsy findings: clinical evidence identifies the regional lymph nodes and subcutaneous tissue as the most common sites of distant metastasis,[6,7] whereas autopsy findings show that death is often due to 'clinically silent' metastases in the lung, heart, liver, brain, bone and other organs.[8] On the other hand, because there is no predictable pattern of melanoma metastasis, surveillance for metastatic melanoma must evaluate the entire body. However, routine surveillance using modern imaging modalities such as computerized tomography (CT) scans is not cost-effective in an asymptomatic patient.[9,10] Moreover, even the most sophisticated imaging techniques cannot detect microscopic disease. Thus, adjunctive blood tests that could detect the presence of microscopic disease would be especially attractive for the management of melanoma patients.

Melanoma is a highly antigenic and metabolically active tumour that releases antigens, enzymes and cytokines into the circulation. These molecules serve as attractive targets for a sensitive and specific serum marker assay that can detect the presence of occult melanoma metastases. Although no serum marker for melanoma has yet proven as useful as carcinoembryonic antigen (CEA) for colon cancer or prostate-specific antigen (PSA) for prostate cancer, several promising serum markers are being actively investigated as potential surveillance tools. Also, as discussed elsewhere in this book, highly sensitive reverse transcriptase polymerase chain reaction (RT-PCR) and PCR techiques to examine the peripheral blood are being developed for the detection of tumour recurrence.

S-100 PROTEIN

S-100, a calcium-binding thermolabile protein with a molecular weight (M_r) of 21 kDa, was originally isolated from bovine brain.[11] Its biological function has not been fully elucidated. S-100 protein is composed of two subunits in three possible combinations: αβ, αα and ββ [α subunit M_r = 10,400; β subunit M_r = 10,500). The β subunit of S-100 protein is found in high concentrations in glial astrocytes, Schwann cells and satellite cells in sympathetic ganglia. The αα isoform of S-100 protein is present only in glial cells. S-100 protein has also been demonstrated in melanocytes and Langerhans' cells.[12,13] Melanoma cells are able to secrete a soluble form of S-100 protein.[14] In addition to melanoma, S-100 protein is expressed in tumours such as glioma, Schwannoma and neuroblastoma.[15] Serum S-100B protein is elevated (>0.15–0.5 μg/l) in 0–8% of patients with AJCC stage I/II melanoma, 8–62% of patients with stage III melanoma and 68–91% of patients with stage IV disease (Table 45.1).[16,17] Its presence in the peripheral blood has been correlated with poor overall survival (OS).[16–23] Several studies have compared the clinical utility of serum S-100B protein with other serum markers. When compared with lipid-associated sialic acid (LASA), S-100B appeared to be superior as a prognostic variable.[20] It was more sensitive than neuron-specific enolase (NSE) in diagnosing AJCC stage IV disease ($P < 0.05$).[24] In stage IV patients, there was a strong correlation between high S-100B and NSE levels.[24,25] When compared with urinary excretion of melanin precursor metabolites, S-100B was superior as a prognostic variable.[22] However, a multivariate analysis considering lactate dehydrogenase (LDH), S-100B and other clinical variables showed that S-100B was not significantly associated with OS, whereas LDH was a statistically significant prognostic variable.[18] In another study, although S-100B level was significantly associated with disease progression in stage IV patients, its prognostic significance did not persist when analyzed with melanoma-inhibiting activity (MIA) and LDH in a multiple logistic regression analysis.[26] In this study, LDH was the only significant marker for progressive disease. Thus, the utility of S-100B may be limited to follow up of patients with a high risk for recurrence. Further longitudinal studies in prospective cohorts are needed to assess the utility of this marker as a surveillance adjunct.

NEURON-SPECIFIC ENOLASE (NSE)

Enolase catalyzes the interconversion of 2-phosphoglycerate and phosphoenolpyruvate in the glycolytic pathway, and participates in the formation of a high-energy phosphate bond. It exists as several dimeric isoenzymes, of which the αγ and γγ dimers are known as NSE. The name was derived from the initial observation that NSE is expressed in neurons, neuroendocrine cells and neoplasms derived from these cells.[27] It is also found in some adenocarcinomas, squamous cell carcinomas and sarcomas.[28] NSE has prognostic value in small cell lung cancer.[29] In melanoma, 10–13% of AJCC stage III patients and 35–48% of stage IV patients have NSE levels >10–15% μg/l (Table 45.2).[24,25,30–32] An elevated NSE level was linked with poor prognosis in one study involving 63 stage III and IV melanoma patients,[32] but a study involving 282 melanoma patients did not demonstrate a correlation between NSE level and survival.[16] When compared with S-100, NSE has a lower diagnostic sensitivity for stage III/IV disease than stage I/II disease.[24] The low sensitivity of NSE in stage IV melanoma limits its utility as a marker for surveillance of high-risk patients.

MELANOMA-INHIBITING ACTIVITY (MIA)

MIA was identified within growth-inhibitory activities purified from tissue culture supernatant of malignant cells in vitro.[33,34] It has an M_r=11,000 and is mapped to human chromosome 19q13.32–13.33.[35,36] MIA was also detected in developing and mature cartilage.[37,38] Serum MIA level is measured by a one-step enzyme-linked immunosorbent assay using monoclonal antibodies to the NH_2 and COOH terminals.[39] MIA is elevated (>6.5 ng/ml) in 13% of AJCC stage I melanoma patients, 23% of stage II melanoma patients, and 88–100% of metastatic patients.[26,39] Elevated serum MIA level has been correlated with disease recurrence in patients with resected melanoma lesions.[39] In patients undergoing therapy for metastatic melanoma, MIA levels were significantly higher in non-responders than in responders.[26,40] However, when MIA was evaluated in combination with S-100 and LDH in a multiple logistic regression analysis, it was not as prognostically significant as LDH.[26]

INTERCELLULAR ADHESION MOLECULE (ICAM)-1

ICAM-1 is a sialylated glycoprotein that binds to the leucocyte integrins LFA-1 (CD11a/CD18) and Mac-1 (CD11b/CD18).[41–43] It supports cell–cell adhesion and

Table 45.1 *Evaluation of serum S-100 protein in melanoma*

Reference (no.)	Assay method*	Cut-off values (μg/l)	Positivity (%)			Correlation with overall survival (OS)
			Stage I/II	Stage III	Stage IV	
Guo et al. (24)	IRMA	0.15	1.3 (1 of 80)	8.7 (2 of 23)	73.9 (17 of 23)	–
Von Schoultz et al. (19)	IRMA		–	–	–	643 stage I–IV patients: ≤0.6 versus >0.6 μg/l (P <0.001)
Miliotes et al. (20)	IRMA		–	–	–	67 stage II–IV patients: ≤0.05 versus >0.05 μg/l (P = 0.0059)
Tofani et al. (25)	IRMA	0.5	0 (0 of 24)	30 (3 of 10)	68 (13 of 19)	–
Karnell et al. (22)	IRMA	0.1	8 (1 of 13)	62 (8 of 13)	74 (48 of 65)	91 stage I–IV patients: ≤0.1 versus 0.11–0.57 versus 0.58–3.23 versus >3.23 μg/l (P <0.001)
Bonfrer et al. (16)	IRMA		–	–	–	74 stage I–IV patients: ≤0.2 versus >0.2 μg/l (P <0.05)
Bosserhoff et al. (39)	IRMA	0.15	0 (0 of 33)	60 (3 of 5)	61 (27 of 44)	–
Buer et al. (18)	IRMA		–	–	–	99 stage IV patients: <3 versus ≤3 μg/l (P <0.001)
Schultz et al. (17)	IRMA	0.3	0 (0 of 36)	31 (4 of 13)	69 (24 of 35)	34 stage IV patients: ≤0.6 versus >0.6 μg/l (P <0.001); <1 versus ≤1 μg/l (P <0.001)
Bonfrer et al. (21)	LIA	0.16	0 (0 of 170)	31 (19 of 62)	79 (15 of 19)	251 stage I–IV patients: ≤0.16 versus >0.16 μg/l (P <0.0001)
Berking et al. (103)	LIA	0.2	2 (7 of 298)	8 (9 of 111)	48 (63 of 131)	–
Hauschild et al. (23)	IRMA	0.2	2 (5 of 286)	19 (14 of 73)	68 (57 of 84)	412 stage I–IV patients: ≤0.2 versus >0.2 μg/l (P <0.001)
Deichmann et al. (26)	LIA	0.12	–	–	91	–

*IRMA, Immunoradiometric assay; LIA, luminescence immunoassay. All assays performed in the above referenced studies were specific for β subunit of S-100 protein.

Table 45.2 *Evaluation of serum NSE in melanoma*

Reference (no.)	Assay method*	Cut-off values (μg/l)	Positivity (%)			Correlation with overall survival (OS)
			Stage I/II	Stage III	Stage IV	
Lorenz (30)	IRMA	15	–	64 (14 of 22)		
Wibe et al. (31)	IRMA	10	–	48 (30 of 63)		
Wibe et al. (32)	IRMA	10	–	–	–	63 stage III and IV patients: ≤10 versus >10 μg/l (P <0.05)
Guo et al. (24)	IRMA	12.5	9 (7 of 80)	13 (8 of 23)	35 (8 of 23)	–
Tofani et al. (25)	IRMA	12.5	17 (4 of 24)	10 (1 of 10)	48 (9 of 19)	–

*IRMA, Immunoradiometric assay. All assays were specific for γ subunit of NSE protein.

induction of effector functions in the immune response. ICAM-1 is expressed on keratinocytes and blood vessels in benign inflammatory disorders, and this expression appears to correlate with the extent of disease.[44] In melanoma, its expression by a primary lesion has been correlated with Breslow thickness and associated with poor disease-free survival.[45–47] ICAM-1 is reportedly found in 50–90% of metastatic melanoma lesions,[45–47] and serum ICAM-1 levels are elevated (>0.2 μg/l) in up to 100% of metastatic melanoma patients.[48] In one study using serum from healthy individuals as a control, 100% (14 of 14) of AJCC stage I/II melanoma patients, 25% (6 of 24 of stage III melanoma patients and 72% (13 of 18) of stage IV melanoma patients had serum ICAM-1 levels >2 SD above mean control (>258.2 ng/ml).[49] In this study, serum ICAM-1 level also correlated with disease-free survival in stage III melanoma patients and with OS in stage IV melanoma patients. However, other investigators have not found a significant correlation between the serum level of ICAM-1 and the extent of melanoma. In contrast to the findings of Harning et al.,[49] Kageshita et al.[48] reported that only patients with stage III and IV melanoma had increased ICAM-1 levels, and there was no significant difference in ICAM-1 levels between 75 melanoma patients and 47 age- and sex-matched healthy controls. Other investigators have reported that serum ICAM-1 level is neither sensitive nor specific for melanoma,[39] and has no correlation with survival on multivariate analysis.[50]

TUMOUR-ASSOCIATED ANTIGEN (TA90)

TA90 is the acronym for a 90 kDa tumour-associated glycoprotein antigen.[51] This antigen is heat stable and has an isoelectric point of 6.1.[52] Its presence in the melanoma cell induces an endogenous immune response against the tumour cells.[53,54] A serum enzyme-linked immunosorbent assay (ELISA) has been developed for measuring the circulating immune complex of TA90 and its immunoglobulin (Ig)-G antibody in melanoma patients.[53] When the cut-off level is >2 SD of mean control serum TA90 immune complex level, this serum TA90 ELISA has a sensitivity of 83% in detecting nodal metastases in melanoma patients undergoing lymphadenectomy.[55] As a predictor of recurrence among patients with early stage melanoma, TA90 ELISA has a sensitivity of 74%. TA90 status is significantly correlated with recurrence of disease in patients who have undergone complete surgical resection of AJCC stage I/II, stage III or stage IV melanoma.[55–57] In a study of 60 patients with stage II melanoma, postoperative TA90 positivity was significantly correlated with disease-free survival (Figure 45.1).[55] In a study of 100 stage III melanoma patients, postoperative TA90 positivity was also the most significant variable influencing disease-free survival (Figure 45.2).[56] TA90 positivity remained significant on multivariate analysis with Cox proportional hazard regression considering other clinical variables (Table 45.3). In a study of 125 stage IV melanoma patients undergoing complete resection of distant metastases, postoperative TA90 positivity was again the most important prognostic variable influencing disease-free survival (Figure 45.3).[57] The significance of TA90 positivity was confirmed by multivariate analysis considering other clinical variables (Table 45.4). These data show that TA90 assay positivity is strongly correlated with recurrence following surgical resection of AJCC stage II, III and IV melanoma. When TA90 assay was combined with positron emission tomography (PET), patients in whom both tests were positive had a much

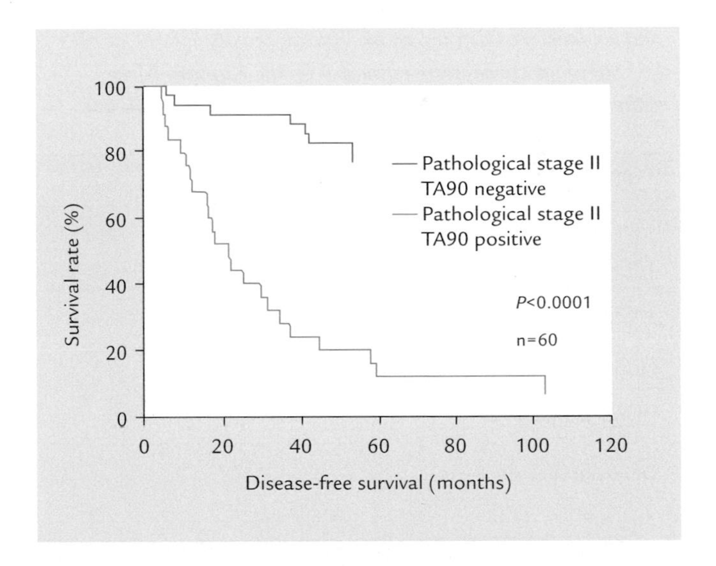

Figure 45.1 *Correlation of TA90 positivity with postoperative disease-free survival in AJCC stage II melanoma patients. Serum samples obtained from 60 AJCC stage II melanoma patients within 3 months of definitive surgery were tested for the presence of TA90 immune complex. A positive TA90 immune complex level was defined as an optical density ≥0.41 at 405 nm. Survival curves were estimated by the Kaplan–Meier method. Univariate analysis was performed by log rank test (P< 0.0001).[55]*

high incidence of recurrence within 6 months of testing than did patients whose test results were negative (Table 45.5).[58] Thus, a combination of diagnostic tests can increase the accuracy of predicting which patients are likely to develop recurrence following surgical resection of melanoma.

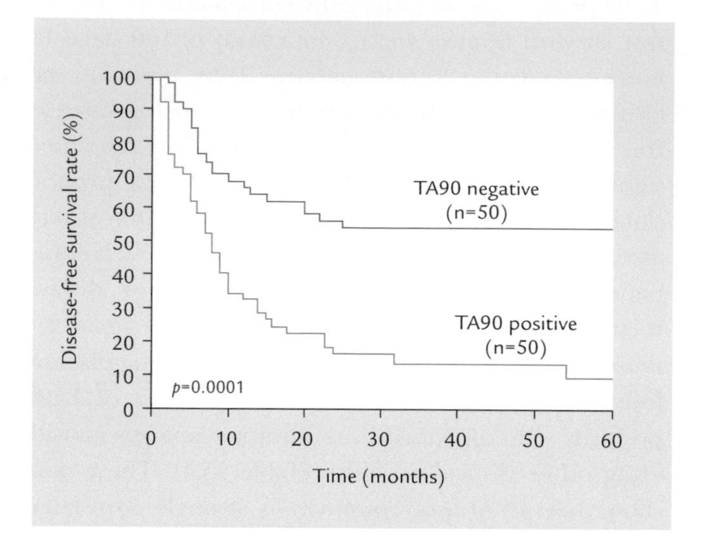

Figure 45.2 *Correlation of TA90 positivity with postoperative disease-free survival in AJCC stage III melanoma patients. Serum samples obtained from 100 AJCC stage III melanoma patients within 3 months of definitive surgery were tested for the presence of TA90 immune complex. A positive TA90 immune complex level was defined as an optical density ≥0.41 at 405 nm. Survival curves were estimated by the Kaplan–Meier method. Univariate analysis was performed by log rank test.*[56]

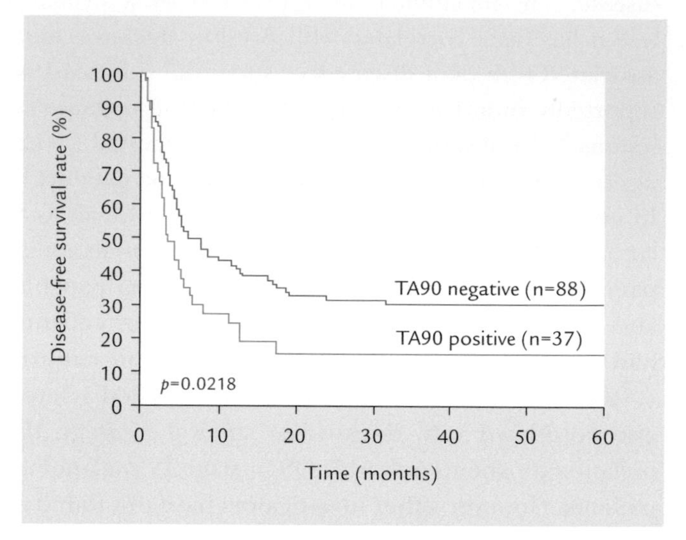

Figure 45.3 *Correlation of TA90 positivity with disease-free survival following complete resection of AJCC stage IV melanoma. Postoperative serum samples obtained from 125 AJCC stage IV melanoma patients were tested for the presence of TA90 immune complex. A positive TA90 immune complex level was defined as an optical density ≥0.41 at 405 nm. Survival curves were estimated by the Kaplan–Meier method. Univariate analysis was performed by log rank test.*[57]

Table 45.3 ***Univariate and multivariate correlation of disease-free survival with TA90 positivity and other clinical variables (AJCC stage III melanoma)***

Variable	Univariate *P* value	Multivariate *P* value
TA90 positivity	0.0001	0.0001
Number of positive nodes	0.0035	0.0028
Disease-free interval	0.3041	0.0120
Ulceration	0.0514	0.0437
Age	0.6367	0.0493
Primary site	0.2415	0.0838
Thickness	0.2290	0.0907
Extranodal extension	0.1619	0.1916
Gender	0.3388	0.3674
Largest node	0.3123	0.4154
Palpable versus non-palpable nodes	0.5169	0.7184

Table 45.4 *Univariate and multivariate correlation of disease-free survival with TA90 positivity and other clinical variables (AJCC stage IV melanoma)*

Prognostic variable	Univariate *P* value	Multivariate *P* value
TA90 positivity	0.0218	0.0031
No. of metastases	0.0657	0.0111
First site of metastases	0.3032	0.1306
Age at diagnosis	0.4250	0.1947
Initial AJCC stage	0.4999	0.2224
Primary site	0.4002	0.5761
Gender	0.2532	0.5884
Disease-free interval	0.8392	0.8987

Table 45.5 *Correlation between the combined results of TA90 assay and PET scan and the clinical evidence of disease recurrence in 87 patients with high-risk melanoma*

	Number of patients at 6 months follow-up		Number of patients at 12 months follow-up	
	Clinical evidence of disease	No clinical evidence of disease	Clinical evidence of disease	No clinical evidence of disease
PET+/TA90+	11	4	13	2
PET+/TA90−	7	1	7	1
PET−/TA90+	4	8	7	5
PET−/TA90−	3	49	6	46
P value*	<0.0001		<0.0001	

*Fisher exact test.

Eighty-seven patients with a history of AJCC stage II–IV melanoma and at high risk for recurrence were evaluated concurrently with TA90 and PET scans. At the time of both tests, patients were deemed clinically disease free. The results of both diagnostic tests were then compared with the patient's subsequent clinical course at 6 and 12 months.

MELANIN PRECURSORS

Melanogenesis (the formation of melanin pigment) is a unique metabolic pathway (Figure 45.4) and is highly elevated in malignant melanoma.[59] Two types of melanin pigments, black eumelanin and reddish-brown pheomelanin, are produced in melanocytes and melanoma cells. Most melanin precursor is oxidized to form the melanin pigments, but a minor portion leaks into the blood stream and thus reflects melanin pigment synthesis.[60] Several of the metabolites have been detected by high-performance liquid chromatography (HPLC) in the plasma and urine of melanoma patients.[59–63] Of the melanogenesis metabolites, 5-*S*-cysteinyldopa (5-*S*-CD) appears to have the most significant association with disease recurrence.[60] In a study of 28 AJCC stage I–III melanoma patients, a 5-*S*-CD level that increased to >10 nmol/l was correlated with disease recurrence following complete resection of melanoma.[60] Serum 6-hydroxy-5-methoxyindole-2-carboxylic acid (6H5MI2C) was also evaluated but did not increase at any stage in most patients.[60,64] In another report, all 11 patients with metastatic melanoma had elevated levels of 5-*S*-CD.[65] However, a study evaluating the use of melanin precursor metabolite in 88 control and melanoma patients noted that 5-*S*-CD did not discriminate between melanoma patients with and without

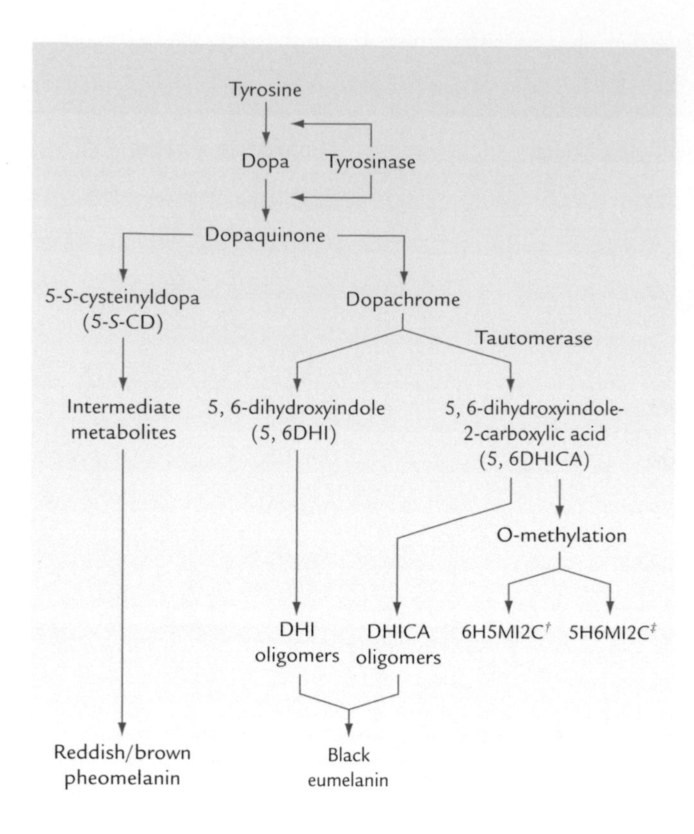

Figure 45.4 *Metabolic pathway for melanogenesis. †6H5MI2C, 6-hydroxy-5-methoxyindole-2-carboxylic acid, ‡5H6MI2C, 5-hydroxy-6-methoxyindole-2-carboxylic acid.*

metastases, but all melanoma patients with metastases had high plasma 6H5MI2C levels (>1.75 ng/ml).[66] The major obstacle to measuring melanin precursors is their release in normal healthy subjects, particularly after ultraviolet (UV) exposure.[67–69] Presently, the measurement of either 5-S-CD or 6H5MI2C in the serum is a rational approach to evaluate the presence of melanoma. However, further study with a larger patient cohort is necessary to determine the role of melanin precursors in the management of melanoma patients.

LIPID-ASSOCIATED SIALIC ACID (LASA)

LASA is derived from the shed lipids of cell membranes. It is present in normal cells but found at higher concentrations in tumour cells.[20] High concentrations of LASA have been identified in patients with leukaemia, Hodgkin's disease, melanoma, sarcoma, advanced ovarian carcinoma and oropharyngeal tumours.[70] Several LASA measurement methods have been proposed.[71–80] Most of these methods measure both lipid- and glycoprotein-bound sialic acid, which includes a significant amount of an acute-phase protein called α1-acid glycoprotein (AGP).[76] Thus, the LASA level may be elevated by an increased concentration of acute-phase proteins produced by the liver as the result of an inflammatory reaction to the liver, and not by an increased concentration of gangliosides from malignant cells. Therefore, while LASA results correlated with tumour burden in melanoma-bearing animals,[81] the serum LASA level reportedly has no significant correlation with survival.[20] Meaningful measurement of sialic acid awaits more sensitive and specific assay techniques.

CYTOKINES

Melanoma expresses multiple cytokines at mRNA as well as protein levels. The RT-PCR technique has identified transcripts of interleukin (IL)-1α, IL-1β, IL-6, IL-8, IL-10 and IL-15 in cultured human melanoma cell lines.[82–84] The RT-PCR technique has also been employed to detect expression of basic fibroblast growth factor (bFGF), IL-1α, IL-1β, IL-6, IL-8 and granulocyte macrophage colony stimulating factor (GM-CSF) in fresh biopsy specimens of primary melanoma and melanoma metastases.[85] Cytokines identified in the culture supernatants include IL-1α, IL-6, IL-8, and tumour necrosis factor (TNF)-α and TNF-β.[82–84,86] Thus, measurements of these cytokines in the serum may correspond with disease progression or tumour-bearing status in melanoma patients. However, the complex interaction of melanoma lesions with endogenous lymphocytes, which are another source of the above-mentioned cytokines, makes this approach difficult. Thus far, only serum IL-6, IL-8 and IL-10 have been studied.[87,88] Serum IL-6 level appeared to correlate with tumour progression in patients undergoing IL-2 therapy and biochemotherapy;[89–91] the higher the serum IL-6 level, the greater the tumour burden. However, for melanoma patiens in general, there is no significant correlation with stage of disease.[92] Serum IL-8 level was elevated (>100 pg/ml) in 21 of 56 (37.5%) metastatic melanoma patients.[87] The presence of IL-8 has been correlated with tumour size: elevated IL-8 was noted in 62% of patients with a tumour burden >250 cm^3 and in only 17% of patients with a tumour burden <250 cm^3 (P = 0.0042). Other investigators reported elevated IL-10 levels in 35% of stage III and 18–75% of stage IV melanoma patients.[93,94]

CATHEPSINS

Tumour invasion and metastasis are associated with various types of proteases. Cathepsins are proteases that have been identified in various tumour types.[95] Aspartic protease cathepsin D, and cystein proteases cathepsins B, H and L have been identified in melanoma tissue.[96,97] Thus, the evaluation of serum cathepsins in relation to disease status has been undertaken in melanoma patients.[98,99] Using median levels as a cut-off, cathepsin B (>4.8 versus <4.8 ng/ml) and cathepsin H (>13.7 versus <13.7 ng/ml) were correlated with survival in 43 patients with metastatic melanoma, whereas cathepsin L was not significantly correlated with survival.[98] Interestingly, while patients with metastatic melanoma had significantly higher serum cathepsin B and cathepsin H levels than did those with non-metastatic melanoma and healthy volunteers, patients with higher cathepsin B and H levels had longer survival times than those with lower cathepsin B and H levels. Although patients with metastatic melanoma had significantly higher serum cathepsin D levels than did healthy individuals and patients with non-metastatic melanoma, these serum levels had no significant correlation with survival.[99]

LACTATE DEHYDROGENASE (LDH)

Serum levels of LDH have been associated with prognosis in patients with AJCC stage IV melanoma.[26,100,101] Because LDH is metabolized at a fairly constant rate, elevated levels of LDH likely represent tumour cell turnover and tumour burden. However, LDH is also elevated in a variety of non-malignant pathologic conditions that involve tissue injury. One study found that LDH was a more significant prognostic variable than S-100 and MIA,[26] and another report confirmed that LDH was prognostically superior to S-100.[18] Its prognostic significance ($P < 0.00001$) was further established in a study of 318 stage IV patients. Recently, the level of LDH was introduced as a new criterion for a subset of stage IV melanoma in the 6th Edition AJCC staging system.[102] Its prognostic value in patients with stage I–III melanoma is limited because most patients with early stage melanoma have normal serum LDH levels.

CONCLUSIONS

There are multiple promising serum marker assays for detection of metastatic melanoma. However, no single tumour marker is expressed by all melanoma lesions. Furthermore, while some serum markers are elevated in most patients with stage IV melanoma, their presence does not add additional clinical value to the existing clinical parameters such as LDH or extent of metastases. Other markers have significant prognostic value but their low prevalence in melanoma precludes their use as a surveillance modality. Currently, the combination of different serum markers as surveillance tools is being actively investigated. Because of the heterogeneity of melanoma cells, an assay that effectively monitors disease recurrence and response to therapy will probably be based on multiple markers.

REFERENCES

1. American Cancer Society (ACS) *Cancer Facts & Figures – 1998 (SEER data)*. ACS: Atlanta, Georgia, 1998.
2. Greenlee RT, Murray T, Bolden S, Wingo PA, Cancer statistics, 2000. *CA Cancer J Clin* 2000; 50: 7–33.
3. Morton DL, Barth A, Vaccine therapy for malignant melanoma. *CA Cancer J Clin* 1996; 46: 225–44.
4. Weiss M, Loprinzi CL, Creagan ET et al, Utility of follow-up tests for detecting recurrent disease in patients with malignant melanomas. *JAMA* 1995; 274: 1703–5.
5. Balch CM, Cutaneous melanoma: prognosis and treatment results worldwide. *Semin Surg Oncol* 1992; 8: 400–14.
6. Morton DL, Essner R, Kirkwood JM, Parker RG, Malignant melanoma. In: *Cancer Medicine*, 4th edn (eds Holland JF, Frei E, Bast R et al). Baltimore: Williams & Wilkins:, MD, 1997 2467–502.
7. Balch CM, Houghton AN, Diagnosis of metastatic melanoma at distant sites. In: *Cutaneous Melanoma*, 2nd edn (eds Balch CM, Houghton AN, Milton GW et al). Philadelpha: Lippincott, 1992: 440.
8. Patel JK, Didolkar MS, Pickren JW, Moore RH, Metastatic pattern of malignant melanoma. A study of 216 autopsy cases. *Am J Surg* 1978; 135: 807–10.
9. Buzaid AC, Tinoco L, Ross MI et al, Role of computed tomography in the staging of patients with local-regional mtastases of melanoma. *J Clin Oncol* 1995; 13: 2104–8.
10. Buzaid AC, Sandler AB, Mani S et al, Role of computed tomography in the staging of primary melanoma. *J Clin Oncol* 1993; 11: 638–43.
11. Moore BW, A soluble protein characteristic of the nervous system. *Biochem Res Commun* 1965; 19: 739–44.
12. Cocchia D, Michetti F, Donato R, Immunochemical and immunocytochemical localization of S 100 antigen in normal human skin. *Nature* 1981; 294: 85–7.
13. Nakajima T, Watanabe S, Sato Y et al, S-100 protein in Langerhans cells, interdigitating reticulum cells and histiocytosis X cells. *Gann* 1982; 73: 429–32.
14. Gaynor R, Irie R, Morton D, Herschman HR, S100 protein is present in cultured human malignant melanomas. *Nature* 1980; 286: 400–1.
15. Cochran AJ, Lu HF, Li PX et al, S-100 protein remains a practical marker for melanocytic and other tumours. *Melanoma Res* 1993; 3: 325–30.
16. Bonfrer JMB, Korse CM, Israels SP, Serum S-100 has prognostic significance in malignant melanoma. *Anticancer Res* 1997; 17: 2975–7.
17. Schultz ES, Diepgen TL, Von Den Driesch P, Clinical and prognostic relevance of serum S-100β protein in malignant melanoma. *Br J Dermatol* 1998; 138: 426–30.
18. Buer J, Probst M, Franzke A et al, Elevated serum levels of S100 and survival in mtastatic malignant melanoma. *Br J Cancer* 1997; 75: 1373–6.

19. Von Schoultz E, Hansson LO, Djureen E et al, Prognostic value of serum analyses of S-100β protein in malignant melanoma. *Melanoma Res* 1996; 6: 133–7.
20. Miliotes G, Lyman GH, Cruse CW et al, Evaluation of new putative tumor markers for melanoma. *Ann Surg Oncol* 1996; 3: 558–63.
21. Bonfrer JM, Korse CM, Nieweg OE, Rankin EM, The luminescence immunoassay S-100: a sensitive test to measure circulating S-100B: its prognostic value in malignant melanoma. *Br J Cancer* 1998; 77: 2210–4.
22. Karnell R, von Schoultz E, Hansson LO et al, S 100B protein, 5-*S*-cysteinyldopa and 6-hydroxy-5-methoxyindole-2-carboxylic acid as biochemical markers for survival prognosis in patients with malignant melanoma. *Melanoma Res* 1997; 7: 393–9.
23. Hauschild A, Engel G, Brenner W et al, S 100B protein detection in serum is a significant prognostic factor in metastatic melanoma. *Oncology* 1999; 56: 338–44.
24. Guo HB, Stoffel-Wagner B, Bierwirth T et al, Clinical significance of serum S100 in metastatic malignant melanoma. *Eur J Cancer* 1995; 31A: 1898.
25. Tofani A, Cioffi RP, Sciuto R et al, S-100 and NSE as serum markers in melanoma. *Acta Oncol* 1997; 36: 761–4.
26. Deichmann M, Benner A, Bock M et al, S100-beta, melanoma-inhibiting activity, and lactate dehydrogenase discriminate progressive from nonprogressive American Joint Committee on Cancer stage IV melanoma. *J Clin Oncol* 1999; 17: 1891–6.
27. Lloyd RV, Warner TF, Immunohistochemistry of neuron-specific enolase. In: *Advances of Immunohistochemistry* (ed DeLellis RA). New York: Masson, 1984.
28. Leader M, Collins M, Patel J, Henry K, Anti-neuron specific enolase staining reactions in sarcomas and carcinomas: its lack of neuroendocrine specificity. *J Clin Pathol* 1986; 39: 1186–92.
29. Jorgensen LGM, Osterlind K, Hansen HH, Cooper EH, The prognostic influence of serum neuron specific enolase in small cell lung cancer. *Br J Cancer* 1988; 58: 805–7.
30. Lorenz J, Neuron-specific enolase – a serum marker for malignant melanoma. *J Natl Cancer Inst* 1989; 81: 1754–5.
31. Wibe E, Paus E, Aamdal S, Neuron specific enolase (NSE) in serum of patients with malignant melanoma. *Cancer Lett* 1990; 52: 29–31.
32. Wibe E, Hannisdal E, Paus E, Aamdal S, Neuron-specific enolase as a prognostic factor in metastatic malignant melanoma. *Eur J Cancer* 1992; 28A: 1692.
33. Bogdahn U, Apfel R, Hahn M et al, Autocrine tumor cell growth-inhibiting activities from human malignant melanoma. *Cancer Res* 1989; 49: 5358–63.
34. Apfel R, Lottspeich F, Hoppe J et al, Purification and analysis of growth regulating proteins secreted by a human melanoma cell line. *Melanoma Res* 1992; 2: 327–36.
35. Blesch A, Bosserhoff AK, Apfel R et al, Cloning of a novel malignant melanoma-derived growth-regulatory protein, MIA. *Cancer Res* 1994; 54: 5695–701.
36. Koehler MR, Bosserhoff A, von Beust G et al, Assignment of the human melanoma inhibitory activity gene (MIA) to 19q13.32-q13.33 by fluorescence in situ hybridization (FISH). *Genomics* 1996; 35: 265–7.
37. Dietz UH, Sandell LJ, Cloning of a retinoic acid-sensitive mRNA expressed in cartilage and during chondrogenesis. *J Biol Chem* 1996; 271: 3311–16.
38. Bosserhoff AK, Kondo S, Moser M et al, Mouse CD-RAP/MIA gene: structure, chromosomal localization, and expression in cartilage and chondrosarcoma. *Dev Dyn* 1997; 208: 516–25.
39. Bosserhoff A-K, Kaufmann M, Kaluza B et al, Melanoma-inhibiting activity, a novel serum marker for progression of malignant melanoma. *Cancer Res* 1997; 57: 3149–53.
40. Dreau D, Bosserhoff AK, White RL et al, Melanoma-inhibitory activity protein concentrations in blood of melanoma patients treated with immunotherapy. *Oncol Res* 1999; 11: 55–61.
41. Marlin SD, Springer TA, Purified intercellular adhesion molecule-1 (ICAM-1) is a ligand for lymphocyte function-associated antigen 1 (LFA-1). *Cell* 1987; 51: 813–19.
42. Springer TA, Adhesion receptors of the immune system. *Nature* 1990; 346: 425–34.
43. Staunton DE, Dustin ML, Erickson HP, Springer TA, The arrangement of the immunoglobulin-like domains of ICAM-1 and the binding sites for LFA-1 and rhinovirus. *Cell* 1990; 61: 243–54.
44. Vejlsgaard GL, Ralfkiaer E, Avnstorp C et al, Kinetics and characterization of intercellular adhesion molecule-1 (ICAM-1) expression on keratinocytes in various inflammatory skin lesions and malignant cutaneous lymphomas. *J Am Acad Dermatol* 1989; 20: 782–90.
45. Johnson JP, Stade BG, Holzmann B et al, De novo expression of intercellular-adhesion molecule 1 in melanoma correlates with increased risk of metastasis. *Proc Natl Acad Sci USA* 1989; 86: 641–4.
46. Natali P, Nicotra MR, Cavaliere R et al, Differential expression of intercellular adhesion molecule 1 in primary and metastatic melanoma lesions. *Cancer Res* 1990; 50: 1271–8.
47. Carrel S, Dore JF, Ruiter DJ et al, The EORTC Melanoma Group exchange program: evaluation of a multicenter monoclonal antibody study. *Int J Cancer* 1991; 48: 836–47.
48. Kageshita T, Yoshii A, Kimura T et al, Clinical relevance of ICAM-1 expression in primary lesions and serum of patients with malignant melanoma. *Cancer Res* 1993; 53: 4927–32.
49. Harning R, Mainolfi E, Bystryn J-C et al, Serum levels of circulating intercellular adhesion molecule 1 in human malignant melanoma. *Cancer Res* 1991; 51: 5003–5.
50. Franzke A, Probst-Kepper M, Buer J et al, Elevated pretreatment serum levels of soluble vascular cell adhesion molecule 1 and lactate dehydrogenase as predictors of survival in cutaneous metastatic malignant melanoma. *Br J Cancer* 1998; 78: 40–5.
51. Euhus DM, Gupta RK, Morton DL, Detection of a tumor-associated glycoprotein antigen in serum and urine of melanoma patients by murine monoclonal antibody (AD1-40F4) in enzyme immunoassay. *J Clin Lab Anal* 1989; 3: 184–90.
52. Euhus DM, Gupta RK, Morton DL, Characterization of a 90–100 kDa tumor-associated antigen in the sera of melanoma patients. *Int J Cancer* 1990; 45: 1065–70.
53. Gupta RK, Morton DL, Monoclonal antibody based ELISA to detect glycoprotein tumor-associated-antigen-specific immune complexes in cancer patients. *J Clin Lab Anal* 1992; 6: 329–36.
54. Hsueh EC, Gupta RK, Yee R et al, Does endogenous immune response determine the outcome of surgical therapy for metastatic melanoma? *Ann Surg Oncol* 2000; 7: 232–8.
55. Kelley MC, Jones RC, Gupta RK et al, Tumor-associated antigen TA-90 immune complex assay predicts subclinical metastasis and survival for patients with early stage melanoma. *Cancer* 1998; 83: 1355–61.
56. Hsueh EC, Gupta RK, Yee R et al, Serum TA 90 immune complex correlates with recurrence following adjuvant immunotherapy for regional metastatic melanoma. *Proc Am Assoc Cancer Res* 1998; 39: 2998.
57. Hsueh EC, Gupta RK, Qi K et al, TA90 immune complex predicts survival following surgery and adjuvant vaccine immunotherapy for stage IV melanoma. *Cancer J Sci Am* 1997; 3: 364–70.
58. Hsueh EC, Gupta RK, GLass EC et al, Positron emission tomography plus serum TA90 immune complex assay for detection of occult metastatic melanoma. *J Am Coll Surg* 1998; 187: 191–7.
59. Jimbow K, Salopek TG, Dixon WT et al, The epidermal melanin unit in the pathophysiology of malignant melanoma. *Am J Dermatopathol* 1991; 13: 179–88.
60. Horikoshi T, Ito S, Wakamatsu K et al, Evaluation of melanin-related metabolites as markers of melanoma progression. *Cancer* 1994; 73: 629–36.
61. Pavel S, Elzinga H, Muskiet FAJ et al, Eumelanin-related indolic compounds in the urine of treated melanoma patients. *J Clin Chem Clin Biochem* 1986; 24: 167–73.
62. Yamada K, Walsh N, Hara H et al, Measurement of eumelanin precursor metabolites in the urine as a new marker for melanoma metastases. *Arch Dermatol* 1992; 128: 491–4.
63. Kagedal B, Lenner L, Arstrand K, Hansson C, The stability of 5-*S*-cysteinyldopa and 6-hydroxy-5-methoxyindole-2-carboxylic acid in human urine. *Pigment Cell Res* 1992; 2 (suppl): 304–7.
64. Horikoshi T, Ito S, Serum 5-*S*-cysteinyldopa (5-*S*-CD) as a marker of melanoma progression. *J Dermatol* 1992; 19: 809–13.

65. Wimmer I, Meyer JC, Seifert B et al, Prognostic value of serum 5-S-cysteinyldopa for monitoring human metastatic melanoma during immunochemotherapy. *Cancer Res* 1997; 57: 5073–6.
66. Hara H, Walsh N, Yamada K, Jimbow K, High plasma level of a eumelanin precursor, 6-hydroxy-5-methoxyindole-2-carboxylic acid as a prognostic marker for malignant melanoma. *J Invest Dermatol* 1994; 102: 501–5.
67. Hansson C, Wirestrand LE, Aronsson A et al, Urinary excretion of 6-hydroxy-5-methoxyindole-2-carboxylic acid and 5-S-cysteinyldopa during PUVA treatment. *Photodermatol* 1985; 2: 52–7.
68. Ito S, Kato T, Fujita K, Seasonal variation in urinary excretion of 5-S-cysteinyldopa in healthy Japanese. *Acta Dermatol Venereol* 1987; 67: 163–5.
69. Stierner U, Rosdahl I, Augustsson A, Kagedal B, Urinary excretion of 5-S-cysteinyldopa in relation to skin type, UVB-nduced erythema, and melanocyte proliferation in human skin. *J Invest Dermatol* 1988; 91: 506–10.
70. Schutter EM, Visser JJ, van Kamp GJ et al, The utility of lipid-associated sialic acid (LASA or LSA) as a serum marker for malignancy. *Tumor Biol* 1992; 13: 121–32.
71. Dnistrian AM, Schwartz MK, Katopodis N et al, Serum lipid-bound sialic acid as a marker in breast cancer. *Cancer* 1982; 50: 1815–19.
72. Katopodis N, Hirshaut Y, Geller NL, Stock CC, Lipid-associated sialic acid test for the detection of human cancer. *Cancer Res* 1982; 42: 5270–5.
73. Raynes JG, Serum concentrations of lipid bound sialic acid and acute phase proteins in patients with cancer and nonmalignant disease. *Biomed Pharmacother* 1983; 37: 136–8.
74. Plucinsky MC, RIley WM, Prorok JJ, Alhadeff JA, Total and lipid-associated serum sialic acid levels in cancer patients with different primary sites and differing degrees of metastatic involvement. *Cancer* 1986; 58: 2680–5.
75. Tautu C, Verazin G, Prorok JJ, Alhadeff JA, Improved procedure for determination of serum lipid-associated sialic acid: application for early diagnosis of colorectal cancer. *J Natl Cancer Inst* 1988; 80: 1333–7.
76. Voigtmann R, Pokorny J, Meinshausen A, Evaluation and limitations of the lipid-associated sialic acid test for the detection of human cancer. *Cancer* 1989; 64: 2279–83.
77. Patel PS, Baxi BR, Adhvaryu SG, Balar DB, Evaluation of serum sialic acid, heat stable alkaline phosphatase and fucose as markers of breast carcinoma. *Anticancer Res* 1990; 10: 1071–4.
78. Dwivedi C, Dixit M, Hardy RE, Plasma lipid-bound sialic acid alterations in neoplastic diseases. *Experientia* 1990; 46: 91–4.
79. Shahangian S, Fritsche HA, Hughes JI et al, Plasma protein-bound sialic acid in patients with colorectal polyps of known histology. *Clin Chem* 1991; 37: 200–4.
80. Ozben T, Elevated serum and urine sialic acid levels in renal diseases. *Ann Clin Biochem* 1991; 28 (Part 1): 44–8.
81. Vedralova E, Borovansky J, Evaluation of serum sialic acid fractions as markers for malignant melanoma. *Cancer Lett* 1994; 78: 171–5.
82. Barzegar C, Meazza R, Pereno R et al, IL-15 is produced by a subset of human melanomas, and is involved in the regulation of markers of melanoma progression through juxtacrine loops. *Oncogene* 1998; 16: 2503–12.
83. Dummer W, Bastian BC, Ernst N et al, Interleukin-10 production in malignant melanoma: preferential detection of IL-10-secreting tumor cells in metastatic lesions. *Int J Cancer* 1996; 66: 607–10.
84. Schadendorft D, Moller A, Algermissen B et al, IL-8 produced by human malignant melanoma cells in vitro is an essential autocrine growth factor. *J Immunol* 1993; 151: 2667–75.
85. Ciotti P, Rainero ML, Nicolo G et al, Cytokine expression in human primary and metastatic melanoma cells: analysis in fresh bioptic specimens. *Melanoma Res* 1995; 5: 41–7.
86. Colombo MP, Maccalli C, Mattei S et al, Expression of cytokine genes, including IL-6, in human malignant melanoma cell lines. *Melanoma Res* 1992; 2: 181–9.
87. Scheibenbogen C, Mohler T, Haefele J et al, Serum interleukin-8 (IL-8) is elevated in patients with metastatic melanoma and correlates with tumour load. *Melanoma Res* 1995; 5: 179–81.
88. Fortis C, Foppoli M, Gianotti L et al, Increased interleukin-10 serum levels in patients with solid tumours. *Cancer Lett* 1996; 104: 1–5.
89. Tartour E, Dorval T, Mosseri V et al, Serum interleukin 6 and C-reactive protein levels correlate with resistance to IL-2 therapy and poor survival in melanoma patients. *Br J Cancer* 1994; 69: 911–13.
90. Mouawad R, Bnhammouda A, Rixe O et al, Endogenous interleukin 6 levels in patients with metastatic malignant melanoma: correlation with tumor burden. *Clin Cancer Res* 1996; 2: 1405–9.
91. Mouawad R, Khayat D, Merle S et al, Is there any relationship between interleukin-6/interleukin-6 receptor modulation and endogenous interleukin-6 release in metastatic malignant melanoma patients treated by biochemotherapy? *Melanoma Res* 1999; 9: 181–8.
92. Boyano MD, Garcia-Vazquez MD, Gardeazabal J et al, Serum-soluble IL-2 receptor and IL-6 levels in patients with melanoma. *Oncology* 1997; 54: 400–6.
93. Dummer W, Becker JC, Schwaaf A et al, Elevated serum levels of interleukin-10 in patients with metastatic malignant melanoma. *Melanoma Res* 1995; 5: 67–8.
94. Sato T, McCue P, Masuoka K et al, Interleukin 10 production by human melanoma. *Clin Cancer Res* 1996; 2: 1383–90.
95. Duffy MJ, Protease as prognostic markers in cancer. *Clin Cancer Res* 1996; 2: 613–18.
96. Otto FJ, Schumann J, Biess B et al, Relevance of ploidy in a battery of prognostic parameters in malignant melanoma. *Anal Cell Pathol* 1997; 13: 97–8.
97. Kageshita T, Yoshii A, Kimura T et al, Biochemical and immunohistochemical analysis of cathepsins B, H, L and D in human melanocytic tumours. *Arch Dermatol Res* 1995; 287: 266–72.
98. Kos J, Stabuc B, Schweiger A et al, Cathepsins B, H, and L and their inhibitors Stefin A and Cystatin C in sera of melanoma patients. *Clin Cancer Res* 1997; 3: 1815–22.
99. Westhoff U, Fox C, Otto FJ, Quantification of Cathepsin D in plasma of patients with malignant melanoma. *Anticancer Res* 1998; 18: 3785–8.
100. Sirott MN, Bajorin DF, Wong GY et al, Prognostic factors in patients with metastatic malignant melanoma. A multivariate analysis. *Cancer* 1993; 72: 3091–8.
101. Eton O, Legha SS, Moon TE et al, Prognostic factors for survival of patients treated systemically for disseminated melanoma. *J Clin Oncol* 1998; 16: 1103–11.
102. Balch CM, Buzaid AC, Atkins MB et al, KM A new American Joint Committee on Cancer staging system for cutaneous melanoma. *Cancer* 2000; 88: 1484–91.
103. Berking C, Schlupen EM, Schrader A et al, Tumor markers in peripheral blood of patients with malignant melanoma: multimarker RT-PCR versus a luminoimmunometric assay for S-100. *Arch Dermatol Res* 1999; 291: 479–84.

46

Surgical treatment of systemic metastases: rationale and principles

John F Thompson, Donald L Morton

INTRODUCTION

Traditional understanding of the process of tumour metastasis has been that once malignant cells have entered the bloodstream and a metastasis at a distant site has been identified, the patient will almost inevitably have multiple sites of metastatic disease. Recent information about the biology of the metastatic process, however, suggests that this may not always be the case. Studies of circulating melanoma cells in the peripheral blood using reverse transcriptase polymerase chain reaction (RT-PCR) techniques (see Chapter 42) indicate that most patients with American Joint Committee on Cancer/International Union against Cancer (AJCC/UICC) stage IV melanoma have melanoma cells circulating in their blood, at least some of which are presumably capable of lodging in an organ or tissue and developing into a metastatic tumour. Moreover, it has been shown that even in patients with stage III disease, i.e. those with only regional lymph node metastases, circulating tumour cells can be identified in almost 75% of them.[1] Yet up to 40% of patients survive for 5 years or more after therapeutic regional lymph node dissection for involved regional nodes,[2] many of them with no evidence of metastatic disease elsewhere. This indicates clearly that the presence of circulating tumour cells in the blood of patients prior to resection is not always synonymous with widespread systemic metastasis.

These concepts help to explain the observation that long-term survival and occasional cure can occur following surgical resection of metastatic deposits in patients with stage IV melanoma. Indeed, the results of surgical resection of distant metastatic deposits in selected patients with stage IV melanoma are considerably better than those achieved using conventional cytotoxic chemotherapy, which is associated with 5-year survival rates of <5%.

Surgery for metastatic disease is generally based on the notion of site-specific organ metastasis. A 'seed-and-soil' hypothesis was proposed by Paget[3] over a century ago to explain the non-random distribution of metastases in patients submitted to autopsy. He observed, for example, a preferential spread of breast cancer to bone and a preferential spread of ocular melanoma to the liver. On the basis of these observations he suggested that certain types of cancer cells would survive and propagate only in certain organs. In the early part of the twentieth century, Ewing[4] proposed an alternative 'mechanical' theory that linked the likelihood of metastasis in a given site to blood flow. According to this theory, circulating malignant cells lodge in the first capillary network that they encounter after leaving the primary tumour. This would explain why colon cancers metastasize preferentially to the liver, whereas sarcomas spread preferentially to the lung.

It is likely that both theories are partially correct, but neither fully acknowledges the undoubted complexity of the metastatic process. The first step in this process is for malignant cells to enter the patient's bloodstream either by invading adjacent capillaries or as a result of the primary tumour developing its own neovascularity. Once they have gained access to the bloodstream, malignant cells can travel to different sites but, for a metastasis to develop, one or more cells must adhere to the vascular endothelium of the target organ. This involves an interaction between site-specific adhesion molecules and organ-specific endothelial receptors. The malignant cells must then produce enzymes which will degrade the basement membrane of the vascular endothelium, so that they can invade the parenchymal tissues of the secondary organ site. Even then, unless the malignant cells can attract specific growth factors and angiogenesis factors from the organ in which they have lodged, or produce their own growth factors and angiogenesis factors, they will remain dormant.[5–9]

It is worthy of note in this discussion that >85% of melanoma patients who present with stage IV disease have demonstrable metastases confined to a single organ site such as the lung or the gastrointestinal tract, although metastases sometimes appear later at other sites. The introduction of positron emission tomography (PET) scanning in recent years to screen for metastatic disease elsewhere (see Chapter 44) has reduced the number of melanoma patients who appear to have genuinely isolated distant metastases, but many still fall into this category. Also to be noted is the fact that the most powerful predictor for survival of melanoma patients with systemic metastasis is the number of organs or tissues containing metastases.[10–12] When metastatic disease is identified at only one site, median survival is of the order of 7 months, but for two sites the median survival is reduced to 4 months, and for three or more sites to only 2 months.[13]

Such considerations have led to a reappraisal of the value of surgical resection of metastatic deposits in patients with AJCC/UICC stage IV melanoma. It has become clear that complete surgical removal of a metastatic melanoma deposit can render selected patients disease-free with a very low surgical morbidity, and substantially improve their survival probability. At the very least, this usually provides excellent palliation of symptoms[14] and can also prevent the development of problems at a later date. However, recent series have demonstrated 5-year survival rates of 20–27% following complete resection of lung metastases[15,16] and 28–41% following complete resection of gastrointestinal metastases.[17–19] Long-term survival has also been reported in many other series of patients who have undergone resection of distant metastases, in some cases when these have been multiple.[20–24] These results indicate that even when multiple metastatic deposits beyond the locoregional lymph node field are present, surgery may still have an important role to play in the management of patients with stage IV melanoma. Alternatively, other methods of complete physical elimination of metastases, such as radiofrequency ablation or cryotherapy, may be used to achieve the same outcome.

Careful patient selection is critically important, however, before recommending surgery for stage IV melanoma. If the metastatic disease is causing no symptoms, surgical intervention, which always has a small risk of causing morbidity, is best avoided unless there is a reasonable prospect of improving outcome. In most cases there is no urgency to proceed with surgery; indeed, a period of observation may provide valuable information. For example, metastatic disease in other sites may become apparent within a few weeks, or a short tumour doubling time (as assessed by sequential imaging studies) may indicate that the rate of progression is very rapid. In either situation, surgical intervention is unlikely to be useful.

Reasons why surgical metastasectomy might be associated with improved survival have not been clearly established, but there is considerable evidence suggesting that cytoreductive surgery of this type is effective because it reduces the overall tumour burden, and thereby allows the host's immunological defence mechanisms to function more efficiently. Even when recurrent metastatic disease is present in a tissue or organ, there is compelling evidence that surgical metastasectomy prolongs survival if all clinically apparent tumour can be resected.[25] The surgical management of metastatic disease in specific visceral sites will be considered in subsequent chapters. Sometimes, prolonged disease-free survival follows surgical resection of single or even multiple distant metastatic deposits. Resection of metastases in distant skin and subcutaneous tissues can be particularly worthwhile.[10,13] The AJCC/UICC staging system recognizes that patients with stage IV disease of this type, i.e. involving only distant skin and subcutaneous tissues, have a significantly better prognosis than is the case when metastatic disease involves visceral organs such as lung, brain, liver and bowel.

So convincing is the evidence that reducing tumour burden in patients with stage IV disease is beneficial in terms of the patient's immune system, that a number of adjuvant vaccine trials have begun which require surgical removal of all detectable metastatic disease before immunological stimulation with a vaccine(s) commences.[26] This strategy of immunotherapy after cytoreductive surgery is discussed in detail in more detail in Chapters 54 and 55.

CONCLUSION

If a patient is found to have a distant melanoma metastasis, this does not mean that widespread metastatic disease is necessarily present. Surgical resection may, therefore, be an appropriate treatment option. The best results have been reported following resection of metastatic deposits in distant skin and subcutaneous tissues, but even in patients with metastases in lung, liver, brain and bowel, 5-year survival figures of 20–40% have recently been reported following complete surgical resection. Even if prolonged survival does not eventuate, resection of these metastases achieves good palliation of symptoms in most patients, and can prevent the later development of troublesome problems. A further advantage of reducing a patient's tumour burden by surgical resection of metastatic disease is that adjuvant immunotherapy is more likely to be successful following the cytoreductive procedure.

REFERENCES

1. Hoon DSB, Wang Y, Dale PS et al, Detection of occult melanoma cells in blood with a multi-marker polymerase chain reaction assay. *J Clin Oncol* 1995; 13: 2109–16.
2. Morton DL, Wanek L, Nizze JA et al, Improved long-term survival after lymphadenectomy of melanoma metastatic to regional lymph nodes. *Ann Surg* 1991; 214: 499–501.
3. Paget S, The distribution of secondary growths in cancer of the breast. *Lancet* 1889; 8: 98–101.
4. Ewing J, *Neoplastic diseases: a treatise on tumours*, 3rd edn. Philadelphia: WB Saunders, 1928.
5. Zetter BR, The cellular basis of site-specific tumour metastasis. *N Engl J Med* 1990; 322: 605–12.
6. Folkam J, Tumor angiogenesis. In: *Cancer Medicine*, 4th edn (eds Holland JF, Frei E, Bast RC et al). Baltimore: Williams & Wilkins, 1997: 165–80.
7. Liotta LA, Steeg PS, Stetler-Stevenson WG, Cancer metastasis and angiogenesis; an imbalance of positive and negative regulation. *Cell* 1991; 64: 327–36.
8. Liotta LA, Kohn EC, Invasion and metastasis. In: *Cancer Medicine*, 4th edn (eds Holland JF, Frei E, Bast RC et al). Baltimore: Williams & Wilkins, 1997: 165–80.
9. Folkman J, The role of angiogenesis in tumor growth. *Semin Cancer Biol* 1992; 3: 65–71.
10. Balch CM, Soong S-J, Murad TM et al, A multifactorial analysis of melanoma: IV. Prognostic factors in 200 melanoma patients with distant metastases (stage III). *J Clin Oncol* 1983; 1: 126–34.
11. Hena MA, Emrich LJ, Nambisan RN et al, Effect of surgical treatment of stage IV melanoma. *Am J Surg* 1987; 153: 270–5.
12. Wong JH, Skinner K, Kim K et al, The role of surgery in the treatment of nonregionally recurrent melanoma. *Surgery* 1993; 113: 389–94.
13. Balch CM, Surgical treatment of advanced melanoma. In: *Cutaneous Melanoma* (eds Balch CM, Houghton AN, Sober AJ, Soong S-J). St Louis: Quality Medical Publishing, 1998: 373–88.
14. Wornom IL, Smith JW, Soong S-J et al, Surgery as palliative treatment for distant metastases of melanoma. *Ann Surg* 1986; 204: 181–5.
15. Harpole Jr D, Johnson CM, Wolfe WG et al, Analysis of 945 cases of pulmonary metastatic melanoma. *J Thorac Cardiovasc Surg* 1992; 103: 743–8.
16. Tafra L, Dale PS, Wanek LA et al, Resection and adjuvant immunotherapy for melanoma metastatic to the lung and thorax. *J Thorac Cardivasc Surg* 1994; 110: 119–29.
17. Ricaniadis N, Konstadoulakis MM, Walsh D et al, Gastrointestinal metastases from malignant melanoma. *Surg Oncol* 1995; 4: 105–10.
18. Ollila DW, Essner R, Wanek LA et al, Surgical resection for melanoma metastatic to the gastrointestinal tract. *Arch Surg* 1996; 131: 975–80.
19. Krige JE, Nel PN, Hudson DA, Surgical treatment of metastatic melanoma of the small bowel. *Am Surg* 1996; 62: 658–63.
20. Wanedo HJ, Chu QQ, Avradopoulos KA et al, Current perspectives on repeat hepatic resection for colorectal carcinoma: a review. *Surgery* 1996; 119: 361–71.
21. Nakamura S, Suzuki S, Baby S, Resection of liver metastases of colorectal carcinoma. *World J Surg* 1997; 21: 741–7.
22. Ollila DW, Morton DL, Surgical resection as the treatment of choice for melanoma metastatic to the lung. *Chest Surg Clin North Am* 1998; 81: 183–6.
23. Putnam Jr JB, Roth JA, Wesley MN et al, Survival following aggressive resection of pulmonary metastases from osteogenic sarcoma; analysis of prognostic factors. *Ann Thorac Surg* 1983; 36: 516–23.
24. McCormack PM, Martini MN, The changing role of surgery for pulmonary metastases. *Ann Thorac Surg* 1979; 28: 139–45.
25. Ollila DW, Hsueh EC, Stern SL, Morton DL, Metastasectomy for recurrent Stage IV melanoma. *J Surg Oncol* 1999; 71: 209–13.
26. Morton DL, Ollila DW, Hsueh EC et al, Cytoreductive surgery and adjuvant immunotherapy: a new management paradigm for metastatic melanoma. *CA Cancer J Clin* 1999; 49: 101–16.

47

Pulmonary resection for metastatic melanoma

David W Ollila, John D Sadoff, Brian C McCaughan

INTRODUCTION

Despite the increased incidence of primary bronchogenic carcinoma, pulmonary metastases remain the most common malignant neoplasms of the lung.[1–4] Certain tumors, including melanoma, metastasize preferentially to the lungs.[5–9] Postmortem studies[10] demonstrated that 70% of melanoma patients had pulmonary metastases whereas antemortem studies demonstrated a 12–16% incidence, suggesting that locoregional therapy, i.e. pulmonary metastasectomy, may be a viable option for some patients.[11–13]

Historically, traditional cytotoxic or cytostatic chemotherapy has been used for patients with pulmonary metastases, but it is usually palliative and rarely achieves a complete response. For patients with unresectable stage IV metastatic melanoma, encouraging non-randomized phase II data[14,15] and randomized phase III data[16] with various combinations of biological therapy, interleukin-2 (IL-2) and interferon alfa-2b (INFα-2b), and chemotherapy have been reported. Immunotherapy may be effective for the control of occult systemic micrometastases following surgical resection of the primary lesion, but it is rarely curative once pulmonary metastases are present. Radiotherapy may be useful for the palliation of symptoms, but it does not significantly extend survival. Currently, complete surgical resection of pulmonary metastases offers the only significant chance for the patient to survive 5 years.[11–13,17–20]

DIAGNOSIS

Pulmonary metastases are most often asymptomatic, with only 25% of patients presenting with symptoms of chronic cough, chest pain, sputum production, hemoptysis, dyspnea and/or fever.[21,22] Most symptoms do not appear until late, and thus are not useful for early detection of pulmonary metastases. The most cost-effective way to follow a patient at risk for pulmonary metastases is by routine chest x ray. It must be emphasized that not all pulmonary lesions appearing on routine chest x ray after definitive treatment of a primary neoplasm are metastases.[23] In melanoma patients, a new solitary pulmonary nodule may represent one of three possible etiologies: metastatic pulmonary disease, a primary bronchogenic tumor, or a benign lesion. In contrast, the appearance of multiple pulmonary nodules is almost always associated with metastatic disease. In fact, there appears to be a >95% chance that patients with known extrathoracic primary tumors and multiple pulmonary nodules have pulmonary metastases.[24]

Routine chest x rays should be obtained in posteroanterior and lateral projections. If a new or suspicious lesion is detected, chest computerized tomography (CT) scans should be obtained, not only to define the characteristics of the newly detected lesion but more importantly to document the presence or absence of multiple lesions. Conventional chest CT scans revealed more pulmonary nodules than conventional linear tomography or routine chest radiographs.[25] However, this increase in sensitivity is accompanied by a decrease in specificity because of benign processes such as fibrotic scar tissue, axial sections of vascular structures, or granulomatous disease.

In an effort to enhance the early detection of pulmonary metastases, several authors have investigated spiral chest CT. With the patient taking and holding a single breath, this technique uses a continuous rotation of the x ray source with concomitant continuous transport of the patient table through the scanning aperture.[26,27] This single breath-hold sequence and continuous rotation of the x ray source decreases movement artifact. Some investigators have demonstrated that spiral CT scanning may be superior to conventional CT scanning for the early detection of pulmonary lesions, revealing up to 20% more lesions than conventional CT scans.[26–28] However, more data are needed to provide clear evidence justifying its routine use in the diagnosis of pulmonary metastases. Unfortunately, all anatomic radiological methods yield less than satisfactory results and regularly underestimate the number of true metastatic lesions.

In contrast to anatomic imaging with CT, positron emission tomography (PET) produces a physiology based imaging with respect to glucose metabolism. PET is a non-invasive modality that attempts to differentiate between a malignant and benign process based upon glucose metabolism.[29,30] Although a variety of radiotracers have been investigated, fluoro-18-2-deoxyglucose (FDG) is the tracer most investigated for pulmonary nodules. FDG is rapidly taken up by malignant cells, which have a higher rate of glucose uptake and glycolysis than most normal cells or metabolically inactive granulomas.[31] FDG accumulates in cancer cells because these cells have very low levels of hexokinase, the dephosphorylating enzyme. PET has been used to define solitary pulmonary nodules, enlarged mediastinal lymph nodes, and extrathoracic metastases. With a reported sensitivity and specificity (for pulmonary nodules) of 97 and 78%, respectively, PET may replace CT as the imaging modality of choice to detect pulmonary metastases.[32,33] However, PET does have significant limitations. Lesions as small as 0.5–0.6 cm have been identified, but many studies have reported false-negative results to be quite high in lesions <1 cm.[34–36] In addition, PET has poor spatial resolution, and thus cannot be used for accurate anatomic information. Thus, at present, PET is most useful when it is combined with another imaging modality such as CT or magnetic resonance imaging (MRI), which provide anatomic correlates. The use of fusion techniques between PET and CT is currently in the investigation stages, but to date has not shown better results than the two modalities performed together but not superimposed.[37]

A novel, non-radiologic tool which may prove useful for the early detection of pulmonary metastases is light-induced fluorescence emission (LIFE) bronchoscopy. Currently being investigated for the early detection of bronchogenic carcinoma, LIFE bronchoscopy is a relatively new technique whereby squamous metaplasia and dysplasia can be detected by autofluorescence. The basic principles of fluorescence bronchoscopy are that when the bronchial surface is illuminated by light, one of four things can happen: reflection, scattering, absorption, or fluorescence.[38] Conventional white-light bronchoscopy makes use of the first three and is called reflectance imaging, while LIFE utilizes innate autofluorescence capabilities of tissues. Tissue autofluorescence is not visible to the unaided eye; however, with suitable instruments the autofluorescence can be seen. Violet or blue light causes normal tissues to have significantly higher fluorescence intensity compared to dysplastic lesions or in situ carcinoma.[38,39] This difference can be viewed with a special light filter mounted on the eyepiece of a bronchoscope, and, when used as an adjunct to standard white-light bronchoscopy, augments the ability to localize intraepithelial lesions (squamous metaplasia, dysplasia or in situ carcinoma). There are, however, no reports in the literature concerning use of this technique for the detection of endobronchial lesions from metastatic melanoma, and its use would not be relevant for the majority of metastatic lesions which are peripheral and not able to be seen at bronchoscopy.

If a patient meets radiologic and physiologic selection criteria for surgical intervention, a preoperative tissue diagnosis of a neoplastic pulmonary lesion is not essential, although a fine-needle aspiration biopsy is readily performed on peripheral lesions in patients in whom there is a doubt concerning the diagnosis. Histologic confirmation of metastatic melanoma can be made at thoracotomy, a procedure that can be both diagnostic and therapeutic.

When a patient is not a candidate for surgical resection, various modalities are used to sample tissue for histologic differentiation between malignant and benign processes. Among these, CT-guided fine-needle biopsy of the suspicious lesion is usually the most appropriate for peripheral lesions. A biopsy yielding a specimen that demonstrates metastatic melanoma confirms the diagnosis, but a specimen demonstrating a benign process or normal pulmonary parenchyma may represent an error in sampling. In this situation, repeat CT-guided biopsy or a more invasive procedure is required if a tissue diagnosis is considered essential. Dowling et al.[40] used thoracoscopic resection for diagnostic resection of presumed metastases. Thoracoscopy is less invasive than thoracotomy for a parenchymal-sparing wedge resection of peripheral lung lesions in patients with a history of malignancy;[41] however, its role in therapeutic metastasectomy remains to be defined, and McCormack et al.[42] have demonstrated that, in a significant number of patients, metastases will be missed if only thoracoscopic examination and resection is performed and not open thoracotomy.

SYSTEMIC THERAPY: CHEMOTHERAPY, BIOTHERAPY AND IMMUNOTHERAPY

For patients with pulmonary metastases, the treatment option which offers the best overall 5-year survival rate is pulmonary metastasectomy with complete microscopic resection of all lesions.[11–13] However, patients chosen as candidates for pulmonary metastasectomy must meet highly selective criteria for the procedure to be of benefit. Only those without evidence of tumor outside the chest (including PET scan evidence), and in whom the pulmonary lesions are resectable within the limits of the patient's cardiopulmonary reserves, should undergo surgery. Patients frequently present with multiple sites of visceral metastases in addition to their pulmonary metastases. For patients with multiple sites of visceral metastases, systemic therapy is not curative. Dacarbazine (DTIC), the most active single agent, produces a partial response (PR) in 18–20% of patients and a complete response (CR) in <5% of patients. The only other single-agent chemotherapy which seems to have equal efficacy to DTIC is fotemustine (FTMU) with a PR of 20–25% and a CR of 5–8%.[43,44] Because of the poor PR and CR rates with single-drug therapy regimens, several multidrug combinations have been tested in phase II and phase III trials. Multidrug DTIC-containing chemotherapeutic regimens, such as cisplatin, vincristine and DTIC (CVD) or the Dartmouth regimen [cisplatin, DTIC, carmustine (BCNU) and tamoxifen], have somewhat higher PR rates (25–40%) but similar CR rates (<5%).[14,45] Furthermore, Chapman et al.[46] recently reported a randomized trial between DTIC and the Dartmouth regimen with no difference in overall survival (median survival 6.3 versus 7.7 months, *P*=not significant). Numerous other multidrug chemotherapy regimens have been proposed; however, none have been demonstrated to be superior to the single agent DTIC.

Recently, several investigators have attempted to improve the low CR rates for multidrug chemotherapy regimens by adding two biologic agents, IFNα-2b and IL-2.[14,15,44,47,48] Attempting to minimize toxicity and expense while maximizing response, these investigators tried various doses, sequences, and combinations of chemotherapeutic and biologic agents, including administration in the outpatient setting.[48] Legha et al.[14] reported a 23% CR rate in patients treated with sequential biochemotherapy (chemotherapy followed immediately by biotherapy). Modifying the IL-2 dosing schedule, O'Day et al.[15] administered biotherapy and chemotherapy concurrently; they reported a 20% CR rate that increased to 30% in 26 chemotherapy naïve patients. Recently, Legha's group presented a single-institution phase III randomized trial of biochemotherapy versus multidrug chemotherapy at the American Society of Clinical Oncology.[16] The response rate for patients receiving biochemotherapy was 48%, as compared to 25% for patients receiving the Dartmouth regimen (*P*=0.001). The median survival for patients receiving biochemotherapy was 11.8 versus 9.5 months for multidrug chemotherapy (*P*=0.005). Other randomized single-institution studies have not demonstrated a survival benefit for patients receiving biochemotherapy.[49] Currently, if a melanoma patient is not a candidate for pulmonary metastasectomy, biochemotherapy appears to offer the best chance for CR. If there is a good PR or a significant slowing of the tumor's growth rate, then the patient can be re-evaluated for pulmonary resection,[50] an approach similar to that used in selecting sarcoma patients for pulmonary metastasectomy.[51]

Immunotherapy in a patient with established pulmonary metastases is palliative unless it slows the tumor's rate of growth enough to qualify the patient for potentially curative surgical intervention.[52,53] This applies to patients with a rapid (<60 days) tumor doubling time (TDT) who might not otherwise be considered surgical candidates.[54] Following complete resection of pulmonary metastases, postoperative adjuvant immunotherapy appears effective against occult micrometastatic disease. Currently, a prospective, randomized, multi-institutional, international trial is investigating whether patients with completely resected stage IV metastatic melanoma benefit from postsurgical adjuvant immunotherapy (a phase III randomized double-blind trial of immunotherapy with a polyvalent melanoma vaccine CancerVax plus BCG versus placebo plus BCG as a postsurgical treatment for stage IV melanoma, Donald L Morton, MD, Principal Investigator). Accrual of 420 patients is projected to be completed by late 2002.

SURGICAL RESECTION

The first surgical resection of a pulmonary metastasis was performed in 1855 by Sedillot.[55] This was followed in 1882 by Weinlechner's report describing the surgical excision of a lung metastasis discovered by chance during surgery to remove a primary sarcoma.[56] The first planned resection of a pulmonary metastasis was reported in 1927 by Divis.[57] Seven years after this successful metastasectomy, Barney and Churchill[58] reported a successful pulmonary lobectomy and nephrectomy for metastatic renal cell carcinoma; the patient survived free of disease for 23 years before succumbing to coronary artery disease. This report stimulated thoracic surgeons to treat solitary pulmonary metastases surgically, regardless of the histology of the primary tumor. However, after reports of unsuccessful pneumonectomies for melanoma patients with pulmonary metastases were published,[59,60] interest waned in resecting melanoma metastatic to the lung. In 1951, however, interest in pulmonary metastasectomy for melanoma was renewed by a report of long-term survival in a patient with an isolated solitary pulmonary metastasis who underwent a pneumonectomy.[61] Since that time, many authors have reported limited success in patients with one or more isolated melanoma pulmonary metastases following complete resection, but an average 5-year survival rate of only 19% has been achieved.[11–13,18–20,22,62]

PATIENT SELECTION

It is widely accepted that pulmonary metastasectomy should not be undertaken if the patient will not be rendered disease free by the surgery.[13,20,22,30,63–68] To maximize the chance of 5-year survival, patients considered for pulmonary metastasectomy should have resectable intrathoracic disease with no extrathoracic sites of tumor. A thorough preoperative evaluation of the patient must reveal no other site of stage IV disease, because patients with extrapulmonary metastatic disease generally do not benefit from pulmonary surgical intervention.[12] The physical examination and work-up should be directed towards anatomic sites known or suspected to be involved in the metastatic cascade. This should include a chest CT scan to evaluate the number of metastatic foci in the thoracic cavity and to investigate possible extrapulmonary intrathoracic involvement. A preoperative chest CT scan correctly predicts resectable intrathoracic disease in *c.* 90% of patients surgically explored.[69] To evaluate potential extrathoracic sites of metastatic disease, CT scans or MRI of the brain, as well as CT scans of the abdomen and pelvis, are frequently used. Whole-body PET scanning is currently the preferred investigation to most accurately exclude extrathoracic disease prior to thoracic surgical intervention.

The preoperative work-up must demonstrate adequate cardiopulmonary reserve and the ability to tolerate the planned surgical procedure. This will exclude patients with severe coronary artery disease, valvular heart disease, or severe chronic obstructive pulmonary disease. If the appearance of the mass, its size, and location suggest a diagnosis other than metastatic neoplasm, fiberoptic bronchoscopy may lend useful additional information for lesions that are centrally located.

In summary, the criteria for selecting patients who may benefit from surgical resection of pulmonary metastases are: (a) control of the primary tumor; (b) no evidence of extrathoracic disease; (c) adequate cardiopulmonary reserve. Additional prognostic factors which are related to patient selection and survival are discussed in the following section.

NUMBER OF PREOPERATIVE LESIONS

The number of metastases is an important prognostic factor. In general, patients with fewer metastases surgically resected have a better 5-year survival rate than those with more metastases.[11,65] In fact, many studies have reported that the 5-year survival rate of patients with a single metastasis was markedly better than that of patients who were found to have multiple metastases.[11,66,67] The International Registry of Lung Metastases study[20] reported that the 5-year survival rate of patients with one metastasis was better than that of patients with two to three metastases or that of patients with four or more metastases.

Currently, resection of an isolated, solitary pulmonary metastasis in a patient with melanoma is widely accepted. Harpole et al.[11] demonstrated a survival advantage in patients undergoing pulmonary metastasectomy for one or two lesions. However, the usefulness of resecting more than two lesions remains somewhat controversial. For patients with multiple metastatic pulmonary foci, other factors, including the disease-free interval (DFI)[68] and the TDT,[12] contribute to the decision whether or not to explore the patient. For patients with multiple pulmonary lesions, a 5-year survival rate of 19% has been reported in patients undergoing pulmonary metastasectomy,[12] suggesting that this approach is still superior to any systemic therapy option currently available for patients with resectable pulmonary disease. Thus, the number of pulmonary metastases is not an absolute contraindication to pulmonary metastasectomy but rather should be considered along with DFI and TDT.

DISEASE-FREE INTERVAL (DFI)

The DFI is defined as the time from the start of therapy for the primary tumor to the diagnosis of metastatic disease. In general, it is regarded as a surrogate for the pace and biology of the patient's metastatic disease, with a prolonged DFI associated with a slow growing, less aggressive neoplasm. Some investigators report a favorable prognosis for patients with a prolonged DFI between excision of the primary tumor and detection of pulmonary metastases.[51,69,70] However, other reports have not always supported this concept.[13,18] While Putnam et al.[71] have demonstrated the cumulative prognostic significance of combining DFI and TDT in sarcoma patients, La Hei et al.,[13] Pogrebniak et al.,[72] and Gorenstein et al.[19] did not find a statistically significant relationship between DFI and prognosis in melanoma patients. The precise DFI which signals a more favorable biology remains in question. The International Registry of Lung Metastases study of patients with all types of cancer found a statistically significant overall survival once the DFI was ≥36 months.[20] In contrast, other recent large institutional reviews of melanoma patients with pulmonary metastases showed a direct correlation betwen improved outcome and a DFI >12 months[11] or 30 months.[12]

TUMOR DOUBLING TIME (TDT)

TDT refers to the time it takes for a metastasis to double in size and represents another surrogate of the biologic aggressiveness of a particular cancer. TDT may in fact be a measurement of a tumor's ability to recruit angiogenic and growth factors necessary to enlarge in relationship to the host's defense mechanisms to inhibit this process. Collins et al.[73] were the first to describe how to calculate TDT by using serial chest radiographs. To calculate TDT, successive chest radiographs are used to measure the changing diameters of each nodule. The greatest perpendicular diameter of each nodule is measured with a ruler on standard 72 inch target film distance posteroanterior chest roentgenograms. Diameters are then plotted versus time on semilogarithmic paper. The slope of the line drawn between the points represents the rate of tumor growth. The horizontal distance between any two doubling points represents the TDT in days. Tumor growth should be measured at intervals of 2 weeks for 1–2 months. When multiple pulmonary metastases are present, the prognosis is determined by the fastest growing lesion.

Morton and associates[17,74] were the first to use TDT to identify possible surgical candidates among patients with pulmonary metastases. In general, patients with a short TDT have a worse prognosis than those with a prolonged TDT.[63,74] Morton's group examined pulmonary resection of metastases in patients with a variety of primary tumor histologies.[17] For patients with a TDT <40 days, there was only a 7 month increase in survival beyond that expected from non-operative management. In contrast, patients whose TDT was >40 days had a 5-year survival rate of 63% following surgical resection of the metastatic lesion(s). Examining TDT in melanoma patients, Ollila et al.[54] found no 5-year survivors if the TDT was <60 days. However, if TDT was ≥60 days, the 5-year survival rate was 20.7%. There is no consensus on the precise TDT which imparts a favorable prognosis. Furthermore, it is very difficult to predict prognosis based on this measurement alone, especially in the light of possible concomitant therapies that may alter tumor cell biology.[75] The present authors believe that the number of lesions, DFI and TDT all contribute to determining the biology of a particular patient's disease, and therefore whether or not surgical exploration is warranted.

TECHNICAL ASPECTS OF THE OPERATIVE PROCEDURE

The operative exposure depends on the number and location of metastatic lesions visualized on the preoperative chest imaging studies; the choice between posterolateral thoracotomy and median sternotomy is left to the discretion of the surgeon. If staged posterolateral thoracotomies are to be used in patients presenting with bilateral metastases, some advocate that resection of the least-involved lung should be performed first. This will enable the surgeon to determine the extent of surgical resection and the remaining pulmonary volume on the side with fewer lesions before undertaking thoracotomy on the side with more metastases, where a major pulmonary resection such as bilobectomy or pneumonectomy may be required.[76] While the surgical principles of pulmonary metastasectomy remain relatively constant, the nuances of exploration and surgical resection at three major cancer facilities are described below.

John Wayne Cancer Institute[79]

A careful visual inspection and bimanual palpation is performed on the pulmonary parenchyma, examining the lung in both the inflated and deflated conditions. The location of each metastasis is marked with a silk suture. After the primary surgeon has completed the exploration, the first assistant also carefully examines the lungs for metastases. All of the metastatic lesions are to be marked with a suture prior to resection of any one lesion, because the resection inevitably results in artifacts at the suture line and atelectasis, which may be mistaken for additional lesions.

After the exploration is completed, and all metastatic lesions have been marked, the type of resection necessary to extirpate all metastases is planned. The majority of metastatic lesions are subpleural, which makes a wedge resection feasible in most instances, unless the metastasis is along a fissure. The mechanical stapling device is extremely useful in patients who need multiple wedge resections. To achieve an adequate margin of normal lung parenchyma surrounding the metastasis (at least 1 cm), Bouie hemorrhoid clamps are placed proximal to the metastasis and the mechanical stapling device is placed beyond the clamps. If multiple wedge resections are not technically feasible, then a lobectomy or pneumonectomy is performed.

University of North Carolina at Chapel Hill

The operation begins with a careful systematic visual inspection of the lung while inflated and then deflated. With the lung deflated, palpation of the entire pulmonary parenchyma is performed. The primary surgeon identifies each pulmonary nodule, creating a diagram of the findings, and the surgical assistant confirms these findings. The surgical plan to excise all the lesions usually entails multiple wedge resections using a stapling device. The endoscopic GIA stapler is used whenever possible. If an area is not amenable to simple wedge resection, formal lobectomy or pneumonectomy is performed in order to completely resect all metastatic foci. There is no difference in survival between patients undergoing wedge resection and those undergoing lobectomy or pneumonectomy, as long as a complete resection is undertaken.[64,77,78] Recognizing that there are no clear data regarding what constitutes an adequate margin for a wedge resection, it is attempted to obtain margins of at least 1 cm. Simple enucleation has been attempted in the past but was abandoned because it resulted in high rates of locoregional recurrence.[79] A few studies recommend at least 0.5 cm margins, but do not provide data to support this advice.[80–82]

In the era of minimally invasive thoracic surgery, i.e., video-assisted thoracic surgery (VATS), a word of caution is necessary. Without palpation of the pulmonary parenchyma, metastases will be missed in *c.* 25% of patients.[47,83,84] Palpation of the entire pulmonary parenchyma is not possible with VATS. Furthermore, good long-term survival data are not available. The present authors cannot advocate performing a pulmonary metastasectomy using VATS outside of a well-designed clinical trial and thus believe that the gold standard for a complete pulmonary metastasectomy is an open procedure with manual palpation of the lungs.

Sydney Melanoma Unit[13]

All patients undergoing surgery for pulmonary metastatic melanoma undergo both PET and CT scanning of the chest. Prior to exploration, all potential lesions are identified and the surgical approach is defined. Thoracoscopy is used only when the diagnosis is in doubt, and thoracoscopic wedge resection and frozen-section examination is performed. If melanoma is suspected on frozen section then thoracotomy is proceeded to directly. The 'miss rate' of thoracoscopic examination alone precludes its use for complete resection of all lesions. Median sternotomy is occasionally utilized for bilateral lesions but sequential thoracotomies are preferred. Contrary to the practice at the John Wayne Cancer Institute, the side with greater disease involvement is explored first to ensure that lung can be cleared of disease, thus avoiding a potentially unnecessary thoracotomy if clearance is not possible.

Irrespective of the surgical approach, at operation the technique is similar to both the John Wayne Cancer Institute and the University of North Carolina. Careful inspection and bimanual palpation of the entire lung in both the deflated and inflated state by both the surgeon and assistant is initially completed. All lesions are identified prior to any resection and the nature of resection planned, incorporating adjacent lesions whenever possible into stapled wedge resections with *c.* 1 cm macroscopic tumor clearance. With large, centrally placed multiple lesions, lobectomy may be required, or even pneumonectomy, to achieve complete surgical clearance. Enucleation is not used. Mediastinal lymph node dissection is not routinely performed unless the preoperative PET scan has revealed evidence of nodal metastatic disease.

SURVIVAL FOLLOWING SURGICAL RESECTION

Following a pulmonary metastasectomy, the primary outcome measure that has been studied is overall 5-year survival rate (Table 47.1). Overall, approximately one-third of patients who undergo complete resection of isolated pulmonary metastases are 5-year survivors.[20] Considerable variation exists in reported survival rates between different primary tumor types, although there is surprisingly little variation between different studies

Table 47.1 *Survival following resection of pulmonary metastases in patients with malignant melanoma*

Author (ref. no.)	No. of patients	Overall 5-year survival rate (%)	Median survival (months)	
			Complete resection	Incomplete resection
Cahan 1973 (85)	29	14	–	–
Mathison et al. 1979 (86)	22	0	12.0	10.5
Dahlback et al. 1980 (87)	8	0	7.0	–
Thayer and Overholt 1985 (88)	18	11	16.5	–
Pogrebniak et al. 1988 (72)	33	6	–	–
Karp et al. 1990 (89)	29	5	11.0	5.0
Gorenstein et al. 1991 (19)	56	25	18.0	–
Harpole et al. 1992 (11)	98*	20	20.4	8.2
Tafra et al. 1995 (12)	106	27	25.0	11.0
La Hei et al. 1996 (13)	83	22	19	–
Pastorino et al. 1997 (90)	328	21	–	–

*Patients undergoing curative resection.

of a single tumor type. Prior to 1973, there were no single-institution reports of melanoma cohorts treated with pulmonary metastasectomy. In 1973, Cahan[85] reported the first single-institution experience of 29 metastatic melanoma patients treated with pulmonary metastasectomy, finding an overall 5-year survival rate of 14%. The enthusiasm for resection dampened when Mathisen et al.[86] reported no 5-year survivors, and no significant difference in survival rates between surgical patients deemed non-resectable (mean survival 10.5 months) and those rendered disease free in the lungs (mean survival 12.0 months). Furthermore, Dahlback's group also reported no long-term survivors, and concluded that lung surgery did not contribute to the survival of melanoma patients with pulmonary metastases.[87]

In the 1990s, however, several single-institution studies[11–13,19] reported more encouraging 5-year survival rate data (20–27%) for patients with pulmonary metastases (Table 47.1). From these reports, several common findings are evident. First, the survival benefit is greatest for patients rendered disease free by complete resection. The survival benefit for patients who had an incomplete resection of intrathoracic disease because of the extent of disease is marginal at best. Morton and colleagues[12] reported a multivariate analysis which demonstrated that complete surgical resection and prolonged DFI (>30 months) before stage IV disease were independent prognostic factors for prolonged survival in melanoma patients with pulmonary metastases.

Harpole's multivariate analysis identified complete resection, DFI >12 months before stage IV disease, chemotherapy, one or two pulmonary nodules, and no intervening stage III disease as independent prognostic factors contributing to the prolonged survival of patients managed surgically.[11] However, the largest and most recent data set comes from the International Registry of Lung Metastases study.[20] Because the registry included such a large number of patients, it represents the best available assessment to date of how to select patients for resection. Four groups were created, based upon the following criteria: resectable with no extrapulmonary disease versus unresectable, the number of lesions (1 versus >1), and DFI (≥36 versus <36 months). Table 47.2 shows the prognostic groupings together with the observed 5-year survival rates. Taken as a group, patients with a single metastasis and prolonged DFI who were completely resected had a very good 5-year survival rate. However, patients with isolated pulmonary metastases from melanoma still fared the worst. The role of pulmonary metastasectomy in this group of patients is still poorly understood and needs to be better defined by well-designed, prospective multi-institution studies.

CONCLUSIONS

The best option for patients with a single focus of metastatic melanoma in the lung remains a pulmonary metastasectomy. Patients who have multiple pulmonary metastases and favorable prognostic features, such as a long DFI and a prolonged TDT, also may benefit from surgical resection. However, if the patient is not a surgical candidate because of extrapulmonary disease, a short DFI or a short TDT, then systemic biochemotherapy offers the patient the best chance for a CR.

Table 47.2 *Survival of 4673 patients with carcinoma, sarcoma and melanoma metastases to the lung, divided into prognostic groups*[19]

Group	Definition*	5-year survival rate (%)
Group I	Resectable, single metastasis, DFI ≥36 months	51
Group II	Resectable, *either* multiple metastases *or* DFI <36 months	37
Group III	Resectable, multiple metastases *and* DFI <36 months	24
Group IV	Unresectable	13

*DFI, Disease-free interval.

REFERENCES

1. Abrams H, Spiro R, Goldstein N, Metastases in carcinoma: analysis of 1000 autopsied cases. *Cancer* 1950; 3: 74.
2. Hammar S, Common neoplasms. In: *Pulmonary pathology* (ed Dail D). New York: Springer Verlag, 1988: 727.
3. Spencer H, *Pathology of the lung*, 4th edn. Oxford: Pergamon Press, 1985.
4. Willis R, *Pathology of tumors*, 4th edn. London: Butterworths, 1967.
5. Hart A, 'Seed and soil' revisited: mechanisms of site-specific metastasis. *Cancer Metastasis Rev* 1982; 1: 5.
6. Paget S, The distribution of secondary growths in cancer of the breast. *Lancet* 1889; 1: 571.
7. Poste G, Gidler I, The pathogenesis of cancer metastasis. *Nature* 283: 139.
8. Sugarbaker E, Cancer metastases: a product of tumor–host interactions. *Curr Probl Cancer* 1979; 3: 1.
9. Viadana E, Bross I, Pickren J, Cascade spread of blood borne metastases in solid and nonsolid cancers of humans. In: *Pulmonary metastasis*, 1st edn. (eds Weiss L, Gilbert H). Boston: GK Hall & Co, 1978: 143.
10. DasGupta T, Brasfield R, Metastatic melanoma: a clinicopathologic study. *Cancer* 1964; 17: 1323–39.
11. Harpole Jr DH, Johnson CM, Wolfe WG et al, Analysis of 945 cases of pulmonary metastatic melanoma. *J Thorac Cardiovasc Surg* 1992; 103: 743–8; discussion 748–50.
12. Tafra L, Dale PS, Wanek LA et al, Resection and adjuvant immunotherapy for melanoma metastatic to the lung and thorax. *J Thorac Cardiovasc Surg* 1995; 110: 119–28; discussion 129.
13. La Hei ER, Thompson JF, McCaughan BC et al, Surgical resection of pulmonary metastatic melanoma: a review of 83 thoracotomies. *Asia Pacific Heart J* 1996; 5: 111–14.
14. Legha SS, Ring S, Bedikian A et al, Treatment of metastatic melanoma with combined chemotherapy containng cisplatin, vinblastine and dacarbazine (CVD) and biotherapy using interleukin-2 and interferon-alpha. *Ann Oncol* 1996; 7: 827–35.
15. O'Day S, Boasberg P, Guo M et al, Phase II trial of concurrent biochemotherapy (c-BC) with decrescendo interleukin-2 (d-IL-2), tamoxifen (T) and G-CSF support in patients with metastatic melanoma (MM). *Proc Am Soc Clin Oncol* 1997; 16: 490a.
16. Eton O, Legha S, Bedikian A et al, Phase III randomized trial of cisplatin, vinblastine and dacarbazine (CVD) plus interleukin-2 (IL2) and interferon-alpha-2b (INF) versus CVD in patients (Pts) with metastatic melanoma. *Proc ASCO* 2000; 19: 2174.
17. Morton DL, Joseph WL, Ketcham AS et al, Surgical resection and adjunctive immunotherapy for selected patients with multiple pulmonary metastases. *Ann Surg* 1973; 178: 360–6.
18. Wong J, Euhus D, Morton D, Surgical resection for metastatic melanoma to the lung. *Arch Surg* 1988; 23: 1091–5.
19. Gorenstein LA, Putnam JB, Natarajan G et al, Improved survival after resection of pulmonary metastases from malignant melanoma [see comments]. *Ann Thorac Surg* 1991; 52: 204–10.
20. Anon, Long-term results of lung metastasectomy: prognostic analyses based on 5206 cases. The International Registry of Lung Metastases. *J Thorac Cardiovas Surg* 1997; 113: 37–49.
21. Morrow C, Vassilopoulous P, Grage T, Surgical resection for metastatic neoplasms of the lung: experience at the University of Minnesota Hospitals. *Cancer* 1980; 45: 2981.
22. Mountain C, McMurtrey M, Hermes K, Surgery for pulmonary metastasis: a 20-year experience. *Ann Thorac Surg* 1984; 38: 323–30.
23. Atkins Jr P, Newman W et al, Thoracotomy on the patient with previous malignancy: metastasis or new primary? *J Thorac Cardiovasc Surg* 1968; 56: 351.
24. Patz Jr EF, Fidler J, Knelson M et al, Significance of percutaneous needle biopsy in patients with multiple pulmonary nodules and a single known primary malignancy. *Chest* 1995; 107: 601–4.
25. Chang AE, Schaner EG, Conkle DM et al, Evaluation of computed tomography in the detection of pulmonary metastases: a prospective study. *Cancer* 1979; 43: 913–16.
26. Remy-Jardin M, Remy J, Giraud F, Marquette CH, Pulmonary nodules: detection with thick-section spiral CT versus conventional CT. *Radiology* 1993; 187: 513–20.
27. Collie DA, Wright AR, Williams JR et al, Comparison of spiral-acquisition computed tomography and conventional computed tomography in the assessment of pulmonary metastatic disease. *Br J Radiol* 1994; 67: 436–44.
28. Paranjpe D, Bergin C, Spiral CT of the lungs: optimal technique and resolution compared with conventional CT. *Am J Roentgenol* 1994; 162: 561–7.
29. Hawkins RA, Hoh C, Glaspy J et al, The role of positron emission tomography in oncology and other whole-body applications. *Semin Nuc Med* 1992; 22: 268–84.
30. Takita H, Edgerton F, Karakousis C et al, Surgical management of metastases to the lung. *Surg Gynecol Obstet* 1981; 152: 191–4.
31. Hughes J, 18F-fluorodeoxyglucose PET scans in lung cancer. *Thorax* 1996; 51 (Suppl 2): 516–22.
32. Lowe VJ, Fletcher JW, Gobar L et al, Prospective investigation of positron emission tomography in lung nodules. *J Clin Oncol* 1998; 16: 1075–84.
33. Graeber G, Gupta N, Murray G, Positron emission tomographic imaging with fluorodeoxyglucose is efficacious in evaluating malignant pulmonary disease. *J Thorac Cardiovasc Surg* 1999; 117: 719–27.
34. Valk PE, Pounds TR, Hopkins DM et al, Staging non-small cell lung cancer by whole-body positron emission tomographic imaging. *Ann Thorac Surg* 1995; 60: 1573–81; discussion 1581–2.
35. Guhlmann A, Storck M, Kotzerke J et al, Lymph node staging in non-small cell lung cancer: evaluation by [18F]FDG positron emission tomography (PET). *Thorax* 1997; 52: 438–41.
36. Dewan NA, Gupta NC, Redepenning LS et al, Diagnostic efficacy of PET-FDG imaging in solitary pulmonary nodules. Potential role in evaluation and management. *Chest* 1993; 104: 997–1002.
37. Vansteenkiste JF, Stroobants SG, De Leyn PR et al, Mediastinal lymph node staging with FDG-PET scan in patients with potentially operable non-small cell lung cancer: a prospective analysis of 50 cases. Leuven Lung Cancer Group. *Chest* 1997; 112: 1480–6.
38. Lam S, Kennedy T, Unger M et al, Localization of bronchial intraepithelial neoplastic lesions by fluorescence bronchoscopy. *Chest* 1998; 113: 696–702.
39. Lam S, Shibuya H, Early diagnosis of lung cancer. *Clin Chest Med* 199; 20: 53–61.
40. Dowling RD, Keenan RJ, Ferson PF, Landreneau RJ, Video-assisted thoracoscopic resection of pulmonary metastases. *Ann Thorac Surg* 1993; 56: 772–5.
41. Dowling R, Ferson P, Landreneau R, Thoracoscopic resection of pulmonary metastases. *Chest* 1992; 102: 1450.
42. McCormack PM, Bains MS, Begg CB et al, Role of video-assisted thoracic surgery in the treatment of pulmonary metastases: results of a prospective trial. *Ann Thorac Surg* 1996; 62: 213–16.
43. Chary KK, Higby DJ, Henderson ES, Swinerton KD, Phase I study of high-dose cis-dichlorodiammiineplatinum (II) with forced diuresis. *Cancer Treat Rep* 1977; 61: 367–70.
44. Khayat D, Avril M, Auclerc G et al, Clinical value of the nitosourea fotemustine in disseminated malignant melanoma: overview of 1022 patients including 144 patients with cerebral metastases. *Proc Am Soc Clin Oncol* 1993; 12: 1343a.
45. McClay EF, Mastrangelo MJ, Berd D, Bellet RE, Effective combination chemo/hormonal therapy for malignant melanoma: experience with three consecutive trials. *Int J Cancer* 1992; 50: 553–6.
46. Chapman PB, Einhorn LH, Meyers ML et al, Phase III multicenter randomized trial of the Dartmouth regimen versus dacarbazine in patients with metastatic melanoma. *J Clin Oncol* 1999; 17: 2745–51.
47. Richards JM, Mehta N, Ramming K, Skosey P, Sequential chemoimmunotherapy in the treatment of metastatic melanoma. *J Clin Oncol* 1992; 10: 1338–43.
48. Thompson J, Gold P, Fefer A, Outpatient chemo-immunotherapy for patients with metastatic melanoma. *Proc Am Soc Clin Oncol* 1996; 15: 433.
49. Rosenberg S, Yang J, Schwartzentruber D et al, Prospective randomized trial of the treatment of patients with metastatic melanoma using chemotherapy with cisplatin, dacarbazine, and tamoxifen alone or in combination with interleukin-2 and interferon alfa-2b. *J Clin Oncol* 1999; 17: 968–75.

50. Ollila D, O'Day S, Esner R et al, Cytoreductive surgery in stage IV melanoma patients with residual metastatic disease following biochemotherapy. World Federation of Surgical Oncology Societies, March, 1998.
51. Huth JF, Holmes EC, Vernon SE et al, Pulmonary resection for metastatic sarcoma. *Am J Surg* 1980; 140: 9–16.
52. Barth A, Irie R, Morton D, Update on immunotherapy for advanced melanoma. *Contemp Oncol* 1994; 4: 52–60.
53. Morton DL, Foshag LJ, Hoon DS et al, Prolongation of survival in metastatic melanoma after active specific immunotherapy with a new polyvalent melanoma vaccine [published erratum appears in *Ann Surg* 1993; 217: 309]. *Ann Surg* 1992; 216: 463–82.
54. Ollila DW, Stern SL, Morton DL, Tumor doubling time: a selection factor for pulmonary resection of metastatic melanoma [see comments]. *J Surg Oncol* 1998; 69: 206–11.
55. Vogt-Moykopf I, Meyer G, Surgical technique in operations on pulmonary metastases. *Thorac Cardiovasc Surg* 1986; 34: 125–32.
56. Weinlechner D, Tumoren an der brustwand und deren behaldlung. Eroffnung der brusthohle und partielle entfernung der lunge. *Wien Med Wochenschr* 1892; 32: 590.
57. Divis G, Ein beitrag zur operativen behandlung der lungengeschwulste. *Acta Chirurgica Scand* 1927; 62: 329.
58. Barney JD, Churchill EJ, Adenocarcinoma of the kidney with metastasis to the lung. *J Urol* 1939; 42: 269–74.
59. Carlucci CA, Schleusser RC, Primary melanoma of the lung: a case report. *J Thorac Surg* 1942; 11: 643–7.
60. Oscher A, DeBakey M, Primary pulmonary malignancy. *Surg Gynecol Obstet* 1939; 68: 435–41.
61. Creech O, Metastatic melanoma of the lung treated by pulmonary resection: a report of a case. *Med Rec Ann* 1951; 45: 4426–7.
62. Marincola FM, Mark JB, Selection factors resulting in improved survival after surgical resection of tumors metastatic to the lungs. *Arch Surg* 1990; 125: 1376–92; discussion 1392–3.
63. Todd TR, Pulmonary metastectomy. Current indications for removing lung metastases. *Chest* 1993; 103 (Suppl 4): 401S–403S.
64. McCormack P, Surgery for pulmonary metastases. In: *Cancer of the colon, rectum and anus* (eds Cohen A, Winawer S). New York: McGraw-Hill, 1995: 857–61.
65. Putnam Jr JB, Roth JA, Prognostic indicators in patients with pulmonary metastases. *Semin Surg Oncol* 1990; 6: 291–6.
66. Mansel JK, Zinsmeister AR, Pairolero PC, Jett JR, Pulmonary resection of metastatic colorectal adenocarcinoma. A ten year experience. *Chest* 1986; 89: 109–12.
67. Girard P, Ducreux M, Baldeyrou P et al, Surgery for lung metastases from colorectal cancer: analysis of prognostic factors. *J Clin Oncol* 1996; 14: 2047–53.
68. Girard P, Baldeyrou P, Le Chevalier T et al, Surgery for pulmonary metastases. Who are the 10-year survivors? *Cancer* 1994; 74: 2791–7.
69. Morton DL, Metastatic tumors in the thorax. In: *Cancer medicine*, 4th edn. (eds Holland JF, Frei E, Bast R et al). Baltimore: Williams & Wilkins, 1997: 1849–60.
70. Putnam Jr JB, Roth JA, Wesley MN et al, Analysis of prognostic factors in patients undergoing resection of pulmonary metastases from soft tissue sarcomas. *J Thorac Cardiovasc Surg* 1984; 87: 260–8.
71. Putnam Jr JB, Roth JA, Wesley MN et al, Survival following aggressive resection of pulmonary metastases from osteogenic sarcoma: analysis of prognostic factors. *Ann Thorac Surg* 1983; 36: 516–23.
72. Pogrebniak HW, Stovroff M, Roth JA, Pass HI, Resection of pulmonary metastases from malignant melanoma: results of a 16-year experience. *Ann Thorac Surg* 1988; 46: 20–3.
73. Collins VP, Loeffler RK, Tivey H, Observations on growth rates of human tumors. *Am J Roentgenol* 1956; 76: 988–1000.
74. Joseph WL, Morton DL, Adkins PC, Prognostic significance of tumor doubling time in evaluating operability in pulmonary metastatic disease. *J Thorac Cardiovasc Surg* 1971; 61: 23–32.
75. Roth JA, Putnam Jr JB, Wesley MN, Rosenberg SA, Differing determinants of prognosis following resection of pulmonary metastases from osteogenic and soft tissue sarcoma patients. *Cancer* 1985; 55: 1361–6.
76. Ollila D, Morton D, Surgical resection as the treatment of choice for melanoma metastatic to the lung. *Chest Surg Clin N Am* 1998; 8: 183–96.
77. Wal Hvd, Verhagen A, Lecluyse A et al, Surgery of pulmonary metastases. *Thorac Cardiovasc Surg* 1986; 34: 153.
78. Cahan W, Castro E, Hajdu S, The significance of a solitary lung shadow in patients with colon carcinoma. *Cancer* 1974; 33: 414–21.
79. Vogt-Moykopt I, Krysa S, Bulzebruck H et al, Surgery for pulmonary metastases: the Heidelberg experience. *Chest Surg Clin N Am* 1994; 4: 85–112.
80. Dresler C, Goldberg M, Surgical management of lung metastases: selection factors and results. *Oncology* 1996; 109: 649–55.
81. Venn G, Sarin S, Goldstraw P, Survival following pulmonary metastasectomy. *Eur J Cardiothorac Surg* 1989; 3: 105–9.
82. Gundry SR, Coran AG, Lemmer J et al, The influence of tumor microfoci on recurrence and survival following pulmonary resection of metastatic osteogenic sarcoma. *Ann Thorac Surg* 1984; 38: 473–8.
83. Ren H, Hruban RH, Kuhlman JE et al, Computed tomography of inflation-fixed lungs: the beaded septum sign of pulmonary metastases. *J Comput Assist Tomogr* 1989; 13: 411–16.
84. Peuchot M, Libshitz H, Pulmonary metastatic disease: radiologic–surgical correlation. *Radiology* 1987; 164: 719–22.
85. Cahan WG, Excision of melanoma metastases to lung: problems in diagnosis and management. *Ann Surg* 1973; 178: 703–9.
86. Mathisen DJ, Flye MW, Peabody J, The role of thoracotomy in the management of pulmonary metastases from malignant melanoma. *Ann Thorac Surg* 1979; 27: 295–99.
87. Dahlback O, Hafstrom L, Jonsson PE, Sundqvist K, Lung resection for metastatic melanoma. *Clin Oncol* 1980; 6: 15–20.
88. Thayer Jr JO, Overholt RH, Metastatic melanoma to the lung: long-term results of surgical excision. *Am J Surg* 1985; 149: 558–62.
89. Karp NS, Boyd A, DePan HJ et al, Thoracotomy for metastatic malignant melanoma of the lung. *Surgery* 1990; 107: 256–61.
90. Anonymous, Long-term results of lung metastasectomy: prognostic analyses based on 5206 cases. The International Registry of Lung Metastases. *J Thorac Cardiovasc Surg* 1997; 113: 37–49.

48

Hepatic surgery for metastatic melanoma

Anton J Bilchik, Richard Essner, John F Thompson, Donald L Morton

HEPATIC RESECTION

The prognosis of patients with American Joint Committee on Cancer (AJCC) stage IV melanoma is dismal, with a median survival of 4–6 months and an actuarial 5-year survival rate of 6%.[1] Although neither chemotherapy nor immunotherapy has yet been shown to improve survival, there is increasing evidence to support the judicious use of surgical resection in appropriately selected patients. Depending on the anatomical site, a median overall survival of 24–49 months has been reported following complete resection of pulmonary,[2–7] gastrointestinal[7–10] and adrenal metastases.[11,12]

The median survival of melanoma patients with initial metastasis to the liver is 4.4 months.[1] Although there are isolated reports of long-term survivors following resection of primary and metastatic hepatic tumours,[13,14] the role of surgery for hepatic metastases of melanoma remains poorly defined. This is partly because liver involvement is identified ante mortem in only 10–20% of patients with AJCC stage IV melanoma – despite the fact that the majority will have autopsy evidence of liver disease.[15] Also, many hepatic metastases are in unresectable locations or in patients with poor hepatic reserve.

The limited data on hepatic resection for metastatic melanoma are derived primarily from subset analysis (Table 48.1).[5,16–26] In 1978, Foster[16] reported a series of 72 patients undergoing liver resections for metastatic disease. He compiled all available contemporary reports and visited 98 hospitals to collect data on hepatic resections. Only 13 patients (18%) underwent surgical resection of melanoma metastatic to the liver. Median survival of these patients was 10 months, with a 5-year survival rate of 8%. Other investigators have reported median survivals of 10–20 months and occasional long-term survival of up to 184 months.[17–21]

Experience of the John Wayne Cancer Institute (JWCI) and the Sydney Melanoma Unit (SMU)

This group has recently reviewed pooled data from the JWCI and the SMU.[27] These major referral centres for the treatment of melanoma have two of the largest prospectively collected melanoma databases in the world. The purpose of this review was to determine the rates of disease-free and overall survival following curative (complete) or palliative surgical resection of hepatic metastases, and to identify the prognostic impact of demographic factors and tumour characteristics.

Of the 26,204 evaluable patients who underwent treatment of melanoma at the two centres between 1971 and 1999, 1750 (6.7%) had hepatic metastases. The study group comprised the 34 (2%) patients who underwent surgical exploration after an extensive staging work-up that included computerized tomographic (CT) scans of the chest, abdomen and pelvis, magnetic resonance imaging (MRI) of the brain, bone scans as clinically indicated, and, more recently, ^{18}fluorodeoxyglucose positron emission tomography (^{18}FDG-PET). A formal abdominal exploration was performed and the liver was completely mobilized. In more recent cases, the number and extent of hepatic lesions were evaluated by intraoperative ultrasonography.

Table 48.1 *Reported outcomes following hepatic resection for metastatic melanoma*

Author (ref. no.)	Year	No. of patients with non-colorectal metastases	Melanoma metastases			
			No. of patients	Overall survival (months)		5-year survival rate (%)
				Median	Range	
Foster (16)	1978	72	13	10	2–72	8
Iwatsuki et al. (25)	1983	19	1			
Papachristou and Fortner (19)	1983		3	16		
Ekberg et al. (20)	1986	8	3	19	5–72	
Olak et al. (26)	1986	30	1			
Stehlin et al. (21)	1988	30	4	13	3–52	
Wolf et al. (22)	1991	10	1			
Karakousis et al. (5)	1994	2	2			
Harrison et al. (23)	1997	96	7			
Lindell et al. (17)	1998	32	3	51	5–184	33
Elias et al. (18)	1998	147	10	20		<20
Lang et al. (24)	1999	140	10			22
JWCI/SMU (27)	2000		24	28	2–147	29

Of the 34 patients, 10 (29%) had extensive intra-abdominal disease identified at laparotomy, and therefore did not undergo resection. The remaining 24 patients (71%) who underwent resection were evenly divided between males and females, and their median age was 57 years (range 26–71 years of age). More than half (63%) of these patients were initially treated for localized disease (AJCC stage I/II melanoma). The median disease-free interval between initial treatment and diagnosis of hepatic metastases was 58 months (range 0–264 months) for all 24 patients.

The most common hepatic resection was lobectomy (14 patients), followed by non-anatomic resection (five patients), segmentectomy (four patients) and extended lobectomy (one patient). Eighteen patients had a single hepatic metastasis, four patients had two metastases and two patients had more than two metastases. The median size of these metastases was 5 cm (range 0.7–22 cm). Twelve patients had synchronous extrahepatic metastases.

Surgical removal of all identified metastatic disease was achieved in 18 (75%) patients, including seven of the 12 patients with synchronous hepatic and extrahepatic metastases (Table 48.2). Six of the 24 patients had residual hepatic and/or extrahepatic metastatic disease (Table 48.3). Of the 18 patients undergoing complete resection, 13 developed recurrent melanoma. The liver was the most common site of recurrence [six patients (33%)]. Three of the 13 patients underwent repeat metastasectomy. In two cases, a second hepatic resection was undertaken 21 and 37 months, respectively, following the initial procedure. One of these patients remains alive and free of disease 76 months following the first resection. A second patient underwent resection of recurrent disease involving the diaphragm 1 year following hepatic resection and remains free of disease at 16 months follow-up.

There were no operative deaths. One patient expired due to multisystem organ failure 2 months following a right hepatic lobectomy. A second patient suffered a fatal cerebrovascular accident 3 months following a right hepatic lobectomy. Autopsy revealed no evidence of intracranial metastatic disease. Both of these patients were free of melanoma at the time of death.

Table 48.2 *Features and outcomes of 18 patients undergoing complete resection of hepatic metastases (JWCI/SMU experience)*

Patient	Extrahepatic sites of resected disease*	Sites of recurrence	Postoperative survival (months)		Clinical status‡
			Disease free	Overall	
1	Diaphragm		147	147	NED
8	None	Lung	24	82	DOD
2	None	Liver+	37	76	NED
6	None	Liver	15	70	AWD
3	Soft tissue		55	55	NED
9	None	Liver, lung	34	44	DOD
10	Mesenteric lymph nodes	Liver, mesenteric lymph nodes	21	38	DOD
4	None		32	32	NED
11	None	GI	15	28	DOD
12	None	Unknown	19	19	DOD
7	Soft tissue	Soft tissue	3	17	AWD
5	None	Diaphragm+	12	16	NED
13	GI, mesenteric lymph nodes	Liver, lung	6	15	DOD
14	None	Brain	4	9	DOD
15	LN	Bone	4	8	DOD
16	None	Liver, omentum	3	7	DOD
17	None		3	3	DOC (CVA)
18	Periportal LN		2	2	DOC (MSOF)

*GI, Gastrointestinal metastases; LN, lymph nodes.
+Patients rendered NED following a second resection.
‡NED, Alive with no evidence of disease; DOD, dead of disease; AWD, alive with disease; DOC, dead of other causes; CVA, cerebrovascular accident; MSOF, multisystem organ failure.

Disease-free and overall survival were determined from the time of operation. The median overall survival for the entire group of 34 patients undergoing exploration was 10 months; corresponding 3- and 5-year estimated overall survival rates were 36 and 20%, respectively. The median disease-free survival in the 24 resected patients was 12 months (range 0–147 months); median overall survival of this group was 28 months (range 2–147 months), with corresponding 3- and 5-year estimated survival rates of 41 and 29%, respectively. The 24 patients undergoing resection had a significantly better survival than the 10 patients undergoing exploration alone (P=0.0009; Figure 48.1). Median overall survival in the latter group was only 4 months. Median survival of 899 JWCI patients undergoing non-operative treatment of hepatic metastases was 6 months, and the estimated 5-year survival rate was only 4%.

Factors analyzed for survival differences included age at diagnosis, gender, initial tumour stage and characteristics, disease-free interval between resection of the

Table 48.3 *Features and outcomes of six patients undergoing incomplete resection of hepatic and extrahepatic metastases (JWCI/SMU experience)*

Patient	Extrahepatic sites of disease at time of operation	Postoperative overall survival (months)	Clinical status*
1	None	37	DOD
2	Lung, omentum	16	DOD
3	Lung, soft tissue	13	DOD
4	Gastrointestinal, omentum, adrenal	7	AWD
5	Mesentery, soft tissue	7	DOD
6	Coeliac lymph nodes	2	DOD

*DOD, dead of disease; AWD, alive with disease.

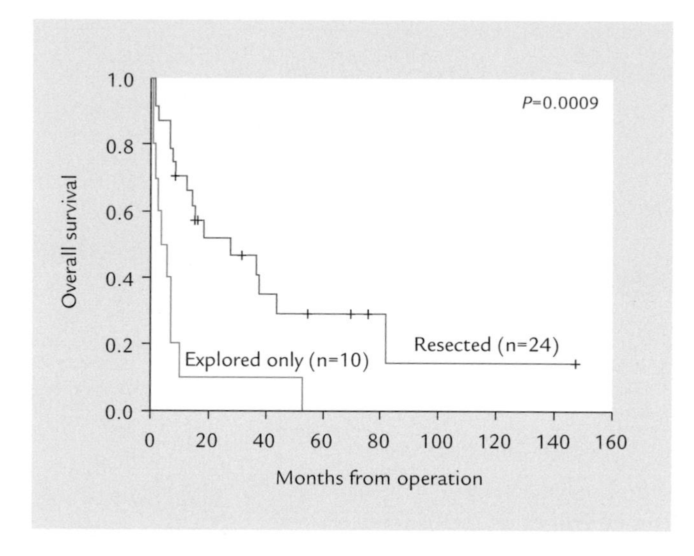

Figure 48.1 *Overall survival following resection of hepatic melanoma metastases versus exploration alone. Patients undergoing hepatic resection had a significantly improved survival (*P*=0.0009).*

primary melanoma and development of hepatic metastases, anatomic extent and location of recurrences, operative details of hepatic resection, pathologic findings, adjuvant therapy, recurrence following resection, and follow-up times. Factors associated with an improved disease-free survival by univariate analysis included macroscopically complete metastasectomy (P=0.001) and a histologically negative resection margin (P=0.03). Patients rendered surgically free of disease tended to have a longer overall survival (P=0.06). Demographic factors, initial tumour characteristics and the use of any adjuvant therapy did not have a significant impact on survival. In addition, no prognostic factor achieved statistical significance for either disease-free or overall survival on multivariate analysis.

Applying prognostic factors to patient selection

Most hepatic metastasectomies have been performed in patients with colorectal carcinoma.[28] The indications for operation are now based on a number of patient and tumour-related factors. Fong et al.[29] made specific recommendations based on number and size of metastases, interval between primary and metastatic disease, presence of lymph node positivity, and preoperative CEA levels. There are fewer reports of hepatic resection for other neoplasms, which makes it difficult to determine indications for resection, but several series suggest that complete resection, a long disease-free interval prior to hepatic metastases, lack of extrahepatic disease and primary tumour type are the most important prognostic factors.[17,18,22,23] Long disease-free interval, complete resection and relative tumour burden have also been identified as prognostic factors following resection of melanoma metastatic to non-hepatic sites.[2–12]

Selection criteria for hepatic resection of metastatic melanoma should be similar to criteria used in patients with metastatic colorectal carcinoma or patients with non-hepatic melanoma metastases. In all cases, selection of appropriate patients for hepatic resection of metastatic melanoma must be individualized and should include an extensive evaluation of the extent of disease. Patients should undergo CT scans of the chest, abdomen and pelvis, CT scanning or MRI of the brain, and whole-body ^{18}FDG-PET scanning.

In the JWCI/SMU experience, improved survival was associated with macroscopically complete metastasectomy, a histologically negative resection margin, the liver as the only initial site of metastatic disease and absence of extrahepatic disease at the time of resection. Not surprisingly, patients undergoing complete surgical resection had a statistically better survival (P=0.0009) than those undergoing exploration alone, and those undergoing complete resection tended to have an improved survival (P=0.06) when compared with patients not rendered free of disease. The importance of complete resection was also noted in the report from Lang et al.[24] on hepatic resection of 140 non-colorectal non-neuroendocrine metastases. These authors suggested that the possibility of complete resection has potentially greater prognostic significance than the presence of extrahepatic tumour. However, seven of the 18 patients (39%) in the JWCI/SMU review had synchronous extrahepatic disease (Table 48.2). Extrahepatic disease is therefore not a contraindication if it can be resected.

The impact of disease-free interval may also be significant in this setting. Patients in the JWCI/SMU database review had a 58 month median disease-free interval prior to presenting with hepatic disease. By contrast, the median disease-free interval of 899 JWCI database patients who underwent non-operative treatment of hepatic metastases was 35 months. At the JWCI, a more aggressive operative approach is favoured for patients with longer disease-free intervals prior to development of hepatic metastases, because the disease-free interval has been identified as an independent prognostic factor in patients with stage IV melanoma.[1]

Repeat metastasectomy has been advocated in selected patients with stage IV melanoma if the patient can be rendered surgically free of disease.[30] Scattered reports of repeat hepatic resection for metastatic melanoma suggest a long-term benefit in these patients.[31] Two patients in the JWCI/SMU experience underwent repeat hepatic resection for isolated recurrent metastatic disease within the liver. The hepatic recurrences appeared 21 and 37 months following resection undertaken with curative intent. One patient lived an additional 17 months before succumbing to systemic disease; the second patient is currently free of disease 3 years following the second hepatic resection. However, repeat metastasectomy should be approached with caution and with attention to the patient's expected quality of life, because survival may be prolonged but cure is unlikely.[32] This procedure should thus be reserved for isolated recurrent disease in carefully screened patients.

ABLATION OF HEPATIC METASTASES

Many patients with hepatic tumours are not eligible for surgical resection because of liver dysfunction, proximity of the tumour to major vascular structures or bile ducts and/or bilobar disease. The remaining patients may be candidates for local ablative techniques (percutaneous ethanol injection, microwave tumour coagulation, interstitial laser photocoagulation, cryosurgical ablation or radiofrequency ablation), hepatic-directed techniques (hepatic artery ligation, transcatheter arterial chemoembolization or hepatic artery infusional chemotherapy) or systemic chemotherapy. Local tumour ablative techniques can destroy unresectable hepatic tumours with only minimal injury to normal hepatic parenchyma.

Cryosurgical ablation (CSA) of hepatic tumours is widely used for patients with unresectable disease.[33–36] CSA can improve overall survival,[37] but it requires a laparotomy and is associated with a relatively high rate of serious complications, including coagulopathy, haemorrhage, pleural effusion, parenchymal cracking, bile duct injury and acute renal failure.[36,38,39] Moreover, its instrumentation is cumbersome and expensive.

Radiofrequency ablation (RFA) destroys tumours by using a high-frequency alternating current to create ionic agitation that results in frictional heating and ultimately cell death. During RFA, high-frequency alternating current causes thermal coagulation and protein denaturation: as the temperature is increased >45°C, cellular proteins denature and cell structure is lost. RFA technology is commonly used for the ablation of aberrant conduction pathways in the heart and has become a primary procedure in the treatment of cardiac dysrhythmias. RFA has increasingly been utilized for unresectable hepatic malignancies.

Unlike CSA, RFA uses relatively inexpensive instrumentation and can be performed in the operating room as an open procedure, or laparoscopically, or in the radiology suite using a percutaneous approach. Its reported complication and recurrence rates are relatively low.[40–42] Preivous reports have demonstrated the utility of RFA for the destruction of small lesions. However, relatively few studies have reported results of RFA in patients with primary and metastatic hepatic malignancies, and its potential complications, optimal approaches and limitations have not been clearly defined.

Radiofrequency ablation (RFA) experience at the John Wayne Cancer Institute (JWCI)

In November 1997, JWCI began its ongoing phase II trial of RFA for patients with unresectable hepatic tumours, including hepatic metastases of malignant melanoma. Patient eligibility for this trial is determined by the presence of multiple hepatic tumours, bilobar involvement, tumours proximal to major vascular and/or biliary structures, and/or attendant co-morbities that would prevent surgical resection. The presence of extrahepatic disease, an exclusion criterion, is ruled out by laparoscopic examination of the abdomen, or by laparotomy if laparoscopy is not possible. A formal assessment of the liver, parietal peritoneum, visceral surfaces of the stomach, small bowel, colon, lesser sac and omentum is performed. The gastrohepatic ligament is divided and the caudate lobe is directly examined. The porta hepatis, coeliac axis and vena cava are examined, and suspicious lymph nodes are biopsied. When there is no evidence of extrahepatic disease, intraoperative ultrasound (IOUS) is performed on all liver segments; the size and location of each lesion are recorded and compared with preoperative imaging results (Figure 48.2). Patients eligible for RFA have a tumour volume <40% of total hepatic volume, as determined by IOUS, and sufficient hepatic reserve to undergo ablation (Childs–Pugh class A or B).

The technique of RFA is the same regardless of the probe used, except for the power and duration of ablation. For lesions ≤2 cm in diameter, the needle is placed into the centre of the lesion under ultrasound guidance (Figure 48.3). This is most easily accomplished by orienting the RFA needle parallel to the plane of the ultrasound probe. Tynes with thermocouples are deployed through the primary channel and 50–200 watts (W) of alternating current is delivered. As soon as the temperature exceeds 90°C, an 8–25 minute

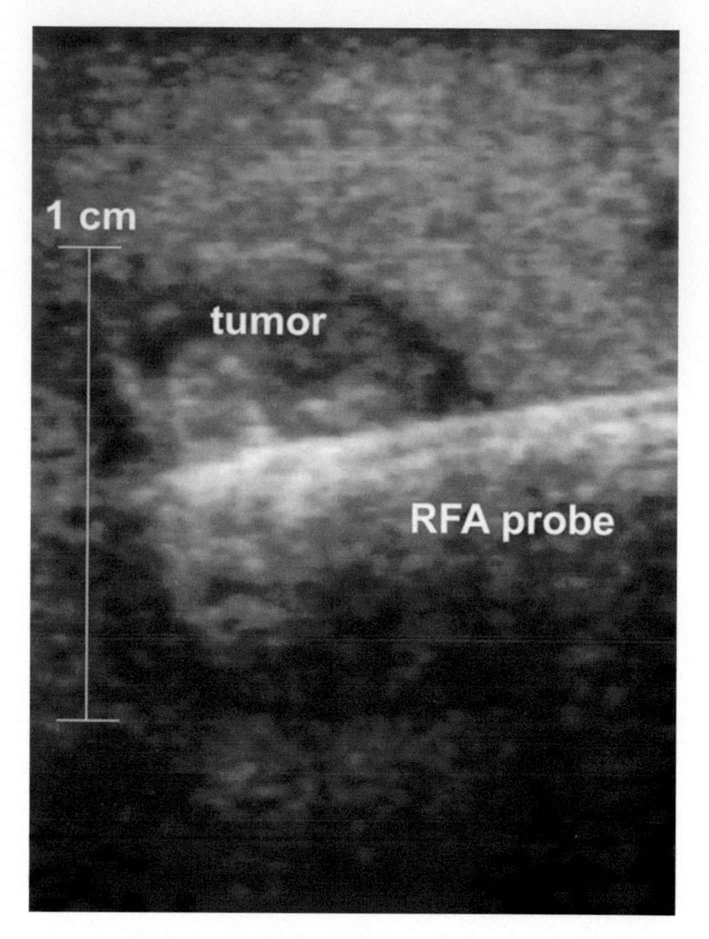

Figure 48.2 *Intraoperative ultrasonogram of a 1.3 cm hepatic tumour not identified on preoperative images.*

ablation is performed, depending upon the probe used. The formation of the heat lesion is monitored with real-time ultrasound (Figure 48.4). The tumour and a 1 cm margin of normal hepatic parenchyma are ablated. The current is terminated and temperatures of the tynes are evaluated 30 seconds later; a temperature of at least 60°C 30 seconds following ablation ensures adequate tissue necrosis. Larger lesions are ablated with multiple overlapping fields. The probe is placed at the deep margin at one side of the tumour. Multiple overlapping ablations are then sequentially performed, progressing superficially and then laterally until the tumour and a 1 cm margin have been successfully ablated. Following ablation, the probe tract is cauterized as the RFA needle is withdrawn. If target temperatures are not reached, as may be the case for lesions near major vascular structures (heat sink), the tynes are withdrawn slightly or rotated *c.* 45° to increase the temperature in the region of ablation. Each tumour is

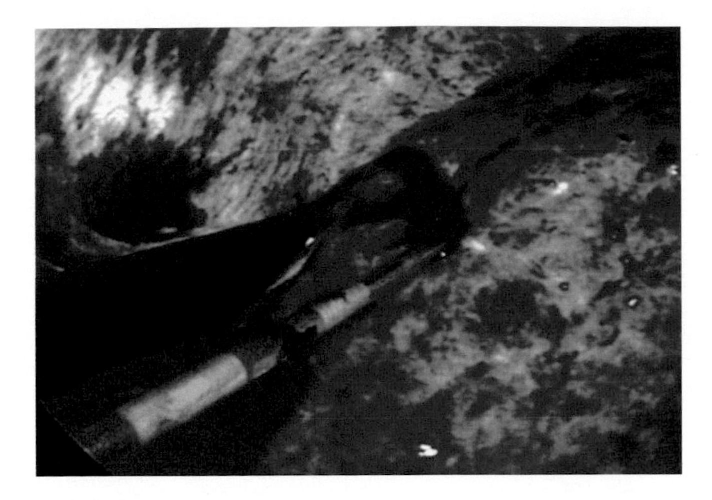

Figure 48.3 *Intraoperative photograph of laparoscopic ultrasound probe and 15-gauge radiofrequency ablation (RFA) probe placed in the tumour.*

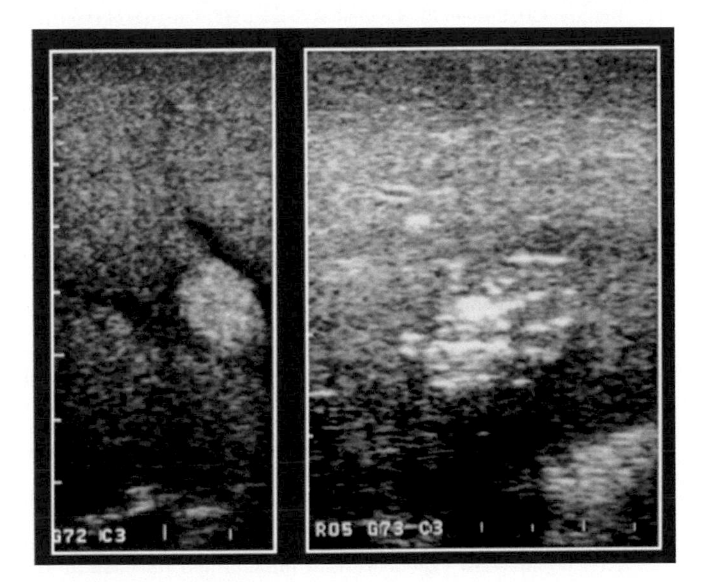

Figure 48.4 *Intraoperative ultrasonogram of hyperechoic heat-ablated tumour.*

ablated under imaging guidance with the goal of complete destruction of the tumour and a 1 cm circumferential margin of parenchyma.

At JWCI, over 150 RFA procedures have been performed in a heterogeneous population of patients with primary and metastatic unresectable hepatic tumours.[43–45] Until mid-1999, the present authors performed RFA using the Model 30 (50 W) probe (RITA Medical Systems, Mountain View, CA). This probe has a 15-gauge needle with a retractable curved-electrode configuration and can ablate an area of tissue that is 2.5–3 cm in diameter. Since mid-1999, RFA has been performed using the Model 70 probe (RITA), the 5 cm Starburst XL needle/150 W electrode (RITA) or a 200 W cluster probe (Cool-tip, Radionics, Burlington, MA). These probes are capable of ablating an area of 4–5 cm in diameter.

Laparoscopic versus percutaneous radiofrequency ablation (RFA)

Much of the published data on RFA originates from Europe, where the majority of ablations are done percutaneously.[46] Although previous reports have shown the utility of percutaneous RFA for the destruction of small, unresectable hepatic tumours,[40,47] this approach has been criticized because it precludes intraoperative exploration and therefore may result in inaccurate staging.

Since laparoscopy and laparoscopic ultrasonography are the most accurate methods of staging intraabdominal neoplasms, the present authors combined this technology with RFA in a select group of patients with melanoma, and found that it was extremely safe and effective. There were no complications, all patients were discharged the following day, and the survival was unexpectedly high considering that the majority of patients had multiple tumours.

Laparoscopic RFA provides surgeons with an invaluable tool in managing patients with unresectable tumours confined to the liver. Laparoscopy is less invastive than laparotomy, and provides accurate staging and effective tumour ablation. Recurrence rates are low, although a longer follow-up is required. Portal inflow occlusion during laparoscopic RFA may further augment the ablation. The protection of vital structures, accurate staging and better patient tolerance provide several advantages of this approach in appropriately selected patients. Of the 84 patients enrolled in the trial as of February 2000, eight patients with metastatic melanoma have undergone laparoscopic RFA. The mean size of the 31 hepatic lesions in these eight patients was 2 cm (range 2–3 cm). Three patients underwent prior treatment with interferon, two with biochemotherapy and three with chemotherapy alone. The median number of lesions treated was four (range one to eight lesions). All patients were discharged the following day with no morbidity. Four patients have died of their disease at a median of 7 months after surgery (range 5–9 months). Two have developed local recurrence at 8 and 15 months after surgery, and two have no evidence of disease 7 months after surgery. However, more patients must be evaluated in a prospective fashion to determine the impact of this treatment modality.

CONCLUSIONS

The growing acceptance of hepatic resection for metastatic disease reflects improvements in operative and anaesthetic techniques, better selection of patients, a significant number of long-term survivors (up to 30 or 40% at 5 years), and low operative morbidity and mortality rates (<5%). In the JWCI/SMU experience, patients with limited metastases who can be rendered surgically free of disease tend to have improved survival. This is similar to results for surgical resection of melanoma metastatic to non-hepatic sites. Some patients will achieve excellent long-term results; however, the majority will progress and eventually die of melanoma. Careful screening and realistic expectations of surgical resection are necessary to achieve optimal outcomes. Because there is no effective systemic therapy, healthy individuals with appropriate prognostic factors should be considered for an aggressive surgical approach. The present authors recommend consideration of hepatic resection in patients who have limited metastatic disease and no co-morbid conditions. These patients should undergo extensive preoperative imaging to determine their candidacy for complete surgical resection. Clearly, the majority of these patients will recur over time; however, this approach does offer the possibility of long-term survival to a select group.

Advances in RFA technology and surgical techniques have allowed ablation of bigger hepatic malignancies with excellent short-term results. However, although RFA offers patients a safe and minimally invasive technique for the destruction of unresectable hepatic tumours, its precise impact on survival is uncertain and its role in combination with systemic therapy remains investigational.

REFERENCES

1. Barth A, Wanek LA, Morton DL, Prognostic factors in 1521 melanoma patients with distant metastases. *J Am Coll Surg* 1995; 181: 193–201.
2. Wong JH, Euhus DM, Morton DL, Surgical resection for metastatic melanoma to the lung. *Arch Surg* 1988; 123: 1091–95.
3. Tafra L, Dale PS, Wanek LA et al, Resection and adjuvant immunotherapy for melanoma metastatic to the lung and thorax. *J Thorac Cardiovasc Surg* 1995; 110: 119–29.
4. Ollila DW, Morton DL, Surgical resection as the treatment of choice for melanoma metastatic to the lung. *Chest Surg Clin North Am* 1998; 8: 183–96.
5. Karakousis CP, Velez A, Driscoll DL, Takita H, Metastasectomy in malignant melanoma. *Surgery* 1994; 115: 295–302.
6. La Hei ER, Thompson JF, McCaughan BC et al, Surgical resection of pulmonary metastatic melanoma: a review of 83 thoracotomies. *Asia Pacific Heart J* 1996; 5: 111–14.
7. Lejeune FJ, Lienard D, Sales F, Badr-el-din H, Surgical management of distant melanoma metastases. *Semin Surg Oncol* 1992; 8: 381–91.
8. Ollila DW, Essner R, Wanek LA, Morton DL, Surgical resection for melanoma metastatic to the gastrointestinal tract. *Arch Surg* 1996; 131: 975–9.
9. Mosimann F, Fontolliet C, Genton A et al, Resection of metastases to the alimentary tract from malignant melanoma. *Int Surg* 1982; 67: 257–60.
10. Khadra MH, Thompson JF, Milton GW, McCarthy WH, The justification for surgical treatment of metastatic melanoma of the gastrointestinal tract. *Surg Gynecol Obstet* 1990; 171: 413–16.
11. Haigh PI, Essner R, Wardlaw JC et al, Long-term survival after complete resection of melanoma metastatic to the adrenal gland. *Ann Surg Oncol* 1999; 6: 633–9.
12. Branum GD, Epstein RE, Leight GS, Seigler HF, The role of resection in the management of melanoma metastatic to the adrenal gland. *Surgery* 1991; 109: 127–31.
13. Schwartz SI, Hepatic resection for noncolorectal nonneuroendocrine metastases. *World J Surg* 1995; 19: 72–5.
14. Foster JH, Lundy J, Liver metastases. *Curr Prob Surg* 1981; 18: 160–202.
15. Meyers ML, Balch CM, Diagnosis and treatment of metastatic melanoma. In: *Cutaneous melanoma*, (eds Balch CM, Houghton AN, Sober AJ, Song S-J). St Louis: Quality Medical Publishing, Inc, 1998: 325–72.
16. Foster JH, Survival after liver resection for secondary tumors. *Am J Surg* 1978; 135: 389–94.
17. Lindell G, Ohlsson B, Saarela A et al, Liver resection of noncolorectal secondaries. *J Surg Oncol* 1998; 69: 66–70.
18. Elias D, Cavalcanti de Albuguerque A, Eggenspieler P et al, Resection of liver metastases from a noncolorectal primary: indications and results based on 147 monocentric patients. *J Am Coll Surg* 1998; 187: 487–93.
19. Papachristou DN, Fortner JJ, Surgical treatment of metastatic melanoma confined to the liver. *Int Surg* 1983; 68: 145–8.
20. Ekberg H, Tranberg K-G, Andersson R et al, Major liver resection: perioperative course and management. *Surgery* 1986; 100: 1–7.
21. Stehlin JS, de Ipolyi PD, Greeff PJ et al, Treatment of cancer of the liver: twenty years' experience with infusion and resection in 414 patients. *Ann Surg* 1988; 208: 23–35.
22. Wolf RF, Goodnight JE, Krag DE, Schneider PD, Results of resection and proposed guidelines for patient selection in instances of noncolorectal hepatic metastases. *Surg Gynecol Obstet* 1991; 173: 454–60.
23. Harrison LE, Brennan MF, Newman E et al, Hepatic resection for noncolorectal nonneuroendocrine metastases: a fifteen-year experience with ninety-six patients. *Surgery* 1997; 121: 625–32.
24. Lang H, Nussbaum K-T, Weimann A, Raab R, Ergebnisse der resektion nichtcolorectaler nicht neuroendokriner lebermetastasen. *Chirurg* 1999; 70: 439–46.
25. Iwatsuki S, Shaw BW, Starzl TE, Experience with 150 liver resections. *Ann Surg* 1983; 197: 247–53.
26. Olak J, Wexler MJ, Rodriguez J, McLean AP, Hepatic resection for metastatic disease. *Can J Surg* 1986; 29: 435–9.
27. Rose DM, Essner R, Hughes TM et al, Surgical resection for metastatic melanoma to the liver: the John Wayne Cancer Institute and Sydney Melanoma Unit experience. *Arch Surg* 136: 950–5.
28. Fong Y, Salo J, Surgical therapy of hepatic colorectal metastasis. *Semin Oncol* 1999; 26: 514–23.
29. Fong Y, Fortner J, Sun RL et al, Clinical score for predicting recurrence after hepatic resection for metastatic colorectal cancer: analysis of 1001 consecutive cases. *Ann Surg* 1999; 230: 309–18.

30. Ollila DW, Hseuh EC, Stern SL, Morton DL, Metastasectomy for recurrent stage IV melanoma. *J Surg Oncol* 1999; 71: 209–13.
31. Mondragon-Sanchez R, Barrera-Franco JL, Cordoba-Gutierrez H, Meneses-Garcia A, Repeat hepatic resection for recurrent metastatic melanoma. *Hepato-gastroenterol* 1999; 46: 459–61.
32. Fong Y, Blumgart LH, Cohen A et al, Repeat hepatic resections for metastatic colorectal cancer. *Ann Surg* 1994; 220: 657–62.
33. Bilchik AJ, Sarantou T, Wardlaw JC, Ramming KP, Cryosurgery causes a profound reduction in tumor markers in hepatoma and noncolorectal hepatic metastases. *Am Surg* 1997; 63: 796–800.
34. Bilchik AJ, Sarantou T, Foshag LJ et al, Cryosurgical palliation of metastatic neuroendocrine tumors resistant to conventional therapy. *Surgery* 1997; 122: 1040–7.
35. Pearson AS, Izzo F, Fleming RY et al, Intraoperative radiofrequency ablation or cryoablation for hepatic malignancies. *Am J Surg* 1999; 178: 592–9.
36. Bilchik AJ, Wood TF, Allegra D et al, Cryosurgery and radiofrequency ablation of unresectable hepatic malignancies: a proposed algorithm. *Arch Surg* 2000; 135: 657–62.
37. Ravikumar TS, Kane R, Cady B et al, A 5-year study of cryosurgery in the treatment of liver tumors. *Arch Surg* 1991; 126: 1520–3.
38. Seifert JK, Morris DL, World survey on the complications of hepatic and prostate cryotherapy. *World J Surg* 1999; 23: 109–113.
39. Sarantou T, Bilchik A, Ramming KP, Complications of hepatic cryosurgery. *Semin Surg Oncol* 1998; 14: 156–62.
40. Rossi S, Di Stasi M, Buscarini E et al, Percutaneous radiofrequency interstitial thermal ablation in the treatment of small hepatocellular carcinoma. *Cancer J Sci Am* 1995; 1: 73.
41. Siperstein AE, Rogers SJ, Hansen PD, Gitomirsky A, Laparoscopic thermal ablation of hepatic neuroendocrine tumor metastases. *Surgery* 1997; 122: 1147–54.
42. Solbiati L, Ierace T, Goldberg SN et al, Percutaneous US-guided radio-frequency tissue ablation of liver metastases: treatment and follow-up in 16 patients. *Radiology* 1997; 202: 195–203.
43. Rose DM, Allegra DP, Bostick PJ et al, Radiofrequency ablation: a novel primary and adjunctive ablative technique for hepatic malignancies. *Am Surg* 1999; 65: 1009–14.
44. Bilchik AJ, Rose DM, Allegra DP et al, Radiofrequency ablation: a minimally invasive technique with multiple applications. *Cancer J Sci Am* 1999; 5: 356–61.
45. Wood TF, Rose DM, Chung M et al, Radiofrequency ablation of 231 unresectable hepatic tumors: indications, limitations, and complications. *Ann Surg Oncol* 2000; 7: 593–600.
46. Rossi S, Di Stasi M, Buscarini E et al, Percutaneous RF interstitial thermal ablation in the treatment of hepatic cancer. *AJR Am J Roentgenol* 1996; 167: 759–68.
47. Curley SA, Izzo F, Delrio P et al, Radiofrequency ablation of unresectable primary and metastatic hepatic malignancies: results in 123 patients. *Ann Surg* 1999; 230: 1–8.

49

Gastrointestinal and other intraabdominal melanoma metastases

Joost M Klaase, Bin BR Kroon

GASTROINTESTINAL METASTASES

Malignant melanoma is one of the most common metastatic lesions to the gastrointestinal tract, representing 50–70% of all gastrointestinal metastases.[1] Most of these metastases are localized in the small intestine (58–71%), with the stomach (27%) and the large bowel (22%) being less frequently involved.[2] Metastases to the oesophagus (5%) and gall bladder are rare (<1%).[2,3] It has been suggested that this pattern is the result of the splanchnic vascular supply. For metastases in the ileum, melanoma is considered to be the principal tumour, apart from primary tumours of the digestive tract itself.[4]

Gastrointestinal metastatic melanoma occurs in several forms. The intramural nodular type is most frequently found in the stomach and its ongoing growth leads to the formation of polypoid masses. Ulceration of these lesions may lead to the typical radiological feature known as a bullseye.[5] Multiple polypoid lesions are mostly encountered in the small intestine but ulcerating lesions can occur (Figure 49.1). Colon metastases are found in a variety of forms.

Post-mortem specimens from patients with melanoma demonstrate gastrointestinal tract involvement in 50–60% of cases.[6] Ante-mortem diagnosis of gastrointestinal tract involvement is made for <5% of patients.[6,7] This difference may be explained by the fact that intestinal metastases usually occur in the course of the disease when other organ systems (such as brain and lungs) are already involved. In such cases, the clinical symptoms resulting from involvement of those organs usually predominate and the intestinal symptoms tend to be non-specific. Only in *c.* 30% of melanoma patients is the gastrointestinal tract the first site of recurrence.[8] The median time from treatment of the primary melanoma to detection of the gastrointestinal metastases ranges from 2 to 4 years.[9–12]

Because patients who develop distant metastases from melanoma have such a poor prognosis, surgical intervention is generally to be avoided, especially in the case of multiple metastases to different sites which cannot be completely resected.[13,14] Occasional studies, however, have demonstrated prolonged survival in selected patients after resection of melanoma metastatic to the gastrointestinal tract.[12,15,16] Traditionally, surgical intervention for gastrointestinal metastases has been reserved for palliation of lesions that are symptomatic

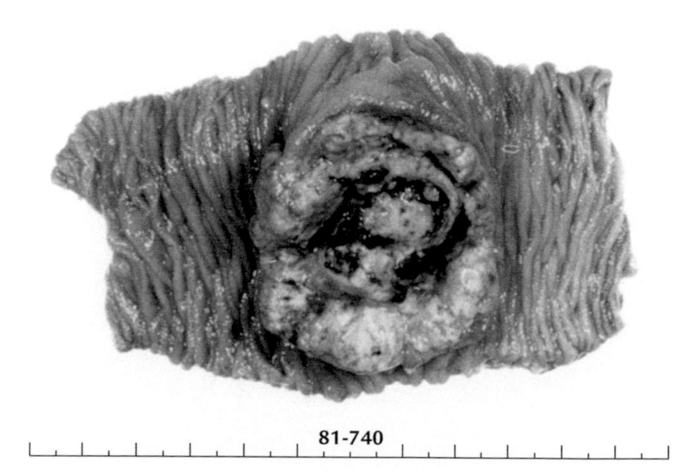

Figure 49.1 *Ulcerating melanoma metastasis in the small bowel.*

(with bleeding, obstruction, pain or perforation).[17] However, several recent studies demonstrating prolonged median survival times for patients with complete resections have renewed interest in surgical resection of gastrointestinal tract metastases.[18]

Symptoms

The clinician should be alerted by non-specific symptoms such as anorexia, nausea and vomiting, signs of anaemia, melaena, periods of diarrhoea and abdominal pain, which sometimes imitate the complaints associated with peptic ulcer disease. In most cases, the diagnosis is made at a late stage when the disease is already advanced and complications have developed. The most common complications requiring surgery are bleeding (acute or chronic) and ileus due to intussusception (Figures 49.2 and 49.3). Bowel perforation and malabsorption are seen less frequently.[10,19]

Diagnostic tests

Because of the high incidence of small bowel metastases, contrast luminal studies and computerized tomography (CT) scanning are the investigations of choice. Ulcerated mucosal tumours may have the classic bullseye appearance, whereas non-ulcerated lesions may appear as luminal indentations or polyps. The roles of CT scanning and luminal radiology are complementary; CT will detect mesenteric masses that minimally affect adjacent bowel; barium studies, in particular enteroclysis, will detect smaller polypoid lesions that would be missed by CT scanning.[20,21] Endoscopic procedures are extremely helpful in the diagnosis of colonic, oesophageal and gastric lesions by offering both visualization and confirmatory biopsies of these tumours.[5,22] Whole-body positron emission tomographic (PET) scans may be employed to identify small bowel metastases, which have a higher metabolic rate than adjacent intestinal epithelium and can easily be differentiated from normal tissue.[16,23,24] Ultrasound may also be of value in assessing hepatic, splenic, pancreatic or renal involvement.

Treatment and results

When metastatic melanoma has been detected in the gastrointestinal tract, the decision to recommend surgery will be influenced by several considerations, including the symptoms, the overall condition of the patient, the presence of concurrent metastases outside the gastrointestinal tract and whether or not the patient has had previous surgical treatment for gastrointestinal melanoma metastases.[11]

The results of surgical intervention for gastrointestinal metastatic melanoma are given in Table 49.1. Palliation of symptoms can be achieved in 80–97% of patients, with a mortality rate ranging from 1.4 to 11%. Survival after surgery ranges from 5.7 to 24 months, with a higher survival rate (10–48.9 months) for patients

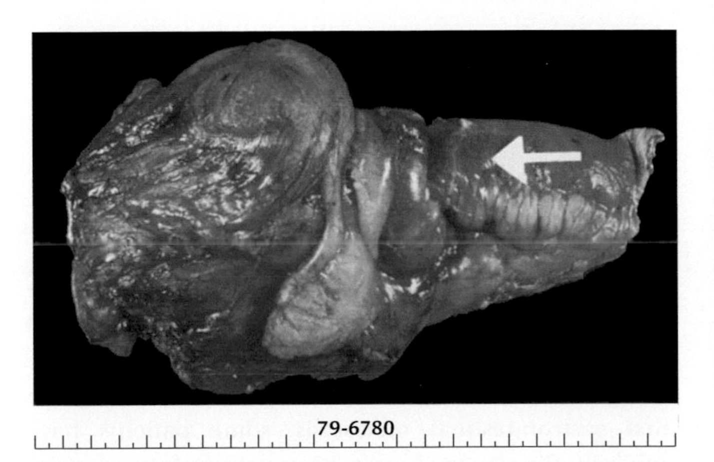

Figure 49.2 *Ileocaecal resection specimen with intussusception due to a polypoid melanoma metastasis in the terminal ileum.*

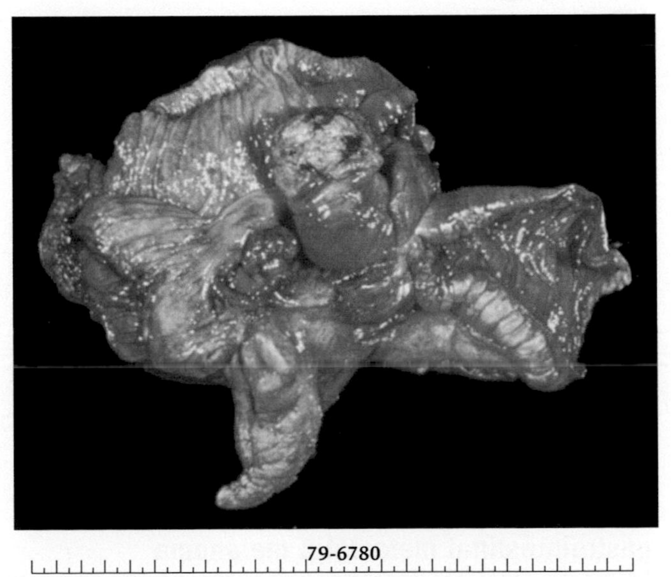

Figure 49.3 *The same specimen as in Figure 49.2, but seen from the inside.*

Table 49.1 *Results of surgical management of melanoma metastatic to the gastrointestinal tract. Only series with more than 20 patients, who were surgically treated in the period of 1980–1999, are included*

Author (ref. no.)	No.	Site (%)				Palliation (%)	Mortality (%)	Survival (months)		
		Stomach	Small bowel	Large bowel	Other			All	CR*	Non-CR*
Ricaniadis et al. 1981 (34)	47	3	47+	25	ns	73	11.0	5.7	27.2	ns
Reintgen et al. 1984 (35)	38	0	100	0	0.0	90	ns	17.3	ns	ns
Overett and Shiu 1985 (36)	25	8	64	16	12.0	ns	ns	9.0	ns	ns
Caputy et al. 1991 (37)	41	27	71	22	5.0	81	5.0	9.5	ns	ns
Ihde and Coit 1990 (38)	32	6	56‡	16	ns	ns	3.0	6.2	10.0	5.3
Khadra et al. 1990 (11)	56	5	89	5	0.0	80	4.0	9.0	ns	ns
Klaase and Kroon 1990 (10)	23	0	74	13	13.0	83	9.0	8.5	ns	ns
Ollila et al. 1996 (16)	69	6	84	26	2.0	97	1.4	24.0	48.9	5.4
Berger et al. 1999 (12)	36	10	80+	49	61.0	ns	3.0	ns	23.5	8.9
Agrawal et al. 1999 (9)	68	3	91	21	1.5	90	2.9	8.2	14.9	6.9

*CR, Complete remission; +Jejunum; ‡Ileum; ns, not specified.

who are macroscopically disease free after surgery compared to those who are not (5.3–8.9 months).

An alternative therapy for bleeding gastrointestinal metastases is radiation therapy [once or twice with 8 gray (Gy) ionizing radiation], which is effective in 50% of patients. Total abdominal perfusion can be considered as a technique of regional chemotherapy which may be used in the treatment of unresectable metastatic melanoma of the abdomen.[25]

Adjuvant therapy after surgery for gastrointestinal metastatic melanoma

No therapy administered after surgical resection of gastrointestinal metastases has been shown to have a demonstrable impact on patient survival. Chemotherapy or chemoimmunotherapy after resection of metastatic lesions seems to be of little or no value.[2]

Recurrence after surgery for gastrointestinal metastatic melanoma

The role of surgical treatment has been shown to be less clear when a second symptomatic gastrointestinal metastasis is detected. With a mean survival time shorter than the mean survival postoperatively for a first gastrointestinal metastasis, some patients have survived for up to 1 year postoperatively, and most have obtained complete relief of gastrointestinal symptoms.[11]

Prognostic factors for survival

The gastrointestinal tract as the initial site of distant metastases, complete resection of gastrointestinal tract metastases, absence of small bowel involvement, metastases at a single site in the gastrointestinal tract, absence of other visceral metastatic disease, adjuvant treatment, disease-free interval >2 years between diagnosis of the primary melanoma and development of gastrointestinal metastases, and a normal level of LDH, have all been mentioned as favourable prognostic factors for survival.[9] However, most of these data were derived from small series, making use of univariate analysis, and confirmation in larger studies using multivariate analysis techniques is required.

Conclusions

In the absence of effective systemic treatment, surgical intervention in selected patients with gastrointestinal metastases from melanoma must be considered as a worthwhile treatment modality. Surgical treatment for symptomatic metastases of melanoma to the gastrointestinal tract offers effective palliation and, in a subset of patients who are rendered disease free, an increase in mean survival time. It is therefore justified in the majority of these patients.

OTHER INTRAABDOMINAL METASTASES

Pancreatic metastases

Though present in more than half of autopsy cases, pancreatic metastases rarely cause symptoms. Only symptomatic lesions should be considered for treatment. Short-term responses have been reported from chemotherapy and radiotherapy. In a few instances, surgical bypass procedures and even pancreaticoduodenectomy have been performed for this patient subgroup. However, this cannot usually be advocated, except in exceptional circumstances.[1]

Splenic metastases

The majority of patients with splenic metastases will also have concomitant synchronous pancreatic or liver spread. Rarely do patients present with haemorrhage from ruptured metastases. In some situations, however, splenectomy may be useful for patients with symptomatic isolated metastases.[1,26–28]

Urinary tract metastases

Only symptomatic or solitary lesions should be considered for treatment and, even then, the severity of symptomatology in relation to the patient's total body tumour load should be evaluated before any surgical treatment is contemplated.[29–31] Renal and bladder metastases commonly occur as multiple deposits and are rarely symptomatic until terminal stages of the disease are reached. A wide spectrum of symptoms can be present. Useful screening tests are physical examination and urinalysis.[32] Despite surgical resection, patient survival is only 4 months. Radiotherapy and chemotherapy are not often useful in these cases.[29–31]

Adrenal gland metastases

Of all the endocrine glands, the adrenal glands are the ones most frequently involved in metastatic melanoma. Metastases in the adrenal glands are reported in 11% of living patients but are present in up to 50% of patients at autopsy.[1] Metastatic disease to the adrenal gland may be unilateral or bilateral. The metastases are variable in size and appearance, but are usually rounded, measuring between 4 and 6 cm in diameter. If the possibility of surgery is entertained, only patients with symptomatic lesions should generally be considered as possible candidates. Radiotherapy or chemotherapy can also serve to palliate some symptoms.[1]

Metastases to the ovary

The diagnosis of melanoma metastatic to the ovary is seldom made in living patients, although *c.* 20% of patients dying of melanoma have ovarian involvement at post-mortem examination. Like gastrointestinal metastatic melanoma, this is because most of these patients have multiorgan metastases and therefore the involvement of the ovary is not clinically significant. Melanoma metastatic to the ovary should be suspected in any patient who presents with an adnexal mass and a history of melanoma. Metastatic melanoma in the ovary may be discovered many years after the diagnosis of the primary lesion. Melanoma metastatic to the vagina, uterus and ovaries can be amenable to surgical excision or irradiation in certain cases. Survival times of up to 2.5 years after diagnosis have been reported following resection. The optimal surgical management has been a subject of debate and has not yet been established. Although total abdominal hysterectomy and bilateral salpingo-oophorectomy has been recommended as the surgical treatment of choice, it seems that unilateral salpingo-oophorectomy is an appropriate and adequate surgical treatment if there is no evidence of involvement of the contralateral ovary. Adjuvant chemo-immunotherapy has recently been applied, but there is no definite evidence that it is beneficial.[33]

Conclusions

For melanoma metastatic to the pancreas and non-gastrointestinal intraabdominal organs like the spleen, the urinary tract, the adrenal glands and the ovary, there is sometimes, and only in selected cases, an indication for surgery. Other treatment options such as radiotherapy and immunochemotherapy can sometimes be useful to palliate symptoms.

REFERENCES

1. Sharpless SM, Das Gupta TK, Surgery for metastatic melanoma. *Semin Surg Oncol* 198; 311–18.
2. Capizzi PJ, Donohue JH, Metastatic melanoma of the gastrointestinal tract: a review of the literature. *Comp Ther* 1994; 20: 20–23.
3. Murphy MN, Lorimer SM, Glennon PE, Metastatic melanoma of the gallbladder: a case report and review of the literature. *J Surg Oncol* 1987; 34: 68–72.
4. MacBeth WASG, Gwynne JF, Jamieson MG, Metastatic melanoma in the small bowel. *Aust NZ J Surg* 1969; 38: 309–15.
5. Morini S, Bassi O, Covolpe V, Malignant melanoma metastatic to the stomach: endoscopic diagnosis and findings. *Endoscopy* 1980; 12: 86–9.
6. Das Gupta TK, Brasfield RD, Metastatic melanoma of the gastrointestinal tract. *Arch Surg* 1964; 88: 969–73.
7. Sharpless SM, Das Gupta TK, Surgery for metastatic melanoma. *Semin Surg Oncol* 1998; 14: 311–18.
8. Adair C, Ro JY, Sahin AA et al, Malignant melanoma metastatic to the gastrointestinal tract: a clinicopathologic study. *Int J Surg Pathol* 1994; 2: 3–10.
9. Agrawal S, Tzy-Jyun Y, Coit DG, Surgery for melanoma metastatic to the gastrointestinal tract. *Ann Surg Oncol* 1999; 6: 336–44.
10. Klaase JM, Kroon BBR, Surgery for melanoma metastatic to the gastrointestinal tract. *Br J Surg* 1990; 77: 60–1.
11. Khadra MR, Thompson JF, Milton GW, McCarthy WH, The justification for surgical treatment of metastatic melanoma of the gastrointestinal tract. *Surg Gynecol Obstet* 1990; 171: 413–16.
12. Berger AC, Buell JF, Venzon D et al, Management of symptomatic malignant melanoma of the gastrointestinal tract. *Ann Surg Oncol* 1999; 6: 155–60.
13. Barth A, Wanek LA, Morton DL, Prognostic factors in 1,521 melanoma patients with distant metastases. *J Am Coll Surg* 1995; 181: 193–201.
14. Hena MA, Emrich LJ, Nambisan RN, Karakousis CP, Effect of surgical treatment on stage IV melanoma. *Am J Surg* 1987; 153: 270–5.
15. Reintgen DR, Surgery for melanoma metastatic to the gastrointestinal tract. Editorial. *Ann Surg Oncol* 1999; 6: 325.
16. Ollila DW, Essner R, Wanek LA, Morton DL, Surgical resection for melanoma metastatic to the gastrointestinal tract. *Arch Surg* 1996; 131: 975–80.
17. Klausner JM, Skornick Y, Lelcuk S et al, Acute complications of metastatic melanoma of the gastrointestinal tract. *Br J Surg* 1982; 69: 195–6.
18. Balch CM, Palliative surgery for stage IV melanoma: is it a primary treatment? *Ann Surg Oncol* 1999; 7: 623–4.
19. Gross E, Hartmann W, Eigler FW, Intraabdominelle melanommetastasen und ihre prognose. *Chirurg* 1981; 52: 89–92.
20. McDermott VG, Low VHS, Keogan MT et al, Malignant melanoma metastatic to the gastrointestinal tract. *Am J Roentgenol* 1996; 166: 809–13.
21. Berman C, Reintgen D, Radiologic imaging in malignant melanoma: a review. *Semin Surg Oncol* 1993; 9: 232–8.
22. Hsu CC, Chen JJ, Chagchien CS, Endoscopic features of metastatic tumors in the upper gastrointestinal tract. *Endoscopy* 1996; 28: 249–53.
23. Kamel IR, Kruskal JB, Gramm HF, Imaging of abdominal manifestations of melanoma. *Crit Rev Diagn Imaging* 1998; 39: 447–86.
24. Holder WD, White RL, Zuger JH et al, Effectiveness of positron emission tomography for the detection of melanoma metastases. *Ann Surg* 1998; 227: 764–71.
25. Klein ES, Davidson B, Apter S et al, Total abdominal perfusion (TAP) in the treatment of abdominal metastatic melanoma. *J Surg Oncol* 1994; 57: 134–7.
26. Kyzer S, Koren R, Klein B, Chaimoff C, Giant splenomegaly caused by splenic metastases of melanoma. *Eur J Surg Oncol* 1998; 24: 336–7.
27. Buzbee TM, Legha SS, Spontaneous rupture of spleen in a patient with splenic metastasis of melanoma. A case report. *Tumori* 1992; 78: 47–8.
28. de Wilt JHW, Thompson JF, McCarthy WH, Surgical treatment of metastatic melanoma of the spleen. *Melanoma Res* 2001; 11: S214.
29. Torok P, Kiss T, Multiple metastases of a malignant cutaneous melanoma in the cavitary system of the upper urinary tract. *Int J Urol Nephrol* 1997; 29: 19–24.
30. Bolkier M, Lichting YG, Levin DR, Metastatic malignant melanoma of the kidney. *Urol Int* 1986; 41: 307–8.
31. Lenisa L, Tragni G, Belli F et al, Solitary melanoma metastasis of the kidney: a case report. *Tumori* 1996; 82: 614–15.
32. Zogno C, Schiaffino E, Boeri R, Schmid C, Cytologic detection of metastatic malignant melanoma in urine. *Acta Cytol* 1997; 41: 1332–6.
33. Piura B, Kedar I, Ariad S et al, Malignant melanoma metastatic to the ovary. *Gynecol Oncol* 1998; 68: 201–5.
34. Ricaniadis N, Lonstadoulakis MM, Walsh D, Karakousis CP, Gastrointestinal metastases from malignant melanoma. *Surg Oncol* 1995; 4: 105–10.
35. Reintgen DS, Thompson W, Garbutt J, Seigler HF, Radiologic, endoscopic, and surgical considerations of melanoma metastatic to the gastrointestinal tract. *Surgery* 1984; 95: 635–9.
36. Overett TK, Shiu MH, Surgical treatment of distant metastatic melanoma. Indications and results. *Cancer* 1985; 56: 1222–30.
37. Caputy GC, Donohue JH, Goellner JR, Weaver AL, Metastatic melanoma of the gastrointestinal tract. Results of surgical management. *Arch Surg* 1991; 126: 1353–8.
38. Ihde JK, Coit DG, Melanoma metastatic to stomach, small bowel, or colon. *Am J Surg* 1991; 162: 208–11.

50

Cerebral melanoma metastases

Graham Stevens, Kate Fife

INTRODUCTION

Involvement of the central nervous system is a frequent manifestation in patients with metastatic melanoma. For most patients this signifies the terminal stage of the disease, with survival usually measured in months. For the vast majority of these patients, management is palliative. The goals of treatment in this setting are to alleviate symptoms resulting from impairment of neurological function and to increase survival. Treatment with curative intent is rarely appropriate but is an important consideration for a highly selected minority of patients.

This chapter commences with a brief account of the incidence of cerebral metastases. This is followed by a summary of the Sydney Melanoma Unit (SMU) experience of cerebral metastases, to provide a backdrop for the subsequent sections concerning particular aspects of patient management.

INCIDENCE

Melanoma ranks third in the incidence of cerebral metastases, behind lung and breast.[1] Up to 75% of all patients with metastatic melanoma develop brain metastases and they are the direct cause of death in 50% of these patients.[2–4] Post-mortem studies indicate that up to 75% of patients with metastatic melanoma harbour brain metastases.[5] This implies that many patients succumb to extracranial metastases before their brain metastases become symptomatic. Therefore, if effective agents become available to control extracranial melanoma, the numbers of patients requiring effective treatment of brain metastases will increase dramatically. It is evident that the management of cerebral metastases from melanoma represents a major issue in melanoma management programmes.

Cerebral metastases are diagnosed following investigation of neurological symptoms, or as a prerequisite for entry into clinical trials, in patients who are intact neurologically. There is no indication for routine brain scans in the follow-up of asymptomatic patients with a past history of melanoma. Cerebral metastases are single in 20–50% of patients and multiple (up to hundreds) in the remainder. There is a predilection for the cerebral hemispheres, but any part of the central nervous system may be involved. Symptoms will vary accordingly. Melanoma brain metastases are frequently haemorrhagic and are second only to choriocarcinoma in the incidence of this complication.[6,7] There is a strong positive correlation between the number of cerebral metastases and the presence of extracranial disease.[8]

Cerebral spread may become apparent at any time during the course of the disease. Patients with a history of a primary melanoma may present with cerebral metastasis as the initial metastatic site. Brain metastasis may also be the first manifestation of melanoma with an occult primary melanoma. One-fifth of patients with metastatic melanoma have the brain as the initial site of metastasis. At the other end of the spectrum, cerebral spread may be the final step in a long history of recurrent or metastatic melanoma. The time from the primary lesion to brain metastasis is logarithmic,[9] bearing no correlation with the depth of the primary melanoma.[8] An increased incidence of brain metastases has been reported with: male gender; head and neck, mucosal or acrolentiginous primary sites; and thick or ulcerated lesions.[10] Commercial airline pilots have a high incidence of melanoma, which is probably related to lifestyle (recreational sun exposure) rather than cosmic radiation.[11] The possibility of sudden neurological deterioration from cerebral metastasis in pilots with a history of melanoma has been addressed.[12] A high incidence has been reported in children with melanoma.[13]

All primary melanomas are potential sources of cerebral metastases. It appears that cerebral metastases result from specific clonal elements within the primary melanoma that have an affinity for neural tissue.[14] It is likely that further investigation of the mechanisms of implantation, angiogenesis and subsequent growth of cerebral metastases will provide novel possibilities for therapeutic intervention.[15]

SYDNEY MELANOMA UNIT (SMU) DATABASE OF CEREBRAL METASTASES

The SMU database was updated in 2001 with respect to patients with cerebral metastases. During the years 1952–2000, 1137 patients who had cerebral metastases were identified in the entire database of *c.* 19,000 patients. Due to the extended time of accrual, there are some missing data. The main patient and tumour characteristics are listed in Table 50.1. Of particular note are the extremely wide ranges recorded for patient age, primary melanoma thickness and time interval from the primary diagnosis to diagnosis of cerebral metastasis. A single cerebral metastasis was present in 30% of patients. The vast majority had extracranial disease, usually in multiple sites. Only 8% of patients had isolated cerebral disease. Management of cerebral disease was surgery in 112 patients, surgery plus postoperative whole-brain radiotherapy (WBRT) in 170 patients, WBRT only in 276 patients and supportive care alone in the remainder.

At the time of analysis, 95% of patients had died of melanoma. The median survival from the time of diagnosis of cerebral metastases was 3.3 months, with a range of 0–25.7 years. Median survival increased with aggressiveness of treatment of cerebral metastases and ranged from 2–9 months (Table 50.2). When a multivariate analysis was performed to identify variables influencing survival, the significant variables for an improved outcome were: treatment with surgery and/or radiation; younger age at diagnosis of cerebral metastases; longer disease-free interval; and lack of active extracerebral metastases. However, as this was a

Table 50.1 *Patient and primary melanoma characteristics*

Gender	
Male	750 (66%)
Female	387 (34%)
Breslow thickness of primary melanoma (768 patients)	2.3 mm (range 0.1–14 mm)
Age at diagnosis of primary	50 years (range 10–89 years of age)
Age at diagnosis of brain metastases	53 years (range 11–90 years of age)
Time from primary to brain metastases	33 months (range 0–40.6 years)
Number of brain metastases	
Solitary	340 (30%)
Multiple	356 (31%)
Unknown	441 (39%)
Other sites of metastases (710 patients)	
None	8%
Active local or regional melanoma	21%
Lung	14%
Other sites	8%
Multiple sites	49%

Table 50.2 *Survival according to treatment*

Treatment	No. (%)*	Median survival (months)
Supportive care	537 (49)	1.9
Radiotherapy alone	276 (25)	3.7
Surgery alone	112 (10)	7.1
Surgery and radiotherapy	170 (16)	9.2

*For 1095 patients with known treatment.

retrospective series, there was undoubtedly a strong selection bias in patient management.

It is of interest to compare this series with 702 patients with cerebral metastases published from the Duke University melanoma database of almost 7000 patients.[10] Patient and tumour characteristics (median age at primary melanoma diagnosis 48 years, median time from primary melanoma to cerebral disease 3.7 years, median primary melanoma thickness 2.8 mm, single cerebral lesion in 39% of patients and visceral metastases in 46% of patients) were all very similar to the SMU data. Outcome was also very similar; the median survival was 3.7 months in the Duke series and 95% died as a consequence of brain metastases. The few 3-year survivors had single cerebral lesions which were resected.

MANAGEMENT OF MULTIPLE CEREBRAL METASTASES

Unfortunately, the majority of patients with metastatic cerebral melanoma are found to have multiple metastases. Extracranial metastases will be present in the majority. In this setting, steroids and WBRT are the mainstays of treatment. Other management options are the treatment of individual lesions by surgery or focused irradiation, and the use of chemotherapy, usually in combination with irradiation.

Role of surgery

Aggressive treatment of individual brain metastases is rarely indicated for these patients. However, surgical resection of a dominant, symptomatic lesion may be undertaken. An example is evacuation of clot following haemorrhage, which is a common complication of melanoma metastases.[16] This is appropriate in highly selected cases. An additional indication for surgery is to obtain a diagnosis when cerebral metastases are the initial presentation of malignancy. The value of this procedure depends on an assessment as to whether the individual patient's management will be affected by knowledge of the histopathology.

Whole-brain radiation therapy (WBRT)

Prompt initiation of high-dose corticosteroid therapy (12–16 mg of dexamethasone daily) will usually lead to a marked improvement in neurological status. Symptomatic response to steroids has significant prognostic value, independent of the amount of surrounding oedema.[1] This is followed by WBRT, unless the patient has a poor performance status. Improvement in neurological function is reported in *c.* 70% of patients following irradiation, with up to 90% of specific neurological symptoms responding.[17,18] Median durations of improvement are *c.* 3 months.

The advantages of steroids plus WBRT when compared with steroids alone are:

- Improved survival – median survivals for steroids alone are 1–2 months (Table 50.2),[19] compared with 2–9 months for the addition of WBRT (see below). These differences may simply reflect patient selection, as there have not been any randomized trials comparing these options.
- The potential to decrease steroid dosage, with a reduction of steroid-related symptoms. Cessation of steroids is possible in *c.* 50% of patients.[20]

The optimal dose schedule for WBRT remains uncertain. The subject has been investigated extensively, predominantly in retrospective series.[8,9,20–26] Survival has been the most common end point, as post-treatment imaging is infrequent. There are few randomized studies and dose schedules vary widely, in relation to both total dose and dose per fraction. Of particular interest is the effect of dose per fraction, as both in vitro and clinical studies have suggested an improved response using hypofractionated, high dose per fraction schedules (see Chapter 51). Most studies have not shown a difference in response according to schedule.[8,9,24,26,27] Survivals of 2–3 months were found for patients treated using either 6 gray (Gy) fractions (to a total of

24–36 Gy) or 1.2–4 Gy fractions (up to 60 Gy).[27] Similarly, there was no survival advantage to treatment using 30–36 Gy in six fractions compared with the standard schedule of 30 Gy in 10 fractions.[24] However, a significant survival difference (9 versus 2 months) was demonstrated according to total dose of ≤30 Gy or >30 Gy (normalized to ten 3 Gy equivalent fractions).[25] An advantage of accelerated fractionation was found in a favourable subgroup in another retrospective series, suggesting the importance of accelerated repopulation.[9]

Median survivals in all these studies are within the range of 2–9 months, with essentially no long-term survivors. Almost all patients with long-term survival were characterized by complete excision of a single metastasis. Treatment schedules of 20 Gy in five fractions over 1 week of 30 Gy in 10 fractions over 2 weeks were standard. Death was due to progressive intracranial melanoma in most cases. Overall, and in keeping with multiple studies of WBRT for brain metastases from various tumour types, no advantage was demonstrated for more intensive treatments in melanoma. Therefore, it is apparent that the doses of radiation that can be delivered to the whole brain are insufficient to control all except the most radiosensitive tumours.

Stereotactic radiosurgery (SRS)

SRS has been used in the treatment of multiple melanoma metastases with encouraging results.[28–30] Whilst these patients were undoubtedly highly selected, the reported local control rates of *c.* 90% and median survivals of 8 months are impressive.[30] Many centres offering SRS for cerebral metastases impose a limit of two or three lesions, although SRS treatment of multiple lesions has been reported.[31] At the SMU, patients accepted for SRS had good performance status, little or no extracranial disease and a maximum of three cerebral lesions (<3 cm maximum diameter), which were progressive after previous WBRT.

The traditional management of multiple brain metastases with steroids and WBRT is being challenged in favour of more aggressive treatment for some patients. In a small randomized trial of WBRT versus WBRT plus SRS boost for patients with two to four cerebral metastases from a range of tumour sites, local control at the metastatic sites was 0% in the WBRT arm, compared with 92% in the SRS arm. Intracranial control was significantly better in the SRS arm, although there was little difference in survivals (7 versus 11 months).[32] If effective treatment of multiple metastases can be achieved with SRS, survival may be improved.[33] This is the subject of several ongoing trials.

Radiation strategies – investigational

Inability to control intracranial disease in the setting of multiple cerebral metastases is a major obstacle to improving the treatment of patients with metastatic melanoma. The use of more intensive radiation schedules has failed to improve short survivals and there are occasional reports of severe, radiation-induced neurotoxicity. It is evident that the therapeutic ratio will not be improved by a further increase in the dose of WBRT.

Efforts to increase the radiation dose selectively to cerebral metastases have included boron-neutron capture therapy (BNCT) and alpha target therapy. In both cases, an inactive carrier moiety with affinity for melanoma cells is used to deliver the active agent into the melanoma cell. For BNCT, the carrier is usually a melanin precursor which is tagged with boron-10 (^{10}B). This should accumulate preferentially in melanin-producing cells, including melanomas. On irradiation with thermal neturons, ^{10}B absorbs a neutron; ^{11}B is unstable and decays with the release of highly damaging, short-range particles (^{7}Li and ^{4}He). In this manner, damage is confined to the approximate diameter of one cell.[34] Some clinical responses have been observed.[35]

In alpha target therapy, the inert carrier is methylene blue, which has a high affinity for melanin. It is tagged with a radioactive isotope. For therapy, the isotope is an α emitter, which also is highly damaging and has a very short range. Preclinical studies have been very encouraging.[36]

SYSTEMIC THERAPY

The poor overall response to conventional treatment with WBRT has led to the investigation of chemotherapy, alone or in combination with radiation. Unfortunately, metastatic melanoma is also usually poorly responsive to systemic agents. However, there have been several reports of interest in relation to cerebral metastases. Response rates of 28 and 12%, respectively, were reported using the nitrosourea fotemustine, either alone[37] or in combination with dacarbazine (DTIC).[38] Temozolomide (TMZ) is an alkylating agent that is able to cross the blood–brain barrier due to its small size and lipophilic nature. Within the brain, it is converted to the active metabolite at *c.* 30% of plasma concentrations. TMZ has been shown to be as effective as DTIC for cerebral metastases.[39] Encouraging results have also been reported with the combination of TMZ and thalidomide.[40] A report of the successful use of interleukin (IL)-2-based therapy for tumours expressing the *P*-glycoprotein pump as a cause of multidrug resistence illustrates the potential role of tailoring therapy to intrinsic tumour properties.[41] The need for this approach is evident; a protocol using cisplatin and etoposide, which had a 38% complete response rate in brain metastases from breast cancer, was ineffective (zero of eight responses) in melanoma.[42]

The combination of systemic agents and radiation has been investigated by several groups. The agents used have included cisplatin,[43] tirapazamine[44] and fotemustine.[45] Although some encouraging responses have been observed (complete responses in 10 of 55 patients with cisplatin and four of 12 patients with fotemustine plus radiation), these methods have remained investigational and have not been compared with radiation alone.

MANAGEMENT OF LIMITED CEREBRAL METASTASES

Up to 50% of patients with cerebral melanoma have only one or two cerebral metastases demonstrated on imaging. These patients, unlike those with multiple cerebral lesions, are less likely to have extracranial metastases. Therefore, aggressive treatment of cerebral metastases, aimed to achieve intracranial disease control, becomes an attractive and appropriate management strategy. Further, as progressive intracranial melanoma is the cause of death in at least 50% of patients with cerebral metastases, control of intracranial melanoma brings with it the possibility of prolonged survival.

With the potential for significantly improved survival, the long-term consequences of treatment modalities become important and relevant considerations. These management issues reach their ultimate consideration in the patient with a solitary cerebral metastasis (see below).

The options for intensive, ablative therapy of individual lesions are surgical resection and SRS; these may be complemented by adjuvant WBRT. Combinations of these modalities have been investigated in both randomized trials and retrospective series.

Surgery

Surgical resection has been the long-standing and predominant modality for local treatment.[46] Patients offered surgery have been highly selected on the basis of factors such as: good general medical status (and anaesthetic risk); limited extent of extracranial metastatic disease (generally excluding hepatic metastases); slow progression of disease; and one or two cerebral lesions (preferably single) located in non-eloquent brain. In contrast to the other local therapy, SRS, surgical extirpation of tumour and clot has advantages of immediate relief of symptoms caused by mass effect and pressure, and confirmation of histopathology. (It was found that 11% of cerebral lesions in patients with known primary malignancies were different tumours or inflammatory processes.[47])

A recent analysis of patients undergoing resection of melanoma brain metastases from the SMU illustrates these features. Over a 20-year period (1979–1999), 147 patients had resection of cerebral metastases from melanoma. This represents the largest series of resection from a single institution. Patients had a mean age of 53 years; 84% of patients had a single cerebral lesion and 56% of patients had extracranial metastases. Most received postoperative WBRT using a schedule of 30 Gy in 10 fractions. Operative mortality was 2%.

The median survival was 8.5 months and 5% of patients survived for 5 years. The median survivals according to number of cerebral metastases is shown in Table 50.3. All long-term survivors had a single resected cerebral metastasis. Of the 23 patients with more than

Table 50.3 ***Survival according to number of cerebral metastases in Sydney Melanoma Unit (SMU) resection series***

No. of cerebral metastases	Median survival (months)
1	9.0
2	6.0
3	3.5

one cerebral lesion, only one survived for 2 years. Progressive cerebral metastases were the cause of death in 25% of patients, with the remainder succumbing to extracranial melanoma. This is the same percentage as that reported for SRS,[48] suggesting similarity in local control rates for the two modalities.

These results are similar to the median survival and 5-year survival rates of 6.7 months and 6%, respectively, in a series of 91 patients from Memorial Sloan–Kettering.[49] The operative mortality was 5%. In this series, infratentorial location of the metastasis carried a worse prognosis. Survival and intracranial recurrence (*c*. 50%) were similar whether patients received WBRT or not.

A prognostic factor that has emerged from the SMU data and other retrospective studies has been the importance of the adequacy of resection.[8,50] Outcomes of patients having incomplete resection or debulking surgery were similar to biopsy alone. Whilst this observation may be related in part to the size of the metastasis, it suggests that debulking may not be a valid goal. In a small series of single cerebral metastases from melanoma, there were no local recurrences in 10 patients whose resection was en bloc.[51]

Non-randomized comparison in melanoma suggests that survival is improved by the addition of resection to WBRT alone. In the SMU database, survival increased from 4 months for WBRT to 9 months for surgery plus WBRT (Table 50.2). In smaller reports of 77[23] and 87[20] patients, overall median survivals in both studies were 4 and 5 months for WBRT and resection plus WBRT, respectively. The survivals for patients who underwent resection of all brain metastases was 9 months in both series. No improved survival was observed in patients with solitary brain metastasis treated by radiotherapy alone.[23] Conversely, survivals of 16 months (surgery plus WBRT) and 4 months (WBRT alone) have been reported.[24] Once again, these variable results presumably relate to selection bias.

Randomized trials assessing the value of adding surgical resection to WBRT have generally shown improved intracranial disease control, but without a survival benefit.[47,52,53] These trials have not been restricted to melanoma. In a series of 740 patients with cerebral metastases, including melanoma, survival at 5 years was correlated strongly with a solitary metastasis treated by resection plus WBRT.[54]

Radiosurgery

Until recently, surgical resection was the only potentially ablative treatment. Over the past decade, however, focused irradiation has become more widely available. The concepts and technology of focused irradiation are summarized in Box 50.1.

Most treatments have used SRS to deliver a high single dose to the lesion. Local control rates, defined as non-progression of the lesion, are quoted at 80–90% for a range of tumour types, including melanoma.[29,48,30,55,56] In a retrospective study of patients with non-radiosensitive tumour types, who had operable cerebral metastases but who were treated instead with SRS plus WBRT, the local control rate was 86%.[48] Excellent response rates are seen with tumours such as melanoma and renal cell carcinoma, which are frequently less responsive to fractionated schedules.[33] As these results are comparable to recent randomized trials of resection plus WBRT, there is considerable discussion of the relative merits of each. SRS has become an attractive alternative for patients with suitable lesions, as it is performed as an outpatient procedure and does not require general anaesthesia. There is an ongoing ECOG randomized comparison of SRS versus surgery for lesions suitable for either technique.[57] This will be an important trial, given the ease with which SRS is delivered. A utility and cost-effectiveness comparison between surgery and SRS for single brain metastases suitable for treatment by either modality showed similar outcomes for quality of life and survival, but that surgery was more expensive by a factor of 1.8 (in a US study).[58] Replacement of SRS by a hypofractionated course of stereotactic radiation therapy (SRT) has also been suggested, based on biological and costing models.[59]

The main limitation of SRS is the size of the lesion. For lesions 1–2 cm in diameter, there is very rapid fall-off of radiation dose outside the lesion, such that high doses can be delivered safely. For lesions >3 cm in diameter, dose fall-off is more gradual; this implies a compromise, with either a lower target dose or a greater risk of complications in the surrounding brain. For melanoma, the response rate was found to be highly dependent on the target volume and independent of the dose.[30] Using a median dose of 18 Gy to the 80% isodose surface, response rates for melanoma metastases were 58 and 11%, respectively, for lesions >1 cm and

Box 50.1 ***Focused irradiation***

Definition: Also called stereotactic irradiation. Irradiation techniques developed to deliver high doses of radiation with great precision to carefully defined intracranial targets using a series of non-coplanar beams. If the dose is delivered in a single fraction, the term stereotactic radiosurgery (SRS) is used. If the dose is delivered as a series of fractions, the term stereotactic radiotherapy (SRT) is used.

Techniques: There are two basic techniques for delivery of radiation. These are based on either the Gammaknife or linear accelerators.

The *Gammaknife* consists of a large number of cobalt-60 radioactive sources which are highly collimated such that the beams from all sources focus onto the same isocentre. SRS treatment is delivered by the Gammaknife.

Linear accelerator-based treatment uses a series of non-coplanar arcs of radiation that all focus on the target at the isocentre. Linear accelerators can deliver either SRS or SRT. In all cases, the patient's head is fixed in a stereotactic frame and the target lesion is located by stereotactic coordinates. The frame is fitted using local anaesthetic.

Advantages: For lesions <3 cm in diameter, there is a very rapid and sharp fall-off in dose beyond the target volume. This means that very high single doses (up to 20–30 Gy) can be delivered to the tumour, with minimal risk of complications in surrounding brain. Doses of this magnitude cause necrosis of the tumour. Control rates for treated metastases are 80–90%, comparable to surgical series. As a craniotomy is not required, the acute risks of SRS and SRT are minimal, and the procedure is performed on an outpatient basis on a single day. It is possible to treat several lesions at the same procedure.

Limitations: The maximum size of lesions treated using stereotactic techniques is *c.* 3 cm in diameter. At greater sizes, an increasing volume of normal surrounding brain is irradiated, increasing the risk of brain necrosis. This size limitation is likely to be overcome by recent advances in radiation dose delivery, particularly intensity modulated radiation therapy (IMRT).

≤1 cm in diameter.[60] Reduction of the SRS dose from 15–16 Gy to 10 Gy, with the addition of WBRT (30 Gy in 10 fractions), led to a reduction in local control.[61] This is not surprising, given the significant dose reduction.

The complications of SRS are acute oedema and late brain necrosis. Oedema is usually self-limiting and controlled by steroids. Necrosis is irreversible and may be progressive, with severe mass effect requiring craniotomy. These adverse effects of SRS are often indistinguishable from tumour recurrence, both in symptomatology and timing after treatment. Distinction may be made by positron emission tomography (PET), magnetic resonance imaging (MRI) or biopsy.[62,63]

Whole-brain radiation therapy (WBRT)

WBRT may be used as an adjunct to localized treatment with either surgery or SRS, or as the sole treatment for cerebral metastases. The most controversial issue relates to the value of postoperative WBRT. This was assessed in a randomized trial of single cerebral lesions (mainly lung cancers), treated either by surgery alone or by surgery plus postoperative WBRT (50.4 Gy in 28 fractions).[64] Intracranial recurrence was markedly reduced at both the excision site and elsewhere in the WBRT group (70% for surgery alone versus 18% for addition of WBRT), with less mortality from progressive brain disease (44% for surgery alone versus 14% for addition of WBRT). Surprisingly, however, there was no difference in overall survival between the treatment arms.

Several non-randomized retrospective comparisons have been reported for melanoma. In 34 patients with resection of a single brain metastasis, nine of 10 patients having surgery alone had intracranial failure, compared with one of 22 patients who received adjuvant WBRT. Survival was improved for patients receiving WBRT.[4] In another small study, 35 patients underwent resection of a single brain metastasis. Death from brain metastases occurred in 85% of those patients receiving surgery alone and in 24% of patients who received postoperative WBRT. Survival was similar in both groups.[65] More recently, in a study of 91 patients, there was no difference in either intracranial recurrence (*c.* 50%) or survival (8–9 months) between those who received surgery alone or postoperative WBRT.[49]

A similar scenerio pertains to the use of WBRT following SRS. Although the concept of using WBRT to sterilize micrometastases outside the stereotactically treated volume is logical, the results of institutional studies have been varied and opinions have been divided regarding its value.[28,29,56,66–68] In retrospective comparisons of patients treated according to physician preference with either SRS alone or SRS plus WBRT, intracranial relapses have been higher in the group not receiving WBRT. In one series, cerebral relapses were 43% for SRS alone versus 22% for SRS plus WBRT. However, there was no survival difference (median *c.* 11 months), as many intracranial relapses could be salvaged.[29] It has been suggested that initial WBRT could be omitted for less than four or four brain metastases.[68] Conversely, the addition of WBRT improved survival for patients with no extracranial disease (8 months for SRS versus 15 months for SRS plus WBRT).[56]

An issue of considerable interest is the possible late neurotoxicity of WBRT. In adults, this manifests clinically as dementia. Atrophy and white matter changes are seen on imaging, and post-mortem studies show diffuse white matter spongiosis, axonal loss and areas of necrosis.[69,70] This is of particular importance in patients with a solitary cerebral metastasis, as they have the greatest potential for long-term survival. The optimal fractionation schedule for WBRT in this setting is uncertain, as both melanoma cell kill and late radiation toxicity have a similar dependence on the size of the dose per fraction as well as the total dose.

For patients with multiple brain metastases, WBRT is probably safe, due to their limited survival. Patients with brain metastases treated with 30 Gy in 10 daily fractions were assessed with the mini mental state examination (MMSE).[71] A score suggesting possible dementia was found in 16% of patients prior to WBRT. With a median survival of 4.2 months, there was no evidence of a reduction in the MMSE score to levels suggesting dementia. On the contrary, an improvement in MMSE was found in long-term survivors.

Of concern, however, is the treatment of patient cohorts with potentially longer survivals. A number of reports have charted the onset of dementia within months of brain irradiation.[69,70] Dementia, ataxia and incontinence commenced after 5 to 36 months in 12 patients who received WBRT using fraction sizes of 3–6 Gy to total doses of 25–39 Gy.[69] Severe dementia was reported in a patient who received WBRT of 45 Gy in 3 Gy fractions.[72] Although the reported cases of dementia represent <5% of treated patients in these series, there is likely to be a gross underestimation of milder cases.

The disparate results from these studies do not allow a firm recommendation to be made regarding the use of adjuvant WBRT following localized treatment with either surgery or SRS. Presumably, the differences between studies relate to patient selection. Based on the results of randomized trials that include melanoma, and show a reduction in intracranial relapse, the policy at the SMU has been to offer adjuvant postoperative WBRT to most patients. Exceptions are patients with either a very poor prognosis, in whom surgery was performed to palliate a distressing symptom, or younger patients with a single cerebral metastasis presenting after a long disease-free interval. Although severe neurotoxicity following WBRT has only been observed rarely, it may be devastating and fatal. The risk is increased with hypofractionation and it may occur within months of WBRT.

Solitary cerebral metastasis

A solitary cerebral metastasis is defined as a single cerebral metastasis in the absence of any other metastatic disease, either intra- or extracranially. This definition is highly dependent on the staging investigations, which have changed markedly over the years. In particular, the wider use of MRI brain scans and whole-body PET scans have improved the detection of metastatic disease. For example, in the SMU craniotomy series, a reduction in intracranial recurrence from 65 to 50% coincided with the availability of MRI brain scanning. Contrast-enhanced MRI brain scans have been reported as being more accurate than both unenhanced MRI and contrast-enhanced CT scanning.[73] The high sensitivity of PET body scans compared with structural imaging has influenced decisions regarding aggressive management.[74,75]

At the SMU, 37 patients who had resection of a single cerebral metastasis, followed by WBRT were identified over an 18-year period (1983–2000). No other metastatic disease was evident in any patient, although nine patients have had previous resection of extracranial metastases. The median survival was 13 months; the 2-, 5- and 10-year survival rates were 37, 20 and 14%, respectively. Surprisingly, those with previous resection of systemic metastases had improved survival. This may relate to selection of patients with more indolent disease. Of patients with disease progression, the brain was the initial site of relapse in *c.* 60%, with recurrence at the resection site identified in half of these cases.

MANAGEMENT OF RECURRENT CEREBRAL METASTASES

A small, highly selected subgroup of patients are considered for retreatment of recurrent cerebral metastases. Selection is multifactorial and is based on features including previous central nervous system treatment, performance status, and both extent and rate of progression of intra- and extracranial disease. The problem of accurate diagnosis of recurrent tumour was discussed above.

Reoperation has been reported as beneficial in selected cases. Reoperation in 48 patients who developed recurrent brain metastases at a median of 7 months from first craniotomy gave an additional median survival of 11.5 months. To facilitate decision-making, a grading scheme was devised, based on the above factors.[76] In the SMU surgical series of 147 patients, 24 patients had subsequent resection of recurrent cerebral disease, either at the initial site (14 patients) or elsewhere for new metastases (10 patients). The median time to reoperation was 8 months following initial surgical and WBRT, and median survival from reoperation was 6 months. Progressive intracranial disease was the direct cause of death in 50% of patients.

For patients whose previous central nervous system treatment had been resection or SRS alone, WBRT is appropriate for recurrent intracranial disease. In this setting, the value of further localized therapy must be individualized. Surgery or SRS may be appropriate for either a single cerebral lesion or a dominant lesion causing symptoms, and survivals of many months are reported.[30] The place of further localized treatment of recurrent disease following previous WBRT needs to be determined on an individual patient basis.

More frequently, there is widespread progression of cerebral metastases following previous WBRT. In most cases there is progressive systemic disease and further active treatment is inappropriate. However, for patients whose cerebral disease responded to initial WBRT and whose extracranial disease is quiescent, whole-brain re irradiation may be considered. In this setting, the high risk of radiation-induced dementia is usually acceptable, due to the anticipated short survival. For 86 patients re-irradiated with 20 Gy WBRT (following initial 30 Gy), 70% had improved in neurological symptoms. The median survival from re-irradiation was 4 months (range 1–72 months) and one patient became demented.[77]

CONCLUSIONS

Patients with cerebral metastases from melanoma present a wide range of management issues for the clinician. Those with multiple lesions and active extracranial disease should receive steroids and a short course of WBRT, as their median survival is a few months and there are almost no long-term survivors. As most patients will die as a direct consequence of uncontrolled intracranial disease, there is an urgent need for improved treatments, consisting of either systemic agents or selective tumour irradiation. The value of a more aggressive approach for patients with less than four metastases is under investigation.

Those patients with one or two cerebral metastases should be considered for more aggressive treatment, particularly if their extracranial disease is of small bulk and slowly progressive. Localized treatments with surgery or SRS appear to be equally effective in controlling individual lesions; each modality has distinct advantages and disadvantages. The use of adjuvant WBRT has not been resolved. Potential advantages to its use are improved intracranial tumour control and survival. Dementia is an uncommon but recognized complication. A randomized trial restricted to melanoma is required to resolve the value of WBRT.

The management of patients with recurrent cerebral metastatic disease is individualized. Further anticancer treatment is inappropriate for most, for whom supportive care is required. A small minority benefit from active treatment, in the form of further wide-field irradiation or localized treatment of specific lesions with surgery or SRS.

ACKNOWLEDGEMENTS

The authors wish to thank: Ms M Colman (Sydney Melanoma Unit) and Dr I Firth (Department of Radiation Oncology, Royal Prince Alfred Hospital) for their invaluable assistance in data collection and analysis; Associate Professor M Besser and Dr D McDowell (Department of Neurosurgery, Royal Prince Alfred Hospital) for critique and discussion regarding the patient management, and collaboration in the stereotactic radiation programme.

REFERENCES

1. Lagerwaard F, Levendag P, Nowak P et al, Identification of prognostic factors in patients with brain metastases: a review of 1292 patients. *Int J Radiat Oncol Biol Phys* 1999; 43: 795–803.
2. Amer MH, Al-Sarraf M, Baker LH, Vaitkevicius VK, Malignant melanoma and central nervous system metastases: incidence, diagnosis, treatment and survival. *Cancer* 1978; 42: 660–8.
3. Zimm S, Wampler GL, Stablein D et al, Intracerebral metastases in solid-tumor patients: natural history and results of treatment. *Cancer* 1981; 48: 384–94.
4. Skibber JM, Soong SJ, Austin L et al, Cranial irradiation after surgical excision of brain metastases in melanoma patients. *Ann Surg Oncol* 1996; 3: 118–23.
5. de la Monte S, Moore G, Hutchins G, Patterned distribution of metastases from malignant melanoma in humans. *Cancer Res* 1983; 43: 3427–33.
6. Byrne TN, Cascino TL, Posner JB, Brain metastasis from melanoma. *J Neurooncol* 1983; 1: 313–17.
7. Graus F, Rogers LR, Posner JB, Cerebrovascular complications in patients with cancer. *Medicine (Baltimore)* 1985; 64: 16–35.
8. Stevens G, Firth I, Coates A, Cerebral metastases from malignant melanoma. *Radiother Oncol* 1992; 23: 185–91.
9. Choi KN, Withers HR, Rotman M, Intracranial metastases from melanoma. Clinical features and treatment by accelerated fractionation. *Cancer* 1985; 56: 1–9.
10. Sampson JH, Carter JH, Friedman AH, Seigler HF, Demographics, prognosis, and therapy in 702 patients with brain metastases from malignant melanoma. *J Neurosurg* 1998; 88: 11–20.
11. Rafnsson V, Hrafnkelsson J, Tulinius H, Incidence of cancer among commercial airline pilots. *Occup Environ Med* 2000; 57: 175–9.
12. Gee MR, Pickard JS, Aeromedical decision-making for aviators with malignant melanoma: an update and review. *Aviat Space Environ Med* 2000; 71: 245–50.
13. Rodriguez-Galindo C, Pappo AS, Kaste SC et al, Brain metastases in children with melanoma. *Cancer* 1997; 79: 2440–5.
14. Fidler IJ, Schackert G, Zhang RD et al, The biology of melanoma brain metastasis. *Cancer Metastasis Rev* 1999; 18: 387–400.
15. Yano S, Shinohara H, Herbst RS et al, Expression of vascular endothelial growth factor is necessary but not sufficient for production and growth of brain metastasis. *Cancer Res* 2000; 60: 4959–67.
16. Maiuri F, D'Andrea F, Gallicchio B, Carandente M, Intracranial hemorrhages in metastatic brain tumors. *J Neurosurg Sci* 1985; 29: 37–41.
17. Borgelt B, Gelber R, Kramer S et al, The palliation of brain metastases: final results of the first two studies by the Radiation Therapy Oncology Group. *Int J Radiat Oncol Biol Phys* 1980; 6: 1–9.
18. Carella RJ, Gelber R, Hendrickson F et al, Value of radiation therapy in the management of patients with cerebral metastases from malignant melanoma: Radiation Therapy Oncology Group Brain Metastases Study I and II. *Cancer* 1980; 45: 679–83.
19. Madajewicz S, Karakousis C, West CR et al, Malignant melanoma brain metastases. Review of Roswell Park Memorial Institute experience. *Cancer* 1984; 53: 2550–2.
20. Ellerhorst J, Strom E, Nardone E, McCutcheon I, Whole brain irradiation for patients with metastatic melanoma: a review of 87 cases. *Int J Radiat Oncol Biol Phys* 2001; 49: 93–7.
21. Retsas S, Gershuny AR, Central nervous system involvement in malignant melanoma. *Cancer* 1988; 61: 1926–34.
22. Seegenschmiedt M, Keilholz L, Altendorf-Hofman A, et al, Palliative radiotherapy for recurrent and metastatic malignant melanoma: prognostic factors for tumour response and long-term outcome: a 20-year experience. *Int J Radiat Oncol Biol Phys* 1999; 44: 607–18.
23. Rate W, Solin L, Turrisi A, Palliative radiotherapy for metastatic malignant melanoma: brain metastases, bone metastases, and spinal cord compression. *Int J Radiat Oncol Biol Phys* 1988; 15: 859–64.
24. Katz H, The relative effectiveness of radiation therapy, corticosteroids and surgery in the management of melanoma metastatic to the central nervous system. *Int J Radiat Oncol Biol Phys* 1981; 7: 897–906.
25. Isokangas O, Mulhonen T, Kajanti M, Pyrhonen S, Radiation therapy of intracranial malignant melanoma. *Radiother Oncol* 1996; 38: 139–44.
26. Ziegler J, Cooper J, Brain metastases from malignant melanoma: conventional vs. high-dose-per-fraction radiotherapy. *Int J Radiat Oncol Biol Phys* 1986; 12: 1839–42.
27. Vlock DR, Kirkwood JM, Leutzinger C et al, High-dose fraction radiation therapy for intracranial metastases of malignant melanoma: a comparison with low-dose fraction therapy. *Cancer* 1982; 49: 2289–94.
28. Grob JJ, Regis J, Laurans R et al, Radiosurgery without whole brain radiotherapy in melanoma brain metastases. Club de Cancerologie Cutanee. *Eur J Cancer* 1998; 34: 1187–92.
29. Mori Y, Kondziolka D, Flickinger JC et al, Stereotactic radiosurgery for cerebral metastatic melanoma: factors affecting local disease control and survival. *Int J Radiat Oncol Biol Phys* 1998; 42: 581–9.
30. Seung SK, Sneed PK, McDermott MW et al, Gamma knife radiosurgery for malignant melanoma brain metastases. *Cancer J Sci Am* 1998; 4: 103–9.
31. Amendola BE, Wolf AL, Coy SR et al, Gamma knife radiosurgery in the treatment of patients with single and multiple brain metastases from carcinoma of the breast. *Cancer J* 2000; 6: 88–92.
32. Kondziolka D, Patel A, Lunsford LD et al, Stereotactic radiosurgery plus whole brain radiotherapy versus radiotherapy alone for patients with multiple brain metastases. *Int J Radiat Oncol Biol Phys* 1999; 45: 427–34.
33. Young RF, Radiosurgery for the treatment of brain metastases. *Semin Surg Oncol* 1998; 14: 70–8.
34. Hawthorne MF, New horizons for therapy based on the boron neutron capture reaction. *Mol Med Today* 1998; 4: 174–81.
35. Mishima Y, Kondoh H, Dual control of melanogenesis and melanoma growth: overview molecular to clinical level and the reverse. *Pigment Cell Res* 2000; 13 (Suppl 8): 10–22.
36. Link EM, Targeting melanoma with 211At/131I-methylene blue: preclinical and clinical experience. *Hybridoma* 1999; 18: 77–82.
37. Jacquillat C, Khayat D, Banzet P et al, Chemotherapy by fotemustine in cerebral metastases of disseminated malignant melanoma. *Cancer Chemother Pharmacol* 1990; 25: 263–6.
38. Chang J, Atkinson H, A'Hern R et al, A phase II study of the sequential administration of dacarbazine and fotemustine in the treatment of cerebral metastases from malignant melanoma. *Eur J Cancer* 1994; 30A: 2093–5.
39. Agarwala SS, Kirkwood JM, Temozolomide, a novel alkylating agent with activity in the central nervous system, may improve the treatment of advanced metastatic melanoma. *Oncologist* 2000; 5: 144–51.
40. Hwu WJ, New approaches in the treatment of metastatic melanoma: thalidomide and temozolomide. *Oncology (Huntingt)* 2000; 14 (12 Suppl 13): 25–8.
41. Savas B, Arslan G, Gelen T et al, Multidrug resistant malignant melanoma with intracranial metastasis responding to immunotherapy. *Anticancer Res* 1999; 19: 4413–20.
42. Franciosi V, Cocconi G, Michiara M et al, Front-line chemotherapy with cisplatin and etoposide for patients with brain metastases from breast carcinoma, nonsmall cell lung carcinoma, or malignant melanoma: a prospective study. *Cancer* 1999; 85: 1599–605.
43. Rosenthal MA, Bull CA, Coates AS et al, Synchronous cisplatin infusion during radiotherapy for the treatment of metastatic melanoma. *Eur J Cancer* 1991; 27: 1564–6.
44. Coates A, Stevens G, Johnston H, A phase I dose-finding study using tirapazamine concurrent with radiotherapy in patients with advanced metastatic melanoma. Clinical Oncology Society Australiasia, Annual Scientific Meeting, Perth, December 1997.
45. Ulrich J, Gademann G, Gollnick H, Management of cerebral metastases from malignant melanoma: results of a combined, simultaneous treatment with fotemustine and irradiation. *J Neurooncol* 1999; 43: 173–8.
46. Lang FF, Wildrick DM, Sawaya R, Management of cerebral metastases: the role of surgery. *Cancer Control* 1998; 5: 124–9.
47. Patchell RA, Tibbs PA, Walsh JW et al, A randomized trial of surgery in the treatment of single metastases to the brain. *N Engl J Med* 1990; 322: 494–500.
48. Auchter RM, Lamond JP, Alexander E et al, A multiinstitutional outcome and prognostic factor analysis of radiosurgery for resectable single brain metastasis. *Int J Radiat Oncol Biol Phys* 1996; 35: 27–35.

49. Wronski M, Arbit E, Surgical treatment of brain metastases from melanoma: a retrospective study of 91 patients. *J Neurosurg* 2000: 93: 9–18.
50. Overett TK, Shiu MH, Surgical treatment of distant metastatic melanoma. Indications and results. *Cancer* 1985; 56: 1222–30.
51. Salvati M, Cervoni L, Caruso R, Gagliardi FM, Solitary cerebral metastasis from melanoma: value of the 'en bloc' resection. *Clin Neurol Neurosurg* 1996; 98: 12–14.
52. Mintz AH, Kestle J, Rathbone MP et al, A randomized trial to assess the efficacy of surgery in addition to radiotherapy in patients with a single cerebral metastasis. *Cancer* 1996; 78: 1470–6.
53. Noordijk EM, Vecht CJ, Haaxma-Reiche H et al, The choice of treatment of single brain metastasis should be based on extracranial tumor activity and age. *Int J Radiat Oncol Biol Phys* 1994; 29: 711–17.
54. Hall WA, Djalilian HR, Nussbaum ES, Cho KH, Long-term survival with metastatic cancer to the brain. *Med Oncol* 2000; 17: 279–86.
55. Cho KH, Hall WA, Gerbi BJ et al, Patient selection criteria for the treatment of brain metastases with stereotactic radiosurgery. *J Neurooncol* 198; 40: 73–86.
56. Pirzkall A, Debus J, Lohr F et al, Radiosurgery alone or in combination with whole-brain radiotherapy for brain metastases. *J Clin Oncol* 1998; 16: 3563–9.
57. Shaw E, Radiotherapeutic management of multiple brain metastases: '3000 in 10' whole brain radiation is no longer a 'no brainer'. *Int J Radiat Oncol Biol Phys* 1999; 45: 253–4.
58. Mehta M, Noyes W, Craig B et al, A cost-effectiveness and cost-utility analysis of radiosurgery vs. resection for single-brain metastases. *Int J Radiat Oncol Biol Phys* 1997; 39: 445–54.
59. Manning MA, Cardinale RM, Benedict SH et al, Hypofractionated stereotactic radiotherapy as an alternative to radiosurgery for the treatment of patients with brain metastases. *Int J Radiat Oncol Biol Phys* 2000; 47: 603–8.
60. Gieger M, Wu JK, Ling MN et al, Response of intracranial melanoma metastases to stereotactic radiosurgery. *Radiat Oncol Invest* 1997; 5: 72–80.
61. Nieder C, Nestle U, Walter K et al, Dose–response relationships for radiotherapy of brain metastases: role of intermediate-dose stereotactic radiosurgery plus whole-brain radiotherapy. *Am J Clin Oncol* 2000; 23: 584–8.
62. Nelson SJ, Imaging of brain tumors after therapy. *Neuroimaging Clin North Am* 1999; 9: 801–19.
63. Nelson SJ, Vigneron DB, Dillon WP, Serial evaluation of patients with brain tumors using volume MRI and 3D 1H MRSI. NMR. *Biomedicine* 1999; 12: 123–38.
64. Patchell RA, Tibbs PA, Regine WF et al, Postoperative radiotherapy in the treatment of single metastases to the brain: a randomized trial. *JAMA* 1998; 280: 1485–9.
65. Hagen NA, Cirrincione C, Thaler HT, DeAngelis LM, The role of radiation therapy following resection of single brain metastasis from melanoma. *Neurology* 1990; 40: 158–60.
66. Vermeulen SS, Whole brain radiotherapy in the treatment of metastatic brain tumors. *Semin Surg Oncol* 1998; 14: 64–9.
67. Chidel MA, Suh JH, Reddy CA et al, Application of recursive partitioning analysis and evaluation of the use of whole brain radiation among patients treated with stereotactic radiosurgery for newly diagnosed brain metastases. *Int J Radiat Oncol Biol Phys* 2000; 47: 993–9.
68. Sneed PK, Lamborn KR, Forstner JM et al, Radiosurgery for brain metastases: is whole brain radiotherapy necessary? *Int J Radiat Oncol Biol Phys* 1999; 43: 549–58.
69. DeAngelis LM, Delattre JY, Posner JB, Radiation-induced dementia in patients cured of brain metastases. *Neurology* 1989; 39: 789–96.
70. Vigliani MC, Duyckaerts C, Hauw JJ et al, Dementia following treatment of brain tumors with radiotherapy administered alone or in combination with nitrosourea-based chemotherapy: a clinical and pathological study. *J Neurooncol* 1999; 41: 137–49.
71. Murray KJ, Scott C, Zachariah B et al, Importance of the mini-mental status examination in the treatment of patients with brain metastases: a report from the Radiation Therapy Oncology Group protocol 91-04. *Int J Radiat Oncol Biol Phys* 2000; 48: 59–64.
72. Hayakawa K, Yamakawa M, Mitsuhashi N et al, Radiotherapeutic management of brain metastases from breast cancer. *Breast Cancer* 1998; 5: 149–54.
73. Sze G, Milano E, Johnson C, Heier L, Detection of brain metastases: comparison of contrast-enhanced MR with unenhanced MR and enhanced CT. *AJNR Am J Neuroradiol* 1990; 11: 785–91.
74. Hicks RJ, Binns DS, Fawcett ME et al, Positron emission tomography (PET): experience with a large-field-of-view three-dimensional PET scanner. *Med J Aust* 1999; 171: 529–32.
75. Damian DL, Fulham MJ, Thompson E, Thompson JF, Positron emission tomography in the detection and management of metastatic melanoma. *Melanoma Res* 1996; 6: 325–9.
76. Bindal RK, Sawaya R, Leavens ME et al, Reoperation for recurrent metastatic brain tumors. *J Neurosurg* 1995; 83: 600–4.
77. Wong WW, Schild SE, Sawyer TE, Shaw EG, Analysis of outcome in patients reirradiated for brain metastases. *Int J Radiat Oncol Biol Phys* 1996; 34: 585–90.

51

Role of radiation therapy in metastatic melanoma: an overview

Graham Stevens

INTRODUCTION

The management of patients with metastatic melanoma presents the radiation oncologist with some of the most challenging problems in oncological practice. The protean pattern of dissemination, to almost any bodily tissue, and the poor response to systemic therapy combine to produce a wide range of distressing symptoms requiring local treatment. Further, the relative insensitivity of many melanomas to radiation and the unpredictable rate of progression of the disease demand that both acute and late tissue tolerances be respected.[1–3]

RADIATION BIOLOGY OF MELANOMA

The optimal dose fractionation for treatment of melanoma has been the subject of research and discussion for decades. Although the main issue has been centred around the optimal dose per fraction, the other parameters of dose scheduling (total dose and overall treatment time) have also been debated. The radiation sensitivity of melanoma was introduced in Chapter 35 in relation to postoperative adjuvant irradiation.

The early clinical reports were confusing. Paterson[4] and Adair[5] concluded that melanoma was insensitive to radiation, while Ellis[6] and Hellriegel[7] obtained some impressive and durable responses. Despite these highly variable results, melanoma gained a reputation as a radioresistant tumour.

An explanation for this radioresistance, and a possible method of circumventing it, were provided by the first in vitro studies with melanoma cell cultures, published by Dewey[8] and Barranco et al.[9] These showed that the single-dose radiation survival curves of several melanoma cell lines were characterized by an initial shoulder (high extrapolation number) that was larger than that found for non-melanoma cell lines. This was interpreted as representing a high capacity for repair. At higher doses the curve had a steep exponential component (low D_0), which was similar to other cell types. Dewey[8] suggested that individual doses >420 cGy (centigray) would be most effective in cell killing, as this would overcome the high repair capacity at lower doses.

These publications are particularly noteworthy for their impact on subsequent thinking that melanoma should be treated using large fractions which would overcome the high repair capacity at lower, more conventional doses. Interestingly, neither Dewey[8] nor Barranco et al.[9] attributed the clinical resistance of melanomas to their in vitro findings. Because the final slopes of their survival curves for melanoma were similar (D_0 = 80–100 rads) to other tumour types that were radioresponsive, they concluded that the reported poor clinical responses were not due to intrinsic radiosensitivity. As Dewey[8] stated: 'It therefore seems as if the reason for the clinical difficulties in curing malignant melanomas probably lies among factors other than the radioresistance of the melanoma cells'. Similarly, Barranco et al.[9] concluded that the differences between in vitro and in vivo responses were due to differences in cell cycling, growth fraction and hypoxia.

Subsequently, the retrospective clinical reports of Hornsey,[10] and Habermalz and Fischer,[11] showed better tumour control using fractions of 400–800 cGy. These studies confirmed the prevailing clinical impression of improved tumour responses using treatment schedules with a small number of large fractions.

The concept that high fractional doses were needed for adequate tumour control was reinforced in a number of publications by Overgaard's group throughout the 1980s.[12–17] They analysed treatment and response data of several hundred soft tissue lesions, and concluded that the dose per fraction was the only significant radiation parameter relating to tumour response. The complete response rate was 59% using fractional doses >400 cGy, compared with 33% for smaller doses.[15] In a small randomized study of two radiation treatment schedules, no differences were observed between three 9 Gy fractions and eight 5 Gy fractions with respect to tumour response or normal tissue damage.[13]

In terms of the linear–quadratic formulism, the survival curves derived for melanoma had low values of α/β, 0.6 Gy in the analysis of Overgaard's data,[16] implying a high sensitivity to the dose per fraction. This is represented graphically in Figure 51.1 as a curvier dose–response curve and quantitatively as a lower α/β ratio in the linear–quadratic mathematical model. However, the risks of late complications from radiation are also characterized by low α/β values. This similarity in the responses of both melanoma and the surrounding normal tissues implies a low potential for a therapeutic gain in the treatment of melanoma.

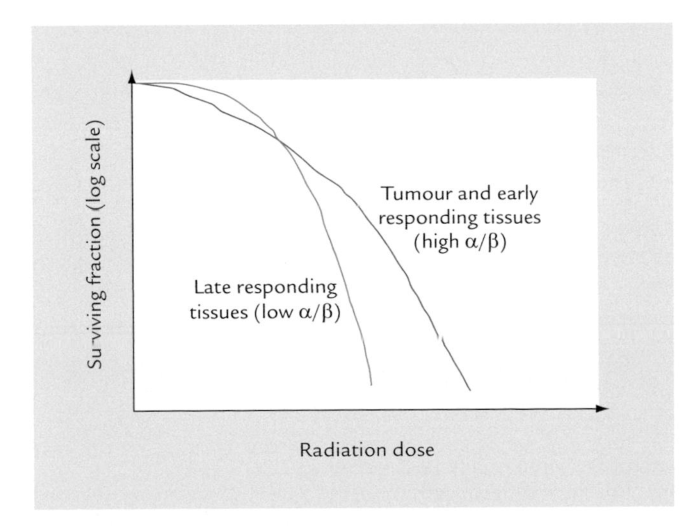

Figure 51.1 *Radiation survival curves for acute and late responding tissues. Some melanomas have curves similar to those of late responding tissues.*

In contrast, other clinical studies have not confirmed the superiority of hypofractionated schedules. Trott et al.[18] analysed the responses of 44 soft tissue lesions and found that overall treatment time, rather than size of dose per fraction, was the most important parameter. In support of the importance of overall time of treatment, Choi et al.[19] found improved survival in subsets of patients with melanoma brain metastases treated using accelerated whole-brain irradiation.

Of greater significance, the single randomized clinical study (RTOG 83-05) comparing hypofractionated and conventionally fractionated schedules failed to demonstrate a difference in either tumour response or in normal tissue toxicity.[20] The schedules were four 8 Gy fractions versus 20 2.5 Gy fractions, with 127 patients randomized. The complete (CR) and partial (PR) tumour response rates were very similar in both arms (CR 24 and 23%, and PR 35 and 34%, respectively). Similarly, as discussed in Chapter 35, local relapse rates following adjuvant postoperative irradiation were identical following conventional[21] or hypofractionated[22] radiation schedules.

Extensive laboratory studies of human melanoma cell lines and xenografts, particularly by Rofstad's group, have demonstrated that the cell survival curves for melanoma are heterogeneous and span the range from the most sensitive to the most resistant tumour types.[23–27] Metastatic lesions tend to be less radiosensitive than primary tumours in in vitro assays.[26] The explanation for this wide spectrum of responses is unknown but is currently under investigation.[28]

Overall, there is a loose correlation between laboratory measures of radiosensitivity (e.g. surviving fraction following 2 Gy (SF2)) and clinical radioresponsiveness for different tumour types. On these parameters, melanomas are, on average, less radiosensitive (i.e. higher SF2) and less radioresponsive than many other common tumour types.[29,30]

To improve the response of melanoma metastases, attempts have been made both to combine radiation with other modalities and to increase the radiation dose delivered to the melanoma cells. Hyperthermia has been demonstrated to be a very effective method of enhancing radiation response in a European randomized clinical trial.[31,32] Local control rates were 28% with radiation alone and 46% for the combined treatment. Unfortunately, there are technical difficulties associated with hyperthermia and it is not widely available, although many superficial lesions would be quite amenable. The combination of radiation with a range of modulating and chemotherapy agents has been reported, with some interesting results.[33,34]

An area of long-standing interest has been attempts to escalate the radiation dose by selective targeting of melanoma cells. A carrier molecule, with selective or preferential uptake into melanoma cells, is tagged with a radioactive isotope. In the case of boron-neutron capture therapy (BNCT), the carrier is a precursor of melanin into which several atoms of boron, specifically boron-10 (^{10}B), have been added. On irradiation with thermal neutrons from a nuclear reactor, ^{10}B decays, liberating highly destructive, short-range particles. A small number of patients have been treated, with good local control,[35] but there are major technical and logistic difficulties with the technique. Alpha target therapy is a simpler technique, in which alpha-emitting isotopes are linked to the carrier. The most intensively investigated system involves tagging astatine-211 to methylene blue, which has a high affinity for melanin.[36] Again, the α particle is highly destructive and has a short range. Early clinical trials are underway. Thirdly, various radioactive isotopes may be linked to bioactive molecules that have an affinity for components of melanoma cells.[37,38]

In summary, melanoma is recognized as one of the less radioresponsive tumour types. The 'average' melanoma is characterized by a low α/β value. The optimal therapeutic ratio is obtained using hypofractionated schedules with a dose per fraction of 4–6 Gy.[16] There is, however, marked intra- and interpatient heterogeneity of response, and prediction of individual tumour radiosensitivity is not yet available. The use of radiation enhancers remains investigational and is not widespread.

ROLE OF RADIATION THERAPY IN METASTATIC MELANOMA

As a result of its relative insensitivity to radiation, moderately high biological doses are usually required for effective palliation of melanoma metastases. As a corollary, palliation of small, single lesions is frequently successful, as higher doses can be delivered to small volumes without excessive acute or late toxicity.

The major indications for palliative irradiation, a brief description of each, and a summary of the uses of radiation in each case is given in Table 51.1.

Cerebral metastases

High radiation doses are required for control of cerebral metastases. Overall, the response of multiple cerebral metastases to whole-brain irradiation using schedules such as ten 30 Gy fractions is disappointing, with only a modest survival improvement compared

Table 51.1 *Uses of radiation therapy in metastatic melanoma*

Site	Use
Central nervous system	
Single cerebral	Stereotactic to lesion ± whole brain
Multiple cerebral	Whole brain
Meningeal	Whole brain (? benefit)
Intrathoracic	
Endobronchial	Bleeding, obstruction
Mediastinal	SVC, tracheal, neural compression
Pulmonary/pleural	Pain, bleeding
Nodal	Pain, vascular/neural compression
Cutaneous/mucosal	Pain, bleeding, infection, obstruction
Skeletal	Pain Spinal cord compression (usually postoperative) Postoperative after internal fixation
Soft tissue	Muscle etc.
Visceral	Rarely indicated

with steroids alone. Schedules utilizing higher fraction sizes have not improved survival for most patients,[39,40] but an accelerated schedule was considered beneficial for subsets with either a resected lesion or no extra-cranial disease.[19]

In contrast, the response rates of lesions treated by stereotactic techniques using singles doses of 15–20 Gy result in local control rates of 90%.[41] The role of adjuvant whole-brain irradiation following treatment of a single cerebral metastasis by resection or stereotactic irradiation remains controversial. Further cerebral relapse is reduced but survival is not affected.[41,42]

Anecdotally, the neurological symptoms from extensive meningeal melanomatosis do not respond well to radiation.

Skeletal metastases

There are few data relating to the palliation of bone pain due to melanoma metastases specifically.[43] The radiation schedules used and the responses in terms of pain relief are similar to other tumour types.[44] The indications for radiation treatment are for relief of bone pain and as postoperative therapy following internal orthopaedic fixation.

The management of malignant spinal cord compression depends on the general state of the patient. For patients with a relatively good prognosis and minimal disease burden, a combination of surgical decompression and postoperative irradiation is preferred, compared with radiation alone.

Intrathoracic metastases

Radiation has a definite role in the palliation of a number of intrathoracic metastatic situations. These include relief of haemoptysis and obstruction from endobronchial lesions, pain from lung or pleural lesions, and the symptoms of mediastinal obstruction from lymph node metastases. Endobronchial lesions may be treated using intracavitary brachytherapy.

Nodal metastases

Lymph node metastases causing pain or compression are usually well palliated by radiation. This includes mediastinal adenopathy causing pressure symptoms on adjacent organs (trachea, oesophagus, SVC, nerves) and peripheral adenopathy causing pain or distal oedema. Paraaortic adenopathy is treated uncommonly with radiation, as it is rarely symptomatic and is usually associated with more widespread dissemination.

Skin and mucosal metastases

Palliation of pain, bleeding, swelling, and fungation of cutaneous and mucosal metastases is quite variable, with marked inter- and intrapatient variability. A common problem is the widespread nature of skin metastases, with the need to treat large areas. This both limits the dose and increases toxicity. Late toxicity is often an issue, as the patient may have extensive cutaneous lesions as the sole site of metastasis and may therefore have a prolonged survival.

Metastases to the upper aerodigestive tract are uncommon; typical sites are the tongue and tonsil. They may give rise to pain, bleeding and, rarely, obstructive symptoms for swallowing and breathing.

Visceral metastases

There is no established role for radiation in the treatment of gastrointestinal, hepatic and other intraabdominal metastases, which are common sites for metastatic melanoma. Radiation has been used to treat a metastasis to the oesophagus causing dysphagia or bleeding.

Other soft tissue metastases

Symptomatic lesions in other tissues are uncommon and may be treated with radiation. These include metastases in muscle, the pelvis, the breast, the genitalia and other tissues.

Adjuvant postoperative therapy

An uncommon situation is the patient with a small metastatic burden in whom a symptomatic lesion has been resected with positive surgical margins. Postoperative radiation has been used in this setting to further reduce local recurrence.

REFERENCES

1. Coates AS, Segelov E, Long term response to chemotherapy in patients with visceral metastatic melanoma. *Ann Oncol* 1994; 5: 249–51.
2. Ollila DW, Hsueh EC, Stern SL, Morton DL, Metastasectomy for recurrent stage IV melanoma. *J Surg Oncol* 1999; 71: 209–13.
3. Hall WA, Djalilian HR, Nussbaum ES, Cho KH, Long-term survival with metastatic cancer to the brain. *Med Oncol* 2000; 17: 279–86.
4. Paterson R, The radical X-ray treatment of the carcinomata. *Br J Radiol* 1936; 106: 671–9.
5. Adair FE, Treatment of melanoma. *Surg Gynecol Obstet* 1936; 62: 406–9.
6. Ellis F, Radiosensitivity of malignant melanomata. *Br J Radiol* 1939; 12: 327–52.
7. Hellriegel W, Radiation therapy of primary and metastatic melanoma. *Ann NY Acad Sci* 1963; 100: 131–41.
8. Dewey DL, The radiosensitivity of melanoma in culture. *Br J Radiol* 1971; 44: 816–17.
9. Barranco SC, Romsdahl MM, Humphrey RM, The radiation of human malignant melanoma cells grown in vitro. *Cancer Res* 1971; 31: 830–3.
10. Hornsey S, The relationship between total dose, number of fractions and fraction size in the response of malignant melanoma in patients. *Br J Radiol* 1978; 51: 905–9.
11. Habermalz HJ, Fischer JJ, Radiation therapy of malignant melanoma. Experience with high individual doses. *Cancer* 1976; 38: 2258–62.
12. Overgaard J, Radiation treatment of malignant melanoma. *Int J Radiat Oncol Biol Phys* 1980; 6: 41–4.
13. Overgaard J, von der Maase H, Overgaard M, A randomized study comparing two high-dose per fraction radiation schedules in recurrent or metastatic malignant melanoma. *Int J Radiat Oncol Biol Phys* 1985; 11: 1837–9.
14. Overgaard J, Overgaard M, Hansen PV, von der Maase H, Some factors of importance in the radiation treatment of malignant melanoma. *Radiother Oncol* 1986; 5: 183–92.
15. Overgaard J, The role of radiotherapy in recurrent and metastatic malignant melanoma: a clinical radiobiological study. *Int J Radiat Oncol Biol Phys* 1986; 12: 867–72.
16. Bentzen SM, Overgaard J, Thames HD et al, Clinical radiobiology of malignant melanoma. *Radiother Oncol* 1989; 16: 169–82.
17. Bentzen SM, Thames HD, Overgaard J, Does variation in the in vitro cellular radiosensitivity explain the shallow clinical dose-control curve for malignant melanoma? *Int J Radiat Biol* 1990; 57: 117–26.
18. Trott KR, von Lieven H, Kummermehr J et al, The radiosensitivity of malignant melanomas part II: clinical studies. *Int J Radiat Oncol Biol Phys* 1981; 7: 15–20.
19. Choi KN, Withers HR, Rotman M, Metastatic melanoma in brain. Rapid treatment or large dose fractions. *Cancer* 1985; 56: 10–15.
20. Sause WT, Cooper JS, Rush S et al, Fraction size in external beam radiation therapy in the treatment of melanoma. *Int J Radiat Oncol Biol Phys* 1991; 20: 429–32.
21. Burmeister BH, Smithers BM, Poulsen M et al, Radiation therapy for nodal disease in malignant melanoma. *World J Surg* 1995; 19: 369–71.
22. Stevens G, Thompson JF, Firth I et al, Locally advanced melanoma: results of postoperative hypofractionated radiation therapy. *Cancer* 2000; 88: 87–93.
23. Rofstad EK, Radiation biology of malignant melanoma. *Acta Radiol* 1986; 25: 1–10 (review).
24. Rofstad EK, Influence of cellular radiation sensitivity on local tumour control of human melanoma xenografts given fractionated radiation treatment. *Cancer Res* 1991; 51: 4609–12.
25. Rofstad EK, Retention of cellular radiation sensitivity in cell and xenograft lines established from human melanoma surgical specimens. *Cancer Res* 1992; 52: 1764–9.
26. Rofstad EK, Radiation sensitivity in vitro of primary tumours and metastatic lesions of malignant melanoma. *Cancer Res* 1992; 52: 4453–7.
27. Rofstad EK, Fractionation sensitivity (alpha/beta ratio) of human melanoma xenografts. *Radiother Oncol* 1994; 33: 133–8.
28. Danielsen T, Smith-Sorensen B, Gronlund HA et al, No association between radiosensitivity and TP53 status, G1 arrest or protein levels of p53, myc, ras or raf in human melanoma lines. *Int J Radiat Biol* 1999; 75: 1149–60.
29. Deacon J, Peckham MJ, Steel GG, The radioresponsiveness of human tumours and the initial slope of the cell survival curve. *Radiother Oncol* 1984; 2: 317–23.
30. Fertil B, Malaise EP, Intrinsic radiosensitivity of human cell lines is correlated with radioresponsiveness of human tumors: analysis of 101 published survival curves. *Int J Radiat Oncol Biol Phys* 1985; 11: 1699–707.
31. Overgaard J, Overgaard M, Hyperthermia as an adjuvant to radiotherapy in the treatment of malignant melanoma. *Int J Hyperthermia* 1987; 3: 483–501.
32. Overgaard J, Gonzalez D, Hulshof MC et al, Randomised trial of hyperthermia as adjuvant to radiotherapy for recurrent or metastatic malignant melanoma. European Society for Hyperthermic Oncology. *Lancet* 1995; 345: 540–3.
33. Zhang M, Stevens, G, Effect of radiation and tirapazamine (SR-4233) on three melanoma cell lines. *Melanoma Res* 1998; 8: 510–15.
34. Ulrich J, Gademann G, Gollnick H, Management of cerebral metastases from malignant melanoma: results of a combined, simultaneous treatment with fotemustine and irradiation. *J Neurooncol* 1999; 43: 173–8.
35. Mishima Y, Kondoh H, Dual control of melanogenesis and melanoma growth: overview molecular to clinical level and the reverse. *Pigment Cell Res* 2000; 13 (Suppl 8): 10–22.
36. Link EM, Targeting melanoma with 211 At/131I-methylene blue: preclinical and clinical experience. *Hybridoma* 1999; 18: 77–82.
37. Kang N, Hamilton S, Odili J et al, In vivo targeting of malignant melanoma by 125iodine- and 99mtechnetium-labeled single-chain Fv fragments against high molecular weight melanoma-associated antigen. *Clin Cancer Res* 2000; 6: 4921–31.
38. Divgi CR, Larson SM, Radiolabeled monoclonal antibodies in the diagnosis and treatment of malignant melanoma. *Semin Nucl Med* 1989; 19: 252–61.
39. Vlock DR, Kirkwood JM, Leutzinger C et al, High-dose fraction radiation therapy for intracranial metastases of malignant melanoma: a comparison with low-dose fraction therapy. *Cancer* 1982; 49: 2289–94.
40. Ziegler JC, Cooper JS, Brain metastases from malignant melanoma: conventional vs. high-dose-per-fraction radiotherapy. *Int J Radiat Oncol Biol Phys* 1986; 12: 1839–42.
41. Mori Y, Kondziolka D, Flickinger JC et al, Stereotactic radiosurgery for cerebral metastatic melanoma: factors affecting local disease control and survival. *Int J Radiat Oncol Biol Phys* 1998; 42: 581–9.
42. Nieder C, Schwerdtfeger K, Steudel WI, Schnabel K, Patterns of relapse and late toxicity after resection and whole-brain radiotherapy for solitary brain metastases. *Strahlenther Onkol* 1998; 174: 275–8.
43. Kirova YM, Chen J, Rabarijaona LI et al, Radiotherapy as palliative treatment for metastatic melanoma. *Melanoma Res* 1999; 9: 611–13.
44. Arcangeli G, Micheli A, Arcangeli G et al, The responsiveness of bone metastases to radiotherapy: the effect of site, histology and radiation dose on pain relief. *Radiother Oncol* 1989; 14: 95–101.

52

Management of the patient with advanced melanoma

Richard F Kefford

INTRODUCTION

Despite continuous research endeavours in chemotherapy, immunotherapy and biological therapy, there is no cure for disseminated melanoma, and only rarely do systemic treatments appear to modify the natural history of the disease. By the time the metastatic phenotype develops, melanoma appears invariably to have evolved into a tumour with a vast number of genetic alterations, conferring cellular proliferative advantages, coupled with resistance to apoptosis and apoptosis-inducing agents like chemotherapy and radiotherapy. Details on the use of those systemic treatments currently in use appear in Chapters 56–59 where encouraging developments on the horizon for the treatment of this disease are reviewed.

Against this background of relative therapeutic impotence, the management of patients with metastatic melanoma presents a special set of challenges. Frequently, the patients are young adults for whom the devastating effects of the disease are compounded by its effects on their ability to meet the demands of work and family. Melanoma is almost unique among cancers for the protean manifestations of its disseminated state. Within these heterogeneous features, certain reproducible patterns can be determined and these provide a basis for a logical approach to special issues in symptom control.

NATURAL HISTORY OF METASTATIC MELANOMA

Melanoma is notoriously variable in its pattern of spread. In selected patients the disease has a propensity to remain confined to locoregional lymphatics for extended periods, and some such patients have achieved long-term remissions even after hindquarter amputation.[1] In others, haematogenous dissemination occurs early and widely. In certain patients, years may pass between the primary presentation and the development of metastases. Certain patients may display serial presentations, each with relatively isolated metastases, remaining in clinical remission for many years between episodes of local (usually surgical) treatment of these exacerbations. Others will suddenly develop fulminant disease in many organs simultaneously, with a very rapid demise. In some patients, the disease displays particular affinity for a particular organ, or organs. Thus, certain individuals may develop extensive pulmonary involvement without ever developing liver metastases. Others will succumb to cerebral metastases without any extracranial disease. This wide spectrum of variability confounds the ability to make an accurate prognosis. However, some broad guidelines may be drawn from statistical analyses of large numbers of patients who have died from metastatic melanoma.

Sites of metastases

A knowledge of the patterns of spread of metastatic melanoma is helpful in guiding follow-up, staging and stratification for clinical trials. In a recent analysis of 114 patients who had died from metastatic melanoma at the Sydney Melanoma Unit, a retrospective analysis of the sites of initial metastasis and sites ever involved with metastatic melanoma was performed. The most common initial sites of metastasis were skin, subcutaneous tissues (29%), distant lymph nodes (41%), lung (18%) and brain (15%) (Table 52.1). This distribution is similar to that in other earlier series, except that liver and bone were more commonly found as initial sites in one series.[2]

Eventually, in the Sydney Melanoma Unit series, 55% of patients followed until the time of death developed involvement of skin and subcutaneous tissue; 56% lymph nodes, 47% lung, 37% brain, 27% liver, 21% bone and 17% gastrointestinal tract (Table 52.2). Similar distributions are seen in other series.[2–4] Approximately 4% of patients present with widespread metastases as the initial manifestation of metastatic disease.[2]

Table 52.1 *Probability of first metastasis at a given site*

Site	Probability	Ninety-five per cent confidence interval
Brain	0.149	0.089–0.228
Lung	0.184	0.117–0.268
Liver	0.053	0.019–0.112
Gastrointestinal tract	0.018	0.006–0.063
Lymph nodes	0.412	0.320–0.509
Bone	0.070	0.030–0.134
Skin and subcutis	0.289	0.207–0.382

Table 52.2 *Probability of ever developing metastases at a given site*

Site	Probability	Ninety-five per cent confidence interval
Brain	0.368	0.279–0.464
Lung	0.474	0.379–0.570
Liver	0.272	0.364–0.192
Gastrointestinal tract	0.167	0.103–0.249
Lymph nodes	0.561	0.464–0.654
Bone	0.211	0.140–0.298
Subcutaneous	0.553	0.457–0.647

In autopsy studies, some have pointed to clustering of metastatic patterns according to the embryological origin of host tissues.[5,6] Such patterns, for example, suggest a strong negative correlation between brain and hepatic metastases, and show that the distribution of melanoma metastases is not random.[5] In autopsy series, the most commonly involved sites are skin, subcutaneous tissues and lymph nodes (50–75%), lung (70–87%), liver (54–75%), brain (36–54%), bone (23–49%) and intestine (26–58%), with each of the following additional sites being involved in 25–45% of autopsies: heart and pericardium, pancreas, spleen, adrenals, kidney and thyroid.[5–7] These figures should be taken only as a rough guide, as there are no studies in the literature which examine the natural history of the disease in a rigorously controlled prospective manner with universal application of scheduled, defined staging investigations.

In addition to those sites mentioned above, unusual sites for melanoma metastases abound, and knowledge of them is essential in diagnosing unusual symptoms. Those clinically relevant include the breast[8] (also a rare site for metastases from ocular melanoma),[9] the testis,[10,11] the epididymis,[12] the endometrium,[13] the placenta,[14] the fetus,[15,16] the ovary,[17] the eye and orbit,[18] the oesphagus,[19] the oral cavity, pharynx and larynx,[20–22] the tongue,[23] the prostate,[24] skeletal muscle,[25] the myocardium and cardiac atria,[26] the synovium,[27] and the internal auditory canal.[28]

Some examples of the clinical manifestations of metastatic melanoma are shown in Figures 52.1–52.4.

Prognosis of metastatic melanoma

Many clinical series have attempted to identify factors that would allow the stratification of patients into different prognostic groups, particularly for the purpose of controlled clinical trials: those factors which have been identified are listed in Table 52.3. The number and site of metastases particularly influence prognosis. For a single metastatic site, the 1-year survival rate was 36%, while it was only 13% for two sites and 0% for three or more sites.[2] The 1-year survival for patients for non-visceral sites (skin, subcutaneous, distant lymph nodes) was 40%, compared to only 11% for visceral metastases and 8% for combined sites.[2]

In a recent revision of the AJCC Staging System for Melanoma,[29] Stage IV melanoma has been subdivided

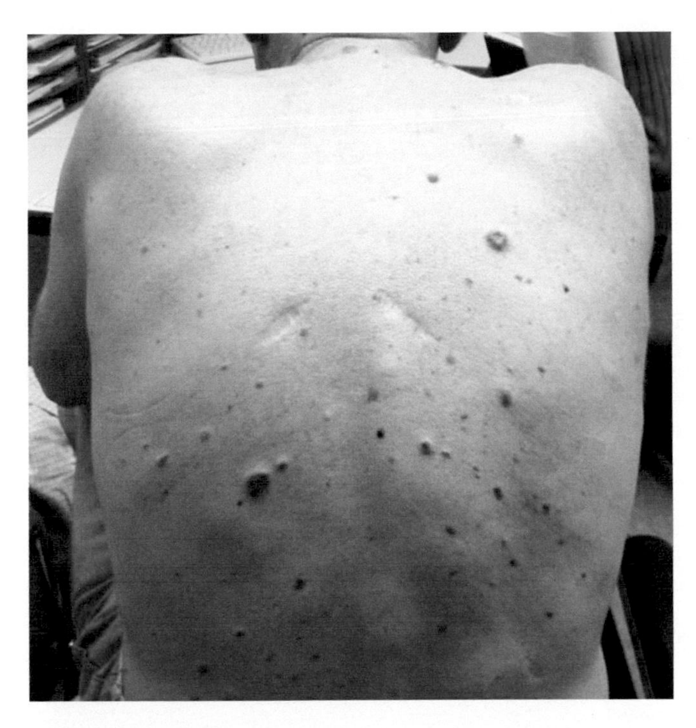

Figure 52.1 *Multiple intracutaneous and subcutaneous melanoma metastases.*

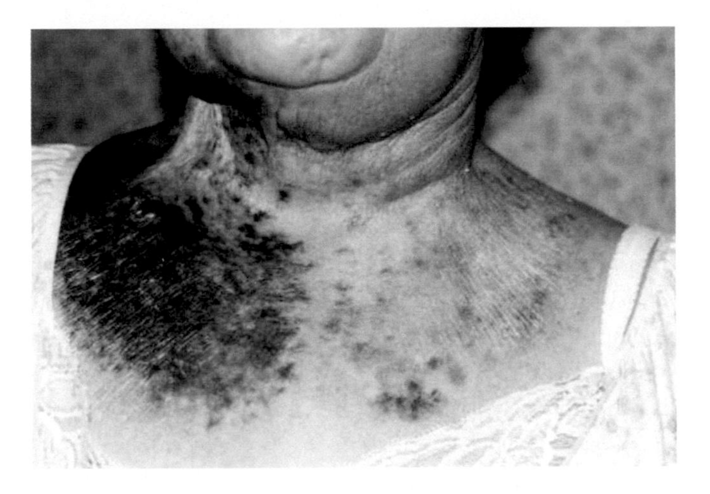

Figure 52.2 *Cutaneous infiltrate of metastatic melanoma. The patient was free of visceral metastases until death.*

into three prognostic groups. The 'M1' category includes those patients with lymph node and/or subcutaneous metastases and has a median survival of >12 months and a 2-year survival of 15–20%. The 'M2' category has pulmonary metastases +/− subcutaneous or lymph node involvement, and has a median survival of 9–12 months and a 2-year survival of 10%. The 'M3' category have other visceral involvement, or any site with an elevated serum LDH. M3 patients have a median survival of 4–6 months and a 2-year survival of 5%.

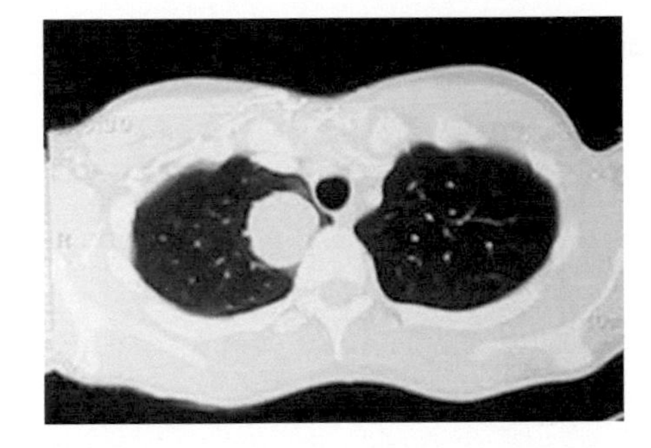

Figure 52.3 *Large right pulmonary melanoma metastasis.*

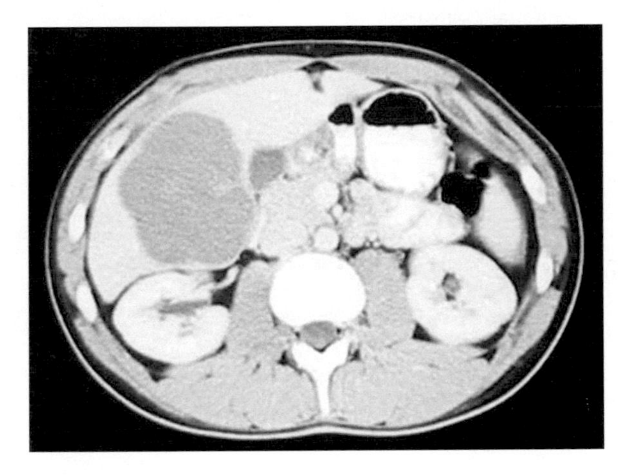

Figure 52.4 *Large hepatic melanoma metastasis.*

Occult primary melanoma was found to have a survival advantage over cutaneous primary melanoma from the time of first metastasis,[30] and patterns of metastasis at autopsy are similar to those of cutaneous primary disease.[31]

Eight patients who remained in long-term remission, 4–15 years after chemotherapy for visceral metastatic melanoma were identified from 1100 patients with visceral melanoma seen at the Sydney Melanoma Unit between 1977 and 1989. All had received single agent dacarbazine (DTIC) or a nitrosourea. This group of apparently 'cured' patients did not differ from the overall group of patients with visceral metastases in baseline characteristics, but six of the eight had nodular lung metastases.[32]

NON-METASTATIC MANIFESTATIONS OF MALIGNANCY

Melanoma is associated with a wide range of paraneoplastic phenomena.[33] The majority of these occur in the context of established metastatic disease. Many are

Table 52.3 *Prognostic factors in metastatic melanoma*

Prognostic factor	Influence on prognosis	Reference no.
Number of sites	More sites; worse prognosis	2,87
Disease-free period	Shorter remission; worse prognosis	2,88,89
Visceral metastases	Visceral metastases; worse prognosis	2
LDH*	High LDH;* worse prognosis	90–92
Albumin	Low albumin; worse prognosis	90,91
Site of initial metastasis	Skin, lymph node, GI‡ > lung > brain, bone	4,89
Performance status	Poor performance status; worse prognosis	87,88,93
Symptoms	Anorexia, fever, emesis; worse prognosis	87
Gender	Females have better prognosis	2,87,93
Serum S-100B	Higher levels; worse prognosis	92,94
Psychosocial predictors	Perceived aim of treatment, minimization and anger independent predictors of survival	68

*LDH, Serum lactate dehydrogenase.
‡GI, Gastrointestinal.

presumed to be the result of cross-reactivity between novel expressed melanoma cell-surface antigens and normal cellular epitopes. Circulating immune complexes can frequently be found in patients with metastatic melanoma.[34]

Some of the paraneoplastic clinical conditions that have been reported include arthritis,[35] the syndrome of inappropriate ADH secretion (SIADH),[36] vitiligo,[37,38] other immunologically mediated dermatoses,[39,40] dermatomyositis,[41,42] cryoglobulinaemia,[34] Sjögren's (sicca) syndrome,[43] hypertrophic pulmonary osteoarthropathy,[44] granulomatous disease,[45] inflammatory neuropathy,[46,47] paraneoplastic eosinophilia[48] and marantic endocarditis.[49]

Melanoma-associated retinopathy is a particularly important paraneoplastic phenomenon. This condition, which may present as night blindness, is characterized by the presence of elevated serum levels of autoantibodies directed against tumour antigen that cross-react with retinal proteins, resulting in rod and cone dysfunction.[50]

Rarely, patients with bulky and widespread metastatic melanoma develop melanosis.[51–54] The entire skin, and internal viscera, develops a grey–blue pigmentation, presumed to be due to the persistent and cumulative dissemination of melanin, via the bloodstream, throughout the body. This, in turn, leads to progressive pigmentation of all internal organs. Dermal deposition is responsible for the change in colour of the skin. Only continuous access to the circulation by neoplastic melanocytes could explain such a phenomenon. In some cases there may be associated melanuria, characterized microscopically by the presence of amorphous, dark-brown casts, which stain positively for melanin pigment, and numerous pigment-laden macrophages.[55] In all but anecdotal instances,[56] melanosis is a terminal event.

Certain patients with metastatic melanoma develop profound cachexia, sometimes out of proportion to the extent and bulk of the metastatic deposits. Cachexia may be associated with pyrexial episodes, nightsweats, myalgia and profound anorexia. This syndrome appears to be cytokine mediated. The cytokines may either be derived directly from the tumour, such as leukaemia inhibitory factor (LIF)[57,58] and proteolysis-inducing factor (PIF),[59] or from activated T cells, such as tumour necrosis factor (TNF).[60] The syndrome may partially respond to megestrol acetate in high doses[61,62] or thalidomide.[63]

Hypercalcaemia occurs in 1–10% of patients with metastatic melanoma.[64,65] It should be routinely sought in patients with extensive bone involvement, but may not be exclusive to this group as tumour-secreted parathyroid hormone (PTH)-related peptide may be responsible.[65–67] Diphosphonates are the treatment of choice. The impact of diphosphonates on the incidence of pathological fractures and bone pain in metastatic melanoma is currently under investigation.

ASSESSMENT OF THE PATIENT WITH DISSEMINATED DISEASE

History

The entire history of the patient's melanoma and it's treatment should be carefully documented. The original histology should be reviewed. The depth of the original primary melanoma and the adequacy of wide excision may influence the likelihood of metastases being present. In a context where other common cancers may sometimes confuse the picture, such information may bear upon the decision to undertake relatively invasive procedures to diagnose metastatic disease. The occurrence of locoregional recurrence and the disease-free interval are relevant to the prognosis of metastatic disease, and possibly to the likelihood of response to systemic therapy. Previous normal x rays and scans may be useful in determining the pace of disease progression.

Careful emphasis should be placed on the patient's current major problems and the symptomatology most urgently calling for relief. The presence of anorexia, significant weight loss and poor performance status are all indicative of an advanced state of the metastatic process, and may bear on prognosis and the prospect of response to therapy.

Symptom review should cover those areas prone to serious medical complication. In particular, questioning should cover the presence or absence of headache, episodic colic with constipation and melaena. The presence of back pain, paraesthesia in the lower limbs, or loss of bowel or bladder control may each signal the possibility of spinal cord compression. Cerebral metastases are so common in patients with advanced melanoma that it is mandatory to enquire about symptoms of raised intracranial pressure (drowsiness, headache, nausea) or fitting. Co-morbities should be reviewed in the light of their impact on therapeutic intervention and a survey of regular medications performed to seek those, such as corticosteroids, that may interfere with systemic therapies, e.g. immunostimulants and cytokines.

Physical examination

Physical examination should include careful palpation of all lymph node sites and palpation of the entire skin surface with the palms of both hands seeking the presence of cutaneous or subcutaneous metastases. The careful documentation of these can be critical in determining response to systemic treatment. Furthermore, such lesions are increasingly useful in providing simple access to tumour material for diagnostic confirmation, and for biochemical and histological monitoring of the cytotoxic effects of new anticancer treatments. Examination of the gastrointestinal system should include careful examination of the oropharynx and a rectal examination. Special attention should be paid to the neurological system, with careful examination of the fundi, and exclusion of the early signs of spinal cord compression, such as peripheral sensory loss, the presence of hyperreflexia and/or an extensor plantar response in the lower limbs.

Investigations

Investigations should only be performed if they are to contribute to clinical management, or if they are in the service of a clinical trial for which the patient has given participation consent.

The full blood count and blood film are simple and informative. Anaemia is common in melanoma and most commonly shows the features of acute or chronic blood loss, the site of which is usually the gastrointestinal tract. A normochromic normocytic picture may also occur in the presence of extensive metastatic disease, without blood loss or marrow involvement. Occasionally, extensive bone marrow replacement is a dominant feature of the metastatic process. In such cases the blood film may or may not show a leucoerythroblastic picture. Bone marrow involvement may first become evident when the positron emission tomography (PET) scan reveals diffuse uptake of isotope throughout the skeleton. Occasionally, microangiopathy may result in haemolytic anaemia and thrombocytopenia.

Clinical chemistry analyses should include an assessment of the hepatic and renal function. The serum LDH, although non-specific, is an independent prognostic indicator in metastatic disease. The serum calcium should be routinely measured, particularly in patients with known extensive bone metastases.

The judicious use of medical imaging investigations should be governed by the clinical situation. For example, if surgery is planned for apparently resectable metastatic disease, the use of a sensitive screen for metastatic disease in other sites, such as PET scanning, may be particularly useful. However, in cases where a clinical examination and simple imaging has established the presence of inoperable metastatic disease then the addition of PET scanning is of questionable value. Serial PET scans are rarely the imaging of choice for assessing response to treatment. The results may simply add to the burden of patient anxiety without contributing to the management plan. Before embarking on a systemic treatment for metastatic melanoma, it is fairly standard practice at the Sydney Melanoma Unit to perform computerized axial tomography (CAT) scanning of the abdomen, pelvis and head. CAT scanning of the head, even in asymptomatic patients prior to the commencement of systemic therapy, is mandated by the high frequency of cerebral metastases in patients with metastatic melanoma, the poor prognosis of cerebral metastases when present and by the failure of certain systemic treatments to penetrate the blood–brain barrier. Certain chemotherapeutic agents, such as lomustine, fotemustine and temozolamide, reach higher levels in the cerebrospinal fluid when administered systemically, and may therefore have a theoretical advantage in patients with central nervous system involvement. Although not routinely recommended for screening, magnetic resonance imaging (MRI) scanning is the most sensitive test for the presence of cerebral metastases, as the combination of haemorrhage and the presence of melanin combine to give a very high signal intensity on T1-weighted images. MRI is also the investigation of choice in screening for spinal cord compression and, when combined with the use of gadolinium, for the detection of leptomeningeal metastases. Bone scans should be performed in patients with symptoms referable to the skeletal system. Hot spots in long bones should be subjected to plain x ray examination to determine the extent of cortical bone erosion, a determinant of the need for prophylactic orthopaedic intervention.

Pathological confirmation of metastatic melanoma

In certain patients, where the nature of the primary melanoma, and the pattern of recurrence and spread, is totally consistent with the pattern of metastatic melanoma, and particularly when a biopsy may be invasive, painful or technically difficult, the diagnosis of metastatic melanoma may be made on the basis of clinical findings and imaging investigations without biopsy confirmation. An example might be an elderly patient with a history of a deep primary melanoma, a relatively short disease-free interval and deep parenchymal lung metastases for which fine-needle aspiration biopsy would carry a risk of inducing a pneumothorax. However, in the majority of patients, biopsy confirmation of metastatic disease is recommended and is most often simply carried out by a fine-needle aspiration biopsy. Most clinical trials demand such confirmation.

Approach to the patient with metastatic melanoma

There are a number of features which distinguish the clinical challenge of managing metastatic melanoma from similar situations in other parallel fields of oncology. Frequently, the patient is a young adult, with the financial, career and family responsibilities and aspirations of mid-life, mid-career and parenthood to teenage children. The devastation of diagnosis is compounded by the gloomy predictions of prior medical attendants and whatever factual material might have been frantically retrieved from the internet. For many, the diagnosis of metastatic disease fulfils the worst nightmare lingering in the recesses of the mind since the very first diagnosis of the sinister 'black cancer'. The medical oncologist is therefore frequently seen as the last hope before traditional medicine is abandoned entirely in a desperate search for solace in the world of alternative and quack therapies.

The initial consultation therefore requires particular attention and skill. A carer or relative should be present. It is helpful for the oncologist to be accompanied by an oncology nurse specialist who will take a key role in case management and in day-to-day follow-up. A principal objective of the initial consultation is to establish an environment of confidence and trust. In most cases, it is more important for the patient to leave this initial consultation with some measure of hope than to take home a statistically accurate, and usually gloomy, prognostic prediction. At this stage of their illness, the dismal prognostic outlook of the disease, and the relative ineffectiveness of current systemic treatments, are usually more than the most pragmatic and stoic young adult can withstand.

Some useful concepts in sustaining patients at this time are: the idea that the oncology medical and nursing team are joining forces with the patient in fighting a battle; the news that certain vital organs are spared on the CAT scans; optimistic anecdotes referring to the successful outcome of the treatment of similar patients in the past; the rapid rate of progress in medical research and the speed with which new treatments are being developed; the fact that the melanoma clinicians are expert, confident and current in their skills and knowledge; the fact that the treatment team are in constant contact with all melanoma clinicians around the world and that patients will therefore immediately receive the benefit of advances in knowledge. It is helpful if these facts are summarized in a brief leaflet aimed at sustaining the patient and carers during the first difficult days and weeks after diagnosis. In this respect, it should be noted that in one study patients who perceived the aim of their treatment to be cure or long-term prolongation of life, who minimized the impact of cancer on their lives and who reported greater anger about their illness survived longer than patients who did not.[68] There is, however, no evidence as yet to suggest that intervention to alter the temperament of patients from a darker to a lighter outlook has any impact on survival, and patients should not have the burden of responsibility for their predicament added to that already rendered by the disease from which they suffer so considerably.

The explicit delineation of a plan of management will do much to allay the fears and anxieties of patients and carers. While it is desirable to involve patients in decision-making, at the time of initial consultation for metastatic melanoma a strength in leadership and direction from the clinical team is often welcomed. The management plan should include specification of investigations, the reasons for them and what they entail. The importance of symptom control, and the objective of rapid absolute relief of pain, require particular attention and time. An emphasis on symptom control and on early engagement of community nursing support will facilitate a smoother transition to palliative care at a later stage of the illness. The initial consultation is rarely a suitable time to arrange formal consultation with palliative care services, but frequently value may be obtained from consultations with multidisciplinary pain clinics, clinical psychologists and, occasionally, psychiatrists. At all times, however, it is essential that the patient knows which clinician is in charge of their overall management. In most cases this is the medical oncologist.

CHOICE AND EVALUATION OF TREATMENTS

Multidisciplinary assessment and management

The clinical challenges posed by the patient with metastatic melanoma cross the whole spectrum of human disease, variously involving every organ system in a manner unique amongst human cancers. Case management should ideally be in the hands of an oncologist/clinical nurse consultant partnership, with regular discussions at multidisciplinary meetings at which the expertise of the surgeon, radiation oncologist, immunologist, medical oncologist and radiologist can be routinely sought. Further specialized care from plastic surgeons, orthopaedic surgeons, thoracic surgeons, neurosurgeons, pain-control experts and palliative-care physicians is commonly required. The assistance of allied health professionals in physiotherapy, occupational therapy, social work, dietetics and clinical psychology is of paramount importance.

Observation

The heterogeneous nature of melanoma and its patterns of spread and progression, together with the fact that no existing form of systemic treatment has been shown to prolong survival in prospective randomized controlled clinical trials, means that, for certain patients, observation may be the most humane and rational choice. Patients best suited to observation are those with relatively low bulk disease who are without symptoms, whose disease has a slow rate of progression, who do not yet display constitutional features of anorexia, weight loss and decline in performance status, and whose temperament is suited to such a plan. Typically, metastatic disease has been detected in these patients by the performance of 'routine' staging investigations. Such patients may be eligible for clinical trials and, in fact, may be the best candidates for certain immunotherapy trials. Patients should be made aware of their potential eligibility for these experimental programmes. Those electing to be observed should be advised to report any new symptoms and should be reviewed at a defined time interval, typically 2 months, with progress imaging investigations aimed at assessing the rate of progression. Patients may be reassured on observation programmes by the knowledge that there is no evidence that delay of initiation of chemotherapy for melanoma jeopardizes response, providing that deterioration in weight and performance status have not intervened. Supportive programmes of counselling, diet and exercise may be useful adjuvants in maintaining morale in this group of patients.

Surgery

Surgery plays a major role in the management of metastatic melanoma. In selected cases, particularly for pulmonary and brain metastases, total resection of metastases may be attempted with the objective of achieving prolonged survival (Chapter 46).[69] Resection of isolated metastases may occasionally result in long-term remissions for 5 years or more.[70,71] PET scanning provides a powerful tool in the staging and selection of patients for metastasectomy. Certain highly selected patients may benefit from repeated metastasectomy. In one study, the 5-year survival rate was 20% for patients undergoing total resection of recurrent metastatic disease after previous metastasectomy.[72] The majority of these patients had isolated metastatic deposits. The two most important prognostic factors for survival following diagnosis of recurrent stage IV melanoma were a prolonged disease-free interval to recurrence and complete surgical resection of the recurrence.

In other settings, the objective of metastasectomy may be palliation by resection of a particular deposit that is responsible for serious symptoms, such as pain, haemorrhage or bowel obstruction.[73] This aggressive surgical approach to disseminated disease is necessitated in part by the relative impotence of current systemic therapies.

Radiotherapy

The role of radiotherapy in the management of metastatic melanoma is discussed in Chapter 35. Radiotherapy is highly valued in the control of symptomatic lesions, particularly those causing pain, haemorrhage, bone destruction, spinal cord compression and obstruction of mediastinal structures. In selected cases, the efficacy of radiation therapy may be enhanced by the synchronous use of radiosensitizers, such as cisplatin.[74] Radiation therapy plays an important role in the management of cerebral metastases.

Clinical trials

Where possible, patients with metastatic cancer should be entered on clinical trials. Despite a long string of disappointments with phase II trials of cytotoxic agents in melanoma, this rule remains highly relevant to the management of this disease. Given recent advances in the rational design of agents which may overcome inherent defences in the melanoma cells against apoptosis, together with major inroads into the molecular abnormalities common to melanoma cells, clinical trials will prove essential in refining the utility of a battery of new potentially potent treatments. New agents under investigation for the treatment of melanoma are reviewed in Chapter 59. The current status of experimentation with immunotherapy for melanoma is reviewed in Chapter 57.

Frequently, the eligibility criteria for participation in phase II and III trials for melanoma select out a small group of patients with good prognosis. For example, most studies require CAT scanning of the brain prior to entry, and few studies regard patients with cerebral metastases as being eligible. Others rule out patients with a poor performance status or even those with slightly elevated levels of LDH. The outcome of this is that, even in units with a high level of commitment to clinical research, there will be a number of patients with metastatic melanoma who are ineligible for treatment with new agents. Such patients may be technically eligible for trials investigating new schedules or new combinations of older agents. However, it must be said that such trials are unlikely to make more than tiny incremental adjustments to the current relatively dismal outlook of systemic treatment with standard agents. Clinician enthusiasm and resource allocation for the conduct of such trials is frequently and understandably low. Consequently, until major advances are made in the introduction of effective agents, there will be a cohort of patients with metastatic melanoma who will justifiably be treated 'off study'.

Systemic chemotherapy with standard agents

Metastatic melanoma is relatively resistant to treatment with cytotoxic drugs. There is no evidence from randomized controlled trials that any form of systemic therapy prolongs overall survival. Partial responses to single agents occur in <25% of treated patients, and complete responses in <5%.[75] The median duration of response is 5–6 months. Only 2% of patients treated with DTIC sustain long-term complete responses.[32] Regrettably, in a disease for which a principal objective of chemotherapy is therefore palliation, there are few studies of the effect of chemotherapy on the quality of life; however, such studies are now in progress. Details of chemotherapy and 'biochemotherapy' for melanoma are considered in Chapter 56.

The current first-line recommendation for patients with symptomatic metastatic disease, outside of clinical trials, is single agent DTIC, which is simple, ambulatory and associated with minimal toxicity when administered with modern antiemetics such as ondansetron.[76] Alopecia does not occur with DTIC therapy, and the drug is minimally myelosuppressive. No combination of cytotoxic drugs has been shown in prospective randomized clinical trials to be reproducibly superior to single agent DTIC in terms of survival. Combinations of cytotoxics and biological agents such as interleukin-2 and interferon-α induce higher response rates, but are significantly more toxic than single agent DTIC. Predictors of response to cytotoxic chemotherapy in metastatic melanoma are shown in Table 52.4.

Table 52.4 ***Predictors of response to cytotoxic chemotherapy in metastatic melanoma***[75,87,95–98]

Response more likely	Response less likely
Subcutaneous metastases	Cerebral metastases
Cutaneous metastases	Liver metastases
Lymph node metastases	Bone metastases
Pulmonary metastases	Leptomeningeal metastases
Good performance status	Poor performance status

Best supportive care

For certain patients, the prospects of response to chemotherapy are so low and/or the risks of toxicity so high that attempts at antitumour therapy are better abandoned and replaced with a policy of best supportive care. Patients who fall into this category include those with a very poor performance status and extensive, or rapidly progressing, metastatic disease in multiple visceral sites. Patients who have failed initial chemotherapy may also fall into this group, as a recent review of the efficacy of salvage chemotherapy for metastatic melanoma at the Sydney Melanoma Unit revealed a response rate of <5%.

SPONTANEOUS REGRESSIONS

Oncologists frequently observe waxing and waning in the size of melanoma metastases. This is most frequently seen in subcutaneous deposits, lymph nodes and pulmonary metastases. Such changes may be heterogeneous, with certain lesions increasing in size while others shrink. Hypotheses for these observations include immunological and inflammatory responses, necrosis induced by out-growth of blood supply, and haemorrhage into highly vascular deposits. This behaviour, which is so characteristic of metastatic melanoma, is one particular reason for the rigorous control necessary in assessing response in clinical trials of new agents.

Complete spontaneous regressions of metastatic melanoma are also well described in the medical literature. About 40% of patients with spontaneous regressions appeared to have had a spontaneous cure, which implies that the disease had not relapsed either during a long period of follow-up or until death from some other cause.[77] Cutaneous metastases are most commonly reported to regress spontaneously but visceral sites have also been reported, including lung, lymph nodes, liver, bone and bowel.[77–85] Whilst patients are naturally prone to attribute this rare event to the supernatural, or to alternative therapies, the mechanism probably relates to immunological events, endocrine alterations, alterations in the metabolism of melanin or nutritional alterations.[77]

DEALING WITH ALTERNATIVE THERAPIES

Motivated by their own desperation, confronted with the inadequacy of medical treatment, fuelled by the exaggerated, and frequently bogus, claims of the unscrupulous in the popular press and on numerous websites, and harassed by the well-meaning attentions of family and friends, the patient with metastatic melanoma frequently seeks alternative therapies. Adoption of an adversarial position by melanoma clinicians is ill-advised and may result in the patient abandoning the skilled professionals so essential to his or her health. In keeping with recent literature on the subject,[86] at the Sydney Melanoma Unit the following points are made in response in discussions about alternative treatments.

- Many proven treatments were derived from careful testing of natural products.
- Many 'alternative' medicines are in uncertain dosage and have unproved toxicity profiles.
- Some treatments carry a high risk of toxicity (e.g. coffee-ground enemas) and should absolutely be avoided.
- When put under scrutiny, none of the exaggerated claims have stood up (e.g. high-dose vitamin C, laetrile).
- Many treatments involve great inconvenience, family disruption and expense.

Patients are advised that although none of these alternative treatments can be medically recommended, those still choosing to pursue them will continue to receive the full support of the melanoma clinical oncology team. Patients are asked, however, to provide full information pertaining to all alternative treatments being used and are strongly counselled against the use of any that are suspected of causing potential harm. Patients and their carers may be assisted by a number of highly informative resources on alternative therapy, such as those available from the American Cancer Society, and those contained in websites such as '*Quackwatch*' (http://www.quackwatch.com/). Certain patients may also be fortified by the provision of safe supportive programmes of sensible dietary and exercise advice, relaxation therapy, and meditation and massage, aimed principally at an improvement in the quality of life and symptom control.

REFERENCES

1. Kourtesis GJ, McCarthy WH, Milton GW, Major amputations for melanoma. *Aust NZ J Surg* 1983; 53: 241–4.
2. Balch CM, Soong SJ, Murad TM, et al, A multifactorial analysis of melanoma. IV. Prognostic factors in 200 melanoma patients with distant metastases (stage III). *J Clin Oncol* 1983; 1: 126–34.
3. Amer MH, Al-Sarraf M, Vaitkevicius VK, Clinical presentation, natural history and prognostic factors in advanced malignant melanoma. *Surg Gynecol Obstet* 1979; 149: 687–92.
4. Barth A, Wanek LA, Morton DL, Prognostic factors in 1,521 melanoma patients with distant metastases. *J Am Coll Surg* 1995; 181: 193–201.
5. de la Monte SM, Moore GW, Hutchins GM, Patterned distribution of metastases from malignant melanoma in humans. *Cancer Res* 1983; 43: 3427–33.
6. Akslen LA, Heuch I, Hartveit F, Metastatic patterns in autopsy cases of cutaneous melanoma. *Invasion Metastasis* 1988; 8: 193–204.
7. Patel JK, Didolkar MS, Pickren JW, Moore RH, Metastatic pattern of malignant melanoma. A study of 216 autopsy cases. *Am J Surg* 1978; 135: 807–10.
8. Majeski J, Bilateral breast masses as initial presentation of widely metastatic melanoma. *J Surg Oncol* 1999; 72: 175–7.
9. Chopra JS, Chandar K, Bilateral breast metastases from malignant melanoma of the eye. *Aust NZ J Surg* 1972; 42: 183–5.
10. Johnson DE, Jackson L, Ayala AG, Secondary carcinoma of the testis. *South Med J* 1971; 64: 1128–30.
11. Segelov E, Coates AS, McCarthy WH, Metastatic melanoma presenting at diagnosis as a testicular mass. *Aust NZ J Med* 1992; 22: 701 (letter).
12. Hammad FA, Metastatic malignant melanoma of the epididymis. *Br J Urol* 1992; 69: 661.
13. Bauer RD, McCoy CP, Roberts DK, Fritz G, Malignant melanoma metastatic to the endometrium. *Obstet Gynecol* 1984; 63: 264–8.
14. Baergen RN, Johnson D, Moore T, Benirschke K, Maternal melanoma metastatic to the placenta: a case report and review of the literature. *Arch Pathol Lab Med* 1997; 121: 508–11.
15. Wong DJ, Strassner HT, Melanoma in pregnancy. *Clin Obstet Gynecol* 1990; 33: 782–91.
16. Squatrito RC, Harlow SP, Melanoma complicating pregnancy. *Obstet Gynecol Clin N Am* 1998; 25: 407–16.
17. Agnello G, Perri G, Cocilovo G, Malignant metastatic ovarian melanoma: a case report. *Eur J Gynaecol Oncol* 1981; 2: 119–20.
18. Ramaesh K, Marshall JW, Wharton SB, Dhillon B, Intraocular metastases of cutaneous malignant melanoma: a case report and review of the literature. *Eye* 1999; 13: 247–50.
19. Eng J, Pradhan GN, Sabanathan S, Mearns AJ, Malignant melanoma metastatic to the esophagus. *Ann Thorac Surg* 1989; 48: 287–8.
20. Henderson LT, Robbins KT, Weitzner S, Upper aerodigestive tract metastases in disseminated malignant melanoma. *Arch Otolaryngol Head Neck Surg* 1986; 112: 659–63.
21. Aydogan LB, Myers JN, Myers EN, Kirkwood J, Malignant melanoma metastatic to the tonsil. *Laryngoscope* 1996; 106: 313–6.
22. Ramamurthy L, Nassar WY, Hasleton PS, Metastatic melanoma of the tonsil and the nasopharynx. *J Laryngol Otol* 1995; 109: 236–7.
23. Stern Y, Braslavsky D, Spitzer T, et al, Metastatic malignant melanoma of the tongue. *J Otolaryngol* 1993; 22: 150–3.
24. Bamberger MH, Romas NA, Clinically significant metastatic melanoma to prostate. *Urology* 1990; 35: 445–7.
25. Yoshioka H, Itai Y, Niitsu M, et al, Intramuscular metastasis from malignant melanoma: MR findings. *Skeletal Radiol* 1999; 28: 714–6.
26. Abraham KP, Reddy V, Gattuso P, Neoplasms metastatic to the heart: review of 3314 consecutive autopsies. *Am J Cardiovasc Pathol* 1990; 3: 195–8.
27. Tandogan RN, Aydogan U, Demirhan B, et al, Intra-articular metastatic melanoma of the right knee. *Arthroscopy* 1999; 15: 98–102.
28. Cervio A, Saadia D, Nogues M, et al, Metastatic melanoma within the internal auditory canal: a case report. *Am J Otolaryngol* 1999; 20: 263–5.
29. Balch C, Buzaid AC, Soong SJ, et al, Final version of the AJCC staging system for cutaneous melanoma. *J Clin Oncol* 2001; 19: 3635–48.
30. Vijuk G, Coates AS, Survival of patients with visceral metastatic melanoma from an occult primary lesion: a retrospective matched cohort study. *Ann Oncol* 1998; 9: 419–22.
31. Akslen LA, Hartveit F, Metastatic melanoma of unknown origin at autopsy. *Eur J Surg Oncol* 1988; 14: 379–82.
32. Coates AS, Segelov E, Long term response to chemotherapy in patients with visceral metastatic melanoma. *Ann Oncol* 1994; 5: 249–51.

33. Wagner Jr RF, Nathanson L, Paraneoplastic syndromes, tumor markers, and other unusual features of malignant melanoma. *J Am Acad Dermatol* 1986; 14: 249–56.
34. Queen WD, Bharwani N, Phillips EA, et al, Biochemical classification of circulating immune complexes in human malignant melanoma and hematologic neoplasms. *Oncology* 1989; 46: 14–25.
35. Speerstra F, Boerbooms AM, van de Putte LB, et al, Arthritis caused by metastatic melanoma. *Arthritis Rheum* 1982; 25: 223–6.
36. Kefford RF, Milton GW, Fatal inappropriate ADH secretion in melanoma. *Med J Aust* 1986; 144: 333–4 (letter).
37. Nordlund JJ, The significance of depigmentation. *Pigment Cell Res* 1992; Suppl 2: 237–41.
38. Lerner AB, The Seiji memorial lecture. Pigment stories: from vitiligo to melanomas and points in between. *Pigment Cell Res* 1992; Suppl 2: 19–21.
39. Snow JL, Muller SA, Malignancy-associated multicentric reticulohistiocytosis: a clinical, histological and immunophenotypic study. *Br J Dermatol* 1995; 133: 71–6.
40. Kaddu S, Soyer HP, Kerl H, Palmar filiform hyperkeratosis: a new paraneoplastic syndrome? *J Am Acad Dermatol* 1995; 33: 337–40.
41. Scerri L, Zaki I, Allen BR, Golding P, Dermatomyositis associated with malignant melanoma—case report and review of the literature. *Clin Exp Dermatol* 1994; 19: 523–5.
42. Sais G, Marcoval J, Juggla A, et al, Dermatomyositis and metastatic malignant melanoma, with complete regression of the primary lesion. *Br J Dermatol* 1994; 130: 796–7.
43. Ritter FN, Salivary gland involvement in systemic diseases. *Otolaryngol Clin N Am* 1977; 10: 371–7.
44. Sethi SM, Saxton GD, Osteoarthropathy associated with solitary pulmonary metastasis from melanoma. *Can J Surg* 1974; 17: 221–4.
45. Robert C, Schoenlaub P, Avril MF, et al, Malignant melanoma and granulomatosis. *Br J Dermatol* 1997; 137: 787–92.
46. Berger JR, Mehari E, Paraneoplastic opsoclonus-myoclonus secondary to malignant melanoma. *J Neurooncol* 1999; 41: 43–5.
47. Rubin DI, Kimmel DW, Cascino TL, Outcome of peroneal neuropathies in patients with systemic malignant disease. *Cancer* 1998; 83: 1602–6 (see comments).
48. Rule SA, Waterhouse P, Costello C, Retsas S, Paraneoplastic eosinophilia in malignant melanoma. *J R Soc Med* 1993; 86: 295.
49. Bouloc A, Wolkenstein P, Authier J, et al, Non-bacterial thrombotic endocarditis complicating metastatic melanoma. *Ann Dermatol Venereol* 1994; 121: 565–7.
50. Solomon SD, Smith JH, O'Brien J, Ocular manifestations of systemic malignancies. *Curr Opin Ophthalmol* 1999; 10: 447–51.
51. Murray C, D'Intino Y, MacCormick R, et al, Melanosis in association with metastatic malignant melanoma: report of a case and a unifying concept of pathogenesis. *Am J Dermatopathol* 1999; 21: 28–30.
52. Tsukamoto K, Furue M, Sato Y, et al, Generalized melanosis in metastatic malignant melanoma: the possible role of DOPAquinone metabolites. *Dermatology* 1998; 197: 338–42.
53. Klaus MV, Shah F, Generalized melanosis caused by melanoma of the rectum. *J Am Acad Dermatol* 1996; 35: 295–7.
54. Konrad K, Wolff K, Pathogenesis of diffuse melanosis secondary to malignant melanoma. Br J Dermatol 1974; 91: 635–55.
55. Valente PT, Atkinson BF, Guerry D, Melanuria. *Acta Cytol* 1985; 29: 1026–8.
56. Ring J, Emslander C, Diffuse melanosis with generalized and ocular metastasis in malignant melanoma. *Hautarzt* 1984; 35: 308–12.
57. Iseki H, Kajimura N, Ohue C, et al, Cytokine production in five tumor cell lines with activity to induce cancer cachexia syndrome in nude mice. *Jpn J Cancer Res* 1995; 86: 562–7.
58. Mori M, Yamaguchi K, Honda S, et al, Cancer cachexia syndrome developed in nude mice bearing melanoma cells producing leukemia-inhibitory factor. *Cancer Res* 1991; 51: 6656–9.
59. Todorov PT, Field WN, Tisdale MJ, Role of a proteolysis-inducing factor (PIF) in cachexia induced by a human melanoma (G361). *Br J Cancer* 1999; 80: 1734–7.
60. Sabatini M, Chavez J, Mundy GR, Bonewald LF, Stimulation of tumor necrosis factor release from monocytic cells by the A375 human melanoma via granulocyte-macrophage colony-stimulating factor. *Cancer Res* 1990; 50: 2673–8.
61. Nathanson L, Meelu MA, Losada R, Chemohormone therapy of metastatic melanoma with megestrol acetate plus dacarbazine, carmustine, and cisplatin. *Cancer* 1994; 73: 98–102.
62. Schacter L, Rozencweig M, Canetta R, et al, Megestrol acetate: clinical experience. *Cancer Treat Rev* 1989; 16: 49–63.
63. Eisen T, Boshoff C, Mak I, et al, Continuous low dose thalidomide: a phase II study in advanced melanoma, renal cell, ovarian and breast cancer. *Br J Cancer* 2000; 82: 812–7.
64. Burt ME, Brennan MF, Hypercalcemia and malignant melanoma. *Am J Surg* 1979; 137: 790–4.
65. Kageshita T, Matsui T, Hirai S, et al, Hypercalcaemia in melanoma patients associated with increased levels of parathyroid hormone-related protein. *Melanoma Res* 1999; 9: 69–73.
66. Yeung SC, Eton O, Burton DW, et al, Hypercalcemia due to parathyroid hormone-related protein secretion by melanoma. *Horm Res* 1998; 49: 288–91.
67. Elias AN, Pandian MR, Jacowatz J, Parathyroid hormone-related protein in patients with malignant melanoma. *Arch Dermatol* 1992; 128: 278–9 (letter).
68. Butow PN, Coates AS, Dunn SM, Psychosocial predictors of survival in metastatic melanoma. *J Clin Oncol* 1999; 17: 2256.
69. Gorenstein LA, Putnam JB, Natarajan G, et al, Improved survival after resection of pulmonary metastases from malignant melanoma. *Ann Thorac Surg* 1991; 52: 204–10 (see comments).
70. Hena MA, Emrich LJ, Nambisan RN, Karakousis CP, Effect of surgical treatment on stage IV melanoma. *Am J Surg* 1987; 153: 270–5.
71. Overett TK, Shiu MH, Surgical treatment of distant metastatic melanoma. Indications and results. *Cancer* 1985; 56: 1222–30.
72. Ollila DW, Hsueh EC, Stern SL, Morton DL, Metastasectomy for recurrent stage IV melanoma. *J Surg Oncol* 1999; 71: 209–13.
73. Wornom ILD, Smith JW, Soong SJ, et al, Surgery as palliative treatment for distant metastases of melanoma. *Ann Surg* 1986; 204: 181–5.
74. Rosenthal MA, Bull CA, Coates AS, et al, Synchronous cisplatin infusion during radiotherapy for the treatment of metastatic melanoma. *Eur J Cancer* 1991; 27: 1564–6.
75. Hill GJD, Krementz ET, Hill HZ, Dimethyl triazeno imidazole carboxamide and combination therapy for melanoma. IV. Late results after complete response to chemotherapy (Central Oncology Group protocols 7130, 7131, and 7131A). *Cancer* 1984; 53: 1299–305.
76. Legha SS, Hodges C, Ring S, Efficacy of ondansetron against nausea and vomiting caused by dacarbazine-containing chemotherapy. *Cancer* 1992; 70: 2018–20.
77. Nathanson L, Spontaneous regression of malignant melanoma: a review of the literature on incidence, clinical features, and possible mechanisms. *Natl Cancer Inst Monogr* 1976; 44: 67–76.
78. O'Connell ME, Powell BW, O'Connell JM, Harmer CL, Spontaneous regression of multiple bone metastases in malignant melanoma. *Br J Radiol* 1989; 62: 1095–100.
79. Bodurtha AJ, Berkelhammer J, Kim YH, et al, A clinical histologic, and immunologic study of a case of metastatic malignant melanoma undergoing spontaneous remission. *Cancer* 1976; 37: 735–42.
80. Bulkley GB, Cohen MH, Banks PM, et al, Long-term spontaneous regression of malignant melanoma with visceral metastases. Report of a case with immunologic profile. *Cancer* 1975; 36: 485–94.
81. Wang TS, Lowe L, Smith 2nd JW, et al, Complete spontaneous regression of pulmonary metastatic melanoma. *Dermatol Surg* 1998; 24: 915–9.
82. Sroujieh AS, Spontaneous regression of intestinal malignant melanoma from an occult primary site. *Cancer* 1988; 62: 1247–50.
83. Mikhail GR, Gorsulowsky DC, Spontaneous regression of metastatic malignant melanoma. *J Dermatol Surg Oncol* 1986; 12: 497–500.
84. Rampen F, Spontaneous regression of metastatic malignant melanoma. *Clin Oncol* 1979; 5: 91–2.
85. McCarthy WH, Shaw HM, Milton GW, Spontaneous regression of metastatic malignant melanoma. *Clin Oncol* 1978; 4: 203–7.
86. Angell M, Kassirer JP, Alternative medicine – the risks of untested and unregulated remedies. *N Engl J Med* 1998; 339: 839–41.
87. Ryan L, Kramar A, Borden E, Prognostic factors in metastatic melanoma. *Cancer* 1993; 71: 2995–3005.

88. Falkson CI, Falkson HC, Prognostic factors in metastatic malignant melanoma. An analysis of 236 patients treated on clinical research studies at the Department of Medical Oncology, University of Pretoria, South Africa from 1972–1992. *Oncology* 1998; 55: 59–64.
89. Nambisan RN, Alexiou G, Reese PA, Karakousis CP, Early metastatic patterns and survival in malignant melanoma. *J Surg Oncol* 1987; 34: 248–52.
90. Eton O, Legha SS, Moon TE, et al, Prognostic factors for survival of patients treated systemically for disseminated melanoma. *J Clin Oncol* 1998; 16: 1103–11.
91. Sirott MN, Bajorin DF, Wong GY, et al, Prognostic factors in patients with metastatic malignant melanoma. A multivariate analysis. *Cancer* 1993; 72: 3091–8.
92. Deichmann M, Benner A, Bock M, et al, S100–Beta, melanoma-inhibiting activity, and lactate dehydrogenase discriminate progressive from nonprogressive American Joint Committee on Cancer stage IV melanoma. *J Clin Oncol* 1999; 17: 1891–6.
93. Brand CU, Ellwanger U, Stroebel W, et al, Prolonged survival of 2 years or longer for patients with disseminated melanoma. An analysis of related prognostic factors. *Cancer* 1997; 79: 2345–53.
94. Hauschild A, Michaelsen J, Brenner W, et al, Prognostic significance of serum S100B detection compared with routine blood parameters in advanced metastatic melanoma patients. *Melanoma Res* 1999; 9: 155–61.
95. Einhorn LH, Burgess MA, Vallejos C, et al, Prognostic correlations and response to treatment in advanced metastatic malignant melanoma. *Cancer Res* 1974; 34: 1995–2004.
96. Luce JK, Chemotherapy of malignant melanoma. *Cancer* 1972; 30: 1604–15.
97. Nathanson L, Wolter J, Horton J, et al, Characteristics of prognosis and response to an imidazole carboxamide in malignant melanoma. *Clin Pharmacol Ther* 1971; 12: 955–62.
98. Costanza ME, Nathanson L, Schoenfeld D, et al, Results with methyl-CCNU and DTIC in metastatic melanoma. *Cancer* 1977; 40: 1010–15.

53

Adjuvant chemotherapy and biochemotherapy for high-risk primary disease and resected metastatic melanoma

Ian N Olver

INTRODUCTION

The concept of using adjuvant systemic therapy to target micrometastatic disease in high-risk primary and resected melanoma is sound, but its potential has yet to be realized in practice. In applying the principles of adjuvant chemotherapy to melanoma, parallels should be drawn with solid tumours such as breast and colon cancer, where adjuvant chemotherapy has been shown to have an impact upon survival.[1,2]

The selection of suitable groups of patients who are likely to benefit from adjuvant therapy is important. It will be difficult to show the additional benefit of any adjuvant therapy in good prognosis disease. The advent of newer staging tests, markers or techniques, such as the multiple sectioning of sentinel nodes in melanoma, may alter the prognostic categories into which patients are placed. This can refine the patient population likely to benefit from systemic adjuvant therapy.

Chemotherapy alone, with both single and multiple drugs, has had no impact on survival when given as systemic adjuvant therapy after definitive local treatment. Whereas biological agents and vaccines alone hold more promise, their combination with chemotherapy (variously called chemoimmunotherapy or, more broadly, biochemotherapy) is being increasingly investigated. Although some systemic adjuvant strategies may result from direct translation of basic research to the clinical setting, most of the adjuvant systemic therapies are first tested in metastatic melanoma. It is here that emerging candidate regimens for testing in the adjuvant setting must be looked for.

SELECTION OF PATIENTS FOR ADJUVANT SYSTEMIC THERAPY

For patients who present with primary cutaneous melanomas without spread to lymph nodes or distant metastases (American Joint Committee on Cancer (AJCC) stage I or II), the major prognostic factors are the depth of invasion of the melanoma and the presence of ulceration.[3] As the depth of invasion increases so the survival rate decreases: this is because of metastatic spread, which is attributed to subclinical micrometastatic disease persisting after resection of the primary tumour.[4] Fifty per cent of patients with thick primaries (>4 mm) will have an overt recurrence, which is what adjuvant therapy attempts to prevent by treating whilst the tumour burden is small.[5,6] For patients who present with local lymph node involvement (stage III disease), the number of lymph nodes is important in determining outcome. However, now that sentinel node biopsies are increasingly common in staging patients with melanomas, the subgroup of patients with micrometastases to sentinel and non-sentinel lymph nodes should identify a subgroup of patients whose worse survival also marks them as a suitable population for trials of adjuvant therapy.[7]

Surgery can be used to palliate localized distant metastatic recurrences of disease and these patients, thereby rendered free of evident disease, are also candidates for trials of systemic adjuvant therapy.[8] Patients with locoregionally recurrent melanoma to the extremities can be treated with adjuvant isolated limb perfusion or infusion chemotherapy after surgery.[9]

CANDIDATE CHEMOTHERAPY STRATEGIES FOR ADJUVANT TREATMENT

Anticancer drugs useful for adjuvant therapy in high-risk resected melanomas are identified from studies in patients with metastatic disease.

Single agents

Few chemotherapy agents have shown activity in metastatic melanoma (Table 53.1). Dacarbazine remains the most active single agent, with a response rate of *c.* 20% and a median duration of response quoted at 5–6 months.[10] Temozolamide is an orally active prodrug of the same alkylating agent as dacarbazine, 5-(3-methyltriazen-1-yl)imidazole-4-carboximide (MTIC), which penetrates into the central nervous system. A randomized phase III study of temozolamide versus dacarbazine in metastatic melanoma showed equal efficacy for the two drugs. The rigorously scrutinized response rates were at the lower end of previously reported ranges, with objective response rates for temozolamide of 13.5% and dacarbazine of 12.1%, including 3% complete responders for each drug. Median survival times were 7.7 and 6.4 months, respectively.[11]

The synthetic nitrosoureas including lomustine (CCNU) and carmustine (BCNU), have well-documented activities that range from 10 to 20%.[12] Fotemustine was synthesized to penetrate better into cells, particularly those of the central nervous system. An objective response rate in a large phase II multicentre study included responders with cerebral metastases.[13]

Other classes of drugs where activity has been recorded include platinum compounds, vinca alkaloids and taxanes.[12,14–16]

Combination chemotherapy

A strategy for improving the response rates to chemotherapy has been to use combinations of active drugs (Table 53.2). Most of these include dacarbazine, although some regimens based on cisplatin have been reported.[17,18] Phase II studies have yielded high response rates, in excess of 40%.[12] However, these increased response rates have not resulted in durable remissions. Randomized trials comparing single agents with combinations have shown the latter to be more toxic than the single agents but have not shown any consistent advantage over dacarbazine, which would warrant using this strategy in the adjuvant setting.[19–21]

Table 53.1 *Single agents for metastatic melanoma*

Drug	Objective response rates (%)
Dacarbazine	20 (12)
Temozolomide	13
Lomustine (CCNU)	13
Carmustine (BCNU)	18
Fotemustine	26
Cisplatin	23
Carboplatin	16
Vincristine	12
Vinblastine	13
Vindesine	14
Paclitaxel	18
Docetaxel	13

Table 53.2 *Selected drug combinations for metastatic melanoma*

Combination	Objective response rates (%)
Dacarbazine Nitrosourea	21
Dacarbazine Vinca alkaloid	18
Dacarbazine Cisplatin	25
Dacarbazine Vinca alkaloid Cisplatin	32
Dacarbazine Cisplatin Carmustine (BCNU)	10
Cisplatin Vinblastine Bleomycin	10

Dose intensity

In metastatic disease, improving the dose intensity of drugs has been tried to overcome resistance. Cisplatin exhibits a dose–response relationship as its dose is escalated. Higher response rates have resulted from cisplatin being given with the chemoprotectant amifostine, but the duration of responses has been disappointing.[22,23] Studies of high-dose chemotherapy with autologous bone marrow rescue include several small trials of alkylating agents, e.g. dacarbazine and nitrosoureas, and combinations which have yielded response rates up to 58% but median response durations have been short.[24–27] This is a suitable approach to investigate for minimal disease in the adjuvant setting in solid tumours.

Regional perfusion

Higher doses of chemotherapy with or without hyperthermia can be delivered to a melanoma by arterial infusion, or isolated perfusion or infusion of an extremity, with in-transit melanoma metastases. Although dacarbazine or cisplatin can be used, melphalan is the drug most commonly reported as being successful.[28–31] This is another strategy suitable for prophylactic or adjuvant use.

Endocrine therapy

Observations of the behaviour of melanomas during pregnancy, their rarity prior to puberty and the improved survival in women as compared to men have suggested that melanomas may be hormonally responsive, perhaps via binding of oestrogen to cell-surface receptors. Tamoxifen, however, demonstrates little objective activity as a single agent.[32,33] An advantage has been shown for the combination of tamoxifen and dacarbazine over dacarbazine alone, particularly in women.[34] There is also a suggestion that tamoxifen increases the sensitivity of melanoma to cisplatin by inhibiting calcium channels.[35,36]

Tamoxifen has been added to melanoma chemotherapy regimens and some phase II trials have suggested favourable response rates.[37] The Dartmouth regimen has been well studied (carmustine, dacarbazine and cisplatin (BCD) plus or minus tamoxifen) but a phase III trial did not show an increased response rate when tamoxifen was added to BCD.[38,39] As with other combinations, a randomized study comparing the Dartmouth regimen to dacarbazine alone has shown no significant survival advantage and more toxicity with the combination regimen, and therefore provides no rationale for testing chemohormonal therapy in the adjuvant setting.[40]

ADJUVANT CHEMOTHERAPY ALONE FOR MELANOMA

The chemotherapy strategies outlined above have been tried in the adjuvant setting for melanoma at high risk of recurrence after definitive local treatment. Chemotherapy has not been successful in the adjuvant setting.

Adjuvant single agent and combination chemotherapy

Dacarbazine

Randomized controlled trials which test dacarbazine in the adjuvant setting include the Central Oncology Group study, which randomized patients with AJCC stages II–IV melanoma to dacarbazine or observation and found that the treated patients' survival was worse than the control group.[41] A World Health Organization (WHO) trial compared dacarbazine with bacille Calmette-Guérin (BCG) or their combination, by observation in 761 patients with AJCC stages I–III melanoma; it was shown that dacarbazine did not alter survival over surgery alone.[42] The European Organization for Research and Treatment of Cancer (EORTC) protocol (trial 18761) compared dacarbazine to levamisole or placebo in 274 AJCC stage II patients, showing no difference for chemotherapy over placebo.[43] In one small trial of only 26 patients with AJCC stage I or II melanoma randomized to dacarbazine, combination chemotherapy with dacarbazine, lomustine and vincristine, or observation, the overall survival was significantly longer than in controls.[44]

Several other trials of dacarbazine alone or in combination have shown no improvement in survival after receiving adjuvant dacarbazine.[45–49]

Lomustine

Lomustine, a single agent nitrosourea, did not improve survival when given to patients with high-risk primary or nodal disease.[50]

Adjuvant high-dose chemotherapy

A trial of high-dose chemotherapy with autologous bone marrow rescue as adjuvant treatment for 39 patients with stage III melanoma with five or more lymph nodes involved, tested the concept of dose intensity in a randomized study against observation. The chemotherapy was high-dose cyclophosphamide (1875 $mg/m^2/day$ for 3 days), 72-hour continuous infusion cisplatin (55 $mg/m^2/day$) and carmustine (600 mg/m^2 on day 4). Although time to progression doubled from 16 to 35 weeks, there was no difference in either the disease-free or overall survival.[51]

Adjuvant regional perfusion chemotherapy

The initial data on the adjuvant use of isolated limb perfusion (ILP) came from retrospective and uncontrolled studies.[52] Three randomized studies have been published. In the first, 107 patients with melanomas of the distal two-thirds of the limbs were randomized to receiving hyperthermic ILP with melphalan or observation after wide local excision and lymphadenectomy. The study was closed after an interim analysis, with a significant improvement in survival in the treatment arm ($P<0.01$) and after a median follow-up of 6 years, 26 recurrences in 54 control patients and only six recurrences in 53 patients in the perfusion arm ($P<0.001$).[53]

In the second study, 69 patients with recurrent malignant melanoma of the extremities were randomly allocated to surgery (36 patients) or surgery plus hyperthermic ILP with melphalan. The tumour-free survival was significantly better for the perfusion group ($P=0.044$), but the difference in median survival was not significant.[9]

The third study was a large, well-planned and carefully conducted multicentre trial of adjuvant ILP conducted jointly by the EORTC, the WHO Melanoma Program and the North American Perfusion Group.[54] A total of 832 patients with melanomas >1.5 mm in thickness were randomized to wide excision only or wide excision plus hyperthermic ILP. No benefit for adjuvant ILP, either in terms of time to distant metastasis or survival, was demonstrated. These trials are discussed in more detail in Chapter 37.

Miscellaneous adjuvant drugs

A number of other agents have been the subject of adjuvant trials.

Megesterol acetate

Based on observations suggesting that hormones have some impact on the natural history of melanoma and the presence of steroid hormone receptors on melanoma cells, the Mayo Clinic performed a randomized trial of megesterol acetate versus placebo in patients with resected high-risk stage II and III melanoma. There was a trend towards a survival advantage at 3 years for the patients receiving megesterol acetate (7.6 versus 2.6 years, $P=0.06$).[55] A second and larger trial was initiated to further investigate this result.

Melatonin

In a small randomized study, 30 patients who were node positive were randomized to melatonin or observation. There was a significant difference in disease-free survival at 31 months in favour of the melatonin-treated group.[56]

Vitamin A and 13-*cis* retinoic acid

Based on the topical activity of vitamin A in non-melanoma skin cancers and activity of retinoids preclinically, the Southwest Oncology Group commenced a large randomized trial of vitamin A given orally in stage I and II melanoma. No disease-free or overall survival advantage was demonstrated, but the study lacked sufficient power for subgroup analyses.[57] A randomized trial of 13-*cis* retinoic acid as adjuvant therapy following resection of melanoma did not reveal a clinically significant benefit.[58]

CANDIDATE BIOLOGICAL THERAPIES TO COMBINE WITH ADJUVANT CHEMOTHERAPY

Along with the trials of chemotherapy in melanoma, there has been an investigation of biological agents. The natural history of melanoma is highly variable and has been thought to be influenced by the body's immune system, particularly following observations of spontaneous regressions of lesions.[59] Biological response modifiers and, more recently, vaccines are being investigated in both metastatic disease and in the adjuvant setting. In the context of this discussion, this creates the potential to add these agents to chemotherapy in the adjuvant setting, so termed biochemotherapy (Table 53.3). Certainly, the toxicity profiles of these biological agents are favourable for combining with chemotherapy and, in many cases, even additive responses would constitute a significant outcome. First, the range of potential agents will be examined and then their use as part of adjuvant biochemotherapy for high-risk melanoma will be considered.

Bacillus Calmette-Guérin (BCG)

Following the observation that intralesional BCG caused regression not only of the cutaneous melanoma metastases injected but also of some non-injected lesions, suggesting a systemic immune response, it was investigated as a postsurgical adjuvant treatment in AJCC stage II and III melanomas.[60] None of 13 randomized trials has shown an impact on either disease-free or overall survival in those patients receiving BCG.[61] In a retrospective analysis of one of these trials it was revealed that, although there was no impact on overall survival, patients with lymph node involvement who initially had a negative BCG skin test showed an improved survival over the observation arm if they received either BCG alone or BCG in combination with dacarbazine.[42] This suggested that a primary response to BCG was necessary for an antitumour response, but this has not been confirmed by other studies. BCG, however, became a candidate for combining with chemotherapy, both in the advanced and adjuvant setting.

Corynebacterium parvum

Heat-killed *Corynebacterium parvum* was also tested for its ability to stimulate an immune response against melanoma. In a study in AJCC stage I and II melanomas the Southeastern Cancer Study Group found no improvement in the 3-year survival for *C. parvum* over placebo, but in patients with melanomas deeper than 3 mm there was an improved disease-free survival.[62] A European trial of *C. parvum* compared to placebo, as adjuvant therapy in node-positive melanoma, showed no benefit.[63] Two further trials compared *C. parvum* with BCG in AJCC stage III disease.[64,65] One showed significantly improved disease-free and overall survival, whereas the other did not. However, retrospective pooled data indicated improvement in both disease-free and overall survival over BCG, particularly for patients younger than 60 years of age.[66]

Table 53.3 *Candidate biological therapies to combine with adjuvant chemotherapy for melanoma*

Bacillo Calmette Guérin
Corynebacterium parvum
Levamisole
Interferon-alfa
Interleukin-2 (IL-2)
Melanoma vaccines

Levamisole

Levamisole is an immunomodulatory agent that restores subnormal T lymphocyte and phagocytic functions.[67] Two randomized studies in node-negative disease could not demonstrate an advantage in either disease-free or overall survival.[43,68] In contrast, one of two large randomized studies which compared adjuvant levamisole with BCG, levamisole alternating with BCG or observation in 543 patients with >0.75 mm thick melanomas, satellite lesions, in-transit metastases or regional lymph node involvement, showed a 29% reduction in both the death rate (P=0.08) and the recurrence rate (P=0.08) at a median follow-up of 8.5 years.[69] In the other double-blind randomized study comparing levamisole and placebo, involving 203 patients with the same characteristics, no difference was seen between the arms after a second analysis at a median of 10.5 years.[70] The first of these studies used higher doses (800 mg for 2 years versus 450 mg for 2 years) but more patients receiving the higher doses needed dose reductions. The role of this agent remains unresolved both as a single agent and in combination with chemotherapy.

Interferon-alfa

Based on the single-agent activity in metastatic disease, where the overall response rate is *c.* 15%, interferon-alfa has been tested in the adjuvant setting.[36] An Eastern Cooperative Oncology Group (ECOG) study (trial 1684) of high-dose interferon (20 MIU/m^2 intravenous (IV) daily × 5 days/week then 10 MIU/m^2

subcutaneous (SC) every 3 weeks for 48 weeks) versus observation in 287 patients with AJCC stage IIB or III melanoma showed that median survival (3.8 versus 2.8 years P=0.002) and 5-year survival (3.8 versus 2.8 years, P=0.02) were significantly better in the high-dose interferon arm.[71] There was no benefit in the node-negative subgroup. The high-dose regimen was toxic but a Q-TWIST analysis showed improvement in the quality-of-life-adjusted survival time.[72] A previous study of the short-term use of high-dose interferon-alfa as adjuvant therapy in node-positive patients with melanoma had shown a disease-free survival advantage.[73] A follow-up trial comparing the ECOG high-dose regimen with low-dose interferon and observation did not reproduce an overall survival advantage for the high-dose interferon, but it did show an improved relapse-free survival at a median follow-up of 52 months.[74] The observation arm did better than in the previous trial; there was no significant effect in the low-dose interferon arm. These results parallel other trials, with two studies showing a disease-free survival benefit in AJCC stage II disease.[75,76] This opens the way for interferon-alfa to be investigated in combination with other biological agents and chemotherapy in the adjuvant therapy of melanoma and advanced disease. Adjuvant therapy with interferon-alfa is discussed in more detail in Chapter 55.

Interferon-gamma

Interferon-gamma is immunomodulatory in that it activates macrophages and upregulates major histocompatability antigens. A randomized study of its use as adjuvant therapy for AJCC stages II and III melanoma performed by the Southwestern Oncology Group was initially stopped early when there was a trend suggesting that the treatment arm may be doing worse, but no increased mortality was evident on longer term follow-up.[77] A study comparing interferon-gamma to low-dose interferon-alfa is ongoing and will need to be completed before combinations of interferon-gamma with chemotherapy can be contemplated.

Interleukin-2 (IL-2)

The cytokine IL-2 had a 15% response rate in an overview of activity in metastatic disease.[78] High-dose IL-2, however, has been reported to yield durable complete remissions.[79] This was the case with the coadministration of lymphocyte-activated killer cells. Later, IL-2 was given with tumour-infiltrating lymphocytes, but the increased toxicity with these has not been matched by sufficient improvements in outcome to warrant them becoming generally applied.[36] Phase II trials of the combination of IL-2 and interferon-alfa have been encouraging, but a randomized trial of IL-2 versus IL-2 and interferon in metastatic disease failed to show a statistically significant difference over IL-2 alone.[80] The results of a small phase II trial of perioperative IL-2 and interferon in patients with high-risk primary disease or resectable recurrences were encouraging.[81] The combinations with chemotherapy when examining adjuvant biochemotherapy will be discussed below.

Transfer factor

Transfer factor was investigated as a postsurgical adjuvant therapy based on reports of transient tumour regressions in melanoma, but none of the controlled randomized studies have shown any significant benefit.[82]

Vaccines

There are many strategies for trying to immunize patients against antigens that will induce an immune response leading to regression of their melanoma. Some vaccines are polyvalent, using whole cells or fractions of cells, while some use more specific peptides as antigens. The initial study of adjuvant vaccine therapy used irradiated allogeneic cells administered either with or without BCG, but this was unsuccessful.[83] The polyvalent melanoma cell vaccine (Cancervax) was given with BCG to 186 patients with AJCC stages IB, IIA and IIB, and these were compared to a surgery only series with 1218 patients. Overall survival was significantly different but a prospectively randomized trial will be required to confirm these findings.[84] A commercial vaccine in cultured tumour cell lines (Melacine) given with the adjuvant Detox is being tested by the Southwest Oncology Group (SWOG 9035) for the adjuvant treatment of T3 melanoma.

Alternatively, vaccines could be prepared from antigens shed into culture media by allogeneic melanomas. A randomized trial in 38 patients with resected AJCC stage III melanoma showed a 2-year mortality rate of 40% for the vaccine versus 23% for the placebo.[85]

A polyvalent vaccine may not target a specific patient's melanoma, so autologous vaccines have been tried. They require sufficient tumour to produce them but in randomized trials postsurgery no objective benefit has been shown.[86] To augment immunogenicity of autologous vaccines, melanoma cells have been transfected with genes encoding cytokines (granulocyte-macrophage-colony-stimulating factor (GM-CSF), interferon-gamma, IL-2) or costimulatory molecules. Heat-shock proteins that carry peptides from tumour antigens have also been used to immunize patients to cause regression and protect from wild-type tumour challenge.[87] Autologous tumour cells have also been modified with the hapten dinitrophenol and tested in the adjuvant setting in lymph-node-positive patients after lymphadenectomy. A phase II trial, recently updated, suggests a better outcome than retrospective surgery only data, and a phase III trial is ongoing, comparing a dinitrophenol (DNP) modified autologous tumour cell vaccine with high-dose interferon-alfa to confirm the efficacy of this approach.[88]

Viral oncolysates have also been created by infecting allogeneic tumour cells with cytolytic viruses, such as vaccinia and Newcastle disease virus, with the aim of initiating an antiviral immune response that will aid in the recognition of tumour-associated antigens. A randomized trial of 217 AJCC stage III patients who received a vaccinia oncolysate or a control of live vaccine failed to demonstrate either an overall or a disease-free survival advantage for the melanoma oncolysate vaccine.[89]

To develop more specific vaccines, the most common tumour-associated antigens were sought. The GM2 ganglioside is a target for antiglycolipid antibodies. In a study of 122 patients with AJCC stage III melanoma, they were randomized to GM2/BCG vaccine or to BCG alone. When patients with prevaccination GM2 antibodies were excluded, an intention-to-treat analysis revealed no improvement in disease-free or overall survival.[90] A subsequently developed vaccine uses GM2 with an immunogenic carrier protein (keyhole limpet haemocyanin (KLH)) and is given with an immunologic adjuvant QS21. Trials are under way comparing this to placebo and high-dose interferon-alfa.

A further approach is to develop peptide vaccines from proteins on the surface of melanomas (gp100, tyrosinase, MART and melanoma antigens Mage 1 and 3) which are all recognized by T cells but are restricted according to the humon leucocyte antigen (HLA) subtype. These peptides have been used to load dendritic cells that present the antigens to induce a primary T cell response.[91]

Adjuvant immunotherapy for melanoma is discussed in more detail in Chapters 54 and 55. The development of vaccines opens up the possibility of combined therapy with biological agents such as interferon-alfa and IL-2, as well as with cytotoxic drugs, where questions of scheduling will be critical.

ADJUVANT BIOCHEMOTHERAPY

Having explored potential biological agents for use in combination with chemotherapy in the adjuvant treatment of melanoma, the trials of biochemotherapy that have been undertaken will now be considered (Table 53.4). Regimens are being developed in metastatic disease and those with promising results tested as adjuvant therapy.

Chemotherapy and bacille Calmette-Guérin (BCG)

Dacarbazine and BCG have been used together in randomized trials in the adjuvant treatment of AJCC stage III melanoma.[42, 92–94] Only a small study suggested an improvement in recurrence and survival.[94] The large WHO trial showed no survival benefit but in the subgroup of patients with AJCC stage III melanoma whose BCG skin test was negative, the BCG and BCG with dacarbazine arms showed a significantly prolonged disease-free and overall survival, even after adjusting for other prognostic factors.[42,95]

Combination chemotherapy has been used with BCG in the adjuvant treatment of melanoma. In a French study of 248 patients there was no difference between BCG and BCG with lomustine, dacarbazine

Table 53.4 *Adjuvant biochemotherapy*

Dacarbazine and BCG
BCG + dacarbazine + CCNU + teniposide
BCNU + hydroxyurea + BCG
C. parvum + BCNU + actinomycin + vinblastine
Dacarbazine + IL-2

BCG, bacille Calmette-Guérin; CCNU, lomustine; BCNU, carmustine; *C. parvum*, *Corynebacterium parvum*.

and teniposide.[96] When carmustine, hydroxyurea and dacarbazine were combined with BCG in a Southwestern Cancer Study Group trial, the chemotherapy alone arm did better than the combination arm with BCG.[94]

Chemotherapy and *Corynebacterium parvum*

C. parvum alone has been compared with dacarbazine and *C. parvum* in combination and no difference has been found. Also, an adjuvant trial combined *C. parvum* and a chemotherapy regimen of carmustine, actinomycin and vinblastine, and compared it to chemotherapy alone. The study was small, with only 77 patients, and no difference between the arms was detected.[46]

Chemotherapy and interferon-alfa

The combination of chemotherapy and interferon is favourable in having non-overlapping toxicities and different mechanisms of activity. After initial reports of favourable activity in phase II trials for the combination, there have been five randomized trials in metastatic disease.[97–101] Only a small study of 61 patients showed a statistically significant improvement in response and survival rate, the others showed no advantage to adding the interferon-alfa to chemotherapy.[98] However, there have also been trials of combination chemotherapy, predominantly the Dartmouth regimen (carmustine, cisplatin, dacarbazine and tamoxifen), BOLD (bleomycin, vincristine, lomustine and dacarbozine) and CVD (cisplatin, vinblastine and dacarbazine), with interferon-alfa: response rates up to 68% have been reported but no survival advantage is apparent.[36,102,103] These results are not encouraging for translation into the adjuvant setting, particularly if contemplating adding the toxicity of chemotherapy to that of high-dose interferon-alfa. There is one small trial of low-dose interferon combined with tamoxifen as a second-line adjuvant treatment for melanoma patients who have relapsed post-adjuvant therapy and then been surgically resected.[104] The hypothesis is that tamoxifen will potentiate interferon activity in the adjuvant setting, but further follow-up is required.

Chemotherapy and interleukin-2 (IL-2)

An overview of 19 trials of IL-2 with chemotherapy in metastatic disease shows very little improvement over chemotherapy alone, although some studies have suggested an additive activity.[105,106] IL-2 with dacarbazine in patients with high-risk primaries or nodal involvement were reported as having a relapse-free survival at 2 years of 65% in 60 patients, which compares favourably with patients treated with adjuvant high-dose interferon on ECOG trial 1684, but will need verifying in a prospectively randomized trial.[107]

Chemotherapy with interferon-alfa and interleukin-2 (IL-2)

In metastatic melanoma, single agents such as cisplatin were given with IL-2 and interferon-alfa, and then combinations (such as cisplatin, vinblastine, dacarbazine or cisplatin, dacarbazine and carmustine) were combined with immunotherapy; durable complete responses were a feature of the reports.[108–110] More recent regimens incorporate GM-CSF to mobilize antigen-presenting cells and also incorporate newer agents such as temozolamide.[111,112]

Randomized studies of biochemotherapy incorporating multiple immunotherapy agents in metastatic disease have yielded variable results. A study by Rosenberg et al.[113] of cisplatin, dacarbazine and tamoxifen, alone or in combination with high-dose interferon-alfa and IL-2, showed more toxicity as a result of adding immunotherapy but no improvement in survival. An interim analysis of the EORTC study of cisplatin, dacarbazine and interferon-alfa, with or without IL-2, showed no difference in response but fewer patients relapsing on the IL-2 arm.[114] A trial from the MD Anderson Cancer Center of cisplatin, vinblastine and dacarbazine, alone or with IL-2 or interferon-alfa-2b, showed significant improvements in response rates, time to progression and overall survival in metastatic disease.[115]

There have been no large trials of immunotherapy agents combined with chemotherapy in the adjuvant setting; however, trials are emerging where immunotherapy is being used in addition to chemotherapy to improve the outcome after the chemotherapy has debulked the disease, or to maintain remission after biochemotherapy in metastatic disease.[116,117] A phase II study of maintenance biotherapy consisting of IL-2 after achieving a complete response or partial response to biochemotherapy has also been reported: five patients (26%) achieved a further response while the progression-free survival was reported as better than that of historical controls.[117]

Sequential or concomitant chemotherapy and immunotherapy as adjuvant therapy requires further exploration.

Chemotherapy and vaccines as adjuvant biochemotherapy

As outlined above, various strategies for developing melanoma vaccines are being trialed in the adjuvant setting. ECOG and the US intergroup are comparing the GM2 vaccine with interferon-alfa, while phase II trials investigate concurrent or sequential use of interferon-alfa and vaccines.[118] Chemotherapy has been used with vaccines. In a trial of adjuvant immunotherapy in high-risk patients with node-positive disease, low-dose cyclophosphamide was administered prior to vaccines of irradiated autologous melanoma cells to reduce the population of T suppressor cells.[119] If chemotherapy is to be used as a cytotoxic with vaccines in melanoma its role may be more to debulk disease before use of a vaccine, or in a sequence of treatments where the immunotherapy is used to prolong remission.

FUTURE ADVANCES IN ADJUVANT CHEMOTHERAPY AND BIOCHEMOTHERAPY

An important advance in adjuvant therapy is an improved ability to predict the prognosis of the disease and to identify patients who require systemic treatment in addition to definitive local treatment. At one level, the prognostic significance of microscopic tumour in sentinel nodes may refine the patient population who require adjuvant therapy. Molecular markers, the assessment of genetic mutations and the increasing ability to detect occult metastases will all impact on the selection of patients for adjuvant therapy.

If chemotherapy is going to be important in the adjuvant therapy of primary or recurrent melanoma, new drugs which impact on survival in metastatic disease will need to be identified. Even then, biochemotherapy has more potential than chemotherapy alone as adjuvant treatment. Melanoma vaccines appear to hold the greatest promise of the adjuvant therapies discussed. The concept of immunotherapy prolonging remissions induced by chemotherapy requires further exploration.

CONCLUSIONS

Chemotherapy or biochemotherapy cannot yet be recommended as standard adjuvant treatment for high-risk primary or resected recurrent melanoma. Patients who are potential candidates for adjuvant systemic treatment should participate in ongoing clinical trials.

REFERENCES

1. Wolmark N, Rockette H, Mamounas E et al, Clinical trial to assess the relative efficacy of fluorouracil and leucovorin, fluorouracil and levamisole, fluorouracil, leucovorin and levamisole in patients with Dukes' B and C carcinoma of the colon: results from the National Surgical Breast and Bowel Project C-04. *J Clin Oncol* 1999; 17: 3553–9.
2. Mansour EG, Gray R, Shatila AH et al, Survival advantage of adjuvant chemotherapy in high-risk node-negative breast cancer: ten year analysis – an intergroup study. *J Clin Oncol* 1998; 16: 3486–92.
3. Agarwala SS, Atkins MB, Kirkwood JM. Current approaches to advanced and high risk melanoma. In: *American Society of Clinical Oncology Fall Educational Book* (ed Perry MC). Alexandria VA: American Society of Clinical Oncology, 1999: 83–97.
4. Morton DL, Davtyan DG, Wanek LA et al, Multivariate analysis of the relationship between survival and the microstage of primary melanoma by Clark level and Breslow thickness. *Cancer* 1993; 71: 3737–43.
5. Barth A, Morton DL, The role of adjuvant therapy in melanoma management. *Cancer* 1995; 75: 726–34.
6. Goldie JH, Scientific basis for adjuvant and primary (neoadjuvant) chemotherapy. *Semin Oncol* 1987; 14: 1–7.
7. Leong S, Achtem T, Miller J et al, Clinical significance of melanoma micrometastases to sentinel lymph nodes and other high risk factors. *Proc ASCO* 2000; 19: 2170a (abstract).
8. Wong H, Skinner KA, Kim KA et al, The role of surgery in the treatment of nonregionally recurrent melanoma. *Surgery* 1993; 113: 389–94.
9. Hafstrom L, Rudenstam CM, Blomquist E et al, Regional hyperthermic perfusion with melphalan after surgery for recurrent malignant melanoma of the extremities. *J Clin Oncol* 1991; 9: 2091–4.
10. Carbone PP, Costello W, Eastern Cooperative Oncology Group studies with DTIC (NSC–45388). *Cancer Treat Rep* 1976; 60: 193–8.
11. Middleton MR, Grob JJ, Aaronson N et al, Randomised phase III study of temozolamide versus dacarbazine in the treatment of patients with advanced metastatic malignant melanoma. *J Clin Oncol* 2000; 18: 158–66.
12. Legha SS, Current therapy for malignant melanoma. *Semin Oncol* 1989; 16: 34–44.
13. Jacquillat C, Khayat D, Banzet P et al, Final report of the French Multicenter phase II study of the nitrosourea fotemustine in 153 evaluable patients with disseminated malignant melanoma including patients with cerebral metastases. *Cancer* 1990; 66: 1873–8.
14. Goodnight JE, Moseley HS, Eilber FR et al, Cis-dichlorodiammineplatinum(II) alone and combined with DTIC for the treatment of disseminated melanoma. *Cancer Treat Rep* 1979; 63: 2007.
15. Evans L, Casper ES, Rosenbluth R, Phase II trial of carboplatin in advanced malignant melanoma. *Cancer Treat Rep* 1987; 71: 171–2.
16. Aamdal S, Wolff I, Kaplan S et al, Docetaxel (Taxotere) in advanced malignant melanoma: a phase II study of the EORTC Early Clinical Trials Group. *Eur J Cancer* 1994; 30A: 1061–4.
17. Costanza ME, Nathanson L, Schoenfeld D et al, Results with methyl-CCNU and DTIC in malignant melanoma. *Cancer* 1977; 40: 1010–15.
18. National Cancer Institute of Canada Melanoma Group. Vinblastine, bleomycin, and cis-platinum for the treatment of metastatic malignant melanoma. *J Clin Oncol* 1984; 2: 131–4.
19. Ahmann DL, Hahn RG, Bisel HF, Evaluation of 1-(2-chloroethyl-3-4-methylcyclohexyl)-1nitrosourea (methyl-CCNU, NSC 95411) versus combined imidazole carboxamide (NSC 45388) and vincristine (NSC 67574) in palliation of disseminated malignant melanoma. *Cancer* 1973; 33: 615–18.

20. Luikart SD, Kennealey GT, Kirkwood JM, Randomised phase III trial of vinblastine, bleomycin and cis-dichlorodiammine-platinum versus dacarbazine in malignant melanoma. *J Clin Oncol* 1984; 2: 164–8.
21. Buziad AC, Legha S, Winn R et al, Cisplatin©, vinblastine (V), and dacarbazine (D) (CVD) versus dacarbazine alone in metastatic melanoma: preliminary results of a phase III cancer community oncology program (CCOP trial). *Proc ASCO* 1993; 12: 389.
22. Chary KK, Higby DJ, Henderson ES, Swinerton KD, Phase I study of high-dose cis-dichlorodiammine platinum(II) with forced diuresis. *Cancer Treat Rep* 1977; 61: 367–70.
23. Glover G, Glick JH, Weiler C et al, WR2721 and high-dose cisplatin: an active combination in the treatment of metastatic melanoma. *J Clin Oncol* 1987; 5: 574–8.
24. Phillips GL, Fay JW, Herzig GP et al, Intensive 1,3-bis(2-chlorethyl)-1-nitrosourea (BCNU), NSC-409962 and cryopreserved autologous marrow transplantation for refractory cancer: a phase I–II study. *Cancer* 1983; 52: 1792–802.
25. Lazarus HM, Herzig RH, Wolff SN et al. Treatment of metastatic malignant melanoma with intensive melphalan and autologous bone marrow transplantation. *Cancer Treat Rep* 1985; 69: 473–7.
26. McElwain TJ, Hedley DW, Burton G et al, Marrow autotransplantation accelerates haematological recovery in patients with malignant melanoma treated with high-dose melphalan. *Br J Cancer* 1979; 40: 72–80.
27. Thatcher N, Lind M, Morgenstern G et al, High dose double alkylating agent chemotherapy with DTIC, melphalan or ifosfamide and marrow rescue for metastatic malignant melanoma. *Cancer* 1989; 63: 1296–302.
28. Savlov ED, Hall TC, Oberfield RA, Intra-arterial therapy of melanoma with dimethyl triazeno imidazole carboxamide (NSC-45388). *Cancer* 1971; 28: 1161–4.
29. Calvo III DB, Patt YZ, Wallace S et al, Phase I–II trial of percutaneous intra-arterial cisdiamminedichloroplatinum(II) for regionally confined malignancy. *Cancer* 1980; 45: 1278–83.
30. Storm FK, Morton DL, Value of therapeutic hyperthermic limb perfusion in advanced recurrent melanoma of the lower extremity. *Am J Surg* 1985; 150: 32–5.
31. Reintgen DS, Cruse CW, Wells KE et al, Isolated limb perfusion for recurrent melanoma of the extremity. *Ann Plast Surg* 1992; 28: 50–4.
32. Creagan ET, Ingle JN, Ahmann DL, Jiang NS, Phase II study of tamoxifen in patients with disseminated malignant melanoma. *Cancer Treat Rep* 1980; 64: 199–201.
33. Papac RC, Kirkwood JM, High-dose tamoxifen in metastatic melanoma. *Cancer Treat Rep* 1983; 67: 1051–2.
34. Cocconi G, Bella M, Calabresi F et al, Treatment of metastatic malignant melanoma with dacarbazine plus tamoxifen. *N Engl J Med* 1992; 327: 516–23.
35. McClay EF, Mastrangelo MJ, Sprandio JD et al, The importance of tamoxifen to a cisplatin-containing regimen in the treatment of metastatic melanoma. *Cancer* 1989; 63: 1292–5.
36. Chowdhurry S, Vaughan MM, Gore ME, New approaches to the systemic treatment of melanoma. *Cancer Treat Rev* 1999; 25: 259–70.
37. Martinez-Cedillo J, Padilla-Rosciano A, Cuellar-Hube M, Maafs-Molina E, Chemo-hormonal therapy in metastatic melanoma. *Proc ASCO* 2000; 19: 2253a (abstract).
38. Del Prete SA, Maurer LH, O'Donnell J et al, Combination chemotherapy with cisplatin, carmustine, dacarbazine and tamoxifen in metastatic melanoma. *Cancer Treat Rep* 1984; 68: 1403–5.
39. Rusthoven JJ, Quirt IC, Iscoe NA et al, Randomised double blind, placebo-controlled trial comparing the response rates of carmustine, dacarbazine and cisplatin with and without tamoxifen in patients with metastatic melanoma. *J Clin Oncol* 1996; 14: 2033–90.
40. Saxman SB, Meyers ML, Chapman PB et al, A phase III multicentre randomised trial of DTIC, cisplatin, BCNU and tamoxifen vs. DTIC alone in patients with metastatic melanoma. *Proc ASCO* 1999; 18: 2068a (abstract).
41. Hill II GJ, Moss SE, Golumb FM et al, DTIC and combination therapy for melanoma: III. DTIC (NSC 45388) Surgical Adjuvant Study COG PROTOCOL 7040. *Cancer* 1981; 47: 2556–62.
42. Veronesi U, Adamus J, Aubert C et al, A randomised trial of adjuvant chemotherapy and immunotherapy in cutaneous melanoma. *N Engl J Med* 1982; 307: 913–16.
43. Lejeune FJ, Macher E, Kleeberg U et al, An assessment of DTIC versus levamisole or placebo in the treatment of high risk stage I patients after surgical removal of a primary melanoma of the skin. A phase II adjuvant study (EORTC protocol 18761). *Eur J Cancer* 1988; 24: S81–S90.
44. Hansson J, Ringborg U, Lagerhof B, Strander H, Adjuvant chemotherapy of malignant melanoma. A pilot study. *Am J Clin Oncol* 1985; 8: 47–50.
45. Karakousis CP, Emrich LJ, Adjuvant treatment of malignant melanoma with DTIC + estracyt or BCG. *J Surg Oncol* 1987; 36: 235–8.
46. Banzet P, Jacquillat C, Civatte J et al, Adjuvant chemotherapy in the management of primary malignant melanoma. *Cancer* 1978; 41: 1240–8.
47. Balch CM, Murray D, Presant C, Bartolucci AA, Ineffectiveness of adjuvant chemotherapy using DTIC and cyclophosphamide in patients with resectable metastatic melanoma. *Surgery* 1984; 95: 454–9.
48. Kaiser LR, Burk MW, Morton DL, Adjuvant therapy for malignant melanoma. *Surg Clin N Am* 1981; 61: 1249–57.
49. Demierre M-F, Koh HK, Adjuvant therapy for cutaneous malignant melanoma. *J Am Acad Dermatol* 1997; 36: 747–64.
50. Fisher RI, Terry WD, Hodes RJ et al, Adjuvant immunotherapy or chemotherapy for malignant melanoma: preliminary report of the NCI randomised trial. *Surg Clin N Am* 1981; 61: 1267–77.
51. Meisenberg BR, Ross M, Vredenburgh JJ et al, Randomized trial of high-dose chemotherapy with autologous bone marrow support as adjuvant therapy for high-risk, multi-node-positive malignant melanoma. *J Natl Cancer Inst* 1993; 85: 1080–5.
52. Krementz ET, Ryan RF, Muchmore JH et al, Hyperthermic regional perfusion for melanoma of the limbs. In: *Cutaneous Melanoma*, 2nd edn (eds Balch CM, Houghton A, Milton GW et al). Philadelphia: Lippincott, 1992: 403–26.
53. Ghussen F, Kruger I, Smalley RV et al, Hyperthermic perfusion with chemotherapy for melanoma of the extremities. *World J Surg* 1989; 13: 598–602.
54. Schraffordt Koops H, Vaglini M, Suciu S et al, Prophylactic isolated limb perfusion for localized, high-risk limb melanoma: results of a multicenter randomized phase III trial. *J Clin Oncol* 1998; 16: 2906–12.
55. Creagan ET, Ingle JN, Schutt AJ, Schaid DJ, A prospective, randomized controlled trial of megesterol acetate among high-risk patients with resected malignant melanoma. *Am J Clin Oncol* 1989; 12: 152–5.
56. Lissoni P, Brivio O, Brivio F et al, Adjuvant therapy with the pineal hormone melatonin in patients with lymph node relapse due to malignant melanoma. *J Pineal Res* 1996; 21: 239–42.
57. Meyskens Jr FL, Liu PY, Tuthill RJ et al, Randomized trial of vitamin A versus observation as adjuvant therapy in high-risk primary malignant melanoma: a Southwest Oncology Group Study. *J Clin Oncol* 1994; 12: 2060–5.
58. Legha SS, Papadopoulos N, Pickett S et al, Adjuvant therapy for high risk local and regional melanoma using 13-cis retinoic acid. In: *Adjuvant Therapy of Cancer IV* (eds Salmon SE, Jones SE). New York: Grune and Stratton, 1984.
59. Sumner WC, Spontaneous regression of melanoma: report of a case. *Cancer* 1953; 6: 1040–3.
60. Morton DL, Eilber FR, Malmgren RA, Wood WC, Immunological factors which influence response to immunotherapy in malignant melanoma. *Surgery* 1970; 68: 158–64.
61. Agarwala SS, Kirkwood JM, Adjuvant therapy of melanoma. *Semin Surg Oncol* 1998; 14: 302–10.
62. Balch CM, Smalley RV, Bartolucci AA et al, A randomised prospective clinical trial of adjuvant *C. parvum* immunotherapy in 260 patients with clinically localised melanoma (stage I): prognostic factors analysis and preliminary results of immunotherapy. *Cancer* 1982; 49: 1079–84.
63. Thatcher N, Mene A, Banerjee SS et al, Randomized study of *Corynebacterium parvum* adjuvant therapy following surgery for (stage II) malignant melanoma. Br J Surg 1986; 73: 111–15 (abstract).
64. Lipton A, Harvey HA, Lawrence B et al, *Corynebacterium parvum* versus BCG adjuvant immunotherapy in human malignant melanoma. *Cancer* 1983; 51: 57–60.

65. Balch CM, Murray DR, Presant C et al, and the Southeastern Cancer Study Group. A randomized prospective comparison of BCG versus *C. parvum* adjuvant immunotherapy in melanoma patients with resected metastatic lymph nodes. *Proc ASCO* 1984; 3: 263.
66. Lipton A, Harvey HA, Balch CM et al, *Corynebacterium parvum* versus bacille Calmette-Guérin adjuvant immunotherapy of stage II malignant melanoma. *J Clin Oncol* 1991; 9: 1151–6.
67. Tripodi D, Parks LC, Brugmans J. Drug-induced restoration of cutaneous delayed hypersensitivity in anergic patients with cancer. *N Engl J Med* 1973; 289: 354–7.
68. Loufti A, Shakr A, Jerry M et al, Double-blind randomized prospective trial of levamisole/placebo in stage I cutaneous malignant melanoma. *Clin Invest Med* 1987; 10: 325–8.
69. Spitler LE, A randomized trial of levamisole versus placebo as adjuvant therapy in malignant melanoma. *J Clin Oncol* 1991; 9: 736–40.
70. Quirt IC, Shelley WE, Pater JL et al, Improved survival in patients with poor-prognosis malignant melanoma treated with adjuvant levamisole: a phase III study by the National Cancer Institute of Canada Clinical Trials Group. *J Clin Oncol* 1991; 9: 729–35.
71. Kirkwood JM, Strawderman MH, Ernstoff MS et al, Interferon alpha-2b adjuvant therapy of high-risk resected cutaneous melanoma: the Eastern Cooperative Oncology Group trial 1684. *J Clin Oncol* 1996; 14: 7–17.
72. Cole BF, Gelber RD, Kirkwood JM et al, A-quality-of-life-adjusted survival analysis of interferon alfa-2b adjuvant treatment for high-risk resected cutaneous melanoma: an Eastern Cooperative Oncology Group Study (E1684). *J Clin Oncol* 1996; 14: 2666–73.
73. Creagan ET, Dalton RJ, Ahmann DL et al, Randomised adjuvant surgical clinical trial of recombinant interferon alpha 2a in selected patients with malignant melanoma. *J Clin Oncol* 1995; 13: 2776–83.
74. Kirkwood JM, Ibrahim J, Sondak V et al, Preliminary analysis of the E1690/S9111/C9190 intergroup postoperative adjuvant trial of high- and low-dose interferon alpha 2b in high-risk primary or lymph node metastatic melanoma. *Proc ASCO* 1999; 18: 537a (abstract).
75. Penhamberger H, Soyer P, Steiner A et al, Adjuvant interferon alpha-2a treatment in resected primary cutaneous melanoma. *Melanoma Res* 1977; 7: 31 (abstract).
76. Grob JJ, Dreno B, Delauney M et al, Randomised trial of interferon alpha 2a as adjuvant therapy in resected primary cutaneous melanoma thicker than 1.5 mm without clinically detectable node metastases. *Lancet* 1998; 351: 1905–10.
77. Meyskens FL, Kopecky KJ, Taylor CW et al, Randomised trial of adjuvant human interferon gamma versus observation in high-risk cutaneous melanoma: a Southwest Oncology Group study. *J Natl Cancer Inst* 1995; 87: 1710–13.
78. Philip PA, Flaherty L, Treatment of malignant melanoma with interleukin-2. *Semin Oncol* 1997; 14: 32–8.
79. Atkins MB, Lotze M, Wiernik P et al, High dose IL 2 therapy alone results in long-term durable complete responses in patients with metastatic melanoma. *Proc ASCO* 1997; 16: 494a (abstract).
80. Sparano JA, Fisher RI, Sunderland M et al. Randomised phase III trial of treatment with high-dose interleukin 2 either alone or in combination with interferon alfa-2a in patients with advanced melanoma. *J Clin Oncol* 1993; 11: 1969–77.
81. Zapas J, Elias E, Beam S, Perioperative adjuvant interleukin-2 and interferon-alpha 2B in patients with cutaneous melanoma. *Proc ASCO* 2000; 19: 2262a (abstract).
82. Miller LL, Spitler LE, Allen RE et al, A randomized double-blinded, placebo controlled trial of transfer factor as adjuvant therapy for malignant melanoma. *Cancer* 1988; 61: 1543–9.
83. Morton DL, Eilber FR, Holmes EC et al, Preliminary results of a randomised trial of adjuvant immunotherapy in patients with malignant melanoma who have lymph node metastases. *Aust NZ J Surg* 1978; 48: 49–52.
84. Shen P, Foshag L, Essner R et al, Postoperative adjuvant therapy using a polyvalent melanoma vaccine improves overall survival of patients with primary melanoma. *Proc ASCO* 2000; 18: 533a (abstract).
85. Bystryn J-C, Oratz R, Shapiro RL et al, Phase III double-blind trial, of a shed polyvalent, melanoma vaccine in stage III melanoma. *Proc ASCO* 1998; 17: 434a (abstract).
86. McIllmurray MB, Embleton MJ, Reeves WG et al, Controlled trial of active immunotherapy in management of stage IIB malignant melanoma. *BMJ* 1977; 1: 540–2.
87. Wolchok JD, Livingston PO, Houghton AN, Vaccines and other adjuvant therapies for melanoma. *Melanoma* 1998; 12: 835–48.
88. Berd D, Maguire HC, Kairys J et al, Post-surgical treatment of stage III melanoma with autologous, hapten-modified vaccine: expanded sample size and long-term follow-up. *Proc ASCO* 2000; 19: 254a (abstract).
89. Wallack MK, Sivanandham M, Balch CM et al, Surgical adjuvant active specific immunotherapy for patients with stage III melanoma: the final analysis of data from a phase III randomised, double blind multicenter vaccinia melanoma oncolysate trial. *J Am Coll Surg* 1998; 187: 69–77.
90. Livingston PO, Wong GY, Adluri S et al, Improved survival in stage III melanoma patients with GM2 antibodies: a randomised trial of adjuvant vaccination with GM2 ganglioside. *J Clin Oncol* 1994; 5: 1036–44.
91. Nestle FO, Alijigac S, Gilliet M et al, Vaccination of melanoma patients with peptide- or tumour lysate-pulsed dendritic cells. *Nat Med* 1998; 4: 328–32.
92. Sterchi JM, Wells HB, Case LD et al, A randomised trial of adjuvant chemotherapy and immunotherapy in stage I and II cutaneous melanoma: an interim report. *Cancer* 1985; 55: 707–12.
93. Morton DL, Adjuvant immunotherapy of malignant melanoma: status of clinical trials at UCLA. *Int J Immunother* 1986; II: 31–6.
94. Wood WC, Cosimi AB, Carey RW, Kaufman SD, Randomised trial of adjuvant therapy for high-risk primary malignant melanoma. *Surgery* 1978; 83: 677–81.
95. Cascinelli N, Rumke P, MacKie R et al, The significance of conversion of skin reactivity to efficacy of bacillus Calmette-Guérin (BCG) vaccinations given immediately after radical surgery in stage II melanoma patients. *Cancer Immunol Immunother* 1989; 28: 543–50.
96. Misset JL, Delgado M, DeVassal F et al, Immunotherapy or chemotherapy as adjuvant treatment for melanoma: a G.I.F. trial. In: *Adjuvant Therapy of Cancer III* (eds Salmon SE, Jones SE). New York: Grune and Stratton, 1981.
97. Kirkwood JM, Ernstoff MS, Giulamo A et al, Interferon alpha 2a and dacarbazine in melanoma. *J Natl Cancer Inst* 1990; 82: 1062–3.
98. Falkson CI, Falkson G, Falkson HC, Improved results with the addition of interferon alpha 2b to dacarbazine in the treatment of metastatic melanoma. *J Clin Oncol* 1991; 9: 1403–8.
99. Thompson DB, Adena M, McLoed GR et al, Interferon alpha 2a does improve response when combined with dacarbazine in metastatic melanoma: results of a multi-institutional Australian randomised trial. *Melanoma Res* 1993; 3: 133–8.
100. Bajetta E, Di Leo A, Zampino MG et al, Multi-centre trial of dacarbazine alone or in combination with two different doses and schedules of interferon alpha 2a in the treatment of advanced melanoma. *J Clin Oncol* 1994; 12: 806–11.
101. Falkson CI, Ibrahim J, Kirkwood JM et al, A phase III trial of dacarbazine versus dacarbazine with interferon α-2b versus dacarbazine with tamoxifen versus dacarbazine with interferon α-2b and tamoxifen in patients with metastatic malignant melanoma: an Eastern Cooperative Oncology Group Study. *J Clin Oncol* 1998; 16: 1743–51.
102. Pyrhoren S, Hahka-Kemppien U, Muhonen T, A promising interferon plus 4 drug chemotherapy regimen for metastatic melanoma. *J Clin Oncol* 1992; 10: 1919–26.
103. Hahka-Kemppinen M, Muhonen M, Virolainen M et al, Response of subcutaneous and cutaneous metastases of malignant melanoma to combined cytostatic plus interferon therapy. *Br J Dermatol* 1995; 132: 973–7.
104. Ascierto P, Daponte A, Parasole R et al, Low dose interferon-alpha + tamoxifen as second line adjuvant treatment for melanoma patients recurred after adjuvant therapy. *Proc ASCO* 2000, 19: 2264a (abstract).
105. Allen IE, Kupelnick B, Kumashiro D et al, The combination of chemotherapy with IL-2 and IFN-A is more active than chemotherapy or immunotherapy alone in patients with metastatic melanoma; a meta-analysis of 7711 patients with metastatic melanoma. *Proc ASCO* 1977; 16: 494a (abstract).

106. Demchak PA, Mier JW, Robert NJ et al, Interleukin-2 and high-dose cisplatin in patients with metastatic melanoma: a pilot study. *J Clin Oncol* 1991; 9: 1821–30.
107. Miller DM, Jones D, Partin M et al, Effective interleukin-2 based adjuvant therapy for high-risk malignant melanoma patients. *Proc ASCO* 1998; 17: 507a (abstract).
108. Keilholz U, Goey SH, Punt CJA et al, Interferon alfa-2a and interlekin-2 with or without cisplatin in metastatic melanoma: a randomised trial of the European Organisation for Research and Treatment of Cancer Melanoma Co-operative Group. *J Clin Oncol* 1997; 15: 1579–88.
109. Legha SS, Ring S, Eton O et al, Development of a biochemotherapy regimen with concurrent administration of cisplatin, vinblastine, dacarbazine, interferon alfa, and interleukin-2 for patients with metastatic melanoma. *J Clin Oncol* 1998; 16: 1752–9.
110. Richards JM, Gale D, Mehta N, Lestingi T, Combination of chemotherapy with interleukin-2 and interferon alfa for the treatment of metastatic melanoma. *J Clin Oncol* 1999; 17: 651–7.
111 Gajewski T, Flickinger S, A phase II study of outpatient chemotherapy using cisplatin and DTIC followed by GM-CSF, Il-2, and IFN-α2b in patients (Pts) with metastatic melanoma. *Proc ASCO* 2000; 19: 2271a (abstract).
112. Gibbs P, O'Day S, Richards J et al, A multicenter phase II study of modified biochemotherapy (BCT) for stage IV melanoma incorporating temozolamide, decrescendo interleukin-2 (IL-2) and GM-CSF. *Proc ASCO* 2000; 19: 2255a (abstract).
113. Rosenberg SA, Yang YC, Schwartzentruber DJ et al, Prospective randomised trial of the treatment of patients with metastatic melanoma using chemotherapy with cisplatin, dacarbazine, and tamoxifen alone or in combination with interleukin-2 and interferon alfa 2b. *J Clin Oncol* 1999; 3: 968–75.
114. Keilholz U, Punt CJ, Gore ME et al, Dacarbazine, cisplatin and interferon alfa with or without interleukin-2 in advanced melanoma: interim analysis of EORTC trial 18951. *Proc ASCO* 1999; 18: 2043.
115. Eton O, Legha S, Bedikian A et al, Phase III randomised trial of cisplatin, vinblastine and dacarbazine (CVD) plus interleukin-2 (IL2) and interferon-alfa-2b (IFN) versus CVD in patients (Pts) with metastatic melanoma. *Proc ASCO* 2000; 19: 2174a (abstract).
116. Kersten M, Boogerd W, Batchelor D et al, Combined immunotherapy with GM-CSF, IL-2 and IFNα allows dose escalation of temozolamide with prevention of lymphocytopenia and brain metastases in metastatic malignant melanoma. *Proc ASCO* 2000; 19: 2244a (abstract).
117. O'Day S, Boasberg P, Kristedja T et al, A phase II study of maintenance biotherapy (MBT) with intermittent high dose decrescendo interleukin-2 (IL-2) for patients with metastatic melanoma (MM) responding to concurrent biochemotherapy (CBC). *Proc ASCO* 2000; 19: 2245a (abstract).
118. Kirkwood JM, Systemic adjuvant treatment of high risk melanoma: the role of interferon alfa-2b and other immunotherapies. *Eur J Cancer* 1998; 34 (Suppl 3): S12–S17.
119. Elias E, Zapas J, Beam S, Long term results of postoperative adjuvant immuno-therapy with irradiated autologous melanoma cells and low dose cyclophosphamide in very high risk patients and the value of revaccination. *Proc ASCO* 2000, 19: 2263a (abstract).

54

Immunotherapy of melanoma: principles

Peter Hersey

INTRODUCTION

The wonderful dream of treating cancer by immunotherapy with vaccines dates from the beginning of the twentieth century, at a time when immunologists were making major gains in the control of infections (such as tetanus and diphtheria) by immunization with bacterial products. The vaccines employed against cancer were autologous or allogeneic tumour cells or extracts and, as early as 1914, physicians were suggesting one of the principles of success of this approach was to select patients with a small tumour burden.[1] Another measure of success was an increase in leucocyte counts in the patients.[1] By 1929, however, Woglom[2] was writing that resistance was 'not connected with any neoplastic qualities of the graft' and that 'while a selective cytolysin for the malignant cell may some day be found, the chances of its discovery are remote'.

Just over 70 years later it is possible to say that Woglom[2] was partially correct, in that the idea of cancers as foreign tissue has been replaced by knowledge that most cancer antigens are also expressed in normal tissue, albeit at different levels or at different developmental stages. This similarity to normal tissue, or lack of 'foreignness', as well as other properties of malignant cells, has meant that effective immunization has proven difficult and progress is slow. New insights into the immune system have shown that exposure to antigen can tolerize lymphocytes rather than stimulate responses. Immune responses can be qualitatively different and vary in their ability to reject tumours. The determinants of these different responses by the immune system are becoming better understood, and attempts are gradually being made to incorporate this information into the design and use of cancer vaccines. There is also a growing awareness of the plasticity and variability of cancer cells, and the need to target the cancer cells with agents that will make them more susceptible to immune attack.

Melanoma remains the model human cancer for development of immunotherapy. There is abundant histopathological and laboratory based evidence for immune responses against the tumour and clinical evidence of regression of primary melanoma is common. Rare instances of regression of metastatic disease are also well documented. Studies on immunotherapy of melanoma should therefore be ideal for the development of principles associated with effective immunotherapy. This chapter outlines some of the progress made in this area.

CONSIDERATIONS UNDERLYING THE DEVELOPMENT OF PRINCIPLES OF IMMUNOTHERAPY

Differences between therapeutic and preventive vaccines

Immunization of patients with cancer differs from immunization against most infectious disease in several respects. Firstly, immunization against infectious organisms is mostly used to prevent the disease, whereas in cancer the aim is to eradicate existing disease and not to prevent it, i.e. the vaccines are intended to be therapeutic not preventive. (In certain infections, such as malaria and leprosy, vaccines may also be used with therapeutic intent.[3,4])

Secondly, vaccines used for prevention are designed principally to establish memory in the immune system, so that subsequent exposure to the infection will lead to rapid expansion of effector mechanisms such as cytotoxic T cells, macrophages and antibodies against the organisms. In patients with cancer, the vaccine is used to induce effector mechanisms against cancer cells and to maintain them for periods of time sufficient to eradicate the tumour, e.g. for periods of 6 months or more. When cancer vaccines are used in an adjuvant setting (i.e. treatment of patients after surgical removal of all clinically evident disease) the aim is similar, but the vaccinations are carried out over a more protracted period, e.g. 1–3 years. Establishment of memory is also critical in cancer patients so that reappearance of the cancer will be met with a rapid expansion of effector mechanisms.

Tolerance in tumour-bearing hosts

Another important difference between therapeutic and preventive vaccines are changes in the immune system that result from prior exposure to the tumour. Several transgenic animal models, which have genetically determined high numbers of T cells that are specific for tumour antigens (e.g. 50% or more) have shown that T cells appear to become rapidly tolerant to the antigens expressed on tumour cells.[5,6] In two of the models, tolerance of CD4 T cells to influenza haemagglutin (HA) on tumour cells appeared to be due to ineffective presentation of antigens by antigen-presenting cells (APC) [5,6] and could be corrected by activation of dendritic cells (DC) with antibodies to CD40 on the DC.[7,8] In another transgenic model, with HA expressed as a transgene under the control of an insulin promoter, exposure of T cells specific for HA resulted in a population of T cells that responded to the antigen but which had low avidity for the antigen measured in tetramer assays.[9] Tolerance to epitopes of the lymphocytic choriomeningitis virus (LCMV) in transgenic mice could also be reversed by activation of APC through the CD40 receptor, improving vaccine efficacy.[8] These models appear instructive for patients with microscopic or macroscopic evidence of tumour and indicate possible measures to counteract tolerance induction.

Studies on tetramers specific for the melanoma antigen tyrosinase in human patients identified circulating T cells that were specific for the antigen but which were unresponsive in cytotoxic or proliferative assays. Similar low responsiveness was found for T cells identified with tetramers for MART-1.[10] High numbers of T cells specific for MART-1 were identified in the circulation and in metastases in another study, but there was no evidence of tumour regression.[11] Similar results were obtained with respect to MART-1 in studies on blood lymphocytes in melanoma patients.[12] These results therefore support the view that tolerance is a central problem in immunity to certain tumour antigens and is a result of deletion of high affinity T cells rather than particular signalling defects. This concept is illustrated in Figure 54.1.

Table 54.1 *Determinants of principles in immunotherapy*

Lack of 'foreignness' of melanoma antigens
Tolerance due to prior exposure to melanoma antigens
Wrong type of immune response, i.e. TH_2TC_2 rather than TH_1TC_1 responses
Immunosuppressive factors released from melanoma cells
Selection of tumour cells which are resistant to apoptosis induced by TNF family ligands.

TH_1 and TH_2, helper T cells, subsets 1 and 2, respectively; TC_1 and TC_2, T cell subsets 1 and 2, respectively; TNF, tumour necrosis factor.

Qualitative differences in immune responses in tumour-bearing patients: helper T cell (TH) subset 1 (TH_1) versus TH_2 responses

It has been known for some time that certain antigens produce predominantly cell-mediated responses or antibody responses.[13,14] However, this phenomenon was poorly understood until the description by Mossman et al.[15] of TH subsets which made different combinations of cytokines that mediated help.[15] So-called TH_1 subsets made interleukin (IL)-2 and interferon-gamma (IFN-γ), which amplified macrophage and cytotoxic T lymphocyte (CTL) responses, and TH_2 subsets made IL-4, IL-5 and IL-10: IL-4 and IL-5 played a key role in antibody

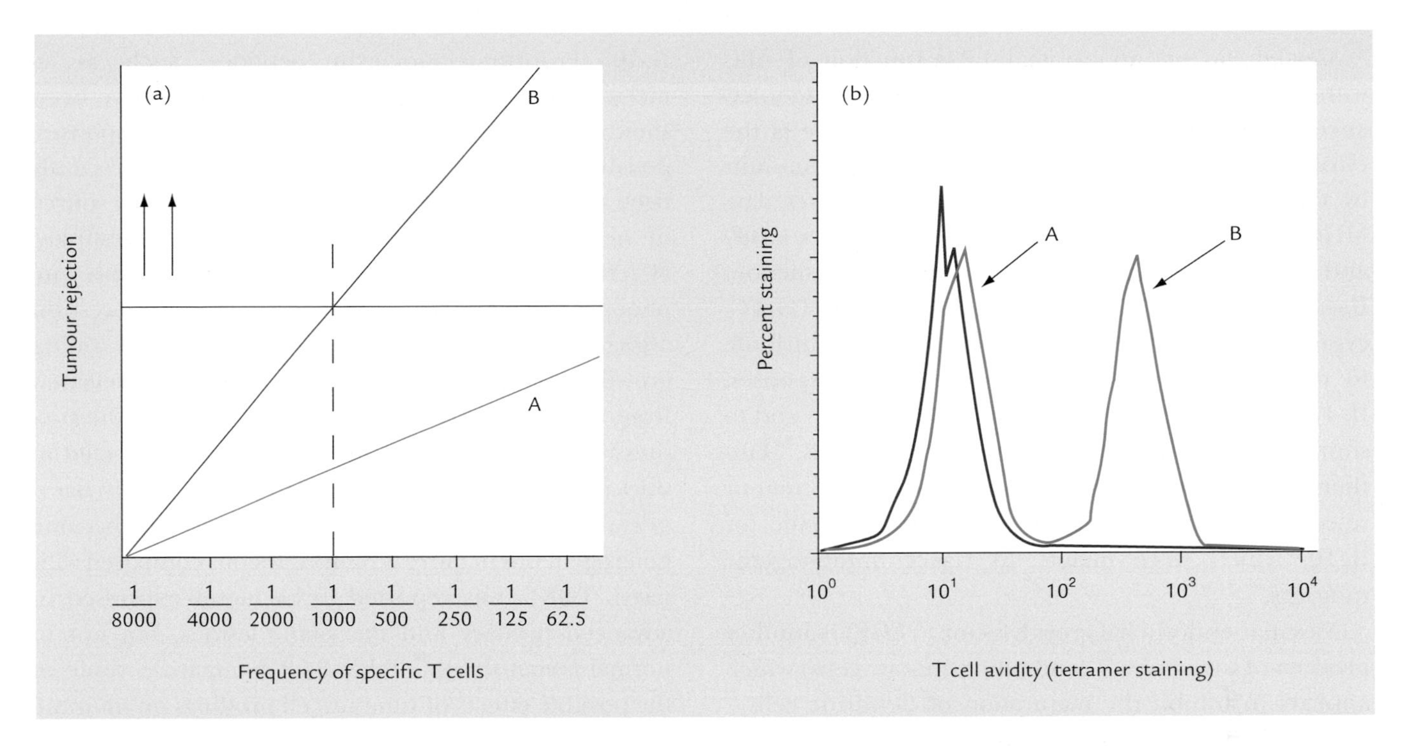

Figure 54.1 *The ability of the immune system to reject tumours depends on the number and affinity of T cells specific to the tumour. Prior exposure to the tumour may delete high affinity T cells as shown by 'A'. There may be insufficient numbers of low affinity T cells to reach the threshold for rejection. Relatively few high affinity T cells may however reach this threshold ('B').*

production. Since then it has become evident that CD8 T cells also exist as T cell subsets (TC_1 and TC_2),[16] which have cytotoxic or immunoregulatory effects on macrophages and surrounding CD8 and CD4 T cells. Rejection of tumour cells is dependent on cell-mediated responses and, in view of this, procedures that induce TH_1TC_1 responses form a key part of new vaccine strategies.

Prolonged exposure to antigens or other factors from tumours is believed to result in a switch of immune responses to the TH_2 pathway, resulting in antibody production rather than cell-mediated responses.[17] Frequent immunization with DC expressing MART-1 was also shown to result in a switch to TH_2 responses.[18] Attempts to switch the response back to cell-mediated responses include use of the cytokine IL-12, as TH_1 but not TH_2 cells express receptors for IL-12.[19]

Immunosuppressive factors from melanoma cells

In addition to induction of tolerance of T cells, tumour cells may also influence immune responses in their microenvironment by the release of factors that act at different stages of the immune response, e.g. it has been known for some time that lymphocytes taken from tumours are often unreactive or anergic to a number of stimuli, such as mitogens and anti-CD3 receptor antibodies.[20] Similar suppressed responses were evident in lymph nodes draining the tumour or adjacent to lymph nodes containing metastases.[21,22] Analysis of cytokine profiles revealed selective defects in the production of IL-2, IL-4 and IFN-γ, whereas IL-10 was present or over-expressed.[23] The unresponsiveness of lymphocytes from these sites was found to be associated with absent or low amounts of several signal transduction molecules, such as CD3γ and CD3ζ, the tyrosine kinases p561ck and p59fyn, and ZAP-70.[24,25]

The cause of these signalling defects is not entirely clear. Proteases have been suggested as one cause of decreased CD3ζ and p561ck levels,[25] whereas hydrogen peroxide (H_2O_2) production by tumour-infiltrating macrophages is another suggested cause of the defects.[26] Irrespective of the cause, there is general agreement that the defects described above: (a) correlate with the stage of tumour growth; (b) show a gradient in severity away from the tumour; (c) do not affect any particular subset of T lymphocytes; and (d) can be reversed by culture in IL-2.[27]

Certain factors appear to inhibit function of APC within or near the tumour cells and contribute to tolerance or anergy to the tumour. One candidate is the cytokine IL-10, which can be released in high amounts by some melanoma.[28] This cytokine can downregulate MHC class II, and the costimulation molecules CD80 and CD86, on APC, thereby inhibiting their function. IL-10 can also inhibit the production of TH_1TC_1 cytokines, IL-2 and IFN-γ, and may thereby contribute to development of TH_2TC_2-type immune responses. IL-10 appears to induce anergy in CD4 T cells [29] and to suppress CTL induction against melanoma cells.[30] Further evidence for its suppressive role against tumour rejection comes from studies on mice transgenic for IL-10, which were unable to reject immunogenic tumours.[31]

Vascular endothelial growth factor (VEGF) is another product of melanoma[32] (and other tumour cells) which appears to inhibit the maturation of dendritic cells,[33] possibly by activation of nuclear factor (NF)-κB,[34] and thereby immune responses to the tumour. VEGF also has the important property of inhibiting expression of vascular adhesion molecule (VCAM) expression on endothelial cells.[35] This has the effect of inhibiting the migration of leucocytes to sites of metastases and may account for the anti-inflammatory effects of some melanoma metastases (Figure 54.2).

Melanoma cells produce several other factors which may act directly on the immune system, or via release of IL-10. Propriomelanocortin peptides, such as α-melanocyte stimulating hormone (α-MSH), have been shown to inhibit contact hypersensitivity responses, possibly by causing the release of IL-10.[36] It has recently been shown that some melanoma cells are a rich source of heavy chain ferritin (H ferritin).[37] Interestingly, H ferritin increases the production of IL-10 from lymphocytes and may contribute to the immunosuppression associated with advanced melanoma. Transforming growth factor (TGF)-β_2 and -β_3 are other factors released from melanoma that have been implicated in the suppression of immune responses. TGF-β_2 was detected in thick primary and metastatic melanoma, but not in naevi or early primaries.[38] TGF-β type II receptors also became heterogeneous in more advanced lesions compared with naevi. TGF-β_3 was reported to be highly expressed in advanced primary and metastatic lesions, but not in normal melanocytes.[39] Table 54.2 summarizes some of the possible effects of tumour cell products on immune responses.

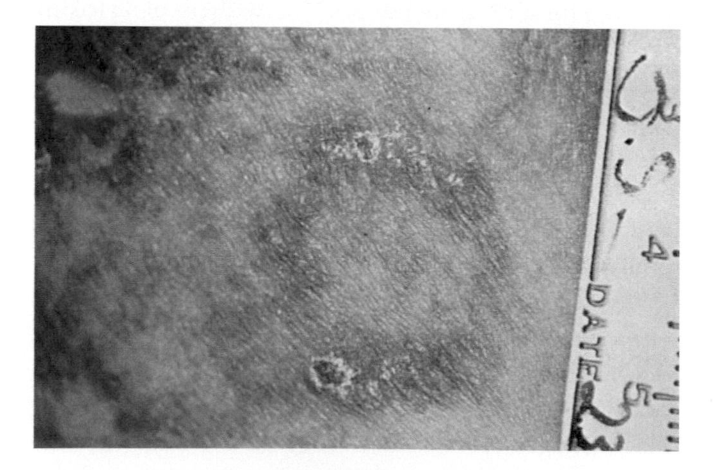

Figure 54.2 *Skin over the thigh of a patient showing an inflammatory response to topically applied dinitrochlorobenzene – except around the small 2–3mm cutaneous melanoma metastases.*

Resistance of melanoma cells to apoptosis

Although it is accepted that many chemotherapy agents mediate their antitumour effects by induction of apoptosis in tumour cells, it is not generally appreciated that a major component of killing by the immune system may also rely on the ability to induce apoptosis of melanoma by transmembrane signalling pathways. This followed from studies which showed that a member of the tumour necrosis factor (TNF) family, TNF-related apoptosis-inducing ligand (TRAIL), appeared to be the main mechanism by which CD4 T cells mediated killing of melanoma. Importantly, it was found that melanoma cells that were resistant to TRAIL were also resistant to killing by CD4 T cells .[40] This did not apply to killing by CD8 T cells, but immunohistological studies show that regression of primary melanoma is usually associated with CD4 T cell infiltrates and not CD8 T cell infiltrates.[41] It is also of much interest to find that sensitivity to TRAIL appears to be predictive of sensitivity to certain chemotherapeutic agents perhaps due to involvement of TRAIL-dependent apoptosis in killing by the chemotherapeutic agents. FasL and TNF-α are two other members of the TNF family that can induce apoptosis in certain cells, but the present author's studies show they have no or little activity against human melanoma.

Table 54.2 *Mechanisms involved in inhibition of immune responses to tumours*

Mechanism	Factors involved
Inhibition of antigen presentation	VEGF, IL-10
Inhibition of cytokine production	IL-10, TGF-β, α-MSH
Tolerance/anergy of T cells	Tumour antigen, H_2O_2, lack of costimulation
Shift of TH_1TC_1 to TH_2TC_2	IL-10, TGF-β, ?FasL
Inhibition of migration of leucocytes from blood vessels	PGE_2, VEGF
Tumour-mediated destruction of T cells	FasL, TRAIL
Resistance of tumour cells to killing	IL-10, immunoselection of HLA and antigen loss variants

VEGF, vascular endothelial growth factor; IL-10, interleukin-10; TGF-β, transforming growth factor; α-MSH, α-melanocyte stimulating hormone; FasL, Fas Ligand; PGE_2, Prostaglandin E_2; TRAIL, tumour-necrosis-factor-related apoptosis-inducing ligand; HLA, human leucocyte antigen; TH_1 and TH_2, helper T cells, subsets 1 and 2, respectively; TC_1 and TC_2, T cell subsets 1 and 2, respectively. (See ref. 39 for additional references.)

Circumstantial evidence for the importance of TRAIL or other TNF family members in immunotherapy also comes from studies in animal models, which show that expression of Flice inhibitory protein (FLIP) protects tumour cells from T cell immunity and results in selection of tumour cells with high FLIP levels.[42,43] The same results were seen in perforin knockout mice. FLIP is known to block FasL- and TRAIL-mediated killing of tumour cells but not perforin granzyme killing.[42] These studies suggest, therefore, that the TNF family may be much more important in the control of tumour growth than at first thought. Melanoma cells in surgical specimens were shown to have high FLIP levels,[44] so it is reasonable to infer that TRAIL may be a major mediator of regression induced by the immune system. Understanding mechanisms of resistance to TRAIL-induced apoptosis may therefore provide new therapeutic approaches based on agents that sensitize melanoma to TRAIL-induced apoptosis.

PRINCIPLES OF IMMUNOTHERAPY (TABLE 54.3)

Reduction of tumour bulk by surgery or chemotherapy and immunization at sites away from the tumour

Given that tumour cells can modulate their microenvironment by release of soluble factors and can induce tolerance in T cells, it appears important to reduce the influence of these factors as much as possible by surgical resection of tumour or reduction in tumour bulk by chemotherapy. Surgical debulking of distant tumour metastases has been championed by a number of surgeons, in particular by Morton and colleagues.[45] A randomized trial to examine whether immunotherapy will prolong life after resection of detectable metastases in stage IV patients is in progress.

Table 54.3 *Principles of immunotherapy*

Principles of immunotherapy
Reduce tumour bulk and immunize away from site of tumour
Provide helper components in the vaccine
Restore high affinity TH_1TC_1 cell-mediated responses
Use adjuvants that increase numbers of APC and processing by APC
Select multiple antigens with high expression per melanoma cell against which there is a high frequency of precursor I cells
Optimize dose, frequency and duration of administration of the vaccine
Induce TRAIL expression on lymphocytes and sensitize melanoma cells to TRAIL-induced apoptosis

TH_1, helper T cells, subset 1; TC, T cells, subset 1; APC, antigen-presenting cells; TRAIL, tumour-necrosis-factor-related apoptosis-inducing ligand.

It appears equally important to immunize away from the tumour, so that APC and draining lymph nodes will not be subject to local effects of tumour-derived products.

Specific inhibitors of some tumour-derived products may be used to inhibit their effects. In this context, the results of clinical trials with monoclonal antibodies (MAbs) to VEGF[46] or VEGF-specific tyrosine kinase inhibitors[47] will be of much interest.

Helper molecules for the generation of optimal immune responses

The design of cancer vaccines has, to a large extent, changed in parallel with advances in the understanding of immune responses. Following the description of T and B cells[48] it was shown that T cells consisted of CD4 helper and CD8 CTL. CD4 T cells provided help to B cells, macrophage responses and CD8+ CTL. These discoveries led to the development of vaccines which incorporated components to stimulate TH_1 cell responses. These included viruses such as vaccinia,[49,50] Newcastle disease virus[51] and influenza.[52]

Other helper strategies include use of chemical haptens such as dinitrophenyl,[52] and foreign proteins such as keyhole limpet haemocyanin (KLH)[53] and tetanus toxoid.[54] Vaccines including helper components remain under evaluation but helper components may differ in their ability to induce cell-mediated compared to antibody responses to tumours. Viruses usually induce strong cell-mediated responses but heterologous proteins, such as tetanus toxoid, may induce help for antibody rather than cell-mediated responses.

Certain proteins, such as tetanus toxoid, contain epitopes which bind to practically all DR class II antigens and are referred to as universal helper epitopes.[55] They can be synthesized to contain class-I-restricted epitopes and so provide help at the site of interaction with CD8 T cells. Helper components in vaccines should, when possible, be derived from melanoma cells so that the helper response can be restimulated on reappearance of the tumour. Unless the helper component is expressed by the tumour, there will be no recall and the tumour may escape detection.[56]

Recent ideas concerning activation of CTL by helper cells are shown in Figure 54.3. This model suggests that helper proteins stimulate CD40 ligand (CD40L) on activated helper T cells and the CD40L then activates dendritic or other APC to a stage where they can activate CTL.[57,58]

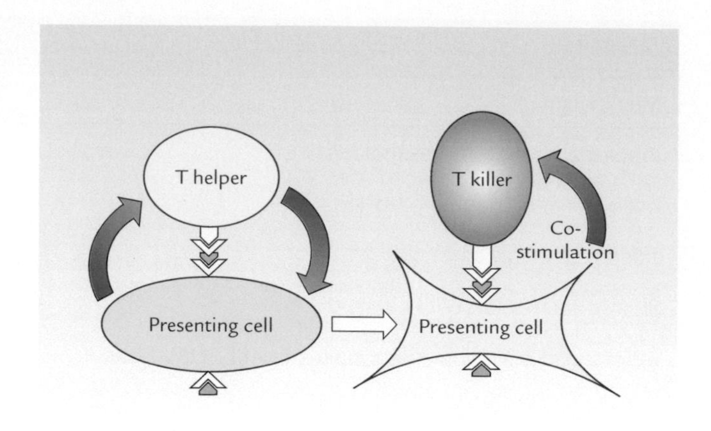

Figure 54.3 *Sequential two-cell interactions.*

Restoration of high-affinity T-cell responses: switching TH_2TC_2 to TH_1TC_1 responses

The studies in animal models referred to above point to the importance of APC and, in particular, DC in converting tolerant responses to effective CTL antitumour responses.[7,8] A number of reagents have been shown to activate DC; these include granulocyte–macrophage colony-stimulating factor (GM-CSF), viruses, lipopolysaccharide, CD40L and so-called CpG oligonucleotides (ODN).[59] Much attention has been given to CD40–CD40L interactions in maturation of DC, as studies in animal models have shown that activation of CD40 on DC can avoid the need for helper proteins to activate DC.[58]

As shown above, helper proteins are believed to function by stimulation of CD4 T cells, which in turn express CD40L and activate DC. Most importantly, it was shown that activation of DC through CD40 overcame tolerance and augmented vaccine efficacy.[8] Activation of DC by CD40L is being tested ex vivo on DC for injection into patients, but so far has not been used in patients receiving vaccines.[60] Similar states of activation may, however, be obtained by inclusion of helper proteins, lipopolysaccharides or CpG ODN. The latter are unmethylated cytosine guanine dinucleotides, which are able to stimulate maturation of DC and enhance their production of TH_1-like cytokines such as IL-12. Their use has been advocated as adjuvants to vaccines and was shown to increase responses to hepatitis B.[59]

Low doses of antigen and intradermal or subcutaneous routes of vaccination are other measures believed to favour the production of high-affinity T cell responses. Vaccination strategies based on immunization with low amounts of antigen (e.g. immunization with DNA) followed by boosting with larger amounts of the protein or peptide antigen have been advocated as a means of obtaining large numbers of high-avidity T cells.[61] For adoptive transfer experiments it was shown that peptide tetramers could be used to select high-avidity CTL that could then be expanded in vitro.[62]

Selection of the right adjuvant

Vaccines are frequently given with an adjuvant to boost the strength of the response. Adjuvants have several roles. One is to act as a depot for slow release of antigens and may, in the case of peptides, also prevent rapid degradation of the antigen. Secondly, they may activate APC, as described above, and induce a microenvironment which favours TH_1TC_1 responses. A detailed discussion of adjuvants is beyond the scope of this chapter but those commonly used with cancer vaccines are listed in Table 54.4. QS21 was reported to be very effective in inducing IgG antibody to the ganglioside GM2,[63] and may have T cell stimulatory properties.[64] Bacille Calmette-Guérin (BCG) is used as an adjuvant in the studies of Morton et al.[65] and presumably activates APC. Detox is used as an adjuvant to a melanoma vaccine

Table 54.4 *Adjuvants for cancer vaccines*

Adjuvant	Manufacturer/investigator
Incomplete Freund's (IFA)	Seppic
Detox	Ribi/Corexa
QS21	Cambridge Biotech
Montanide ISA 720	Seppic
MF59	Chiron Corporation
Bacille Calmette-Guérin (BCG)	Morton et al.[65]
GM colony-stimulating factor (GM-CSF)	Jager et al.[71]
Interleukin (IL)-12	Schmidt and Mescher[72]
IL-2	Shrikant et al.,[75] Rosenberg et al.[83]

prepared from an ultrasonicate of two melanoma cell lines.[66] It has cell walls from a mycobacterium and monophosphoryl lipid A from *Salmonella*, which may activate macrophages. Montanide ISA720 is a water-in-oil adjuvant containing a metabolizable oil which was shown to be effective in induction of T cell responses to cytomegalovirus (CMV) peptides in murine models and to proteins from malaria in human studies.[67,68] The water-in-oil composition was found to be important in the induction of CTL. Incomplete Freund's (IFA) is composed of mineral oil, Arlacel A (emulsifier) and pristine oil. Although widely used for induction of immune responses to peptides,[69] it induces granuloma formation and skin reactions at the site of injections. MF59 is an oil-in-water biodegradable adjuvant which has been used to increase immune responses to peptides.[70]

Several cytokines have been used as adjuvants. GM-CSF was used to increase the number of APC at the injection site and was found to increase responses to melanoma peptides.[71] IL-12 was shown to reverse tolerance to peptides,[72] and has been used in studies by Gajewski et al.[73] and Weber et al.[74] to induce TH_1TC_1 responses to melanoma peptides. IL-2 at low doses, or anti-CTLA-4 Mab, were shown to reverse T cell tolerance in transgenic models with T cells against ovalbumin as a tumour antigen.[75] Similar results were obtained in adoptive transfer models in patients with CMV and melanoma.[76] In the latter studies, IL-2 at doses of 500,000 $IU/m^2/day$ were needed to maintain CD8 T cell responses to the antigens. CpG ODN as adjuvants are discussed above, and may be an effective, well-defined and non-toxic adjuvant.

Selection of the right combination of melanoma antigens

The introduction of gene transfection and limiting dilution techniques[77,78] to screen cDNA libraries with T cells, and the use of serological screening of expression libraries (SEREX) with antisera from patients,[79] has led to the identification of a large number of melanoma antigens recognized by T cells, as summarized in Table 54.5. It is not yet clear, however, which of these antigens are able to induce immune responses that cause regression of melanoma. Factors that are known to influence the development of effective T cell responses are the density of the antigen on the melanoma, avidity of the T cells for the antigen and the

Table 54.5 *Melanoma antigens recognized by T cells*

Antigen category	
Tumour-specific antigens (TSA)	MAGE 1–4, 6, 9–12, MAGE C1
Cancer testis (CT) antigens	BAGE, GAGE, DAM, LAGE, NY-ESO-1, SSX2 (Hom-mel-40), SCP1, CT7, *N*-acetylglucosaminyl transferase
Differentiation antigens	Tyrosinase, MART-1, gp100, Tyrosinase-related protein (TRP)-1, TRP2
Individual specific/mutated genes	N ras, CDK4, caspase 8, β-catenin, MUM-1, MUM-2
Overexpressed genes	p15, PRAME, CD63

(See ref. 111 for additional references to the above antigens.)

frequency of the T cells that can respond to the antigen.[80] The importance of the latter is born out by alloresponses that can reject organ transplants and, in some unusual cases, allografts of melanoma.[81] The frequencies of alloantigens range from *c.* 1:200 to 1:400,[82] whereas frequencies against melanoma antigens appear much lower, e.g. 1:2000–1:10,000, for the most frequently recognized MART-1 antigen.[11]

Differentiation antigens

Some indication of the importance of certain antigens in causing tumour rejection may be derived from the phase I and II studies on melanoma peptide vaccines or DC vaccines plus peptides summarized in Table 54.6. When the peptides from differentiation antigens are given alone they appear relatively ineffective[83,84] unless they are given with cytokines such as GM-CSF,[71] IL-2[83] or IL-12.[85] However, responses were seen in patients immunized with these peptides on DC[86] and adoptive transfer of tumour-infiltrating lymphocytes (TIL) with specificity for gp100 appeared to mediate tumour regression.[87] Responses to gp100 209 2M peptides were mainly seen in patients receiving IL-2 as well.[83,88] A randomized trial is now in progress to establish whether the clinical effects were due to IL-2 alone or the combination with the peptides. Jager et al.[89] reported that differentiation antigens could be lost during immunotherapy with peptides.

Tumour-specific antigens (TSA)

Impressive responses were seen in some patients who were immunized with human leucocyte antigen (HLA)-A1-restricted peptides from MAGE-3, a member of the cancer testis (CT) antigen family.[90] Responses were also seen in patients immunized with this peptide on DC.[91] It is possible that these clinical responses may reflect higher avidity of the T cells for this class of antigen than to the differentiation antigens. The main limitation of the TSA/CT family may be the low frequency of T cells available to respond to the CT antigens.[92] Other potential advantages of the TSA is their higher expression in metastatic lesions compared to primary melanoma, perhaps because of demethylation associated with malignancy.[93] Coordinate expression of several of the family has been noticed, such as MAGE, GAGE, LAGE and NY-ESO-1,[94] which would increase the number of T cells responding to the melanoma cells.

Individual specific antigens

A number of animal studies[80,95] have shown that individual specific antigens were much more effective in inducing regression of tumours than antigens common to tumours. It is quite possible that the same may apply in melanoma, e.g. it was reported that immune responses against the MUM-2 antigens were associated with long periods of remission in the patient concerned.[96] It is generally thought that the main reason for the effectiveness of individual neoantigens is their generation of highly avid T cell responses.[80] Their strength as tumour rejection antigens, however, is still dependent on the density of expression on melanoma cells and the frequency of responding T cells. The main limitation of immunization with individual specific antigens is the practical difficulty of obtaining a supply of

Table 54.6 *Melanoma peptide vaccine trial*

Investigators	Peptide	Adjuvant	No. of patients	Clinical response
Marchand et al.[90]	MAGE-1, 3A.1	Nothing	25	7
Ludwig Institute	MAGE-3A.1 MAGE-3A.2 MAGE-3 protein	MPL and QS21 Nothing MPL and QS21		
Rosenberg et al.[83]	MART-1 gp100 154, 209, 280	IFA IFA	23 28	
Rosenberg et al.[83]	gp100 209 2M	IFA IFA, IL-2	11 31	3 Mixed 13/1 CR, 12 PR
Ranieri et al.[110]	MART-1, gp100, tyrosinase 368	MF59 or local IL-12	28 28	0 0
Jaeger et al.[84]	MART-1, gp100, tyrosinase 1, 368	GM-CSF (three patients)	10	3/1 CR, 2 PR
Weber et al.[74]	MAGE-3A.1	IFA	18	n.a.
Wang et al.[111]	MART-1	IFA	25	n.a.
Cebon et al.[85]	MART-1	IL-12	20	1 CR, 1 PR
Scheibenbogen et al.[112]	Tyrosinase 234, 368, 206, 192	GM-CSF	18	1 MR, 2 SD
Hersey et al.[113]	MART-1, 26, 2L Tyrosinase, MAGE-3A.2 gp100 209, 2M; 280, 9V	Montanide ISA720 PPD ± GM-CSF	16	3 SD

MPL, monophosphoryl lipid A (modified lipopolysaccharide); QS21, carbohydrate extract of *Quillaja saponaria*; IFA, incomplete Freund's adjuvant; IL, interleukin; MF59, oil (squalene) in water emulsion with muramyldipeptide from bacterial cell walls; GM-CSF, GM colony-stimulating factor; Montanide ISA720, water in (metabolizable) oil emulsion; PPD, purified protein derivative; CR, complete response; PR, partial response; n.a, not available; MR, mixed response; SD, stable disease.

such antigens. At present, the only source is from the patient's own tumour, which limits this approach to patients with bulky tumours. Given that sentinel node biopsy techniques are leading to early resection of tumour-involved lymph nodes, the number of patients that can be treated with autologous vaccines now, and in the future, is low. However, trials based on immunization with autologous melanoma are being conducted by Berd et al.[97] and the results of these trials are awaited with much interest.

Combinations of multiple antigens in vaccines

A potentially serious problem is the loss of antigens and other recognition structures from melanoma cells under the selection pressure of the immune system. The loss of HLA antigens on melanoma cells has been well publicized,[98] but the frequency with which it occurs is debated.[99] It is also well documented that antigens related to differentiation molecules may be downregulated, or lost, during immunotherapy.[89,100] In some instances, the immune system has adapted to this loss by recognition of less dominant antigens associated with other major histocompatibility complex (MHC) antigens.[101] There are, so far, few reports of loss of the tumour specific CT antigens during immunotherapy, but whether this means that they are more stable is unknown. In any case, it would appear prudent to include a number of different antigens in vaccines to minimize the potential for selection of antigen loss variants and to span a range of common HLA class I and class II antigens, e.g. A1 (35%), A2 (49%), A3 (26%), A24 (17%), DR1 (19%), DR2 (25%), DR3 (30%), DR4 (29%) and DR13 (20%).

Optimizing dose and administration in vaccine protocols

There are large variations in dose of the vaccines in current use, ranging (per dose) from 40 μg protein,[102] 100 μg protein,[50] 2 mg protein[49] and 20–25 million melanoma cells.[64,66] Substantiation of the dose has received very little attention, except in the studies of Mitchell[103] who measured precursor T cell responses to different doses of the vaccine. To the extent that large antigen doses were shown in experimental studies to produce antibody rather than cell-mediated responses[14] and low avidity T cells,[61] it would appear preferable to use small rather than large doses of antigen.

There are equally large variations in the timing of vaccine injections between different studies. Two objectives underlie the timing of injections. One is to generate high numbers of CTL to clear residual melanoma cells from tissues and circulation. The other is to obtain high numbers of circulating memory cells which can be reactivated should they be exposed to melanoma antigens again. Given that the life of CTL is relatively short, it seems reasonable to have an initial period of frequent immunization and follow this with repeat immunizations at less frequent intervals to maintain high memory T cell numbers. Wallack et al.[49] administered their vaccine at multiple sites weekly for 12 weeks then fortnightly to 1 year. The present author's group administered vaccina melanoma cell lysates (VMCL) intradermally (id) every 2 weeks for four doses, then every 3 weeks for six doses and monthly thereafter to 2 years.[50] Morton et al.[65] administered Cvax every 2 weeks for four doses then monthly to 1 year, and then at increasing intervals up to 5 years. Melacine (Ribi/Mitchell) vaccines were given subcutaneously (s.c.) weekly for four injections then one injection after an interval of 4 weeks, and then every 8 weeks to 4 years.[66] Bystryn[104] gave injections i.d. every 3 weeks for four injections, then every 4 weeks for three injections and at fixed intervals to 5 years. Berd et al.[97] gave injections each week for 6 weeks and repeated this after an interval of 4 weeks; a booster was given at 6 months.

Some guidance concerning optimization of schedules may be gained from studies on memory T cell responses to lymphochoriomeningitis infection in mice, where it was shown that the level of memory T cells is set by the height of the initial response and that following the first booster injection.[105] Subsequent injections had no additive effect on memory T cell numbers. In certain animal models, frequent immunizations were shown to result in a switch to TH_2 responses, which is widely believed to be an undesirable outcome.[18]

Recruitment of the tumour necrosis factor (TNF) family of ligands to induce apoptosis of melanoma during immunotherapy

The objective of inducing apoptosis by the TNF family of ligands has received very little attention as a therapeutic strategy in immunotherapy but may hold the key to successful immunotherapy. As discussed above, CD4 T cells may have direct effects on melanoma via expression of TRAIL on their surface and this may account for the frequent association of CD4 T cells with regression of melanoma.[41] Importantly, the present author's group and Kayagaki et al.[106] have shown that IFN-α2 is able to induce TRAIL on a variety of different lymphocytes, such as CD4 T cells, natural killer (NK) cells and monocytes. This provides a rational basis for combining IFN-α2 with vaccines. Variation in IFN-α2-induced expression of TRAIL on leucocytes is seen between patients and understanding the basis for this may assist in selecting patients that may respond to IFN-α2. Furthermore, a number of agents appear to sensitize melanoma cells to apoptosis induced by TRAIL. These include the chemotherapy agents temozolomide and cisplatin,[107] and newly described proteasome inhibitors, such as PS341.[108] Combining these agents with IFN-α2 or TRAIL in patients undergoing immunotherapy may allow a higher percentage of patients to respond to this form of therapy.

VACCINE DELIVERY SYSTEMS

Figure 54.4 illustrates the different forms of vaccines in use or under development. The randomized trials in progress are based on the use of whole melanoma cells or melanoma cell lysates, but as more information becomes available it is probable that vaccine delivery systems will be based on immunization with well-defined antigens in the form of whole protein, peptide epitopes, naked DNA or viral vectors containing DNA for one or more melanoma antigens. Further details of the different vaccine delivery systems are given elsewhere.[109]

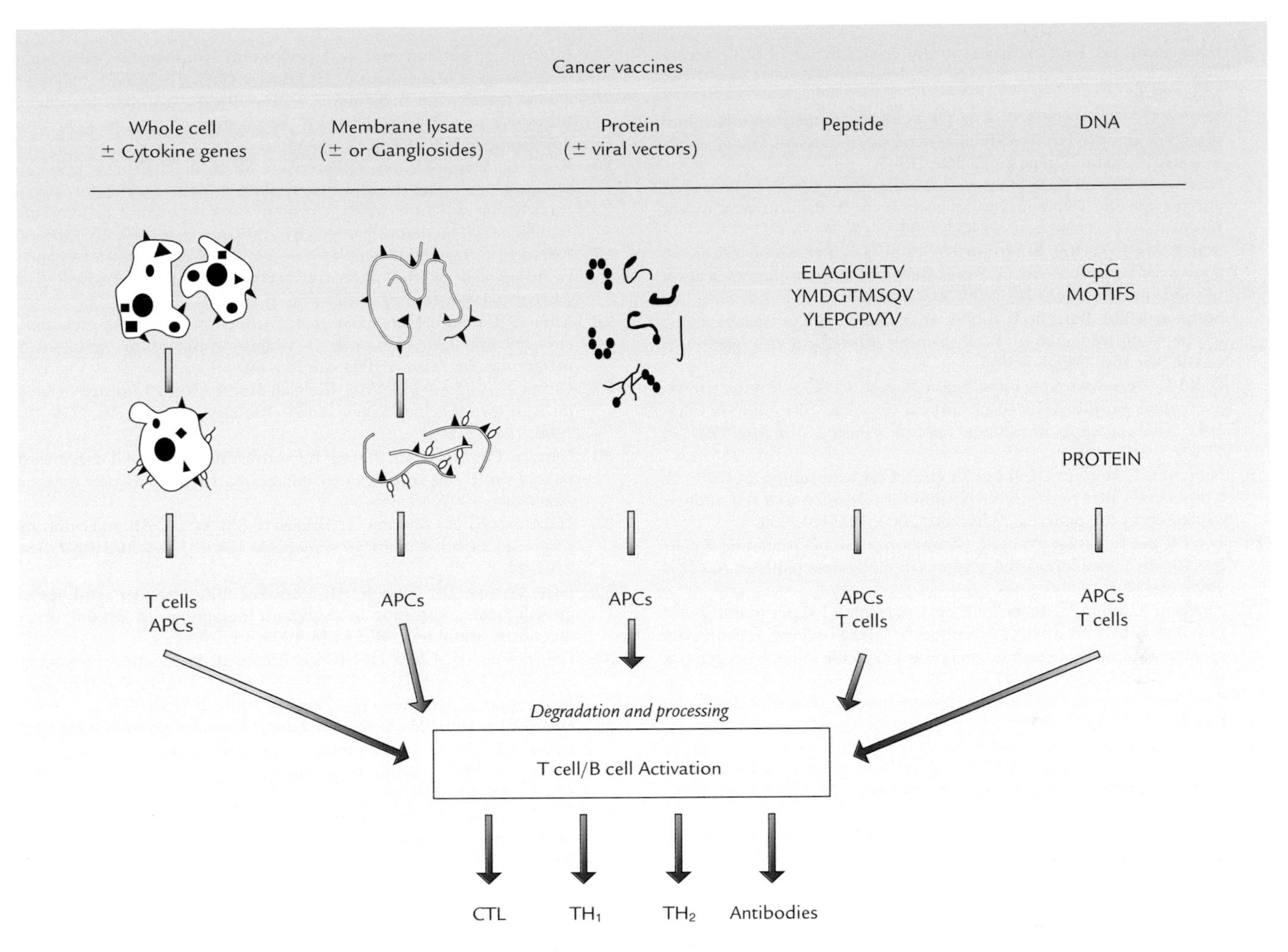

Figure 54.4 *Diagrammatic representation of different vaccine approaches used in treatment of cancer. The APCs referred to in the diagram may be those naturally occurring in the patient or dendritic cells generated ex vivo and primed with the antigen preparations shown in the diagram.*

CONCLUSIONS

Studies over the past few years suggest that tolerance of T cells to melanoma antigens and immunosuppressive factors released from melanoma cells are major hurdles for immunization against melanoma. The most effective strategy may be presentation of melanoma antigens (i.e. having maximum 'foreignness') on antigen-presenting cells (e.g. DC) that have been conditioned to generate TH_1TC_1 CTL responses. Judicious use of cytokines such as IL-12, IL-2 and GM-CSF may assist in obtaining the 'right' TH_1TC_1 response. The protocol should aim at obtaining maximum response in the first two injections to set the immune response at high levels. Inclusion of multiple antigens in the vaccine is desirable to minimize selection of antigen loss variants. Helper determinants in the vaccine are needed to recruit CD4 T cell responses and to maintain CD8 CTL responses. Adjuvants should be included that act as a depot for antigen and which condition antigen-presenting cells. Greater attention to apoptosis inducing mechanisms in immunotherapy and susceptibility of melanoma cells to apoptosis is required. Judicious use of agents that sensitize melanoma cells to apoptosis and which induce expression of apoptosis-inducing ligands may add to the effectiveness of immunotherapy of melanoma, and help select patients who are suitable for this treatment.

REFERENCES

1. Vaughan HW, Cancer vaccine and anti-cancer globulin as an aid in the surgical treatment of malignancy. *JAMA* 1914; 63: 1258–68.
2. Woglom WH, Immunity to transplantable tumours. *Cancer Rev* 1929; 4: 129–40.

3. Ponnighaus JM, Fine PEM, Sterne JAC et al, Efficacy of BCG vaccine against leprosy and tuberculosis in northern Malawi. *Lancet* 1992; 339: 636–9.
4. Nosten F, Luxemburger C, Kyle DE et al, Randomised double-blind placebo-controlled trial of SPf66 malaria vaccine in children in northwestern Thailand. *Lancet* 1996; 348: 701–7.
5. Staveley-O'Carroll K, Sotomayor E, Montgomery J et al, Induction of antigen-specific T cell anergy: an early event in the course of tumor progression. *Proc Natl Acad Sci USA* 1998; 95: 1178–83.
6. Marzo AL, Lake RA, Robinson BW et al, T-cell receptor transgenic analysis of tumor-specific CD8 and CD4 responses in the eradication of solid tumors. *Cancer Res* 1999; 59: 1071–9.
7. Sotomayor EM, Borrello I, Tubb E et al, Conversion of tumor-specific CD4+ T-cell tolerance to T-cell priming through in vivo ligation of CD40. *Nat Med* 1999; 5: 780–7.
8. Diehl L, Den Boer A, Schoenberger P et al, CD40 activation in vivo overcomes peptide-induced peripheral cytotoxic T-lymphocyte tolerance and augments anti-tumor vaccine efficacy. *Nat Med* 1999; 5: 774–9.
9. Nugent CT, Morgan DJ, Biggs JA et al, Characterization of CD8+ T lymphocytes that persist after peripheral tolerance to a self antigen expressed in the pancreas. *J Immunol* 2000; 164: 191–200.
10. Lee PP, Yee C, Savage PA et al, Characterization of circulating T cells specific for tumor-associated antigens in melanoma patients. *Nat Med* 1999; 5: 677.
11. Anichini A, Molla A, Mortarini R et al, An expanded peripheral T cell population to a cytotoxic T lymphocyte (CTL)-defined, melanocyte-specific antigen in metastatic melanoma patients impacts on generation of peptide-specific CTLs but does not overcome tumor escape from immune surveillance in metastatic lesions. *J Exp Med* 1999; 190: 651–67.
12. Pittet MJ, Valmori D, Dunbar PR et al, High frequencies of naive melan-A/MART-1 specific CD8+ T cells in a large proportion of human histocompatibility leukocyte antigne (HLA)-A2 individuals. *J Exp Med* 1999; 190: 705–15.
13. Parish CR, The relationship between humoral and cell-mediated immunity. *Transpl Rev* 1972; 13: 35–66.
14. Parish CR, Immune deviation: a historical perspective. *Immunol Cell Biol* 1996; 74: 449–56.
15. Mosmann TR, Cherwinski H, Bond MW et al, Two types of murine helper T cell clone. I. Definition according to profiles of lymphokine activities and secreted proteins. *J Immunol* 1986; 136: 2348–57.
16. Seder RA, Le Gros GG, The functional role of CD8+ T helper type 2 cells. *J Exp Med* 1995; 181: 5–7.
17. Guilloux Y, Viret C, Gervois N et al, Defective lymphokine production by most CD8+ and CD4+ tumor-specific T cell clones derived from human melanoma-infiltrating lymphocytes in response to autologous tumor cells in vitro. *Eur J Immunol* 1994; 24: 1966–73.
18. Ribas A, Butterfield LH, McBride WH et al, Characterization of antitumor immunisation to a defined melanoma antigen using genetically engineered murine dendritic cells. *Cancer Gene Ther* 1999; 6: 523–36.
19. Rogge L, Barberis-Maino L, Biffi M et al, Selective expression of an interleukin-12 receptor component by human T helper 1 cells. *J Exp Med* 1997; 185: 825–31.
20. Miescher S, Stoeck M, Qiao L et al, Proliferative and cytolytic potentials of purified human tumor-infiltrating T lymphocytes. Impaired response to mitogen-driven stimulation despite T-cell receptor expression. *Int J Cancer* 1988; 42: 659–66.
21. Cochran AJ, Wen DR, Farzad Z et al, Immunosuppression by melanoma cells as a factor in the generation of metastatic disease. *Anticancer Res* 1989; 9: 859–64.
22. Farzad Z, Cochran AJ, McBride WH et al, Lymphocyte subset alterations in nodes regional to human melanoma. *Cancer Res* 1990; 50: 3585–8.
23. Luscher U, Filgueira L, Juretic A et al, The pattern of cytokine gene expression in freshly excised human metastatic melanoma suggests a state of reversible anergy of tumor-infiltrating lymphocytes. *Int J Cancer* 1994; 57: 612–19.
24. Matsuda M, Petersson M, Lenkei R et al, Alterations in the signal-transducing molecules of T cells and NK cells in colorectal tumor-infiltrating, gut mucosal and peripheral lymphocytes: correlation with the stage of the disease. *Int J Cancer* 1995; 61: 765–72.
25. Zier K, Gansbacher B, Salvadori S, Preventing abnormalities in signal transduction of T cells in cancer: the promise of cytokine gene therapy. *Immunol Today* 1996; 17: 39–45.
26. Kono K, Salazar-Onfray F, Petersson M et al, Hydrogen peroxide secreted by tumor-derived macrophages down-modulates signal-transducing zeta molecules and inhibits tumor-specific T cell- and natural killer cell-mediated cytotoxicity. *Eur J Immunol* 1996; 26: 1308–13.
27. Salvadori S, Zier K, Molecular basis of T cell dysfunction in cancer is influenced by the paracrine secretion of tumor-derived IL-2. *J Immunol* 1996; 156: 2927–32.
28. Chen Q, Daniel V, Maher DW et al, Production of IL-10 by melanoma cells: examination of its role in immunosuppression mediated by melanoma. *Int J Cancer* 1994; 56: 755–60.
29. Groux H, Bigler M, deVries JE et al, Interleukin-10 induces a long-term antigen-specific anergic state in human CD4+ T cells. *J Exp Med* 1996; 184: 19–29.
30. Nguyen TD, Smith MJ, Hersey P, Contrasting effects of T cell growth factors on T cell responses to melanoma in vitro. *Cancer Immunol Immunother* 1997; 43: 345–54.
31. Hagenbaugh A, Sharma S, Dubinett SM et al, Altered immune responses in interleukin 10 transgenic mice. *J Exp Med* 1997; 185: 2101–10.
32. Bayer-Garner IB, Hough AJJ, Smoller BR, Vascular endothelial growth factor expression in malignant melanoma: prognostic versus diagnostic usefulness. *Mod Pathol* 1999; 12: 770–4.
33. Gabrilovich DI, Chen HL, Girgis KR et al, Production of vascular endothelial growth factor by human tumors inhibits the functional maturation of dendritic cells. *Nat Med* 1996; 2: 1096–103.
34. Gabrilovich D, Ishida T, Oyama T et al, Vascular endothelial growth factor inhibits the development of dendritic cells and dramatically affects the differentiation of multiple hematopoietic lineages in vivo. *Blood* 1998; 92: 4150–66.
35. Griffioen AW, Damen CA, Mayo KH et al, Angiogenesis inhibitors overcome tumor induced endothelial cell anergy. *Int J Cancer* 1999; 80: 315–19.
36. Grabbe S, Bhardwaj RS, Mahnke K et al, alpha-Melanocyte-stimulating hormone induces hapten-specific tolerance in mice. *J Immunol* 1996; 156: 473–8.
37. Gray CP, Arosio P, Hersey P, Heavy chain ferritin activates regulatory T cells by induction of changes in dendritic cells. *Blood* 2002; 99: 3326–34.
38. Schmid P, Itin P, Rufli T, In situ analysis of transforming growth factor-beta (TGF-beta 1, TGF-beta 2, TGF-beta 3), and TGF-beta type II receptor expression in malginant melanoma. *Carcinogenesis* 1995; 16: 1499–503.
39. Hersey P, Impediments to successful immunotherapy. *Pharmacol Ther* 1999; 81: 111–19.
40. Thomas WD, Hersey P, TRAIL induces apoptosis in Fas ligand resistant melanoma cells and mediates CD4 T cell killing of target cells. *J Immunol* 1998; 161: 2195–200.
41. Tefany FJ, Barnetson RS, Halliday GM et al, Immunocytochemical analysis of the cellular infiltrate in primary regressing and non-regressing malignant melanoma. *J Invest Dermatol* 1991; 97: 197–202.
42. French LE, Tschopp J, Inhibition of death receptor signaling by FLICE-inhibitory protein as a mechanism for immune escape of tumors. *J Exp Med* 1999; 190: 891–3.
43. Medema JP, de Jong J, van Hall T et al, Immune escape of tumors in vivo by expression of cellular FLICE-inhibitory protein. *J Exp Med* 1999; 190: 1033–8.
44. Irmler M, Thome M, Hahne M et al, Inhibition of death receptor signals by cellular FLIP. *Nature* 1997; 388: 190–5.
45. Balch CM, Palliative surgery for stage IV melanoma: is it a primary treatment? *Ann Surg Oncol* 1999; 6: 623–4.
46. Gabrilovich DI, Ishida T, Nadaf S et al, Antibodies to vascular endothelial growth factor enhance the efficacy of cancer immunotherapy by improving endogenous dendritic cell function. *Clin Cancer Res* 1999; 5: 2963–70.
47. Shaheen RM, Antiangiogenic therapy targeting the tyrosine kinase receptor for vascular endothelial growth factor receptor inhibits the

growth of colon cancer liver metastasis and induces tumor and endothelial cell apoptosis. *Cancer Res* 1999; 59: 5412–6.

48. Raff MC, T and B lymphocytes and immune responses. *Nature* 1973; 242: 19–23.
49. Wallack MK, Sivanandham M, Balch CM et al, Surgical adjuvant active specific immunotherapy for patients with stage III melanoma: the final analysis of data from a phase III, randomised, double-blind, multicenter vaccinia melanoma oncolysate trial. *J Am Coll Surg* 1998; 187: 69–77.
50. Hersey P, Edwards A, Coates A et al, Evidence that treatment with vaccinia melanoma cell lysates (VMCL) may improve survival of patients with stage II melanoma. *Cancer Immunol Immunother* 1987; 25: 257–65.
51. Cassel WA, Murray DR. A ten-year follow-up on stage II malignant melanoma patients treated postsurgically with Newcastle Disease Virus oncolysate. *Med Oncol Tumor Pharmacother* 1992; 9: 169–71.
52. Berd D, Murphy G, Maguire HC Jr et al, Immunization with haptenized, autologous tumor cells induces inflammation of human melanoma metastases. *Cancer Res* 1991; 51: 2731–4.
53. Livingston PO, Approaches to augmenting the immunogenicity of melanoma gangliosides: from whole melanoma cells to ganglioside–KLH conjugate vaccines. *Immunol Rev* 1995; 145: 147–66.
54. Livingston BD, Crimi C, Grey H et al, The hepatitis B virus-specific CTL responses induced in humans by lipopeptide vaccination are comparable to those elicited by acute viral infection. *J Immunol* 1997; 159: 1383–92.
55. O'Sullivan D, Arrhenius T, Sidney J et al, On the interaction of promiscuous antigenic peptides with different DR alleles. *J Immunol* 1991; 147: 2663–9.
56. Ossendorp F, Mengede E, Camps M et al, Specific T helper cell requirement for optimal induction of cytotoxic T lymphocytes against major histocompatibility complex class II negative tumors. *J Exp Med* 1998; 187: 693–702.
57. Ridge JP, Di Rosa F, Matzinger P, A conditioned dendritic cell can be a temporal bridge between a CD4+ T-helper and a T-killer cell. *Nature* 1998; 393: 474–8.
58. Bennett SR, Carbone FR, Karamalis F et al, Help for cytotoxic-T-cell responses is mediated by CD40 signalling. *Nature* 1998; 393: 478–80.
59. Hartmann G, Weeratna RD, Ballas ZK et al, Delineation of a CpG phosphorothioate oligodeoxynucleotide for activating primate immune responses in vitro and in vivo. *J Immunol* 2000; 64: 1617–24.
60. Morse MA, Lyerly HK, Gilboa E et al, Optimization of the sequence of antigen loading and CD40–ligand-induced maturation of dendritic cells. *Cancer Res* 1998; 58: 2965–8.
61. Ramsey AJ, Kent SJ, Strugnell RA et al, Genetic vaccination strategies for enhanced cellular, humoral and mucosal immunity. *Immunol Rev* 1999; 171: 27–44.
62. Yee C, Savage PA, Lee PP et al, Isolation of high avidity melanoma-reactive CTL from heterogeneous populations using peptide–MHC tetramers. *J Immunol* 1999; 162: 2227–34.
63. Helling F, Zhang S, Shang A, GM2–KLH conjugate vaccine: increased immunogenicity in melanoma patients after administration with immunological adjuvants QS-21. *Cancer Res* 1995; 55: 2783–8.
64. Rhodes J, Covalent chemical events in immune induction: fundamental and therapeutic aspects. *Immunol Today* 1996; 17: 436–41.
65. Morton DL, Foshag LJ, Hoon DSB et al, Prolongation of survival in metastatic melanoma after active specific immunotherapy with a new polyvalent melanoma vaccine. *Ann Surg* 1992; 216: 463–82.
66. Mitchell MS, Harel W, Kempf RA et al, Active-specific immunotherapy for melanoma. *J Clin Oncol* 1990; 8: 856–69.
67. Scalzo AA, Elliott SL, Cox J et al, Induction of protective cytotoxic T cells to murine cytomegalovirus by using a nonapeptide and a human-compatible adjuvant (Montanide ISA 720). *J Virol* 1995; 69: 1306–9.
68. Lawrence GW, Saul A, Giddy AJ et al, Phase I trial in humans of an oil-based adjuvant SEPPIC MONTANIDE ISA 720. *Vaccine* 1997; 15: 176–8.
69. Salgaller ML, Marincola FM, Cormier JN et al, Immunization against epitopes in the human melanoma antigen gp100 following patient immunization with synthetic peptides. *Cancer Res* 1996; 56: 4749–57.
70. O'Hagan DT, Ott GS, Van Nest G, Recent advances in vaccine adjuvants: the development of MF59 emulsion and polymeric microparticles. *Mol Med Today* 1997; 3: 69–75.
71. Jager E, Ringhoffer M, Dienes HP et al, Granulocyte-macrophage-colony-stimulating factor enhances immune responses to melanoma-associated peptides in vivo. *Int J Cancer* 1996; 67: 54–62.
72. Schmidt CS, Mescher MF, Adjuvant effect of IL-12: conversion of peptide antigen administration from tolerizing to immunizing for CD8+ T cells in vivo. *J Immunol* 1999; 163: 2561–7.
73. Gajewski TF, Fallarino F, Vogelzang N et al, Effective melanoma antigen vaccination without dendritic cells (DC): a phase I study of immunization with Mage3 or Melan-A peptide-pulsed autologous PBMC plus RhIL-12. *Proc ASCO* 1999; 18: 539a (abstract).
74. Weber JS, Hua FL, Spears L et al, A phase I trial of an HLA-A1 restricted MAGE-3 epitope peptide with incomplete Freund's adjuvant in patients with resected high-risk melanoma. *J Immunother* 1999; 22: 431–40.
75. Shrikant P, Khoruts A, Mescher MF, CTLA-4 blockade reverses CD8+ T cell tolerance to tumor by a CD4+ T cell- and IL-2-dependent mechanism. *Immunity* 1999; 11: 483–93.
76. Walter EA, Greenberg PD, Gilbert MJ et al, Reconstitution of cellular immunity against cytomegalovirus in recipients of allogeneic bone marrow by transfer of T-cell clones from the donor. *N Engl J Med* 1995; 333: 1038–44.
77. Boon T, van der Bruggen P, Human tumor antigens recognized by T lymphocytes. *J Exp Med* 1996; 183: 725–9.
78. Rosenberg SA, A new era for cancer immunotherapy based on the genes that encode cancer antigens. *Immunity* 1999; 10: 281–7.
79. Old LJ, Chen Y-T, New paths in human cancer serology. *J Exp Med* 1998; 187: 1163–7.
80. Gilboa E, The makings of a tumor rejection antigen. *Immunity* 1999; 11: 263–70.
81. Elder GJ, Hersey P, Branley P, Remission of transplanted melanoma – clinical course and tumour cell characterisation. *Clin Transpl* 1997; 11: 565–8.
82. Klein J, Nature of alloreactivity. In: *Natural history of the major histocompatibility complex*. New York: Wiley & Sons, 1986: 417–22.
83. Rosenberg SA, Yang JC, Schwartzentruber DJ et al, Immunologic and therapeutic evaluation of a synthetic peptide vaccine for the treatment of patients with metastatic melanoma. *Nat Med* 1998; 4: 321–7.
84. Jaeger E, Bernhard H, Romero P et al, Generation of cytotoxic T-cell responses with synthetic melanoma-associated peptides in vivo: implications for tumor vaccines with melanoma-associated antigens. *Int J Cancer* 1996; 66: 162–9.
85. Cebon JS, Jaeger E, Gibbs P et al, Phase I studies of immunization with Melan-A and IL-12 in HLA A2+ positive patients with stage III and IV malignant melanoma. *Proc ASCO* 1999; 18, 434a (abstract).
86. Nestle FO, Alijagic S, Gilliet M et al, Vaccination of melanoma patients with peptide- or tumor lysate-pulsed dendritic cells. *Nat Med* 1998; 4: 328–32.
87. Kawakami Y, Eliyahu S, Delgado CH et al, Identification of a melanoma antigen recognised by tumour infiltrating lymphocytes associated with in vivo tumour rejection. *Proc Natl Acad Sci USA* 1994; 91: 6458–62.
88. Rosenberg SA, Yang JC, Schwartzentruber DJ et al, Impact of cytokine administration on the generation of antitumor reactivity in patients with metastatic melanoma receiving a peptide vaccine. *J Immunol* 1999; 163: 1690–5.
89. Jager E, Ringhoffer M, Altmannsberger M et al, Immunoselection in vivo: independent loss of MHC class I and melanocyte differentiation antigen expression in metastatic melanoma. *Int J Cancer* 1997; 71: 142–7.
90. Marchand M, van Baren N, Weynants P et al, Tumor regressions observed in patients with metastatic melanoma treated with an antigenic peptide encoded by gene MAGE-3 and presented by HLA-A1. *Int J Cancer* 1999; 80: 219–30.
91. Thurner B, Haendle I, Roder C et al, Vaccination with Mage-3A1 peptide-pulsed mature, monocyte-derived dendritic cells expands specific cytotoxic T cells and induces regression of some metastases in advanced stage IV melanoma. *J Exp Med* 1999; 190: 1669–78.

92. Chaux P, Vantomme V, Coulie P et al, Estimation of the frequencies of anti-MAGE-3 cytolytic T-lymphocyte precursors in blood from individuals without cancer. *Int J Cancer* 1998; 77: 538–42.
93. Brasseur F, Rimoldi D, Lienard D et al, Expression of MAGE genes in primary and metastatic cutaneous melanoma. *Int J Cancer* 1995; 63: 375–80.
94. Dalerba P, Ricci A, Russo V et al, High homogeneity of MAGE, BAGE, GAGE, tyrosinase and Melan-A/MART-1 gene expression in clusters of multiple simultaneous metastases of human melanoma: implications for protocol design of therapeutic antigen-specific vaccination strategies. *Int J Cancer* 1998; 77: 200–4.
95. Hellstrom I, Hellstrom KE. Tumor immunology: an overview. In: *Specific immunotherapy of cancer with vaccines* (eds Bystryn J-C, Ferrone S, Livingston P). *Ann NY Acad Sci* 1993; 690: 24–33.
96. Chiari R, Foury F, De Plaen E et al, Two antigens recognized by autologous cytolytic T lymphocytes on a melanoma result from a single point mutation in an essential housekeeping gene. *Cancer Res* 1999; 59: 5785–92.
97. Berd D, Maguire HC, Schuchter LM et al, Autologous hapten-modified melanoma vaccine as postsurgical adjuvant treatment after resection of nodal metastases. *J Clin Oncol* 1997; 15: 2359–70.
98. Ferrone S, Marincola FM. Loss of HLA class I antigens by melanoma cells: molecular mechanisms, functional significance and clinical relevance. *Immunol Today* 1995; 16: 487–94.
99. Cormier JN, Hijazi YM, Abati A et al, Heterogeneous expression of melanoma-associated antigens and HLA-A2 in metastatic melanoma in vivo. *Int J Cancer* 1998; 75: 517–24.
100. Riker A, Cormier J, Panelli M et al, Immune selection after antigen-specific immunotherapy of melanoma. *Surgery* 1999; 126: 112–20.
101. Ikeda H, Lethe B, Lehmann F et al, Characterization of an antigen that is recognized on a melanoma showing partial HLA loss by CTL expressing an NK inhibitory receptor. *Immunity* 1997; 6: 199–208.
102. Bystryn J-C, Oratz R, Shapiro RL et al, Double-blind, placebo-controlled, trial of a shed, polyvalent, melanoma vaccine in stage III melanoma. *Proc ASCO* 1999; 18: 434a (abstract).
103. Mitchell MS, Attempts to optimize active specific immunotherapy for melanoma. *Int Rev Immunol* 1991; 7: 331–47.
104. Brstryn JC, Zeleniuch-Jacquotte A, Oratz R et al, Double-blind trial of a polyvalent, shed antigen, melanoma *Clin Cancer Res* 2001; 7: 1882–7.
105. Murali-Krishna K, Lau LL, Sambhara S et al, Persistence of memory CD8 T cells in MHC class I-deficient mice. *Science* 1999; 286: 1377–81.
106. Kayagaki N, Yamaguchi N, Nakayama M et al, Type I interferons (IFNs) regulate tumor necrosis factor-related apoptosis-inducing ligand (TRAIL) expression on human T cells: a novel mechanism for the antitumor effects of type I IFNs. *J Exp Med* 1999; 189: 1451–60.
107. Thomas W, Van Berkel E, Franco A et al, Temozolomide and cisplatin sensitize melanoma cells to TRAIL induced apoptosis. *AACR* 2000; 41: A451.
108. Teicher BA, Ara G, Herbst R et al, The proteasome inhibitor PS-341 in cancer therapy. *Clin Cancer Res* 1999; 5: 2638–45.
109. Hersey P, Advances in non-surgical treatment of melanoma. *Expert Opin Invest Drugs* 2002; 11: 75–85.
110. Ranieri E, Kierstead LS, Zarour H et al, Dendritic cell/peptide cancer vaccines: clinical responsiveness and epitope spreading. *Immunol Invest* 2000; 29: 121–5.
111. Wang F, Bade E, Kuniyoshi C et al, Phase I trial of a MART-1 peptide vaccine with incomplete Freund's adjuvant for resected high-risk melanoma. *Clin Cancer Res* 1999; 5: 2756–65.
112. Scheibenbogen C, Schmittel A, Keilholz U et al, Vaccination with tyrosinase peptides and GM-CSF in metastatic melanoma: a phase II trial *Proc ASCO* 1999; 18: 436a (abstract).
113. Hersey P, Will vaccines really work for melanoma? In: *Melanoma: critical debates*, (eds Newton-Bishop JA, Gore M). Oxford: Blackwell Science, 2002: 212–29.

55

Adjuvant immunotherapy for high-risk primary melanoma and resected metastatic melanoma

Peter Hersey, Donald L Morton, Alexander MM Eggermont

INTRODUCTION

Melanoma differs from the other common forms of skin cancer in that it has a propensity to spread from its site of origin in the skin to other body organs. The risk of such systemic spread is related to the thickness of the primary tumour, whether it is ulcerated and whether there is involvement of regional lymph nodes. Recurrence of melanoma after apparently complete surgical removal implies that metastasis to other sites had already occurred prior to, or at the time of, removal of clinically evident melanoma. Implementation of treatment in the postoperative period would be expected to provide the greatest chance of eradicating residual foci of disease, but a variety of different treatments have not had significant effects on survival.[1,2]

The basis for suggesting that immunotherapy may prove effective in eradicating residual micrometastases stems from clinical observations of regression of primary melanomas associated with lymphoid infiltration,[3–5] and more rarely of regression of metastatic disease. Numerous studies have reported laboratory evidence of antibody and T cell responses to melanoma, and adoptive transfer of tumour-infiltrating lymphocytes has been associated with regression of melanoma.[6]

The question remains, however, whether immunotherapy with vaccines or cytokines will recruit host-effector mechanisms to eradicate micrometastases and influence the survival of patients with high-risk resectable melanoma. Chapter 54 outlines some of the principles involved in immunotherapy and some of the inherent obstacles to this approach. The present chapter reviews some of the clinical trials that have been initiated to test the efficacy of the vaccine approach, and discusses possible merits and shortcomings of the different trials. The use of interferon-alfa (IFN-α) as an adjuvant to surgery in various trials is also reviewed and suggestions made for more forward-looking evaluation of this reagent. Several trials have also been conducted on levamisole as an adjuvant in melanoma but these are not discussed further.[7,8]

WHO SHOULD BE CONSIDERED FOR ADJUVANT THERAPY?

The traditional criteria for selection of patients for adjuvant therapy have been based on thickness of the primary melanoma and whether or not the melanoma has metastasized to regional lymph nodes.[9] As shown in Table 55.1, patients with American Joint Committee on Cancer (AJCC) stage IIA have the lowest risk and patients with resected stage IV disease the highest risk. The degree of risk has an important bearing on the type of treatment being considered for adjuvant therapy. Those with low risk disease have high survival rates from treatment with surgical removal alone and it is considered unwarranted to expose them to toxic long-term treatments such as high-dose IFN-α2 (HDI). Most vaccine treatments are relatively non-toxic and hence appropriate for treatment of low- and moderate-risk patients.

As discussed elsewhere in this book, the new AJCC/Union Internationale Contre le Cancer (UICC)

Table 55.1 *Melanoma patients considered for adjuvant treatment*

Risk	AJCC* stage	10-year survival (%)
Moderate	IIA (primary melanoma 1.5–4 mm thick)	50–70
High	IIB (primary melanoma >4 mm thick)	30–50
	III (regional lymph node metastases)	20–40
Very high	IV (resected distant metastases)	<20

*AJCC, American Joint Committee on Cancer.

staging system for melanoma places emphasis on the importance of ulceration of the primary melanoma on prognosis, which at most thickness levels reduces 5- and 10-year survival rates by 10%.[9] In view of this, it would appear justifiable in future adjuvant therapy trials to include T2b (i.e. 1–2 mm thick primaries with ulceration).[10] Staging of patients by the sentinel lymph node biopsy technique (SLNB)[11,12] has proved to be a valuable predictor of prognosis[13,14] and, in future trials, it may become mandatory to include SLNB for accurate staging of the patients. This technique can be made more sensitive by inclusion of polymerase chain reaction (PCR) assays for tyrosinase to detect low numbers of melanoma cells. The survival of patients with PCR-positive lymph nodes (LN) but histologically negative LN for melanoma appears worse than those with the PCR-negative LN,[15] but the performance of PCR tests on nodes remains controversial, mainly because the tests do not discriminate between naevus cells and melanoma cells in LN and because the extraction procedure destroys tissue that may be needed for histopathological review.

Detection of melanoma cells in the circulation, by PCR tests for tyrosinase and MART-1, has also been shown to be associated with an adverse prognosis and was a more powerful prognostic indicator than LN status.[16–18] The tests were, however, associated with a 30% false-negative rate,[16,17] which will probably limit their application in the selection of patients for adjuvant therapy.

MELANOMA VACCINES BEING TESTED IN PHASE III TRIALS

The melanoma vaccines which have progressed through to phase III trials are summarized in Table 55.2. Five studies have now been completed by: Wallack et al.,[19] Livingston et al.,[20] Sondak et al.[21] (the Southwest Oncology Group (SWOG) trial 9035), Kirkwood et al.[22] (Intergroup trial E1694) and Hersey et al.[23,24] There was a non-significant trend in favour of the vaccine treatment in studies by Wallack et al.[19] and Livingston et al.,[20] but patient numbers were relatively small and their power to exclude clinically significant benefits was therefore low. SWOG[21] used Melacine and Detox in a randomized trial involving 689 patients with stage IIA primary melanoma (i.e. 1.5–4.00 mm in thickness). The median follow-up was 4.1 years and the minimum follow-up was 3 years. The results showed an overall improvement in disease-free survival (DFS) (P=0.04) when results were analyzed on an intention-to-treat basis, but not when patients with protocol violations were excluded.[19] There was no effect on overall survival (OS). The subgroup of patients with primary melanomas <3 mm in thickness accounted for most of the improvement in DFS (P=0.06). These results are regarded by most investigators as not sufficiently impressive to warrant routine use in this subgroup of patients. However, analysis of the results in terms of human leucocyte antigen (HLA) typing showed that there were fewer relapses in patients who were HLA-A2 and HLA-C3; these differences were highly significant.[25]

The Intergroup trial E1694[22] in patients with stage IIB and stage III melanoma compared HDI with immunization versus GM2/keyhole limpet haemocyanin (KLH) in the QS21 adjuvant; 880 patients were entered and 774 were considered eligible. The trial was stopped at the second interim analysis after a median follow-up of 16 months because patients in the HDI arm had a significantly better DFS than those in the vaccine arm (DFS, P=0.0009; OS, P=0.046). These results need to be confirmed after a longer follow-up period, but appear to suggest that immunization with the ganglioside GM2 is ineffective. The absence of a control group also makes interpretation difficult, as the improved survival of the HDI group may represent improved survival of all patients in the group with time, as seen in the Intergroup trials E1694[22] and E1690.[26]

The trial by Hersey et al.[23,24] used vaccinia viral lysates as an adjuvant following surgery in patients with stage

Table 55.2 *Randomized trials with melanoma vaccines*

Investigators – clinical stage of trial*	Melanoma vaccine	Trial design	Protocol	No. of patients – status
Hersey et al.[23,24] – IIB and III	Vaccinia lysates of one allogeneic melanoma cell	Control untreated	id: q2w × 4, then q3w × 6, then q4w × 18	700 (closed 2/98) – *P*=0.077 in favour of vaccines
Wallack et al.[19] – III	Vaccinia lysates of three allogeneic melanoma cells	Control vaccinia alone	id: q1w × 13, then q2w × 40	250 – non-significant trend
Livingston et al.[20] – III	GM2 + Cyclo and BCG vaccine	Control BCG/Cyclo	4–5 × over 6 months	122 – non-significant trend
Intergroup trial E1694[22] (Schering/Bristol Myers) – IIB and III	GM2/KLH/QS21	Control HDI	sc: q1w × 4, then every 12 weeks for 2 years	880 (closed 11/99) – significant difference in favour of HDI; *P*=0.009 for survival, *P*=0.0015 for DFS
EORTC trial 18961[32] (Bristol Myers) – IIA and IIB	GM2/KLH/QS21	Control untreated	sc: q1w × 4, then every 12 weeks for 2 years and every 6 months for year 3	1300–1500 (projected)
Morton et al.[27] (NCI) – IIB and III	Three allogeneic melanoma cells + BCG vaccine	Control HDI or BCG alone	id: q2w × 3, then monthly × 12, then 3 monthly × 4, then 6 monthly × 6	825 (projected) – in progress
Morton et al.[27] (NCI) – IV	Three allogeneic melanoma cells + BCG vaccine	Control HDI or BCG alone	id: q2w × 3, then monthly × 12, then 3 monthly × 4, then 6 monthly × 6	420 projected – in progress
Mitchell et al.[27] (Corixa/Schering) – IIB and III	Two allogeneic melanoma cells + Detox + IFN 5×10^6	Control HDI	sc: q1w × 4, then q2w × 1, then monthly with repeat courses 6 monthly	315/400 accrued as of 2/2000 – in progress
Sondack et al.[21] (SWOG 9035/Ribi/Corixa) – IIA	Two allogeneic melanoma cells + Detox	Control untreated	sc: q1w × 4, then q4w × 1, then q8w × 5, then 6 monthly to 2 years	689 (closed 11/96) – DFS, *P*=0.04. in subset <3 mm, DFS, *P*=0.06
Berd et al.[30] (Avax) – III	Cyclo Autol Mel/ DNP/BCG	Control HDI	sc: q1w × 6 booster at 6 months	400 projected
Bystryn et al.[52] – III	Shed antigens from tour melanoma + Alum	Placebo [ALB] + Alum	id: q3w × 4 then monthly × 3, then to 5 years	36 significant DFS; non-significant survival

*American Joint Committee on Cancer (AJCC) stages III and IV refer to patients with lymph node metastases and disseminated metastases, respectively. Stage IIA and IIB refer to localized melanoma >1.5 and >4.00 mm thick, respectively. NCI, National Cancer Institute (USA).

BCG, Bacillus Calmette-Guérin; Cyclo, cyclophosphamide; id, intradermal; IFN, interferon; HDI, high dose IFN-α2b; KLH, keyhole limpet haemocyanin; q*x*w, every *x* weeks; sc, subcutaneous; DNP, dinitrophenyl; DFS, disease-free survival; Autol Mel, autologous melanoma; Alum, aluminium hydroxide; NCCTG, North Central Cancer Treatment Group; DKG; Deutsche Krebsgesellschaft.

IIB and stage III melanoma; 700 patients were entered and the median follow-up was 8 years. There was a marked improvement in OS of all patients in the study, with a median OS of 88 months compared to an historical median OS of 32–36 months; the median OS of the treated group had not been reached but was >100 months. The survival at 5 years was 55.1, and 59.6% for control and vaccine-treated patients, respectively; survival at 10 years was 41.9 and 52.7%, respectively. The percentage improvement at 5 and 10 years survival was 11 and 17%, respectively. The *P* value for these differences, however, was 0.07. There was no significant toxicity associated with the treatment.[24]

The other trials in Table 55.2 remain in progress, but some indication of possible benefit comes from studies on patients with stage IV metastatic disease. Morton et al.[27] reported apparent improvements in the survival of patients with stage IV disease treated with a mixed allogeneic whole-cell vaccine. Although the study was non-comparative, the patient numbers were relatively large. A high number of patients (26%) survived for 5 years, which is unusual for this disease. These results have prompted a trial of Cancervax in patients with resected stage IV disease, and in patients with resected and regional lymph node disease.

Mitchell[28] used vaccines prepared from a pool of ultrasonicated melanoma cell lines and a novel adjuvant (Detox; Ribi Immunochemical Co., Montana, USA). Treatment with this vaccine was reported to induce response rates that were equivalent to, or higher than, those seen with chemotherapy with dacarbazine (DTIC) alone, and was associated with longer remission periods.[28] This particular vaccine, referred to as Melacine, is now produced commercially (in a freeze-dried form) by Ribi Immunochemical Co. and Corixa, and is licensed for use in Canada. The US National Cancer Institute (NCI) sponsored a controlled trial with this vaccine in patients with stage IV disease, comparing Melacine with the Dartmouth chemotherapy regime (tamoxifen, dacarbazine, cisplatin (Cis-DPP) and carmustine (BCNU)). There was no significant difference in survival of the patients in the two groups, i.e. the vaccine-treated patients fared no worse than those treated with chemotherapy.[28]

Berd et al.[29,30] attempted to increase the effectiveness of melanoma vaccines by coupling a chemical hapten, dinitrofluorobenzene (DNFB), to autologous melanoma cells. The immune response to DNP on the tumour cells is believed to induce a strong response to the adjacent tumour antigens, analogous to the helper effect of viral antigens in vaccinia viral lysates of melanoma cells. These investigators showed that the DNP-coupled melanoma cells induced a strong inflammatory response to distant metastases in 26 of 46 patients, and that 21 of 24 patients had histological evidence of a marked CD8+ T cell infiltrate.[29] Information about the clinical response rate is preliminary, but partial responses were seen in five of 46 patients. Subsequent adjuvant studies in patients with bulky LN metastases were also encouraging.[30]

These studies therefore provide encouraging, but not conclusive, evidence that melanoma vaccines may be of benefit in the treatment of melanoma. Whether this promise is substantiated by phase III trials should be known over the next few years. It is important to note that most of the ideas involved in the design of these trials were generated in the 1980s and are not based on the more up-to-date information that was accumulated during the 1990s. It is therefore of interest to scrutinize these existing studies to see, with the benefit of hindsight, whether there are major flaws in the design of the vaccines or in the administration protocols.

GANGLIOSIDE VACCINES IN THE TREATMENT OF MELANOMA

Adoptive transfer studies in animal models have indicated that lymphocytes, rather than antibodies, are responsible for tumour rejection.[31] Nevertheless, two large randomized studies were based on the premise that antibody responses have an important role against melanoma. These include the Intergroup trial E1694[22] and possibly the European Organization for Research and Treatment of Cancer (EORTC) trial 18961,[32] both of which aimed to stimulate antibody responses to the GM2 ganglioside expressed on most melanomas. There are relatively few animal studies to support this approach, except for the study by Zhang et al.[33] on antibodies to the GD2 ganglioside. Immunization of mice with GD2/KLH/QS21 was found to reduce the incidence of liver metastases from subcutaneous transplants of the EL4 lymphoma. Passive infusion of MAb to GD2 was, however, only effective in reducing metastases if given shortly after injection of the tumour and had no effect on the growth of tumour at the inoculation site. In this model, the antibody therefore appeared to act by limiting blood-borne metastasis.

The main evidence in melanoma patients for a possible benefit of GM2 antibodies is the association of the latter with improved survival in patients with resected stage IIB or III disease.[19,34,35] However, this does not prove that the antibodies are directly responsible and it may merely be an indicator of more relevant mechanisms. It seems unlikely that antibodies to GM2 would have a direct effect on solid tumours because of poor penetration into the tumour and the presence of molecules on the tumour cells such as CD55 (DAF) and CD59 (protectin), which degrade complement and inhibit complement-mediated lysis.[36,37]

The use of the ganglioside vaccines is therefore controversial and the results of the Intergroup trial E1694[22] suggest that further preclinical studies may be needed. Similar vaccines have been prepared against GD3, GD2 and fucosylated GM1,[38] and immunization of 31 patients with vaccines against both GM2 and GD2 was reported to be well tolerated.[39] Immunization against GD3 has been more difficult but was reported with KLH conjugates given with the adjuvant QS21.[40] The use of anti-idiotype antibodies to induce immune responses is an interesting approach designed to circumvent the low immunogenicity of the gangliosides. Forty-seven patients were immunized with an anti-idiotype against GD2. One patient had a complete response and 18 patients had stabilization of their disease. Adjuvant studies were in progress on 44 of the patients.[41]

VACCINES BASED ON INDUCTION OF T CELL RESPONSES TO MELANOMA

As discussed in Chapter 54, a large number of melanoma antigens recognized by T cells have now been described. These are classified as: (a) differentiation antigens; (b) tumour-specific antigens (TSA), cancer-testis (CT) antigens; (c) overexpressed antigens; and (d) individual specific antigens. Allogeneic vaccines will not usually contain individual specific antigens. It can also be assumed that all of the allogeneic vaccines will contain melanoma differentiation antigens to varying degrees and that major differences in responses to these antigens would not be expected. Any differences would therefore depend on their content of TSA (CT antigens), e.g. MAGE, GAGE etc. Information on this point is not freely available. In the case of the MM200 melanoma cell used in the Hersey et al.[23,24] vaccine study, it is known to express MAGE-3 and -10, XAGE, BAGE and GAGE, but not CT7, NY-ESO-1 and NA17. Typing has not been carried out for the other members of the CT family. From Table 55.3, it may be seen that the MAGE family have high levels of expression in melanoma lines and it is quite likely that most allogeneic melanoma vaccines will contain some of these antigens.[42] It is also clear from ongoing studies that the major histocompatibility complex (MHC) restriction of the MAGE family is wide and includes helper CD4 T cell epitopes.[43–45]

It is therefore unlikely that there are major differences between the allogeneic vaccines in their content of TSA or differentiation antigens. If differences in results from clinical trials do appear, it is probable that they are due to the adjuvant used with the vaccine, or the dose, timing and frequency of administration of the injections. Possible limitations of allogeneic vaccines are reviewed by Mitchell[46] and include suppression of responses to weak antigens due to the strong alloresponse or antigenic competition from too many foreign antigens occupying antigen-presenting cells.

Very few studies have yet been initiated to test adjuvant immunotherapy with purified peptides. The exceptions are the trials initiated by ECOG in which HLA-A2 patients are immunized with peptides from MART-1, gp100 and tyrosinase, given alone or with GM colony-stimulating factor (GM-CSF) or IFN-α2 (Intergroup trial E1696). The optimum therapy in terms of T cell responses will then be tested in resected stage IIIC or IV patients with or without GM-CSF (Intergroup trial E4697).

A number of animal studies have shown that individual specific antigens were much more effective in inducing regression of tumours than antigens common to tumours.[31,47–49] It is quite possible that the same may apply in melanoma, e.g. it was reported that immune responses against the MUM-2 antigens were associated with long periods of remission in the patients concerned.[50] MUM-3 was also associated with high precursor frequencies.[51] It is generally thought that the main reason for the effectiveness of individual neoantigens is that they may generate highly avid T cell responses.[49] The main limitation of immunization with individual specific antigens is the practical difficulty of obtaining a supply of such antigens. Given that SLNB techniques are leading to early resection of tumour-involved LN,

Table 55.3 *Expression of tumour-specific antigens in melanoma*

	Cell Lines (%)[71]	Melanoma tissue		HLA* restriction
		Primary (%)	Metastases (%)	
MAGE-A1[a[75,76]]	53	16	48	A1, A3, B37, Cw1601
MAGE-A2	89	41	70	A3, B37
MAGE-A3[[77–79]]	94	36	76	A1,A2, A3, A24, B37, B44, DR11, DR13
MAGE-4A[a]	55	11	22	
MAGE-A6	89	?	?	
MAGE-A10	53	16	48	A2
MAGE-A12	89	?	?	
MAGE-C1 (CT7)		37	53	
BAGE			22	Cw1601
GAGE			24	Cw6
LAGE			50	
SSX-2			43	
NY-ESO-1			20–40	A2, A31
DAM				A2
Glucosaminyl transferase V NA17-1			50	A2

[a]MAGE-9 and -11 are expressed only weakly in melanoma. References to studies in the table are given elsewhere.[42,45]
*HLA, human leucocyte antigen.

the number of patients that can be treated with autologous vaccines now and in the future is likely to be low. As indicated in Table 55.2, however, trials based on this approach are being conducted by Berd et al.[30] and results of these trials are awaited with much interest.

Table 55.2 also indicates that there has been a wide variation in the timing of vaccine administration and in the dose of the vaccines used; e.g. Bystryn et al.[52] administered 40μg protein per dose, Wallack et al.[19] 2 mg per dose and Hersey et al.[24] 100μg per dose. Relatively large doses (20–25 × 10 cells) of whole cells are used in studies by Morton et al.,[27] Berd et al.[53] and Mitchell et al.[28] As discussed in Chapter 54, these differences in amounts and the timing of vaccine administration may be important determinants of the immune response.

INTERFERON-ALFA 2 (INF-α2) AS ADJUVANT THERAPY FOR MELANOMA

IFN-α2 as a single agent has a response rate similar to chemotherapy with darcarbazine in the treatment of metastatic disease. In view of this, it has received considerable attention as a possible adjuvant treatment for melanoma. The results of these studies are summarized in Tables 55.4 and 55.5. Much enthusiasm was generated by the results of a relatively small randomized trial conducted by the Intergroup trial (E1684),[23] which showed modest improvements in DFS and OS (from 2.8 to 3.8 years).[54] The dose of IFN-α2 used in these studies was high and associated with considerable toxicity. A follow-up larger confirmatory trial by this group (Intergroup trial E1690)[26] failed to show any effects on OS and only a small effect on DFS. Nevertheless, a further trial (Intergroup trial E1694) has shown a highly significant difference in patients with stage IIB and stage III melanoma treated with HDI compared to immunization with the GM2/KLH vaccine (see above).[23] The latter result could be due to worsening of OS in the group treated with the ganglioside vaccine, but this was considered unlikely because the survival of the latter group was comparable to that of the control, untreated patients in the previous Intergroup trial E1690.

The survival of patients treated with HDI in the Intergroup trial E1694 appeared to be superior to that of patients treated with HDI in the Intergroup trial E1690. The reasons for this may become clearer with further analysis of subgroups in the two trials. The main limitation of the Intergroup trial E1694 results is the absence of an untreated control group. It is therefore possible that the improved results may reflect improved survival of all patients in the study and a negative impact of treatment with the GM2 vaccine.

Finally, another, but quite important, word of caution regarding the interpretation of the Intergroup trial E1694 early analysis is that there is evidence from Intergroup trials E1684 and E1690 that a survival benefit after HDI does not last. The differences in Intergroup trial E1694 were reported at a median follow-up of only 1.3 years, which makes it virtually impossible to make solid claims on impact on OS. In a pooled analysis of the Intergroup trials E1684 and E1690, presented at the American Society for Clinical Oncology (ASCO) in 2001, the impact on OS by HDI was not so evident when one realizes that 198 patients in the observation arms of Intergroup trials E1684 and E1690 had died thus far, whereas 201 patients had died in the HDI arms.[55]

Lower doses of IFN-α2, as used in the World Health Organization (WHO) trial 16,[56] Intergroup trial E1690[26] and EORTC trial 18871,[57] had no impact on the DFS of patients with high-risk (stage IIB and stage III) melanoma. The latter trial used 1 MIU of IFN-α2 on alternate days and included studies on IFN-γ and

Table 55.4 *Outcome of studies on IFN-α2 as adjuvant to surgery in patients with melanoma*

STAGE II (A + B) or IIB (T3-4N0M0)				STAGE III (any TN1-2M0)			
No. of patients	Trial	DFS	OS	No. of patients	Trial	DFS	OS
High dose IFN							
122	NCCTG	−	−	160	NCCTG	−	−
31	Intergroup E1684	−	−	249	Intergroup E1684	+	+ at 5 years − at 10 years
112	Intergroup E1690	−	−	314	Intergroup E1690	+	+
Low dose IFN							
107	Intergroup E1690	−	−	318	Intergroup E1690	−	−
499	French	+	+ at 5 years − at 8 years	427	WHO 16	−	−
311 95	Austrian Scottish	+ +/−	− +/−				
340	EORTC 18871 /DKG-80	−	−	490	EORTC 18871 /DKG-80	−	−

DFS, disease-free survival; OS, overall survival; NCCTG, North Central Cancer Treatment Group; WHO, World Health Organization; EORTC, European Organization for Research and Treatment of Cancer; DKG, Deutsche Krebsgesellschaft.

Table 55.5 *All trials of adjuvant IFN-α2 in melanoma*

Investigators*	AJCC† clinical stage	Dose/schedule	No.	Results
Intergroup E1684[54]	IIB/III	HDI	280	OS 2.8–3.8 years
NCCTG 837052	IIA and B, III	20 MU/m^2/day im tiw × 3 months	262	No effect
Intergroup E1690[26]	IIB, III	HDI 3 MU/day sc tiw × 2 years	642	No effect on survival Small effect on DFS
WHO 16[56]	III	3 MU/day sc tiw × 3 years	427	No effect
EORTC 18871[57]	IIA and B, III	1 MU/day sc × 1 year versus IFN-γ 0.2 mg/day sc × 1 year	830	No effect
EORTC 18952[61]	IIB, III	10 MU/day sc × 1 month; then IFNα-2b 10MU/day sc tiw × 1 year IFNα-2b 5MU/day sc tiw × 2 year versus observation	1418	Accrual complete on 06/2000: 1 year: DMFI: no effect 2 year: DMFI, *P*=0.0145 OS: too early
Intergroup E1694[22]	IIB, III	HDI versus GM2/KLH/QS21 vaccine	774	Benefit for HDI DFS, (*P*=0.0009) OS, (*P*2=0.046)
Austrian[58] Trial	IIA and B	3 MU/day sc × 3 weeks then tiw × 11 months	311	Significant improvement in DFS but not OS
French[59] Trial	IIA and B	3 MU sc tiw × 18 months	499	Significant improvement DFS, *P*=0.038; OS, 0.059
Scottish[60] Trial	IIA and B	3 MU sc tiw × 6 months	95	Transient effect on DFS and OS; same size too small
Intergroup E1697	IIA	20 MU/m^2/days IV × 1 month	1420	In progress
EORTC 18991	III	PEG-Intron 6.0 μg/kg/week for 8 weeks then 3.0 μg/kg/ week for 5 years	900	In progress
Sunbelt	III by SNB (IIIA)	HDI	3000 projected	In progress
UKCCCR[62]	III	3 MU sc tiw × 2 years	654	Not significant (early report)

*NCCTG, North Central Cancer Treatment Group; WHO, World Health Organization; EORTC, European Organization for Research and Treatment of Cancer; UKCCCR, United Kingdom Co-ordinating Committee on Cancer Research.
†American Joint Committee on Cancer.

HDI: high dose IFN-α2b (20 MU/m^2/day intravenous (iv) × 1 month, 10 MU/m^2 subcutaneous (sc) tiw for 11 months); im, intramuscular; tiw, three times per week; OS, overall survival; DFS, disease-free survival; DMFI, distant-metastasis-free interval; SNB, sentinel node biopsy.

Iscador, a mistletoe extract. IFN had no effect on survival but Iscador was associated with an adverse effect on survival.[57] Three trials, one in Austria,[58] one in France[59] and one in Scotland,[60] have suggested that low dose IFN-α may have some benefit in the treatment of patients at moderate risk from recurrent melanoma (AJCC stage IIA + IIB). All three trials showed an increase in DFS but an effect on OS has not yet been confirmed (Tables 55.4 and 55.5).

Several other trials are being conducted to examine whether mid-range doses of IFN-α2 alone (EORTC trial 18952)[61] or in combination with vaccines may improve the results (Tables 55.2, 55.5 and 55.6).[28] The largest trial by far in high-risk melanoma patients (stage IIB–III) is the EORTC trial 18952 in 1418 patients. This trial evaluated the impact of intermediate doses of IFN-α where, after an induction period of 4 weeks, for 5 days per week, 10 MU, subcutaneously (sc) was followed by a maintenance period of 10 MU, sc, three times per week (tiw) for 1 year, versus 5 MU, sc, tiw for 2 years, versus observation. The first analysis of EORTC trial 18952 was reported at the 37th Annual Meeting of ASCO.[61] The analysis indicated that duration of treatment was more important than dose of IFN-α, since the higher dose of 10 MU for 1 year had no significant impact on distant-metastasis-free interval (DMFI), the primary end point in this trial, whilst the lower dose of 5 MU for 2 years showed a significant impact on DMFI (P=0.0145).[61] Again, just as with the short follow-up of Intergroup trial E1694, these data should be interpreted with great caution as many early positive reports have seen the light in the history of phase III trials. Yet, these results support the trial design of the currently ongoing EORTC trial 18991, which evaluates the impact of long-term maintenance therapy of 5 years with Pegylated-IFN-α (PEG-Intron) as compared to observation in 900 stage III patients. The mature results of the EORTC trial 18952 on intermediate dose INF (IDI) are awaited great interest, as IDI has an acceptable toxicity profile (*c.* 10% grade III–IV toxicity events in contrast to 78% with HDI). If the reported early impact on DMFI translates into an OS benefit, IDI may, because of its acceptable toxicity profile, be considered as a reasonable candidate for adjuvant therapy in high-risk melanoma patients.

Taking into account the early report of the United Kingdom Co-ordinating Committee on Cancer Research (UKCCCR) low-dose IFN trial (3 MU, sc, tiw for 2 years in stage IIB–III patients)[62] and the early report on the EORTC trial 18952,[61] a meta-analysis was presented at ASCO in 2001. This showed clearly that IFN therapy in the adjuvant setting has a consistent impact on DFS for all doses ≥3 MU, but no significant impact on OS.[63]

Table 55.6 *Interferon (INF) trials with insufficient follow-up or still in progress*

No. of patients	Trial*	DFS	OS median follow-up
High dose IFN (HDI)			
774	Intergroup E1694	+ P=0.0009	+ P=0.046 at 1.3 years
1420	Intergroup E1697	In progress	In progress
Intermediate dose IFN (IDI)			
1418	EORTC 18952	DMFI P=0.0145 For treatment with 5 MU IFN for 2 years	Too early at 1.5 years
Low dose IFN (LDI)			
654	UK-MCG ('Aim High')	–	– at 1.2 years

*EORTC, European Organization for Research and Treatment of Cancer; UK-MCG, UK Melanoma Cooperative Group, DFS, disease-free survival; OS, overall survival; DMFI, distant-metastases-free interval.

The EORTC is conducting a further trial (trial 18991) using slow release PEG-Intron in patients with stage III melanoma, given sc each week over a 5-year period. The Eastern Co-operative Oncology Group (ECOG) is also testing whether 1 month of high dose IFN-α2b will be an effective treatment in patients with stage IIA–B melanoma (Intergroup trial E1697). A further trial – Intergroup trial E2001 – is planned to compare 1 month of high dose IFN-α2b with the standard high-dose regime given over 1 year.

On the basis of the Intergroup trial E1684, IFN-α2 was licensed for use in the USA as adjuvant treatment for melanoma and remains so. Similarly, low dose IFN-α2 has been licensed for use in Europe for treatment of patients with stage IIA–B melanoma, but its use has been questioned.[64]

NEW DIRECTIONS IN USE OF INTERFERON-ALFA-2 (IFN-α2) AS ADJUVANT THERAPY OF MELANOMA

Once the results of the EORTC trial 18952 on intermediate doses of IFN are known, large trials on the use of IFN-α2 as a single agent as adjuvant therapy of melanoma over a range of doses will have been completed. The PEG-Intron trial will further show whether prolonged high levels of IFN-α2b given over a long period will be of benefit. There are, at present, very few initiatives to extend the use of IFN-α2, either by selection of patients who may be more likely to respond or to investigate combinations with IFN-α2. Mitchell et al.[65] are, however, evaluating whether IFN-α2b will enhance response to a melanoma vaccine.

New insights into the possible mechanism of action of IFN-α2b have been provided by studies on apoptosis of melanoma induced by a member of the tumour necrosis factor (TNF) family, referred to as TNF-related apoptosis-inducing ligand (TRAIL).[66] The latter molecule appears to induce apoptosis in a wide range of melanomas.[67,68] Most importantly, studies by this group and others have shown that IFN-α2 and, to a lesser extent, IFN-γ are potent inducers of TRAIL in T cells[69] and monocytes.[70] It has also been shown that the ability to induce TRAIL on lymphocytes from melanoma patients varies from patient to patient, and can be inhibited by supernatants from melanoma cultures.[71] These studies do not prove that IFN-α2 mediates its effect through TRAIL-induced apoptosis but it certainly raises this possibility. Further studies to assess induction of TRAIL by IFN-α2 in individual patients, and to determine whether their melanoma cells are sensitive to TRAIL-induced apoptosis, should assist in establishing this hypothesis and facilitate a new approach to use of IFN-α2. It has been shown, for example, that proteasome inhibitors sensitize some melanoma cells to TRAIL-induced apoptosis, probably by inhibiting the activation of the transcription factor, nuclear factor kappa B (NF-κB),[72] which is known to induce antiapoptotic mechanisms.[73] Should IFN-α2 mediate its effects through TRAIL, the combination of IFN-α2 and proteasome inhibitors, such as PS-341[74] may be a promising combination to test in future trials.

CONCLUSIONS

Although many trials have been conducted, the results show very little gain in survival of patients over that expected from surgery alone. The Australian trial in particular, but also those by ECOG, illustrate very forcefully that controlled trials are essential in evaluating adjuvant treatments. This is illustrated in Table 55.7, which compares the median survival of control groups in a number of recent trials. In the case of the Australian trials, there was an increase in median overall survival from 32 to 88 months and in the ECOG studies from 34 to 72 months. In the absence of randomized controls, these increases would have been attributed to the treatment.

Several large trials of immunotherapy with cancer vaccines and treatment with IFN-α2 at medium doses will be completed over the next few years and results of these studies are awaited with much interest. Irrespective of their results, there is a continuing need for studies on new approaches in treatment, such as the use of agents able to induce apoptosis, as referred to above. It is also important to define different categories of melanoma that are responsive to different forms of therapy. The latter initiative will require development in phase I–II studies and hopefully lead to more substantial gains in survival in subsequent multi-institutional trials.

Table 55.7 ***Median overall survival (OS) of patients in control and treated groups in recent melanoma vaccine and interferon (INF) adjuvant trials***

Trial	Stage	No.	Median survivals (months)	
			Control	Treated
Historical controls (1980–1984)[23]	IIB, III	151	32	
Wallack et al.[19]	III	217	41	50
Hersey et al.[24]	IIB, III	700	88	>100
WHO 16[56]	III	427	31	36
Intergroup E1684[22]	IIB, III	280	34	46
Intergroup E1690[26]	IIB, III	642	72	61

REFERENCES

1. Hersey P, Balch CM, Current status and future prospects for adjuvant therapy of melanoma. *Aust NZ J Surg* 1984; 54: 303.
2. Barth A, Morton DL, The role of adjuvant therapy in melanoma management. *Cancer* 1995; 75: 726.
3. McGovern VJ, Spontaneous regression of malignant melanoma. In: *Melanoma: histological diagnosis and prognosis* (ed Blaustein A). New York: Raven Press 1982; 138–47.
4. Hersey P, Murray E, Grace J, McCarthy WH, Current research on immunopathology of melanoma: analysis of lymphocyte populations in relation to antigen expression and histological features of melanoma. *Pathology* 1985; 17: 385.
5. Tefany FJ, Barnetson RS, Halliday GM et al, Immunocytochemical analysis of the cellular infiltrate in primary regressing and non-regressing malignant melanoma. *J Invest Dermatol* 1991; 97: 197.
6. Rosenberg SA, Yannelli JR, Yang JC et al, Treatment of patients with metastatic melanoma with autologous tumour-infiltrating lymphocytes and interleukin 2. *J Natl Cancer Inst* 1994; 86: 1159.
7. Spitler LE, A randomized trial of levamisole versus placebo as adjuvant therapy in malignant melanoma. *J Clin Oncol* 1991; 9: 736.
8. Quirt IC, Shelley WE, Pater JL et al, Improved survival in patients with poor-prognosis malignant melanoma treated with adjuvant levamisole: a phase III study by the National Cancer Institute of Canada Clinical Trials Group. *J Clin Oncol* 1991; 9: 729.
9. Balch CM, Soong S-J, Shaw HM et al, An analysis of prognostic factors in 8500 patients with cutaneous melanoma. In: *Cutaneous melanoma* (eds Balch CM, Houghton AN, Milton GW et al). Philadelphia: JB Lippincott, 1992; 165–87.
10. Balch CM, Buzaid AC, Atkins MB et al, A new American Joint Committee on Cancer staging system for cutaneous melanoma. *Cancer* 2000; 88: 1484.
11. Morton DL, Wen DR, Cochran AJ, Management of early-stage melanoma by intra-operative lymphatic mapping and selective lymphadenectomy. *Surg Oncol Clin N Am* 1992; 1: 247.
12. Morton DL, Thompson JF, Essner R et al, Validation of the accuracy of intraoperative lymphatic mapping and sentinel lymphadenectomy for early-stage melanoma: a multicenter trial. Multicenter Selective Lymphadenectomy Trial Group. *Ann Surg* 1999; 230: 453.
13. Gershenwald JE, Thompson W, Mansfield PF et al, Multi-institutional melanoma lymphatic mapping experience: the prognostic value of sentinel lymph node status in 612 stage I or II melanoma patients. *J Clin Oncol* 1999; 17: 976.
14. Gadd MA, Cosimi AB, Yu J et al, Outcome of patients with melanoma and histologically negative sentinel lymph nodes. *Arch Surg* 1999; 134: 381.
15. Shivers SC, Wang X, Li W et al, Molecular staging of malignant melanoma: correlation with clinical outcome. *JAMA* 1998; 280: 1410.
16. Curry BJ, Myers K, Hersey P, Polymerase chain reaction detection of melanoma cells in the circulation: relation to clinical stage, surgical treatment, and recurrence from melanoma. *J Clin Oncol* 1998; 16: 1760.
17. Curry BJ, Myers K, Hersey P, MART-1 is expressed less frequently on circulating melanoma cells in patients who develop distant compared to locoregional metastases. *J Clin Oncol* 1999; 17: 2562.
18. Ghossein RA, Coit D, Brennan M et al, Prognostic significance of peripheral blood and bone marrow tyrosinase messenger RNA in malignant melanoma. *Clin Cancer Res* 1998; 4: 419.
19. Wallack MK, Sivanandham M, Balch CM et al, Surgical adjuvant active specific immunotherapy for patients with stage III melanoma: the final analysis of data from a phase III, randomized, double-blind, multicenter vaccinia melanoma oncolysate trial. *J Am Coll Surg* 1998; 187: 69.
20. Livingston PO, Wong GY, Adluri S et al, Improved survival in stage III melanoma patients with GM2 antibodies: a randomized trial of adjuvant vaccination with GM2. *J Clin Oncol* 1994; 12: 1036.
21. Sondak VK, Liu P-Y, Tuthill RJ et al, Adjuvant immunotherapy of resected, intermediate-thickness node-negative melanoma with an allogeneic tumor vaccine. I. Overall results of a randomized trial of the Southwest Oncology Group. *J Clin Oncol* 2002; 20: 2058–66.
22. Kirkwood JM, Ibrahim JG, Sosman JA et al, High-dose interferon alfa-2b significantly prolongs relapse-free and overall survival compared with the GM2–KLH/QS-21 vaccine in patients with resected stage IIB–III melanoma: results of intergroup trial E1694/S9512/C509801. *J Clin Oncol.* 2001; 19: 2370.
23. Hersey P, Edwards A, Coates A et al, Evidence that treatment with vaccinia melanoma cell lysates [VMCL] may improve survival of patients with stage II melanoma. *Cancer Immunol Immunother* 1987; 25: 257.
24. Hersey P, Coates AS, McCarthy WH et al, Adjuvant immunotherapy of patients with high risk melanoma using vaccinia viral lysates of melanoma. Results of a randomized trial. *J Clin Oncol* (in press).
25. Sosman JA, Unger JM, Liu P-Y et al, Adjuvant immunotherapy of resected, intermediate-thickness node-negative melanoma with an allogeneic tumor vaccine. II. Impact of HLA class I antigen expression on outcome. *J Clin Oncol* 2002; 20: 2067–75.
26. Kirkwood JM, Ibrahim JG, Sondak VK et al, High- and low-dose interferon alpha-2b in high-risk melanoma: first analysis of intergroup trial E1690/S9111/C9190. *J Clin Oncol* 2000; 18: 2444.
27. Morton DL, Foshag LJ, Hoon DSB et al, Prolongation of survival in metastatic melanoma after active specific immunotherapy with a new polyvalent melanoma vaccine. *Ann Surg* 1992; 216: 463.
28. Mitchell MS, Perspective on allogeneic melanoma lysates in active specific immunotherapy. *Semin Oncol* 1998; 25: 623.
29. Berd D, Murphy G, Maguire Jr HC, Mastrangelo MJ, Immunization with haptenized, autologous tumor cells induces inflammation of human melanoma metastases. *Cancer Res* 1991; 51: 2731.

30. Berd D, Maguire HC, Schuchter LM et al, Autologous hapten-modified melanoma vaccine as postsurgical adjuvant treatment after resection of nodal metastases. *J Clin Oncol* 1997; 15: 2359.
31. Hellstrom I, Hellstrom KE, Tumor immunology: an overview. In: *Specific immunotherapy of cancer with vaccines* (eds Bystryn J-C, Ferrone S, Livingston P). *NY Acad Sci* 1993; 690: 24–33.
32. Eggermont AM, Strategy of the EORTC–MCG trial programme for adjuvant treatment of moderate-risk and high-risk melanoma. *Eur J Cancer* 1998; 34: S22–S26.
33. Zhang H, Zhang S, Cheung N-KV et al, Antibodies against GD2 ganglioside can eradicate syngeneic cancer micrometastases. *Cancer Res* 1998; 58: 2844.
34. Jones PC, Sze LL, Liu PY, Prolonged survival for melanoma patients with elevated IgM antibody to oncofetal antigen. *J Natl Cancer Inst* 1981; 66: 249.
35. Takahashi H, Johnson TD, Nishinaka Y et al, IgM anti-ganglioside antibodies induced by melanoma cell vaccine correlate with survival of melanoma patients. *J Invest Dermatol* 1999; 112: 205.
36. Cheung NK, Walter EI, Smith-Mensah WH et al, Decay-accelerating factor protects human tumor cells from complement-mediated cytotoxicity in vitro. *J Clin Invest* 1988; 81: 1122.
37. Brasoveanu LI, Altomonte M, Fonsatti E et al, Levels of cell membrane CD59 regulate the extent of complement-mediated lysis of human melanoma cells. *Lab Invest* 1996; 74: 33.
38. Livingston P, Ganglioside vaccines with emphasis on GM2. *Semin Oncol* 1998; 25: 636.
39. Israel RJ, Chapman PB, Hamilton WB et al, Phase I/II dose-ranging clinical trials of the ganglioside conjugate cancer vaccines GM2-KLH/QS-21 [GMK] and GM2-KLH/GD2-KLH/QS-21 [MGV]. *Proc ASCO* 1999; 18: 437a (abstract).
40. Ragupathi G, Meyers M, Adluri S et al, Induction of antibodies against GD3 ganglioside in melanoma patients by vaccination with GD3–lactone–KLH conjugate plus immunological adjuvant QS-21. *Int J Cancer* 2000; 85: 659.
41. Foon KA, Sen G, Hutchins L et al, Antibody responses in melanoma patients immunized with an anti-idiotype antibody mimicking disialoganglioside GD2. *Clin Cancer Res* 1998; 4: 1117.
42. Hersey P, Will vaccines really work for melanoma? In: *Challenges in melanoma* (eds Newton-Bishop JA, Gore M). Oxford: Blackwell Science, 2002: 212–29.
43. Chaux P, Vantomme V, Stroobant V et al, Identification of MAGE-3 epitopes presented by HLA-DR molecules to $CD4^+$ T lymphocytes. *J Exp Med* 1999; 189: 767.
44. Manici S, Sturniolo T, Imro MA et al, Melanoma cells present a MAGE-3 epitope to $CD4^+$ cytotoxic T cells in association with histocompatibility leukocyte antigen DR11. *J Exp Med* 1999; 189: 871.
45. Renkvist N, Castelli C, Robbins PF, Parmiani G, A listing of human tumor antigens recognized by T cells. *Cancer Immunol Immunother* 2001; 50: 3.
46. Mitchell MS, Active specific immunotherapy of cancer: therapeutic vaccines ['Theraccines'] for the treatment of disseminated malignancies. In: *Biological approaches to cancer treatment* (ed Mitchell MS). New York: McGraw-Hill, 1993; 326–51.
47. Boon T, van der Bruggen P, Human tumor antigens recognized by T lymphocytes. *J Exp Med* 1996; 183: 725–9.
48. Rosenberg SA, A new era for cancer immunotherapy based on the genes that encode cancer antigens. *Immunity* 1999; 10: 281–7.
49. Gilboa E, The makings of a tumor rejection antigen. *Immunity* 1999; 11: 263–70.
50. Chiari R, Foury F, De Plaen E et al, Two antigens recognized by autologous cytolytic T lymphocytes on a melanoma result from a single point mutation in an essential housekeeping gene. *Cancer Res* 1999; 59: 5785.
51. Baurain J-F, Colau D, van Baren N et al, High frequency of autologous anti-melanoma CTL directed against an antigen generated by a point mutation in a new helicase gene. *J Immunol* 2000; 164: 6057.
52. Bystryn J-C, Oratz R, Shapiro RL et al, Double-blind, placebo-controlled, trial of a shed, polyvalent, melanoma vaccine in stage III melanoma. *Proc ASCO* 1999; 18: 434a (abstract).
53. Berd D, Maguire HC, Schuchter LM et al, Autologous hapten-modified melanoma vaccine as postsurgical adjuvant treatment after resection of nodal metastases. *J Clin Oncol* 1997; 15: 2359.
54. Kirkwood JM, Strawderman MH, Ernstoff MS, Interferon-alpha-2b adjuvant therapy of high-risk resected cutaneous melanoma; the Eastern Cooperative Oncology Group Trial EST 1684. *J Clin Oncol* 1996; 14: 7.
55. Kirkwood JM, Manola J, Ibrahim JG et al, Pooled analysis of four ECOG-Intergroup trials of high-dose interferon alfa-2b (HDI) in 1916 patients with high-risk resected cutaneous melanoma. *Proc ASCO* 2001; 20: 1395 (abstract).
56. Cascinelli N, Belli F, Mackie RM, Effect of long-term adjuvant therapy with interferon alpha-2a in patients with regional node metastases from cutaneous melanoma: a randomized trial. *Lancet* 2001; 358: 866–9.
57. Kleeberg U, Broecker EB, Chartier C, EORTC 18871 adjuvant trial in high risk melanoma patients IFNα vs IFNgamma vs Iscador vs observation. *Eur J Cancer* 1999; 35: S4.
58. Pehamberger H, Soyer HP, Steiner A et al, Adjuvant interferon alfa-2a treatment in resected primary stage II cutaneous melanoma. *J Clin Oncol* 1998; 16: 1425.
59. Grob JJ, Dreno B, de la Salmoniere P et al, Randomised trial of interferon α-2a as adjuvant therapy in resected primary melanoma thicker than 1.5 mm without clinically detectable node metastases. *Lancet* 1998; 351: 1905.
60. Cameron DA, Cornbleet MC, MacKie RM et al, Adjuvant interferon alpha in high risk melanoma: the Scottish study. *Br J Cancer* 2001; 84: 1146–9.
61. Eggermont AMM, Kleeberg UR, Ruiter DJ, Suciu S, The European Organization for Research and Treatment of Cancer Melanoma Group trial experience with more than 2000 patients, evaluating adjuvant therapy treatment with low or intermediate doses of interferon alpha-2b. In: *American Society of Clinical Oncology , 2001 Educational Book* (ed Perry MC). Alexandria, Virginia: American Society of Clinical Oncology, 2001: 88.
62. Hancock BW, Wheatley K, Harrison G, Gore M, Aim high-adjuvant interferon in melanoma (high risk), a United Kingdom Co-ordinating Committee on Cancer Research (UKCCCR) randomised study of observation versus adjuvant low dose extended duration interferon alfa-2a in high risk resected malignant melanoma. *Proc ASCO* 2001; 20: 1393 (abstract).
63. Wheatley K, Hancock B, Gore M et al, Interferon-α as adjuvant ther apy for melanoma: a meta-analysis of the randomised trials. *Proc ASCO* 2001; 20: 1394A (abstract); Kofler R, Binder M, Mischer P et al, Adjuvant interferon α-2a treatment in resected primary stage II cutaneous melanoma. *J Clin Oncol* 1998; 16: 1425.
64. Groenewegen G, Osanto S, van der Rhee HJ, Punt CJA, Interferon as an adjuvant treatment for melanoma: registered but not indicated. *Ned Tijdschr Geneesk* 2000; 144: 2160.
65. Mitchell MS, Jakowatz J, Harel W et al, Increased effectiveness of interferon alfa-2b following active specific immunotherapy for melanoma. *J Clin Oncol* 1994; 12: 402.
66. Griffith TS, Lynch DH, TRAIL: a molecule with multiple receptors and control mechanisms. *Curr Opin Immunol* 1998; 10: 559.
67. Thomas WD, Hersey P, TNF-related apoptosis-inducing ligand [TRAIL] induces apoptosis in Fas ligand-resistant melanoma cells and mediates CD4 T cell killing of target cells. *J Immunol* 1998; 161: 2195.
68. Zhang XD, Franco A, Myers K et al, Relation of TNF-related apoptosis-inducing ligand [TRAIL] receptor and FLICE-inhibitory protein expression to TRAIL-induced apoptosis of melanoma. *Cancer Res* 1999; 59: 2747.
69. Kayagaki N, Yamaguchi N, Nakayama M et al, Type I interferons [IFNs] regulate tumor necrosis factor-related apoptosis-inducing ligand [TRAIL] expression on human T cells: a novel mechanism for the antitumor effects of type I IFNs. *J Exp Med* 1999; 189: 1451.
70. Griffith TS, Wiley SR, Kubin MZ et al, Monocyte-mediated tumoricidal activity via the tumor necrosis factor-related cytokine, TRAIL. *J Exp Med* 1999; 189: 1343.
71. Nguyen T, Thomas W, Zhang, XD et al, Immunologically-mediated tumour cell apoptosis: the role of TRAIL in T cell and cytokine-mediated responses to melanoma. *Forum [Genova]* 2000; 10: 243.
72. Franco AV, Zhang XD, Van Berkel E et al, The role of NF-κB in TRAIL induced apoptosis of melanoma cells. *J Immunol* 2000; 166: 5337.

73. Wang C-Y, Cusack JC, Liu R, Baldwin AS, Control of inducible chemoresistance: enhanced anti-tumor therapy through increased apoptosis by inhibition of NF-κB. *Nat Med* 1999; 5: 412.
74. Teicher BA, Ara G, Herbst R et al, The proteasome inhibitor PS-341 in cancer therapy. *Clin Cancer Res* 1999; 5: 2638.
75. Zakut R, Topalian SL, Kawakami Y et al, Differential expression of MAGE-1, 2, and -3 messenger RNA in transformed and normal human cell lines. *Cancer Res* 1993; 53: 5.
76. McIntyre CA, Rees RC, Platts KE et al, Identification of peptide epitopes of MAGE-1, -2, -3 that demonstrate HLA-A3-specific binding. *Cancer Immunol Immunother* 1996; 42: 246.
77. van der Bruggen P, Szikora J-P, Boel P et al, Autologous cytolytic T lymphocytes recognize a MAGE-1 nonapeptide on melanomas expressing HLA-Cw*1601*. *Eur J Immunol* 1994; 24: 2134.
78. Valmori D, Gileadi U, Servis C et al, Modulation of proteasomal activity required for the generation of a cytotoxic T lymphocyte-defined peptide derived from the tumor antigen MAGE-3. *J Exp Med* 1999; 189: 895.
79. Chaux P, Vantomme V, Stroobant V et al, Identification of MAGE-3 epitopes presented by HLA-DR molecules to $CD4^+$ T lymphocytes. *J Exp Med* 1999; 189: 767.
80. Manici S, Sturniolo T, Imro MA, Melanoma cells present a MAGE-3 epitope to $CD4^+$ cytotoxic T cells in association with histocompatibility leukocyte antigen DR11. *J Exp Med* 1999; 189: 871

56

Systemic chemotherapy and biochemotherapy for non-resected and metastatic melanoma

David Khayat, Jean-Baptiste Meric, Olivier Rixe

INTRODUCTION

Although very curable when diagnosed at an early stage, malignant melanoma becomes one of the most aggressive and resistant tumours as soon as the first distant metastasis appears. Indeed, the median survival of patients with systemic disease ranges from 6 to 8 months and <5% of these patients will survive 5 years (Table 56.1).[1] One of the reasons that can explain such a bad prognosis is the relative lack of active treatment that can overcome the natural resistance mechanisms of this tumour. For >30 years, tens of chemotherapeutic agents and biological response modifiers, both alone and in combination, have been tested but very few have yet shown any activity that would significantly alter the classical poor outcome of this disease.

Table 56.1 *Average survival with metastatic melanoma*[1]

	Site alone	Other sites
Skin, soft tissue, distant lymph node	7.2	5.0
Lung	11.4	4.0
Brain	5.0	1.4
Liver	2.4	2.0
Bone	6.0	4.0
Other	2.2	2.0
Widespread	2.4	2.4

CHEMOTHERAPY

Single agents

As shown in Table 56.2, very few agents have shown any significant activity in metastatic malignant melanoma.[1–12] The classic active agent is dacarbazine (DTIC), and it has been the most widely tested single agent since its discovery by Shealy and colleagues in 1970. The main mechanism of action of dacarbazine is based on its alkylating properties. It has been tested on >1800 melanoma patients in various phase II studies, with an overall response rate of 18–20%. Several concerns may be raised regarding these figures. Firstly, most of these studies were performed before the use of the World Health Organization's (WHO) guidelines for evaluation and reporting of responses and toxicities. Many of the responses reported would most probably not reach today's standard of objective response and, indeed, the most recent evaluations of the clinical activity of dacarbazine in advanced malignant melanoma are rather less impressive. Secondly, dacarbazine achieves a relatively low complete response rate, usually <5%, and complete responders are the only candidates for long-term survival or cure. Finally, dacarbazine is mainly active on skin, soft tissue and lymph node metastases, and does not show any significant activity on visceral (i.e. hepatic) or cerebral sites. The median duration of response does not exceed 6 months.

Temozolamide, a new compound which is a precursor of dacarbazine, has recently been evaluated and

Table 56.2 *Single drug activity in metastatic melanoma*

Drug	No. of patients	Overall response (%)
DTIC	1868	20
FTMU	153	24
BCNU	122	18
CCNU	270	13
Met-CCNU	347	16
CDDP	114	15
CBDCA	30	11
TXL	34	15
TXT	43	14
VDS	273	14
VLB	62	13
VCR	52	12
BRS	15	7
	34	3

Drug abbreviations used in Tables 56.2–56.6, 56.9, 56.11, 56.12 and 56.14–56.17

Abbreviation	Drug
AraC	Cytosine-aralinoside
B	Belustine
BCD	Carmustine, cisplatinum and dacarbazine (Dartmouth regimen)
BCDT	Carmustine, cisplatinum, dacarbazine and tamoxifen (Dartmouth regimen)
BCNU	Carmustine
BLM	Bleomycin
BRS	Bryostatin
CBDCA	Carboplatinum
CCNU	Lomustine
CDDP	Cisplatinum
CVD	Cisplatinum, vindesine or vinblastine and dacarbazine
DTIC	Dacarbazine
FTMU	Fotemustine
5FU	Fluorouracil
IL-2	Interleukin-2
INF-α	Interferon-alfa
Met-CCNU	Semustine
RA	Retinoic acid
T	Tamoxifen
TMZ	Temozolamide
TXL	Paclitaxel
TXT	Docetaxel
TZP	Tirazapamine
VCR	Vincristine
VDS	Vindesine
VLB	Vinblastine

compared to dacarbazine in a large randomized study: it did not show any significant improvement in terms of response rate or survival, and only a slight increase in progession-free survival (1.9 versus 1.7 months).

Among the platinum salts, only cisplatinum showed some activity at doses ≥100 mg/m^2; carboplatinum was relatively inactive, as was oxaliplatinum.

The early nitrosoureas carmustine (BCNU) and lomustine (CCNU) have shown response rates of 13–18%. More interestingly, fotemustine (FTMU), a more modern nitrosourea, has repeatedly shown response rates of 20–24%, with a 5–8% complete response rate and a *c.* 20% response rate on cerebral metastases.[8] However, this drug is not yet available in many countries.

All of the other drugs studied are of very limited interest (e.g. vinca alkaloids, taxanes etc.).[13]

Drug combinations

Although it is unlikely that the combination of poorly active drugs will overcome the natural resistance of metastatic melanoma, a number of phase II studies have tested two-, three- and four-drug regimens.[14–22]

Table 56.3 shows some of the most frequently tested combinations. Among them, three have been widely used:

- The combination of carmustine, cisplatinum and dacarbazine, minus or plus tamoxifen (BCD or BCDT, respectively, also called the Darmouth regimen).[15]
- The combination of cisplatinum, vinca alkaloid, either vindesine or vinblastine, and dacarbazine (CVD, also called the MD Anderson regimen).[16]
- The combination of fotemustine, dacarbazine and vindesine (FDV; mostly used in Europe).[18]

However, it is not certain that these combinations are any better than single agents. When compared retrospectively to historical controls, these combinations seem to achieve slightly increased objective response rates, 30–45%, but all the prospective randomized phase III studies aimed at comparing these multidrug

Table 56.3 Drug combinations

Authors (ref.)	Year	Combination*	No. of patients	CR (%)	PR (%)	OR (%)
Young (97)	1974	DTIC/CCNU/VDS/BLM	20	15	30	45
Seigler (98)	1980	DTIC/CCNU/VCR/BLM (BOLD)	72	9	31	40
Mulder (99)	1982	CDDP/VDS	61	3	18	21
Del Prete et al. (14)	1984	CDDP/DTIC/BCNU/T	20	20	35	55
Ringborg (100)	1987	CDDP/DTIC/VDS	40	8	30	38
York (101)	1988	DTIC/CCNU/VCR/BLM	46	11	11	22
Avril (102)	1989	DTIC/FTMU	103	11	27	38
Buzaid (103)	1989	CDDP/DTIC/VLB	52	10	38	48
McClay et al. (15)	1989	CDDP/DTIC/BCNU/T	21	9.5	43	52.5
Comella (104)	1991	VLB/BCNU/CDDP	46	7	21	28
Fletcher (105)	1991	CDDP/DTIC	30	7	30	37
Icli (106)	1991	CDDP/DTIC	20	5	15	20
Murren (107)	1991	CDDP/DTIC	22	14	18	32
Steffens et al. (19)	1991	CDDP/DTIC	30	0	17	17
Olver (108)	1992	CDDP/5FU	29	0	3	3
Richards (109)	1992	CDDP/DTIC/BCNU/T	20	0	55	55
Khayat (110)	1994	DTIC/VDS/FTMU	38	10	34	44
Bedikian (111)	1997	CDDP/TZP	48	0	19	19
Schultz (112)	1997	CDDP/DTIC/BCNU/T	24	13	25	38
Hoffmann (113)	1998	CDDP/DTIC/BCNU/T	69	10	29	39
Margolin (114)	1998	CDDP/DTIC/BCNU/T	69	6	10	16
Richard (115)	1998	CDDP/DTIC/FTMU/T	19	0	10.5	10.5
Seeber (116)	1998	DTIC/FTMU	63	5	6	11
Semb (117)	1998	CDDP/FTMU/T	69	6	16	22.7
Gander (118)	1999	TML/FTMU sequential	24	4	12	16

CR, complete response; PR, partial response; OR, overall response.

regimens to dacarbazine alone have failed to demonstrate any significant response rate and/or overall survival benefit. The last reported study, published in 1999 by Chapman et al.,[23] on 240 patients randomized between dacarbazine alone or the BCDT regimen, showed an equivalent response rate (10 versus 18%) with no difference in overall survival (6.3 versus 7.7 months).[23] Other randomized studies are described in Table 56.4.[21–25]

The role of tamoxifen has been debated for *c.* 10 years, since McClay et al.[26] reported, in 1987, a phase II study where 20 evaluable patients were treated with the BCDT regimen and achieved a 50% response rate. Two years later, the same author published the results of two

Table 56.4 *Randomized studies of dacarbazine (DTIC) versus drug combinations*

Author (ref.)	Year	Combination	No. of patients	OR (%)	OS (months)
Moon (24)	1975	DTIC versus BCNU/VCR	130	24/16 ns	–
Bellet (25)	1976	DTIC versus BCNU/VCR	50	29/23 ns	–
Luikart (22)	1984	DTIC versus CDDP/VDS/BLM	57	14/10 ns	–
Ringborg (21)	1989	DTIC versus DTIC/VDS	119	18/25 ns	4/5.7 ns
Chapman (23)	1999	DTIC versus BCDT	240	10/18 ns	6.3/7.7 ns

OR, overall response; OS, overall survival; ns, not significant.

consecutive non-randomized studies where the first one used the BCD regimen, i.e. minus tamoxifen, and achieved a relatively disappointing 10% response rate on 20 evaluable patients, and the second used the BCDT regimen (i.e. plus tamoxifen) and achieved a remarkable 52% response rate, including a 10% complete response on 21 patients.[15]

Based on these promising results, a large number of investigators looked at the effect of the addition of tamoxifen to a single cytotoxic drug or to drug combinations; the results are shown in Table 56.5.[13,27] Although benefit had not been proved, the addition of tamoxifen to treatment regimens became fashionable in many parts of the world until two large prospective randomized studies clearly showed the lack of benefit of tamoxifen in the treatment of metastatic melanoma. Rusthoven et al.[28] randomized 211 patients either to BCD or to BCDT regimens and found no difference in either the objective response rates or the overall survival. Falkson et al.[29] randomized 271 patients in a study with four arms: dacarbazine versus dacarbazine/interferon-alfa (INF-α) versus dacarbazine/tamoxifen versus dacarbazine/INF-α/tamoxifen. No benefit was found in the addition of tamoxifen to DTIC or to DTIC/INF-α on the response rate, the time-to-treatment failure or overall survival. Three other smaller studies are shown in Table 56.6 and they also seem to indicate that tamoxifen plays no role in the treatment of metastatic melanoma.[31,32] Only one small randomized study has supported the use of tamoxifen in combination with dacarbazine. This study, conducted by Cocconi et al.,[33] included 117 patients who were randomized between dacarbazine alone or in combination with tamoxifen. A difference in favour of the tamoxifen group was observed only in women, i.e. no difference was reported for men. At the time this paper was published, in 1992, an accompanying editorial called for great caution in interpreting these results, as bias could have accounted for the gender difference.

In conclusion, combination chemotherapy does not seem to induce a dramatic improvement in the outcome of patients with metastatic melanoma. If a slight increase in response rate is achieved, then this is most probably relatively limited and may need larger studies to prove it. The second conclusion that can be drawn is that tamoxifen is ineffective and its use should clearly be abandoned.[27] Lastly, one can still observe that the most likely active single agent, fotemustine, has not yet been thoroughly tested in combination therapy and fotemustine-based multidrug regimens may improve upon the results achieved with dacarbazine combinations.

IMMUNOTHERAPY

The concept that immune effectors could be active in metastatic malignant melanoma is based on: the observation of objective spontaneous remissions; the presence of activated lymphocytes in tumoral tissues; and the prognostic value of vitiligo in the outcome of patients with this disease.

Interferon-alfa (INF-α)

Since their description and the demonstration of their activity as an antiviral defence mechanism in the 1970s, the interferons (α, β and γ) have been extensively tested in different pathological conditions. Among the interferon group molecules, INF-α is the most active in clinical practice in cancer patients. Two forms,

Table 56.5 *Phase II studies of tamoxifen-containing combinations*

Author (ref.)	Year	Drugs*	No. of patients	Response rate (%)
McClay (26)	1987	BCDT	20	50
McClay (15)	1989	BCDT	21	52
Thomson (119)	1993	DTIC + T	27	15
McKeage (120)	1993	DTIC + T	14	29
Flaherty (121)	1993	CDDP/DTIC + T	55	18
Schultz (122)	1997	BCDT + INF-α	22	29
Feun (123)	1995	BCDT + INF-α	16	50
Gause (124)	1998	CDDP + CBDCA + T + INF-α	10	20
McClay (125)	2001	CDDP(w) + T (HD)	14	35
O'Neill (126)	1996	CBDT + INF-α	34	27
Nathan (127)	2000	TXL + T	23	22
Margolin (128)	1997	BCDT	79	15
Saba (129)	1993	BCDT	48	37
Lattanzi (130)	1993	BCDT	24	50
Spitler (131)	1994	BCDT	18	44

*w, weekly; HD, high dose.

Table 56.6 *Randomized studies comparing cytotoxic drugs with or without tamoxifen (T)*

Author (ref.)	Year	Drugs*	No. of patients	Response rate −T/+T	*P* value†
Cocconi (33)	1992	DTIC ± T (R)	112	2/28	0.03
Legha (132)	1993	CVD ± T (R)	69	47/30	ns
Agarwala (133)	1999	CBDCA ± T (R)	51	12/21	ns
Bajetta (134)	1995	CBDCA-AraC ± T (R)	46	19/8	ns
Rusthoven (28)	1996	CBD ± T (R)	195	21/30	ns
Chiaron-Sileni (135)	1997	CBD ± T (R)	58	6/22	na

*R, randomized.
†ns, not significant; na, not available.

produced through genetic recombination technologies, which differ by a single amino acid (INF-α2a and INF-α2b), are available. The mechanism of action of INF-α is still not fully understood but it seems that it can slow down the cell cycle by slowing entry into the S phase. It can also stimulate natural killer (NK) cell activity, and the expression and stabilization of the major histocompatibility complex (MHC) antigens, as well as tumour-associated antigens. It can also increase monocyte/macrophage activity.

Several studies have been reported since the mid-1980s and have shown that INF-α can produce an average 15% response rate, including <5% complete response. The median duration of response ranged from 6 to 9 months, with a maximum of 12 months in the best series.[34,35] However, some of these responses have been remarkably durable. There is no widely accepted consensus regarding the optimal dose and schedule. However, the moderate dose of 9–18 MIU (million international units), given as a subcutaneous injection three times per week, is most probably the most popular regimen in metastatic melanoma. Side effects, which include fatigue, malaise, fever, chills, myalgias, headaches, anorexia and a decrease in blood counts, are common, but always reversible and of short duration.[1]

Interleukin-2 (IL-2)

IL-2 is a naturally occurring immunomodulatory cytokine produced by activation of CD4+ T lymphocytes. It can stimulate both the growth and the level of activity of T lymphocytes. It was isolated in 1976 by Gallo and colleagues and cloned in 1983. The molecule used nowadays in metastatic melanoma is produced through recombinant techniques. As far as cytotoxic properties of IL-2 are concerned, several authors have established that IL-2 stimulates human-leucocyte-antigen (HLA)-restricted and HLA-non-restricted cytotoxic T cell populations, and induces the production of a cascade of other cytokines such as tumour necrosis factor (TNF), INF-γ or IL-1.[36]

The first report of clinical activity of IL-2 in metastatic melanoma was by Rosenberg et al.[37] who, at the National Cancer Institute (NCI), initiated the concept that the combination of the transplantation of ex vivo IL-2 autologous lymphocyte-activated killer (LAK) cells and recombinant high-dose intravenous (IV) IL-2 may be an efficient way to use, in the clinical setting, the potential antitumour properties of IL-2. In 1985, he achieved a 15% response rate, which has been confirmed by several authors. The toxicity reported using high-dose bolus IV injections was quite significant, including cardiovascular, renal, pulmonary, neurologic and haematologic acute side effects, usually rapidly reversible upon cessation of the treatment but which may be associated with a 1–2% mortality rate (mainly due to myocardial infarction or sepsis). In 1987, West et al.[38] reported another regimen where IL-2 was given as a continuous IV infusion. The doses were smaller and the toxicity, although identical in nature, was considerably less intense and frequent. Other toxic side effects, related to chronic administration, include (as for INF) fatigue, myalgia, fever, chills, anorexia and endocrine effects or vitiligo, and have been seen using both IV and continuous infusion regimens.[1] The question of the clinical utility of combining LAK cells with IL-2 has been subject to debate, but the numerous randomized[39–43] and non-randomized[26,44–54] studies recently reported have clarified this point (Tables 56.7–56.9), and demonstrated that LAK cells do not add any benefit to IL-2 alone. Another way to combine IL-2 to conditioned cells is based on the use of ex vivo IL-2-activated tumour-infiltrating lymphocytes (TIL). Administered together, or with cyclophosphamide, TIL and IL-2 have produced reproducible responses in metastatic melanoma (Table 56.10). However, the necessity of combining IL-2 and TIL remains to be demonstrated and prospective randomized trials are awaited.

In conclusion, IL-2 alone, or combined with autologous activated lymphocyte, is active in metastatic melanoma, with response rates in the range of those achieved with chemotherapy. However, a trend towards an increase in the complete response rate and the repeated observation of long-lasting, unmaintained remissions, as well as the lack of cross-resistance with cytotoxic drugs, tend to favour this approach.

Attempts have been made, as with cytotoxic drugs, to combine IL-2 and INF-α. The rationale was based on the idea that INF-α could increase the recognition and the destruction of tumour cells by IL-2-activated lymphocytes through its induction of MHC and tumour-associated membrane antigens.[55] Several studies have been reported but all failed to demonstrate any clinical relevance of this theoretical concept.[56,57]

BIOCHEMOTHERAPY

Biochemotherapy is the combined use of cytotoxic drug(s) and one or several biological response modifiers such as IL-2 and INF-α. Preclinical data suggest that a synergy may exist between these two different classes of molecules. Several hypotheses have been raised based on these preclinical experiments[58–62] but the true relevance of these concepts is still controversial:

Table 56.7 *Non-randomized studies of interleukin-2 (IL-2)/lymphocyte-activated killer (LAK) cell combinations*

Author (ref.)	Year	IL-2*	No. of patients	Complete response (%)	Overall response (%)
Rosenberg (37)	1987	BIV	48	8	21
Dutcher (44)	1989	BIV	36	3	17
West (45)	1989	CIV + BIV	22	0	36
Gaynor (46)	1989	CIV	30	0	3
Bar (47)	1990	BIV + CIV	50	2	14
Richards (39)	1990	CIV	35	0	6
Parkinson (48)	1990	BIV	46	4	22
Dillman (49)	1991	CIV	33	6	12
Dutcher (50)	1991	CIV	33	3	7
McCabe (40)	1991	BIV	49	6	12
Rosenberg (41)	1993	BIV	28	11	22

*BIV, bolus intravenous; CIV, continuous intravenous.

Table 56.8 *Non-randomized studies of interleukin-2 (IL-2) alone*

Author (ref.)	Year	IL-2*	No. of patients	CR (%)	OR (%)	MDR (months)	OS (months)
Rosenberg (37)	1987	BIV	42	0	24	10	–
Thatcher (51)	1989	BIV	31	0	13	–	–
Parkinson (48)	1990	BIV	46	4	22	8	–
Richards (39)	1990	CIV	33	0	9	4	–
Dorval (52)	1991	CIV	37	3	22	4	–
Perez (53)	1991	CIV	17	0	6	4	–
Whitehead (54)	1991	BIV	42	0	10	–	8
McCabe (40)	1991	BIV	45	4	16	5	–
Koretz (42)	1991	CIV	9	0	0	–	–
Rosenberg (41)	1993	BIV	26	0	23	8	–
Sparano (43)	1993	BIV	44	0	5	11	10

*BIV, bolus intravenous; CIV continuous intravenous.
CR, complete response; OR, overall response; MDR, median response rate; OS, overall survival.

- The sensitivity to immunotherapy may be increased by the cytoreduction achieved with cytotoxic drugs.
- Chemotherapy may increase the immunogenicity of tumour cells through its effects on cell membranes.
- Chemotherapy may induce the stabilization of antigenic targets on membrane cells and therefore stimulate an IL-2-mediated immune response.
- Chemotherapy may have direct immunomodulatory

Table 56.9 Randomized studies comparing interleukin-2 (IL-2) and IL-2/lymphocyte-activated killer (LAK) combinations

Author (ref.)	Year	Regimen*	No. of patients	Overall response (%)	Survival (2 years)
Richards (39)	1990	IL2 (CIV) IL2/LAK	33 35	9 6	– –
Koretz (42)	1991	IL2 (CIV) IL2/LAK	9 10	0 0	– –
McCabe (40)	1991	IL2 (BIV) IL2/LAK	45 49	16 12	– –
Rosenberg (41)	1993	IL2 (BIV) IL2/LAK	26 28	27 28	15 32 (*P*=0.064)

BIV, bolus intravenous; CIV, continuous intravenous.

Table 56.10 Studies using interleukin-2 (IL-2) combined with tumour-infiltrating lymphocytes (TIL) in the treatment of malignant melanoma

Author (ref.)	Evaluable patients		RR (%)	IL-2 administration*
	CR	PR		
Rosenberg (136)	1/20	10/0	55	BIV
Hanson (13)	0/6	2/6	33	BIV
Topalian (13)	0/6	1/6	17	BIV
Dillman (137)	1/21	4/21	24	CIV
West (13)	0/13	3/13	23	CIV
Kradin (138)	0/13	3/13	23	CIV

CR, complete response; PR, partial response; RR, response rate.
* BIV, bolus intravenous; CIV, continuous intravenous.

effects, i.e. decreasing T lymphocyte suppressor activity or activating NK cells.

- Immunotherapy may alter the pharmacokinetic profile of cytotoxic drugs such as temozolamide through increased capillary permeability and metabolic modifications.
- The secondary cytokine cascade activated by IL-2 may increase the cytotoxic activity of anticancer drugs such as cisplatinum.

It has been shown, for instance, that biotherapy can stimulate the production of nitric oxides by monocytes or, maybe more importantly, by endothelial cells, which may ultimately lead to direct cytotoxic effects in addition to chemotherapy.[62] It can also, through the production of reactive oxygen metabolites by TIL, affect the capacity of tumour cells to repair cisplatinum-induced DNA damage.

Combination of interferon-alfa (INF-α) and cytotoxic drugs

Several cytotoxic drugs have been combined with INF-α in phase II and III trials on metastatic melanoma patients. Among them, dacarbazine is the most frequently tested drug combined with INF-α either as a single agent or combined with one or several other drugs (Table 56.11). Although promising when reported from single arm non-randomized studies, the results achieved in large multicentre randomized phase

Table 56.11 Studies combining interferon-alfa (INF-α) to cytotoxic drugs

Author (ref.)	Year	Drug	No. of patients	Response rate (%)
Richner (139)	1990	CDDP + INF-α	15	20
Margolin (64)	1992	CDDP + INF-α	42	24
Stark (140)	1993	CDDP/B/DTIC + INF-α	34	35
Bajetta (32)	1990	DTIC + INF-α	75	25
Breier (13)	1990	DTIC + INF-α	17	52
Michiewicz (13)	1990	DTIC + INF-α	37	29
Mulder (141)	1991	DTIC + INF-α	12	66
Daponte (142)	1996	DF + INF-α	43	40
Bruno (13)	1996	DTIC + INF-α	24	54
Meyskens (143)	1997	RA + INF-α	52	10
Kirkwood (144)	1997	TMZ + INF-α	12	25

III studies do not show any significant advantage (Table 56.12). Among the four phase III studies, only one, that by Falkson et al.,[30] showed a statistically significant benefit in favour of the combination of dacarbazine with high-dose INF-α over dacarbazine alone. The difference was observed in terms of complete response, overall response, median duration of response and median survival. These results were achieved in a study which included only 30 patients in each arm. Moreover, the other randomized studies did not confirm these results,[31,32] including a later study from the same authors.[29]

Several studies have tested the combination of cisplatinum and INF-α. Five of them, reported in patient samples of 14–42, did not show results exceeding 26%; therefore, not suggesting any advantage compared to cisplatinum or INF-α alone (Table 56.13).[13,63–66]

Other drugs have also been tested in combination with INF-α, e.g. temozolamide and retinoic acid, but results have not been impressive.[13]

Combination of interleukin-2 (IL-2) and cytotoxic drugs

Cyclophosphamide was combined with IL-2 in 88 patients, with an average response rate of 15%.[67,68] Dacarbazine was also combined with IL-2 in several phase II studies.[69,70] Different doses and schedules of both compounds were tested with or without LAK cells. Response rates ranged from 0 to 33%, with a median survival of *c.* 6–8 months, i.e. not apparently any better than the results achieved with either drug alone.

Cisplatinum/interleukin-2 (IL-2)-based biochemotherapy

In 1991, three independent phase II studies using a cisplatinum (CDDP)/IL-2-based chemotherapeutic regimen were reported.[71–73] All used a high-dose bolus schedule of IL-2 and one study added INF-α to IL-2. All used the administration of CDDP, although two of them combined it with dacarbazine. The three studies reported objective response rates ranging from 37 to 82%, including complete response rates ranging from 11 to 25%. At the same time, several investigators were testing similar CDDP/IL-2-based biochemotherapeutic regimens. This group's experience is based on three consecutive trials.[74] A total of 129 evaluable patients were treated. In the first trial, CDDP was administered at a dose of 100 mg/m^2 on day 0 of each cycle, and immunotherapy consisted of a continuous infusion of IL-2 from days 3 to 6 and days 17–21 at a dose of 18 MIU/m^2/day, and subcutaneous injections of INF-α at a dose of 9 MIU/three times per week throughout

Table 56.12 *Dacarbazine (DTIC) plus interferon-alfa (INF-α) versus DTIC alone*

Author (ref.)	Year	Regimen*	No. of patients	CR (%)	OR (%)	MDR (months)	OS (months)
Falkson (30)	1991	DTIC/IFN-α (HD)	30	40†	53†	8.9†	17.5†
		DTIC	30	7	20	2.5	9.5
Thompson (31)	1992	DTIC/IFN-α (LD)	87	7	23	8.6	7.6
		DTIC	86	2	17	9.5	8.9
Bajetta (32)	1994	DTIC/IFN-α (HD)	76	8	28	8.4	13.0
		DTIC/IFN-α (LD)	84	7	23	5.5	11.0
		DTIC	82	5	20	2.6	11.0
Falkson (29)	1998	DTIC/IFN-α (HD)	68	6	21	2.9	9.3
		DTIC	69	2	15	2.3	10.0
		DTIC/T	66	2	18	1.8	8.0
		DTIC/T/IFN-α (HD)	68	3	19	2.6	9.5

CR, complete response; OR, overall response; MDR, median duration of response; OS, overall survival.
*HD, high dose; LD, low dose.
†Statistically significant.

Table 56.13 *Phase II studies of cisplatinum (CDDP) and interferon-alfa (INF-α) combinations*

Author (ref.)	Year	No. of patients	CR (%)	OR (%)
Richner (63)	1992	15	7	26
Oratz (65)	1987	15	7	7
Schuchter (66)	1992	14	0	14
Margolin (64)	1992	42	7	24

CR, complete response; OR, objective response.

the cycle. Cycles were repeated every 28 days for two cycles; 94 patients were included. A lower dose maintenance treatment was given to patients who responded and showed good tolerance (39 patients). The initial study was modified for the addition of high-dose tamoxifen (160 mg/day) from day −5 to day +5; 24 patients were included. In the third study, cycles were shortened to 3 weeks, only one period of IL-2 was scheduled (days 3–7), and CDDP and INF-α were given at day 0 and throughout the cycle, respectively; 12 patients were included. Eighty per cent of these patients were heavily pretreated (Table 56.14) and 70% had two or more metastatic sites, including 58 versus 42% of visceral versus non-visceral metastases.

The overall response rates were very consistent from one study to another (48, 54 and 46%), including an

Table 56.14 *Patient characteristics*

Characteristics	No. of patients
Male/female	78/51
Median age, years (range)	44 (18–69)
ECOG* performance status	
0	78 (60%)
1	27 (21%)
2	24 (19%)
Prior treatment	
Chemotherapy	95 (80%)
Adjuvant	40 (42%)
Metastatic	55 (58%)
Drugs	
DTIC and/or FTMU	72 (76%)
CDDP	23 (34%)
IFN-α	47 (45%)
No treatment	23 (20%)

*ECOG, Eastern Cooperative Oncology Group.

8–10% complete response rate (Table 56.15). Interestingly, nine patients (7%) were noted to have long-lasting unmaintained remission. Median survival was 11 months; the median survival was 17 months for responders versus 7 months for non-responders. Among responders, those achieving a complete response had both a significant survival and disease-free survival advantage compared with patients who achieved a partial response.[13] Interestingly, the presence of visceral versus non-visceral metastases and

Table 56.15 Response rates (RR)

	PI2	PI2 + T	PI2/3w	Total
PR	34 (37%)	11 (46%)	4 (36%)	49 (39%)
CR	10 (11%)	2 (8%)	1 (10%)	13 (10%)
RR	44 (48%)	13 (54%)	5 (46%)	62 (49%)

PR, partial response; CR, complete response; OR, overall response; w, weekly.

pretreatment status were not significantly correlated with either response or survival. The occurrence of vitiligo, but not of thyroid dysfunction (which may be another autoimmune-induced disorder), was found to be significantly correlated to response, disease-free survival and survival. The toxicity was very similar to that observed with doses of IL-2 and INF-α alone, and only the addition of tamoxifen suggested induction of a more important haematotoxicity.

More than 10 other studies using this CDDP/IL-2-based regimen have been reported (Table 56.16), using bolus IV or continuous IL-2 infusions. Doses, schedules, number and type of cytotoxic drugs, as well as the addition of INF-α, were very variable.[71–87]

Two studies in addition to these used CDDP as the sole cytotoxic agent. One randomized study looked at the role of INF-α (CDDP/IL-2/INF-α versus CDDP/IL-2) and found no benefit for the addition of INF-α (response rate of 26 versus 17%; median duration of response similar at 11 months).[75] Another study looked at the last sequence between cytotoxic drugs and immunotherapy, and found that the best results were achieved when the CDDP-containing chemotherapy regimen preceded immunotherapy, or was given concurrently.[80]

Another group of studies looked at the use of lower dose subcutaneous IL-2 (Table 56.17),[88–95] with results that look slightly lower than those achieved with higher dose IV IL-2.

Table 56.16 Studies of cisplatinum (CDDP)- and interleukin-2 (IL-2)-based biochemotherapy combinations

Author (ref.)	Year	Regimen	No. of patients	CR (%)	PR (%)	OR (%)
Blair (72)	1991	CDDP/DTIC/IL-2	28	18	25	43
Demchak (71)	1991	CDDP/IL-2	27	11	26	37
Hamblin (73)	1991	CDDP/DTIC/IL-2/INF-α	12	25	58	83
Richards (76)	1992	BCD ± T/IL-2/INF-α	74	15	40	55
Flaherty (78)	1993	CDDP/DTIC/IL-2	32	16	26	41
Atkins (82)	1994	CDDP/DTIC/T/IL-2	38	8	34	42
Dorval (75)	1994	CDDP/IL-2 ± INF-α	101	3 2	5 11	16 24
Khayat (74)	1997	CDDP/IL-2/INF-α	127	10	39	49
Rosenberg (83)	1999	CDDP/DTIC/T ± IL-2/INF-α	102	4 3	10 19	27 44
Keilhotz (84)	1999	DTIC/CDDP/INF-α ± IL-2	118	5 5	23 17	28 22
Legha (85)	1998	CDDP/VLB/DTIC/INF-α/IL-2	53	21	43	64
Richards (86)	1999	CDDP/DTIC/BCNU/IL-2/INF-α	83	14	31	55
Proebstle (87)	1998	CDDP/DTIC/INF-α/IL-2	42	0	24	24
O'Day (90)	1999	CVD/IL2/INF-α	35	20	37	57

CR, complete response; PR, partial response; OR, overall response.
IL-2 administered intravenously.

Table 56.17 Cisplatinum (CDDP)-based biochemotherapy with subcutaneous interleukin-2 (IL-2)

Author (ref.)	Year	Regimen	No. of patients	CR (%)	PR (%)	OR (%)
Atzpodien (77)	1995	DTIC/CBDCA IL-2/INF-α	40	7.5	27.5	35
Atzpodien (77)	1995	BCDT IL-2/INF-α	27	11	44	55
Bernengo (88)	1996	CDDP/T IL-2/INF-α	36	14	33	47.2
Dreno (89)	1996	CDDP IL-2/INF	38	5.2	32.1	37.3
Dillman (95)	1999	CDDP/DTIC/BCNU/INF-α/IL-2	30	10	24	34
Andres (92)	1998	CDDP/INF-α/IL-2	33	10	20	30
Kamanabrou (94)	1999	CDDP/DTIC/BCNU/INF-α/IL-2	109	11	27.5	38.5
McDermott (93)	1997	CVD/IL-2/INF-α	21	0	43	43
Thompson (91)	1997	BCD ± T/IL-2/INF-α	53	19	23	42
Honeycut (145)	1998	BCD ± T/IL-2/INF-α	19	5	21	26

CR, complete response; PR, partial response; OR, overall response.

The question of the real benefit of CDDP-based biochemotherapy compared to biotherapy alone is the matter of an interesting, although as yet unanswered, debate. A study conducted by the European Organization for Research and Treatment of Cancer (EORTC),[84] compared a combination of IL-2/INF-α with or without CDDP. In this study, the addition of CDDP doubled the response rate from 18 to 35%. The progression-free survival was also increased (53 versus 92 days), but overall survival was similar. A meta-analysis of 15 phase II–III trials performed between 1988 and 1995, comprising 522 patients, was recently reported.[96] The response rates ranged from 33% in the IL-2/INF-α/chemotherapy group to 9% in the IL-2-only group. A difference was seen in survival between the IL-2 ± INF-α group (7.5 months) and the IL-2/chemotherapy ± INF-α group (10.1 months), suggesting a benefit for biochemotherapy.

The only available information that seems to indicate a lack of benefit for biochemotherapy comes from a recently randomized study where CDDP/dacarbazine/tamoxifen was compared to the same regimen combined with IL-2 and INF-α.[83] No statistical difference was observed either in response rates or in survival parameters; however, this study may be biased for several reasons. Firstly, the study was designed to accrue 67 patients in each arm with a primary end point based on response rates (80% power to identify a 25% improvement in response rates with a 0.05 alpha level). The study included only 50 and 52 patients instead of the 67 scheduled in each arm. The study, which was prematurely interrupted, seemed to be shorter at an interim analysis, although this difference never reached statistical significance. Finally, patients randomized to biochemotherapy received less than half the IL-2 theoretical dose in 30% of cases. Therefore, this study cannot exclude the hypothesis that biochemotherapy does better than chemotherapy or immunotherapy alone.

Large randomized, well-designed phase III studies are still needed before any conclusions can be drawn. In the meantime, despite the long-term unmaintained remissions achieved with biochemotherapy, 90–95% of patients with metastatic melanoma do not survive >3 years.

REFERENCES

1. Balch CM, Houghton AN, Peters LJ, Cutaneous melanoma. In: *Cancer: principles and practice of oncology* (eds De Vita VT, Hellman S, Rosenberg SA). Philadelphia: JB Lippincott, 1993: 1612–61.
2. Middleton MR, Gore M, Tilgen W et al, A randomized phase III study of temozolomide (TMZ) versus dacarbazine (DTIC) in the treatment of patients with advanced metastatic melanoma. *Proc ASCO* 1999; 2069 (abstract).

3. Hill GJ, Krementz ET, Hill HZ, Dimethyl triazeno imidazole carboxamide and combination therapy for melanoma stage IV. Late results after complete response to chemotherapy. *Cancer* 1984; 53: 1299–305.
4. Al-Sarraf M, Fletcher W, Oishi N et al, Cisplatin hydratation with and without mannitol diuresis in refractory disseminated malignant melanoma: a South-West Oncology Group Study. *Cancer Treat Rep* 1982; 66: 31–3.
5. Schilcher RB, Wessens M, Niderle M et al, Phase II evaluation of fractionated low and single high-dose cisplatinum in various tumors. *J Cancer Res Clin Oncol* 1984; 107: 57–60.
6. Song SY, Chary KK, Higby DJ et al, Cisdiamminedichloride platinum(II) in the treatment of metastatic malignant melanoma. *Clin Res* 1977; 25: 411.
7. Jacquillat C, Khayat D, Banzet P et al, Final report on a French multicenter phase II study of the nitrosourea fotemustine in 153 evaluable patients with disseminated malignant melanoma including patients with cerebral metastases. *Cancer* 1990; 66: 1873–8.
8. Khayat D, Avril MF, Auclerc G et al, Clinical value of the nitrosourea fotemustine in disseminated malignant melanoma: overview on 1022 patients including 144 patients with cerebral metastases. *Proc ASCO* 1993; 12: 1343.
9. Retsas S, Peat E, Ashford R et al, Updated results of vindesine as a single agent in the therapy of advanced malignant melanoma. *J Cancer Clin Oncol* 1982; 18: 1293–5.
10. Rowinsky EK, McGuire WP, Taxol: present status and future prospects. *Contemp Oncol* 1991; 29–36.
11. Aamdal S, Wolff I, Kaplan S et al, Docetaxel (Taxotere) in advanced malignant melanoma: a phase II study of the EORTC Early Clinical Trials Group. *Eur J Cancer* 1994; 8: 1061–4.
12. Bedikian A, Legha S, Genkins J et al, Phase II trial of docetaxel in patients (pts) with advanced melanoma previously untreated with chemotherapy. *Proc ASCO* 1995; 14: 1304.
13. Khayat D, Coeffic D, Antoine EC, Overview on medical treatments of metastatic malignant melanoma. In: (ed). American Society of Clinical Oncology, 2000: 414–27.
14. Del Prete SA, Maurer LH, O'Donnel J et al, Combination chemotherapy with cisplatinum, carmustine, dacarbazine and tamoxifen in metastatic melanoma. *Cancer Treat Rep* 1984; 68: 1403–5.
15. McClay EF, Mastrangelo MJ, Sprandio JD et al, The importance of tamoxifen to a cisplatinum-containing regimen in the treatment of metastatic melanoma. *Cancer* 1989; 63: 1292–5.
16. Buzaid AC, Legha S, Winn R et al, Cisplatin, vinblastine and dacarbazine alone in metastatic melanoma: preliminary results of a phase III Cancer Community Oncology Program (CCOP) trial. *Proc ASCO* 1993; 12: 1328.
17. Avril MF, Bonneterre J, Cupissol D et al, Fotemustine plus dacarbazine for malignant melanoma. *Eur J Cancer* 1992; 11: 1807–11.
18. Khayat D, Borel C, Benhammouda A et al, Active three drugs (fotemustine, dacarbazine and vindesine) outpatient combination in advanced malignant melanoma. *Proc ASCO* 1992; 33: 1336.
19. Steffens T, Bajorin DF, Chapman PB et al, A phase II trial of high-dose cisplatinum and dacarbazine. *Cancer* 1991; 68: 1230–7.
20. Carey RW, Anderson JR, Green M et al, Treatment of metastatic malignant melanoma with vinblastine, dacarbazine, and cisplatinum: a report from the Cancer and Leukemia Group B. *Cancer Treat Rep* 1986; 70: 329–31.
21. Ringborg U, Rudenstam CM, Hansson J et al, Dacarbazine versus dacarbazine–vindesine in disseminated malignant melanoma: a randomized phase II study. *Med Oncol Tumor Pharmacother* 1989; 6: 285–9.
22. Luikart SD, Kennealey GT, Kirkwood JM, Randomized phase III trial of vinblastine, bleomycin, and cisdichlorodiammine-platinum versus dacarbazine in malignant melanoma. *J Clin Oncol* 1984; 2: 164–8.
23. Chapman PB, Einhorn LH, Meyers ML et al, Phase III multicenter randomized trial of the Dartmouth regimen versus dacarbazine in patients with metastatic melanoma. *J Clin Oncol* 1999; 7: 2745–51.
24. Moon JH, Gailani S, Cooper MR et al, Comparison of the combination of 1,3-bis(2-chloroethyl)-1-nitrosourea (BCNU) and vincristine with two dose schedules of 5-(3,3-dimethyl-1-triazino) imidazole 4-carboxamide (DTIC) in the treatment of disseminated malignant melanoma. *Cancer* 1975; 35: 368–71.
25. Bellet RE, Mastrangelo MJ, Laucius JF et al, Randomized prospective trial to DTIC (NSC-45388) alone versus BCNU (NSC-409962) plus vincristine (NSC-67574) in the treatment of metastatic malignant melanoma. *Cancer Treat Rep* 1976; 60: 595–600.
26. McClay EF, Mastrangelo MJ, Bellet RE, Berd D, Combination chemotherapy and hormonal therapy in the treatment of malignant melanoma. *Cancer Treat Rep* 1987; 71: 465–9.
27. Rusthoven JJ, The evidence for tamoxifen and chemotherapy as treatment for metastatic melanoma. *Eur J Cancer* 1998; 34 (Suppl 3): S31–S36.
28. Rusthoven JJ, Quirt IC, Iscoe NA et al, Randomized, double-blind, placebo-controlled trial comparing the response rates of carmustine, dacarbazine, and cisplatinum with and without tamoxifen in patients with metastatic melanoma. National Cancer Institute of Canada Trials Group. *J Clin Oncol* 1996; 14: 2083–90.
29. Falkson CI, Ibrahim J, Kirkwood JM et al, Phase III trial of dacarbazine versus dacarbazine with alpha-interferon-2b versus dacarbazine with tamoxifen versus dacarbazine with alpha-interferon-2b and tamoxifen in patients with metastatic melanoma: an Eastern Cooperative Oncology Group study. *J Clin Oncol* 1998; 16: 1743–51.
30. Falkson CI, Falkson G, Falkson HC, Improved results with the addition of interferon alfa-2b to dacarbazine in the treatment of patients with metastatic malignant melanoma. *J Clin Oncol* 1991; 9: 1403–8.
31. Thompson DB, Adena M, McLeod GRC et al, Alpha-interferon does not improve response or survival when added to dacarbazine in metastatic melanoma: results of a multiinstitutional Australian randomised tiral QMP8704. *Proc ASCO* 1992; 11: 1177.
32. Bajetta E, Di Leo A, Zampino MG et al, Multicenter randomized trial of dacarbazine alone or in combination with two different doses and schedules of interferon alfa-2a in the treatment of advanced melanoma. *J Clin Oncol* 1994; 12: 806–11.
33. Cocconi G, Bella M, Calabresi F et al, Treatment of metastatic malignant melanoma with dacarbazine plus tamoxifen. *N Engl J Med* 1992; 327: 516–23.
34. Kirkwood JM, Studies of interferons in the therapy of melanoma. *Semin Oncol* 1991; 18: 83–9.
35. Legha S, Current therapy for melanoma. *Semin Oncol* 1989; 16:34–44.
36. Lindemann A, Brossart P, Hoffken K et al, Immunomodulatory effects of ultra-dose interleukin-2 in cancer patients: a phase IB study. *Cancer Immunol Immunother* 1993; 37: 307–15.
37. Rosenberg SA, Lotze MT, Muul LM et al, A progress report on the treatment of 157 patients with advanced cancer using lymphokine-activated killer cells and interleukin-2 or high-dose interleukin-2 alone. *N Engl J Med* 1987; 16: 889–97.
38. West WH, Tauer KW, Yannelli JR et al, Constant-infusion recombinant interleukin-2 in adoptive immunotherapy of advanced cancer. *N Engl J Med* 1987; 15: 898–905.
39. Richards JM, Bajorin DF, Vogelzang N et al, Treatment of metastatic melanoma with continuous intravenous IL2 +/- LAK cells: a randomized trial. *Proc ASCO* 1990; 9: 1080.
40. McCabe MS, Stablein D, Hawkins MJ, The modified group C experience – phase III randomized trials of interleukin-2 vs interleukin-2/LAK in advanced renal cell carcinoma and advanced melanoma. *Proc ASCO* 1991; 10: 714.
41. Rosenberg SA, Lotze MT, Yang JC et al, Prospective randomized trial of high-dose interleukin-2 alone or in conjunction with lymphokine-activated killer cells for the treatment of patients with advanced cancer. *J Natl Cancer Inst* 1993; 85: 622–32.
42. Koretz MJ, Lawson DH, York RM et al, Randomized study of interleukin-2 versus interleukin-2-LAK for treatment of melanoma and renal cell cancer. *Arch Surg* 1991; 126: 898–903.
43. Sparano JA, Fisher RI, Sunderland M et al, Randomized phase III trial of treatment with high-dose interleukin-2 either alone or in combination with interferon alfa-2a in patients with advanced melanoma. *J Clin Oncol* 1993; 11: 1969–77.
44. Dutcher JP, Creekmore S, Weiss GR et al, A phase II study of interleukin-2 and lymphokine-activated killer cells in patients with metastatic malignant melanoma. *J Clin Oncol* 1989; 7: 477–85.
45. West WH, Clinical application of continuous infusion of recombinant interleukin-2. *Eur J Cancer Clin Oncol* 1989; 25 (Suppl 3): S11–S15.
46. Gaynor ER, Weiss GR, Margolin KA et al, Phase I study of high-dose continuous-infusion recombinant interleukin-2 and autologous

lymphokine-activated killer cells in patients with metastatic or unresectable malignant melanoma and renal cell carcinoma. *J Natl Cancer Inst* 1990; 82: 1397–402.
47. Bar MH, Sznol M, Atkins MB et al, Metastatic malignant melanoma treated with combined bolus and continuous infusion interleukin-2 and lymphokine-activated killer cells. *J Clin Oncol* 1990; 8: 1138–47.
48. Parkinson DR, Abrams JS, Wiernik PH et al, Interleukin-2 therapy in patients with metastatic malignant melanoma: a phase II study. *J Clin Oncol* 1990; 8: 1650–6.
49. Dillman RO, Oldham RK, Tauer KW et al, Continuous interleukin-2 and lymphokine-activated killer cells for advanced cancer: a National Biotherapy Study Group trial. *J Clin Oncol* 1991; 9: 1233–40.
50. Dutcher JP, Gaynor ER, Boldt DH et al, A phase II study of high-dose continuous infusion interleukin-2 with lymphokine-activated killer cells in patients with metastatic melanoma. *J Clin Oncol* 1991; 9: 641–8.
51. Thatcher N, Dazzi H, Johnson RJ et al, Recombinant interleukin-2 (rIL-2) given intrasplenically and intravenously for advanced malignant melanoma. A phase I and II study. *Br J Cancer* 1989; 60: 770–4.
52. Dorval T, Mathiot C, Brandely M et al, Lack of effect of tumour infiltrating lymphocytes in patients with metastatic melanoma who failed to respond to interleukin 2. *Eur J Cancer* 1991; 27: S99.
53. Perez EA, Scudder SA, Meyers FA et al, Weekly 24-hour continuous infusion interleukin-2 for metastatic melanoma and renal cell carcinoma: a phase I study. *J Immunother* 1991; 10: 57–62.
54. Whitehead RP, Kopecky KJ, Samson MK et al, Phase II study of intravenous bolus recombinant interleukin-2 in advanced malignant melanoma: Southwest Oncology Group study. *J Natl Cancer Inst* 1991; 83: 1250–2.
55. Brunda MJ, Bellantoni D, Sulich V, In vivo anti-tumor activity of combinations of alpha-interferon and interleukin-2 in a murine model. Correlation of efficacy with the induction of cytotoxic cells resembling natural killer cells. *Int J Cancer* 1989; 40: 365–71.
56. Whitehead RP, Figlin R, Citron ML et al, A phase II trial of concomitant human interleukin-2 and interferon-alpha-2a in patients with disseminated malignant melanoma. *J Immunother* 1993; 13: 117–21.
57. Rosenberg SA, Lotze MT, Yang JC et al, Combination therapy with interleukin-2 and alpha-interferon for the treatment of patients with advanced cancer. *J Clin Oncol* 1989; 7: 1863–74.
58. Cameron RB, Spiess PJ, Rosenberg SA, Synergistic antitumor activity of tumor-infiltrating lymphocytes, interleukin 2, and local tumor irradiation. Studies on the mechanism of action. *J Exp Med* 1990; 171: 249–63.
59. Ehrke MJ, Mihich E, Berd D, Mastrangelo MJ, Effects of anticancer drugs on the immune system in humans. *Semin Oncol* 1989; 16: 230–53.
60. Berd D, Maguire Jr HC, Mastrangelo MJ, Potentiation of human cell-mediated and humoral immunity by low-dose cyclophosphamide. *Cancer Res* 1984; 44: 5439–43.
61. Chabot GG, Flaherty LE, Valdivieso M et al, Alteration of dacarbazine pharmacokinetics after interleukin-2 administration in melanoma patients. *Cancer Chemother Pharmacol* 1990; 27: 157–60.
62. Buzaid AC, Anderson CM, Ali Osman F et al, Biochemotherapy in the treatment of advanced melanoma: clinical results and potential mechanisms of anti cancer activity. *Prog Anti-cancer Treat* 1997; 68–87.
63. Richner J, Joss RA, Goldhirsch A, Brunner KW, Phase II study of continuous subcutaneous interferon-alfa combined with cisplatinum in advanced malignant melanoma. *Eur J Cancer* 1992; 28: 1044–7.
64. Margolin KA, Doroshow JH, Akman SA et al, Phase II trial of cisplatinum and alpha-interferon in advanced malignant melanoma. *J Clin Oncol* 1992; 10: 1574–8.
65. Oratz R, Speyer JL, Green M et al, Treatment of metastatic malignant melanoma with dacarbazine and cisplatin. *Cancer Treat Rep* 1987; 71: 877–8.
66. Schuchter LM, Wohlganger J, Fishman EK et al, Sequential chemotherapy and immunotherapy for the treatment of metastatic melanoma. *J Immunother* 1992; 12: 272–6.
67. Mitchell MS, Kempf RA, Harel W et al, Effectiveness and tolerability of low-dose cyclophosphamide and low-dose intravenous interleukin-2 in disseminated melanoma. *J Clin Oncol* 1988; 6: 409–24.
68. Mitchell MS, Principles of combining biomodulators with cytotoxic agents in vivo. *Semin Oncol* 1992; 19: 51–6.
69. Papadopoulos NEJ, Howard JG, Murray JL et al, Phase II DTIC and interleukin-2 trial for metastatic malignant melanoma. *Proc ASCO* 1990; 277: 1072a (abstract).
70. Dillman RO, Oldham RK, Barth NM, Recombinant interleukin-2 and adoptive immunotherapy alternated with dacarbazine therapy in melanoma: a National Biotherapy Study Group trial. *J Natl Cancer Inst* 1990; 82: 1345–9.
71. Demchak PA, Mier JW, Robert NJ et al, Interleukin-2 and high-dose cisplatinum in patients with metastatic melanoma: a pilot study. *J Clin Oncol* 1991; 9: 1821–30.
72. Blair S, Flaherty L, Valdiviaso M et al, Comparison of high dose interleukin-2 with combined chemotherapy low-dose IL2 in metastatic malignant melanoma. *Proc ASCO* 1991; 10: 1031.
73. Hamblin TJ, Davies B, Sadullah S et al, A phase II study of the treatment of metastatic malignant melanoma with a combination of dacarbazine, cisplatinum, interleukin-2 and alpha-interferon. *Proc ASCO* 1991; 10: 1029.
74. Antoine EC, Benhammouda A, Bernard A et al, Salpetriere Hospital experience with biochemotherapy in metastatic melanoma. *Cancer J Sci Am* 1997; 3: S16–S21.
75. Dorval T, Négrier S, Chevreau C et al, Results of a French multicentric randomized trial of chemoimmunotherapy with or without interferon in metastatic malignant melanoma. *Proc ASCO* 1994; 13: 1347.
76. Richards JM, Mehta N, Ramming K et al, Sequential chemoimmunotherapy in the treatment of metastatic melanoma. *J Clin Oncol* 1992; 10: 1338–43.
77. Atzpodien J, Lopez Hanninen E, Kirchner H et al, Chemoimmunotherapy of advanced malignant melanoma: sequential administration of subcutaneous interleukin-2 and interferon-alpha after intravenous dacarbazine and carboplatin or intravenous dacarbazine, cisplatinum, carmustine and tamoxifen. *Eur J Cancer* 1995; 31: 876–81.
78. Flaherty LE, Robinson W, Redman BG et al, A phase II study of dacarbazine and cisplatinum in combination with outpatient administered interleukin-2 in metastatic malignant melanoma. *Cancer* 1993; 71: 3520–5.
79. Atkins MB, O'Boyle KR, Sosman JA et al, Randomized phase III trial of treatment with high-dose interleukin-2 either alone or in combination with interferon alfa-2a in patients with advanced melanoma. *J Clin Oncol* 1993; 11: 1969–77.
80. Legha SS, Ring S, Bedikian A et al, Treatment of metastatic melanoma with combined chemotherapy containing cisplatinum, vinblastine and dacarbazine (CVD) and biotherapy using interleukin-2 and interferon-alpha. *Ann Oncol* 1996; 827–35.
81. Legha SS, Buzaid AC, Role of recombinant interleukin-2 in combination with interferon-alfa and chemotherapy in the treatment of advanced melanoma. *Semin Oncol* 1993; 20: 27–32.
82. Atkins MB, O'Boyle KR, Sosman JA et al, Multiinstitutional phase II trial of intensive combination chemoimmunotherapy for metastatic melanoma. *J Clin Oncol* 1994; 12: 1553–60.
83. Rosenberg SA, Yang JC, Schwartzentruber DJ et al, Prospective randomized trial of the treatment of patients with metastatic melanoma using chemotherapy with cisplatin, dacarbazine, and tamoxifen alone or in combination with interleukin-2 and interferon alfa-2b. *J Clin Oncol* 1999; 17: 968–75.
84. Keilholz U, Punt C, Gore M et al, Dacarbazine, cisplatin and interferon alpha with or without interleukin-2 in advanced melanoma: interim analysis of EORTC trial 18951. *Proc ASCO* 1999; 18: 530a (abstract).
85. Legha SS, Ring S, Eton O et al, Development of a biochemotherapy regimen with concurrent administration of cisplatin, vinblastine, interferon alfa, and interleukin-2 for patients with metastatic melanoma. *J Clin Oncol* 1998; 16: 1752–9.
86. Richards JM, Gale D, Mehta N, Lestingi T, Combination of chemotherapy with interleukin-2 and interferon alfa for the treatment of metastatic melanoma. *J Clin Oncol* 1999; 17: 651–7.
87. Proebstle TM, Fuchs T, Scheibenbogen C et al, Long-term outcome of treatment with dacarbazine, cisplatin, interferon-alpha and intravenous high dose interleukin-2 in poor risk melanoma patients. *Melanoma Res* 1998; 8: 557–63.

88. Bernengo MG, Doveil GC, Bertero M et al, Low-dose integrated chemoimmuno-hormonotherapy with cisplatinum, subcutaneous interleukin-2, alpha-interferon and tamoxifen for advanced metastatic melanoma. A pilot study. *Melanoma Res* 1996; 6: 257–65.
89. Dreno B, Cupissol B, Gillot B et al, Subcutaneous interleukin-2 (IL2) and cisplatinum and alpha-interferon 2a (INF alpha 2a) for metastatic melanoma. *Sixth International Congress on Anti-cancer Treatment* 1996: 107.
90. O'Day SJ, Gammon G, Boasberg PD et al, Advantages of concurrent biochemotherapy modified by decrescendo interleukin-2, granulocyte colony-stimulating factor, and tamoxifen for patients with metastatic melanoma. *J Clin Oncol* 1999; 17:2752–61.
91. Thompson JA, Gold PJ, Fefer A, Outpatient chemoimmunotherapy for the treatment of metastatic melanoma. *Semin Oncol* 1997; 24: S44–8.
92. Andres P, Cupissol D, Guillot B et al, Subcutaneous interleukin-2 and interferon-alpha therapy associated with cisplatin monochemotherapy in the treatment of metastatic melanoma. *Eur J Dermatol* 1998; 8: 235–9.
93. McDermott DF, Mier JW, Lawrence DP et al, A phase II pilot trial of concurrent biochemotherapy with cisplatin, vinblastin, dacarbazine (CVD) interleukin-2 and interferon alpha-2b in patients with metastatic melanoma. *Proc ASCO* 1997; 16: 490a (abstract).
94. Kamanabrou D, Straub C, Heinsch M et al, Sequential biochemotherapy of INF-a/IL-2, cisplatin (CDDP), dacarbazine (DTIC) and carmustine (BCNU). Results of a monocenter phase II study in 109 patients with advanced metastatic malignant melanoma (MMM). *Proc ASCO* 1999; 18: 530a (abstract).
95. Dillman R, Soori G, Schulof R et al, Cancer Biotherapy Research Group (CBRG) trial 94-11: outpatient subcutaneous interleukin-2 [Proleukin®] and interferon-a2b [Intron® A] with combination chemotherapy plus tamoxifen in the treatment of metastatic melanoma. *Proc ASCO* 1999; 18: 530a (abstract).
96. Maral J, Long-term follow up of patients with metastatic malignant melanoma treated with continuous infusion-IL-2 alone or in combination. *Eight International Congress on Anti-cancer Treatment* 1998: 1560.
97. Young RC, Canellos GP, Chabner BA et al, Treatment of malignant melanoma with methyl CCNU. *Clin Pharmacol Ther* 1974; 15: 617–22.
98. Seigler SA, Lucas VR Jr, Pickett NJ et al, DTIC, CCNU, Bleomycin and Vincristine (BOLD) in metastatic melanoma. *Cancer* 1980; 46: 2346–8.
99. Mulder JH, Dodion P, Cavalli P et al, Cisplatin and vindesine combination chemotherapy in advanced malignant melanoma: an EORTC phase II study. *Eur J Cancer Clin Oncol* 1982; 18: 1297–301.
100. Ringborg U, Rudenstam CM, Hansson J et al, Dacarbazine versus dacarbazine-vindesine in disseminated malignant melanoma: a randomized phase II study. *Med Oncol Tumor Pharmacother* 1989; 6: 285–9.
101. York RM, Foltz AT, Bleomycin, vincristine, lomustine, and DTIC chemotherapy for metastatic melanoma. *Cancer* 1988; 61: 2183–6.
102. Avril MF, Bonneterre J, Cupissol D et al, Fotemustine plus dacarbazine for malignant melanoma. *Eur J Cancer* 1992; 11: 1807–11.
103. Buzaid AC, Legha S, Winn R et al, Cisplatin, vinblastin and dacarbazine alone in metastatic melanoma: Preliminary results of a phase III Cancer Community Oncology Program (CCOP) trial. *Proc Am Soc Clin Oncol* 1993; 12: 1328a.
104. Comella G, Daponte A, Comella P et al, Combination chemotherapy with vinblastine, BCNU and cisplatin in advanced metastatic melanoma. *Tumori* 1991; 77: 216–18.
105. Fletcher WS, Green S, Fletcher JR et al, Evaluation of *cis*-platinum and DTIC combination chemotherapy in disseminated melanoma. A Southwest Oncology Group Study. *Am J Clin Oncol* 1988; 11: 589–93.
106. Icli F, Karaoguz H, Dincol D et al, Treatment of metastatic malignant melanoma with 24 hours continuous venous infusion of dacarbazine and cisplatin. *J Surg Oncol* 1991; 48: 199–201.
107. Murren JR, DeRosa W, Durivage HJ et al, High-dose cisplatin plus dacarbazine in the treatment of metastatic melanoma. *Cancer* 1991; 67: 1514–17.
108. Olver IN, Bishop JF, Geen M et al, A phase II study of cisplatinum and continuous infusion 5-fluorouracil for metastatic melanoma. *Am J Clin Oncol* 1992; 15: 503–5.
109. Richards JM, Mehta N, Raming K et al, Sequential chemoimmunotherapy in the treatment of metastatic melanoma. *J Clin Oncol* 1992; 10: 1338–43.
110. Khayat D, Borel C, Benhammouda A et al, Active three drugs (fotemustine, dacarbazine and vindesine) outpatient combination in advanced malignant melanoma. *Proc Am Soc Clin Oncol* 1992; 11: 1336a.
111. Bedikian AY, Legha SS, Eton O et al, Phase II trial of tyrapazamine combined with cisplatin in chemotherapy of advanced malignant melanoma. *Ann Oncol* 1997; 8: 363–7.
112. Schultz MZ, Buzaid AC, Poo WJ et al, A phase II study of interferon-alpha 2b with dacarbazine, carmustine, cisplatin and tamoxifen in metastatic melanoma. *Melanoma Res* 1997; 7: 147–51.
113. Hoffman R, Muller I, Neuber K et al, Risk and outcome in metastatic malignant melanoma patients receiving DTIC, cisplatin, BCNU and tamoxifen followed by immunotherapy with interleukin 2 and interferon alpha 2a. *Br J Cancer* 1998; 78: 1076–80.
114. Margolin KA, Liu PY, Flaherty L et al, Phase II study of carmustine, dacarbazine cisplatin, and tamoxifen in advanced melanoma: a Southwest Oncology Group study. *J Clin Oncol* 1998; 16: 664–9.
115. Richard MA, Grob JJ, Zarrour H et al, Combined treatment with dacarbazine, cisplatin, fotemustine and tamoxifen in metastatic malignant melanoma. *Melanoma Res* 1998; 8: 170–4.
116. Seeber A, Binder M, Steiner A et al, Treatment of metastatic malignant melanoma with dacarbazine plus fotemustine. *Eur J Cancer* 1998; 34: 2129–31.
117. Semb KA, Aamdal S, Bohmann T et al, Clinical experience of fotemustine, cisplatin and high dose tamoxifen in patients with metastatic malignant melanoma. *Melanoma Res* 1998; 8: 565–72.
118. Gander M, Leyvraz S, Decorsterd L et al, Sequential administration of temozolomide and fotemustine: depletion of O6-alkyl guanine-DNA transferase in blood lymphocytes and in tumours. *Ann Oncol* 1999; 10: 831–8.
119. Thomson DB, Adena M, McLeod GR et al, Interferon-alpha 2a does not improve response or survival when combined with dacarbazine in metastatic malignant melanoma: results of a multi-institutional Australian randomized trial. *Melanoma Res* 1993; 3: 133–8.
120. McKeage MJ, Lorentzos A, Gore ME et al, Tamoxifen and chemotherapy for refractory metastatic malignant melanoma. *N Engl J Med* 1993; 328: 140–1.
121. Flaherty LE, Robinson W, Redman BG et al, A phase II study of dacarbazine and cisplatin in combination with outpatient administered interleukin-2 in metastatic malignant melanoma. *Cancer* 1993; 71: 3520–5.
122. Schultz MZ, Buzaid AC, Poo WJ et al, A phase II study of interferon-alpha 2b with dacarbazine, carmustine, cisplatin and tamoxifen in metastatic melanoma. *Melanoma Res* 1997; 7: 147–51.
123. Feun LG, Savaraj N, Moffat F et al, Phase II trial of recombinant interferon-alpha with BCNU, cisplatin, DTIC and tamoxifen in advanced malignant melanoma. *Melanoma Res* 1995; 5: 273–6.
124. Gause BL, Sharfman WH, Janik JE et al, A phase II study of carboplatin, cisplatin, interferon-alpha, and tamoxifen for patients with metastatic melanoma. *Cancer Invest* 1998; 16: 374–80.
125. McClay EF, McClay MT, Monroe L et al, A phase II study of high dose tamoxifen and weekly cisplatin in patients with metastatic melanoma. *Melanoma Res* 2001; 11: 309–13.
126. O'Neill P, Hersh E, Warneke J et al, Phase II trial of combination chemotherapy and biological response modification in metastatic melanoma. *Proc Am Soc Clin Oncol* 1996; 432b: A 1338.
127. Nathan FE, Berd D, Sato T et al, Paclitaxel and tamoxifen: An active regimen for patients with metastatic melanoma. *Cancer* 2000; 88: 79–87.
128. Margolin K, Liu PY, Flaherty L et al, Low antitumor activity of BCNU, DTIC cisplatin (DDP) and tamoxifen (TAM) in advanced melanoma: a Southwest Oncology Group study. *Proc Am Soc Clin Oncol* 1997; 495a: A 1783.
129. Saba HI, Klein C, Reintgen D, Management of advanced stage IV metastatic melanoma with a platinol based chemotherapy regimen: a University of South Florida and H. Lee Moffitt Melanoma Center Study. *Proc Am Soc Clin Oncol* 1993; 397a: A 1359.
130. Lattanzi SC, Tosteson T, Maurer LH et al, Dacarbazine (D), Cisplatin (C), and Carmustine (B), +/− Tamoxifen (T), in the treatment of

patients (PTS) with metastatic melanoma (MM): results of a 5-year follow-up. *Proc Am Soc Clin Oncol* 1993, 390: A 1333.
131. Spitler L, Good J, Jacobs M et al, The use of high dose tamoxifen to potentiate the anti-tumor effects of cytotoxic chemotherapy in patients with metastatic melanoma. *Proc Am Soc Clin Oncol* 1994; 397: A 1353.
132. Legha S, Ring S, Bedikian A et al, Lack of benefit from Tamoxifen (T) added to a regimen of Cisplatin (C), Vinblastine (V), DTIC (D) and alpha-Interferon (IFN) in patients (PT) with metastatic melanoma (MM). *Proc Am Soc Clin Oncol* 1993; 388: A 1325.
133. Agarwala SS, Ferri W, Gooding W et al, A phase III randomized trial of dacarbazine and carboplatin with and without tamoxifen in the treatment of patients with metastatic melanoma. *Cancer* 1999; 85: 1979–84.
134. Bajetta E, Buzzoni R, Vicario G et al, Combined carboplatin and cytosine arabinoside in metastatic melanoma refractory to dacarbazine. *Tumori* 1995; 81: 238–40.
135. Chiaron Sileni V, Nortilli R, Medici M et al, BCNU (B), Cisplatin (C), Dacarbazine (D), and Tamoxifen (T) (BCDT) in metastatic melanoma (MM): results of a randomized phase II study. *Proc Am Soc Clin Oncol* 1997, 495a: A 1782.
136. Rosenberg SA, Yannelli JR, Yang JC et al, Treatment of patients with metastatic melanoma with autologous tumor-infiltrating lymphocytes and interleukin 2. *J Natl Cancer Inst* 1994; 86: 1159–66.
137. Dillman RO, Oldham RK, Barth NM, et al, Continuous interleukin-2 and tumor-infiltrating lymphocytes as treatment of advanced melanoma. A national biotherapy study group trial. *Cancer* 1991; 68: 1–8.
138. Kradin RL, Kurnick JT, Lazarus DS et al, Tumour-infiltrating lymphocytes and interleukin-2 in treatment of advanced cancer. *Lancet* 1989; 1: 577–80.
139. Richner J, Joss RA, Goldhirsch A et al, Phase II study of continuous subcutaneous interferon-alfa combined with cisplatin in advanced malignant melanoma. *Eur J Cancer* 1992; 28A: 1044–7.
140. Stark JJ, Dillman RO, Schulof R et al, Interferon-alpha and chemohormonal therapy for patients with advanced melanoma: final results of a phase I–II study of the Cancer Biotherapy Research Group and the Mid-Atlantic Oncology Program. *Cancer* 1998; 82: 1677–81.
141. Mulder NH, Willemse PH, Schraffordt Koops H et al, Dacarbazine (DTIC) and human recombinant interferon alpha 2a (Roferon) in the treatment of disseminated malignant melanoma. *Br J Cancer* 1990; 62: 1006–7.
142. Daponte A, Ascierto PA, Gravina A et al, Cisplatin, dacarbazine, and fotemustine plus interferon alpha in patients with advanced malignant melanoma. A multicenter phase II study of the Italian Oncology Group. *Cancer* 2000; 89: 2630–6.
143. Sondak VK, Liu PY, Flaherty LE et al, A phase II evaluation of all-trans-retinoic acid plus interferon alfa-2a in stage IV melanoma: a Southwest Oncology Group study. *Cancer J Sci Am* 1999; 5: 41–7.
144. Kirkwood JM, Agarwala SS, Diaz B et al, Phase I study of temozolomide in combination with interferon alfa-2b in metastatic malignant melanoma. *Proc Am Soc Clin Oncol* 1997; 491a: A 1767.
145. Dillman RO, Soori G, Wiemann MC et al, Phase II trial of subcutaneous interleukin-2, subcutaneous interferon-alpha, intravenous combination chemotherapy, and oral tamoxifen in the treatment of metastatic melanoma: final results of Cancer Biotherapy Research Group 94-11. *Cancer Biother Radiopharm* 2000; 15: 487–94.

57

Immunotherapy of non-resected melanoma

Peter Hersey

INTRODUCTION

When melanoma metastases become established at distant body sites they have acquired a number of properties which potentially limit immunotherapeutic approaches to treatment. Not only have the melanoma cells acquired properties of invasion and motility but they also now have the ability to grow at different body sites because of the production of their own growth factors or inherent ability to divide independently of host tissues.[1] Migration through lymphatics or via the blood also suggests the adaptive and non-adaptive immune defence mechanisms have failed to eradicate the tumour cells, either because of loss of key recognition and antigenic molecules from the tumour cells,[2,3] or because they have acquired intracellular mechanisms that protect them from apoptotic and other death pathways resulting from contact with the lymphocytes.[4,5] In addition, a number of other barriers are acquired by established metastases, including downregulation of recognition molecules on endothelial cells in the vicinity of the tumour[6] and the release of factors that inhibit the function of antigen-presenting cells and lymphocyte responses.[7]

Given this long list of possible limitations to immunotherapy of established metastatic melanoma, it is not surprising that these approaches have met with limited success. Nevertheless, over the last 20 years a number of studies using different vaccine approaches have been carried out which have achieved perhaps more success than would be anticipated. The approaches used have mirrored the evolution of developments in immunology. Hence, in the early 1980s the main strategy involved recruitment of helper responses and the use of various adjuvants.[8–10] Street and Mosmann[11] described different subsets of T lymphocytes that could be generated by different cytokines, which resulted in the employment of cytokines in vaccines. Studies by Townsend et al.[12] also showed that T cells recognized internally processed antigens on major histocompatibility complex (MHC) antigens, which led to the discovery of a large number of antigens in melanoma recognized by T cells. This, in turn, has ushered in the development of vaccines based on known melanoma antigens. This chapter describes the progress made in studies using these approaches in patients with metastatic melanoma.

TRADITIONAL MELANOMA VACCINE APPROACHES

The simplest vaccines for treatment of melanoma are those prepared from allogeneic melanoma cell lines.[9,10] These have the advantage of being readily available for use and are readily standardized for cell dose, antigenic content and sterility.[9] Perhaps the best known of the vaccines that are currently under evaluation is the CVax vaccine, prepared by Morton et al.,[10] and Melacine, produced originally by Mitchell and colleagues.[9,13] Table 57.1 summarizes results from phase II studies with these vaccines and smaller studies with a variety of other vaccines. The study by Hollinshead et al.[14] was not evaluated by accepted response criteria but nevertheless is

Table 57.1 *Results from studies with traditional vaccines made from whole cells, cell lysates or cell extracts*

Authors (ref.)	Vaccine*	Adjuvant†	No. of patients	Results‡ (%)
Morton et al. (10)	Three allog mel lines	BCG	40	CR 8, PR 15, SD 10
Mitchell (9, 13)	Ultrasonicate of two allog mel lines	Detox	106	CR 4.7, PR 14.1, MR 8.5
Weisenburger et al. (55)	Three allog mel lines	Intralymphatic administration	34	CR 6, PR 21, SD 6
Phillips et al. (56)	Autol mel *n*-butanol extracts	Liposomes	13	CR 23, PR 14
Hollinshead et al. (14)	Allog mel extracts ± dacarbazine	Complete Freund's	51	CR 23
Eton et al. (57)	Autol mel UVB irradiation	Detox	24	CR 12.5
Adler et al. (58)	Extracts of six allog mel lines	IL-2 in liposomes	10	CR 30, PR 30

* Allog, allogeneic; autol, autologous; mel, melanoma.
† BCG, bacille Calmette-Guérin.
‡ CR, MR, PR, complete, mixed and partial responses respectively; SD, stable disease.

included as an indicator of the considerable thought and enterprise of studies at that time.

It is clear that many responses were seen in these phase I–II studies but whether they are indicative of responses in stage IV patients overall is not known, as in most studies it is likely that patients were selected with low tumour volume or slow tumour progression. Some indication that the results of immunotherapy may be at least no worse than chemotherapy came from a multicentre randomized trial comparing Melacine with the Dartmouth chemotherapy regimen (cisplatin, dacarbazine and carmustine plus or minus tamoxifen); 70 patients were enrolled in each group. Median survivals were not significantly different (Melacine 9.4 months versus chemotherapy 12.3 months, $P=0.16$). Quality-of-life measures were superior in the immunotherapy treated patients.[15,16]

HAPTEN-CONJUGATED MELANOMA CELL VACCINES

During the 1970s, treatment of cutaneous and subcutaneous tumours by topical application of dinitrochlorobenzene (DNCB) became popular.[17,18] These studies led in two directions, one of which was to combine topical application of DNCB with systemic chemotherapy – usually dacarbazine (DTIC). Large phase II studies suggested that the response was greater than would be expected from dacarbazine alone (59 patients, complete response (CR) 25%, partial response (PR) 12%).[19] On this basis, a randomized study is in progress in Europe to test whether the combination is better than dacarbazine alone.

The other direction has been the development of autologous vaccines haptenized with dinitrofluorobenzene (DNFB), which, like DNCB, puts a dinitrophenyl group on to melanoma cells. The rationale for this approach is based on the helper T cell strategy in which T cell responses to strong antigens are believed to increase immune responses to weak tumour antigens.[8] This formed the basis for the use of viral antigens and foreign proteins, as well as chemical haptens, in tumour vaccines.

Berd et al.[20,21] reported that such vaccines induced inflammatory responses in distant cutaneous metastases and clinical responses in patients with metastatic melanoma. Of 40 patients with measurable disease there were four CR and one PR, and some responses were seen in another six patients. These vaccines are now being evaluated in a randomized trial in patients with bulky American Joint Committee on Cancer (AJCC) stage III disease and in phase II studies in patients with stage IV metastatic melanoma.

GENE-TRANSFECTED MELANOMA CELL VACCINES

Studies by Street and Mosmann[11] indicated that there were different subsets of T cells and that differentiation along different pathways was determined by the presence of cytokines in the local environment. In view of this, attempts have been made to incorporate these findings into the development of tumour vaccines.

Studies in animal models have indicated that transfection of tumour cells with cytokine genes can increase T cell responses to the tumour and mediate rejection of non-transfected tumour cells.[22] In view of this, a number of phase I–II studies have been carried out in patients with melanoma to test this approach in humans; the results of published studies are shown in Table 57.2. Immunization with granulocyte macrophage colony-stimulated factor (GM-CSF) transfected melanoma cells has received much attention and has been associated with several marked clinical responses associated with lymphocytic infiltration into tumours.[23–25] In one study, immunization with GM-CSF-transfected melanoma cells was associated with adoptive immunotherapy with regional lymph node lymphocytes taken after the injections and expanded in vitro.[26]

Similarly, immunization with interleukin (IL)-2-gene-transfected autologous melanoma cells has been the focus of several trials.[27,28] No definite clinical responses were seen but stabilization of disease was recorded in a number of patients. Somewhat similar results were seen in studies with autologous melanoma transfected with interferon-gamma (IFN-γ),[29] IL-7[30] or IL-12[31] genes. Immunization with allogeneic melanoma cells transfected with IL-2[32,33] or IL-4[34] genes was examined in several studies. Immunological responses were seen but there were no major clinical responses.

Another approach to gene therapy has been to transfect alloantigens directly into melanoma metastases in the hope that a strong response against the alloantigen will act as a helper response for induction of responses against autologous melanoma antigens.[33] The delivery system was based on use of a cationic lipid vector to deliver plasmids containing the gene for human leucocyte antigen (HLA)-B7. The product has now been

Table 57.2 *Gene-transfected melanoma vaccines in treatment of American Joint Committee on Cancer (AJCC) stage IV melanoma*

Authors (ref.)	Vaccine*	No. of patients	Outcome†
Soiffer et al. (23)	Autol mel + GM-CSF genes	21	Lymphoid infiltrates
Mastrangelo et al. (24)	Autol mel + intratumoral VV GM-CSF injection	7	1 CR, 1 PR, 3 MR
Chang et al. (25)	Autol mel + GM-CSF injections Adoptive transfer of VPLN	5	1 CR
Palmer et al. (27)	Autol mel + IL-2 genes	12	3 SD
Schreiber et al. (28)	Autol mel + IL-2 genes	15	5 SD
Fujii et al. (29)	Intratumoral retroviral IFN-γ: 1 cycles 6 cycles	9 8	1 SD 3 PR, 5 SD
Moller et al. (30)	Autol mel + IL-7 genes	10	2 minor responses
Sun et al. (31)	Autol mel + IL-12 genes	6	1 minor response
Belli et al. (32)	Allog mel + IL-2 genes	12	2 MR, 4 SD
Osanto et al. (33)	Allog mel + IL-2 genes	33	2 PR, 7 SD
Arienti et al. (34)	Allog mel + IL-4 genes	12	2 MR
Stopeck et al. (59)	Intratumoral DNA-Liposome HLA-B7	17	7 patients had a decrease in size of injected metastases

*Allog, allogeneic; autol, autologous; GM-CSF, granulocyte macrophage colony-stimulating factor; HLA, human leucocyte antigen; IL, interleukin; INF-γ, interferon-gamma; mel, melanoma; VPLN, vaccine primed lymph nodes; VV, vaccinia virus.
†CR, MR, PR, complete, mixed and partial responses respectively; SD, stable disease.

tested in a large number of patients and shown to be safe. Phase II studies have shown both local and systemic responses, and a phase III study is in progress comparing the product (allovectin) to chemotherapy with dacarbazine.

CYTOKINES GIVEN IN ASSOCIATION WITH VACCINES OR PERITUMORALLY

One of the questions arising from studies on gene-transfected tumour cells as vaccines is whether the cytokine genes needed to be transfected into the tumour cells, or whether similar effects could be achieved by injection of the cytokines directly into the tumour or together with the vaccines. In an animal model, a slow-release preparation of GM-CSF was reported to induce similar responses to immunization with gene-transfected tumour cells.[35] It was found that intralesional injection of GM-CSF was associated with PR in non-injected lesions in three of 13 patients.[36] GM-CSF was injected with the autologous melanoma cells by Dillman et al.,[37] who reported two PR in 25 patients. Leong et al.[38] gave GM-CSF with autologous melanoma and bacille Calmette-Guérin (BCG) as an adjuvant. They reported two CR, two PR and three with stable disease (SD) in a group of 20 patients. Fifteen patients given the autologous vaccine plus BCG alone showed no responses. Direct intralesional injections of IFN-alfa (α) was reported to induce systemic responses in nine of 51 patients and local responses in 24 patients.[39] Similarly, IL-2,[40] but not tumour necrosis factor (TNF)-α with IFN-γ,[41] was reported to induce local responses when injected intratumorally into subcutaneous metastases (Table 57.3).

WELL-DEFINED MELANOMA ANTIGEN VACCINES

As discussed in Chapter 54, a large number of melanoma antigens recognized by T cells have been defined at the genetic and peptide epitope level. This has provided the opportunity to test the efficacy of individual antigens either by direct administration of peptide epitopes or by administration on dendritic cells (DC). The results of these trials are summarized in Tables 57.4 and 57.5. Many of the studies are ongoing and, therefore, some results are preliminary. Nevertheless, there are a number of responses which provide encouragement for this approach, e.g. the studies by Guilloux et al.[42] using NA17-A2 peptides in saline are particularly promising, as were the studies by Marchand[60] with the MAGE-3A.1 peptides. Both of these peptide epitopes are from tumour-specific antigens and may indicate that these antigens are more likely to stimulate the high-affinity T cells needed for rejection. Much interest is also focused on peptides from MAGE-A10, which is frequently recognized by patients with melanoma.[43] In contrast, administration of peptides from differentiation antigens has so far been disappointing, and may indicate that T cells against these antigens are of low affinity and relatively ineffective. The exception has been studies by Rosenberg et al.[44] when IL-2 was administered as well as the peptide

Table 57.3 *Cytokines given in association with vaccines or given intratumorally*

Authors (ref.)	Vaccine/Cytokine*	No. of patients	Outcome†
Si et al. (36)	GM-CSF intratumoral	13	3 PR
Dillman et al. (37)	Autol mel + GM-CSF injections	25	2 PR
Leong et al. (38)	Autol mel + BCG + GM-CSF injections Autol mel + BCG	20 15	2 CR, 2 PR, 3 SD 0
Von Wussow et al. (39)	IFN-α intratumoral	51	9 PR, 29 local CR or PR
Gutwald et al. (40)	IL-2 intratumoral	2	2 PR at local site
Retsas et al. (41)	TNF-α and IFN-γ intratumoral	7	0

*Allog, allogeneic; autol, autologous; BCG, bacille Calmette-Guérin; GM-CSF, granulocyte macrophage colony-stimulating factor; IL, interleukin; INF-γ, interferon-gamma; mel, melanoma; TNF, tumour necrosis factor.
†CR, MR, PR, complete, mixed and partial responses respectively; SD, stable disease.

Table 57.4 *Melanoma peptide vaccine trials*

Authors (ref.)	Peptide	Adjuvant*	No. of patients	Clinical response†
Marchand et al. (60)	MAGE-1, 3A.1 MAGE-3A.1 MAGE-3A.2	Nothing MPL + QS21 Nothing	25	7
Kruit et al.	MAGE-3 protein	MPL + QS21	49	2 PR, 3 MR ISD
Rosenberg et al. (44) (61)	MART-1 gp100 154, 209, 280	IFA IFA	23 28	
Rosenberg et al. (44)	gp100 209 2M	IFA IFA, IL-2	11 31	3 Mixed 13–1 CR, 12 PR
Ranieri et al. (70)	MART-1, gp100, Tyrosinase 368	MF59 or Local IL-12	28 28	0 0
Jaeger et al. (62)	MART-1, gp100, Tyrosinase 1, 368	GM-CSF (3 patients)	10	3–1 CR, 2 PR
Weber et al. (63)	MAGE-3A.1	IFA	18	n.a.
Wang et al. (64)	MART-1	IFA	25	n.a.
Cebon et al. (65)	MART-1	IL-12	20	1 CR, 1 PR
Scheibenbogan et al. (66)	Tyrosinase 234, 368, 206, 192	GM-CSF	18	1 MR, 2 SD
Hersey et al.	MART-1, 26, 2L, Tyrosinase, MAGE-3A.2	Montanide ISA720, PPD + GM-CSF	16	3 SD
Brichard et al.	gp100 209, 2M; 280, 9V NA17–1		14	1 CR, 2 PR, 3 SD

*GM-CSF, granulocyte macrophage colony-stimulating factor; IFA, incomplete Freund's adjuvant; IL, interleukin; MF59, oil (squalene) in water emulsion with muramyldipeptide from bacterial cell walls; montanide ISA720, water in (metabolizable) oil emulsion; MPL, monophosphoryl lipid A (modified LPS); PPD, purified protein derivative; QS21, Carbohydrate extract of *Quillaja Saponaria*.

†CR, MR, PR, complete, mixed and partial responses respectively; n.a., not available; SD, stable disease.

injections. Responses in a group of 31 patients were impressive and may indicate that IL-2 is important, either in restoring competency to the T cells or in allowing them to migrate into the tumour.

DISCUSSION

Evaluation of the efficacy of vaccines in the treatment of non-resected melanoma is difficult because most have been tested in small phase I or II trials and it is likely that patients were highly selected. There is also a growing sentiment that the usual response criteria may be inadequate to assess treatment with vaccines. Overall survival or progression-free survival are thought, by some investigators, to be more appropriate for the assessment of efficacy. This said, the above results show no major differences in outcomes, irrespective of whether traditional vaccines or cytokine gene-transfected vaccines were used. Much the same may be said about the initial results from the early trials using purified melanoma antigen vaccines. It is, however, heartening that similar results are being obtained with the pure antigen vaccines, as they provide much more scope for improvement of results than is possible with the traditional vaccines, e.g. it is possible to select antigens that are known to be expressed on the patient's tumour. Secondly, it is possible to measure the response to individual antigens and select protocols that maximize T cell responses.

An even more healthy development is the growing realization that the outcome of immune responses against melanoma is the result of a two-way interaction

Table 57.5 *Dendritic cell vaccines against melanoma*

Authors (ref.)	Source of antigen*	Route†	No. of patients	Response‡
Nestle et al. (67)	Melanoma tumour lysates or peptides + KLH helper protein	Lymph nodes	16	2 CR, 3 PR
Hu et al. (68)	MAGE-1	id and iv	3	–
Chakraborty et al. (69)	Melanoma lysates	id	15	1 PR
Ranieri et al. (70)	gp100, MART-1, tyrosinase	iv	28	3 PR
Thurner et al. (71)	MAGE-3A.1	sc and id × 3 iv × 3	11	6 PR or MR
Gajewsky et al. (72)	MAGE-3 MART-1	sc + IL-12 sc	15	1 PR, 3 MR
Panelli et al. (73)	MART-1, gp100	iv	17	
Hersey et al.	Lysates Peptides	Intranodal	13 7	1 PR, 1 MR, 2 SD 3 SD

* Peptides were tyrosinase, gp100 or MART-1 for human leucocyte antigen (HLA)-A2 patients and MAGE-1A.1 for HLA-A1 patients.
† id, iv, intradermal and intravenous, respectively; IL, interleukin; sc, subcutaneous.
‡ CR, MR, PR, complete, mixed and partial responses, respectively; SD, stable disease.

between immune responses and the patient's tumour. A number of reviews have drawn attention to loss of antigens and recognition structures on melanoma during the course of melanoma growth,[3,7] but so far relatively little attention has been given to resistance of melanoma cells to apoptosis. Our interest in this area was stimulated by the finding that CD4 T cells killed melanoma by interaction of TNF-related apoptosis-inducing ligand (TRAIL) on their surface with TRAIL receptors on the melanoma cells.[45] Of great interest was the finding that TRAIL-induced apoptosis via the mitochondrial pathway is commonly involved in apoptosis induced by chemotherapeutic agents.[46] Even more surprising were recent studies showing that granzyme B from CD8 cytotoxic T lymphocytes (CTL) induces apoptosis via the same mitochondrial pathway.[47,48] These results imply that the mechanism of cell death is similar between CD4 TRAIL-mediated killing, chemotherapy and CD8 CTL killing. They may also explain why melanoma often exhibits sensitivity or resistance to different forms of treatment and why it is that many agents seem to induce the same response rate.

An important consequence of these findings is that there is already much information about factors involved in inhibition of the mitochondrial pathway to apoptosis and some of these are amenable to therapy,[49] e.g. one of the proteins involved in inhibition of this pathway is Bcl-2 and clinical trials are already in progress using antisense oligonucleotides to inhibit Bcl-2 production.[50] Cisplatin is believed to induce apoptosis via the mitochondrial pathway and was shown to sensitize melanoma to killing by T cells.[51] Some chemotherapy agents, such as actinomycin D, are also effective in vitro in blocking production of apoptosis inhibitors and have been shown to sensitize tumour cells to killing by TRAIL.[52] Another approach is the use of proteasome inhibitors, such as PS341, which are being tested in clinical trials.[53] These prevent activation of the transcription factor NF-κB, which upregulates many inhibitors of apoptosis in melanoma.[54]

It can therefore be anticipated that in addition to maximizing T cell responses by well-characterized vaccines, treatments that sensitize melanoma cells to apoptosis may lead to a major increase in response of the melanoma to therapy. The next few years therefore promise to be a most exciting time, which may see clinical response rates ⩾50% as a realistic goal.

REFERENCES

1. Herlyn M, Berking C, Li G, Satyamoorthy K, Lessons from melanocyte development for understanding the biological events in naevus and melanoma formation. *Melanoma Res* 2000; 10: 303–12.
2. Houghton AN, Gold JS, Blachere NE, Immunity against cancer: lessons learned from melanoma. *Curr Opin Immunol* 2001; 13: 134–40.
3. Marincola FM, Jaffee EM, Hicklin DJ, Ferrone S, Escape of human solid tumors from T-cell recognition: molecular mechanisms and functional significance. *Adv Immunol* 2000; 74: 181–273.
4. Nguyen T, Thomas W, Zhang XD, Gray C, Hersey P, Immunologically-mediated tumour cell apoptosis: the role of TRAIL in T cell and cytokine-mediated responses to melanoma. *Forum (Genova)* 2000; 10: 243–52.
5. Raisova M, Bektas M, Wieder T et al, Resistance to CD95/Fas-induced and ceramide-mediated apoptosis of human melanoma cells is caused by a defective mitochondrial cytochrome c release. *FEBS Lett* 2000; 473: 27–32.
6. Piali L, Fichtel A, Terpe HJ et al, Endothelial vascular cell adhesion molecule 1 expression is suppressed by melanoma and carcinoma. *J Exp Med* 1995; 181: 811–16.
7. Hersey P, Impediments to successful immunotherapy. *Pharmacol Ther* 1999; 81: 111–19.
8. Mitchison NA, Immunologic approach to cancer. *Transpl Proc* 1970; 2: 92–103.
9. Mitchell MS, Attempts to optimize active specific immunotherapy for melanoma. *Int Rev Immunol* 1991; 7: 331–47.
10. Morton DL, Foshag LJ, Hoon DS et al, Prolongation of survival in metastatic melanoma after active specific immunotherapy with a new polyvalent melanoma vaccine. *Ann Surg* 1992; 216: 463–82.
11. Street NE, Mosmann TR, Functional diversity of T lymphocytes due to secretion of different cytokine patterns. *FASEB J* 1991; 5: 171–77.
12. Townsend AR, Rothbard J, Gotch FM et al, The epitopes of influenza nucleoprotein recognized by cytotoxic T lymphocytes can be defined with short synthetic peptides. *Cell* 1986; 44: 959–68.
13. Mitchell MS, Perspective on allogeneic melanoma lysates in active specific immunotherapy. *Semin Oncol* 1998; 25: 623–35.
14. Hollinshead A, Arlen M, Yonemoto R et al, Pilot studies using melanoma tumor-associated antigens (TAA) in specific-active immunochemotherapy of malignant melanoma. *Cancer* 1982; 49: 1387–404.
15. Mitchell MS, Von Eschen KB, Phase III trial of Melacine® melanoma theraccine versus combination chemotherapy in the treatment of stage IV melanoma. *Proc ASCO* 1997.
16. Elliott GT, McLeod RA, Perez J, Von Eschen KB, Interim results of a phase II multicenter clinical trial evaluating the activity of a therapeutic allogeneic melanoma vaccine (theraccine) in the treatment of disseminated malignant melanoma. *Semin Surg Oncol* 1993; 9: 264–72.
17. Klein E, Holtermann OA, Helm F et al, Immunologic approaches to the management of primary and secondary tumors involving the skin and soft tissues: review of a ten-year program. *Monograph* 1976; Nov 01: 159–77.
18. Budzanowska E, Pawlicki M, An attempt at topical DNCB immunomodulation in advanced malignant melanoma. *Tumori* 1988; 74: 519–22.
19. Strobbe LJ et al, Topical dinitrochlorobenzene combined with systemic dacarbazine in the treatment of recurrent melanoma. *Melanoma Res* 1997; 7: 507–12.
20. Berd D, Murphy G, Maguire HC Jr, Mastrangelo MJ, Immunization with haptenized, autologous tumor cells induces inflammation of human melanoma metastases. *Cancer Res* 1991; 51: 2731–4.
21. Berd D, Maguire HC Jr, McCue P, Mastrangelo MJ, Treatment of metastatic melanoma with an autologous tumor-cell vaccine: clinical and immunologic results in 64 patients. *J Clin Oncol* 1990; 8: 1858–67.
22. Dranoff G, Jaffee E, Lazenby A et al, Vaccination with irradiated tumor cells engineered to secrete murine granulocyte-macrophage colony-stimulating factor stimulates potent, specific, and long-lasting anti-tumor immunity. *Proc Natl Acad Sci USA* 1993; 90: 3539–43.
23. Soiffer R, Lynch T, Mihm M et al, Vaccination with irradiated autologous melanoma cells engineered to secrete human granulocyte-macrophage colony-stimulating factor generates potent antitumor immunity in patients with metastatic melanoma. *Proc Natl Acad Sci USA* 1998; 95: 13,141–6.
24. Mastrangelo MJ, Maguire HC Jr, Eisenlohr LC et al, Intratumoral recombinant GM-CSF-encoding virus as gene therapy in patients with cutaneous melanoma. *Cancer Gene Ther* 1999; 6: 409–22.
25. Chang AE, Li Q, Bishop DK et al, Immunogenetic therapy of human melanoma utilizing autologous tumor cells transduced to secrete granulocyte-macrophage colony-stimulating factor. *Hum Gene Ther* 2000; 11: 839–50.
26. Ellem KA, O'Rourke MG, Johnson GR et al, A case report: immune responses and clinical course of the first human use of granulocyte-macrophage-colony-stimulating-factor-transduced autologous melanoma cells for immunotherapy. *Cancer Immunol Immunother* 1997; 44: 10–20.
27. Palmer K, Moore J, Everard M et al, Gene therapy with autologous, interleukin 2-secreting tumor cells in patients with malignant melanoma. *Hum Gene Ther* 1999; 10: 1261–8.
28. Schreiber S, Kampgen E, Wagner E et al, Immunotherapy of metastatic malignant melanoma by a vaccine consisting of autologous interleukin 2-transfected cancer cells: outcome of a phase I study. *Hum Gene Ther* 1999; 10: 983–93.
29. Fujii S, Huang S, Fong TC et al, Induction of melanoma-associated antigen systemic immunity upon intratumoral delivery of interferon-gamma retroviral vector in melanoma patients. *Cancer Gene Ther* 2000; 7: 1220–30.
30. Moller P, Sun Y, Dorbic T et al, Vaccination with IL-7 gene-modified autologous melanoma cells can enhance the anti-melanoma lytic activity in peripheral blood of patients with a good clinical performance status: a clinical phase I study. *Br J Cancer* 1998; 77: 1907–16.
31. Sun Y, Jurgovsky K, Moller P et al, Vaccination with IL-12 gene-modified autologous melanoma cells: preclinical results and a first clinical phase I study. *Gene Ther* 1998; 5: 481–90.
32. Belli F, Arienti F, Sule-Suso J et al, Active immunization of metastatic melanoma patients with interleukin-2 transduced allogeneic melanoma cells: evaluation of efficacy and tolerability. *Cancer Immunol Immunother* 1997; 44: 197–203.
33. Osanto S, Schiphorst PP, Weijl NI et al, Vaccination of melanoma patients with an allogeneic, genetically modified interleukin 2-producing melanoma cell line. *Hum Gene Ther* 2000; 11: 739–50.
34. Arienti F, Belli F, Napolitano F et al, Vaccination of melanoma patients with interleukin 4 gene-transduced allogeneic melanoma cells. *Hum Gene Ther* 1999; 10: 2907–16.
35. Golumbek PT, Azhari R, Jaffee EM et al, Controlled release, biodegradable cytokine depots: a new approach in cancer vaccine design. *Cancer Res* 1993; 53: 5841–4.
36. Si Z, Hersey P, Coates AS, Clinical responses and lymphoid infiltrates in metastatic melanoma following treatment with intralesional GM-CSF. *Melanoma Res* 1996; 6: 247–55.
37. Dillman RO, Nayak SK, Barth NM et al, Clinical experience with autologous tumor cell lines for patient-specific vaccine therapy in metastatic melanoma. *Cancer Biother Radiopharmacol* 1998; 13: 165–76.
38. Leong SP, Enders-Zohr P, Zhou YM et al, Recombinant human granulocyte macrophage-colony stimulating factor (rhGM-CSF) and autologous melanoma vaccine mediate tumor regression in patients with metastatic melanoma. *J Immunother* 1999; 22: 166–74.
39. von Wussow P, Block B, Hartmann F, Deicher H, Intralesional interferon-alpha therapy in advanced malignant melanoma. *Cancer* 1988; 61: 1071–4.
40. Gutwald JG, Groth W, Mahrle G, Peritumoral injections of interleukin 2 induce tumour regression in metastatic malignant melanoma. *Br J Dermatol* 1994; 130: 541–2.
41. Retsas S, Leslie M, Bottomley D, Intralesional tumour necrosis factor combined with interferon gamma in metastatic melanoma. *BMJ* 1989; 298: 1290–1.
42. Guilloux Y, Lucas S, Brichard VG et al, A peptide recognized by human cytolytic T lymphocytes on HLA-A2 melanomas is encoded by an intron sequence of the *N*-acetylglucosaminyltransferase V gene. *J Exp Med* 1996; 183: 1173–83.
43. Valmori D, Dutoit V, Rubio-Grody V et al, Frequent cytolytic T-cell responses to peptide MAGE-A10(254–262) in melanoma. *Cancer Res* 2001; 61: 509–12.

44. Rosenberg SA, Yang JC, Schwartzentruber DJ et al, Immunologic and therapeutic evaluation of a synthetic peptide vaccine for the treatment of patients with metastatic melanoma. *Nat Med* 1998; 4: 321–7.
45. Thomas WD, Hersey P, TNF-related apoptosis-inducing ligand (TRAIL) induces apoptosis in Fas ligand-resistant melanoma cells and mediates CD4 T cell killing of target cells. *J Immunol* 1998; 161: 2195–200.
46. Thomas WD, Zhang XD, Franco AV, Nguyen T, Hersey P, TNF-related apoptosis-inducing ligand-induced apoptosis of melanoma is associated with changes in mitochondrial membrane potential and perinuclear clustering of mitochondria. *J Immunol* 2000; 165: 5612–20.
47. MacDonald G, Shi L, Vande Velde C, Lieberman J, Greenberg AH, Mitochondria-dependent and -independent regulation of granzyme B-induced apoptosis. *J Exp Med* 1999; 189: 131–43.
48. Sutton VR, Davis JE, Cancilla M et al, Initiation of apoptosis by granzyme B requires direct cleavage of bid, but not direct granzyme B-mediated caspase activation. *J Exp Med* 2000; 192: 1403–13.
49. Nicholson DW, From bench to clinic with apoptosis-based therapeutic agents. *Nature* 2000; 407: 810–16.
50. Jansen B, Schlagbauer-Wadl H, Brown BD et al, bcl-2 antisense therapy chemosensitizes human melanoma in SCID mice. *Nat Med* 1998; 4: 232–4.
51. Frost PJ, Butterfield LH, Dissette VB, Economou JS, Bonavide B, Immunosensitization of melanoma tumor cells to non-MHC Fas-mediated killing by MART-1-specific CTL cultures. *J Immunol* 2001; 166: 3564–73.
52. Matsuzaki H, Schmied BM, Ulrich A et al, Combination of tumor necrosis factor-related apoptosis-inducing ligand (TRAIL) and actinomycin D induces apoptosis even in TRAIL-resistant human pancreatic cancer cells. *Clin Cancer Res* 2001; 7: 407–14.
53. Teicher BA, Ara G, Herbst R, Palombella VJ, Adams J, The proteasome inhibitor PS-341 in cancer therapy. *Clin Cancer Res* 1999; 5: 2638–45.
54. Franco AV, Zhang XD, Van Berkel E et al, The role of NF-κB in TNF-related apoptosis-inducing ligand (TRAIL)-induced apoptosis of melanoma cells. *J Immunol* 2001; 166: 5337–45.
55. Weisenburger TH et al, Active specific intralymphatic immunotherapy in metastatic malignant melanoma: evidence of clinical response. *J Biol Response Modifiers* 1982; 1: 57–66.
56. Phillips NC, Loutfi A, A-Kareem AM, Shibata HR, Baines MG, Clinical evaluation of liposomal tumor antigen vaccines in patients with stage-III melanoma. *Cancer Detec Prev* 1990; 14: 491–5.
57. Eton O, Kharkevitch DD, Gianan MA et al, Active immunotherapy with ultraviolet B-irradiated autologous whole melanoma cells plus DETOX in patients with metastatic melanoma. *Clin Cancer Res* 1998; 1: 619–27.
58. Adler A, Schachter J, Barenholz Y et al, Allogeneic human liposomal melanoma vaccine with or without IL-2 in metastatic melanoma patients: clinical and immunobiological effects. *Cancer Biother* 1995; 10: 293–306.
59. Stopeck AT, Hersh EM, Akporiaye ET et al, Phase I study of direct gene transfer of an allogeneic histocompatibility antigen, HLA-B7, in patients with metastatic melanoma. *J Clin Oncol* 1997; 15: 341–9.
60. Marchand M, van Baren N, Weynants P et al, Tumor regressions observed in patients with metastatic melanoma treated with an antigenic peptide encoded by gene MAGE-3 and presented by HLA-A1. *Int J Cancer* 1999; 80: 219–30.
61. Rosenberg SA, Zhai Y, Yang JC et al, Immunizing patients with metastatic melanoma using recombinant adenoviruses encoding MART-1 or gp100 melanoma antigens. *J Natl Cancer Inst* 1998; 90: 1894–900.
62. Jaeger E, Bernhard H, Romero P et al, Generation of cytotoxic T-cell responses with synthetic melanoma-associated peptides in vivo: implications for tumor vaccines with melanoma-associated antigens. *Int J Cancer* 1996; 66: 162–9.
63. Weber JS, Hua FL, Spears L et al, A phase I trial of an HLA-A1 restricted MAGE-3 epitope peptide with incomplete Freund's adjuvant in patients with resected high-risk melanoma. *J Immunother* 1999; 22: 431–40.
64. Wang F, Bade E, Kuniyoshi C et al, Phase I trial of a MART-1 peptide vaccine with incomplete Freund's adjuvant for resected high-risk melanoma. *Clin Cancer Res* 1999; 5: 2756–65.
65. Cebon JS, Jaeger E, Gibbs P et al, Phase I studies of immunization with Melan-A and IL-12 in HLA A2+ positive patients with stage III and IV malignant melanoma. *Proc ASCO* 1999; 18: 434a (abstract).
66. Scheibenbogen C, Schmittel A, Keilholz U et al, Vaccination with tyrosinase peptides and GM-CSF in metastatic melanoma: a phase II trial. *Proc ASCO* 1999; 18: 436a (abstract).
67. Nestle FO, Alijagic S, Gilliet M et al, Vaccination of melanoma patients with peptide- or tumor lysate-pulsed dendritic cells. *Nat Med* 1998; 4: 328–32.
68. Hu X, Chakraborty NG, Sporn JR et al, Enhancement of cytolytic T lymphocyte precursor frequency in melanoma patients following immunization with the MAGE-1 peptide loaded antigen presenting cell-based vaccine. *Cancer Res* 1996; 56: 2479–83.
69. Chakraborty N, Tortora A, Sporn J et al, Melanoma cell lysate loaded autologous antigen presenting cell (APC) as a vaccine in melanoma. *Proc Am Assoc Cancer Res* 1997; 38: 400.
70. Ranieri E, Kierstead LS, Zarour H et al, Dendritic cell/peptide cancer vaccines: clinical responsiveness and epitope spreading. *Immunol Invest* 2000; 29: 121–5.
71. Thurner B, Haendle I, Roder C et al, Vaccination with Mage-3A1 peptide-pulsed mature, monocyte-derived dendritic cells expands specific cytotoxic T cells and induces regression of some metastases in advanced stage IV melanoma. *J Exp Med* 1999; 190: 1669–78.
72. Gajewski TF, Fallarino F, Vogelzang N et al, Effective melanoma antigen vaccination without dendritic cells (DC): a phase I study of immunization with Mage3 or Melan-A peptide-pulsed autologous PBMC plus RhIL-12. *Proc ASCO* 1999; 18: 539a (abstract).
73. Panelli MC, Wunderlich J, Jeffries J et al, Phase I study in patients with metastatic melanoma of immunization with dendritic cells presenting epitopes derived from the melanoma-associated antigens MART-1 and gp100. *J Immunother* 2000; 23: 487–98.

58

Gene therapy of melanoma

Giorgio Parmiani, Piero Dalerba

INTRODUCTION

Over the last decade techniques have become available that allow the transfer of genes from one cell to another, along with the control of expression of such genes. These techniques, and the information acquired on the molecular mechanisms of neoplastic transformation, have made it possible to introduce normal genes into tumour cells that have lost or mutated their oncosuppressor gene(s) or other genes involved in the control of proliferation and progression. This represents the more direct form of gene therapy of cancer, so-called gene replacement therapy, aimed at restoring normal mechanisms of cell growth control. Such an approach, however, suffers from the difficulty of having to identify the appropriate genes in at least a fraction of human tumours. In fact, while loss or mutation of genes like p53 and p16 are common, and their replacement in tumour cells may result in growth inhibition in vitro or in vivo, e.g. with non-small cell lung cancer (NSCLC) or head-and-neck (H/N) cancers, for a variety of other neoplasms, e.g. melanoma, it is not clear which gene(s) should be replaced.

In such a situation, an alternative therapeutic approach has been devised in which target neoplastic cells are transduced with genes encoding non-mammalian enzymes endowed with the property of metabolizing a prodrug into a cytotoxic compound. These enzymes are absent or inefficient in both normal and neoplastic mammalian cells (enzyme/prodrug or 'suicide' gene therapy).

A third possible strategy, conceptually similar to suicide gene therapy, is the modulation of susceptibility to anticancer drugs by gene transfer.

In all these approaches, however, the major limitation lies in the in vivo targeting or delivery of gene expression. Reaching each individual tumour cell of a metastatic lesion growing in a visceral organ, such as lung or liver, remains an almost impossible task, and even when the tumour is targeted there is no guarantee that 100% of cells will receive the therapeutic transgene. Such an apparent drawback appears less dramatic at the single-cell level in the enzyme/prodrug strategy thanks to the bystander effect, a phenomenon by which even cells that did not receive the gene coding for the metabolizing enzyme can be killed by the activated drug that diffuses from nearby gene-transduced cells.

An additional indirect strategy to hit tumour cells, even at distant sites, without killing normal counterparts is that of eliciting an immune response against tumours, since the immune system is equipped with effector lymphocytes endowed with the ability to travel throughout the body and discriminate molecules (antigens) expressed by neoplastic cells and not by normal tissues. To help the immune system of cancer patients to react against tumour cells that usually escape the immune attack, genes can be inserted into neoplastic or normal cells in order to increase their immunogenicity. Such cells will then be used to construct cellular vaccines. Most studies have focused on gene manipulation of either tumour cells or dendritic cells (DC). Moreover, genetic manipulations are possible that can modify normal patients' lymphocytes to make them more specific for tumour cells, allowing these reagents to be used in the adoptive immunotherapy of cancer. Overall, these approaches are known as immunological gene therapy of cancer.

To transfer the gene of interest (transgene) into target cells one needs an appropriate vector, which can be viral (such as adenovirus, adeno-associated virus, retrovirus, herpesvirus, pox virus) or non-viral (such as cationic liposomes, plasmid DNA, etc.). Several types of vectors have been constructed with different features and these are used according to the genetic profile of the tumour, site of tumour growth and gene therapy approach. In addition to direct in vivo administration, genes can be transduced either in vitro or ex vivo, i.e. removing the prospective recipient's cells from the body, culturing them in vitro and reinjecting the gene-modified cells into the patient.

STRATEGIES FOR VARIOUS STAGES OF DISEASE

Several stages have been defined by histopathology and biomolecular markers in the progression of melanoma, starting from early cutaneous lesions (with horizontal tumour growth) through to vertical tumour growth and metastases.[1] Since the vast majority of primary melanomas are cured by surgery, only metastases in stage IV patients are usually the focus of therapeutic interventions. Needless to say, visceral metastases or in transit subcutaneous lesions represent the most dangerous, and often incurable, forms of the disease. Considering the many possible strategies of gene therapy, one should select the most appropriate for each step of melanoma progression or, more importantly, for the localization of the lesions that need to be attacked. The situation is complicated by the fact that frequently both visceral and subcutaneous lesions are simultaneously present in the same patient and different organs can be involved, including the brain.

One may thus consider an approach that includes a direct injection of the transgene into inoperable subcutaneous or other easily accessible lesions by different vectors or plasmid DNA, a procedure which has been shown to result in regression of human melanoma tumours growing in nude mice after adenovirus-mediated herpes simplex thymidine kinase (HSV-tk) intratumour gene transfer and ganciclovir (GCV) administration.[2] Direct intratumoral gene transfer using cationic lipid-complexed plasmid DNA coding for interleukin (IL)-2 has been performed by Clark and co-workers,[3] who injected human melanomas growing in severe combined immunodeficiency (SCID) mice and found that IL-2 transgene expression increased in a DNA dose-dependent manner.

Clinical studies (see Table 58.1) have been carried out by the intratumour route using an allogeneic *HLA-B7* gene with the aim of inducing an alloimmune reaction at the tumour site that could translate into a destruction of autologous tumour cells as well. The authors showed that the anti-allo reaction against HLA-B7 was accompanied by systemic T cell reactivity in a proportion of patients.[4] However, no major clinical responses were noted in this small study. A subsequent trial with the use of HLA-B7 in a larger group of metastatic melanoma patients was then carried out. This study recorded one complete and six mixed responses out of 17 treated melanoma patients; toxicity at the injection site included pain and haemorrhage.[5] In another small trial, seven melanoma patients received intratumoral granulocyte macrophage colony-stimulating factor (GM-CSF) by means of a recombinant vaccinia virus that resulted in one complete, one partial and three mixed responses.[6] Using a similar approach, IL-2 or interferon (IFN)-γ genes have been given intratumorally by different vectors, again with negligible clinical results.[7–9] Overall, the local clinical response in these trials was limited, even though it was possible to inject melanoma metastases directly.

More difficult is to devise an efficient method of transferring a therapeutic gene into distant, visceral lesions given the unsolved problem of in vivo targeting (see below). However, animal models have shown that by using a tissue-specific promoter of melanocyte-specific genes like tyrosinase, one can obtain a fairly good expression of the transgene (e.g. HSV-tk) by using either retroviral or adenoviral vectors.[10,11] (For further details see below.)

GENE REPLACEMENT

Animal models and clinical trials

The possibility of restoring normal growth in melanoma cells by interfering with cancer genes, or replacing mutated or deleted tumour-suppressor genes,

Table 58.1 *Summary of clinical responses observed in melanoma patients treated in immunological gene therapy trials based on gene manipulation of tumour cells*

Transduction strategy	Transduced gene*	Study phase	No. of patients	Local response†	Clinical responses‡						Reference number
					PD	SD	MNR	MXR	PR	CR	
Intratumour injection	HLA-B7	I	5	1	4			1§			4
	HLA-B7	I	14	7	13					1‖	5
	IL-2	I	15	5	15						7
	IL-2	I–II	16	4	12	3			1‖		8
	IFN-γ	I	17	4	8	8		1§			9
	GM-CSF	I–II	7	5	2			3§	1§	1§	6
Total			74	26	54	11		5	2	2	
Autologous cell line	IL-2	I	12		8	4					41
	IL-2	I	14		9	4		1			42
	IL-7	I	8		2	4		2			43
	IL-12	I	6		2	3	1				44
	IFN-γ	I	5		4	1¶					45
	GM-CSF	I–II	21		13	3	3	1	1		46
Allogeneic cell line	IL-2	I–II	12		7	2		3			47
	IL-2	I–II	33		21	7		3	1	1	48
	IL-4	I–II	12		9	1		2			49
Total			123		75	29	4	12	2	1	

* HLA, human leucocyte antigen; IL, interleukin; IFN, interferon; GM-CSF, granulocyte–macrophage colony-stimulating factor;
† Response of the injected tumour lesion.
‡ PD, progression of disease; SD, stable disease; MNR, minor response; MXR, mixed response; PR, partial response; CR, complete response.
§ Complete response of the injected tumour lesion and of one or more untreated metastases.
‖ Complete or partial response due to a local response only.
¶ Stable disease after surgical resection of multiple visceral metastases.

appears difficult at the present time insomuch as no genes have been identified that are involved with high frequency in the neoplastic transformation of melanocytes. For example, *p16 (INK4A)* has been reported to be deleted or altered in familial and, much less frequently, sporadic human melanomas, but such an event usually occurs in <10% of cases,[12] whereas *N-Ras* mutations have been described in up to 15% of sporadic tumours, particularly in those originating in heavily ultraviolet (UV) irradiated body sites.[13] The role of p53 deletion, mutation or overexpression has not been clearly defined in human melanoma, where these alterations are usually rare or absent in primary lesions but possibly have an increased frequency in metastases.[14,15] Even in animal models, melanocyte neoplastic transformation is difficult to achieve. Only recently, melanomas have been induced by complex genetic manipulations of mice, such as in H-RasVal12 (mutated at position 12) transgenic (tg) animals in which the oncogene was placed under the tyrosinase promoter, leading to the selective expression of the *ras* transgene in melanocytes. However, even these animals failed to develop melanomas unless treated with a chemical carcinogen. Only by mating these mice with another mouse line in which the homozygous *p16* genes had been knocked out, could a high frequency of melanoma be obtained; however, the maintenance of *H-Ras* expression was required.[16] Studies with these animals suggest that neoplastic transformation of melanocytes is a multifactorial process involving different genes, most of which are still to be identified. Thus, at the moment, neither human nor animal studies provide sufficient information as to whether deletion of a specific, well-known gene (or genes) occurs during melanomagenesis, thus preventing the implementation of an efficient strategy of gene replacement therapy in such a disease.

Clinical application of this approach therefore appears premature. However, a small study in which an adenoviral vector was used to reintroduce wild-type p53 by intratumour injections in p53 functionally altered lesions of five melanoma patients has recently been carried out.[17] After 48 hours from the last injection, metastases of four out of five patients were found to express the transgene, but this was not accompanied by a clinically relevant effect.

ENZYME PRODRUG ACTIVATION

Animal studies

As described in the above sections, genes coding for specific enzymes can be inserted into tumour cells to confer the ability to metabolize a prodrug into a tumour cytotoxic compound, leading to the 'suicide' of cancer cells. The most common systems of enzyme/prodrug combinations that have been adopted in the gene therapy of different types of experimental and human cancers are HSV-tk/GCV and cytosine deaminase/5-fluorocytosine (CD/5-FC). In the first system, GCV is phosphorylated by tk and converted to an intermediate that blocks DNA synthesis and kills proliferating cells. This killing is then amplified by the bystander effects by which surrounding tumour cells can be destroyed, even when not targeted by the *tk* gene, due to diffusion of the phosphorylated GCV from gene-transduced tumour cells.[18] In the CD/5-FC system, the CD enzyme converts the non-toxic 5-FC into the potent anticancer drug 5-fluorouracil (5-FU).

Mouse studies have been carried out to test the efficacy of the HSV-tk/GCV combination in the B16 murine melanoma. Of particular interest are the results reported by Vile and co-workers,[10] who used the HSV-tk gene driven by a tyrosinase (i.e. melanocyte-specific) promoter that allowed not only a local treatment but also a systemic therapy to be carried out with high titred retroviral supernatants that rendered lung melanoma metastases sensitive to the drug, leading to a significant tumour growth inhibition after injection of GCV. It was also noted that the extent of the therapeutic effect was dependent on a functional immune system, since cures were reduced in athymic mice. This effect was further explored by the same group of investigators, who showed that a local destruction of murine melanoma nodules through the HSV-tk/GCV combination can generate a systemic immune response mediated by the local release of T cell helper (Th)1-type cytokines that, in turn, can cause the rejection of distant, non-transduced metastases.[19] Similar results were obtained by transducing the B16 melanoma with the *HSV-tk* gene by an adenoviral vector, either in vitro or in vivo by local intratumour administration followed by systemic GCV.[2]

Another system, which includes the *Escherichia coli* purine nucleoside phosphorylase and the non-toxic drug 6-methylpurine-deoxyriboside converted into the toxic 6-methylpurine, was tested in human melanoma cells in vitro. This study showed a strong tumour cell killing with a bystander toxicity estimated to be of at least 100 untransduced cells killed by each cell expressing the enzyme driven by a tyrosinase-specific promoter region.[20] Human melanoma lines were also used after xenotransplantation into athymic nude mice as targets of adenoviral vectors bearing the *HSV-tk* gene: systemic administration of GCV to melanoma-bearing animals resulted in significant, though often not complete, tumour regression,[21] even when the vector contained melanocyte-specific promoters.[11]

Clinical trials

With this kind of rationale a phase I–II clinical study was carried out by Klatzmann and co-workers.[22] They used a retroviral vector to insert the *HSV-tk* gene into subcutaneous nodules of metastatic melanoma patients who then received GCV systemically for 14 days. The transgene was detected in the injected melanoma lesions, but only in three of the six patients treated. No clear clinical responses were observed, but in three patients >50% necrosis was detected on histological examination of the resected metastases. The authors concluded that the weak clinical response was likely to be due to poor gene transfer efficiency.

Modulation of susceptibility to anticancer drugs by gene transfer

This is an entirely new approach in the gene therapy of cancer. Based on the new knowledge that several genes can affect susceptibility of tumour cells to anticancer drugs, attempts have been made to increase the response of melanoma cells to compounds to which this tumour is usually rather resistant. In fact, Pehamberger and coworkers[23] have shown that inhibition of Bcl-2 expression by antisense oligonucleotides substantially increases the susceptibility of human melanoma lines growing in SCID mice to cisplatin. Moreover, transduction of IFN-α into melanoma lines upregulates p53, decreases Bcl-2 expression and enhances cisplatin-induced apoptosis.[24] In this study, cisplatin administration to nude mice bearing 3-day-old human melanoma producing IFN-α resulted in complete regression, while only a partial tumour inhibition was observed upon cisplatin treatment of mice bearing parental tumours. Thus, it appears that a better knowledge of mechanisms that influence the reaction of tumour cells to various chemicals may be exploited to increase, by gene manipulation, the susceptibility of melanoma to anticancer drugs.

GENE-MODIFIED TUMOUR CELL VACCINES

Animal models

In mouse models, cellular vaccines have proved effective in immunization against cancer when strongly immunogenic neoplasms were used, such as chemically induced sarcomas or virus-induced tumours. However, spontaneous tumours of mice and rats were found to be weakly immunogenic or non-immunogenic in in vivo transplantation assays. Therefore, strategies were devised to increase such low or absent immunogenicity, which is thought to occur with most human tumours. Hitherto, two systems based on gene modification of prospective cellular vaccines have proved particularly effective: (a) transduction of tumour cells with cytokines (i.e. IL-2, IL-3, IL-4, IL-5, IL-7, IL-12, IFN-α or -γ, IL-12, GM-CSF, G-CSF); (b) transduction of tumour cells with costimulatory molecules (i.e. B7.1, B7.2, CD40 ligand (L)). Some authors have also envisaged a synergistic combination of the two approaches (reviewed in reference 25).

Tumour cells transduced with cytokines display powerful immunizing properties in mice. After in vivo injection of living tumour cells, cytokine release leads to recruitment of inflammatory cells that cause a direct or indirect destruction of at least a fraction of the tumour cells. It is noteworthy that the kinetics and cellular composition of the inflammatory infiltrate may vary significantly with different cytokines (see reference 26). The end result, however, is similar in most tumour models, with regression of the growing tumour, accompanied by a systemic immunization against both transduced and parental neoplastic cells, the degree of such immunization being dependent on the antigenic strength of the tumour (see reference 27). Debulking of the primary cytokine-secreting tumour is strongly dependent on neutrophils and other non-specific effectors, whereas systemic immune memory is mediated by CD8+ T lymphocytes.[26] Systemic immunization appears to rely on an indirect mechanism of cross-priming, with the debulking inflammatory reaction elicited by the cytokine allowing tumour destruction and subsequent antigen release. Antigens are then taken up by professional antigen-presenting cells (APC) that activate a protective CD8+ T cell memory response (Figure 58.1).

This approach has proved effective in the prophylactic setting, where different tumours releasing cytokines like IL-2, IL-4 and IL-12 displayed good immunizing properties and provided full protection against subsequent challenges with the same tumour. Results have been less convincing in the therapeutic setting, where mice are immunized after tumour cell injection. Cytokines that, once secreted by certain tumours, show the most powerful therapeutic activity are IL-2, IL-12 and GM-CSF.[26,28–30] In most cases, however, the therapeutic success is difficult to define, since vaccination with cytokine-engineered tumour cells was able to eradicate only small, 3–10-day-old tumours and only in a fraction of treated animals.

An alternative strategy to enhance tumour immunogenicity is to provide neoplastic cells with costimulatory molecules, i.e. membrane proteins usually expressed by APC and able to facilitate activation of naive T cells upon simultaneous encounter with the appropriate major histocompatibility complex (MHC)–peptide complex. The aim of this approach is to confer to tumour cells the properties of APC that can prime and/or boost tumour-specific naive or memory T lymphocytes. Gene transduction with B7.1 has proved effective in several mouse models.[31] Disappointing results have been reported with the B16 murine melanoma or MCA102 sarcoma that do not express, or have downregulated expression of class I MHC molecules and are thus resistant to T cell attack.[31] It is

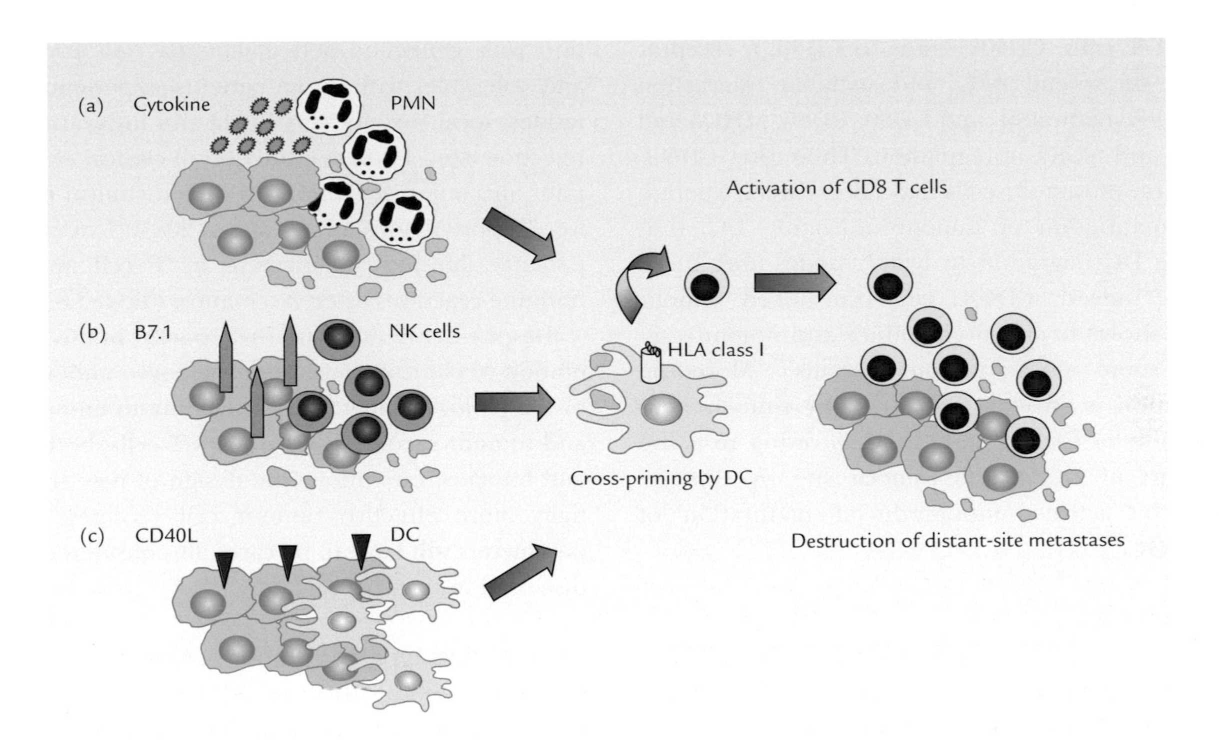

Figure 58.1 *Vaccination strategies based on gene manipulation of tumour cells all rely on the activation of a memory CD8 T cell response through cross-priming by antigen presenting cells, like dendritic cells (DC). (a) Tumour cells (green cells) transduced with cytokines (purple stars) recruit a powerful inflammatory infiltrate, usually composed of neutrophils (PMN). The cytokine-induced inflammatory reaction destroys the cytokine-producing tumour mass, releasing antigens that are captured by DC, processed and presented to CD8 T cells in association with human leucocyte antigen (HLA) class I molecules. (b) A similar mechanism is probably involved in the case of B7.1–transduced tumour cells, where B7.1 (orange pikes) activates natural killer (NK) cells and promotes tumour cell lysis and antigen release, followed by cross-priming by DC. (c) In the case of CD40 ligand (L) -transduced tumour cells, tumour cells directly induce maturation of tumour-infiltrating DC through CD40L (red triangles), and thus promote their migration to lymph nodes. Once CD8 T cells are primed by DC, they can reach distant-site metastases through blood circulation and can provide systemic protection against the parental tumour to the vaccinated host.*

noteworthy that B7.1 molecules can directly activate a subset of natural killer (NK) cells through binding of CD28,[32] leading to speculation that B7.1 may work through NK cell-mediated tumour destruction followed by APC presentation of tumour antigens and cross-priming of T cells (Figure 58.1).[33] B7.1 Transduction in human melanoma cells was also able to increase their immunogenicity in vitro.[34]

Similar to B7.1 in molecular structure, but different in function, B7.2 has also been used, but conflicting data have been reported on its ability to increase immunogenicity of tumour cells.[35,36] This makes it difficult to assess the use of this molecule in the construction of cellular gene-modified vaccines.

Tumour cells transduced with CD40 ligand (CD40L).

CD40L is a membrane protein expressed mainly by activated CD4 T cells. CD40L binds to CD40, a receptor expressed on several APC, and such an interaction induces APC maturation and CD80, CD86, MHC-I and -II, CD83 and CCR7 upregulation. Therefore, CD40L transduction of tumour cells may allow direct, tumour-induced maturation of tumour-infiltrating DC, thus promoting DC migration to lymph nodes and T cell activation. Indeed, CD40L gene-transduced tumour cells were shown to effectively induce antitumour resistance in some mouse tumour systems.[37] Moreover, immunization is strongly enhanced by simultaneous coexpression of CD40L and GM-CSF, owing to active recruitment of DC at the tumour site by GM-CSF followed by active tumour-induced maturation of recruited DC.[38]

Clinical studies

Several clinical trials based on gene-modified cellular vaccines have been performed or are underway in melanoma patients.[39] Hitherto, two main approaches have been pursued, focusing on transduction of cytokine genes into either autologous or allogeneic melanoma lines. Autologous cell lines have some important advantages insomuch as they do not induce immunization against allo-HLA and potentially express the full repertoire of tumour antigens of a patient's cancer cells, including 'unique' antigens that have been shown to be the most immunogenic, at least in mouse models.[40] However, the use of autologous gene-modified melanoma cells as a vaccine is seriously limited by the low frequency of success (40–50%) and the high cost of vaccine production. Many patients eventually cannot be treated, either because the tumour line cannot be established or because of disease progression during vaccine preparation. On the contrary, the use of allogeneic melanoma lines allows preventive safety certification and careful standardization of their biological and pharmacological properties (i.e. antigenic profile, transgene expression, level of cytokine production), thus securing rapid treatment of all patients. A disadvantage of allogeneic lines may lie in the lack of immunogenic, unique antigens.

Results are available from clinical trials based on: (a) autologous cell lines transduced with genes coding for IL-2,[41,42] IL-7,[43] IL-12,[44] IFN-γ[45] or GM-CSF;[46] (b) on allogeneic lines transduced with genes coding for IL-2[47,48] or IL-4[49] (see Table 58.1). In all these studies, vaccination with gene-modified melanoma cells proved safe and tolerable, with most patients experiencing only modest local toxicity (erythema and induration at the injection site). However, the overall clinical efficacy was poor and only a few minor or mixed clinical responses were reported, with an average of 20–30% of vaccinated patients showing an increase in T cell antitumour immune reactions after vaccination (Table 58.1).[39]

Despite the limited success reported in this first generation of clinical trials, the progressive understanding of the biological mechanisms leading to immunization and tumour recognition by host's T cells, both in mice and humans, now allows the design of new and potentially more effective tumour cell vaccines.[50] Several parameters will have to be carefully considered and are discussed in turn below.

Amount and type of tumour antigens

New cellular vaccines should be selected for high expression of known tumour antigens, especially of the most immunogenic ones, either shared or individual. Vectors encoding tumour antigens could be used to increase the load of tumour-specific antigens. However, no clear information is available on a dose-dependent effect of vaccination with cellular vaccines.

Amount and type of cytokine

Vaccines should be designed to produce high quantities of selected cytokines that have shown powerful immunizing activity and high efficacy in the therapeutic setting in mouse models. Hitherto, cytokines that have shown the most promising immunological and therapeutic profile in mouse models are IL-2, IL-12 and GM-CSF. Since the use of living tumour cells is unacceptable in humans, future efforts should focus on strategies to obtain high levels of cytokine production by irradiated tumour cells. Levels of cytokine production should be carefully assessed, and vectors should be designed to obtain maximal release, since irradiated cytokine gene-engineered tumour cells are less effective than living ones, probably because of the lack of tumour growth and lower in vivo cytokine production.[28] However, it has been reported in a mouse model that an excess of IL-2 release by gene-transduced tumour cells may impair the antitumour efficacy of the vaccine,[51] although it is difficult to extrapolate from animal models to humans in terms of the dose effect of cytokine release.

Costimulatory molecules

Tumour cell vaccines could also be engineered to express costimulatory molecules such as B7.1. The true mechanism of the increased immunogenicity conferred by such molecules is not completely clear (see above). However, the expression of B7.1 can provide the tumour cell with functions leading to expansion of melanoma-specific T cells at the local site, at least in those melanoma patients (40–50%) who appear to have been previously primed by tumour antigens.[52]

Selection of patients

Future clinical trials should enrol patients whose tumours express a detectable level of class I human leucocyte antigen (HLA) in the lesions to be targeted by T cells. In fact, HLA loss or downregulation is commonly observed in human melanoma,[53] though its clinical impact remains uncertain[54] and, therefore, patient selection is necessary for a clear evaluation of the clinical efficacy of vaccines.

GENE-MODIFIED DENDRITIC CELL VACCINES

DC are professional APC particularly effective in stimulating naive T cells. Since DC play a key role in the process of immunization against tumour antigens, several authors have envisaged the use of DC transduced with genes coding for tumour-associated antigens (TAA) as a strategy to obtain direct, rapid and efficient activation of tumour-specific T lymphocytes (reviewed in reference 55). *In vitro* studies clearly show that human DC transduced with genes encoding TAA can process and present the antigen in association with both class I and II HLA, and efficiently trigger activation and proliferation of antigen-specific CD4 and CD8 T cell clones. In vivo studies in mice showed that TAA gene-transduced DC efficiently immunized against related TAA, and that immunization could protect mice from subsequent challenges with TAA-bearing tumour cells and also be effective in a therapeutic setting.[56] DC transduced with TAA genes appear more effective than TAA-bearing tumour cells transduced with GM-CSF,[57] or than protein- or peptide-pulsed DC,[58] because gene transduction allows stable expression of both MHC class I and class II epitopes and, therefore, optimal CD4 T cell activation. Since DC pulsed with tumour lysates or TAA peptide epitopes have been used in melanoma patients with encouraging preliminary results,[59] the next step will be to assess immunizing and therapeutic potential of TAA-transduced DC. Hitherto, however, no data from clinical trials with DC genetically engineered to express human TAA are available.

ADOPTIVE IMMUNOTHERAPY WITH GENE-MODIFIED LYMPHOCYTES

Adoptive transfer of T cells has shown remarkable antitumour activity in animal models[60] and a certain activity even in cancer patients.[61,62] Tumour responses, however, are difficult to obtain reproducibly in high numbers of patients, especially in solid tumours like melanoma or renal cancer. High variability in functional properties of infused T cells,[63] low frequency of antitumour T cells in lymphocyte preparations,[61] defective trafficking of infused T cells to tumour sites and escape of the T cell response by the tumour owing to antigen-loss variants,[53] are all possible explanations of the high rate of failures observed in adoptive immunotherapy of melanoma. Recent developments in gene-transfer technology have offered new tools both to control undesired effects and to enhance tumour-specific targeting of adoptively transferred T cells.

Three main approaches aimed at modifying T cells for therapeutic purposes are currently under investigation, namely transduction of T cells with: (a) suicide genes; (b) genes coding for tumour-specific T cell receptors (TCR); and (c) genes encoding chimeric receptor molecules (Figure 58.2).

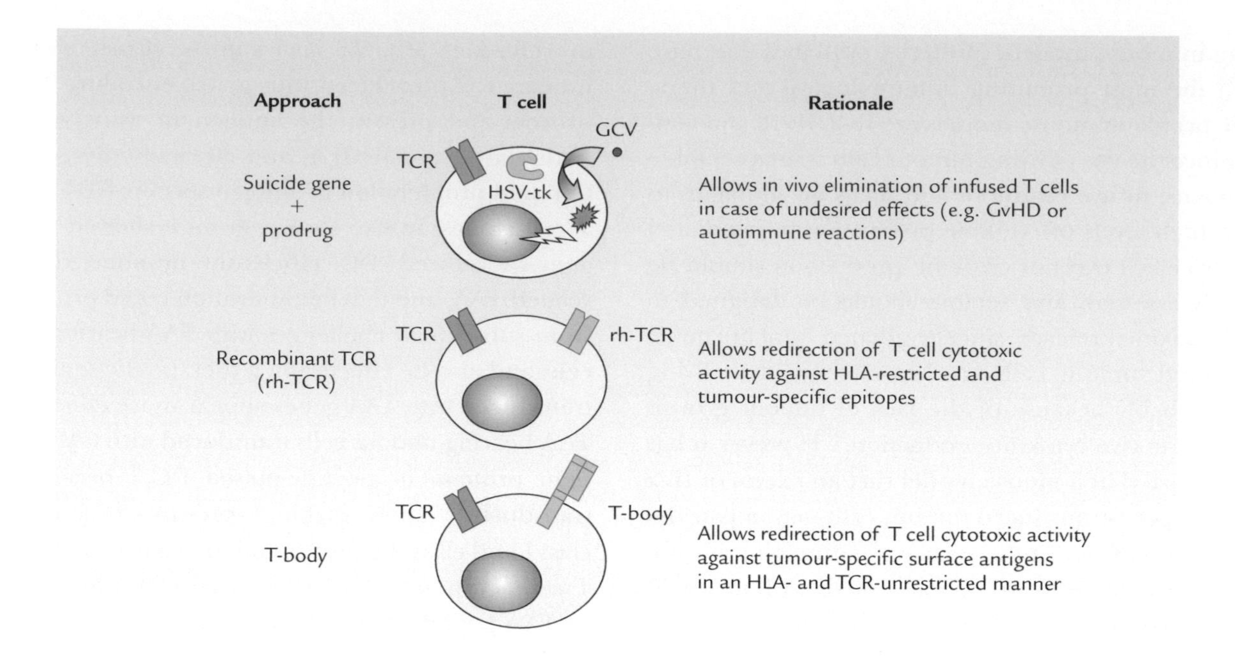

Figure 58.2 *Different approaches in adoptive immunotherapy with gene-modified lymphocytes.*

T cells engineered with suicide genes

One of the few clinical settings where adoptive T cell immunotherapy has gained a clear role in cancer treatment involves donor lymphocyte infusion (DLI) for the treatment of leukaemic relapse or Epstein-Barr virus-induced B cell lymphoproliferative disorders (EBV-BLPD) after allogeneic stem cell transplant (allo-SCT). DLI can induce complete molecular remission in 60–70% of relapsed chronic myeloid leukaemias, in 15–29% of relapsed acute myeloid leukaemias and in most EBV-BLPD.[62] The antitumour effect of DLI, however, is clearly correlated with graft versus host disease (GvHD), a severe and potentially life-threatening complication, where infused T cells of the donor recognize and attack normal tissues of the recipient.

An approach to obtain control of GvHD is the transduction of donor lymphocytes with a suicide gene encoding the HSV-tk that allows selective elimination of transduced cells upon administration of the prodrug GCV.[64]

In the long run, this approach could also be used in adoptive immunotherapy of melanoma and other solid tumours, especially if future developments allow the adoptive transfer of high numbers of tumour-specific T cells directed against self differentiation antigens. In such a case, the suicide gene technology could be useful in the control of potential and undesired autoimmune responses. Moreover, the idea to exploit graft-versus-tumour responses as a therapeutic tool in the context of allo-SCT is also currently under evaluation in solid tumours. A preliminary report in renal cancer shows the great potential of this approach.[65]

T cells engineered with recombinant T cell receptors

One of the major limitations of adoptive immunotherapy of solid tumours is the difficulty in obtaining high numbers of tumour-specific T cells to be infused into the patient. One possible strategy to circumvent the problem of specificity is to transduce unselected lymphocytes with genes encoding tumour antigen-specific TCR in an attempt to redirect against the tumour the cytotoxic activity of high numbers of T cells. Transduction of a gene coding for a functional TCR was obtained in a murine system, although it involved a tumour-unrelated antigen.[66] More recently, HLA-A2 transgenic mice were immunized with a human p53 peptide to generate T cells that recognized human tumours over-expressing mutated *p53*. Subsequently, a p53-specific murine TCR was cloned and expressed in naive recipient T cells, conferring upon them the ability to recognize tumours over-expressing p53 but not normal human fibroblasts.[67]

The experimental validation of this idea in a full human system has proven to be, technically, a difficult task. However, a retroviral vector has recently been designed that allows efficient transfer to peripheral blood lymphocytes (PBL) of a recombinant HLA-A2-restricted, Melan-A/MART-1_{27-35}-specific αβTCR, originally derived from a tumour-reactive T cell clone isolated from tumour-infiltrating lymphocytes (TIL) of a melanoma patient.[68] PBL transduced with the recombinant TCR acquired Melan-A/MART-1_{27-35}-specific reactivity, secreting IFN-γ and lysing target cells upon encounter with the target epitope. Similar results were obtained by using the TCR of a MAGE-3-specific T cell clone, although in this case the functional transgene was expressed in the Jurkat T cell lymphoma line.[69] Animal models and human clinical trials to evaluate in vivo activity of adoptive transfer of TCR gene-modified T cells are now eagerly awaited.

T cells engineered with chimeric T bodies

Tumour cells frequently downregulate expression of HLA class I molecules, thus avoiding recognition by tumour-specific T cells.[53] One interesting strategy to overcome immune escape by tumour cells could lie in providing T cells with artificial receptors, in an attempt to allow recognition of tumour cell-surface molecules which do not require presentation by HLA nor antigen-specific TCR. One of the best characterized examples of such artificial receptors are the so-called T bodies, chimeric receptors composed of antibody-derived single-chain variable fragments (scFv) as extracellular recognition domains, joined to the intracellular domains of the signalling subunits of different lymphocyte antigen receptors (e.g. the ζ chain of TCR, or the γ chain of Fc receptors).[70] The design of simple and functional T bodies that could easily be expressed in T cells and could effectively mediate T cell activation upon binding with target antigen, has required a long period of in vitro studies and testing of several different constructs.[70] The T body approach has also shown interesting activity in at least two animal tumour models.[71,72] Recent work by Bolhuis's group[73] has demonstrated that this approach is feasible, even in the human system. No published data are currently available on the use of T bodies in clinical trials but the time is now ripe for the first studies in melanoma patients.

However, the problem of harvesting in vitro the billions of T cells necessary to reach a number which may have a chance to target tumour cells growing in distant organs without impairing their function is not completely solved, although the use of antibodies, which help in triggering costimulatory molecules in addition to TCR, may expand tumour-specific T cells to clinically significant numbers.[74] Moreover, the use of tetramers now allows the selection and expansion of specific subsets of T cells, though it is not yet clear whether these effectors will maintain their function in vivo.[75]

CONCLUSIONS

Gene therapy of human melanoma has been carried out using several different approaches, outlined above. Overall results of the first generation of clinical trials with a limited number of patients are disappointing in terms of clinical response rates, although such studies have provided several useful pieces of information. Gene replacement therapy and modulation of susceptibility to anticancer drugs by gene manipulation remain important therapeutic options, as assessed from preclinical animal studies. However, the limited knowledge of the molecular mechanisms of melanomagenesis does not yet allow such approaches to be applied in the clinic in an effective way. Enzyme/prodrug suicide gene therapy remains a valid approach that is being tested more extensively in clinical trials. The limitations here are those of in vivo gene therapy in general, i.e. the in vivo targeting and specific delivery of the genes, which confer the prodrug metabolizing activity to melanoma cells. Further progress is expected from the immunological approaches of gene therapy, thanks to the remarkable advances in the understanding of the basic mechanisms of antitumour immunization and in vivo tumour killing by gene-modified T lymphocytes. Therefore, it is believed that gene therapy of melanoma remains a crucial area of investigation both at preclinical and clinical levels, with a realistic prospect of becoming a useful tool for the clinical management of this disease. The key points discussed in this chapter are listed in Box 58.1.

Box 58.1 ***Key points in the gene therapy of melanoma as discussed in this chapter***

Different approaches have been considered in the gene therapy of melanoma
Gene replacement therapy is not yet feasible due to a limited knowledge of genes involved in melanomagenesis
Enzyme/prodrug (suicide gene) therapy has been found to be effective in animal models but its clinical application in humans remains limited and needs further experimental validation. The same holds true for modulation of susceptibility to anticancer drugs by gene transfer
The largest number of gene therapy trials in melanoma patients deals with immunological gene therapy
Vaccination with gene (cytokine)-modified tumour cells has been applied in several trials, but with limited success at both the clinical and immunological level. However, recent progress in the understanding of the immune system's cellular and molecular circuitry today allows the design of a second generation of more effective cellular vaccines
A promising approach involves the use of gene-modified T lymphocytes to be used in adoptive immunotherapy. However, no clinical data are yet available in melanoma patients

REFERENCES

1. Meier F, Satyamoorthy K, Nesbit M et al, Molecular events in melanoma development and progression. *Front Biosci* 1998; 3: 1005–10.
2. Bonnekoh B, Greenhalgh DA, Bundman DS et al, Inhibition of melanoma growth by adenoviral-mediated HSV thymidine kinase gene transfer in vivo. *J Invest Dermatol* 1995; 104: 313–17.
3. Clark PR, Stopeck AT, Ferrari M et al, Studies of direct intratumoral gene transfer using cationic lipid-complex plasmid DNA. *Cancer Gene Ther* 2000; 7: 853–60.
4. Nabel GJ, Nabel EG, Yang Z-Y et al. Direct gene transfer with DNA-liposome complexes in melanoma: expression, biological activity, and lack of toxicity in humans. *Proc Natl Acad Sci USA* 1993; 90: 11307–11.
5. Stopeck AT, Hersh EM, Akporiaye ET et al, Phase I study of direct gene transfer of an allogeneic histocompatibility antigen, HLA-B7, in patients with metastastic melanoma. *J Clin Oncol* 1997; 15: 341–9.
6. Mastrangelo MJ, Maguire HC Jr, Eisenlohr LC et al, Intratumoral recombinant GM-CSF-encoding virus as gene therapy in patients with cutaneous melanoma. *Cancer Gene Ther* 1999; 6: 409–22.
7. Stewart AK, Lassam NJ, Quirt IC et al, Adenovector-mediated gene delivery of interleukin-2 in metastatic breast cancer and melanoma: results of a phase I clinical trial. *Gene Ther* 1999; 6: 350–63.
8. Galanis E, Hersh EM, Stopeck AT et al, Immunotherapy of advanced malignancy by direct gene transfer of an interleukin-2 DNA/DMRIE/DOPE lipid complex: Phase I/II experience. *J Clin Oncol* 1999; 17: 3313–23.
9. Nemunaitis J, Fong T, Burrows F et al, Phase I trial of interferon gamma retroviral vector administered intratumorally with multiple courses in patients with metastatic melanoma. *Hum Gene Ther* 1999; 10: 1289–98.
10. Vile RG, Nelson JA, Castleden S et al, Systemic gene therapy of murine melanoma using tissue specific expression of HSV/tk gene involves an immune component. *Cancer Res* 1994; 54: 6238–4.
11. Siders WM, Halloran PJ, Fenton RG, Melanoma-specific cytotoxicity induced by a tyrosinase promoter-enhancer/herpes simplex virus thymidine kinase adenovirus. *Cancer Gene Ther* 1998; 5: 281–91.
12. Castellano M, Parmiani G, Genes involved in melanoma: an overview of *INK4a* and other loci. *Melanoma Res* 1999; 9: 421–32.
13. van Elsas A, Zerp S, van der Flier S et al, Relevance of UV-induced N-ras oncogene point mutations in development of primary human cutaneous melanoma. *Am J Pathol* 1996; 149: 883–93.
14. Lubbe J, Reichel M, Burg G et al, Absence of p53 gene mutations in cutaneous melanoma. *J Invest Dermatol* 1994; 102: 819–21.
15. Akslen LA, Monstad SE, Larsen B et al, Frequent mutations of the p53 gene in cutaneous melanoma of the nodular type. *Int J Cancer* 1998; 79: 91–5.
16. Chin L, Tam A, Pomerantz J et al, Essential role for oncogenic Ras in tumour maintenance. *Nature* 1999; 400: 468–72.
17. Dummer R, Bergh J, Karlsson Y et al, Biological activity and safety of adenoviral vector-expressed wild type *p53* after intratumoral injection in melanoma and breast cancer patients with *p53*-overexpressing tumors. *Cancer Gene Ther* 2000; 7: 1069–76.
18. Freeman SM, Abboud CN, Whartenby KA et al, The 'bystander effect': tumor regression when a fraction of the tumor mass is genetically modified. *Cancer Res* 1993; 53: 5274–83.
19. Vile RG, Castleden S, Marshall J et al, Generation of an antitumour immune response in a non-immunogenic tumour: HSVtk killing in vivo stimulates a mononuclear cell infiltrate and a Th1–like profile of intratumoural cytokine expression. *Int J Cancer* 1997; 71: 267–74.
20. Hughes BW, Wells AH, Bebok Z et al, Bystander killing of melanoma cells using the human tyrosinase promoter to express the *Escherichia coli* purine nucleoside phosphorylase gene. *Cancer Res* 1995; 55: 3339–45.
21. Bonnekoh B, Greenhalgh DA, Bundman DS et al, Adenoviral-mediated herpes simplex virus-thymidine kinase gene transfer in vivo for treatment of experimental human melanoma. *J Inves Dermatol* 1996; 106: 1163–8.
22. Klatzmann D, Cherin P, Bensimon G et al, and Study Group on Gene Therapy of Metastatic Melanoma, A phase I/II dose-escalation study of herpes simplex virus type 1 thymidine kinase 'suicide' gene therapy for metastatic melanoma. *Hum Gene Ther* 1998; 9: 2585–94.
23. Jansen B, Schlagbauer-Wadl H, Brown BD et al, bcl-2 Antisense therapy chemosensitizes human melanoma in SCID mice. *Nat Med* 1998; 4: 232–4.
24. Mecchia M, Matarrrese P, Malorni W et al, Type I consensus interferon (CIFN) gene transfer into human melanoma cells up-regulates p53 and enhances cisplatin-induced apoptosis: implications for new therapeutic strategies with IFN-α. *Gene Ther* 2000; 7: 167–79.
25. Kuiper M, Sanches R, Bignon YJ et al, B7.1 and cytokines. Synergy in cancer gene therapy. *Adv Exp Med Biol* 2000; 465: 381–90.
26. Musiani P, Modesti A, Giovarelli M et al, Cytokines, tumour-cell death and immunogenicity: a question of choice. *Immunol Today* 1997; 18: 32–6.
27. Parmiani G, Colombo MP, Melani C et al, Cytokine gene transduction in the immunotherapy of cancer. *Adv Pharmacol* 1997; 40: 259–307.
28. Allione A, Consalvo M, Nanni P et al, Immunizing and curative potential of replicating and non replicating murine mammary adenocarcinoma cells engineered with interleukin (IL)-2, IL-4, IL-6, IL-7, IL-10, tumor necrosis factor-α, granulocyte-macrophage colony-stimulatng factor, and δ-interferon gene or admixed with conventional adjuvants. *Cancer Res* 1994; 54: 6022–6.
29. Dranoff G, Jaffee E, Lazenby A et al, Vaccination with irradiated tumor cells engineered to secrete murine granulocye-macrophage colony-stimulating factor stimulates potent, specific, and long-lasting anti-tumor immunity. *Proc Natl Acad Sci USA* 1993; 90: 3539–43.
30. Tahara H, Zitvogel L, Storkus WJ et al, Effective eradication of established murine tumors with IL-12 gene therapy using a polycistronic retroviral vector. *J Immunol* 1995; 154: 6466–74.
31. Chen L, McGowan P, Ashe S et al, Tumor immunogenicity determines the effect of B7 costimulation on T cell-mediated tumor immunity. *J Exp Med* 1994; 179: 523–32.

32. Azuma M, Cayabyab M, Buck D et al, Involvement of CD28 in MHC-unrestricted cytotoxicity mediated by a human natural killer leukemia cell line. *J Immunol* 1992; 149: 1115–23.
33. Huang AY, Bruce AT, Pardoll DM et al, Does B-7 expression confer antigen-presenting cell capacity to tumors in vivo? *J Exp Med* 1996; 183: 769–76.
34. Sulé-Suso J, Arienti F, Melani C et al, A B7–1 transfected human melanoma line stimulates proliferation and cytotoxicity of autologous and allogeneic lymphocytes. *Eur J Immunol* 1995; 25: 2737–42.
35. Matulonis FM, Dosiou C, Freeman G et al, B7–1 is superior to B7–2 costimulation in the induction and maintenance of T cell-mediated antileukemia immunity. Further evidence that B7–1 and B7–2 are functionally distinct. *J Immunol* 1996; 156: 1126–31.
36. Takahashi T, Hirano N, Chiba S et al, Immunogene therapy against mouse leukemia using B7 molecules. *Cancer Gene Ther* 2000; 144–50.
37. Grossman ME, Brown MP, Brenner MK, Antitumor responses induced by transgenic expression of CD40 ligand. *Human Gene Ther* 1997; 8: 1935–43.
38. Chiodoni C, Paglia P, Stoppacciaro A et al, Dendritic cells infiltrating tumors cotransduced with granulocyte-macrophage colony-stimulating factor (GM-CSF) and CD40 ligand genes take up and present endogenous tumor-associated antigens, and prime naive mice for a cytotoxic T lymphocyte response. *J Exp Med* 1999; 190: 125–33.
39. Parmiani G, Arienti F, Melani C et al, Gene therapy of melanoma methods in molecular medicine. In: *Melanoma methods and protocols* (ed Nickoloff BJ). Loyola University Medical Center, Maywood, IL: Humana Press Inc., 2001, vol 61: 203–22.
40. Dudley ME, Roopenian DC, Loss of a unique tumor antigen by cytotoxic T lymphocyte immunoselection from a 3-methylcholanthrene-induced mouse sarcoma reveals secondary unique and shared antigens. *J Exp Med* 1996; 184: 441–7.
41. Palmer K, Moore J, Everard M et al, Gene therapy with autologous, interleukin 2–secreting tumor cells in patients with malignant melanoma. *Hum Gene Ther* 1999; 10: 1261–8.
42. Schreiber S, Kampgen E, Wagner E et al, Immunotherapy of metastatic malignant melanoma by a vaccine consisting of autologous interleukin 2–transfected cancer cells. *Hum Gene Ther* 1999; 10: 983–93.
43. Moller P, Sun Y, Alijagic S et al, Vaccination with IL-7 gene-modified autologous melanoma cells can enhance the anti-melanoma lytic activity inperipheral blood of patients with a good clinical performance status: a clinical phase I study. *Br J Cancer* 1998; 77: 1907–16.
44. Sun Y, Jugovsky K, Moller P et al, Vaccination with IL-12 gene-modified autologous melanoma cells: preclinical results and first clinical phase I study. *Gene Ther* 1998; 5: 481–90.
45. Nemunaitis J, Bohart C, Fong T et al, Phase I trial of retroviral vector-mediated interferon (IFN)-gamma transfer into autologous tumor cells in patients with metastatic melanoma. *Cancer Gene Ther* 1998; 5: 292–300.
46. Soiffer R, Lynch T, Mihm M et al, Vaccination with irradiated autologous melanoma cells engineered to secrete human granulocyte-macrophage colony-stimulating factor generates potent antitumor immunity in patients with metastatic melanoma. *Proc Natl Acad Sci USA* 1998; 95: 13, 141–6.
47. Belli F, Arienti F, Sulé-Suso J et al, Active immunization of metastatic melanoma patients with interleukin-2–transduced allogeneic melanoma cells: evaluation of efficacy and tolerability. *Cancer Immunol Immunother* 1997; 44: 197–203.
48. Osanto S, Schiphorst PP, Weijl NI et al, Vaccination of melanoma patients with an allogeneic, genetically modified interleukin 2–producing melanoma cell line. *Hum Gene Ther* 2000; 11: 739–50.
49. Arienti F, Belli F, Napolitano F et al, Vaccination of melanoma patients with interleukin 4 gene-transduced allogeneic melanoma cells. *Hum Gene Ther* 1999; 2907–16.
50. Parmiani G, Rodolfo M, Melani C, Immunological gene therapy with ex vivo gene-modified tumor cells: a critique and a reappraisal. *Hum Gene Ther* 2000; 11: 1269–75.
51. Schmidt W, Schweighoffer T, Herbst E et al, Cancer vaccines: the interleukin 2 dosage effect. *Proc Natl Acad Sci USA* 1995; 4711–14.
52. Anichini A, Molla A, Mortarini R et al, An expanded peripheral T cell population to a cytotoxic T lymphocyte (CTL)-defined, melanocyte-specific antigen in metastatic melanoma patients impacts on generation of peptide-specific CTLs but does not overcome tumor escape from immune surveillance in metastatic lesions. *J Exp Med* 1999; 190: 651–67.
53. Marincola F, Jaffee EM, Hicklin DJ et al, Escape of human solid tumors from T cell recognition: molecular mechanisms and functional significance. *Adv Immunol* 2000; 74: 181–273.
54. Giacomini P, Giorda E, Fraioli R et al, Low prevalence of selective human leukocyte antigen (HLA)-A and HLA-B epitope losses in early-passage tumor cell lines. *Cancer Res* 1999; 59: 2657–67.
55. Kirk CJ, Mulè JJ, Gene-modified dendritic cells for use in tumor vaccines. *Hum Gene Ther* 2000; 11: 797–806.
56. Song W, Kong H-L, Carpenter H et al, Dendritic cells genetically modified with an adenovirus vector encoding the cDNA for a model antigen induce protective and therapeutic antitumor immunity. *J Exp Med* 1997; 186: 1247–56.
57. Klein C, Bueler H, Mulligan RC, Comparative analysis of genetically modified dendritic cells and tumor cells as therapeutic cancer vaccines. *J Exp Med* 2000; 191: 1699–708.
58. Schnell S, Young JW, Houghton AN et al, Retrovirally transduced mouse dendritic cells require CD4+ T cell help to elicit antitumor immunity: implications for the clinical use of dendritic cells. *J Immunol* 2000; 164: 1243–50.
59. Nestle F, Alijagic S, Gilliet M et al, Vaccination of melanoma patients with peptide- or tumor lysate-pulsed dendritic cells. *Nat Med* 1998; 4: 328–32.
60. Melief CJM, Kast M, T-cell immunotherapy of tumors by adoptive transfer of cytotoxic T lymphocytes and by vaccination with minimal essential epitopes. *Immunol Rev* 1995; 146: 167–77.
61. Rosenberg SA, Yannelli JR, Yang JC et al, Treatment of patients with metastatic melanoma with autologous tumor-infiltrating lymphocytes and interleukin-2. *J Natl Cancer Inst* 1994; 86: 1159–66.
62. Dazzi F, Goldman J, Donor lymphocyte infusions. *Curr Opin Hematol* 1999; 6: 394–9.
63. Parmiani G, An explanation of the variable clinical response to interleukin 2 and LAK cells. *Immunol Today* 1990; 11: 113–15.
64. Bonini C, Ferrari G, Verzeletti S et al, HSV-TK gene transfer into donor lymphocytes for control of allogeneic graft-versus-leukemia. *Science* 1997; 276: 1719–24.
65. Childs R, Chernoff A, Contentin N et al, Regression of metastatic renal carcinoma after nonmyeloablative allogeneic peripheral blood stem cell transplantation. *N Engl J Med* 2000; 343: 750–8.
66. Sensi M. Dembic Z, Steinmetz M, Transcription of a T cell receptor B chain gene in L cell fibroblasts following DNA-mediated gene transfer. *Eur J Immunol* 1987; 17: 1371–4.
67. Liu X, Peralta EA, Ellenhorn JDI et al, Targeting of human p53, over-expressing tumor cells by an HLA-A*0201-restricted murine T-cell receptor expressed in Jurkat T cells. *Cancer Res* 2000; 60: 693–701.
68. Clay TM, Custer MC, Sachs J et al, Efficient transfer of a tumor antigen-reactive TCR to human peripheral blood lymphocytes confers anti-tumor reactivity. *J Immunol* 1999; 163: 507–13.
69. Calogero A, Hospers GA, Kruse KM et al, Retargeting of a T cell line by anti-MAGE-3/HLA-A2 α β TCR gene transfer. *Anticancer Res* 2000; 20: 1793–9.
70. Eshhar Z, Tumor-specific T-bodies: toward clinical application. *Cancer Immunol Immunother* 1997; 45: 131–6.
71. Morritz D, Wels W, Mattern J et al, Cytotoxic T lymphocytes with a grafted recognition specificity for ERBB2-expressing tumor cells. *Proc Natl Acad Sci USA* 1994; 91: 4318–22.
72. Hwu P, Yang JC, Cowherd R et al, In vivo antitumor activity of T cells redirected with chimeric antibody/T-cell receptor genes. *Cancer Res* 1995; 55: 3369–73.
73. Willemsen RA, Debets R, Hart E et al, A phage display selected fab fragment with MHC class I-restricted specificity for MAGE-A1 allows for retargeting of primary human T lymphocytes. *Gene Ther* 2001; 8: 1601–8.
74. Maccalli C, Farina C, Sensi M et al, TCR β chain variable region-driven selection and massive expansion of HLA-class I-restricted anti-tumor CTL lines from HLA-A*0201+ melanoma patients. *J Immunol* 1997; 158: 5902–13.
75. Valmori D, Pittet MJ, Rimoldi D et al, An antigen-targeted approach to adoptive transfer therapy of cancer. *Cancer Res* 1999; 59: 2167–73.

59

New anticancer agents: possibilities for improving the therapy of metastatic melanoma

Michael Millward

INTRODUCTION

Patients with non-localized metastatic melanoma have few useful treatment options. While dacarbazine has been considered the 'reference' drug, it produces response rates of no more than 15–20%.[1] In phase III trials, where lower response rates are generally seen, the response rate to dacarbazine is closer to 10%.[2] In the past two decades, only two new cytotoxic agents, temozolamide and fotemustine, have been extensively investigated in metastatic melanoma. Temozolamide, an orally active methylating agent, spontaneously converts to the active species 5-(3-methyltriazen-1-yl) imidazole-4-carboxamide (MTIC), unlike dacarbazine that requires metabolic activation in the liver to MTIC. Temozolamide essentially has the same level of antitumour activity and toxicity in metastatic melanoma as dacarbazine.[2] Fotemustine, a chlorethyl nitrosourea, showed response rates of *c.* 20% in large phase II studies conducted in Europe in the 1980s.[3] The addition of an aminophosphonate onto the nitrosurea molecule increases the permeability of fotemustine through the blood–brain barrier, and may account for its activity in cerebral metastases from melanoma being equivalent to its activity at other visceral sites.[3] However, there are no direct phase III trials reported comparing fotemustine to dacarbazine or temozolamide to draw any firm conclusion on its potential superiority.

Therefore, there is an urgent need to develop new agents for systemic therapy of disseminated melanoma. Advances in understanding the molecular mechanisms that underlie the development and progression of malignant disease have led to new therapeutic targets. The central roles of aberrant cell-cycle regulation, overexpression of transmembrane signalling factors and the requirement for tumour-induced angiogenesis are now well recognized. Drugs that specifically inhibit these critical pathways have been isolated or synthesized and have started to enter clinical trials. This chapter will outline some of the most interesting of these new agents. While there are few published phase II (or later) studies examining their therapeutic potential in melanoma, these will be forthcoming in the not too distant future. Before embarking on these areas though, it is timely to review some of the recent studies looking at newer, but still more 'traditional', cytotoxic agents in melanoma.

NEW CYTOTOXIC AGENTS

A survey of phase II studies of new cytotoxic agents for metastatic melanoma published since 1993 is summarized in Table 59.1.[4–27] Selected phase II combination studies are summarized in Table 59.2.[28–34] No new cytotoxic agent shows remarkable activity in metastatic melanoma; however, some promise is evident for taxanes and platinum agents.

Two taxanes, paclitaxel and docetaxel, were investigated in metastatic melanoma based on their activity against B16 melanoma in preclinical testing and their promise in other tumour types. As part of its initial clinical development, four phase II studies of paclitaxel given as a 24-hour infusion in varying doses were performed.

Table 59.1 *Recent phase II trials of new cytotoxics in metastatic melanoma*

Drug	No. of patients	Prior chemotherapy	Responses (%)	Reference no.
Paclitaxel	15	Yes	13	4
KW2189	15	Yes	0	5
KW2189	30	No	17	5
Dolastatin 10	12	No	0	6
LU103793	80	No	6	7
Bryostatin	15	Yes	7	8
Bryostatin	16	Yes	0	9
CI980	24	No	0	10
Doxil	32	Yes	6	11
Melphalan	17	No	0	12
Zilascorb	16	Yes	6	13
Zeniplatin	24	No	14	14
Zeniplatin	21	No	10	15
Topotecan	17	No	0	16
Docetaxel	37	No	6	17
Docetaxel	40	No	12.5	18
Docetaxel	38	No	17	19
Rhizoxin	26	No	0	20
Merbarone	35	No	6	21
Piroxantrone	46	No	5	22
CB10-277	28	No	4	23
Gemcitabine	39	No	3	24
Didemnin B	14	No	0	25
Paclitaxel*	73	No	16	26
Carboplatin	30	No	11	27

*Combined data from four studies.

In 73 evaluable patients,[26] responses occurred in 16.4%, while another 26% had unconfirmed responses, minor responses or stable disease. Interestingly, two complete responses were reported as being very durable, with the patients having no recurrence at 33+ and 46+ months.[26] Despite this, paclitaxel was not further tested in melanoma, perhaps because the 24-hour infusion produced substantial myelosuppression, and perhaps because the resources required for the drug's development were used in other malignancies.

More recently, Nathan et al.[29] used a 3-hour infusion of 225 mg/m^2 paclitaxel with tamoxifen 40 mg/day in

Table 59.2 *Recent phase II trials of new agent combinations in metastatic melanoma*

Drugs	No. of patients	Prior chemotherapy	Responses (%)	Reference no.
Vinorelbine/tamoxifen	31	Some	20	28
Paclitaxel/tamoxifen	21	Yes	24	29
Paclitaxel/vinorelbine	15	No	20	30
Paclitaxel/dacarbazine	16	Some	12.5	31
Paclitaxel/carboplatin	17	Some	20	32
Tirapazamine/cisplatin	48	No	20	33
Tirapazamine/cisplatin	48	Some	19	34

patients who had progressed after the multiagent Dartmouth regimen (carmustine, cisplatin and dacarbazine, plus or minus tamoxifen). The rationale for using tamoxifen was its potential to modulate P-glycoprotein-associated multidrug resistance, although the dose used was substantially lower than that required to produce plasma levels capable of this.[35] Consequently, the response rate of 24% is likely to be attributable to the paclitaxel alone and suggests at least some potential non-cross-resistance with dacarbazine. An even more recent study, using a weekly schedule of paclitaxel, reported a 13% response rate in previously treated melanoma patients.[4] However, a phase II trial in melanoma patients combining paclitaxel and dacarbazine, using a variety of paclitaxel doses and infusion durations of 24 and 3 hours, produced only limited responses.[31]

Three phase II studies of docetaxel have been performed in metastatic melanoma.[9–11] All used a dose of 100 mg/m^2 every 3 weeks and the response rates ranged from 6 to 17%. Again, like paclitaxel, two of the studies documented patients with prolonged responses lasting from 14+ to 24+ months.[17,18] Combination studies utilizing docetaxel with either dacarbazine or temozolamide are being performed, but have not yet been reported.

Based on the results seen with paclitaxel and docetaxel, it will be worthwhile evaluating new agents of this class in metastatic melanoma patients. Paclitaxel and docetaxel are tubulin-interacting drugs that bind to a defined taxane binding site on β tubulin and cause microtubule stabilization. A large number of chemical entities have been discovered that can interact with tubulin and appear, preclinically, to have advantages over paclitaxel and docetaxel. These advantages include greater potency, more favourable formulation not requiring solvents, and, more importantly, retained activity against paclitaxel-resistant cell lines. New tubulin-interacting agents can be divided into new taxanes that retain the basic taxane structure and bind to the taxane-binding site, conjugates of taxanes to liposomes or other attempts to improve tumour targeting and pharmacology, and drugs that have new tubulin targets. Some of the most promising agents are listed in Table 59.3.[36–51] The latter group are perhaps the most interesting, with agents such as BMS247550 able to overcome all known molecular mechanisms of paclitaxel resistance.[46]

Of the other agents listed in Table 59.1, only zeniplatin, carboplatin and KW2189 produced response rates ≥10%. The high incidence of haematological, gastrointestinal and, in one study,[15] renal toxicity following zeniplatin led to its abandonment. Although carboplatin has moderate single-agent activity in melanoma, comparable to cisplatin,[27] nearly all contemporary multiagent regimens have preferred cisplatin. A recent phase II study of paclitaxel and carboplatin reported a response rate of 20%, including some patients with prior chemotherapy.[32] In two phase II trials totalling 96 patients,[33,34] the addition of the hypoxic cell cytotoxin tirapazamine to cisplatin produced response rates higher than would be expected with cisplatin alone, but tirapazamine does not appear to have been investigated further in melanoma, despite a phase III study in non-small cell lung cancer showing the value of this approach.[52] KW2189, a semisynthetic antitumour antibiotic, has recently been reported to have moderate activity in previously untreated

Table 59.3 *Selected new tubulin-interacting agents*

Drug	Manufacturer	Current development	Reference no.
New taxanes			
BMS184476	Bristol-Myers Squibb	Phase II	36,37
BMS188797	Bristol-Myers Squibb	Phase II	38
TXD258	Aventis	Late preclinical	39
RPR109881	Aventis	Phase I	40
IDN5109	Indena	Phase I	41
Taxol conjugates			
PNU166945	Pharmacia & Upjohn	Phase II	42
Taxaprexin	ProTarga	Phase I	43
Liposome encapsulated paclitaxel (LEP)	NeoPharm	Phase I	44
Poly(L-glutamic acid) paclitaxel conjugate	Cell Therapeutics	Late preclinical	45
Novel entities			
BMS247550	Bristol-Myers Squibb	Late preclinical	46
Epothilone B (EP0906)	Novartis	Phase I	47
LY355703	Eli Lilly	Phase I–II	48
Discodermolide	Novartis	Late preclinical	49
T138067	Tularik	Phase I–II	50
T900607	Tularik	Late preclinical	51

melanoma patients, but not in patients who had prior chemotherapy.[5] However, myelosuppression was substantial and often required dose modification. Further studies would be of interest. The other agents listed in Table 59.1 warrant no further testing in melanoma patients.

CYCLIN-DEPENDENT KINASE (CDK) INHIBITORS

The CDK are the primary regulators of the cell cycle in eukaryotes.[53] Passage of a cell through critical checkpoints at G1/S and G2/M requires a coordinated series of interactions between CDK, cyclins and natural inhibitors. Activation of CDK2 by cyclin A, or CDK4 or CDK6 by cyclin D, is required for progression from G1 to S. This is inhibited by $p16^{INK4A}$, $p21^{WAF/CIP1}$ or $p27^{Kip1}$. Transition from G2 to M requires complexing of CDK1 and cyclin B (or cyclin A), which can be inhibited by $p21^{WAF/CIP1}$ or $p27^{Kip1}$. Loss of cell-cycle control regulation due to alteration of the p16 gene is frequently encountered in melanomas and, therefore, drugs that inhibit CDK are of great interest.

The first CDK modulators to enter clinical trials were flavopiridol and UCN-01. Flavopiridol inhibits multiple CDK including CDK2, CDK4, CDK1 and CDK7.[54] Although it can inhibit multiple other protein kinases, including protein kinase A, protein kinase C and the epidermal growth factor receptor (EGFR) tyrosine kinase, the levels required to do this in vivo are substantially higher than those required for CDK inhibition. The initial phase I trial indicated unusual toxicities, including dose-limiting diarrhoea, hypotension and inflammatory serositis.[55] Subsequent phase II trials in renal, gastric and non-small cell lung cancer have shown only minimal activity, and substantial toxicity.[56–58] In addition, UCN-01 has produced unusual toxicities and also unpredictable pharmacokinetics due to extensive protein binding.[59]

Advances in molecular drug design, high-throughput screening and genomics have been applied to discover new potent, specific small molecule CDK inhibitors. By screening purine-based chemical libraries, a highly potent CDK2 inhibitor, purvalanol A, was selected and several derivatives synthesized.[60] Because these agents inhibit both human CDK2 and the *S. cerevisiae* CDK Cdc28p, changes in gene expression following exposure of *S. cerevisiae* were measured using a microarray of 6400 genes.[26] Downregulation of transcription genes associated with progression through the cell cycle was found, consistent with CDK inhibition. The combination of CDK inhibitors and cytotoxics may be expected to be synergistic on tumour cells, as has been shown for flavopiridol.[61]

Rather than the broad-spectrum CDK inhibition seen with flavopiridol, the emphasis is now on developing specific inhibitors of one or two members of the CDK family. In theory, combined CDK2 and CDK1 inhibitors are attractive, as they could block the cell cycle at both G1/S and G2/M. CDK4 inhibitors would be a rational choice for testing in melanomas with loss of $p16^{INK4A}$ function. Some recently described CDK inhibitors are listed in Table 59.4.[62–69] Of these, only E7070, a novel sulphonamide derivative, has progressed as far as phase I trials. Initial results suggest that myelosuppression will be dose limiting.[62] Interestingly, some of the preclinical data suggest that the combination of CDK inhibitors and certain cytotoxics leads to less toxicity on normal cells than seen with cytotoxics alone.[66] Thus, with potentially synergistic effects on tumour cells and protection of normal tissues, such combinations may have an excellent therapeutic index in the clinic.

Table 59.4 *New agents targeting cyclin-dependent kinases (CDK)*

Agents	Primary target(s)	Reference no.
E7070	CDK2	62
Alsterpaullone	CDK1	63
PD0183812	CDK4	64
GW8510/GW2059	CDK2	65,66
Fascaplysin	CDK4	67
NU2058/NU6027	CDK1/CDK2	68
CGP79807	CDK1/CDK2	69

AGENTS BLOCKING SIGNAL TRANSDUCTION PATHWAYS

Normal cells require complex mechanisms to respond to signals from the extracellular environment. Critically important for malignant cells is the overexpression and, in some cases, dependence on transmembrane growth factor receptors that contain an intracellular tyrosine kinase domain. Binding of a growth factor or other ligand to the extracellular portion of the receptor leads to dimerization of receptors and to activation of the kinase. Activated kinase can then phosphorylate intracellular second messenger pathways, that ultimately lead to the nucleus, and transcription of appropriate genes to mediate the response to the extracellular signal. Blockage of these signal transduction pathways can lead to cell death or cessation of cell division. There are many families of growth factor receptors, including the EGFR, the platelet-derived growth factor receptor (PDGFR) and the fibroblast growth factor receptor (FGFR) families. In addition to these transmembrane molecules, there are many intracellular proteins involved in signal transduction containing tyrosine kinase domains, including Abl, Src and Yes.

There are three principal ways that new agents have been developed to block signal transduction: (a) synthesis of antibodies that bind to the extracellular portion of a receptor and prevent binding of growth factors, thus blocking receptor function; (b) design of small molecule inhibitors of the tyrosine kinase domain; and (c) inhibiting downstream second messengers.

The monoclonal antibody trastuzumab (Herceptin) has been the first specific drug designed to block a growth factor receptor to demonstrate significant benefit for patients with solid tumours, in this case women with advanced breast cancer who had tumours overexpressing its target, HER2. For these patients, herceptin has activity as a single agent and markedly enhances the effectiveness of chemotherapy.[70,71] Of the small molecule tyrosine kinase inhibitors, Iressa (ZD1839), targeting the EGFR, has shown encouraging responses in phase I trials in patients with metastatic non-small cell lung cancer, and head and neck cancers,[72,73] and has rapidly been taken to phase III trials. Even more exciting has been the effectiveness of the Abl tyrosine kinase inhibitor STI571 (CGP57148) that has produced remission in the majority of patients with chronic myeloid leukaemia, a disease characterized by an abnormal Abl protein (the product of the Bcr–Abl translocation) with uncontrolled tyrosine kinase activity.[74] Other molecules in the process of development as antibodies or tyrosine kinase inhibitors are listed in Table 59.5.

Translating this knowledge into potential therapies for melanoma requires understanding of the signal transduction pathways characteristic of melanoma cells. There has been relatively little work in this area compared to that undertaken in breast, prostate and other common solid tumours. Investigations should concentrate on analysis of samples of advanced stages of melanoma from patients (i.e. resected distant metastases or regional nodes) rather than primary melanomas or melanoma cell lines. Additionally, protein levels (immunohistochemistry), mRNA overexpression and gene amplification (by fluorescent in situ hybridization, FISH) need to be assessed, as discordant results may occur.[75]

It appears that the FGFR pathway is important in melanoma, while other growth factors involved in growth and division of normal melanocytes are repressed in melanomas (reviewed in reference 76). The intracellular tyrosine kinase c-Yes is also a potential target for development of new therapies for melanoma,[77] and two studies have also suggested that EGFR may have a role too.[78,79]

The drugs in Table 59.5 consist of both specific inhibitors of one tyrosine kinase and inhibitors of multiple tyrosine kinases. There are no specific FGFR inhibitors in current clinical development but SU6668,[80] developed by Sugen Inc, is in phase I trials. As this drug also targets the vascular endothelial growth factor receptor (VEGFR), it is likely that antiangiogenesis will be responsible for at least part of any antitumour efficacy seen (see below). Another multiple tyrosine kinase inhibitor, PD166285, developed by Parke-Davis Medical, and a specific FGFR inhibitor, SU5402 (Sugen Inc), have been described and preclinical data presented.[81,82] If EGFR can be confirmed as a useful target in melanoma, then Iressa and other EGFR inhibitors should be investigated too.

Of the downstream second messengers, the one that has been most actively pursued as a therapeutic target is the family of small GTP-binding proteins, Ras. Activating oncogenic mutations in one of three *ras* genes (K-*ras*, N-*ras* or H-*ras*) are frequent in some tumour types. Unlike some solid tumours and leukaemias, melanomas are not reported to frequently harbour *ras* mutations.

Table 59.5 ***Drugs affecting signal-transduction pathways***

Drug	Target/pathway	Development
Monoclonal antibodies		
Trastuzumab	HER2	Licenced Breast, Phase III other
Cetuximab	EGFR	Phase III
ABX-EGF	EGFR	Preclinical
Kinase inhibitors		
Leflunomide	PDGFR	Phase III
Iressa	EGFR	Phase III
STI571	Abl, PDGFR, c-kit	Phase II
PKI166	EGFR	Phase I
CP358774	EGFR	Phase I
SU6668	PDGF/VEGFR/FGFR	Phase I
BIBX1382	EGFR	Phase I
PD183805	EGFR	Phase I
CEP751, CEP701	Trk	Phase I
PD166285	FGFR/EGFR/PDGFR/src	Preclinical
PD184352	Mek	Preclinical
CL387785	EGFR	Preclinical
PD183805	HER2	Preclinical
CT052923	PDGFR	Preclinical
SB238039	EGFR/Lck, Jak2	Preclinical
AG1478	HER2	Preclinical
SU5402	FGFR	Preclinical

EGFR, epidermal growth factor receptor; FGFR, fibroblast growth factor receptor; PDGFR, platelet-derived growth factor receptor; VEGFR, vascular endothelial growth factor receptor.

Of 50 melanoma studies, eight (16%) had mutations, principally in N-*ras* (data from reference 83).

Abnormal Ras proteins produced by these mutations remain active in the absence of upstream growth factor receptor stimulation. However, all Ras proteins, including products of mutated *ras* genes, must undergo post-translational addition of a farnesyl group to a cysteine residue. This step is controlled by the enzyme farnesyltransferase and many drugs that are potent inhibitors of this enzyme have been developed. However, the importance of Ras as being fundamental to the antitumour activity of farnesyltransferase inhibitors is doubtful. Although inhibitors can block oncogenic signalling in *ras*-transformed cells, they inhibit the farnesylation of many other proteins, and are preclinically active against both *ras*-transformed tumour cells and tumour cells without *ras* mutations.[84] Additionally, drugs that inhibit farnesyltransferase not only block the activity of abnormal Ras but would also be expected to block Ras-mediated signal transduction from abnormally stimulated or overexpressed growth factor receptors, independent of the presence of *ras* mutations. Therefore, evaluation of farnesyltransferase inhibitors in melanoma seems warranted.

To date, four farnesyltransferase inhibitors have progressed to phase I trials, R115777 (Janssen), SCH66336 (Schering-Plough), L778123 (Merck) and BMS214662 (Bristol-Myers Squibb).[85–88] All of these agents are oral, facilitating long-term chronic dosing, although briefer schedules have also been tested. The toxicities experienced in the phase I trials have included myelosuppression, nausea/vomiting, fatigue and diarrhoea. Elegant pharmacodynamic studies in the phase I trials have demonstrated that the doses associated with acceptable toxicity produce inhibition of protein farnesylation in vivo in humans. Other farnesyltransferase inhibitors have been developed by Parke-Davis Medical, Rhône-Poulenc Rorer (now Aventis) and academic groups.

ANTI-ANGIOGENIC AND ANTI-VASCULAR AGENTS

No other area of developmental therapeutics in oncology has caused the same degree of excitement as angiogenesis inhibition. It is now accepted that a solid mass of tumour cells cannot grow >1–2 mm in size because this is the diffusion limit for oxygen. Consequently, tumours must be associated with the ingrowth and development of new blood vessels,[89] a process termed tumour angiogenesis. In breast cancer and several other tumour types, tumour angiogenesis, as assessed by microvessel density, is an important negative prognostic marker (reviewed in reference 90).

Agents affecting angiogenesis can be subdivided into five classes (Table 59.6). Firstly, there are agents that act directly on endothelial cells to inhibit angiogenesis. These negative regulators of angiogenesis are very attractive potential anticancer drugs because the endothelium is not subject to the genetic diversity and mutation frequency that characterizes malignant cells. Therefore, drug resistance to this class of drugs should be much slower to develop, or not develop at all. Second are inhibitors of angiogenesis-promoting factors. As these are secreted by tumour cells in response to hypoxic stimulation, it is possible that blockading these may lead to malignant cells activating alternative pathways. The most important of these factors are vascular endothelial growth factor (VEGF) and basic fibroblast growth factor (bFGF). Both small molecules and antibodies have been developed to inhibit VEGF angiogenic signalling in the same way as other signal transduction pathways have been targeted. Third are inhibitors of the matrix metalloproteinase enzymes. These enzymes are important for the breaking down of the extracellular matrix that is required for the ingress of new blood vessels. The fourth group are drugs that are selectively toxic to formed tumour vasculature. The fifth group consists of agents where the mode of action in producing anti-angiogenesis is unknown.

There are no features of angiogenesis that are known to be specific to melanoma. Indeed, recently it has been reported that uveal melanomas can grow and metastasize without the formation of new endothelial-lined vessels. This phenomenon, termed vasculogenic mimicry, results from the melanoma cells themselves forming structures analogous to blood vessels lined by pluripotent cells derived from the malignant melanoma cells.[91,92] Should this pathway be confirmed as being a general property of melanomas, then many of the anti-angiogenic drugs would be expected to have limited applicability in this disease, particularly agents that block signalling through VEGF. However, other agents, e.g. matrix metalloproteinase inhibitors, would still be potentially active.

Thalidomide is the anti-angiogenic drug with the most widespread experience, in part due to its easier availability, as it has been used sporadically over the past

Table 59.6 *Anti-angiogenic drugs*

Drugs acting directly on endothelial cells	
TNP470	Synthetic analogue of antibiotic fumagillin secreted by *Aspergillus* (TAP Pharmaceuticals)
Platelet factor 4	Natural polypeptide found in platelet granules, recombinant form synthesized
Squalamine lactate	Natural aminosterol isolated from liver of dogfish shark (Magainin Pharmaceuticals)
Endostatin	C-terminal proteolytic product of collagen (EntreMed)
EMD121974	Small molecule inhibitor of $\alpha V\beta 3$ integrin (Merck)
Vitaxin	Humanized monoclonal antibody to $\alpha V\beta 3$ integrin (Ixsys Inc)
Angiostatin	Internal fragment of plasminogen containing kringle domains 1–4 (EntreMed)
Drugs blocking activators of angiogenesis	
SU5416	VEGF receptor tyrosine kinase inhibitor (Sugen Inc)
SU6668	VEGF, FGF, PDGF receptors tyrosine kinase inhibitor (Sugen Inc)
PTK787	VEGF receptor tyrosine kinase inhibitor (Novartis)
Anti-VEGF Ab	Humanized monoclonal antibody (Genentech)
Anti-VEGFR Ab	Antibody to VEGF receptor KDR (ImClone)
Angiozyme	Hammerhead ribozyme targeting VEGF receptor (Chiron)
Tecogalan sodium	Sulphated polysaccharide from bacterial cell wall, inhibits bFGF signalling (Daiichi Pharmaceuticals)
Matrix metalloproteinase (MMP) inhibitors	
Marimastat	Synthetic MMP inhibitor (British Biotech)
BAY12–9566	Synthetic MMP inhibitor (Bayer)
AG3340	Synthetic MMP inhibitor (Agouron Pharmaceuticals)
AE941	Naturally occurring MMP inhibitor from shark cartilage (Aeterna)
CGS27023A	Synthetic MMP inhibitor (Novartis)
BMS275291	Synthetic MMP inhibitor (Bristol-Myers Squibb)
Antivascular agents	
Combretastatin A4 prodrug	Tubulin agent that causes apoptosis of proliferating tumour vasculature (Oxigene)
CM101/ZD0101	Toxin from group B streptococcus, targets capillary endothelium of tumours (AstraZeneca)
Unknown mechanism of action	
CAI	?Inhibitor of calcium-influx channels (NCI)
IM862	Synthetic dipeptide
Tetrathiomolybdate	Depletes copper stores
Thalidomide	?Integrin antagonist, many other possible actions (commercially available)

bFGF, basic FGF; FGF, fibroblast growth factor; PDGF, platelet-derived growth factor; VEGF, vascular endothelial growth factor.

two decades for erythema nodosum leprosum, Behçet's syndrome, severe graft versus host disease and other conditions. Dating back to the 1960s are anecdotal reports of thalidomide producing benefit in patients with malignancy.[93] The demonstration that thalidomide has potent in vivo anti-angiogenic activity[94] provided a strong rationale for controlled trials, and very promising results have been reported in patients with multiple myeloma resistant to other forms of treatment.[95] Phase II trials of thalidomide have been reported in a number of solid tumours, including gliomas, breast cancer, and head and neck cancers, with some hints of activity.[96–98] No 'pure' phase II studies in melanoma are available, but two groups have included melanoma patients in broad-based studies of thalidomide in cancer patients.[99,100] Eisen et al.[99] treated 17 patients with melanoma using a low dose of thalidomide (100 mg/day): no responses occurred, although one melanoma patient had symptomatic improvement in tumour-related pain. While some benefit in certain quality-of-life parameters were documented, only a small number of the total patient group completed the questionnaires and it is not possible to discern whether there was any benefit for the melanoma patients.[99] No specific details on outcome of thalidomide in melanoma patients can be obtained from the other report. It is therefore unlikely that low-dose thalidomide will be of substantial value in metastatic melanoma. While higher doses, up to 1200 mg/day, have been used in some trials, such doses are associated with troublesome fatigue and somnolence in many patients. Other toxicities of thalidomide include skin rashes, peripheral neuropathy and constipation.

Of the agents acting directly on endothelial cells, that with the most clinical experience is TNP-470, a synthetic analogue of the antibiotic fumagillin. Phase I trials using a brief intravenous infusion given weekly or three times per week identified neurological toxicity (including ataxia, vertigo, and disturbed higher functions) as dose limiting, but this was reversible.[101,102] Of four melanoma patients, one with lymph node and bone metastases that were progressing despite chemotherapy and immunotherapy had stabilization of disease for 27 weeks.[101] Because of the short half-life of TNP-470 and its major metabolite, and the possibility that neurological toxicity may be reduced by avoiding high peak plasma levels produced by a short infusion, more recent trials have examined a continuous infusion schedule.[103] With the continuous infusion, patients' plasma achieved biological activity capable of inhibiting endothelial cell function, even at low TNP-470 doses.[103] Other agents listed in Table 59.6 are in phase I studies, and some preliminary results have been reported.[104–107] No activity was noted in two melanoma patients treated with squalamine;[104] the natural substances endostatin and angiostatin have demonstrated very promising activity as angiogenesis inhibitors but there are no clinical results available for these agents.[108]

Small molecule inhibitors of the tyrosine kinase domain of the VEGF receptor are a particularly promising approach for anti-angiogenic therapy. There are two receptor subtypes, VEGF1 (also called Flt-1) and VEGF2 (also called Flk-1/KDR). The leading candidate VEGF inhibitors have been developed by Sugen Inc (now part of Pharmacia). SU5416 is a specific inhibitor of VEGF2,[109] whereas SU6668 inhibits multiple receptors (see above).[80] The preclinical evaluation of both agents shows that they are highly effective inhibitors of angiogenesis and result in tumour regression in distant sites in multiple tumour types.[80,109] Phase I studies of SU5416 given as a twice weekly or weekly infusion identified an unusual toxicity of severe headaches and vomiting,[110–112] however, at lower doses this was not a significant problem in most patients. Although only a small number of true responses were seen in these phase I trials, more patients had prolonged stabilization of their disease. Unfortunately, no melanoma patients were included in the published trials of SU5416. This drug is now in phase III studies in colorectal cancer and non-small cell lung cancer, where patients receive either standard chemotherapy or the same chemotherapy with SU5416. Melanoma has not been included in this first round of phase III studies. SU6668, an orally active agent, has only recently entered phase I trials.[113]

An alternative way of inhibiting the VEGF pathway is by using monoclonal antibodies directed against VEGF. Such an antibody functions to bind VEGF and prevent access to the VEGF receptor by VEGF secreted by the malignant cells, thus preventing angiogenesis. A high-affinity antibody has been developed by Genentech Inc and appears particularly promising. Most noteworthy is a report of chemotherapy resistant metastatic breast cancer patients achieving a response to administration of this antibody as a single agent.[114] Small randomized trials in advanced colorectal cancer and advanced non-small cell lung cancer have been performed where patients were randomized to a standard chemotherapy regimen alone or the same chemotherapy regimen plus anti-VEGF antibody.[115,116] In both trials there was evidence of higher responses and longer time to disease progression in the antibody treated patients, although neither study was powered to specifically examine these end points, which will require confirmation in formal phase III studies. A low but definite incidence of tumour-related haemorrhagic complications was seen in patients with lung tumours, where fatal haemoptysis was reported.[116] While this complication may be specific to lung cancers, it is of concern for melanoma trials, given the highly vascular nature of many melanoma metastases.

Inhibitors of the matrix metalloproteinase enzyme system have been considered as anti-angiogenic because the ingrowth of new vessels requires breakdown of the extracellular matrix. As the same breakdown is required for the liberation of potentially metastatic cells from a primary tumour mass, this class of drugs has also been investigated as so-called anti-metastatic agents in patients. Of all the classes listed in Table 59.6, matrix metalloproteinase inhibitors are the furthest into clinical development, although again there has been little attention given to starting trials in melanoma patients. Nevertheless, large phase III trials of Marimastat, BAY12-9566 and AG3340 have been commenced in lung, ovarian, pancreatic, gastric, colorectal and other cancers. These trials have been done using a variety of designs. In relatively resistant malignancies, such as pancreatic cancer, patients have been randomized to the matrix metalloproteinase inhibitor or a standard cytotoxic. For more responsive tumours, such as non-small cell lung or gastric cancers, patients have been randomized to standard cytotoxics alone or with a matrix metalloproteinase inhibitor. For tumours very sensitive to chemotherapy, such as small cell lung or ovarian cancers, patients have been randomized to observation or an adjuvant matrix metalloproteinase inhibitor after response to chemotherapy has been achieved. No convincing positive results have been reported, apart from one trial of Marimastat in gastric cancer where a borderline significant benefit to the combination of Marimastat plus chemotherapy over chemotherapy alone occurred.[117] Disappointing results have been obtained with BAY12-9566, which seems inferior to standard management,[118] and this compound has now been withdrawn from clinical development. The future of matrix metalloproteinase inhibitors as a class of drugs is currently unclear.

True antivascular agents act on formed blood vessels rather than preventing the formation of new vessels. The lead compound in this class is combretastatin A4 prodrug. This is a synthetic phosphate analogue that is converted, in vivo, to the active agent combretastatin A4, a compound isolated from the African willow tree. While combretastatin A4 functions as a tubulin-binding agent through the colchicine binding site, its administration to tumour-bearing animals results in immediate collapse of the tumour vasculature with haemorrhagic necrosis of the tumour, despite no effect on vessels in normal organs.[119] The precise reason for this striking effect is unknown. Initial clinical trials with combretastatin A4 prodrug have shown evidence for the same phenomenon in humans, with tumour pain and reduced blood flow as assessed by serial dynamic magnetic resonance imaging (MRI).[120,121] Much interest was aroused because of one patient with chemotherapy resistant metastatic anaplastic thyroid cancer achieving a pathological complete response in this phase I trial.[122] Further results are eagerly awaited.

TRIALS OF NOVEL NON-CYTOTOXIC AGENTS IN MELANOMA

The recent emphasis in drug development for treatment of malignant disease has been away from cytotoxics towards compounds that target specific pathways in signal transduction, cell-cycle regulation and angiogensis. For all these new classes of drugs, questions have been raised as to whether the paradigms of clinical testing used for cytotoxics are appropriate.[123] The traditional pathway of phase I dose escalation to establish the maximum tolerated dose and dose-limiting toxicities, followed by phase II testing to determine whether responses occur in patients with advanced disease, followed by phase III testing in advanced disease by randomized comparison against best standard therapy, followed by testing as adjuvant treatment in disease-free patients, may not be appropriate for these new drugs.

In particular, it has been argued that these agents may not produce substantial shrinkage of established bulky metastatic disease (and so would be considered 'inactive' on phase II testing), but could have a marked effect in slowing tumour growth (producing prolonged disease stabilization in advanced disease). They could also be potentially active in delaying or preventing recurrence when given to patients with minimal disease in the adjuvant situation. In either situation, efficacy is likely to require protracted administration of the drug (hence the particular attraction of orally absorbed agents) rather than the brief cyclical exposure produced by the traditional chemotherapy schedules. Given this, together with the very high potency of many of these new agents against their target, it is argued that efficacy may not require drug doses that are close to a maximally tolerated dose. Hence, phase I trials should aim primarily to document that the desired effect at a biological level is being achieved with a particular dose, rather than focus on whether limiting toxicity to normal tissues is produced. Consequently, initial clinical trials (i.e. phases I and II) are accompanied by detailed studies such as MRI scans to assess tumour vascularity, positron emission tomography (PET) scans to assess tumour metabolism, and tumour biopsies to assess biochemical and molecular changes consistent with the desired effect of the drug.

Experience to date with the compounds discussed above has not fully supported this conceptual framework. Unpredictable and unusual toxicities to non-proliferative normal tissues can occur.[55,101,110] True (and in some cases quite dramatic) responses have been documented in patients with advanced chemotherapy resistant cancers.[73,114]

What does this mean for trials in melanoma patients? One group of patients that is particularly sought for initial clinical trials is that with easily accessible disease amenable to repeated biopsy. Melanoma patients with multiple cutaneous and subcutaneous metastases are ideal, and enrolment of these patients in early trials of new agents should be encouraged. The converse though is that these patients, who do not also have visceral metastases, fall into a good prognosis group, and the finding of prolonged disease stability or even responses should not lead to the assumption that the drug being tested will be of value in more aggressive metastatic melanoma. There is still a role for formal phase II testing, both in previously untreated metastatic melanoma patients and previously treated patients who remain of good performance status.

In the adjuvant situation, there is scope for testing new compounds in patients with resected stage IV melanoma and poor prognosis stage III patients, e.g. those presenting with palpable nodes or having multiple involved nodes. These patients have a high risk of further distant disease and an appropriate study would be a randomized phase II versus observation, or an approved adjuvant therapy with an initial end point of tolerability of the new agent when given for a prolonged period to disease-free patients. Should satisfactory tolerability be shown, and an encouragingly low short-term recurrence rate noted, then a phase III study could rapidly follow.

This is an exciting period for new drug development. Many of the recent discoveries in cancer biology are resulting in potential new treatments. There is real reason for optimism that substantially better results in advanced melanoma patients will be achievable in the future than is possible with standard treatments today.

REFERENCES

1. Comis RL, DTIC in malignant melanoma: a perspective. *Cancer Treat Rep* 1985; 60: 165–76.
2. Middleton MR, Grob JJ, Aaronson N et al, Randomized phase III study of temozolamide versus dacarbazine in the treatment of patients with advanced metastatic malignant melanoma. *J Clin Oncol* 2000; 18: 158–66.
3. Jacquillat C, Khayat D, Banzet P et al, Final report of the French multicentre phase II study of the nitrosurea fotemustine in 153 evaluable patients with disseminated malignant melanoma including patients with cerebral metastases. *Cancer* 1990; 66: 1873–8.
4. Zonder JA, LoRusso P, Heilbrun L et al, Phase II trial of weekly paclitaxel as 2nd line treatment of metastatic malignant melanoma. *Proc ASCO* 2000; 19: 571a (abstract).
5. Markovic SN, Creagan ET, Suman VJ, Vukov A, Phase II trial of KW2189 in patients with advanced malignant melanoma. *Proc ASCO* 2000; 19: 570a (abstract).
6. Margolin KA, Longmage J, Gandara DR et al, Dolastatin 10 in metastatic melanoma: a phase II trial of the California Cancer Consortium. *Proc ASCO* 2000; 19: 569a (abstract).
7. Bonneterre M-E, Schellens JHM, Aamdal S et al, Final results of a phase II trial with LU103793 in metastatic melanoma. *Proc Am Ass Cancer Res* 2000; 41: 511 (abstract).
8. Bedikian A, Plager N, Papadopoulos N et al, Phase II trial of bryostatin-1 in patients with melanoma. *Proc ASCO* 1999; 18: 532a (abstract).
9. Propper DJ, Macaulay V, O'Byrne KJ et al, A phase II study of bryostatin 1 in metastatic melanoma. *Br J Cancer* 1998; 78: 1337–41.
10. Whitehead RP, Unger JM, Flaherty LE et al, Phase II trial of CI-980 in patients with disseminated melanoma: a Southwest Oncology Group Study. *Proc ASCO* 1999; 18: 554a (abstract).
11. Ellerhorst JA, Bedikian A, Ring S et al, Phase II trial of doxil for patients with metastatic melanoma refractory to frontline therapy. *Oncol Rep* 1999; 6: 1097–9.
12. Hochster H, Strawderman MH, Harris JE et al, Conventional dose melphalan is inactive in metastatic melanoma: results of an Eastern Cooperative Oncology Group trial. *Anti-Cancer Drugs* 1999; 10: 245–8.
13. Semb KA, Aamdal S, Mette E et al, Zilascorb(2H), a low toxicity protein synthesis inhibitor that exhibits signs of activity in malignant melanoma. *Anti-Cancer Drugs* 1998; 9: 797–802.
14. Aamdal S, Bruntsch U, Kerger J et al, Zeniplatin in advanced malignant melanoma and renal cancer: phase II studies with unexpected nephrotoxicity. *Cancer Chemother Pharmacol* 1997; 40: 439–43.
15. Olver I, Green M, Peters W et al, A phase II trial of zeniplatin in metastatic melanoma. *Am J Clin Oncol* 1995; 18: 56–8.

16. Kraut EH, Walker MJ, Staubas A et al, Phase II trial of topotecan in malignant melanoma. *Cancer Invest* 1997; 15: 318–20.
17. Einzig AI, Schuchter LM, Recio A et al, Phase II trial of docetaxel (Taxotere) in patients with metastatic melanoma previously untreated with cytotoxic chemotherapy. *Med Oncol* 1996; 13: 111–17.
18. Bedikian AY, Weiss GR, Legha SS et al, Phase II trial of docetaxel in patients with advanced cutaneous melanoma previously untreated with chemotherapy. *J Clin Oncol* 1995; 13: 2895–9.
19. Aamdal S, Wolff I, Kaplan S et al, Docetaxel (Taxotere) in advanced malignant melanoma: a Phase II study of the EORTC Early Clinical Trials Group. *Eur J Cancer* 1994; 30A: 1061–4.
20. Hanauske AR, Catimel G, Aamdal S et al, Phase II clinical trials with rhizoxin in breast cancer and melanoma: the EORTC Early Clinical Trials Group. *Br J Cancer* 1996; 73: 397–9.
21. Slavik M, Liu PY, Kraut EH et al, Evaluation of merbarone (NSC336628) in disseminated malignant melanoma. A Southwest Oncology Group study. *Invest New Drugs* 1995; 13: 143–7.
22. Sosman JA, Flaherty LE, Liu PY et al, A phase II trial of piroxantrone in disseminated malignant melanoma. A Southwest Oncology Group study. *Invest New Drugs* 1995; 11: 83–7.
23. Bleehan NM, Calvert AH, Lee SM et al, A Cancer research Campaign (CRC) phase II trial of CB10–277 given by 24 hour infusion for malignant melanoma. *Br J Cancer* 1994; 70: 775–7.
24. Sessa C, Aamdal S, Wolff I et al, Gemcitabine in patients with advanced malignant melanoma or gastric cancer: phase II studies of the EORTC Early Clinical Trials Group. *Ann Oncol* 1994; 5: 471–2.
25. Sondak VK, Kopecky KJ, Liu PY et al, Didemnin B in metastatic malignant melanoma: a Phase II trial of the Southwest Oncology Group. *Anti-Cancer Drugs* 1994; 5: 147–50.
26. Wiernik PH, Einzig AI, Taxol in malignant melanoma. *Monogr Natl Cancer Inst* 1993; 15: 185–7.
27. Chang A, Hunt M, Parkinson DR et al, Phase II trial of carboplatin in patients with metastatic melanoma. A report from the Eastern Cooperative Oncology Group. *Am J Clin Oncol* 1993; 16: 152–5.
28. Feun LG, Savaraj N, Hurley J et al, A clinical trial of intravenous vinorelbine tartrate plus tamoxifen in the treatment of patients with advanced malignant melanoma. *Cancer* 2000; 88: 584–8.
29. Nathan FE, Berd D, Sato T, Mastrangelo MJ, Paclitaxel and tamoxifen: an active regimen for patients with metastatic melanoma. *Cancer* 2000; 88: 79–87.
30. Retsas S, Mohith A, Mackenzie H, Taxol and vinorelbine: a new active combination for disseminated malignant melanoma. *Anti-Cancer Drugs* 1996; 7: 161–5.
31. Feun LG, Savaraj N, Schwartz M et al, Phase II trial of taxol and DTIC with fligrastim administration in advanced malignant melanoma. *Proc ASCO* 1997; 16: 505a (abstract).
32. Hodi FS, Soiffer RJ, Clark J et al, Phase II study of paclitaxel and carboplatin for metastatic melanoma. *Proc ASCO* 1999; 18: 551a (abstract).
33. Bedekian AY, Legha SS, Eton O et al, Phase II trial of escalated dose of tirapazamine combined with cisplatin in advanced malignant melanoma. *Anti-Cancer Drugs* 1999; 10: 735–9.
34. Bedekian AY, Legha SS, Eton O et al, Phase II trial of tirapazamine combined with cisplatin in chemotherapy of advanced malignant melanoma. *Ann Oncol* 1997; 8: 363–7.
35. Millward MJ, Cantwell BMJ, Lien EA et al, Intermittent high-dose tamoxifen as a potential modifier of multidrug resistance. *Eur J Cancer* 1992; 28: 805–10.
36. Hidalgo M, Aylesworth C, Baker S et al, A Phase I and pharmacokinetic (PK) study of the taxane analogue BMS 184476 administered as a 1-hour IV infusion every 3 weeks. *Cancer Res* 1999; 5 (Suppl): 68 (abstract).
37. Highley M, Sessa C, Hughes A et al, Phase I and pharmacokinetic (PK) study of BMS-184476, a new taxane analogue, given weekly in patients with advanced malignancies. *Proc ASCO* 1999; 18: 169a (abstract).
38. Sullivan D, Rago R, Garland L et al, A phase I study of BMS-188797, a new taxane analogue. *Cancer Res* 1999; 5 (Suppl): 68 (abstract).
39. Bissery M-C, Bouchard H, Riou JF et al, Preclinical evaluation of TXD258, a new taxoid. *Proc Am Ass Cancer Res* 2000; 41: 214 (abstract).
40. Sessa C, Caldiera S, De Jong J et al, Phase I study of RPR109881A, a new taxoid administered as a three hour intravenous infusion to patients with advanced solid tumours. *Ann Oncol* 1998; 9 (Suppl 4): 125 (abstract).
41. Nicoletti MI, Colombo T, Rossi C et al, IDN5109, a taxane with oral bioavailability and potent antitumor activity. *Cancer Res* 2000; 60: 842–6.
42. Nanna Panday VR, Meerum Terwogt JM, ten Bokkel Huinink WW et al, Phase I and pharmacologic study of water soluble polymer-conjugated paclitaxel (PNU 166945) administered as a 1-hour infusion in patients with advanced solid tumours. *Proc ASCO* 1998; 17: 193a (abstract).
43. Bradley MO, Webb NL, Anthony FA, Swindell CS, Increased therapeutic index by conjugation of a natural fatty acid to paclitaxel. *Proc Am Ass Cancer Res* 2000; 41: 303 (abstract).
44. Treat JA, Zrada S, Kesslehelm S et al, A Phase I trial in advanced malignancies with liposome encapsulated paclitaxel (LEP). *Proc ASCO* 1999; 18: 230a (abstract).
45. Li C, Yu D-F, Newman RA et al, Complete regression of well-established tumors using a novel water-soluble poly(L-glutamic acid)–paclitaxel conjugate. *Cancer Res* 1998; 58: 2404–9.
46. Lee FYF, Vite GD, Borzilleri RM et al, BMS-247550 – An epothilone analog possessing potent activity against paclitaxel-sensitive and -resistant human tumors. *Proc Am Ass Cancer Res* 2000; late-breaking Abstract 34, (http://aacr.edoc.com/2000_latebreaking/ch00001.html).
47. Gianakakou P, Gussio R, Nogales E et al, A common pharmacophore for epothilone and taxanes: molecular basis for drug resistance conferred by tubulin mutations in human cancer cells. *Proc Natl Acad Sci USA* 2000; 97: 2904–9.
48. Pagani O, Greim G, Weigang K et al, Phase I clinical and pharmacokinetic (PK) study of the cryptophycin analog LY 355703 administered on an every 3 weeks schedule. *Cancer Res* 1999; 5 (Suppl): 2–3 (abstract).
49. Sorensen E, Wang B, Lassota P et al, Discodermolide, a potent microtubule stabilising agent, is not cross-resistant with paclitxel in vitro and in vivo. *Proc Am Ass Cancer Res* 2000; 41: 554 (abstract).
50. Berg WJ, Vongphrachanh P, Motzer RJ et al, A phase I study of T138067-sodium in patients with advanced malignancy. *Proc ASCO* 1999; 18: 203a (abstract).
51. Schwendner S, Hoffman LA, Thoolen M, Efficacy of the novel tubulin binding agent T900607 against human tumor xenografts in mice. *Proc Am Ass Cancer Res* 2000; 41: 302 (abstract).
52. von Pawel J, von Roemeling R, Gatzemeier U et al, Tirapazamine plus cisplatin versus cisplatin in advanced non-small cell lung cancer: a report of the international CATAPULT 1 Study Group. *J Clin Oncol* 2000; 18: 1351–9.
53. Sherr CJ. Cancer cell cycles. *Science* 1996; 274: 1672–7.
54. Carlson BA, Dubay MM, Sausville EA et al, Flavopiridol induces G1 arrest with inhibition of cyclin dependent kinases (CDK)2 and CDK4 in human breast carcinoma cells. *Cancer Res* 1996; 56: 2973–8.
55. Senderowicz AM, Headlee D, Stinson SF et al, Phase I trial of continuous infusion flavopiridol, a novel cyclin-dependent kinase inhibitor, in patients with refractory neoplasms. *J Clin Oncol* 1998; 16: 2986–99.
56. Stadler WM, Vogelzang NJ, Amato R et al, Flavopiridol, a novel cyclin-dependent kinase inhibitor, in metastatic renal cancer: a University of Chicago phase II consortium study. *J Clin Oncol* 2000; 18: 371–5.
57. Werner JL, Kelson DP, Karpeh M et al, The cyclin-dependent kinase inhibitor flavopiridol is an active and unexpectedly toxic agent in advanced gastric cancer, *Proc ASCO* 1998; 17: 234a (abstract).
58. Shapiro G, Patterson A, Lynch C et al, A phase II trial of flavopiridol in patients with stage IV non-small cell lung cancer. *Proc ASCO* 1999; 18: 522a (abstract).
59. Fuse E, Tanii H, Kurata N et al, Unpredicted clinical pharmacology of UCN-01 caused by specific binding to human α_1-acid glycoprotein. *Cancer Res* 1998; 58: 3248–53.
60. Gray NS, Wodicka L, Thunnison A-MWH et al, Exploiting chemical libraries, structure and genomics in the search for kinase inhibitors. *Science* 1998; 281: 533–8.
61. Bible KC, Kaufmann SH, Cytotoxic synergy between flavopiridol (NSC 649890, L86–8275) and various antineoplastic agents: the importance of sequence of administration. *Cancer Res* 1997; 57: 3375–80.

62. Fumoleau P, Punt CJA, Priou F et al, Phase I clinical and pharmacokinetic (PK) trial of E7070, a novel sulphonamide, administered daily × 5 days every 3 weeks in patients with solid tumours. *Clin Cancer Res* 1999; 5 (Suppl): 2(abstract).
63. Lahusen JT, Singh S, Sausville EA, Senderowicz AM, Alsterpaullone (ALP) blocks cell cycle progression at G1/S and G2/M with altered expression of G1 and G2 cyclins. *Proc Am Ass Cancer Res* 2000; 41: 30 (abstract).
64. Fry DW, Harvey PJ, Keller PR et al, Cell cycle and biochemical effects of PD0183812, a specific inhibitor of cyclin-dependent kinase 4. *Proc Am Ass Cancer Res* 2000; 41: 314 (abstract).
65. Watkins PJ, Bramson HN, Davis ST et al, The novel cyclin dependent kinase inhibitor GW8510 potentiates adriamycin cytotoxicity by abrogation of a G2/M checkpoint. *Proc Am Ass Cancer Res* 2000; 41: 30 (abstract).
66. Knick VB, Bramson N, Davis ST et al, Novel substituted oxindole inhibitors of cyclin-dependent kinases arrest and protect normal cells from chemotherapy-induced toxicity in vitro. *Proc Am Ass Cancer Res* 2000; 41: 31 (abstract).
67. Fretz H, Soni R, Muller L et al, Fascaplysin, an unusual pigment from marine sponges, inhibits CDK4-dependent RB phosphorylation. *Proc Am Ass Cancer Res* 2000; 41: 249 (abstract).
68. Newell DR, Arris CE, Boyle FT et al, Antiproliferative cyclin dependent kinase inhibitors with distinct molecular interactions and tumor cell growth inhibition profiles. *Clin Cancer Res* 1999; 5 (Suppl): 27 (abstract).
69. Ruetz S, Imbach P, Solf R et al, Effect of CGP79807 on cell cycle dependent kinases, cell cycle progression and onset of apoptosis in in-vitro as well as in-vivo models. *Proc Am Ass Cancer Res* 2000; 41: 560 (abstract).
70. Cobleigh MA, Vogel CL, Tripathy D et al, Multinational study of the efficacy and safety of humanized anti-HER2 monoclonal antibody in women who have HER-2 overexpressing metastatic breast cancer that has progressed after chemotherapy for metastatic disease. *J Clin Oncol* 1999; 17: 2639–48.
71. Norton L, Slamon D, Leyland-Jones B et al, Overall survival advantage to simultaneous chemotherapy plus the humanized anti-HER2 monoclonal antibody Herceptin in HER2-overexpressing metastatic breast cancer. *Proc ASCO* 1999; 18: 127a (abstract).
72. Baselga J, LoRusso P, Herbst R et al, A pharmacokinetic/pharmacodynamic trial of ZD1839 (Iressa), a novel oral epidermal growth factor receptor tyrosine kinase inhibitor, in patients with five selected tumour types. *Clin Cancer Res* 1999; 5 (Suppl): 7 (abstract).
73. Kris M, Ranson M, Ferry D et al, Phase I study of ZD1839 (Iressa), a novel inhibitor of epidermal growth factor receptor tyrosine kinase: evidence of good tolerability and activity. *Clin Cancer Res* 1999; 5 (Suppl): 21–2 (abstract).
74. Druker BJ, Sawyers CL, Talpaz M et al, Phase I trial of a specific ABL tyrosine kinase inhibitor, CGP 57148, in interferon refractory chronic myelogenous leukemia patients. *Proc ASCO* 1999; 18: 7a (abstract).
75. Jacobs TW, Gowan AM, Yadzi H et al, Specificity of HercepTest in determining HER2/neu status of breast cancers using the United States Food and Drug Administration-approved scoring system. *J Clin Oncol* 1999; 7: 1983–7.
76. Halaban R, Growth factors and melanomas. *Semin Oncol* 1996; 23: 673–81.
77. Loganzo Jr F, Dosik JS, Zhao Y et al, Elevated levels of protein tyrosine kinase c-Yes, but not c-Src, in human malignant melanoma. *Oncogene* 1993; 8: 2637–44.
78. De Wit PE, Moretti S, Koenders PG et al, Increasing epidermal growth factor receptor expression in human melanocytic tumor progression. *J Invest Dermatol* 1992; 99: 168–73.
79. Sparrow LE, Heenan PJ, Differential expression of epidermal growth factor receptor in melanocytic tumours demonstrated by immunohistochemistry and mRNA in situ hybridisation. *Australas J Dermatol* 1999; 40: 19–24.
80. Shaheen RM, Davis DW, Liu W et al, Antiangiogenic therapy targeting the tyrosine kinase receptor for vascular endothelial growth factor receptor inhibits the growth of colon cancer liver metastases and induces tumor and endothelial cell apoptosis. *Cancer Res* 1999; 59: 5412–6.
81. Mohammadi M, McMahon G, App H et al, Structure of the tyrosine kinase domain of fibroblast factor receptor in complex with inhibitors. *Science* 1997; 276: 955–60.
82. Patmore SJ, Atkinson BA, Bradford LA et al, In vivo activity of the broadly active tyrosine kinase inhibitor PD166285. *Proc Am Ass Cancer Res* 1999; 40: 723–4 (abstract).
83. Rowinsky EK, Windle JJ, Von Hoff DD, Ras protein farnesyltransferase: a strategic target for anticancer drug development. *J Clin Oncol* 1999; 17: 3631–52.
84. Sepp Lorinzino L, Ma Z, Rands E et al, A peptidomimetic inhibitor of farnesyl–protein transferase blocks the anchorage-dependent and -independent growth of human tumor cell lines. *Cancer Res* 1995; 55: 5302–9.
85. Zujewski J, Horak ID, Bol CJ et al, Phase I and pharmacokinetic study of farnesyl protein transferase inhibitor R115777 in advanced cancer. *J Clin Oncol* 2000; 18: 927–41.
86. Hudes GR, Schol J, Baab J et al, Phase I clinical and pharmacokinetic trial of farnesyltransferase inhibitor R115777 on a 21-day dosing schedule. *Proc ASCO* 1999; 18: 156a (abstract).
87. Brittan CD, Rowinsky E, Yao S-L et al, The farnesyl protein transferase inhibitor L-778,123 in patients with solid cancers. *Proc ASCO* 1999; 18: 155a (abstract).
88. Awada A, Eskens F, Piccart MJ et al, A clinical, pharmacodynamic and pharmacokinetic phase I study of SCH66336 an oral inhibitor of the enzyme farnesyl transferase given once daily in patients with solid tumors. *Clin Cancer Res* 1999; 5 (Suppl): 5 (abstract).
89. Folkman J, What is the evidence that tumours are angiogensis dependent? *J Natl Cancer Inst* 1990; 82: 4–6.
90. Craft PS, Harris AL. Clinical prognostic significance of angiogenesis. *Ann Oncol* 1994; 5: 305–11.
91. Maniotis AJ, Folberg R, Hess A et al, Vascular channel formation by human melanoma cells in vivo and in vitro: vasculogenic mimicry. *Am J Pathol* 1999; 155: 739–52.
92. Bissel MJ, Tumor plasticity allows vasculogenic mimicry, a novel form of angiogenic switch: a rose by any other name?. *Am J Pathol* 1999; 155: 675–9 (commentary).
93. Olsen KB, Hall TC, Horton K et al, Thalidomide (N-phthaloyl-glutamimide) in the treatment of advanced cancer. *Clin Pharmacol Ther* 1965; 6: 292–7.
94. D'Amato RJ, Loughnan MS, Flynn E et al, Thalidomide is an inhibitor of angiogenesis. *Proc Natl Acad Sci USA* 1994; 91: 4082–5.
95. Singhal S, Mehta J, Desikan R et al, Antitumor activity of thalidomide in refractory multiple myeloma. *N Engl J Med* 1999; 341: 1565–71.
96. Fine HA, Figg WD, Jaeckle K et al, Phase II trial of the antiangiogenic agent thalidomide in patients with recurrent high grade gliomas. *J Clin Oncol* 2000; 18: 708–15.
97. Baidas SM, Winer EP, Fleming GF et al, Phase II evaluation of thalidomide in patients with metastatic breast cancer. *J Clin Oncol* 2000; 18: 2710–17.
98. Tseng JE, Glisson BS, Khuri FR et al, Phase II trial of thalidomide in the treatment of recurrent and/or metastatic squamous cell carcinoma of the head and neck. *Proc ASCO* 2000; 19: 417a (abstract).
99. Eisen T, Boschoff C, Mak I et al, Continuous low dose thalidomide: a phase II study in advanced melanoma, renal cell, ovarian and breast cancer. *Br J Cancer* 2000; 82: 812–17.
100. Marx GM, Levi J, Bell DR et al, A phase I/II trial of thalidomide as an antiangiogenic agent in the treatment of advanced cancer. *Proc ASCO* 1999; 18: 454a (abstract).
101. Bhargava P, Marshall JL, Rizvi N et al, A phase I and pharmacokinetic study of TNP-470 administered weekly to patients with advanced cancer. *Clin Cancer Res* 1999; 5: 1989–95.
102. Kudelka AP, Levy T, Verschraegen CF et al, A phase I study of TNP-470 administered to patients with advanced squamous cell carcinoma of the cervix. *Clin Cancer Res* 1997; 3: 1501–5.
103. Bhargava P, Rizvi N, Baidas S et al, Phase I study and assessment of bioactivity of 120-hour infusion of TNP-470 in patients with advanced cancer. *Proc ASCO* 2000; 19: 176a (abstract).
104. Bhargava P, Trocky N, Marshall J et al, A phase I safety, tolerance and pharmacokinetic study of rising dose, rising duration continuous infusion of MSI-1256F (squalamine lactate) in patients with advanced cancer. *Proc ASCO* 1999; 18: 162a (abstract).

105. Amita P, Rowinsky E, Hammond L et al, A phase I and pharmacokinetic study of the unique angiogenesis inhibitor squalamine lactate (MSI-1256F). *Clin Cancer Res* 1999; 5 (Suppl): 4 (abstract).
106. Posey J, Del Grosso A, Khazaeli MB et al, A pilot trial of vitaxin, an antiangiogenic humanized antibody in patients with advanced solid tumors. *Clin Cancer Res* 1999; 5 (Suppl): 21 (abstract).
107. Eskens F, Dumez H, Verweij et al, Phase I and pharmacologic study of EMD121974, an $\alpha_v\beta_3$ and $\alpha_v\beta_5$ integrin inhibitor that perturbs tumor angiogenesis, in patients with solid tumors. *Proc ASCO* 2000; 19: 206a (abstract).
108. Boehm T, Folkman J, Browder T, O'Reilly MS, Antiangiogenic therapy of experimental cancer does not induce acquired drug resistance. *Nature* 1997; 390: 404–7.
109. Fong TAT, Shawver LK, Sun L et al, SU5416 is a potent and selective inhibitor of the vascular endothelial growth factor receptor (Flk-1/KDR) that inhibits tyrosine kinase catalysis, tumor vascularization, and growth of multiple tumor types. *Cancer Res* 1999; 59: 99–106.
110. Rosen L, Mulay M, Mayers A et al, Phase I dose-escalating trial of SU5416, a novel angiogenesis inhibitor in patients with advanced malignancies. *Proc ASCO* 1999; 18: 161a (abstract).
111. O'Donnell AE, Trigo JM, Banerji U et al, A phase I trial of the VEGF inhibitor SU5416, incorporating dynamic contrast MRI assessment of vascular permeability. *Proc ASCO* 2000; 19: 177a (abstract).
112. Stopeck A, Results of a phase I dose-escalating study of the antiangiogenic agent SU5416 in patients with advanced malignancies. *Proc ASCO* 2000; 19: 206a (abstract).
113. Rosen L, Hannah A, Rosen P et al, Phase I dose-escalating trial of oral SU00668, a novel multiple receptor tyrosine kinase inhibitor in patients with advanced malignancies. *Proc ASCO* 2000; 19: 182a (abstract).
114. Sledge G, Miller K, Novotny J et al, A phase II trial of single-agent rhuMAb VEGF (recombinant humanized monoclonal antibody to vascular endothelial cell growth factor) in patients with relapsed metastatic breast cancer. *Proc ASCO* 2000; 19: 3a (abstract).
115. Bergsland E, Hurwitz H, Fehrenbacher L et al, A randomized phase II trial comparing rhuMAb VEGF (recombinant humanized monoclonal antibody to vascular endothelial cell growth factor) plus 5-fluorouracil/leucovorin (FU/LV) to FU/LV alone in patients with metastatic colorectal cancer. *Proc ASCO* 2000; 19: 242a (abstract).
116. DeVore RF, Fehrenbacher L, Herbst RS et al, A randomized phase II trial comparing rhuMAb VEGF (recombinant humanized monoclonal antibody to vascular endothelial cell growth factor) plus carboplatin/paclitaxel (CP) to CP alone in patients with stage IIIB/IV NSCLC. *Proc ASCO* 2000; 19: 485a (abstract).
117. Fielding J, Scholefield J, Stuart R et al, A randomized double-blind placebo-controlled study of marimastat in patients with inoperable gastric cancer. *Proc ASCO* 2000; 19: 240a (abstract).
118. Moore MJ, Hamm J, Eisenberg P et al, A comparison between gemcitabine and the matrix metalloproteinase inhibitor BAY12-9566 in patients with advanced pancreatic cancer. *Proc ASCO* 2000; 19: 240a (abstract).
119. Dark GG, Hill SA, Prise VE et al, Combretastatin A-4, an agent that displays potent and selective toxicity toward tumor vasculature. *Cancer Res* 1997; 57: 1829–34.
120. Rustin GJS, Galbraith SM, Taylor NJ et al, Combretastatin A4 phosphate selectively targets vasculature in animal and human tumors. *Clin Cancer Res* 1999; 5 (Suppl): 4 (abstract).
121. Remick SC, Dowlati A, Lewin J et al, A phase I pharmacokinetic study of single dose intravenous combretastatin A4 prodrug in patients with advanced cancer. *Proc ASCO* 2000; 19: 180a (abstract).
122. News, *J Natl Cancer Inst* 2000; 92: 520.
123. Gelmon KA, Eisenhauer EA, Harris AL et al, Anticancer agents targeting signalling molecules and cancer cell environment: challenges for drug development? *J Natl Cancer Inst* 1999; 91: 1281–7

60

Melanoma of the urogenital tract

Michael A Henderson, John F Thompson

INTRODUCTION

Melanomas arising from the mucosal surfaces of the respiratory, digestive and genitourinary tracts are rare, accounting for *c.* 1% of all melanomas. Melanomas of the urogenital tract (vulva, vagina, external urethral meatus and glans penis) account for only 25% of all mucosal melanomas. The majority of patients are female, as there is no male counterpart to the vulva or vagina, which account for the majority of genitourinary melanomas. It is generally held that mucosal melanomas are different from cutaneous melanomas because of dissimilar tumour characteristics, poor prognosis and clear lack of a relationship to sun exposure. Mucosal melanomas, along with melanomas of the palm of the hand and the sole of the foot, are the usual (but still rare) forms of melanoma found amongst non-Caucasians.

Although urogenital melanomas are commonly considered as mucosal melanomas, many do not arise from a true mucosal surface. The surface of the vulva changes from macroscopically and histologically normal skin, with hair follicles overlying the labia majora, to glabrous skin, lacking hair follicles and sebaceous glands over the labia minora, then merging with typical mucosa at the vaginal introitus.[1] Not infrequently, the exact histological site of origin of a melanoma cannot be determined when it is adjacent to more than one type of skin or the mucosa.

The skin of the glans penis is histologically glabrous skin similar to most of the vulva. Lesions arising from this part of the penis have many clinical similarities to vulval melanomas and are therefore included in the urogenital group of melanomas.[2] Melanomas arising from the shaft of the penis and scrotum are very uncommon but appear to behave as typical cutaneous melanomas and will not be considered further.

Melanomas thought to arise from the distal urethra or urethral meatus, in either the male or female, can be very difficult to distinguish from melanomas arising from the adjacent vulva or glans penis. There is little to be gained by distinguishing lesions arising around the female urethral meatus, which merges with the vaginal mucosa, or the male urethral meatus, which merges with the glabrous skin of the glans penis, because the treatment and behaviour of these lesions is no different from that of lesions located adjacent to, but unequivocally not related, to the urethral meatus. Melanomas elsewhere in the urinary tract (in the urethra and bladder) are extraordinarily rare.

Melanoblasts are found in increased numbers in the glabrous skin of the external genitalia of both sexes compared to normal skin. The mucosa of the female genital tract is sparsely populated with melanoblasts and may explain the rarity of melanoma at this site. It has been suggested that the poor prognosis of urogenital melanoma is related to specific histological features of the environment in which they arise. Glabrous skin lacks a well-formed reticular dermis while mucosa lacks both a dermo–epidermal junction and a reticular dermis, and is closely supplied with blood vessels and lymphatics. The absence of a barrier to vertical growth and early access to the lymphatic/vascular system may provide an avenue for early invasion and metastasis.

Staging of urogenital melanomas remains problematic because of the very limited data available and lack of a useful staging system. Clark level microstaging is not possible and experience with tumour thickness as a prognostic factor is limited. Clinical staging (stage I, local disease only; stage II, spread to regional lymph nodes only; and stage III, metastatic disease) is of some value as many patients present with regional or distant disease.

MELANOMA OF THE FEMALE UROGENITAL TRACT – VULVA

The vulva is the commonest site for melanomas arising in the urogenital region. They account for <10% of all malignancies affecting the vulva. It is a rare disease entity and consequently most reported series of this disease are small, usually representing the experience of large centres (with possible referral bias) and rarely with the numbers to evaluate treatment options. The largest and most comprehensive study of vulvar melanoma is a series of 219 cases, representing nearly all the vulvar melanomas occurring in Sweden over a 25-year period, treated in 60 hospitals.[1] In comparison with cutaneous melanoma, which increased in frequency during that period, the incidence of vulvar melanoma actually fell. There are no recognized aetiological factors for vulvar melanoma. In a report from a large North American centre, black females were equally represented among patients with vulvar melanoma but not among women with cutaneous melanoma.[3]

Most patients present with symptomatic disease, while a few are found during routine gynaecological examination. It is typically a disease of elderly females, with few women under the age of 50 being affected.[4] The majority of patients report the presence of a mass and/or bleeding.[1] Pruritis and pain are common symptoms at presentation, while urinary difficulties are less commonly reported.[3] An example of a vulval melanoma in an elderly vulvar patient is shown in Figure 60.1.

Box 60.1 ***Melanoma of the vulva***

Presentation:	Mass/vaginal bleeding, 25% of patients present with inguinal lymphadenopathy
Treatment:	Complete excision, consider adjuvant radiotherapy
Outcome:	Five-year survival 25–35%

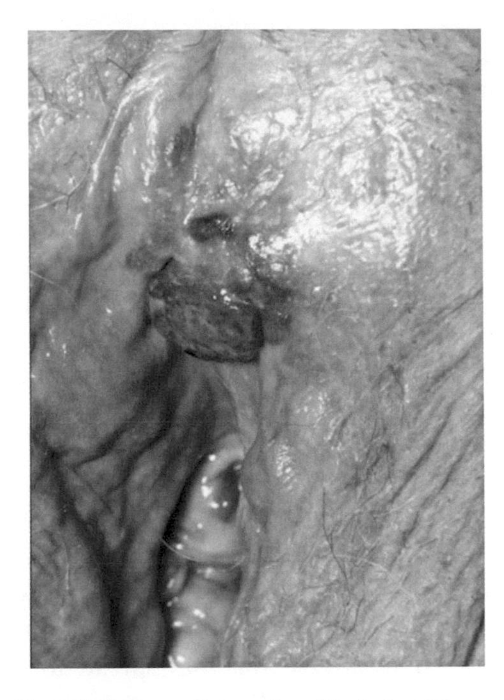

Figure 60.1 *Melanoma of the vulva. Typical appearance of a central vulva melanoma. The lesion is pigmented and nodular in appearance.*

Vulvar melanomas arise predominantly from two specific areas, laterally over the labia majora (31%) and near the midline from the clitoris (31%), the periurethral region (11%) and the vaginal introitus (4%). The characteristics of vulvar melanomas vary with the histological site of origin. Melanomas arising in the hair-bearing skin over the labia majora are characteristically flat pigmented lesions with serpiginous margins, accounting for 12% of all vulvar melanomas and not infrequently arising from a pre-existing naevus (35%). The majority of vulvar melanomas arise from glabrous type skin; these lesions are not associated with a pre-existing naevus and are amelanotic in nearly one-quarter of all cases. In one-third of cases the melanomas extended to both types of skin; the features of these lesions represent a mix of both skin types. It has been suggested that melanomas arising from the hair-bearing skin of the lateral labia majora occur at a rate consistent with their surface area compared to other sites in the body. In contrast more medially placed lesions arising from glabrous skin occur *c.* 2.5 times more frequently than would be expected on the basis of their surface area.[1]

The histology of vulvar melanoma is quite characteristic and differs markedly from that of cutaneous melanoma. The commonest type is mucosal lentiginous melanoma (57%), which is similar to acral lentiginous melanoma, the specific form of melanoma arising from the glabrous skin of the palms, soles and subungual areas. Nodular melanoma is the next most common type (22%) and superficial spreading melanoma the least common (4%). Nearly all vulvar melanomas have a vertical growth phase and more than 80% of lesions are ulcerated. Nearly all vulvar melanomas are characteristically thick lesions – most (even clinical stage I lesions) >4 mm in thickness. Thin tumours (<1 mm) account for less than 5% of the total.[1]

Staging and prognosis

In the absence of a useful and widely accepted staging system that specifically addresses the unique features of vulvar melanoma, a simple clinical staging system is used by most authors. Stage I disease is local disease only, stage II is disease that has spread to regional lymph nodes and stage III is metastatic disease. The major limitation of this system is that for patients with localized disease (stage I), it fails to account for the major differences in survival between patients with thick or thin lesions. In an attempt to redress this problem, many reports in recent years have included tumour thickness in describing their patients. International Federation for Gynecology and Obstetrics (FIGO) staging, devised for the more common vulvar malignancies, is of little prognostic or clinical value. A staging system specifically designed for vulvar melanomas has been described, but is yet to be validated and has not achieved widespread usage.[5]

Approximately one-quarter of patients present with involved inguinal lymph glands and another 5–10% with distant metastatic disease.[1,6,7] Survival for all patients at 5 years is a consistent 25–35%.[1,4,7–9] For patients with stage I disease at presentation, survival is much improved (up to 50% at 5 years) but even within this group there is considerable heterogeneity.[1,3] Most clinically localized melanomas would be regarded as thick with an average thickness of 4 mm but less than one-third of patients have thin, good prognosis lesions.[1,3,6] Although the survival of patients with thin, clinically localized disease is considerably higher than it is for most patients with vulvar melanoma (>50% alive at 5 years), their outcome falls far short of that for patients with cutaneous melanomas of similar thicknesses. In summary, clinical stage is a good predictor of outcome. For patients with localized, thin melanomas, tumour thickness is important. Older age, mitotic rate, ulceration and tumour site have also been associated with a poorer prognosis.[8,10–12] In a large multivariate analysis, clinical stage and ulceration were the only factors found to be independently predictive of outcome for all patients with vulvar melanoma. For patients with localized disease, tumour thickness, tumour ulceration and clinical amelanosis were independently associated with outcome.[13]

Treatment

For many years, radical surgery (vulvectomy and inguinal lymphadenectomy) was the standard approach because of the often extensive nature of the primary lesion, surrounding in situ changes and the advanced nature of the disease.[14] Overall, one-third of patients will experience local recurrence.[3] Major procedures such as bilateral radical vulvectomy do not appear to confer any survival benefit over less radical procedures such as hemivulvectomy or complete local excision. Limited surgical procedures are associated with a higher local recurrence rate but this does not appear to translate into a poorer overall outcome.[3,6,13,15] Similarly, prophylactic lymphadenectomy (which should be bilateral for centrally located lesions) has also not been shown to affect outcome. The role of sentinel lymph node biopsy, whilst a theoretically attractive option, has yet to be evaluated.

For the patient requiring a major surgical approach, the patient refusing surgery or the patient presenting with extensive primary or recurrent disease, palliative local radiotherapy is a reasonable option. Radiotherapy may be combined either in association with a limited resection or as primary therapy.[16] Generally, radiation therapy has been thought to have limited effectiveness in melanoma, however, hypofractionation techniques (higher than conventional doses per treatment) appear to be more effective.[17]

MELANOMA OF THE FEMALE UROGENITAL TRACT – VAGINA

Vaginal melanomas account for *c.* one-third of urogenital melanomas.[2,3] Primary vaginal melanomas, however, account for <5% of all vaginal malignancies. Melanomas occurring elsewhere in the female genital tract are exceedingly rare. There are a handful of

Box 60.2 ***Melanoma of the vagina***

Very rare tumour	
Presentation:	Mass/vaginal bleeding
Appearance:	Usually amelanotic
Management:	Radical resection (pelvic exenteration)
Outcome:	Five-year survival 15–25%

isolated reports of melanoma involving the cervix and even fewer of melanoma involving the uterus.[2,3,14]

Typically, vaginal melanomas are located in the lower one-third of the vagina, in contrast to other malignant lesions which typically involve the upper vagina, and the patients are usually younger than women with vulvar melanomas. One small series reported an average age of 43 years, with the youngest patient aged 25.[18] A small proportion of patients are identified on routine gynaecological examination but most patients present with symptoms, the most common being vaginal bleeding. Discharge is also commonly reported, along with palpation of a mass.[19] Urinary symptoms may be prominent in cases with lesions close to the bladder neck.[20] Many vaginal melanomas are amelanotic and they may measure several centimetres in size.[19] More advanced lesions may be polypoid in appearance and ulceration is not uncommon. Satellite lesions around the primary tumour may also be seen.

Because of the rarity of vaginal melanomas, there is very little objective experience on which to base treatment recommendations. Approximately one-third of patients will have evidence of regional and/or distant disease at presentation.[14] Generally, radical approaches to treatment (pelvic exenteration plus regional node resection) are justified by the high rates of local recurrence after limited surgery and the observation that the majority of patients dying with distant disease also have locoregional failure.[21,22] Less aggressive local surgery with adjuvant radiotherapy appears to offer a reasonable compromise between operative morbidity and outcome.[22]

There are very few cases available to investigate factors predictive for survival. Clinical stage at presentation and the presence of regional node metastases found at operation are predictive of outcome. Tumour thickness is of limited value as most tumours are deeply invasive at presentation.[19] The prognosis for vaginal melanomas is significantly worse than for vulvar melanomas, with most patients succumbing within 2 years of diagnosis, and long-term survival is rare.[14,19,22,23]

MELANOMAS OF THE MALE URETHRAL MEATUS AND GLANS PENIS

Lesions in this site are extraordinarily rare and there is little objective evidence on which to base treatment recommendations. These lesions present as a flat pigmented lesion, typically brown; in most cases the lesion arises de novo. The patients are usually elderly. Presentation is often delayed and a significant proportion of lesions are ulcerated at the time of presentation. An example of a melanoma arising in the region of the urethral meatus and extending onto the glans penis is shown in Figure 60.2.

The few series reported all describe experiences with only a handful of patients. Not surprisingly, studies reporting patients with thicker lesions demonstrate a higher rate of regional and distant disease at presentation, more aggressive surgical procedures and poorer survival.[24–26] In a recent report of six cases from the Sydney Melanoma Unit all were stage I at presentation, with an average melanoma thickness of 1.78 mm. Even among this good prognosis group, three have since died of the disease.[2] In contrast, others have reported

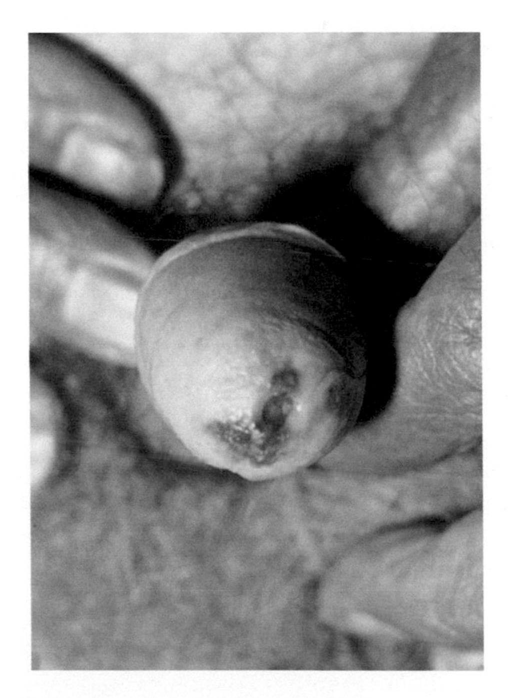

Figure 60.2 *Melanoma of the glans penis. The lesion is typically flat and pigmented.*

Box 60.3 ***Melanoma of glans penis***

Very rare tumour	
Appearance:	Flat brown pigmented lesion
Treatment:	Complete excision
Outcome:	Poor

significantly more advanced disease at presentation, with a predictable decrease in survival.[24–26] Survival of patients with lesions >1.50 mm in thickness is particularly poor. For thin lesions, complete local excision is indicated. Except in the most extraordinary situations, total penectomy with bilateral groin and suprainguinal node dissections, which has been practised in the past, does not appear to be justified. Elective lymphadenectomy, which should be bilateral, is associated with significant morbidity, with no convincing evidence of any effect on survival. The role of sentinel node biopsy is yet to be determined. Patients with positive inguinal nodes at presentation should undergo dissection of both the inguinal and the iliac lymph nodes.[2]

REFERENCES

1. Ragnarsson-Olding BK, Kanter-Lewensohn LR, Lagerlof B et al, Malignant melanoma of the vulva in a nationwide, 25-year study of 219 Swedish females: clinical observations and histopathologic features. *Cancer* 1999; 86: 1273–84.
2. Larsson KBM, Shaw HM, Thompson JF et al, Primary mucosal and glans penis melanomas: the Sydney Melanoma Unit experience. *Austr N Z J Surg* 1999; 69: 121–26.
3. DeMatos P, Tyler DS, Seigler HF, Malignant melanoma of the mucous membranes: a review of 119 cases. *Ann Surg Oncol* 1998; 5: 733–42.
4. Piura B, Egan M, Lopes A, Monaghan JM, Malignant melanoma of the vulva: a clinicopathologic study of 18 cases. *J Surg Oncol* 1992; 50: 234–40.
5. Chung AF, Woodruff JM, Lewis Jr JL, Malignant melanoma of the vulva: a report of 44 cases. *Obstet Gynecol* 1975; 45: 638–46.
6. Phillips GL, Bundy BN, Okagaki T et al, Malignant melanoma of the vulva treated by radical hemivulvectomy. A prospective study of the Gynecologic Oncology Group. *Cancer* 1994; 73: 2626–32.
7. Look KY, Roth LM, Sutton GP, Vulvar melanoma reconsidered. *Cancer* 1993; 72: 143–6.
8. Bradgate MG, Rollaston TP, McConkey CC, Powell J, Malignant melanoma of the vulva: a clinicopathological study of 50 women. *Br J Obstet Gynaecol* 1990; 97: 124–33.
9. Rogo KO, Anderrson R, Edborn G, Stendahl U, Conservative surgery for vulvovaginal melanoma. *Eur J Gynaecol Oncol* 1991; 12: 113–9.
10. Tasseron EW, van der Esch EP, Hart A et al, A clinicopathological study of 30 melanomas of the vulva. *Gynecol Oncol* 1992; 46: 170–5.
11. Trimble EL, Lewis JL, Williams LL et al, Management of vulvar melanoma. *Gynecol Oncol* 1992; 45: 254–8.
12. Rose PG, Piver MS, Tsukada Y, Lau T, Conservative therapy for melanoma of the vulva. *Am J Obstet Gynecol* 1988; 159: 52–5.
13. Ragnarsson-Olding BK, Nilsson BR, Kanter-Lewensohn LRK et al, Malignant melanoma of the vulva in a nationwide 25-year study of 219 Swedish females. *Cancer* 1999; 86: 1285–93.
14. Ariel IM, Malignant melanoma of the female genital system: a report of 48 patients and review of the literature. *J Surg Oncol* 1981; 16: 371–83.
15. Scheistroen M, Trope C, Karen J et al, Malignant melanoma of the vulva FIGO stage I: evaluation of prognostic factors in 43 patients with emphasis on DNA ploidy and surgical treatment. *Gynecol Oncol* 1996; 61: 253–8.
16. Slevin NJ, Pointon RC, Radical radiotherapy for carcinoma of the vulva. *Br J Radiol* 1989; 62: 145–7.
17. Harwood AR, Cummings BJ, Radiotherapy for mucosal melanomas. *Int J Rad Oncol Biol Phys* 1982; 8: 1121–6.
18. Liu LY, Hou YJ, Li JZ, Primary malignant melanoma of the vagina: a report of seven cases. *Obstet Gynecol* 1987; 70: 569–72.
19. Borazjani G, Prem KA, Okagaki T et al, Primary malignant melanoma of the vagina: a clinicopathological analysis of 10 cases. *Gynecol Oncol* 1990; 37: 264–7.
20. Johnston Jr GA, Klotz J, Boutselis JG, Primary invasive carcinoma of the vagina. *Surg Gynecol Obstet* 1983; 156: 34–40.
21. Van Nostrand KM, Lucci III JA, Schell M et al, Primary vaginal melanoma: improved survival with radical pelvic surgery. *Gynecol Oncol* 1994; 55: 234–7.
22. Irvin Jr WP, Bliss SA, Rice LW et al, Malignant melanoma of the vagina and locoregional control: radical surgery revisited. *Gynecol Oncol* 1998; 71: 476–80.
23. Geisler JP, Look KY, Moore DA, Sutton GP, Pelvic exenteration for malignant melanomas of the vagina or urethra with over 3 mm of invasion. *Gynecol Oncol* 1995; 59: 338–41.
24. Manivel JC, Fraley EE, Malignant melanoma of the penis and male urethra: 4 case reports and literature review. *J Urol* 1988; 139: 813–6.
25. Stillwell TJ, Zincke H, Gaffey TA, Woods JE, Malignant melanoma of the penis. *J Urol* 1988; 140: 72–5.
26. Oldbring J, Mikulowski P, Malignant melanoma of the penis and male urethra. Report of nine cases and review of the literature. *Cancer* 1987; 59: 581–7.

61

Primary pulmonary melanoma

John F Thompson, Johannes HW de Wilt

INTRODUCTION

Primary melanoma of the lung is undoubtedly a very rare condition, with only a few reports of it in the literature, but the exact incidence of this disease is a subject of continuing debate. Some investigators are convinced that it does not exist and simply represents a melanoma that has metastasized to the lung from an unknown or totally regressed primary tumour. Without a visible primary lesion, a lung metastasis could continue to grow and eventually present as an apparently isolated focus of melanoma.[1,2] Since melanocytes have not been demonstrated in the normal tracheobronchial tree it is difficult to explain the histogenesis of a primary lung melanoma. Moreover, metastases to the lung from a primary cutaneous melanoma are very common, with *c.* 70% of patients who die of metastatic melanoma having involvement of the lungs at autopsy.[3–6] Metastatic disease involving the lung typically presents as multiple pulmonary nodules, but can occur as a solitary nodule as well. In 7–9% of patients, pulmonary metastases are the only clinically detectable foci of metastatic disease.[7]

Despite this controversy, the literature contains a number of reports of patients with melanomas which seem to be of primary lung origin. In these patients, their history and subsequent follow-up appear to exclude the possibility of metastasis to the lung from a primary site elsewhere.[3,8–39] Supporting evidence for a diagnosis of primary lung melanoma may be obtained from histopathological features of the tumour, as well as a pattern of subsequent regional lymph node involvement that is consistent with that of other tumours of primary bronchial origin. Failure to find a primary melanoma elsewhere, either during life or at the time of autopsy, is another piece of evidence suggesting a diagnosis of primary pulmonary melanoma.

Primary melanomas most commonly present as neoplasms of the skin but their occasional origin in non-cutaneous sites is comprehensively documented in the literature.[11,40,41] Ocular and conjunctival melanomas are the most common, but non-cutaneous melanomas are also well recognized to arise in the nasopharynx, the oropharynx, the leptomeninges, the adrenal gland, the urethra, the vulva, the ovaries, the vagina and, occasionally, in parts of the gastrointestinal tract, including the oesophagus, the stomach, the gall bladder, the small bowel, the large bowel and the anal canal.[42] An important difference from melanoma of the tracheobronchial tree, however, is that melanocytes have been identified in most of these sites in normal individuals, providing a plausible histogenetic basis for the origin of the melanomas.

CRITERIA FOR DIAGNOSIS

Jensen and Egedorf[15] were the first to propose minimal criteria on which a diagnosis of primary lung melanoma could be made with certainty. Other authors have since adjusted these criteria, proposing minor variations and additions.[16,23,27,35,36,43] Although such strict criteria are undoubtedly appropriate and desirable, there are instances in which they cannot all be satisfied and yet the likelihood is high that a lung tumour is a primary melanoma.[32] The criteria currently used for the diagnosis of primary lung melanoma are given in Box 61.1.

INCIDENCE OF PRIMARY LUNG MELANOMA

The majority of primary lung malignancies are squamous cell carcinomas, small cell carcinomas, large cell carcinomas, adenocarcinomas and carcinoid tumours; these account for >99% of all primary lung neoplasms.[33,44] Reviewing 10,134 patients with primary lung tumours treated at the Mayo Clinic over a 10-year period, three patients with primary lung melanomas were reported.[33] These figures emphasize the rarity of primary lung melanomas but cannot be used to quantify incidence, since the patients seen at the Mayo Clinic were referred for treatment and the data are therefore not population based. Other uncommon lung tumours have usually been described as single case reports or in small series.

A diagnosis of primary lung melanoma has been claimed in numerous publications, but in many early reports patients did not fulfil the criteria subsequently accepted as being necessary to definitively establish the diagnosis. The first two recorded cases, reported in 1888 by Todd,[8] were certainly based on insufficient evidence to warrant the diagnosis. Similarly, other early reports, e.g. Kunkel and Torrey[9] in 1916 and Carlucci and Schleussner[10] in 1942, were deficient because full autopsies were not performed to exclude the possibility of a primary melanoma elsewhere. It was not until 1963 that a patient fulfilling subsequently accepted criteria for the diagnosis of primary lung melanoma was reported by Salm.[3] In a 1987 publication, Alghanem et al.[27] considered it appropriate to accept only seven previously reported cases as true primary lung melanomas on the basis of stringent criteria for diagnosis. Reporting a further patient in 1990, Jennings et al.[32] suggested that only 19 previous cases in the literature could be regarded as fulfilling minimal criteria for the diagnosis of primary lung melanoma. As far as could be determined from a comprehensive review of the literature by the present authors, the total number of reported cases in the English literature for which the diagnosis had been established by appropriate criteria stood at 38 in 2001 (see Table 61.1).

Box 61.1 ***Criteria that suggest a primary pulmonary melanoma***

- A solitary, central tumour in the lung or surgical specimen
- No previous history of excision or fulguration of a cutaneous, ocular or mucous membrane lesion that could have been melanoma
- No demonstrable melanoma in any other organ at the time of diagnosis
- Tumour morphology compatible with a primary malignant tumour by immunohistochemistry and/or electron microscopy (considerable polymorphism will argue in favour of metastatic disease)
- No evidence at autopsy of a primary melanoma elsewhere in the body

HISTOGENESIS

Although melanocytes are predominantly localized in the basal portions of the epidermis at the dermo-epidermal junction of the skin, they have also been described in other organs. Migration of melanocytes to other organs during embryogenesis is a plausible theory for the existence of these cells in parts of the body other than the skin. Melanocytes have been demonstrated in the mucosa of the oropharynx, the larynx (including the glottis) and the oesophagus,[45–48] and the presence of these potential precursor cells could explain the occasional occurrence of primary melanomas in these sites. The trachea, bronchi and lungs develop as a tubular outgrowth from the primitive foregut during embryogenesis. This outgrowth arises anteriorly at a point between the oropharynx and the oesophagus, in the region of the larynx.[15] No systematic study has demonstrated melanocytes in the bronchial mucosa, but because the bronchi and lungs are structures that are embryologically so closely related to the oropharynx, larynx and oesophagus, and are of similar endodermal derivation, it is surprising that melanocytes are not found in them. However, it is thought that they may indeed migrate to the bronchial mucosa and be present on rare occasions.

Although this explanation would seem to provide the most likely histogenetic basis for the development of primary lung melanomas, alternative explanations have been proposed. One is that they result from a process of metaplasia, a suggestion supported by the

Table 61.1 *Published reports of patients with primary melanomas of the trachea, bronchi, lungs and pleura fulfilling most or all of the currently accepted diagnostic criteria*

Authors/year (ref. no.)	Sex/age*	Site†	Outcome‡
Salm/1963 (3)	M/45	LL	Died 6 months postoperatively
Reed and Kent/1964 (13)	M/71	LL	Alive 10 years postoperatively
Reid and Mehta/1966 (14)	F/60	Trachea	Alive 11 years postoperatively
	M/35	LL	NA
Jensen and Egedorf/1967 (15)	F/61	UL	Died 7 months postoperatively
Allen and Drash/1968 (16)	F/40	LL	NA
Taboada et al./1972 (17)	M/56	LL	Died 14 months postoperatively
	M/40	UL	NA
Mori et al./1977 (18)	F/47	Trachea	Alive 1 year postoperatively
Smith and Opipari/1978 (19)	M/49	Pleura	Died 10 months postoperatively
Adebonojo et al./1979 (20)	F/55	UL	Alive 3 years postoperatively
Robertson et al./1980 (21)	F/70	Carina	Died 9 weeks after diagnosis
Gephardt/1981 (22)	M/47	MSB	Died at time of diagnosis
Verweij et al./1982 (23)	M/46	Trachea, MSB	Died 2 months postoperatively
Angel and Prados/1984 (24)	F/41	ML	NA
Cagle et al./1984 (25)	M/80	ML	Died 5 months after diagnosis
Carstens et al./1984 (26)	F/29	UL	Died 1 month postoperativly
Alghanem et al./1987 (27)	F/42	LL	Alive 2.5 years postoperatively
Demeter et al./1987 (28)	M/56	UL	Died 1 month postoperatively
Santos et al./1987 (29)	M/58	LL	Alive 18 months postoperatively
Bagwell et al./1989 (30)	M/62	UL	Died 2 months postoperatively
Bertola et al./1989 (31)	F/30	LL	Died 5 months postoperatively
Jennings et al./1990 (32)	F/34	LL	Alive 19 months postoperatively
Miller and Allen/1993 (33)	M/56	LL	Died 4 months postoperatively
	M/67	ML	Died 14 months postoperatively
	F/77	LL	Died 18 months postoperatively
Pasquini et al./1994 (34)	F/66	LL	NA
Farrell et al./1996 (35)	F/66	LL	NA
Wilson and Moran/1997 (36)	F/55	UL	Died 18 months postoperatively
	M/71	LL	Alive 9 years postoperatively
	M/45	UL	Alive 4 months postoperatively
	M/NA	ML	Died 4 months postoperatively
	M/52	UL	Died 32 months postoperatively
	M/64	UL	Died 4 months postoperatively
	M/48	UL	Died 14 months postoperatively
	M/50	UL	Alive 30 months postoperatively
Duarte et al./1998 (37)	F/NA	Trachea	Died 13 months postoperatively
Ost et al./1999 (38)	M/90	UL	Died at time of diagnosis

*M, male; F, female; NA, not available.
†LL, lower lobe; ML, middle lobe; MSB, main stem bronchus; UL, upper lobe.

frequent finding of squamous metaplasia around the site of a tracheobronchial melanoma.[14] In mucous glands in the oral cavity, a condition described as melanogenic metaplasia has been reported,[49] and the possibility has been raised that a similar process might occur in the mucous glands of the tracheobronchial tree. Another proposal is that precursor cells (Kulchitsky cells) have the potential to undergo melanocytic differentiation as well as neuroendocrine differentiation.[32] Also of possible relevance in a consideration of the possible histogenetic origin of primary lung melanomas is the observation that melanin is present in some carcinoid tumours, indicating that it is possible for the epithelium of the lower respiratory tract to undergo melanocytic differentiation.[50] Carcinoid tumours and melanomas share many biological and histopathological features,[28,51] and it is well documented that both peripheral and central carcinoid tumours occasionally contain melanosomes as well as neurosecretory granules.[50–52]

A similar problem exists in seeking to explain the origin of primary adrenal melanomas,[26,53–55] since melanocytes have not been identified in this location either. However, it may be relevant to note that melanocytes are of neural crest origin and are thus clearly related to the cells in the adrenal medulla from which phaeochromocytomas arise.

CLINICAL PRESENTATION AND DEFINITIVE DIAGNOSIS

The cases of lung melanoma reported in the literature are divided approximately equally into those which presented as a polypoid obstructing lesion within the tracheobronchial tree and those which presented as a mass within the lung parenchyma. The tumour is almost always unifocal, but multifocal primary lung melanomas have been described.[23,56] Four cases of tracheal melanoma[14,18,23,37] and one case of primary pleural melanoma have also been reported.[19]

As expected, the presenting symptoms of a patient with a primary lung melanoma are determined by the site and size of the tumour. A wide variety of clinical manifestations of primary lung melanoma have been described. In the previously published reports patients' symptoms included cough (50%), haemoptysis (40%), postobstructive pneumonia (25%), lobar collapse or atelectasis (25%), and constitutional symptoms of weight loss, night sweats, or fever (25%).[38] In one-third of the patients the lesion was diagnosed as an incidental finding on chest radiography for an unrelated reason.[17,31] A definitive histological diagnosis of melanoma for endobronchial lesions can usually be obtained by bronchoscopy and biopsy, and for lesions in the lung parenchyma by fine needle aspiration biopsy. However, a diagnosis of primary (rather than metastatic) lung melanoma is unlikely to be made at this time and may not be reached until after full staging investigations, pathological examination of the resected tumour, an appropriate period of follow-up and, possibly, at autopsy.

PATHOLOGY

In 1968, Allen and Drash[16] suggested that the surgical pathologist must 'think' melanoma when examining a lung tumour if the diagnosis is not to be missed.[16] Over three decades later this advice may still be appropriate, as melanoma remains 'the great imitator'. It may be confused with more conventional types of lung cancer, such as large cell carcinoma, sarcoma or poorly differentiated small cell carcinoma of the lung or a carcinoid tumour. Having considered the possibility of a melanoma diagnosis, confirmation or exclusion of this possibility should then be achievable by careful examination for the classical features of melanoma, with support from immunohistochemistry and electron microscopy. The particular histological features recognized as being indicative of a primary lung melanoma are summarized in Box 61.2.[16,24,31,37]

Box 61.2 ***Histological criteria suggesting a diagnosis of primary pulmonary melanoma***

- Obvious melanoma cells, confirmed by immunohistochemical staining for S-100 and HMB-45 and possibly electron microscopy
- Evidence of junctional change (atypical melanocytic hyperplasia and mitoses) in the mucosa with 'dropping off' of melanoma cells
- 'Nesting' of melanoma cells beneath the bronchial epithelium
- Invasion of the intact (i.e. non-ulcerated) bronchial epithelium by melanoma cells

PATTERNS OF METASTASIS

Primary melanoma of the lung metastasizes in a pattern consistent with that of other primary lung tumours; indeed, this is one of the points of evidence raised in support of the existence of lung melanoma as an entity (see Box 61.1). Thus, involvement of regional lymph nodes in the lung hilum and mediastinum is likely to be observed. As with primary cutaneous melanomas, there is the additional possibility of systemic dissemination via the bloodstream to sites such as the brain, the liver, the adrenal gland, the mesentery and bone. Metastatic disease involving the pleura, pericardium and heart also occurs.[30,31]

TREATMENT

Based on experience with primary melanomas arising in other sites, the treatment of choice for primary lung melanoma is radical surgical excision. This will usually involve formal lobectomy or pneumonectomy. For primary cutaneous melanomas the prognosis for the patient does not appear to be significantly worse if regional lymph node dissection is delayed until metastatic disease in regional nodes becomes clinically apparent. For primary lung melanoma, however, there is little possibility of performing a satisfactory delayed regional lymph node clearance in the lung hilum and mediastinum following a lobectomy or pneumonectomy. It therefore seems logical to clear these nodes at the time of the initial definitive lung surgery whenever possible. The major difficulty with this theoretically ideal approach is that the diagnosis of primary rather than secondary lung melanoma may not be established with reasonable certainty until after detailed pathological examination of the resected tumour (see Box 61.2).

In the absence of any evidence to indicate otherwise, the treatment of locally recurrent melanoma from a lung primary must be based on the same standard treatment principles that have been established for other forms of melanoma. If radical surgical excision is possible, it provides the best form of palliation, and may even achieve cure. If whole-body imaging by computerized tomography (CT) scanning or, more reliably, by positron emission tomography (PET) scanning does not reveal any evidence of metastatic disease elsewhere, radical surgery is certainly indicated. Because melanoma tissue invariably has a very high glucose uptake, whole-body PET scanning with fluorine-18-fluorodeoxyglucose has largely replaced CT and MRI scanning as the staging investigation of choice in several major melanoma treatment centres.[57–62] This imaging modality is therefore likely to assist in determining whether a focus of melanoma in a lung is a primary or secondary tumour. If a diagnosis of primary lung melanoma is confirmed, PET scanning should also demonstrate whether distant metastasis has occurred and, if it has, should allow inappropriate surgery as treatment for the primary lung melanoma to be avoided.[62]

If surgical clearance of the recurrent disease is not feasible, systemic chemotherapy may be considered, or radiotherapy if the tumour mass in the chest is causing troublesome symptoms. Foci of metastatic disease outside the chest must similarly be treated on their merits, according to general principles for the treatment of metastatic melanoma, since there are no data for primary lung melanomas to indicate that any different form of treatment is likely to be more effective in this situation.

PROGNOSIS

Although information is very limited, previous reports of patients with primary lung melanomas indicate that the prognosis is generally very poor, with most patients succumbing to the disease within 16 months. The principal determinant of outcome is the presence or absence of local (peribronchial and hilar) lymph node metastases. However, there have been a number of long-term survivors after treatment by radical surgery that was apparently curative.[13,14,20,27,29,32,36] Long-term survival after treatment of primary lung melanoma by chemotherapy, immunotherapy or radiotherapy alone has not been reported.

As previously explained, it is possible that some tumours diagnosed as primary lung melanomas may actually be metastases from a totally regressed primary cutaneous melanoma. Thus, the results of treating foci of metastatic melanoma from an occult primary site warrant review. It is clear that, in general, the survival outcome for patients with metastatic disease from an occult primary tumour is no worse than the outcome for patients with metastatic disease from a known primary site.[63–66] Some authors have even demonstrated an improved outcome for patients with visceral metastases from an occult primary compared to those from a known primary lesion.[67] The treatment of choice for melanoma metastases, regardless of primary site, is therefore radical surgical resection whenever possible.

La Hei et al.[68] reported a 22% actuarial 5-year survival following surgical resection of pulmonary metastatic melanoma in 83 patients at the Sydney Melanoma Unit, with a median survival of 19 months. Similar results following resection of pulmonary metastases have been reported by other groups,[69,70] with occasional long-term survivors in several published series.[71–74] A recent study described 15 patients with an unknown primary (cutaneous) melanoma who underwent resection of a pulmonary melanoma mass;[75] histopathological review of 13 resection specimens could not differentiate these lesions from a primary pulmonary melanoma. During follow-up, six patients developed cutaneous or lymph node recurrences, suggesting that these pulmonary lesions were metastatic; however, the remaining seven patients were without a primary cutaneous lesion after long-term follow-up or at the time of death. Overall survival in the total group of patients operated upon for these pulmonary melanoma lesions with no evidence of a primary cutaneous melanoma was remarkably good, with a 42% 5-year survival rate.

Thus, if a lung tumour is identified and shown on biopsy to be melanoma, with no other focus of melanoma demonstrable elsewhere in the body by relevant imaging techniques, the possibility that this tumour is a primary lung melanoma needs to be considered. Radical surgical excision then becomes an appropriate treatment option, offering the patient the best, and probably the only, chance of cure, even if it is subsequently shown to have been a deposit of metastatic melanoma.

REFERENCES

1. Smith JL, Stehlin JS, Spontaneous regression of primary malignant melanomas with regional metastases. *Cancer* 1965; 18: 1399–415.
2. Milton GW, Lane Brown MM, Gilder M, Malignant melanoma with an occult primary lesion. *Br J Surg* 1967; 54: 651–8.
3. Salm R, A primary malignant melanoma of the bronchus. *J Path Bact* 1963; 85: 121–6.
4. Das Gupta T, Brasfield R, Metastatic melanoma: a clinicopathological study. *Cancer* 1964; 17: 1323–39.
5. Webb WR, Gamsu G, Thoracic metastasis in malignant melanoma. A radiographic survey of 65 patients. *Chest* 1977; 71: 176–81.
6. Sutton FD, Vestal RE, Creagh CE, Varied presentations of metastatic pulmonary melanoma. *Chest* 1974; 65: 415–9.
7. Gromet MA, Ominsky SH, Epstein WL, Blois MS, The thorax as the initial site for systemic relapse in malignant melanoma: a prospective survey of 324 patients. *Cancer* 1979; 44: 776–84.
8. Todd FW, Two cases of melanotic tumors in the lungs. *JAMA* 1888; 11: 53–4.
9. Kunkel OF, Torrey E, Report of a case of primary melanotic sarcoma of lung presenting difficulties in differentiating from tuberculosis. *NY State J Med* 1916; 16: 198–201.
10. Carlucci GA, Schleussner RC, Primary (?) melanoma of the lung; case report. *J Thorac Surg* 1942; 11: 643–9.
11. Allen AC, Spitz S, Malignant melanoma; clinicopathological analysis of the criteria for diagnosis and prognosis. *Cancer* 1953; 6: 1–45.
12. Hsu CW, Wu SC, Ch'En CS, Melanoma of lung. *Chin Med J* 1962; 81: 263–6.
13. Reed RJ, Kent EM, Solitary pulmonary melanomas: two case reports. *J Thorac Cardiovasc Surg* 1964; 48: 226–31.
14. Reid JD, Mehta VT, Melanoma of the lower respiratory tract. *Cancer* 1966; 19: 627–31.
15. Jensen OA, Egedorf J, Primary malignant melanoma of the lung. *Scand J Respir Dis* 1967; 48: 127–35.
16. Allen SM, Drash EC, Primary melanoma of the lung. *Cancer* 1968; 21: 154–9.
17. Taboada CF, McMurray JD, Jordon RA, Seybold WD, Primary melanoma of the lung. *Chest* 1972; 62: 629–31.
18. Mori K, Cho H, Som M, Primary 'flat' melanoma of the trachea. *J Pathol* 1977; 121: 101–5.
19. Smith S, Opipari M, Primary pleural melanoma. A first reported case and literature review. *J Thorac Cardiovasc Surg* 1978; 75: 827–31.
20. Adebonojo SA, Grillo IA, Durodola JI, Primary malignant melanoma of the bronchus. *J Natl Med Ass* 1979; 71: 579–81.
21. Robertson AJ, Sinclair DJ, Sutton PP, Guthrie W, Primary melanocarcinoma of the lower respiratory tract. *Thorax* 1980; 35: 158–9.
22. Gephardt GN, Malignant melanoma of the bronchus. *Hum Pathol* 1981; 12: 671–3.
23. Verweij J, Breed WP, Jansveld CA, Primary tracheo-bronchial melanoma. *Neth J Med* 1982; 25: 163–6.
24. Angel R, Prados M, Primary bronchial melanoma *J LA State Med Soc* 1984; 136: 13–15.
25. Cagle P, Mace ML, Judge DM et al, Pulmonary melanoma. Primary vs metastatic. *Chest* 1984; 85: 125–6.
26. Carstens PH, Kuhns JG, Ghazi C, Primary malignant melanomas of the lung and adrenal. *Hum Pathol* 1984; 15: 910–14.
27. Alghanem AA, Mehan J, Hassan AA, Primary malignant melanoma of the lung *J Surg Oncol* 1987; 34: 109–12.
28. Demeter SL, Fuenning C, Miller JB, Primary malignant melanoma of the lower respiratory tract: endoscopic identification. *Cleve Clin J Med* 1987; 54: 305–8.
29. Santos F, Entrenas LM, Sebastian F et al, Primary bronchopulmonary malignant melanoma. Case report. *Scand J Thorac Cardiovasc Surg* 1987; 21: 187–9.
30. Bagwell SP, Flynn SD, Cox PM, Davison JA, Primary malignant melanoma of the lung. *Am Rev Respir Dis* 1989; 139: 1543–7.
31. Bertola G, Pasquotti B, Morassut S et al, Primary lung melanoma. *Ital J Surg Sci* 1989; 19: 187–9.
32. Jennings TA, Axiotis CA, Kress Y, Carter D, Primary malignant melanoma of the lower respiratory tract. Report of a case and literature review. *Am J Clin Pathol* 1990; 94: 649–55.
33. Miller DL, Allen MS, Rare pulmonary neoplasms. *Mayo Clin Proc* 1993; 68: 492–8.
34. Pasquini E, Rastelli E, Muretto P et al, Primary bronchial malignant melanoma. A case report. *Pathologica* 1994; 86: 546–8.
35. Farrell DJ, Kashyap AP, Ashcroft T, Morritt GN, Primary malignant melanoma of the bronchus. *Thorax* 1996; 51: 223–4.
36. Wilson RW, Moran CA, Primary melanoma of the lung: a clinicopathologic and immunohistochemical study of eight cases. *Am J Surg Pathol* 1997; 21: 1196–202.
37. Duarte IG, Gal AA, Mansour KA, Primary malignant melanoma of the trachea. *Ann Thorac Surg* 1998; 65: 559–60.
38. Ost D, Joseph C, Sogoloff H, Menezes G, Primary pulmonary melanoma: case report and literature review. *Mayo Clin Proc* 1999; 74: 62–6.
39. Thompson JF, Bishop JF. Primary melanoma of the lung. In: *Textbook of uncommon cancer,* 2nd edn. (eds Raghaven D, Brechner ML, Johnson DH et al.): John Wiley & Sons Ltd 1999; 537–41.
40. DasGupta TK, Brasfield RD Paglia MA, Primary melanomas in unusual sites. *Surg Gynecol Obstet* 1969; 128: 841–8.

41. Scotto J, Fraumeni JF, Lee JA, Melanomas of the eye and other non-cutaneous sites: epidemiologic aspects. *J Natl Cancer Inst* 1976; 56: 489–91.
42. Ross MI, Stern SJ, Mucosal melanomas. In: *Cutaneous melanoma* 3rd edn. (eds Balch CM, Houghton AN, Sober AJ, Soong S-J). St Louis, Missouri: Quality Medical Publishing Inc, 1998: 195–206.
43. Carter D, Eggleston JC,Tumors of the lower respiratory tract. In: *Atlas of tumor pathology, Series 2, Fascile 17.* Washington DC Armed Forces Institute Pathology: 1979: 220.
44. Sekine I, Kodama T, Yokose T et al, Rare pulmonary tumors – a review of 32 cases. *Oncology* 1998; 55: 431–4.
45. Fowler M, Sutherland HD'A, Malignant melanoma of the oesophagus. *J Path Bact* 1952; 64: 473–8.
46. Goldman JL, Lawson W, Zak FG, Roffman JD, The presence of melanocytes in the human larynx. *Laryngoscope* 1972; 82: 824–35.
47. Busuttil A, Dendritic pigmented cells within human laryngeal mucosa. *Arch Otolaryngol* 1976; 102: 43–4.
48. Batsakis JG, Regezi JA, Solomon AR, Rice DH, The pathology of head and neck tumors: mucosal melanomas, part 13. *Head Neck Surg* 1982; 4: 404–8.
49. Shivas AA, MacLennan WD, 'Melanogenic metaplasia' of mucous glands. *Br J Cancer* 1963; 17: 411–14.
50. Cebelin MS, Melanocytic bronchial carcinoid tumor. *Cancer* 1980; 46: 1843–8.
51. Gould VE, Memoli VA, Dardi LE et al, Neuroendocrine carcinomas with multiple immunoreactive peptides and melanin production. *Ultrastruct Pathol* 1981; 2: 199–217.
52. Grazer R, Cohen SM Jacobs JB, Lucas P, Melanin-containing peripheral carcinoid of the lung. *Am J Surg Pathol* 1982; 6: 73–8.
53. Kniseley RM, Baggenstoss AH, Primary melanoma of the adrenal gland. *Arch Pathol* 1946; 42: 345–9.
54. Dick JC, Ritchie GM, Thompson H, Histological differentiation between phaeochromocytoma and melanoma of suprarenal gland. *J Clin Pathol* 1955; 8: 89–98.
55. Sasidharan K, Babu AS, Pandey AP et al, Primary melanoma of the adrenal gland: a case report. *J Urol* 1977; 117: 663–4.
56. Rosenberg LM, Polanco GB, Blank S. Multiple tracheobronchial melanomas with ten-year survival *JAMA* 1965; 192: 717–19.
57. Damian DL, Fulham MJ, Thompson E, Thompson JF, Positron emission tomography in the detection and management of metastatic melanoma. *Melanoma Res* 1996; 6: 325–9.
58. Gritters L, Francis IR, Zasadny KR, Wahl RL, Initial assessment of positron emission tomography using 2–fluorine-18–fluoro-2–deoxy-D-glucose in the imaging of malignant melanoma. *J Nucl Med* 1993; 34: 1420–27.
59. Boni R, Boni RA, Steinert H et al, Staging of metastatic melanoma by whole-body positron emission using 2–fluorine-18–fluoro-2–deoxy-D-glucose. *Br J Dermatol* 1995; 132: 556–62.
60. Rigo P, Paulus P, Kaschten BJ et al, Oncological applications of positron emission tomography with fluorine-18-fluorodeoxyglucose. *Eur J Nucl Med* 1996; 23: 1641–74.
61. Valk PE, Pounds TR, Tesar RD et al, Cost-effectiveness of PET imaging in clinical oncology. *Nucl Med Biol* 1996; 23: 737–43.
62. Tyler DS, Onaitis M, Kherani A et al, Positron emission tomography scanning in malignant melanoma. *Cancer* 2000; 89: 1019–25.
63. Das Gupta T, Bowden L, Berg JW, Malignant melanoma of unknown origin. *Surg Gynecol Obstet* 1963; 117: 341–5.
64. Guiliano AE, Moseley HS, Morton DL, Clinical aspects of unknown primary melanoma. *Ann Surg* 1980; 191: 98–104.
65. Reintgen DS, McCarty KS, Woodard B et al, Malignant melanoma with an unknown primary. *Surg Gynecol Obstet* 1983; 156: 335–40.
66. Norman J, Cruse CW, Wells KE et al, Metastatic melanoma with an unknown primary. *Ann Plast Surg* 1992; 28: 81–4.
67. Vijuk G, Coates AS, Survival of patients with visceral metastatic melanoma from an occult primary lesion: a retrospective matched cohort study. *Ann Oncol* 1998; 9: 419–22.
68. La Hei ER, Thompson JF, McCaughan BC et al, Surgical resection of pulmonary metastatic melanoma: a review of 83 thoracotomies. *Asia Pacific Heart J* 1996; 5: 111–4.
69. Harpole DH, Johnson CM, Wolfe WG et al, Analysis of 945 cases of pulmonary metastatic melanoma. *J Thorac Cardiovasc Surg* 1992; 103: 743–50.
70. Gorenstein LJ, Putnam Jr JB, Natarajan G et al, Improved survival after resection of pulmonary metastases from malignant melanoma. *Ann Thorac Surg* 1991; 52: 204–10.
71. Leo F, Cagini L, Rocmans P et al, Lung metastases from melanoma: when is surgical treatment warranted? *Br J Cancer* 2000; 83: 569–72.
72. Pogrebniak HW, Stovroff M, Roth JA, Pass HI, Resection of pulmonary metastases from malignant melanoma: results of a 16–year experience. *Ann Thorac Surg* 1988; 46: 20–3.
73. Thayer JO, Overholt RH, Metastatic melanoma to the lung: long-term results of surgical excision. *Am J Surg* 1985; 149: 558–62.
74. Wong JH, Euhus DM, Morton DL, Surgical resection for metastatic melanoma to the lung. *Arch Surg* 1988; 123: 1092–5.
75. de Wilt JHW, Farmer SEJ, McCaughan BC, Thompson JF, Surgical treatment of metastatic melanoma of the lung in patients with an unknown primary site. *Melanoma Res* 2001; 11: S215.

62

Primary melanoma of the gastrointestinal tract

B Mark Smithers

INTRODUCTION

This chapter will deal with melanoma arising in the gastrointestinal (GI) tract from the oesophagus to the anorectal region. Melanomas of the upper aerodigestive tract are considered elsewhere in this book.

Non-cutaneous primary melanoma has been reported to occur in 15% of all cases of melanoma.[1] Melanoma arising in mucosa occurred in 1.3% of all cases of primary melanoma reported over a 10-year period to the National Cancer Database Report on cutaneous and non-cutaneous melanoma.[2] The most common GI form of primary melanoma occurs in the anorectum, accounting for 23.8% of mucosal melanomas and 0.2–0.3% of all melanomas.[2,3] In Queensland, Australia, from the State Cancer Registry nine cases of anorectal melanoma were reported amongst 21,391 cases of primary melanoma from all other sites, an incidence of 0.04%.[4]

Following anorectal melanoma, the next most common GI melanoma occurs in the oesophagus. In an American College of Surgeons patient-care survey there were no oesophageal melanomas reported from 681 hospitals and 5000 patients in 1981, and there were only three reported from 844 hospitals and 6900 patients in 1987, an incidence of 0.04%.[5] An earlier report suggested that primary melanoma of the oesophagus accounted for 0.5% of all melanomas.[6] Primary melanoma at other sites in the GI tract is even more rare, with the literature comprising only single or collective case reports. As well as in oesophagus and anorectum, melanoma of the GI tract has been reported in the gall bladder, biliary tract, pancreas, small intestine and colon. There is continuing controversy as to the real existence of primary melanoma in these regions.

MELANOCYTES AND THEIR ORIGIN IN RELATION TO THE GASTROINTESTINAL TRACT

During early embryogenesis, melanoblasts migrate into the epidermis, hair follicles, uvea, choroid, leptomeninges, substantia nigra, oral cavity and nasopharynx.[7] It is reasonable to accept that melanocytes will exist in the oesophageal and anal canal epithelium, given their ectodermal origin during fetal development. The origin of melanocytes and thus primary melanoma in the endodermal organs is less clear.

The concept of a primary melanoma arising in the oesophagus was in doubt until 1962, when de la Pava et al.[8] reported a 4% incidence of normal melanocytes in the basal layer of the oesophageal epithelium in autopsy specimens. The areas of microscopic collections measured between 1 and 3 cm and were not visible as macroscopic pigmentation. This finding has been confirmed by others,[9,10] with one study finding an 8% incidence of normal melanocytes in the basal layer of the oesophageal epithelium.[11] The latter authors suggested that melanocytes migrate from the neural crest to the oesophagus in the same way as they migrate to the skin and other organs, with subsequent developmental differentiation into melanocytes or argyrophil cells from suitable stimuli.[11] Indeed, melanosis has now been recognized to occur in one-quarter of the cases of patients with primary melanoma of the oesophagus[11–14] and melanosis of the entire oesophagus has been reported.[15] Patients may show appearances in the surrounding mucosa suggestive of in situ melanoma.[16]

In relation to melanomas arising in the anorectal region, melanocytes were demonstrated below the dentate line as long ago as 1958.[17] More recently, melanocytes have been clearly demonstrated in the various epithelial zones of the anal canal.[18] The normal anal canal contained melanocytes in the squamous and transitional zones in a sporadic fashion, however, none were found in the colorectal zone. In a group of patients with primary melanoma of the anal canal, melanocytes were found in the epithelium, separate to the malignancy, in the squamous, transitional and rectal zones. The authors of this study felt that this supported the observation that melanoma may have its origin above as well as below the dentate line.[18] It had been considered that all the primary melanomas of the lower rectum had their origin from the junctional zone. The lower rectal tumour was considered to represent an extension of a tumour derived from anal melanocytes that had undergone malignant transformation.[19,20] The melanocytes in the rectum adjacent to the primary lesion, and the increased number and proliferation of melanocytes seen on histology, were postulated to have been induced by the primary melanoma.[18] However, that group only looked at the histology of 16 normal anal canals. It is possible that there may be sporadic melanosis above the dentate line, but it is likely to be uncommon and one would need to examine a large number of normal anorectal regions to confirm or deny its presence. However, there is clear evidence that primary melanoma can occur above and separate to the dentate line, which, along with the findings of benign melanocytes in this area, allow primary melanoma of the lower rectum to be accepted as a true entity.[18,21,22]

Nicholson et al.[22] suggested three possible mechanisms for melanocytes being present in the rectum: (a) some form of heterotopia via dedifferentiation from primitive stem cells; (b) migration of melanocytes from the anal mucosa into the rectum; (c) migration of melanocytes into the rectum during fetal development, perhaps as a result of inexact targeting of the migrating melanoblasts.[22] If the first postulate was correct, then heterotopic melanocytes would be expected to be found with equal frequency throughout the large intestine, which has not been shown. Thus, it would seem that one of the two last postulates is most likely. The majority of reports of anorectal melanoma include patients with tumours in the lower rectum. Reports of primary melanoma in the mid- and upper rectum are uncommon. There is one report of a melanoma 5 cm above the dentate line[23] and two reports of lesions higher in the sigmoid,[24,25] although there remains doubt that the lesion at the rectosigmoid was a primary melanoma because there were secondaries at the time of diagnosis and the lesion was submucosal on histological sections.[24] There has been one Russian report of a primary melanoma of the caecum[26] which, along with the other two sigmoid reports, are the only reports of colonic primary lesions in the literature.

In exploring the origin of melanocytes in the glandular epithelial regions of the remainder of the GI tract, a number of observations and postulations have been made. Early studies, without the advantage of specialized immunohistochemistry and stains, found melanoblasts only in the skin and mucous membrane of ectodermal origin.[27] At that time, it was felt that melanomas in other areas were all likely to be secondary rather than primary, arising from a primary cutaneous melanoma that had regressed. In experimental animals melanoblasts were seen to arise from the neural crest and migrate to peripheral parts of the body. It was suggested that the melanoblasts would migrate along outgoing sensory plates to ectodermal as well as endodermal organs.[7] Non-neoplastic melanocytes have been reported in the gall bladder,[28,29] and in normal[30] and abnormal biliary tract mucosa.[31] Indeed, at other sites, it has been postulated that there may be ectopic migration of the melanocyte precursors occurring in the embryo to sites where melanocytes would not normally be found, thus giving the potential to develop a primary melanoma.[32]

It has been suggested that melanocytes, particularly within the small bowel and possibly in other areas of glandular epithelium, may belong to the amine-precursor uptake and decarboxylation (APUD) cell system.[33] Given that APUD cells have a common ancestral origin in the neural crest, it is reasonable that in addition to the parent cells, e.g. enterochromaffin cells in the small intestine, melanoblasts may occasionally be present, thus giving rise to malignant melanoma. The melanoblasts, unlike the APUD cells, do not produce hormones but melanomas, like their parent cells the melanoblasts, can produce melanin and protein.[34] It has been suggested that, in the small intestine, the melanocytic tumours may arise from 'Schwannian neuroblasts' associated with the autonomic innervation of the gut.[35] Despite these proposals for the presence of normal melanocytes in the small intestine they have only been demonstrated, using immunoperoxidase studies, in Meckel's diverticula.[36,37] This would suggest there should be a predominance of tumours in the ileum if primary melanoma were to occur in the small intestine.

In summary, it appears reasonable to presume that the melanocytes that occur in the oesophagus and the anal canal are derived from a source similar to the epidermis, i.e. by migration of melanocytes from the neural crest. Indeed, as observed by Iverson and Robins,[38] because the melanocyte is primarily an integumental component, it is not surprising that mucosal melanomas are most frequent near mucocutaneous junctions. With respect to the glandular epithelium and endodermal organs, if primary melanoma exists, the origin may be either as a result of normal migration of melanoblasts from the neural crest or because of inexact targeting of melanoblasts during migration from the neural crest during fetal development. Alternatively, there may be a relationship between the melanocyte and the APUD system, particularly in the intestine.

PATHOLOGICAL CONSIDERATIONS

In 4–8% of patients, a melanoma may be found within a lymph node or as a solitary lesion in a viscus with no historical, clinical or pathological evidence of a cutaneous, mucosal or ocular melanoma – so-called melanoma with unknown primary.[30,39] Given the concept that a primary cutaneous melanoma may exist, then regress completely and subsequently present with metastatic disease, this sequence needs to be considered in all patients who present with a solitary lesion in the GI tract.

The pathological criterion used to consider a melanoma of mucosal origin as a primary lesion was initially outlined by Allen and Spitz[40] to be the presence of junctional change at the site of the 'primary' lesion. They believed that these lesions were preceded by an activated junctional naevus and stated that one could not depend upon the presence of melanin to make a diagnosis of melanoma. In the oesophagus, Raven and Dawson[41] expanded this to a number of criteria to allow the diagnosis of a primary oesophageal melanoma and these criteria have been confirmed by others.[42] The criteria recommended were: the lesion has the characteristic structure of melanoma and contains melanin pigment; the tumour is polypoid; melanocytes are found in the adjacent epithelium; and the tumour arises in an area of junctional change in the adjacent epithelium. Due to the presence of ulceration, or because of the size of the lesion, junctional change or associated melanocytes may be absent. Raven and Dawson[41] felt that one of those two criteria should be present to make a diagnosis of primary melanoma of the oesophagus. It has been suggested that the above criteria can be extrapolated to make the diagnosis of primary melanoma in all GI melanomas.[1] However, not all tumours are polypoid, notably in the anorectum, and a number of tumours will be amelanotic. It seems reasonable to expand the criteria previously proposed to include the modern use of immunohistochemistry and clinical information relating to the absence of any other primary melanoma. This will increase the potential to correctly differentiate a primary from a secondary melanoma of the GI tract; the proposed criteria are outlined in Box 62.1. Finally, it is difficult to accept a lesion as a primary melanoma if the presentation includes the presence of other metastatic disease, especially if the histological criteria are absent.

HISTOLOGY

The cells in a primary melanoma of the GI tract have a similar appearance to those of their cutaneous counterparts. Clark et al.[43] reported melanoma of mucosal origin to have a similar pattern to volar-subungual

Box 62.1 ***Proposed clinicopathological criteria to diagnose primary melanoma of the gastrointestinal (GI) tract***

- The lesion has the characteristic structure of melanoma and contains melanin pigment, or stains for S-100 or HMB-45 confirm the nature of an amelanotic tumour
- The tumour is polypoid
- Melanocytes are found in the adjacent epithelium
- The tumour arises in an area of junctional change in the adjacent epithelium
- No other primary site has been established – cutaneous, ocular or mucosal

melanoma, with a radial growth phase followed by a vertical growth phase. However, the appearances typical of superficial spreading and nodular melanoma can also be found.[43] Cellular pleomorphism is considerable. Microscopic pigment is present in 90% of cases. There are usually nests and sheets of epithelioid cells characterized by round to polygonal cells with abundant clear to amphophilic cytoplasm. The cells normally contain round to oval vesicular nuclei with a single, centrally located, prominent nucleolus. Areas of spindle cells exhibiting identical nuclear features of epithelioid cells may be present. The presence of a lentiginous growth pattern in the adjacent mucosa has been described in both the oesophagus and the anorectum.[12,44] There tends to be a pushing margin, especially in the submucosa, with infiltration of the margins into the muscularis mucosae and outside the organ.[12] Malignant cells may infiltrate the mucosa singly or in nests, especially in the anorectum.

In patients with amelanotic lesions, immunohistochemistry looking for the presence of the proteins S-100 and HMB-45, along with electron microscopy, will assist in making the diagnosis and also in distinguishing primary from secondary disease.[12] Electron microscopy of these lesions in the oesophagus has shown large, loosely cohesive cells with variable shapes. The cytoplasm showed pre-melanosomes exhibiting a lattice-like arrangement and melanin pigment. The endoplasmic reticulum, both rough and smooth, was abundant and there were a few desmosomes.[12]

EVIDENCE CONFIRMING PRIMARY MELANOMA – SPECIFIC SITES

Oesophagus

In the oesophagus, benign melanosis and benign melanocytes have been associated with primary melanoma.[12–15,45] There may be changes adjacent to the tumour consistent with melanoma in situ, as well as appearances resembling superficial spreading melanoma (SSM).[46] Muto et al.[46] suggested that the radial growth phase gave the SSM appearance whilst the vertical growth phase produced the polypoidal melanoma. With the presence of lentiginous spread, there will be melanocytes along the basal layer of the mucosa in a confluent arrangement. Melanosis is characterized by scattered pigment cells of small diameter with small uniform nuclei and inconspicuous nucleoli. Foci of benign mucosal melanocytes are usually noted microscopically.[12]

Junctional changes will be absent in 60% of primary oesophageal melanomas.[14] Given the large size of these lesions at the time of diagnosis, it is likely that these features, if present, were obliterated by the tumour growth. Other clinical and histological criteria will assist in making the diagnosis of a primary melanoma. The differential diagnosis in the oesophagus is squamous cell carcinoma with spindle cell features, sarcoma, small cell carcinoma, carcinosarcoma or metastatic melanoma. Distinguishing between these entities may be difficult from biopsy specimens; the addition of immunohistochemistry and electron microscopy should resolve the issue.[12]

Gall bladder

There are case reports confirming the pathological criteria allowing the diagnosis of a primary melanoma to be made. However there are still questions about the true existence of this entity.[47,48] Heath and Womack,[49] examined the world literature in 1988, when 20 cases of primary melanoma of the gall bladder had been reported. Using the clinical and pathological criteria previously proposed,[41] they felt that six patients fulfilled the requirements to confirm a diagnosis of primary gall bladder melanoma, however, they did state that the tumours might have overgrown the evidence of junctional activity. They felt that they could not say that the other cases were not primary melanomas of the gall bladder but did cast some doubt on those reports. Higgins and Strutton[47] reported a case of metastatic melanoma to the gall bladder that displayed all the pathological features required to make a diagnosis of a primary lesion, but the patient was known to have disseminated melanoma from a previous primary lesion. Others have stated that, even with cutaneous melanoma, the presence of atypical melanocytes within the epidermis at the sides of an invasive tumour does not necessarily define the lesion to be a primary, given that secondary cutaneous deposits may simulate in situ melanoma.[50] Naguib and Aterman[51] carefully established reasons why their patient had a primary gall bladder melanoma, only to subsequently discover good evidence that the patient was likely to have had a regressed primary cutaneous melanoma.[51]

In a number of the case reports of primary melanoma of the gall bladder, there has been repeated emphasis on the absence of another primary melanoma and the presence of a single polypoidal lesion in the gall bladder. In the reports the open gall bladder usually reveals a dark, polypoidal or papillary mucosal nodule. Histologically, the lesion rarely involves the muscular layer. However, all these appearances grossly and on histology have also been described with secondary melanoma of the gall bladder.[47,51] In addition, it is difficult to accept many of the previously reported cases of primary melanoma of the gall bladder where there is evidence of metastasis at the time of diagnosis of the polypoidal gall bladder melanoma. Despite the doubts about some of the case reports, it is reasonable to accept that primary melanoma of the gall bladder exists because melanocytes have been demonstrated in the gall bladder, and there are patients with solitary lesions in the gall bladder that have fulfilled the clinicopathological criteria and who have survived long term after cholecystectomy.[52]

Bile ducts

If one is prepared to accept primary melanoma of the gall bladder as an entity then it is sensible to consider that the biliary tree could also be a source of a primary melanoma because of the common embryological origin. Metastasis to the major bile ducts is well recognized[53] and there are only six cases of primary melanoma of the biliary tree reported to date,[54] which leads to the suspicion that the condition may not be real. Only one case clearly reported the presence of junctional change within the mucosa of the bile duct adjacent to the tumour.[55] One patient had an associated primary melanoma of the gall bladder[56] and there has been a report of a gall bladder primary melanoma with subsequent presentation of a common bile duct melanoma.[57] The latter was considered by the authors to be distal implantation because the operative cholangiogram at the time of the cholecystectomy was normal. It seems reasonable to consider the possible reality of primary biliary melanoma, given the common epithelial origin with the gall bladder, but there must still be some doubt.

Pancreas

There are three reports in the literature of possible primary melanomas of the pancreas.[58–60] There are elements in each case that lead to doubt as to the primary or secondary nature of the pancreatic lesions. The report from Bianca et al.[58] is more consistent with a lesion based on the distal common bile duct; however, the exact origin is impossible to confirm and there were no histological features to support the conclusions that it was a primary lesion.[58] The patient subsequently had recurrence in axillary nodes. Rutter et al.[59] reported on a patient with a solitary lesion in the head of the pancreas who was subsequently found to have a lesion with similar pathology in the nasal mucosa.[59] Finally, the report from Petiot and Raynal[60] presented a patient with a pancreatic head lesion who also had a second mass of melanoma in the left mesocolon at the time of presentation, which suggested these may both have been secondary lesions. Although it seems reasonable to expect that melanocytes might exist in pancreatic ductal mucosa if they occur in the biliary mucosa, they have never been demonstrated at this site. With the discrepancies in the three reports cited above and the known reports of secondary melanoma in the pancreatic head, the existence of primary melanoma of the pancreas remains an uncertainty.

Stomach

The literature carries five case reports of primary melanomas of the stomach.[61–65] In support of the potential for melanocytes to be present in the stomach, there is a case report of a patient with a primary melanoma of the oesophagus with associated melanosis in both the oesophagus and the stomach.[66] In a large series of oesophageal and cardia malignancies, Aagaard et al.[65] reported a single primary melanoma of the gastric cardia out of 332 cancers. There is one other report of a patient with a lesion in the cardia,[63] whilst the other three were tumours in the body of the stomach.[61,62,64] The authors of these reports accept the possibility that the gastric lesions may have been metastatic to the gastric wall from an unknown primary site.[61–64] The case against the diagnosis of primary melanoma in these reports includes the presence of secondaries at other sites at the time of diagnosis and the absence of any histological evidence of melanocytic activity in the gastric mucosa, adjacent to the potential primary lesion.

Gastric secondaries from melanoma are a relatively common manifestation in the gastrointestinal tract,[53,67] with one report of resection with prolonged survival.[68] Thus, presently, the evidence for the existence of primary melanoma of the stomach is not strong.

Small intestine

The features of primary melanoma of the small bowel are found in case reports. The histological features have been summarized earlier. In the case reports there is no mention of the histology of the adjacent mucosa or junctional change associated with the primary lesion. Because these lesions will be diagnosed late, when patients present with a mass, obstruction or bleeding, the subtle adjacent mucosal changes may be lost. There is one case where the small bowel lesion was not too large because it was found incidentally at the time of laparotomy for other reasons.[69] In that patient there were multiple foci of melanoma in the mucosa around the 3 × 2 cm 'primary' lesion. The presence of atypical melanocytes or junctional change was not mentioned.

In a summary of a number of reports on surgery for GI symptoms from melanoma the reported incidence of an occult primary was 20–27%,[70] whereas the incidence of an occult primary in a series of patients with palpable axillary nodes was 10%.[71] It was felt that this discrepancy offered supportive evidence that primary small bowel melanoma does exist.[70] Elsayed et al.[72] examined a series of patients with metastatic melanoma to the small intestine and reported that in 103 patients the primary lesion preceded metastasis by an average of 5.6 years in those patients who were fit to proceed to resection. When comparing patients with a known primary melanoma and small intestinal metastasis with patients without a primary lesion but with a small bowel melanoma, there was no difference between the age of those who presented with the primary cutaneous lesion and those who presented without a primary cutaneous lesion. It was felt that melanoma in the small intestine was most likely to be a secondary from an unknown primary site.[72]

Most reports conclude that the lesion in question was a primary melanoma because no ocular or cutaneous lesion was found. However, the small intestine is the most common GI site for metastatic melanoma[73,74] and thus a number of authors believe that all melanomas in this region are secondary.[73,75] Many of the patients in the case reports have secondaries elsewhere which, in the absence of supportive histological evidence, makes the diagnosis of a primary lesion unlikely.

Sachs et al.[76] recently reported a case of a jejunal melanoma with long-term survival after resection and proposed the following specific criteria to allow a diagnosis of primary small bowel melanoma to be made: biopsy proven melanoma from the small intestine at a single focus; no evidence of disease in any other organs, including skin, eye and nodes outside of the regional drainage at the time of diagnosis, and a disease-free interval of at least 12 months after diagnosis. Using the stated criteria and examining the literature they found two previous cases that were considered to be consistent with primary melanoma of the ileum.[36,73] Using survival as a criterion for differentiation between a primary and secondary tumour ignores a large number of tumour-versus-host variables that may be relevant in an individual. Although it may seem reasonable to consider that an increased survival following resection of a solitary lesion offers a greater chance that the lesion was a primary, long-term survivors do occur after resection of solitary visceral metastases when there was a known cutaneous primary lesion. As well, if these criteria were added to the list of clinicopathological criteria previously mentioned, a number of patients with oesophageal and anorectal lesions that were clearly primary melanomas, yet who died within 12 months, would be excluded.

Only two case reports of possible duodenal primary melanoma could be found in the literature.[77,78] The possibility of a primary melanoma of the small intestine would appear more acceptable if melanocytes were demonstrated throughout the small intestine or if, on histology, the presence of junctional change was demonstrated and atypical melanocytes were found in the mucosa adjacent to the solitary deposit of melanoma. With the available evidence it seems reasonable to agree with Sachs et al.[76] that 'Whether small bowel melanoma exists is an unanswered question'

Anorectum

In a literature review of primary melanoma of the anorectum, 77% of the tumours contained melanin.[20] Separate reviews have also reported pigment in 71[79] and 83%[80] of cases. Spindle and naevoid cells forming patterns reminiscent of acral lentiginous melanoma are commonly observed.[40] There is often a junctional pattern or an in situ component in the mucosa beside the main lesion.[80] This was seen in 23% of one large review but these cases were from some time ago when it was probably not formally reported. Recent series have reported junctional changes in 63–73% of patients. There is usually a nesting growth pattern that may be helpful in making the diagnosis in non-pigmented lesions.[20] Mucosal extension occurs and may extend proximally into the anorectal region,[20] more so than squamous cell carcinoma (SCC) of the anal canal.[79]

It has been stated that the histological criteria that suggest the diagnosis of an anorectal melanoma are: the presence of melanin; junctional change; nesting growth pattern; submucosal spread into the rectum.[20] Because of the lack of a papillary dermis in this region, Clark's levels are irrelevant.[81] However, Breslow thickness, from the mucosal surface or ulcer base, can be measured: the thinner lesions having a better prognosis.[44] The median thickness in one large series was 7.5 mm (range 0.5–20 mm).[79] However, many lesions are polypoid, making measurement of thickness difficult. As in polypoidal cutaneous melanoma, the prognosis is poor.

With respect to the rest of the colon, the evidence for the existence of primary melanoma is minimal, being restricted to three case reports with at least one, on review, having very little evidence to support the diagnosis of primary melanoma.[24]

CLINICAL FEATURES – SPECIFIC SITES

Oesophagus

Primary malignant melanoma of the oesophagus represents <1% of all oesophageal neoplasms.[82] A Danish unit reported the incidence of primary melanoma amongst oesophageal cancers to be 0.5%.[6] The Upper GI Unit at the Princess Alexandra Hospital, Brisbane, has a prospective database of 645 oesophageal cancers with one case of primary malignant melanoma (a local incidence of 0.15%). In a series of 1918 patients with primary oesophageal cancer, over 42 years, two patients had primary melanoma, an incidence of 0.1%.[83] Since the first report in 1906[84] there have been over 200 cases reported. Recently, there has been a higher rate of case reporting, with an average of eight cases per year in the international literature between 1996 and 1998.

Clinical picture

This has been well summarized by DeMatos et al.[85] A population study in the United States suggested a male: female ratio of 1:1,[86] however, from summaries of the case reports, there seemed to be a male predominance over females by 2:1.[87] Patients had a mean age of 60 years, although there is one report in a child.[88] The tumour occurs predominantly in Caucasians. Patients will present in a similar fashion to other oesophageal malignancies, with symptoms such as dysphagia, vague retrosternal pain or discomfort, regurgitation and weight loss. Usually, these symptoms are short-lived, of the order of a few weeks or months. The primary lesions are usually in the lower two-thirds of the oesophagus.[13]

Diagnosis

At endoscopy the tumour is usually a polypoidal nodule, which may be covered, to a degree, by normal oesophageal mucosa. There may be associated stenosis and focal ulceration. The nodule will be pigmented with colours ranging from brown to black in 75–90% of cases and there may be associated black pigment within the mucosa around the nodule. Figure 62.1 is an example of a primary oesphageal melanoma treated by the present author. The features seen on barium swallow have been summarized by Yoo et al.[89] All the tumours were bulky, presenting as polypoidal, intraluminal masses with an average length of 8 cm (range 5–12 cm) and a diameter of 3.7 cm (range 3–5 cm). The

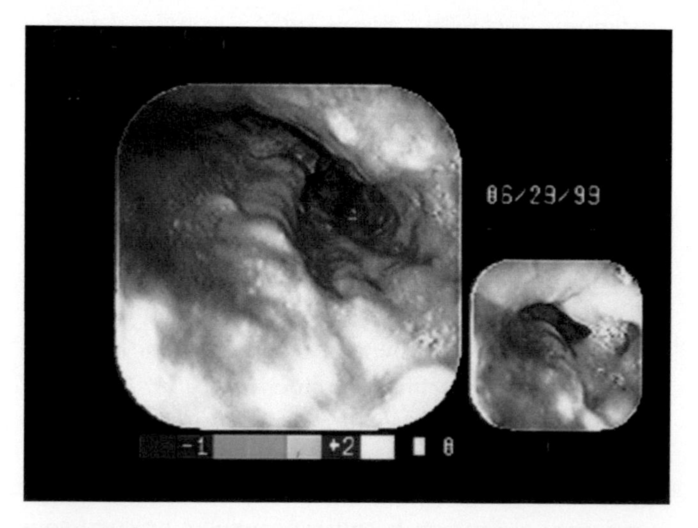

Figure 62.1 *Endoscopic appearance of a primary oesophageal melanoma. Diagnosis confirmed at subsequent oesophageal resection. Note the pigment on the polypoidal tumour and in the mucosa in the foreground.*

radiological differential diagnoses of such a large polypoidal mass are: a spindle cell carcinoma; lymphoma; Kaposi's sarcoma; leiomyosarcoma. Adenocarcinoma and squamous cell carcinoma (SCC) will have these appearances only rarely.[89]

Staging

Endoscopic ultrasound has been used to assess the nature of the lesion and, in particular, to accurately evaluate the depth of invasion into the oesophageal wall.[85,90] Patients with this tumour should be staged with computerized tomography (CT) scans of the chest and abdomen, assessing the oesophagus and any mediastinal mass, the associated lymph nodes in the mediastinum, left gastric and coeliac regions, and the presence or absence of systemic metastases. Fifty per cent of patients with primary melanomas of the oesophagus will present with some form of metastasis, either within surrounding lymph nodes or within viscera.[13]

Management

Surgical resection offers the only chance of cure. On review of the literature, by 1995 there were four reported long-term survivors (>5 years) following oesophageal resection.[91] Surgery should include resection of the primary tumour with a clear margin of the oesophagus, including pigmented areas, along with associated mediastinal and left gastric lymph nodes. There was a report of a long-term survivor who was treated with radiotherapy alone;[92] however, there is no clear role for consideration of this modality in the primary management of patients with melanoma of the oesophagus. Radiation may offer good palliation of dysphagia in patients who have metastatic disease or who are not fit for resection.

Prognosis

A review of 139 patients reported a median survival of 9.8 months and a 5-year survival rate of 1.69%: only 30% of patients were alive 1 year after diagnosis.[13] Following resection of the tumour, the mean survival was 14 months and the 5-year survival rate was 4.2%. The results published in 1956 were compared to those published in 1980,[12] with little difference seen over that time. There have been reports of major resectional surgery for metastatic disease but follow-up was short.[93]

Alternative therapies

Both radiotherapy and chemotherapy, using single or multiple agents, have been used with no influence on survival.[94] The single agent darcarbazine (DTIC) did not have any marked effect as an adjuvant treatment. Combinations of chemotherapeutic agents, post-surgery, have been reported in Japan,[95] as have pre- and postoperative therapy which, in two reports, showed a tumour response prior to resection. In both cases, follow-up was short and the long-term results are unknown.[96,97] In a post-mortem study the most common site of metastatic disease was the liver (31%); this was followed by the mediastinum and mediastinal lymph nodes (29%), the lung (17.7%) and the brain (13.2%). It was less common to see metastases to bone and to other intraabdominal organs.[87]

Summary

Primary melanoma of the oesophagus is uncommon, occurring in <1% of patients with oesophageal malignancy. Surgery remains the treatment of choice but the overall outcome is poor, with the 5-year survival rate following resection reported to be 4.2%.

Gall bladder

Clinical

There have been few reports of primary melanoma in the gall bladder since the first description in 1907,[98] as previously discussed. Patients usually present with abdominal pain, as a manifestation of acute cholecystitis or an attack of biliary colic. Some patients have presented with jaundice and perforation following an acutely obstructed gall bladder. Patients have been between 40 and 60 years of age, with an equal sex incidence.

Radiology

Ultrasound will usually define a solid mass within the gall bladder; this will typically be solitary and large with a polypoidal or papillary appearance. CT scans may show some contrast enhancement within the mass. Only two of the 20 patients reported in the literature review by Heath and Womack[49] had gallstones and in both of these cases the authors were doubtful that the lesion was a primary melanoma.

Treatment

In most cases, the tumour is localized to the mucosa and submucosa, making a simple cholecystectomy the treatment of choice. In recent times, laparoscopic cholecystectomy[99] has been used, but the decision on approach should be made in each individual case. Liver resection has not been necessary. Aside from cholecystectomy, there are no other therapeutic guidelines that can be recommended at this stage. There is one report of a patient with a lesion considered to be a primary melanoma with multiple metastasis localized to the peripancreatic region. The patient was treated with a cholecystectomy and total pancreatectomy with postoperative chemotherapy. The follow-up was short, 21 months, thus the long-term result is not clear.[100] To date, there is no evidence that adjuvant therapy has been worthwhile.

Prognosis

It has been stated that distinguishing a primary from a secondary melanoma of the gall bladder is an academic exercise,[49] as a patient with a localized lesion in this site and no other evidence of metastatic disease should have a resection anyway. There has been a long-term survivor reported following cholecystectomy[52] but overall the prognosis is poor.

Bile ducts

Clinical

Patients will present with symptoms consistent with obstruction of the biliary tree, such as painless jaundice and pruritus. Investigation will follow the guidelines used for patients with suspected biliary or pancreatic malignancy, using CT scanning to look for a local mass and the evidence of visceral and nodal secondaries. Endoscopic retrograde cholangiopancreatography (ERCP) or magnetic resonance cholangiopancreatography may be used to define the ductal anatomy and the site of the obstruction.

Treatment

Resection should be performed for any localized lesion in a patient who is fit for pancreaticoduodenectomy or a liver resection with radical resection of the biliary tree. As in the four reported cases to date, diagnosis will be made from the histology of the resected specimen, not as a clinical diagnosis preoperatively.

Small intestine

Primary melanoma of the small intestine has been reported to occur in 2.6%[101] and 5%[102] of patients with primary malignant tumours of the small bowel. However, in a large review of 2144 collected cases of small bowel primary malignancies, no melanomas were reported. There was no mention of the possibility of a primary melanoma amongst the pathological groups, suggesting that the authors did not believe that the entity was real.[103]

Clinical presentation

Patients present with symptoms suggestive of acute or subacute obstruction. Intussusception has been commonly reported. There may be evidence of occult or overt GI bleeding or just a palpable mass. The lesion found in the small bowel at the time of surgery is usually pigmented and polypoidal, varying in size but averaging *c.* 3 cm. Diagnosis has been made at the time of histology of the resected specimen.

Treatment

Treatment is surgical resection with a margin of normal bowel. There have been four long-term survivors following the resection of a solitary lesion in the small bowel considered to be a primary melanoma.[36,70,73,76] However, the prognosis of a solitary melanoma within the small bowel is poor.

Anorectum

The first case report of a primary anal melanoma was in 1857.[104] In a review of the literature in 1982 there had been 199 reports from 1857 to 1966 and 258 reports from 1966 to 1981.[105] The anorectum is usually described as a single entity in most reports. The incidence of primary melanoma, when compared with other tumours in this region, has been reported to be 0.2%.[3] With respect to tumours confined to the anal canal, the incidence is 4–5%.[106–109] In a large series of rectal malignancies, the incidence of primary melanoma of the rectum was 0.04%.[110] There has been a suggestion that the incidence of primary melanoma of the anorectum is higher in cultures with increased skin pigmentation and that sun exposure may be protective.[3] Certainly, the incidence with respect to cutaneous melanoma is different in different races but the population incidence rates per 100,000 people for anorectal melanoma were similar in four different cultural groups: white population, United States (US), 0.017; US Native Americans, 0.015; North Pakistanis, 0.01; Queensland, Australia, 0.028.[4] The conclusion was that sunshine was neither causative nor protective for melanoma in the anorectal region.

Anatomical considerations

Anatomical definitions of anal canal tumours in the literature are varied. The majority of tumours arise at the junctional zone or below in the squamous epithelium. Tumours also arise in the columnar lined upper third of the anal canal or lower rectum.[1,44] In a large, single institution series 92% were seen to arise from or below the dentate line and the remaining 8% above it.[79] The anatomical distinction may be quite subjective, with a number of authors convinced that the tumours in the glandular epithelium have come from below.[19,20] However, there are recent reports of primary rectal melanomas seen quite separate to the dentate line.[18,21,111] At the distal end of the anal canal, anal margin tumours arise outside the anal verge. The natural history of anal canal tumours differs from that of anal margin tumours and they should be considered as different entities.[112]

The anatomical site of the tumour will influence presenting symptoms. A small tumour in the lower anal canal is more amenable to earlier diagnosis, whereas within the upper anal canal and lower rectum, there is a greater potential to have a larger, more locally advanced lesion. This possible distinction is not addressed in the case reports or reviews.

Diagnosis and staging

The disease usually occurs in patients over 60 years of age and is more common in females than males, in some series by a factor of two. There are no pathognomonic symptoms. Patients may present with bleeding (54%), mass (13–15%), pain (14%), haemorrhoid pathology (8%) or pruritis (4%).[79,80] When examined, there will typically be a polypoidal mass and the lesion will be pigmented in two-thirds of patients.[20] The mean diameter in most studies is *c.* 3–4 cm. Figure 62.2 shows an example of this tumour managed at the Princess Alexandra Hospital, Brisbane.[4]

Endoanal ultrasound has been used to accurately assess the depth of invasion and to examine the perirectal lymph nodes.[108] On sigmoidoscopy or colonoscopy the blue-black or dark brown appearance of a polypoidal lesion at or near the dentate line is characteristic.[113,114]

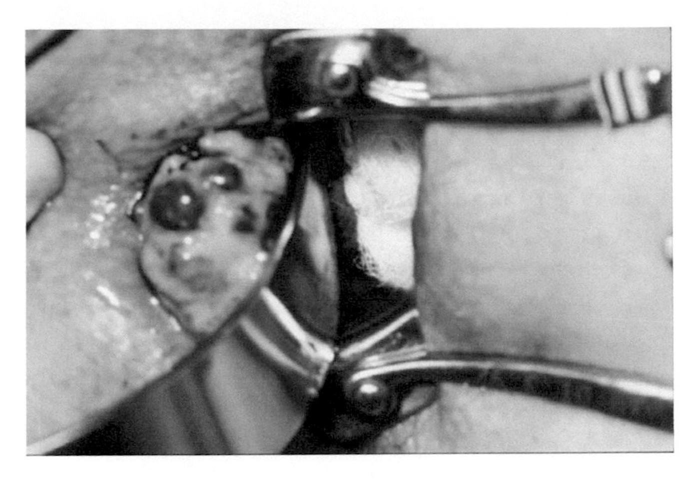

Figure 62.2 *Malignant melanoma of the anal canal. Diagnosis on biopsy and local excision. Subsequent management with abdominoperineal resection (APR).*

The larger reports have found that one-third of patients will have definite evidence of metastasis at presentation. Staging CT scans of the chest and abdomen should be performed routinely. Recently magnetic resonance imaging (MRI) has been performed in patients with anorectal melanoma.[115,116] On the fat-saturation MRI scans the lesions had high signal intensities and the margins of the melanoma were clearly demonstrated. Given the other available modalities for local and metastatic staging, the role for routine MRI would appear limited.

Although the use of positron emission tomography (PET) has not been reported for this condition it seems likely to be a worthwhile investigation. PET has a high sensitivity for melanoma and, given the high incidence of metastasis in this condition, a positive result may influence the clinician's decision towards more conservative therapy.

Treatment

The overall prognosis is poor, with a median survival of 12 months and a 5-year survival rate, if resected, of 6.4%. Surgical removal offers the only chance of cure. The options for removal are local excision (LE) or an abdominoperineal resection (APR) of the rectum and anus. Most series have shown no difference in survival between these two procedures, although there is a higher incidence of local recurrence after local excision. Because the reports are either collected literature reviews or series from institutions collected over many years, there is no easy way to gain definitive comparisons. There is a sparsity of pathological details, along with inconsistent reporting, with poor definitions of local therapy (LE versus wide local excision (WLE)), case selection and other factors that may have influenced the decision (tumour size and position in the anorectum) for therapy. Thus it is difficult to establish guidelines for management with any degree of confidence. It seems reasonable to use the literature to assess the information that may assist in individualizing care for these patients.

Management of local disease: local factors

For patients with local disease, on clinical and radiological assessment, where the aim is cure, the issues influencing treatment are as follows:

- The site of the tumour in the anal canal or rectum and the size or thickness of the tumour.
- More distal tumours are likely to be more amenable to local resection.
- Tumours at the dentate line or above will be harder to resect locally with normal margins and maintain normal anal function – this group of patients is generally elderly.

The size of the tumour and depth of invasion have been implicated as prognostic factors. Goldman et al.,[109] in a collected series from Sweden, found a better survival in patients with smaller lesions: patients with lesions 0–1.9 cm in size had a median survival of 50 months; those with 2–3.9 cm lesions 12 months; those with 4–5.9 cm lesions 9 months; those with lesions >6 cm 8 months. Brady et al.[79] reported their long-term survivors to have a median lesion size of 2.5 cm compared with 4.0 cm for the non-survivors. However, Cooper et al.,[20] in their review, found that tumour size and configuration, e.g. polypoid shape, had no influence on survival – survival was the same for tumours $>$ or <4 cm – but patients having local excision had smaller tumours (3.5 cm). Using tumour thickness as a guide to prognosis, Wanebo et al.[44] had a number of long-term survivors in patients where the tumour was <2 mm thick. Others have reported patients, in whom thickness was measured, with melanomas <2 mm, who have survived long term.[49]

Management of local disease: technical factors – the margin of excision

The margin of excision is not usually defined in series reporting local excision as the definitive surgical procedure. Ward et al.[117] had no local recurrences in a group of nine patients that had wide local excision with a stated margin of 2 cm. As mentioned earlier, a larger tumour may not be adequately excised locally. When treating for cure it seems pointless to use local excision unless one is clear of disease as well as being able to maintain sphincter function. The presence of proximal submucosal extension that occurs with these tumours is a factor to be considered in those patients in whom local excision is being considered.

Management of local disease: oncological factors – stage of local disease, local control and potential for cure

Malignant tumours at this site have the potential for lymphatic spread to both inguinal regions and to the pelvis. Because of this risk, bilateral inguinal dissection has been advocated, along with management of the primary tumour.[79] Metastasis to the inguinal region is more common with SCC of the anal canal, with reports as high as 42% compared with primary melanoma of 14%. Melanoma is more likely to spread to the pelvic mesenteric nodes, with an incidence of 33% compared with 15% for SCC.[118] The observation that the mesenteric nodes were more likely to be involved with melanoma when compared with SCC has been confirmed by Brady et al.[79] It is likely that the tumours found in the rectum or upper anal canal have a low incidence of inguinal node involvement, although no one has specifically examined this point. Iliac nodal disease is rare and, if it occurs, it is usually in the late stages of disease and is rarely symptomatic.[119] Brady et al.[79] reported the inguinal region to be the site of metastatic involvement in four of 43 patients (9.3%) after an APR and in three of 13 patients (23%) who had a WLE; one of the latter patients had a therapeutic node dissection and was a long-term survivor. Ross et al.[119] reported the inguinal region to be the site of first recurrence in nine of 23 patients (39%). To date, there is little evidence to justify routine elective lymph node dissection in patients with cutaneous melanoma and, given the potential added morbidity of a bilateral groin dissection,[120] it seems reasonable to watch the groins and perform a dissection only if a secondary node develops.

The rate of mesenteric nodal metastasis varies between series, probably because of the differing locations of the primary tumour and the different stages of disease in patients having an APR.[119,121] Brady et al.[79] reported 42% of patients undergoing APR to have positive mesenteric nodes, with one long-term survivor in that group. Patients with negative mesenteric nodes following APR had a better survival rate than those with positive nodes.[79] Unlike SCC of the anus, this is a common site of metastasis and there are no positive data for chemotherapeutic regimens as an adjunct to local therapy, as is seen in the management of SCC of the anal canal.

To gain a little more insight into the local control of disease by the surgical options of APR , LE or WLE, it is useful to examine the larger series that clearly define the presence and absence of local recurrence after surgical therapy for cure, where adequate follow-up information was available.[79,80,109,117,119,122] Some have not defined the extent of LE.[109,119] Radiotherapy has been used postoperatively as an adjuvant in two series but there is not enough information to extract any meaningful message.[79,122] Local recurrence occurred in 13 of 89 patients (14.6%) after APR, four of 24 patients (16.6%) after WLE and 29 of 49 patients (59%) after LE (margin undefined). Patients with local recurrence after LE will often require APR for symptom relief and local control.[80] Clearly, surgery aimed at total local eradication of disease should be performed, i.e. either APR or WLE.

When examining patient survival, all authors agree that there are no data showing an advantage of APR over LE and such recommendations for therapy tend to relate to the local experience or bias at the particular time of the report. The majority of recurrent disease manifests as visceral metastasis, with local or pelvic recurrence often a manifestation of widespread disease. Brady et al.[79] reported a subgroup of patients with early, localized disease, or favourable biology, in whom surgical cure is possible. The 5-year survival rate was 27% after APR and 5% after LE. It is of interest that all of the long-term survivors were women.[79] However, Ross et al.[119] had one survivor (3%) after LE and none following APR, with an overall median survival of 18.6 months and disease-free survival of 6 months; however, there was a trend for a longer disease-free interval following APR. The overall median survival rates were between 12 and 19 months. There is only one study in which the survival times for primary rectal and primary anal melanomas have been examined separately, reporting a median survival of 5 months for rectal tumours and 20 months for anal tumours ($P < 0.05$).[122]

In summary, APR removes the mesenteric nodes that are a common source of metastasis. It clearly offers a better potential for local control of disease over LE but not necessarily over WLE. The benefit of local control achieved by APR may be overshadowed by the rapid progression of systemic disease and death, and thus Ross et al.[119] have reasonably recommended sphincter sparing (wide) local excision when technically feasible, reserving APR for bulky local disease that can not be removed by LE alone and for salvage local control. In a situation where very few patients live long term, it will not take many extra survivors to gain improved survival rates in a disease where surgery is the only modality offering a potential for cure. In those patients with small localized lesions in the lower rectum and/or the upper anal canal it is difficult to ignore the pelvic mesentaric nodes as a potential site of recurrence, and the possibility of cure if the nodes are resected by doing an APR. The role of elective inguinal dissection is unclear, but it is unlikely to offer any benefit over careful observation of both inguinal regions.

Palliation

Palliation is usually provided by various local therapy modalities for the patients who present with metastatic disease or who are unfit for major surgery. The options for therapy include local excision, fulguration, radiotherapy and/or proximal stoma bypass. Therapies need to be tailored for each individual patient. The median survival in this group is 6 months.[79,109]

Radiotherapy

There has been a study of radiotherapy for patients with mucosal melanoma, with reports of a reasonable response in patients who had the treatment as the primary treatment modality.[123] Brady et al.[79] used radiotherapy as a postoperative adjuvant in patients after APR, WLE and biopsy with or without fulguration; they did not comment on its role, or the presence or absence of local recurrence, in relation to the radiotherapy. There were no long-term survivors who had radiotherapy. One other study reported patients having radiotherapy after APR without comment on the possible effects.[122]

Ross et al.[119] suggested that radiotherapy might be a useful adjuvant to treat the groins after LE of the primary tumour. It also seems reasonable to consider this modality as an adjuvant in any patient having LE where the margins are < 2 cm. All reasonable efforts should be made to try to avoid symptomatic local recurrence in these patients.

Chemotherapy

Adjuvant chemotherapy has been used,[124] but there is no evidence of a benefit in this group of patients.

CONCLUSIONS

Clearly, primary melanoma of the oesophagus and the anorectal region are definite entities. They tend to present late with locally advanced tumours that carry a poor prognosis. For patients who are able to undergo a resection of the primary lesion, the 5-year survival rate is 4–6% for both groups. The existence of primary melanoma of the rest of the GI tract would appear theoretically possible using a number of postulates relating to embryological development. However, using strict clinical and histological criteria, it is difficult to accept many of the case reports, especially with the acknowledged possibility of regression of a primary cutaneous melanoma and subsequent appearance of a visceral metastasis. There appear to be reasonable data indicating that primary melanoma occurs in the gall bladder and possibly the bile ducts, although on very rare occasions. Whether primary melanoma does occur in the small intestine and other GI sites is still questionable.

Despite the uncertainty of the existence of primary melanoma in a number of the GI regions, the principle remains that the best treatment, aiming for cure, whether the tumour is primary or a solitary metastasis, is surgical resection of all the disease. All other considerations remain an interesting academic exercise.

REFERENCES

1. Mills SE, Cooper PH, Malignant melanoma of the digestive system. *Pathol Ann* 1983; 18: 1–26.
2. Chang AE, Karnell LH, Menck HR, The National Cancer Data Base report on cutaneous and noncutaneous melanoma: a summary of 84,836 cases from the past decade. The American College of Surgeons Commission on Cancer and the American Cancer Society. *Cancer* 1998; 83: 1664–78.
3. Weinstock MA, Epidemiology and prognosis of anorectal melanoma. *Gastroenterology* 1993; 104: 174–8.
4. Miller BJ, Rutherford LF, McLeod GRC et al, Where the sun never shines: anorectal melanoma. *Aust NZ J Surg* 1997; 67: 846–8.
5. Sutherland CM, Chmiel JS, Henson DE et al, Patient characteristics, methods of diagnosis, and treatment of mucous membrane melanoma in the United States of America. *J Am Coll Surg* 1994; 179: 561–6.
6. Scotto J, Fraumeni Jr JF, Lee JAH, Melanoma of the eye and other noncutaneous sites: epidemiologic aspects. *J Natl Cancer Inst* 1976; 56: 489–91.
7. Rowles ME, Origin of mammalian pigment cell and its role in pigmentation of hair. In: *Pigment cell growth.* (ed Gordon, M) New York: Academic Press, 1953: 1–15.
8. de la Pava S, Nigogosyan G, Pickren JW et al, Melanosis of the esophagus. *Cancer* 1963; 16: 48–50.
9. Ladouch A, Fabre M, Quillard J et al, Melanoblasts in the esophageal mucosa and their relationship to malignant melanoma. *Arch Anat Cytol Pathol* 1976; 24: 473–6.
10. Shibata T, Distribution of melanocytes in human stratified squamous epithelium. *Ochanomizu Med J* 1973; 21: 87.
11. Tateishi R, Tanigushi H, Wade A et al, Argyrophil cells and melanocytes in oesophageal mucosa. *Arch Pathol* 1974; 98: 87–9.
12. DiCostanzo DP, Urmacher C, Primary malignant melanoma of the esophagus. *Am J Surg Pathol* 1987; 11: 46–52.
13. Sabaratnam S, Jibah E, Gautam NP, Primary malignant melanoma of the esophagus. *Am J Gastroenterol* 1989; 84: 1475–81.
14. Kreuser ED, Primary malignant melanoma of the esophagus. *Virchows Arch A Pathol Pathol Anat* 1979; 385: 49–59.
15. Piccone VA, Klopstock R, Laveen HH et al, Primary malignant melanoma of the oesophagus associated with melanosis of the entire oesophagus: first case report. *J Thorac Cardiovasc Surg* 1970; 59: 864–70.
16. De Mik JI, Kosijman CD, Hockstrom JBC et al, Primary malignant melanoma of the oesophagus. *Histopathology* 1992; 20: 77–9.
17. Walls EW, Observations on the microscopic anatomy of the human anal canal. *Br J Surg* 1958; 45: 504–12.
18. Clemmensen OJ, Fenger C, Melanocytes in the anal canal epithelium. *Histopathology* 1991; 18: 237–41.
19. Morson BC, Dawson JMP. *Malignant epithelial tumours in the gastro-intestinal pathology.* Oxford: Blackwell Scientific Publications. 1972: 132–60.
20. Cooper PH, Mills SE, Allen MS, Malignant melanoma of the anus: report of 12 patients and analysis of 255 additional cases. *Dis Colon Rectum* 1982; 25: 693–703.
21. Werdin C, Limas C, Knodell RG, Primary malignant melanoma of the rectum. Evidence for origination from rectal mucosal melanocytes. *Cancer* 1988; 61: 1364–70.
22. Nicholson AG, Cox PM, Marks CG et al, Primary malignant melanoma of the rectum. *Histopathology* 1993; 22: 261–4.
23. Hambrick E, Abcarian H, Smith D et al, Malignant melanoma of the rectum in a Negro man: report of a case and review of the literature. *Dis Colon Rectum* 1974; 17: 360–4.
24. Behrend M, Behrend A, Melanosarcoma (malignant melanoma) of the rectosigmoid: report of a unique case. *Gastroenterology* 1949; 12: 142
25. Mester E, Juhasz J, Primares malignes melanom des sigma. *Zentralbl Chir* 1968; 93: 1514
26. Zimouskii VL, Melanoblastoma slepoi kishki. *Klin Khir (Kiev)* 1968; 8: 54
27. Laidlow FG, Melanoma studies. *Am J Pathol* 1932; 8: 477–90.
28. Breathreach AS, Normal and abnormal melanin pigmentation of the skin. In: *Pigments in pathology.* (ed Wolman M) London: Academic Press. 1969: 3555.
29. Carle G, Lessels AM, Best PV, Malignant melanoma of the gall bladder. *Cancer* 1981; 48: 2318–22.
30. Das Gupta T, Bowden L, Berg JW, Malignant melanoma of unknown primary origin. *Surg Gynaecol Obstet* 1963; 117: 341–5.
31. Yamamoto M, Takahashi I, Iwamoto T et al, Endocrine cells in extrahepatic bile duct carcinoma. *J Cancer Res Clin Oncol* 1984; 108: 331–5.
32. Le Douarin NM, Cell migrations in embryos. *Cell* 1984; 38: 353–60.
33. Whitman JG, APUD cell and apendomas. *Anaesthesia* 1977; 32: 879–88.
34. Rost FWD, Polak JM, Pearce AGE, The melanocyte. Its cytochemical and immunological relationship to cells of the endocrine polypeptide (APUD) series. *Virchows Arch Abt B Zellpath* 1969; 4: 93–106.
35. Mishima Y, Melanocytic and neuroctic malignant melanomas. Cellular and subcellular differentiation. *Cancer* 1967; 20: 632–49.

36. Amar A, Jougon J, Edouard A et al, Melanome malin primitif de litestin grele. *Gastroenterol Clin Biol* 1992; 16: 365–7.
37. Bloch T, Tejada E, Brodhecker C, Malignant melanoma in Meckel's diverticulum. *Am J Clin Pathol* 1986; 84: 231–4.
38. Iverson K, Robins RE, Mucosal melanoma. *Am J Surg* 1980; 139: 660–64.
39. Jonk A, Kroon BBR, Runke P et al, Lymph node metastasis from melanoma with unknown primary site. *Br J Surg* 1990; 77: 665–8.
40. Allen AC, Spitz S, Malignant melanoma: a clinocopathological analysis of the criteria for diagnosis and prognosis. *Cancer* 1953; 6: 1–45.
41. Raven RW, Dawson I, Malignant melanoma of the oesophagus. *Br J Surg* 1964; 51: 551–5.
42. Mansson T, Berge T, Primary malignant melanoma of the oesophagus. *Acta Pathol Microbiol Scand* 1977; 85: 395–8.
43. Clark WH, Ainsworth AM, Bernardino CE et al, The developmental biology of primary tumour malignant melanomas. *Semin Oncol* 1975; 2: 83–103.
44. Wanebo HJ, Woodruff JN, Farr GH et al, Anorectal melnoma. *Cancer* 1981; 47: 1891–900.
45. Guzeman RP, Wightman R, Ravinsky E et al, Primary malignant melanoma of the esophagus with melanocytic atypia and melanoma in situ. *Am J Clin Pathol* 1990; 92: 802–4.
46. Muto M, Saito Y, Koike T et al, Primary malignant melanoma of the oesophagus with diffuse pigmentation resembling superficial spreading melanoma. *Am J Gastroenterol* 1997; 92: 1936–7.
47. Higgins CM, Strutton GM, Malignant melanoma of the gall bladder – does primary melanoma exist? *Pathology* 1995; 27: 312–14.
48. McFadden PM, Krementz ET, McKinnon WMP et al, Metastatic melanoma of the gallbladder. *Cancer* 1979; 44: 1802–8.
49. Heath DI, Womack C, Primary malignant melanoma of the gall bladder. *J Clin Pathol* 1988; 41: 1073–7.
50. Abernathy JL, Soyer HP, Kerl H et al, Epidermotropic metastatic malignant melanoma stimulating melanoma in situ. *Am J Surg Pathol* 1994; 18: 1140–9.
51. Naguib SE, Aterman K, Presumed primary malignant melanoma of the gallbladder. Report of a case and a review of the literature. *Am J Dermatopathol* 1984; 6 Supp: 231–43.
52. Walsh TS, Primary melanoma of the gallbladder with cervical metastasis and 14½ years survival. *Cancer* 1956; 6: 518–22.
53. Das Gupta T, Brasfield R, Metastatic melanoma: a clinico pathological study. *Cancer* 1964; 10: 1323–9.
54. Washburn WK, Noda S, Lewis WD et al, Primary malignant melanoma of the biliary tract. *Liver Transpl Surg* 1995; 1: 103–6.
55. Carstens PHB, Ghazi C, Carnighan RH et al, Primary melanoma of the common bile duct. *Hum Pathol* 1986; 17: 1282–4.
56. Zhang Z, Myles J, Pai RP et al, Malignant melanoma of the biliary tract: a case report. *Surgery* 1991; 109: 323–7.
57. Verbanck JJ, Rutgeerts LJ, Van Aelst FI et al, Primary malignant melanoma of the gallbladder metastatic to the common bile duct. *Gastroenterology* 1986; 91: 214–8.
58. Bianca A, Carboni N, Di Carlo V et al, Pancreatic malignant melanoma with occult primary lesion – a case report. *Pathologea* 1991; 83: 531–7.
59. Rutter JE, De Graaf PW, Kooyman CD et al, Malignant melanoma of the pancreas: primary tumour or unknown primary? *Eur J Surg* 1994; 160: 119–20.
60. Petiot JM, Raynal JN, Melanosacome de la tete du pancreas en apparence primitive. *J Chir (Paris)* 1995; 132: 322–3.
61. Banzet F, Delarue J, Chappellart P et al, Un cas de melanom a localisations gastrointestinales multiples apparemment primitives. *Presse Med* 1953; 82: 1732–42.
62. Hofmann GO, Primares malignes Melanom des Magens? Eine literaturegestuzte Kasuistik. *Chirurg* 1990; 61: 77–80.
63. Liang JT, Yu SC, Lee PH et al, Endoscopic diagnosis of malignant melanoma in the gastric cardia. Report of a case without a detectable primary lesion. *Endoscopy* 1995; 27: 409.
64. Macak J, Melanoma of the stomach: reality or fiction? *Pathologica* 1998; 90: 388–90.
65. Aagaard MT, Kristensen IB, Lund O et al, Primary malignant nonepithelial tumours of the thoracic oesophagus and cardia in a 25-year surgical material. *Scand J Gastroenterol* 1990; 25: 876–82.
66. Alberti JE, Bodor J, Torres AD et al, Primary melanoma of the esophagus associated with melanosis of the oesophagus and the stomach. *Acta Gastroenterol Latinoam* 1984; 14: 139–48.
67. Backman H, Davidson L, Metastases of malignant melanoma in the stomach and small intestine. *Acta Med Scand* 1965; 178: 329.
68. Pector JC, Crokaert F, Lejeune F et al, Prolonged survival after resection of a malignant melanoma metastatic of the stomach. *Cancer* 1988; 61: 2134.
69. Kadivar TF, Vanek VW, Krishnan EU, Primary malignant melanoma of the small bowel: a case study. *Am Surg* 1992; 58: 418–22.
70. Wade TP, Goodwin MN, Countryman DM et al, Small bowel melanoma: extended survival with surgical management. *Eur J Surg Oncol* 1995; 21: 90–1.
71. Karakousis CP, Goumas W, Rao U et al, Axillary node dissection in malignant melanoma. *Am J Surg* 1991; 162: 202–7.
72. Elsayed AM, Albahra M, Nzeako UC et al, Malignant melanomas in the small intestine: a study of 103 patients. *Am J Gastroenterol* 1996; 91: 1001–6.
73. Wilson BG, Anderson JR, Malignant melanoma involving the small bowel. *Postgrad Med J* 1986; 62: 355–7.
74. Das Gupta TK, Braasfield RD, Metastatic melanoma on the gastrointestinal tract. *Arch Surg* 1964; 88: 969–73.
75. Willbanks OC, Fogelman MJ, Gastrointestinal melanosarcoma. *Am J Surg* 1970; 120: 602–6.
76. Sachs DL, Lowe L, Chang AE et al, Do primary small intestinal melanomas exist? Report of a case. *J Am Acad Dermatol* 1999; 41: 1042–4.
77. Calso F, Carpani G, Fiora U, A case of malignant melanoma of apparent primary duodenal localization. *Minerva Chir* 1984; 15: 919–21.
78. Nedjabat T, Paquet KJ, Klammer H-L et al, Primares malignes melanom des dunndarm. *Med Welt* 1975; 26: 1093.
79. Brady MS, Kavolius JP, Quan SHQ, Anorectal melanoma. A 64–year experience at the Memorial Sloan-Kettering Cancer Centre. *Dis Colon Rectum* 1995; 38: 146–51.
80. Slingluff CL, Vollmer RT, Seigler HF, Anorectal melanoma: clinical characteristics and results of surgical management in twenty-four patients. *Surgery* 1990; 107: 1–9.
81. Chui YS, Umni KK, Beart RW, Malignant melnoma of the anorectum. *Dis Colon Rectum* 1980; 23: 122–4.
82. Caldwell CB, Bains MS, Bust M, Unusual malignant neoplasms of the oesophagus: oatcell carcinoma, melanoma and sarcoma. *J Thorac Cardiovasc Surg* 1991; 101: 100–7.
83. Turnbull AD, Rosen P, Goodner JT, Beattie EJ, Primary malignant tumors of the esophagus other than typical epidermoid carcinoma. *Ann Thorac Surg* 1973; 15: 463–73.
84. Baur EH, Fin fall von primäten melanoma des oesophagus. *Aub ad Gep d path. Anat Inst Zu Tubingen* 1906; 5: 343–54.
85. DeMatos P, Wolfe WG, Shea CR et al, Primary malignant melanoma of the esophagus. *J Surg Oncol* 1997; 66: 201–6.
86. Pollack ES, Horn JW, Trends in cancer incidence and mortality in the United States. *J Natl Cancer Inst* 1980; 64: 1091–103.
87. Chalkiadakis G, Wihlm JM, Morand G et al, Primary malignant melanoma of the oesophagus. *Ann Thorac Surg* 1985; 39: 472–5.
88. Basque CJ, Boline TE, Holyoke JB, Malignant melanoma of the oesophagus. First reported case in a child. *Am J Clin Pathol* 1970; 53: 609–11.
89. Yoo CC, Levine MS, McLarney JK, Lowry MA, Primary malignant melanoma of the oesophagus; radiographic findings in seven patients. *Radiology* 1998; 209: 455–9.
90. Kanamoto K, Aoyagi K, Nakamura S et al, The value of endoscopic ultrasonography in primary malignant melanoma of the esophagus. *Gastrointest Endosc* 1997; 46: 88–9 (letter).
91. Joob AW, Haines GK, Kies MS et al, Primary malignant melanoma of the oesophagus. *Ann Thorac Surg* 1995; 60: 217–22.
92. McCormack P, Nasumento A, Bains M et al, Primary melanocarcinoma of the esophagus. *Memorial Sloan-Kettering Cancer Bull* 1979; 9: 162–4.
93. Mukaiya M, Hirata K, Tarumi K et al, Surgical treatment for recurrent tumours of primary malignant melanoma of the oesophagus: a case report and review of literature. *Hepatogastroenterology* 1999; 46: 295.

94. Jawalekar K, Tretter P, Primary malignant melanoma of the oesophagus. *J Surg Oncol* 1979; 12: 19–25.
95. Kato H, Watanabe H, Tachimori Y et al, Primary malignant melanoma of the oesophagus. Report four cases. *Jpn J Clin Oncol* 1991; 21: 306–13.
96. Yano M, Shiozaki H, Murata A et al, Primary malignant melanoma of the esophagus associated with adenocarcinoma of the lung. *Surg Today* 1998; 28: 405–8.
97. Naomoto Y, Perdomo JA, Kamikawa Y et al, Primary malignant melanoma of the esophagus: report of a case successfully treated with pre- and post-operative adjuvant hormone-chemotherapy. *Jpn J Clin Oncol* 1998; 28: 758–61.
98. Weitung H, Hamdi, Uber die physiologische und pathologische melanin pigmentierung und den epithelialen usprung der melanoblastome ein primares melanoblastome der gallen blase. *Biete Path Anat* 1907; 42: 73–84.
99. Velez AF, Penetrante RB, Spellman JE et al, Malignant melanoma of the gall bladder: a report of a case and review of the literature. *Am Surg* 1995; 61: 1095–8.
100. Hatanaka N, Miyata M, Kamiike W et al, Radial resection of primary malignant melanoma of the gallbladder with multiple metastasis: report of a case. *Surg Today* 1993; 23: 1023–6.
101. Mittal VK, Bodzin JH, Primary malignant tumors of the small bowel. *Am J Surg* 1980; 140: 396–9.
102. Reyes EL, Talley RW, Primary malignant tumours of the small intestine. *Am J Gastroenterol* 1970; 54: 30–43.
103. Wilson JM, Melvin DB, Gray GF et al, Primary malignancies of the small bowel: a report of 96 cases and review of the literature. *Ann Surg* 1974; 180: 175–9.
104. Moore W, Recurrent melanoma of the rectum after previous removal from the verge of the anus in a man aged sixty-five. *Lancet* 1857; 1: 290.
105. Bolivar JC, Harris JW, Branch W, Sherman R, Melanoma of the anorectal region. *Surg Gynaecol Obstet* 1982; 154: 337–41.
106. Longo WE, Vernava AM, Wade TP et al, Rare anal canal cancers in the U.S. Veteran: patterns of disease and results of treatment. *Am Surg* 1995; 61: 495–500.
107. Boman BM, Moertel CG, O'Connell MJ et al, Carcinoma of the anal canal: a clinical and pathologic study of 188 cases. *Cancer* 1984; 54: 114–25.
108. Klas JV, Rothenberger DA, Wong WD et al, Malignant tumors of the anal canal. The spectrum of disease, treatment, and outcomes. *Cancer* 1999; 85: 1686–93.
109. Goldman S, Glimelius B, Pahlman L, Anorectal melanoma in Sweden. Report of 49 patients. *Dis Colon Rectum* 1990; 33: 874–7.
110. Slaney G, Cancer of the large bowel. In: *Clinical cancer monographs.* (eds Slaney G, Powell J, McConkey C et al) London: Macmillan Press, 1991: 62.
111. Remacle G, Havt J, Kartheuser A, Detry R, Primary melanosarcoma of the rectum. *Acta Chir Belg* 1993; 93: 63–6.
112. Hermanek P, Sobin LH, *International Union Against Cancer. TNM classification of malignant tumors*, 4th edn. New York: Springer-Verlag, 1987; 50–2.
113. Amano K, Iida M, Matsumoto T et al, A case of malignant melanoma in the anorectal region: colonoscopic features. *Gastrointest Endosc* 1997; 45: 536–7.
114. Rubin KP, Ghanekar D, Friedrick IA, Panella VS, Endoscopic diagnosis of anorectal melanoma. *N J Med* 1992; 89: 309–10.
115. Ojima Y, Nakatsuka H, Haneji H et al, Primary anorectal malignant melanoma: report of a case. *Surg Today* 1999; 29: 170–3.
116. Ishida J, Sugimura K, Okizuka H, Kaji Y, Malignant anorectal melanoma: usefulness of fat saturation MR imaging. *Eur J Radiol* 1997; 16: 195–7.
117. Ward MWN, Romano G, Nicholls RJ, The surgical treatment of anorectal malignant melanoma. *Br J Surg* 1986; 73: 68–9.
118. Quan SH, Deddish MR, Non cutaneous melanoma: malignant melanoma of the rectum. *Cancer* 1966; 16: 111–14.
119. Ross M, Pezzi C, Pezzi T et al, Patterns of failure in anorectal melanoma. *Arch Surg* 1990; 125: 313–16.
120. Urist MM, Maddox WA, Kennedy JE, Balch CM, Elective bilateral groin dissection carries significant morbidity. *Cancer* 1983; 51: 2151–6.
121. Paradis P, Douglass HO, Holyoke ED, The clinical implications of a staging system for carcinoma of the anus. *Surg Gynecol Obstet* 1975; 141: 411–16.
122. Abbas JS, Karakousis CP, Holyoke ED, Anorectal melanoma: clinical features, recurrence and patient survival. *Int Surg* 1980; 65: 423–6.
123. Harwood AR, Cummings BJ, Radiotherapy for mucosal melanomas. *Int J Radiat Oncol Biol Phys* 1982; 8: 1121–6.
124. Banner WP, Quan SHQ, Woodruff JM, Malignant melanoma of the anorectum. *Surg Rounds* 1990; 13: 28–32.

63

Ocular melanoma

Michael E Giblin, Jerry A Shields, Carol L Shields

INTRODUCTION

Under the term ocular melanomas are included intraocular (uveal) melanomas, conjunctival melanomas, eyelid melanomas, orbital melanomas and melanomas metastatic to the ocular area. These will be considered separately.

UVEAL MELANOMA

The uvea is the vascular coat within the eye that includes the iris, ciliary body and choroid. Uveal melanoma is a malignant neoplasm arising from neuroectodermal melanocytes in the choroid, ciliary body or iris and is the most common primary intraocular malignant neoplasm in adults.[1]

Melanomas involving the posterior uveal tract arise more commonly from the choroid rather than from the ciliary body. A posterior segment melanoma can extend into the anterior segment and the reverse is also true. Posterior uveal melanomas are generally more malignant, both clinically and cytologically, than iris melanoma.[2]

Aetiology

The incidence of uveal melanoma is <1:100,000 of the Caucasian population per year. About one in 2500 whites will develop a uveal melanoma during their lifetime and the risk increases with age. Most posterior uveal melanomas are diagnosed when the patient is older than 50 years of age and iris melanomas are diagnosed somewhat earlier.[3,4]

Although a probable link exists between sunlight exposure and melanoma of the conjunctiva and iris, this relationship is less clear for melanoma arising in the posterior segment of the eye. Evidence that sunlight may cause uveal melanoma lies in its extreme rarity in dark-skinned races and the increased incidence in patients with light coloured irides.[5] Most iris melanomas are located in the inferior portion of the iris, which has greater exposure to sunlight than does the superior portion.

Genetic factors specific for ocular melanoma have been identified. The most commonly encountered chromosomal abnormalities involve chromosomes 3, 6, 8 and 9.[6] Occasionally, one elicits either a past history or family history of dysplastic cutaneous naevi or cutaneous melanoma in patients with primary uveal melanoma, but the exact nature of this relationship remains to be established.[7–10]

It is not uncommon for a primary uveal melanoma patient to have had another primary cancer or else to have a separate malignant neoplasm when the uveal melanoma is first discovered, or subsequent to treatment for the melanoma.[11,12]

Ocular melanocytosis is a specific predisposing factor for the development of uveal melanoma, the cumulative lifetime risk for the development of which in the presence of that condition is estimated at 1:400.[13] Ocular melanocytosis describes the congenital hyperpigmentation of the episclera and uveal tract, the histological counterpart of which is a dense concentration of heavily pigmented, plump melanocytes in the iris, ciliary body and choroid. In this usually unilateral, but sometimes bilateral, condition, the sclera of the involved eye has a characteristic patchy, slate-grey to brown appearance, with the involved iris and fundus appearing darker than the fellow, uninvolved eye. The periocular skin may also be involved, in which case the term oculodermal melanocytosis or naevus of Ota is used.

Clinical features

Iris melanomas do not usually cause visual symptoms, but rather present as a mass lesion on the iris noted on routine ophthalmic examination or, less often, noted by the patient. These tumours can result in a darkening of the involved iris so that the irides are of different colours (heterochromia iridis).

The typical iris melanoma is a discrete mass which may be seen on the front surface of the iris as well as on the back surface, where the tumour can elevate the iris off the underlying lens. The degree of pigmentation is variable. When an iris tumour is very large at presentation, or is associated with a rapid growth pattern, the index of suspicion of malignancy is heightened, likewise if the tumour is associated with visual loss or spontaneous hyphaema.

Secondary glaucoma, sector cataract and distortion of the pupil (ectropion uveae) are of less help clinically in distinguishing an iris melanoma from a naevus.[14] Less often, melanomas of the iris assume a more diffuse, flatter clinical appearance with the sudden onset of hyperchromia of the involved iris and a rapid growth pattern which usually leads to enucleation.[15]

Melanomas arising primarily from the ciliary body frequently attain a large size before detection because of their increased distance from the macula. Also, routine ophthalmic examination is less likely to detect smaller tumours in the periphery of the eye than those situated in the posterior pole.

The clinical appearance of a ciliary body melanoma has much in common with that of a choroidal melanoma (see below). Extrascleral extension of a ciliary body melanoma is more easily seen clinically than with a choroidal melanoma, due to the more anterior tumour location, and manifests as a small dark lobulated mass on the outside of the eye. So-called sentinel vessels, which are dilated, tortuous episcleral vessels overlying the involved sector of a large ciliary body melanoma, are sometimes seen.

A choroidal melanoma may be asymptomatic and detected as part of a routine ophthalmic examination. Symptoms include reduced visual acuity, flashing lights (photopsia), floaters, distortion of vision (metamorphopsia) and visual field defects. Pain is not a characteristic presenting feature of posterior uveal melanoma, but can occur in the case of a very advanced tumour with secondary glaucoma, or occasionally with inflammation associated with tumour necrosis.[16]

A choroidal melanoma typically appears as an elevated, nodular or dome-shaped, usually melanotic, but occasionally amelanotic mass. When the tumour has broken through Bruch's membrane it assumes a characteristic mushroom shape. Subretinal fluid often surrounds the melanoma or lies in a dependent position inferiorly. Haemorrhage in association with a posterior uveal melanoma is not characteristic, but may be seen occasionally, especially if the melanoma has broken through Bruch's membrane. Orange pigment over the surface of the tumour is common and correlates with the histopathologic finding of lipofuscin pigment within macrophages.

Approximately 5% of malignant melanomas of the uveal tract are characterized by diffuse growth in the plane of the uvea. Such tumours often present late, are difficult to diagnose, are frequently associated with extraocular extension and carry a poor systemic prognosis.[17,18]

Diagnostic methods

Baseline iris or fundus photographs facilitate detection of tumour growth in patients being followed with uveal naevi and presumed inactive melanomas, and assist the examiner to monitor the regression of locally treated melanomas.

Fluorescein angiography is indicated in selected patients with suspected uveal melanoma, particularly those involving the posterior uvea. The variations in the angiographic appearance of posterior uveal melanoma are numerous. The simultaneous fluorescence of the retinal and choroidal vasculature has been referred to as the double-circulation pattern, which is highly characteristic of many choroidal melanomas and is due to the intrinsic tumour circulation.

Transillumination of iris melanomas involving the angle of the eye can detect posterior segment extension. Transillumination of ciliary body melanomas assists in determining if the tumour base is small enough for plaque radiation therapy or local resection.

Ultrasonography is occasionally helpful diagnostically, but is of most benefit in documenting regression of posterior uveal melanomas in the form of thickness reduction following tumour irradiation. The typical ultrasonographic feature of a posterior uveal melanoma is acoustic hollowness due to the tumour's uniform internal structure. The commonest regression pattern is one of gradual shrinkage over several years. Rapid regression has been found to be associated with a worse systemic prognosis.[19]

In occasional patients with uveal tumours, fine needle aspiration biopsy may be appropriate.[20,21] The chance of tumour development along the needle tract is minimized if definitive treatment is performed after the biopsy. Open surgical incisional biopsy also has a role to play, but must be employed with caution because of the risk of local tumour recurrence.

Pretreatment systemic investigations include liver function tests as well as a liver scan for large melanomas. The liver is preferentially involved with metastases in 90% of cases. Only 2% of uveal melanoma patients have detectable metastatic disease at initial presentation.[22]

Pathology (Figures 63.1 and 63.2)

Evidence indicates that the vast majority of uveal malignant melanomas arise from pre-existing naevi. In rare cases, choroidal melanomas have been observed to arise de novo from areas previously examined and found to be normal.[23]

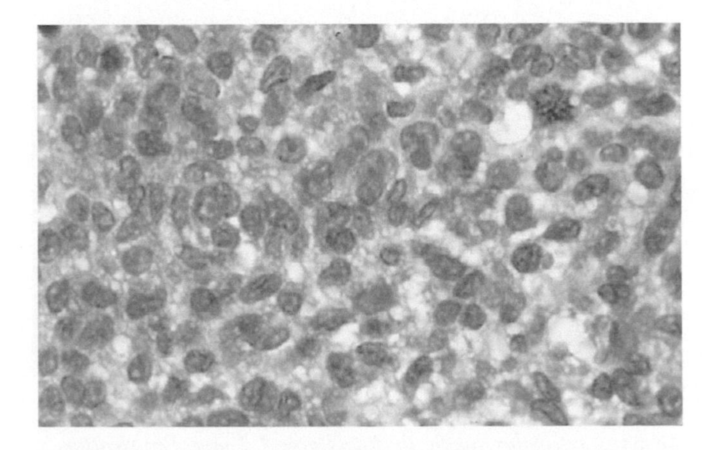

Figure 63.1 *Predominantly spindle cell iris melanoma.*

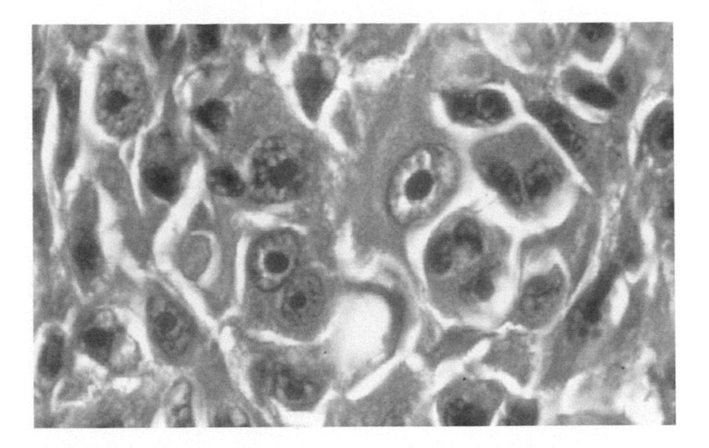

Figure 63.2 *Predominantly epithelioid cell posterior uveal melanoma.*

Melanoma of the uveal tract, including iris melanoma, may be categorized histopathologically, according to the Callender classification,[24] depending on the cell type as follows:

- Spindle A cells (now regarded as benign): cohesive cells with small, spindled nuclei with a central, dark nuclear stripe, but no distinct nucleoli.
- Spindle B cells: more common. Cohesive cells with prominent nuclei and distinct nucleoli. Both spindle A and spindle B cells have indistinct cell borders. The cell pattern is described as fasicular if in palisade formation.
- Epithelioid cells: non-cohesive cells, large round nuclei, prominent nucleoli and distinct cells borders.
- Mixed: spindle and epithelioid.
- Necrotic: cell types cannot be identified.

The Callender classification of ciliary body and choroidal melanomas is not applicable to iris melanomas as far as assessment of systemic prognosis is concerned. For example, mixed and epithelioid iris melanomas may have a more benign course when compared with posterior uveal melanomas of a similar cell type.

Management (Figures 63.3–63.9)

In the great majority of patients with pigmented uveal tumours and, indeed, in a considerable number with amelanotic mass lesions, the differential diagnosis rests between naevus and melanoma. Biopsy of such tumours is not as straightforward as for cutaneous lesions and

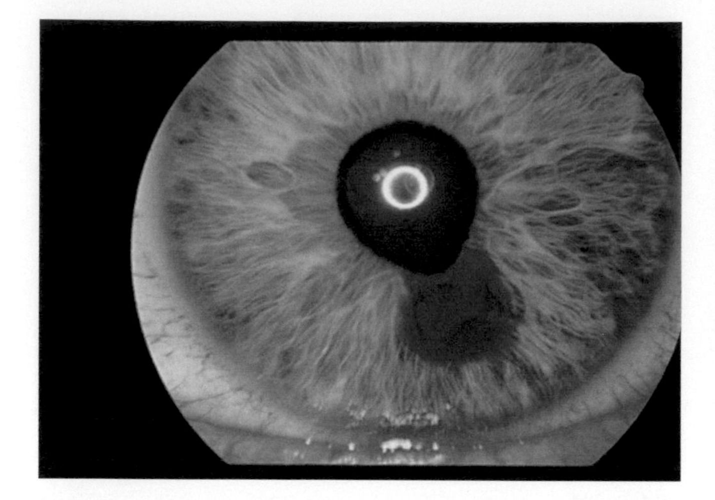

Figure 63.3 *Iris melanoma in a 25-year-old white male.*

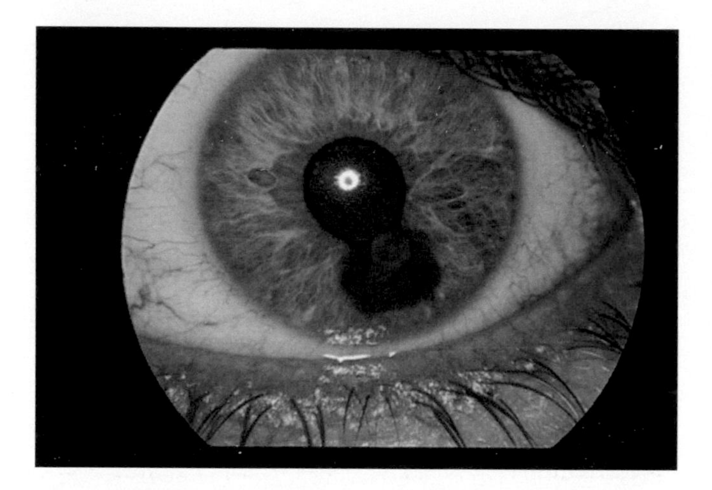

Figure 63.4 *Same patient as in Figure 63.3, after 18 months, showing significant growth. Histopathology showed spindle B melanoma.*

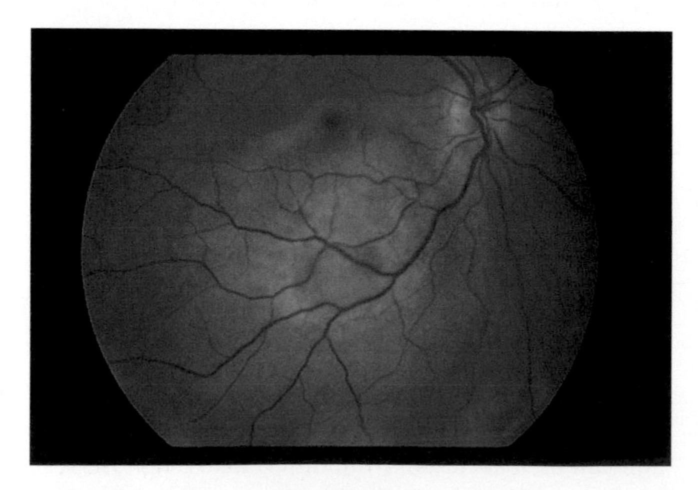

Figure 63.5 *Choroidal melanoma prior to episcleral plaque radiation therapy.*

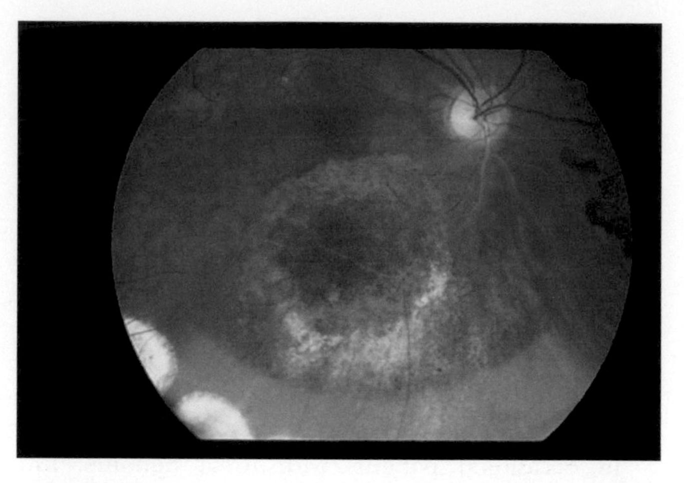

Figure 63.6 *Same patient as in Figure 63.5 showing melanoma regression.*

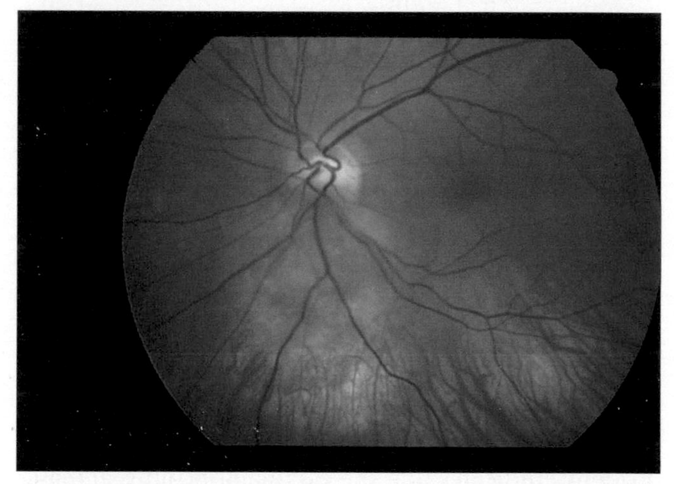

Figure 63.7 *Small peripapillary choroidal melanoma, 1.5 mm thick, managed initially by observation.*

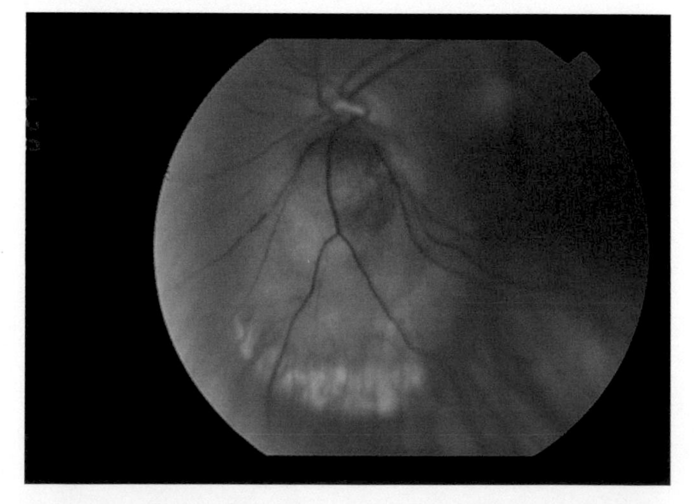

Figure 63.8 *Same patient as in Figure 63.7, 7 years later, showing extensive growth, thickness now 4.7 mm. Enucleation recommended but declined.*

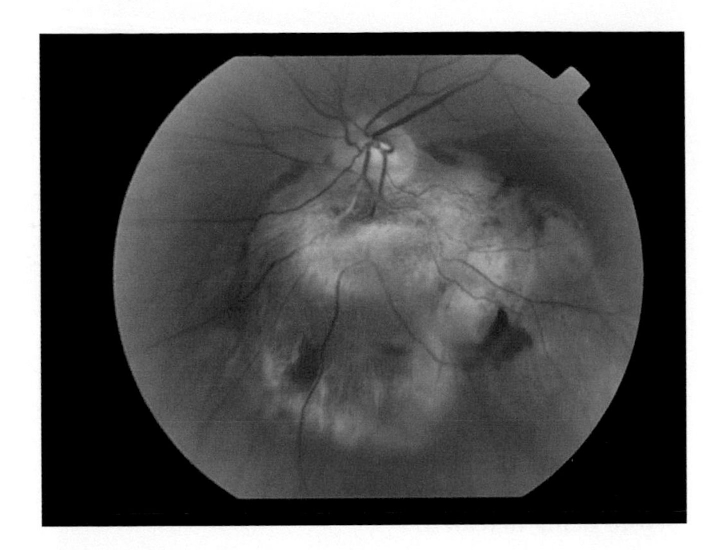

Figure 63.9 *Same patient as in Figures 63.7 and 63.8, showing response 2 months after two sessions of laser thermotherapy, thickness now 1.4 mm.*

carries with it possible visual consequences. For this reason, selected patients with uveal tumours are managed by observation and treatment is undertaken if definitive growth is documented.[12]

This is especially true for iris tumours, most of which are managed by periodic observation. Surgical treatment of larger or actively growing melanomas involves excision of the tumour using either iridectomy or, if there is extension of the melanoma into the angle or the posterior segment of the eye, an iridocyclectomy.

Radioactive plaques also play a role in the primary treatment of iris melanomas[25] and can also be employed to supplement a local resection operation. Some eyes with extensive iris melanoma require enucleation.

Posterior uveal melanomas are also treated by enucleation of the eye if too large or if optic nerve involvement is too extensive for an eye-sparing alternative. Pre-enucleation radiotherapy has not been found to significantly alter the systemic prognosis.[26,27]

It is not entirely clear whether enucleation improves the systemic prognosis as patients with large melanomas are not routinely managed by observation, which makes comparative analysis difficult. Furthermore, the finding of a peak in mortality some 18 months after enucleation raises the possibility that removal of an eye containing a uveal melanoma may actually worsen survival.[28] One possible explanation of this observation relates to the phenomenon of inhibition of tumour growth by tumour mass, in which a tumour-dependent circulating angiogenesis inhibitor has been found to play a role in the prevention of metastases in an experimental animal model.[29] The argument in favour of eye-saving treatment alternatives to enucleation has been strengthened by such evidence which, however, remains contentious.[30,31]

Suitably sized posterior uveal melanomas may be handled with the application of a radioactive episcleral plaque.[32] The plaque is usually left in place until a dose of 80–100 gray (Gy) has been delivered to the apex of the tumour. Plaque radiation therapy is most appropriate for melanomas whose thickness is <8 mm; however, thicker tumours may sometimes be irradiated. The principal limiting factor for the use of plaque brachytherapy is the maximal basal dimension of the melanoma, which should be at least 2 mm less than the diameter of the radioactive plaque being used to ensure that the entire melanoma is adequately treated.

The most commonly used radioactive isotopes are iodine-125 and ruthenium-106. These lower energy plaques have largely replaced those containing cobalt-60, which is a higher energy isotope. Other isotopes in use include iridium-192 and palladium-103. A commonly employed plaque diameter is 15 mm.[2]

Charged particle external beam irradiation, most often in the form of protons[33] or helium ions,[34,35] is also employed, but this treatment modality is currently much less widely available than plaque radiotherapy. With this technique the tumour base is first localized using radio-opaque tantalum rings, which are sutured to the surrounding sclera. The treatment is fractionated over 4–7 days.

Selected melanomas involving the posterior segment may be amenable to local resection.[36] During the operation a scleral flap is usually raised and the tumour then excised with the assistance of hypotensive anaesthesia to minimize haemorrhage. This technique lends itself well to melanomas situated anterior to the equator of the eye and with a relatively narrow base. The presence of subretinal fluid facilitates tumour removal, as the fluid acts as a protective buffer between the melanoma and the overlying retina. Plaque brachytherapy, on the other hand, is better suited for the more posterior melanoma with a larger base and smaller thickness, because such tumours are more difficult to resect and require relatively less radiation than do thicker melanomas.

Transpupillary thermotherapy using a diode laser with an operating wavelength of 810 nm is a newer treatment modality which is suited for selected small choroidal melanomas situated behind the equator of the eye and having a thickness of <4 mm.[37–42] The more pigmented the tumour the greater the uptake of the laser energy and hence the greater the treatment effect. This technique works by heating the melanoma to 20°C or more above body temperature.

Laser thermotherapy is useful as a primary form of treatment either on its own or in conjunction with the application of an episcleral plaque. Thermotherapy also has a role to play as a secondary form of treatment if there has been inadequate regression following tumour irradiation. Laser photocoagulation has also been used in the treatment of selected small choroidal melanomas in the posterior pole of the eye, although its effect is limited by coagulation and traction of the overlaying retina, and tissue penetration is in the order of only 1 mm, significantly less than with laser thermotherapy.

Prognosis

The overall survival after treatment for uveal melanoma seems to be similar regardless of the treatment method employed for patients with equivalent tumour parameters. The 5-year survival rate for patients whose eyes have been enucleated for posterior uveal melanoma is *c.* 70% and the 10-year survival rate is 50%.[43–45] The higher survival rate after eye-sparing treatment reflects, at least in part, the smaller size of those melanomas. The mortality rate for iris melanoma is significantly better, with an overall mortality rate of <4%.[46,47]

Metastases from uveal melanoma result from haematogenous spread and are usually a late manifestation. A significant difference between uveal and cutaneous melanoma is the rarity of lymphatic spread in the former, whereas early regional lymph node metastasis is characteristic of the latter. This observation is not totally explained by the lack of lymphatics in the uveal tract and orbit, as lymphatic involvement is not observed even in those cases in which uveal melanoma is associated with extraocular extension to the conjunctiva where lymphatics are present.[48]

The mortality rates of cutaneous and uveal melanoma may be comparable when tumour volumes are compared. Survival rates in patients whose posterior uveal melanomas are <300 mm^3 are similar to those in cutaneous melanoma patients with equivalent-sized tumours.[49]

As well as the adverse finding of extraocular extension,[50,51] there are several other systemic prognostic variables[44] which have been found to be significant for posterior uveal melanoma, i.e. patient age,[52] tumour location, largest tumour dimension and cell type.[52,53] The older the age of the patient the worse the prognosis, as is also the case the more anterior the melanoma is in the posterior segment, presumably because tumours in this location have greater access to the extraocular circulation and can attain a larger size before being detected.

The greater bulk of a larger melanoma imposes an increased burden on the patient's tumour defences. Moreover, there is a higher chance that a larger melanoma will be associated with a more unfavourable cell type; the higher the epithelioid cell content, the worse the systemic prognosis. The standard deviation of the nucleolar area has been measured using computerized histopathologic assessment in eyes enucleated for uveal melanoma and this calculation correlates closely with systemic prognosis when combined with the largest dimension of the tumour.[54–56]

The detection of microvascular loops and networks in choroidal and ciliary body melanomas has more recently been found to be an accurate prognostic indicator,[57–59] as has the presence of monosomy of chromosome 3 in melanoma tissue.[6]

CONJUNCTIVAL MELANOMA

Conjunctival melanoma is a distinctly different entity from uveal melanoma and has a cell type more closely connected with that of cutaneous melanoma.[60] Seventy-five per cent of conjunctival melanomas arise from primary acquired conjunctival melanosis, while the remainder of cases arise either from pre-existing conjunctival naevi or de novo.[61,62] Conjunctival melanomas are extremely rare in dark-skinned races and in individuals under the age of 20. An example is shown in Figure 63.10.

The tumour is characteristically a brown, nodular, elevated, vascularized mass on the conjunctiva, but may be amelanotic, especially if recurrent.

Conjunctival and cutaneous melanomas are not classified according to cell type as are uveal melanomas,

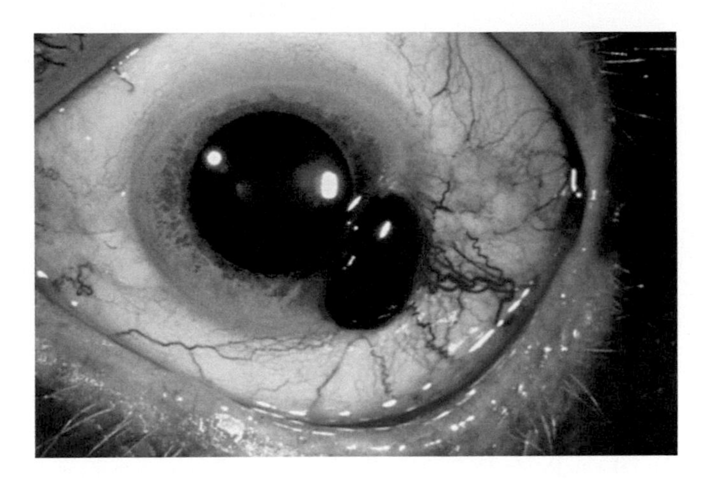

Figure 63.10 *Conjunctival melanoma.*

although conjunctival, dermal and uveal melanocytes are most probably all derived from the neural crest. Conjunctival melanoma pathology is similar to that of cutaneous melanoma. The majority of conjunctival melanomas are most closely analagous to superficial spreading melanoma of the skin.

Conjunctival melanoma has a propensity for local seeding from intraoperative tissue manipulation. Treatment for localized tumours consists of local excision, using a minimal touch technique with double freeze–thaw cryotherapy to the cut conjunctival margins.[63] Absolute alcohol on a surgical sponge may be employed to remove areas of melanoma involving the limbus and cornea. Orbital exenteration is sometimes necessary in those patients whose tumour is too extensive for local excision.

The use of chemotherapeutic agents, e.g. 5-fluorouracil and mitomycin C, topically as supplemental treatment of primary acquired conjunctival melanosis with atypia has recently been introduced.[64] Recurrent conjunctival melanoma, which might otherwise necessitate orbital exenteration, has also occasionally been successfully treated in this manner.

The overall mortality from conjunctival melanoma is *c.* 25%.[61] Tumour spread is both local and via the regional lymphatics, which provides an opportunity for subsequent haematogenous spread. Tarsal conjunctival melanoma has a worse systemic prognosis than does bulbar conjunctival melanoma. A thickness of *c.* 1.5 mm was found in one study to separate most lethal from non-lethal conjunctival melanomas, although one can not exclude a fatal outcome in flatter lesions.[65,61]

EYELID MELANOMA

Cutaneous melanoma involving the eyelid follows the same classification as cutaneous melanoma in general. An example is shown in Figure 63.11. Management is usually surgical,[60] but with generally smaller excision margins than for cutaneous melanoma elsewhere because of the confined anatomy of the eyelid and the need to maintain protection of the underlying globe. Like cutaneous melanoma elsewhere, the depth of the tumour invasion is an important prognostic factor.

ORBITAL MELANOMA

Most primary orbital melanomas arise from cellular blue naevi or from ocular melanocytosis.[66–68] The melanoma that arises from either of these congenital conditions is generally circumscribed, even though the underlying congenital pigmentation is diffuse and not circumscribed.

In some instances, orbital melanoma apparently arises de novo without clinical evidence of pre-existing blue naevus or ocular melanocytosis. The tumour is generally circumscribed. It is important to remove an orbital melanoma intact by way of an excisional biopsy. A full cutaneous and systemic evaluation should be done to exclude the possibility that a primary melanoma elsewhere could have metastasized to the orbit.

MELANOMA METASTATIC TO THE OCULAR AREA

Primary cutaneous melanoma occasionally metastasizes to the eye and/or the ocular adnexae. The posterior uveal tract is more commonly involved than the iris but

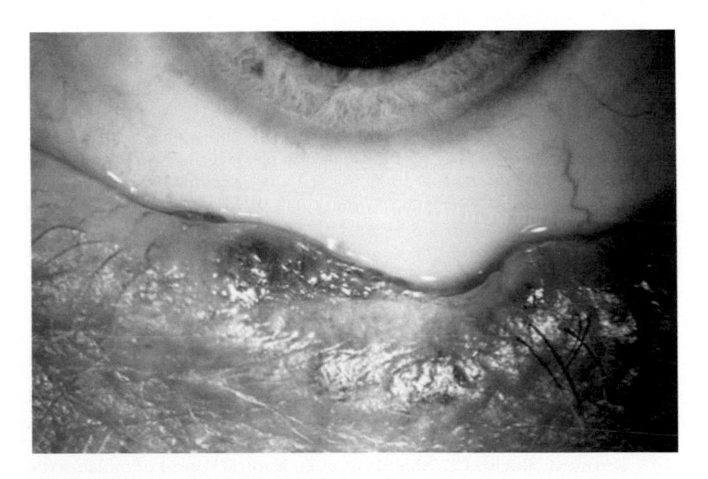

Figure 63.11 *Eyelid melanoma.*

metastases can involve almost any part of the eye, including the retina and vitreous.[2]

Usually, the diagnosis of secondary ocular melanoma is clear cut on the basis of clinical findings and history of a prior primary cutaneous melanoma, but not uncommonly a patient with a primary uveal melanoma will give a past history of primary cutaneous melanoma.

Cutaneous melanoma metastatic to the posterior uveal tract characteristically has a rather sudden onset and relatively rapid growth rate, and may be multifocal and/or bilateral, which helps to distinguish it from primary uveal melanoma. Liver involvement is commonly seen at the time of ocular involvement from metastatic cutaneous melanoma, whereas this is exceptional at the time of initial presentation of primary uveal melanoma.

Secondary ocular melanoma, like primary uveal melanoma, is poorly responsive to chemotherapy. Treatment of sight-threatening intraocular metastases usually consists of external beam irradiation. Plaque brachytherapy may also be employed for selected, circumscribed, secondary posterior uveal melanomas.

REFERENCES

1. Shields JA, Shields CL, *Atlas of intraocular tumours*. Philadelphia: Lippincott, 1999.
2. Shields JA, Shields CL, *Intraocular tumours: a text and atlas*. Philadelphia: WB Saunders, 1992.
3. Egan KM, Seddon JM, Glynn R et al, Epidemiologic aspects of uveal melanoma. *Surv Ophthalmol* 1988; 32: 239–51.
4. Tucker MA, Hartge P, Shields JA, Epidemiology of intraocular melanoma. Recent results. *Cancer Res* 1986; 102: 159–65.
5. Tucker MA, Hartge P, Shields JA, Sunlight exposure as a possible risk factor for intraocular malignant melanoma. *N Engl J Med* 1985; 313: 789–92.
6. Singh AD, Boghosian-Sell L, Wary KK et al, Cytogenetic findings in primary uveal melanoma. *Cancer Genet Cytogenet* 1994; 72: 109–15.
7. Abramson DH, Rodriguez-Sains RS, Rubman RB, B-K mole syndrome: cutaneous and ocular melanoma. *Arch Ophthalmol* 1980; 98: 1397–9.
8. Albert DM, Chang MA, Lamping K et al, The dysplastic naevus syndrome. A pedigree with malignant melanomas of the choroid and skin. *Ophthalmology* 1985; 92: 1728–34.
9. Bellet RE, Shields JA, Soll DB et al, Primary choroidal and cutaneous melanomas occurring in a patient with the B-K mole syndrome phenotype. *Am J Ophthalmol* 1980; 89: 567–70.
10. Rodriguez-Sains RS, Ocular findings in patients with dysplastic naevus syndrome. *Ophthalmol* 1986; 93: 661–5.
11. Lischko AM, Seddon JM, Gragoudas ES et al, Evaluation of prior primary malignancy as a determinant of uveal melanoma. *Ophthalmology* 1989; 96: 1716–21.
12. Gass JD, Observation of suspected choroidal and ciliary body melanomas for evidence of growth prior to enucleation. *Ophthalmology* 1980; 87: 523–8.
13. Singh AD, De Potter P, Fijal BA et al, Lifetime prevalence of uveal melanoma in Caucasian patients with ocular (dermal) melanocytosis. *Ophthalmology* 1998; 105: 195–8.
14. Territo C, Shields CL, Shields JA et al, Natural course of melanocytic tumours of the iris. *Ophthalmology* 1988; 95: 1251–5.
15. Shields JA, Shields CL, Hepatic metastasis of low grade iris melanoma seventeen years after enucleation. *Am J Ophthalmol* 1988; 106: 749–50.
16. Shields CL, Shields JA, Santos CM et al, Incomplete spontaneous regression of choroidal melanoma associated with inflammation. *Arch Ophthalmol* 1999; 117: 1245–7.
17. Shields CL, Shields JA, De Potter P et al, Diffuse choroidal melanoma: clinical features predictive of metastasis. *Arch Ophthalmol* 1996; 114: 956–63.
18. Font RL, Spaulding AG, Zimmerman LE, Diffuse malignant melanoma of the uveal tract. A clinicopathologic report of 54 cases. *Trans Am Acad Ophthalmol Otolaryngol* 1968; 72: 877–94.
19. Ausburger JJ, Gamel JW, Shields JA et al, Post irradiation regression of choroidal melanomas as a risk factor for death from metastatic disease. *Ophthalmology* 1987; 94: 1173–7.
20. Ausburger JJ, Shields JA, Folberg R et al, Fine needle aspiration biopsy in the diagnosis of intraocular cancer. Cytologic–histologic correlations. *Ophthalmology* 1985; 92: 39–49.
21. Shields JA, Shields CL, Ehya H et al, Fine needle aspiration biopsy of suspected intraocular tumours. The 1992 Urwick Lecture. *Ophthalmology* 1993; 100: 1677–84.
22. Zimmerman LE, Malignant melanoma of the uveal tract. In: *Opthalmic pathology: an atlas and textbook, volume 3*, 3rd edn. (eds Spencer WH, Font RL, Green WR et al). Philadelphia: WB Saunders, 1985: 2118, 2135–6.
23. Sahel JA, Pesavento R, Frederick AR et al, Melanoma arising de novo over a 16 month period. *Arch Ophthalmol* 1988; 106: 381–5.
24. Callender GR, Malignant melanotic tumours of the eye: a study of histologic types in 111 cases. *Trans Am Acad Ophthalmol Otolaryngol* 1931; 36: 131–42.
25. Shields CL, Shields JA, De Potter P et al, Treatment of non-resectable malignant iris tumours with custom designed plaque radiotherapy. *Br J Ophthalmol* 1995; 79: 306–12.
26. Augsburger JJ, Eagle RC, Chiu M, Shields JA, The effect of pre-enucleation radiotherapy on mitotic activity of choroidal and ciliary body melanomas. *Ophthalmology* 1987; 94: 1627–30.
27. Collaborative Ocular Melanoma Study Group, The Collaborative Ocular Melanoma Study (COMS) randomised trial of pre-enucleation radiation of large choroidal melanomas II: initial mortality findings. COMS report no.10. *Am J Ophthalmol* 1998; 125: 779–96.
28. Zimmerman LE, McLean IW, Foster WD, Does enucleation of an eye containing a malignant melanoma prevent or accelerate the dissemination of tumour cells? *Br J Ophthalmol* 1978; 62: 420–5.
29. O'Reilly MS, Holmgren L, Shing Y et al, Angiostatin: a novel angiogenesis inhibitor that mediates the suppression of metastases by a Lewis lung carcinoma. *Cell* 1994; 79: 315–28.
30. Seigel D, Myers M, Ferris III F, et al, Survival rates after enucleation of eyes with malignant melanoma. *Am J Ophthalmol* 1979; 87: 761–5.
31. Manschot WA, van Peperzeel HA, Choroidal melanoma: enucleation or observation? A new approach. *Arch Ophthalmol* 1980; 98: 71–7.
32. Shields CL, Shields JA, Gunduz K et al, Radiation therapy for uveal malignant melanoma. *Opthal Surg Lasers* 1998; 29: 397–409.
33. Gragoudas ES, Goitein M, Verhey L et al, Proton beam irradiation: an alternative to enucleation for intraocular melanomas. *Ophthalmology* 1980; 87: 571–81.
34. Char D, Castro JR, Quivey JM et al, Helium ion charged particle therapy for choroidal melanoma. *Ophthalmology* 1980; 87: 565–70.
35. Char DH, Saunders W, Castro JR et al, Helium ion therapy for choroidal melanoma. *Ophthalmology* 1983; 90: 1219–25.
36. Shields JA, Shields CL, Shah P, Sivalingam V, Partial lamellar sclerouvectomy for ciliary body and choroidal tumours. *Ophthalmology* 1991; 98: 971–83.
37. Journee-de Korver JG, Oosterhuis JA, Van Best JA, Fakkel J, Xenon arc photocoagulator used for transpupillary hyperthermia. *Doc Ophthalmol* 1991; 78: 183–7.
38. Journee-de Korver JG, Oosterhuis JA, Kakebeeke-Kemme HM, de Wolff-Rouendaal D, Transpupillary thermotherapy (TTT) by infrared irradiation of choroidal melanoma. *Doc Ophthalmol* 1992; 82: 185–91.
39. Journee-de Korver JG, Verburg-van de Marel EH, Oosterhuis JA et al, Tumoricidal effect of hyperthermia by near infrared irridiation on pigmented hamster melanoma. *Lasers Light Ophthalmol* 1992; 4: 175–80.

40. Oosterhuis JA, Journee-de Korver JG, Kakebeeke-Kemme HM, Bleeker JC, Transpupillary thermotherapy in choroidal melanomas. *Arch Ophthalmol* 1995; 113: 315–21.
41. Shields CL, Shields JA, De Potter P, Kheterpal S, Transpupillary thermotherapy in the management of choroidal melanoma. *Ophthalmology* 1996; 103: 1642–50.
42. Shields CL, Shields JA, Cater J et al, Transpupillary thermotherapy for choroidal melanoma. Tumour control and visual outcome in 100 consecutive cases. *Ophthalmology* 1998; 105: 581–90.
43. Jensen OA, Malignant melanomas of the human uvea. Recent follow-up of cases in Denmark, 1943–1952. *Acta Ophthalmol* 1970; 48: 1113–28.
44. Paul EV, Parnell BL, Fraker M, Prognosis of malignant melanomas of the choroid and ciliary body. *Int Ophthalmol Clin* 1962; 2: 387–402.
45. Zimmerman LE, McLean IW, An evaluation of enucleation in the management of uveal melanomas. *Am J Ophthalmol* 1979; 87: 741–60.
46. Arentsen JJ, Green WR, Melanoma of the iris: report of 72 cases treated by surgically. *Ophthalmic Surg* 1975; 6: 23–37.
47. Rones B, Zimmerman LE, The prognosis of primary tumours of the iris treated by iridectomy. *Arch Ophthalmol* 1958; 60: 193–205.
48. Zimmerman LE, Malignant melanoma of the uveal tract. In: *Opthalmic pathology: an atlas and textbook, volume 3*, 3rd edn. (eds Spencer WH, Font RL, Green WR et al). Philadelphia: WB Saunders, 1985: 2112–13.
49. Davidorf FH, The melanoma controversy. A comparison of choroidal, cutaneous and iris melanomas. *Surv Ophthalmol* 1981; 25: 373–7.
50. Shammas HF, Blodi FC, Prognostic factors in choroidal and ciliary body melanomas. *Arch Ophthalmol* 1977; 95: 63–9.
51. Shammas HF, Blodi FC, Orbital extension of choroidal and ciliary body melanomas. *Arch Ophthalmol* 1977; 95: 2002–5.
52. McLean IW, Foster WD, Zimmerman LE, Prognostic factors in small malignant melanomas of the choroid and ciliary body. *Arch Ophthalmol* 1977; 95: 48–58.
53. Flocks M, Gerende JH, Zimmerman LE, The size and shape of malignant melanomas of the choroid and ciliary body in relation to prognosis and histologic characteristics: a statistical study of 210 tumours. *Trans Am Acad Ophthalmol Otolaryngol* 1955; 59: 740–58.
54. Gamel JW, McLean IW, Greenberg RA et al, Computerised histopathologic assessment of malignant potential: a method for determining the prognosis of uveal melanomas. *Hum Pathol* 1982; 13: 893–7.
55. Gamel JW, McLean IW, Computerised histopathologic assessment of malignant potential II. A practical method for predicting survival following enucleation for uveal melanoma. *Cancer* 1983; 52: 1032–8.
56. Gamel JW, McLean IW, Computerised histopathologic assessment of malignant potential III. Refinements of measurement and data analysis. *Analyt Quant Cytol* 1984; 6: 37–44.
57. Folberg R, Pe'er J, Gruman LM et al, The morphologic characteristics of tumour blood vessels as a marker of tumour progression in primary human uveal melanoma. A matched case–control study. *Hum Pathol* 1992; 23: 1298–305.
58. Folberg R, Rummelt V, Parys-Van Ginderdeuren R et al, The prognostic value of tumor blood vessel morphology in primary uveal melanoma. *Ophthalmology* 1993; 100: 1389–98.
59. Makiti T, Summanen P, Tarkkanen A, Kivela T, Microvascular loops and networks as prognostic indicators in choroidal and ciliary body melanomas. *J Natl Cancer Inst* 1999; 91: 359–67.
60. Shields JA, Shields CL, *Atlas of eyelid and conjunctival tumours*. Philadelphia: Lippincott, 1999.
61. Folberg R, McLean IW, Zimmerman LE, Malignant melanomas of the conjunctiva. *Hum Pathol* 1985; 16: 136–43.
62. Jakobiec FA, Bronstein S, Albert W et al, The role of cryotherapy in the management of conjunctival melanoma. *Ophthalmology* 1982; 89: 502–15.
63. Shields JA, Shields CL, De Potter P, Surgical approach to conjunctival tumours. The 1994 Lynn B. McMahan Lecture. *Arch Ophthalmol* 1997; 115: 808–15.
64. Frucht-Pery J, Pe'er J, Use of mitomycin C in the treatment of conjunctival primary acquired melanosis with atypia. *Arch Ophthalmol* 1996; 114: 1261–4.
65. Silvers D, Jakobiec FA, Freeman T et al, Melanoma of the conjunctiva: a clinicopathologic study. In: *Ocular and adnexal tumours* (ed Jakobiec FA). Birmingham AL: Aesculapius Publishing Co, 1978: 583–9.
66. Shields JA, Shields CL, *Atlas of orbital tumours*. Philadelphia: Lippincott, 1999.
67. Jakobiec FA, Ellsworth R, Tannenbaum M, Primary orbital melanoma. *Am J Ophthalmol* 1974; 78: 24–39.
68. Drews RC, Primary malignant melanoma of the orbit in a Negro. *Arch Ophthalmol* 1975; 93: 335–6.

64

Guidelines for the management of melanoma

William H McCarthy, Bin BR Kroon

INTRODUCTION

Practice guidelines are systematically developed statements to assist practitioners in making decisions about appropriate health care for patients in specific clinical circumstances. The development of clinical practice guidelines has expanded markedly over the past 10 years. Many practice guidelines and practice parameters have been published by numerous professional organizations. An increasing interest in the concept of evidence-based medicine has given impetus to guideline development in recent years.

Guidelines for melanoma management have been published in the United States, various countries in Europe, including The Netherlands,[1] France and Italy, and in Australia. The most detailed guidelines document has been produced by the Australian Cancer Network[2] and promulgated worldwide on the website of the Australian National Health and Medical Research Council.[3] Review of all the published guidelines reveals a remarkable degree of consensus on the management of melanoma.

In all published guidelines, it is noted that the recommendations are based on current knowledge and may be altered with the passage of time. It is also stressed that guidelines are not 'cookbooks' prescribing the only way to manage a patient with melanoma, and that individual circumstances and situations may necessitate a practice plan individualized to the specific patient. The general thrust of all the guidelines is that the recommendations presented are the options best supported by current available evidence.

In some guidelines, levels of evidence are specifically stated using the following criteria:

Level I	Evidence obtained from a systematic review of all relevant randomized controlled trials
Level II	Evidence obtained from at least one properly designed randomized controlled trial
Level III-1	Evidence obtained from well-designed pseudo-randomized controlled trials (alternate allocation or some other method)
Level III-2	Evidence obtained from comparative studies with concurrent controls and allocation not randomized (cohort studies), case–control studies, or interrupted time series with a control group
Level III-3	Evidence obtained from comparative studies with historical control, two or more single arm studies, or interrupted time series without a parallel control group
Level IV	Evidence obtained from case series, either post-test or pretest/post-test

It is stressed by most guidelines committees that practice guidelines must be reviewed and updated on a regular basis if they are to remain useful documents for contemporary clinical practice. The most recent published practice guidelines vary with regard to the degree in which all aspects of melanoma management are detailed. However, all include sections on prevention, early diagnosis, biopsy of pigmented lesions, appropriate investigations for primary, nodal and metastatic melanoma, the classification of melanoma, including the new staging system recently approved by the American Joint Committee on Cancer (AJCC) and the Union Internationale Contre le Cancer (UICC) (see Table 17.1), the treatment of primary melanoma based on tumour thickness, the management of lymph nodes including biopsy, elective lymphadenectomy (sentinel node biopsy), elective and therapeutic lymph node dissection, the management of in-transit recurrence, the management of disseminated melanoma, follow-up programmes and skin surveillance programmes for melanoma patients and their families.

Some guidelines include discussions of pregnancy; hormone replacement therapy and hormonal contraception; management of congenital naevi; management of melanoma in unusual sites (e.g. subungual and the sole of the foot); the reporting, by pathologists, on the primary lesion and lymph nodes.

PRIMARY PREVENTION

Consensus is evident in all published guidelines that a most important aspect of the management of melanoma is to minimize the major known risk factor by taking appropriate precautions to limit ultraviolet damage to the skin. Prevention is based on a hierarchy of effective measures, with physical protection being more important than the use of sunscreens, i.e. it is more important to avoid the higher levels of ultraviolet light in sunshine around the 4-hour period based on solar noon, and to utilize appropriate sun-protective clothing such as hats and long-sleeved shirts during the hottest months of the year. It is noted that dark clothes offer the best protection, particularly if closely woven, and that some of the lightweight T-shirts popular in most communities have a sun protection factor (SPF) <10.[4–7]

Sunscreens are advised as an adjunct to physical protection. Sunscreens with an SPF of at least 15 are highly recommended and the very high protection sunscreens, SPF 30+, are recommended for people with sun-sensitive skin or those who expect to have a long period of sunlight exposure. Sunscreens containing broad-spectrum protection, i.e. protection against ultraviolet A as well as ultraviolet B, are recommended, as are sunscreens that have a high degree of water resistance, particularly for those undertaking water-related recreational activities. Sun beds and sun-tanning salons are noted to be associated with an increased risk of melanoma.[8]

EARLY DIAGNOSIS (SECONDARY PREVENTION)

The major reduction in melanoma mortality apparent in most white-skinned populations is undoubtedly due to community education, leading to earlier diagnosis. Community education programmes directing attention to new or changing lesions on the skin, particularly if pigmented, are encouraged. The recognition of early melanoma is stressed in most guidelines.

Very important in the diagnosis and management of the patient with a possible melanoma is the taking of a careful history of the specific lesion, a history of exposure to excessive sunlight, a family history of melanoma and a previous history of skin lesion excision. In evaluating the history presented by the patient, specific emphasis should be placed on changes in colour, shape and surface characteristics, and, in many cases, it is important to acquire historical information from the patient's partner. The only specific symptom that may be mentioned by patients is an intermittent itch. Pain and bleeding are not features of early melanoma. Some guidelines remind the clinician that quite a large number of melanomas arise in previously normal skin rather than pre-existing melanocytic naevi, and that a proportion of melanomas are not pigmented (i.e. amelanotic melanomas). In these patients, only a history of a new or changing lesion may provide the clue that biopsy may be necessary.

Examination of the specific lesion with good lighting and magnification is important. The use of surface microscopy (dermatoscopy, dermoscopy, epiluminescence microscopy) is recommended, with recent studies suggesting a substantial improvement in the accuracy of diagnosis by clinicians undertaking training and gaining experience in this technique.[9–12]

The clinical examination of a patient with a suspected melanoma includes examination of the patient's other pigmented lesions, palpation of the draining lymph node fields and a general assessment of the skin type of the patient, i.e. hair colour, eye colour, freckling and evidence of previous skin damage.

Clinical diagnosis of melanoma based on the A (asymmetry), B (border), C (colour), D (diameter) system of Friedman et al.,[13] provides a good basis for the diagnosis of melanoma. An important factor in the clinical diagnosis of a pigmented melanoma is irregularity of the lesion. Irregularity of colour (C) is the most important, and the presence of a variety of colours is very important. Black or blue-black is the most common colour noted by patients, but many other shades of colour, including brown, blue, red, grey and white, are often seen. Depigmentation of one area of the lesion is also important, as is a slight red flare around the outside of the lesion. In contrast to a dysplastic naevus, where the border (B) of the lesion is indistinct, most melanomas have a well-demarcated border, at least in part of the lesion (see Figures 17.4–17.7).

The second important feature is irregularity of the outline, or asymmetry (A), such as a coastline appearance, with bays and promontories, as on a map. The diameter (D) of a melanoma is usually >6 mm but it should be noted that melanoma, particularly nodular melanoma, can be diagnosed at considerably <6 mm.[14] Elevation (E) was then added to the A,B,C,D system;[15] it is also important but this will not be present in the earliest of lesions. The formation of a nodule implies an invasive melanoma and therefore a more dangerous lesion. The E of this system can also be used to remind the clinician to *e*xamine and compare the suspect lesion with the patient's other moles. Occasionally, such examination not only confirms the diagnosis of melanoma but also detects a second primary lesion.

Other features helpful in the diagnosis of melanoma are an amorphous glass appearance in part of the lesion (i.e. areas where the skin lines have been destroyed), a shiny light-reflecting surface, small flakes of keratin on the surface or loss of hairs in the lesion (see Figure 17.13). It is important to palpate the lesion. A melanoma is firm in consistency, without the excessive keratinization of a pigmented seborrhoeic keratosis. Haemangiomas are soft and compressible and the 'waxy' feel of a seborrhoeic keratosis can be helpful.

The differential diagnosis of melanoma includes dysplastic naevus, Spitz naevus, pigmented basal cell carcinoma, blue naevus, haemangioma, seborrhoeic keratosis and some rare adnexal tumours.

The practitioner should make the diagnosis of melanoma both by recognition of the lesion and by exclusion of these other pigmented lesions. By thinking of all the alternative diagnoses and excluding them, as well as recognizing some of the characteristics listed above, 90% of melanomas can be accurately diagnosed, particularly if surface microscopy is used as an adjunct to a normal clinical examination.[16]

BIOPSY OF PIGMENTED LESIONS

Consensus is reached in all guideline documents that excisional biopsy is preferred over any form of partial biopsy, e.g. punch biopsy or shave biopsy. Shave and punch biopsies may lead to incorrect or inadequate evaluation of the entire lesion. However, it is noted that an incisional biopsy or punch biopsy may be appropriate for very large lesions, and for lesions on the finger, palm, sole, face and ear because of the deformities which may follow complete excision of larger lesions in these areas.

INVESTIGATIONS FOR PRIMARY MELANOMA PATIENTS

Published guidelines recommend against extensive investigation of the patient with primary melanoma because of the cost-ineffective nature of these procedures. Except with very thick melanomas (T4+), a positive finding from routine investigations is rarely reported.[17] All major guidelines suggest only full blood counts, liver function tests, particularly serum lactic dehydrogenase (LDH), and a chest x ray. More extensive investigations may be undertaken for T4+ tumours and for patients with positive lymph nodes, but even in these situations the tests are usually negative. However, for this group of patients, such investigation may provide baseline studies for subsequent repeat investigations initiated by specific symptoms.

TREATMENT OF PRIMARY MELANOMA

Treatment policies recommended in all published guidelines are based on the Breslow tumour thickness measurement. This measurement is the maximum vertical diameter of the tumour from the granular cell layer of the epidermis to the deepest malignant cell discernible, ignoring infiltration by the tumour along hair follicles. The new classification system developed by a committee of the AJCC, and also adopted by the UICC (see Table 17.1) is the basis for excision margins.

The morphological classification of melanoma (superficial spreading melanoma, nodular melanoma, lentigo maligna melanoma and acral lentiginous melanoma) is no longer used in clinical management decisions. The histopathological criteria of radial versus vertical growth phase[18] are mentioned in some guidelines but Breslow thickness remains the major parameter on which therapeutic decision making is based. Microscopic ulceration is also considered in the new classification system. Level of invasion is an important prognostic parameter only for T1 tumours.

All guidelines show a remarkable consensus for the excision margins appropriate for each tumour classification. Recommended margins of excision for each of the T classification groups are:

- pTis – 5 mm clearance
- pT1, pT2 – 1 cm clearance
- pT3 – minimum margin 1 cm, maximum margin 2 cm
- pT4 – minimum margin 2 cm, maximum margin 3 cm.

However, it is noted that there is no conclusive evidence that any margins >1 cm influence survival, although wider excision may diminish the rate of local recurrence.

TREATMENT OF LYMPH NODES

The risk of a melanoma patient developing metastatic disease in regional lymph nodes is related to the Breslow tumour thickness, with <5% of T1 tumours metastasizing to the lymph nodes while T4 tumours have >50% risk of metastatic nodal involvement.

All recent guidelines indicate that the question of elective lymph node dissection has become less relevant with the development of lymphatic mapping and the sentinel node biopsy procedure. It is clear from all recent studies of lymph node dissection that the benefit of dissection occurs only in those patients with positive lymph nodes, and that the identification of these patients by sentinel node biopsy will allow radical dissection to be performed for patients proven to have metastastic disease in the lymph nodes. Elective lymph node dissection is thus not recommended in any of the published guidelines for the majority of melanoma patients. However, it is noted that two recent international controlled clinical trials (Intergroup Melanoma Surgical trial[19] and World Health Organization (WHO) Melanoma Group Trial #14[20]) provide evidence that elective lymph node dissection may be appropriate for certain subsets of melanoma patients if sentinel node biopsy is not available.

The technique of lymphatic mapping and sentinel node biopsy, with selective complete regional lymphadenectomy, is detailed in Chapter 30. Published guidelines note that a survival benefit for sentinel node biopsy has yet to be demonstrated, pending completion and analysis of a large international multicentre randomized controlled trial. Sentinel node biopsy may, however, be useful in the selection of patients for inclusion in adjuvant studies.

LYMPH NODE BIOPSY

Ultrasound evaluation of lymph node fields is helpful in determining the possible need for lymph node biopsy. Fine needle aspiration is preferable to open biopsy of a clinically palpable lymph node in a patient who has had a primary melanoma. Fine needle biopsy minimizes the risk of tumour cell spillage and subsequent recurrence in the lymph node field. Should the patient subsequently have a therapeutic node dissection, minimal disturbance of the operative field will have been produced by needle biopsy. If needle biopsy is not diagnostic and clinical suspicion remains, open biopsy should be performed as a first step in a planned therapeutic lymph node dissection, i.e. the node biopsy should be undertaken with the patient prepared for immediate therapeutic node dissection if the frozen section diagnosis confirms the presence of metastatic melanoma.

THERAPEUTIC LYMPH NODE DISSECTION

If regional lymph node metastases are confirmed, a complete node dissection is considered to be mandatory and the entire lymph node field should be cleared. Therapeutic node dissection for melanoma carries a considerable risk of recurrence in the node field if the dissection is not performed adequately by a surgeon trained in these procedures.[21] Neck dissections have a particularly high rate of local recurrence,[22,23] but even in the axilla and the groin, local recurrence poses a considerable risk if a dissection is incomplete or inadequate. Recurrence in a lymph node field is almost always associated with a fatal outcome. A thorough, formal dissection will substantially lower the risk of recurrence in a dissected field. Techniques of therapeutic node dissection are discussed in Chapters 24–26.

Prior to therapeutic lymph node dissection, staging procedures should be undertaken to determine if the patient has metastatic disease elsewhere apart from the node field. However, in most instances a therapeutic node dissection will still be necessary to minimize the local problems associated with persistent or progressive enlargement of the involved lymph nodes. Where extensive systemic metastases are apparent, local radiotherapy may be an acceptable alternative to node dissection. The role of adjuvant radiotherapy following lymph node dissection remains controversial, although some centres advocate radiotherapy for node fields where multiple positive nodes are present or extranodal extension is detected.

LOCOREGIONAL (IN-TRANSIT) RECURRENT MELANOMA

A relatively common site for recurrence of melanoma in a limb is in the skin and subcutaneous tissues between the primary lesion site and the regional lymph node field or fields (in-transit recurrences). If a single, easily resectable local recurrence is present, or alternatively a small number of such lesions, surgical removal should be performed and regional lymph node dissection considered. These resected specimens may be used to produce vaccines for use in clinical trials of adjuvant therapy. However, for repeated episodes of recurrence in a limb, or for extensive in-transit metastases, isolated limb perfusion or infusion with cytotoxic agents, with or without node dissection, is the treatment of choice. Where no systemic metastases are detected by computerized tomography (CT) scanning or positron emission tomography (PET), node dissection (if not previously performed) with perfusion/infusion is appropriate. Isolated limb perfusion is the gold standard for this type of recurrence but it has considerable morbidity, and is expensive and time consuming. An alternative to isolated limb perfusion is isolated limb infusion,[24] which is less morbid and costly, and has almost the same therapeutic outcome. Detailed descriptions of isolated limb perfusion and isolated limb infusion therapy are given in Chapters 36–39.

DISSEMINATED MELANOMA

At the present time, there is no effective therapeutic protocol which achieves good long-term control of disseminated melanoma. Although occasional complete responses can be achieved with chemotherapy and/or immunotherapy, $<5\%$ of patients with melanoma disseminated beyond the lymph nodes are alive 5 years after the first systemic recurrence is detected.[25] Due to the lack of effective treatment modalities for patients with disseminated melanoma, clinicians are advised to refer such patients to specialized melanoma centres for inclusion in clinical trials of new therapeutic modalities, both cytotoxic and immunotherapeutic. Many such trials are currently recruiting patients and their results may provide more effective approaches for disseminated melanoma in the future. These trials include combination chemotherapy, immunotherapy and biochemotherapy. The longest remissions, and even the occasional cure, for disseminated melanoma can be achieved by surgical removal where the patient presents with isolated metastatic lesions, especially in the brain, lung or abdomen. The advent of high quality scanning (i.e. CT, magnetic resonance imaging (MRI) and PET) has enabled detailed evaluation of the patient with systemic disease and allowed specific treatments, such as surgery, radiotherapy and isolated regional chemotherapy, to be appropriately applied to the individual patient with metastatic melanoma. However, all these advanced imaging techniques should be undertaken only in situations where the outcome will influence patient therapy and in consultation with a major melanoma centre.

FOLLOW-UP

All patients with invasive melanoma should enter a follow-up programme. Follow-up should also be arranged for patients with non-invasive melanoma (melanoma in situ) who have a significant number of naevi, particularly if the naevi are clinically dysplastic. All patients, even those not being specifically followed up, should be advised that recurrence of a melanoma, particularly in lymph nodes, remains a remote possibility, even many years after the primary tumour has been removed. Any change in a naevus, any lump on or under the skin, or any enlarged lymph node draining the area of a previously excised melanoma should be regarded as melanoma until a histopathological diagnosis confirms or excludes this possibility.

A considerable risk for the development of a second primary melanoma exists for people who have multiple naevi. Thus, a lifetime surveillance programme should be organized for people in this situation. In the absence of other risk factors, a follow-up period of 5 years is generally considered sufficient for patients with thin melanomas, i.e. <1.0 mm in thickness. A follow-up period of 10 years is recommended for patients with thicker melanomas. Melanoma patients with a family history of melanoma or dysplastic naevi, whether sporadic or familial, should be followed up for life because of their high risk of developing a second melanoma.

It is important to actively involve patients in the follow-up programme. They should be instructed to look for changes in the area between the primary lesion site and the regional nodes, to examine the regional nodes and to report quickly any lump that occurs anywhere in the body, particularly in the lymph node field. They should also be taught how to monitor their naevi.

Extensive follow-up investigations have not been shown to be beneficial for the majority of patients with melanoma (see Chapter 41). A yearly chest x ray for the first 5 years may be helpful because early metastatic melanoma in the lung is asymptomatic and the lungs are the most common site for systemic metastatic disease. The development of other symptoms, or the finding of nodal metastases, necessitate staging investigations, including CT scans of the brain, chest and abdomen. Scanning by MRI and PET may also be useful for staging patients with suspected metastatic melanoma. However, these investigations should be undertaken after consultation with a melanoma treatment centre.

SKIN SURVEILLANCE PROGRAMMES

Skin surveillance programmes should be provided for all people with multiple naevi. If there is melanoma in the family pedigree, skin surveillance programmes should also be introduced for other family members, particularly if the family members have multiple dysplastic or banal naevi.

Approximately 10% of melanoma patients will have at least one first-degree relative who has had a melanoma. Most of these apparently familial melanomas are due to chance, e.g. in a high-incidence community such as Australia. However, strict analyses have shown that at least 1 in 5 (i.e. 20% of familial clusters or 2% of all melanoma cases) represent genuine risk resulting from inheritance of uncommon major melanoma susceptibility genes. These patients require close surveillance throughout life.

ADJUVANT THERAPY

As yet, there is no conclusive evidence that adjuvant therapy is beneficial for anyone with melanoma. However, in view of the known poor prognosis for patients with melanomas >4 mm in thickness and/or with involved nodes, it may be appropriate to refer these patients to a melanoma centre for inclusion in clinical trials of immunotherapy, chemotherapy or gene therapy. Only in this way will the value of new therapies be established.

OCCULT PRIMARY MELANOMA

Occult primary melanoma comprises 4–12% of clinical presentations to major melanoma centres. Occult primary melanoma patients usually present with a palpable lymph node or, in rare cases, a systemic metastasis, in the absence of recognizable coincident primary melanoma and with no past history of melanoma. The treatment for cryptogenic metastatic melanoma in lymph nodes is exactly the same as that for lymph node recurrence in patients with a previous or existing primary tumour.[26,27] There is no difference in survival between those patients with known or unknown primary tumours, providing that they present with a comparable number of involved lymph nodes.[28,29]

HORMONES AND MELANOMA

Pregnancy

Major reviews of studies on this subject have found no conclusive evidence that melanoma during or near the time of pregnancy adversely affects the clinical course or prognosis of the disease.[30,31] A recent large study indicated that although melanomas detected during pregnancy were thicker than those in non-pregnant women, these lesions were not associated with a less favourable prognosis for a given tumour thickness.[32] Where nodal involvement occurs during pregnancy there is a moderately worse prognosis than in the non-pregnant patient.[33] Melanoma has been reported to cross the placenta but this appears to occur only rarely in mothers with very advanced melanoma. Cases have been reported where melanoma metastasis was detected in a surviving baby and the melanoma in the baby regressed spontaneously shortly after birth.

While there is no specific evidence that pregnancy adversely affects the prognosis, a consensus view is that pregnancy is not advisable for at least 2 years after the excision of a clinically significant melanoma, i.e. a tumour >1.5 mm in thickness, where the risk of occult metastasis is moderately high. Pregnancy in a woman with occult metastases may promote earlier appearance of metastatic melanoma. Avoiding pregnancy for some years may add reassurance that a subsequent pregnancy will be less likely to be associated with recurrent melanoma. Advice to women with stage III melanoma, i.e. melanoma in lymph nodes, should be that pregnancy is inadvisable for at least 5 years because of the high risk (>50%) of systemic disease. The treatment of primary melanoma does not differ because a woman is pregnant. However, in the late stages of pregnancy, where node dissection is contemplated, it may be advisable to delay the dissection to allow the pregnancy to be completed or to initiate early delivery to allow the operation to proceed.

Hormone replacement therapy

There is no conclusive evidence that either hormone replacement therapy or the use of the oral contraceptive pill play any role in the natural history of melanoma. Indeed, several studies have shown a marginal benefit, while others have suggested no association between these hormones and survival.[34,35]

REFERENCES

1. Kroon BBR, Nieweg OE, Hoekstra HJ, Lejeune FJ, Principles and guidelines for surgeons: management of cutaneous malignant melanoma. *Eur J Surg Oncol* 1997; 23: 550–68.
2. Australian Cancer Network. *The management of cutaneous melanoma.* Canberra: NHMRC, 1999.
3. http://www.health.gov.au/nhmrc/publicat/pdf/cp68.pdf.
4. Hill D, White V, Marks R et al, Changes in sun-related attitudes and behaviours, and reduced sunburn prevalence in a population at high risk of melanoma. *Eur J Cancer Prev* 1993; 2: 447–56.
5. IARC Monograph on the evaluation of carcinogenic risks to humans. *Solar Ultraviolet Rad* 1992; 55: 95–122.
6. Swerdlow AJ, English J, MacKie RM et al, Benign melanocytic naevi as a risk factor for malignant melanoma. *Br Med J Clin Res* 1986; 292: 1555–9.
7. Holman CD, Armstrong BK, Cutaneous malignant melanoma and indicators of total accumulated exposure to the sun: an analysis separating histogenetic types. *J Natl Cancer Inst* 1984; 73: 75–82.
8. Westerdahl J, Olsson H, Masback A et al, Use of sunbeds or sunlamps and malignant melanoma in southern Sweden. *Am J Epidemiol* 1994; 140: 691–9.
9. Steiner A, Pehamberger H, Wolff K, In vivo epiluminescence microscopy of pigmented skin lesions. II Diagnosis of small pigmented skin lesions and early detection of malignant melanoma. *J Am Acad Dermatol* 1987; 17: 584–91.
10. Pehamberger H, Binder M, Steiner A et al, In vivo epiluminescence microscopy: improvement of early diagnosis of melanoma. *J Invest Dermatol* 1993; 100: 356S–362S.
11. Stoltz W, Braun-Falco O, Lanthaler M et al (eds), *Color atlas of dermatoscopy.* Oxford: Blackwell Science, 1994.
12. Westerhoff K, McCarthy WH, Menzies SW, Increase in the sensitivity for melanoma diagnosis by primary care physicians using skin surface microscopy. *Br J Dermatol* 2000; 143: 1–6.
13. Friedman RJ, Rigel DS, Kopf AW, Early detection of malignant melanoma: the role of physician examination and self-examination of the skin. *CA Cancer J Clin* 1985; 35: 130–51.
14. Fitzpatrick TB, Rhodes AR, Sober AJ et al, Primary malignant melanoma of the skin: the call for action to identify persons at risk: to discover precursor lesions: to detect early melanomas. *Pigment Cell* 1988; 9: 110–17.
15. Shaw HM, McCarthy WH, Small-diameter malignant melanoma: a common diagnosis in New South Wales, Australia. *J Am Acad Dermatol* 1992; 27: 679–82.
16. Menzies SW, Igvar C, Crotty KA, McCarthy WH, Frequency and morphologic characteristics of invasive melanomas lacking specific microscopic features. *Arch Dermatol* 1996; 132: 1178–82.
17. Weiss M, Loprinzi CL, Creagan ET et al, Utility of follow-up tests for detecting recurrent disease in patients with malignant melanoma. *JAMA* 1995; 274: 1703–5.
18. McGovern VJ, Cochran AJ, Van der Esch EP et al, The classification of malignant melanoma, its histological reporting and registration: a revision of the 1972 Sydney classification. *Pathology* 1986; 18: 12–21.
19. Drepper H, Kohler CO, Bastian B et al, Benefit of elective lymph node dissection in subgroups of melanoma patients. Results of a multicenter study of 3616 patients. *Cancer* 1993; 72: 741–9.
20. Cascinelli N, Morabito A, Santinami A et al on behalf of the WHO Melanoma Programme, Immediate or delayed dissection of regional nodes in patients with melanoma of the trunk: a randomised trial. *Lancet* 1998; 351: 793–6.
21. Calabro A, Singletary SE, Balch CM, Patterns of relapse in 1001 consecutive patients with melanoma nodal metastases. *Arch Surg* 1989; 124: 1051–5.
22. Jonk A, Kroon BBR, Mooi WJ et al, Value of therapeutic neck dissection in patients with melanoma. *Diagnos Oncol* 1993; 3: 268–70.
23. O'Brien CJ, Gianoutsos MP, Morgan MJ, Neck dissection for cutaneous malignant melanoma. *World J Surg* 1992; 16: 222–6.
24. Thompson JF, Waugh RC, Saw RPM et al, Isolated limb infusion with melphalan for recurrent limb melanoma: a simple alternative to isolated limb perfusion. *Reg Cancer Treat* 1994; 7: 188–92.
25. Coates AS, Systemic chemotherapy for malignant melanoma. *World J Surg* 1992; 16: 277–81.
26. Balch CM, Houghton AN, Diagnosis of metastatic melanoma at distant sites. In: *Cutaneous melanoma.* (eds Balch CM, Houghton AN, Milton GW et al) Philadelphia: Lippincott, 1992: 439–67.
27. Velez A, Walsh D, Karakousis CP, Treatment of unknown primary melanoma. *Cancer* 1991; 68: 2579–81.
28. Milton GW, Shaw HM, McCarthy WH, Occult primary malignant melanoma: factors influencing survival. *Br J Surg* 1977; 64: 805–8.
29. Norman J, Cruse CW, Wells KE et al, Metastatic melanoma with an unknown primary. *Ann Plast Surg* 1992; 28: 81–4.
30. Driscoll MS, Grin-Jorgensen CAM, Grant-Kels JM, Does pregnancy influence the prognosis of malignant melanoma? *J Am Acad Dermatol* 1993; 29: 619–30.
31. Holly EA, Cress RD, Melanoma and pregnancy. In: *Epidemiological aspects of cutaneous malignant melanoma.* (eds Gallagher RP, Elwood JM). Boston: Kluwer, 1994: 209–21.
32. Travers RL, Sober AJ, Berwick M et al, Increased thickness of pregnancy-associated melanoma. *Br J Dermatol* 1995; 132: 876–83.
33. Mansfield PF, Lee JE, Balch CM, Cutaneous melanoma: current practice and surgical controversies. *Curr Prob Surg* 1994; 31: 253–374.
34. Holly EA, Cress RD, Ahn DK, Cutaneous melanoma in women: ovulatory life, menopause, and use of exogenous estrogens. *Cancer Epidemiol Biomarkers Prev* 1994; 3: 661–8.
35. Holly EA, Cress RD, Ahn DK, Cutaneous melanoma in women. III Reproductive factors and oral contraceptive use. *Am J Epidemiol* 1995; 141: 943–50.

FURTHER READING

The Australian Guidelines[2] provide a comprehensive overview of melanoma management and are consistent with guidelines from other countries. The Australian Guidelines are available on the Internet at the Australian National Health and Medical Research Council Website.[3]

Index